The Art and Science of Diabetes Self-Management Education Desk Reference

Third Edition

Editor in Chief
Carolé Mensing, RN, MA, CDE, FAADE

Associate Editors
Susan Cornell, BS, PharmD, CDE, FAPhA, FAADE
Cindy Halstenson, RD, LD, CDE

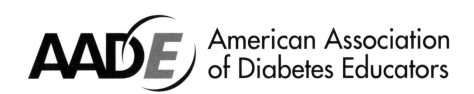

American Association of Diabetes Educators©

TABLE OF CONTENTS

SECTION 1
The Art of Diabetes Self-Management Education

SECTION 2
The Science of Diabetes Self-Management Education

DEDICATION

Dedicated to Richard Rubin and his family.

In recognition of the time and energy they devoted to the pursuit of living well with diabetes through the art and science of diabetes education.

PREFACE

Develop your thoughts, for they become words.
Choose your words, for they become actions.
Understand your actions, for they become habits.
Study your habits, for they will become your character.
Develop your character, for it becomes . . .
Your destiny!

Anonymous

Introduction

As we began the task of revising *The Art and Science of Diabetes Self-Management Education Desk Reference* for the third edition, it again secured my belief in the power of education, the educator, and the vast repository of "science" that lays the foundation and shapes our diabetes educator character and our destiny. This third edition will continue to be a powerful symbol of the commitment educators, and the organization, have for the profession of diabetes educators and the process of education.

Words

This third edition reinforces a focus based on the chronic care model[1] and guided by the revised National Standards for Diabetes Self-Management Education and Support (NSDSMES[2]), and the professional practice positions outlined by the American Association of Diabetes Educators (AADE[3]), and incorporates a more public health view of diabetes and how it affects all our lives. The *Art and Science Desk Reference* continues to be unique among publications, focusing on educational approaches based in science and provided in the individualized application (truly the art and style of each unique educator) and the assessed need of each of the person(s) affected by diabetes.

The first and second editions have provided a respected reference and resource in identifying and driving professional practice. The third edition carries this philosophy further and continues to maintain its presence as an authoritative reference, reflecting the unique and distinct body of knowledge developed for, and applied by, diabetes educators with the valued outcome of behavior change for the medical provider, educators, patients, and our extended communities.[4]

This edition continues to serve as a guide for both the experienced and the new educator. Section 1 reviews the art of diabetes self-management education and support (DSMES), and section 2 lays the groundwork and addresses the science of this professional practice. Unique to the third edition is the revamping of chapter 1, introducing newer concepts related to the process of education and more clarity to the role of the educator, both in content and practice level. It also supports the role of those in the health professions and community who serve people affected by diabetes (families, friends, colleagues, health care professionals) in a variety of roles, by providing support, information, clarity, problem solving.

Chapters 6, 18, and 19 update the reader with the wider variety of medications available to our providers, offering a menu of choices for the best possible clinical management of the person with diabetes and all its ramifications.

Chapter 7 offers a broader review of all the monitoring essential to managing diabetes, and expands on the concept of "lnowing (all) your numbers." Chapter 11 includes the revised standards for DSMES2 and, along with chapters 8, 9, and 10, focuses on support, coping, problem solving, and risk reduction skills for our "patients" and ourselves.

Chapter 4, 16, and 20 review the updated nutritional guidelines and how to apply the information. Included in chapters 5 and 17 are resources for improving on and supporting a more active lifestyle. Diabetes management across the lifespan, acute and chronic complications are discussed in the remaining chapters in section 2, offering the reader a review and strong foundation in recommended practice.

As is the routine practice of our editors, the content of each and every chapter is carefully reviewed, guided by our authors (previous and current), editor discussion, fact finding, peer reviewers, and staff. Several new authors are introduced in this third edition. We are thankful for all the time and energy each one offered to see this publication through to the end. Their collective contributions and dedication to accuracy and relevance (the science) and application (the art) make this publication the revered reference and resource as intended.

Actions, Habit, and Character

The *action* plan for this reference is to provide the reader with a condensed professional desktop practice guide and a source for a variety of additional educational strategies and delivery options. Each chapter continues to offer *action* steps, delivery alternatives, and pearls of wisdom to the reader. It is the readers' responsibility to take action, apply these options to their practice (forming more comfortable *habits*) and thus, building and broadening their *characters'* foundation.

Destiny

I am astonished at how each of our destinies as diabetes clinicians and educators has lead us to a most fulfilling life's work, and for me, how quickly time passed. As editor, I reflect upon my actions and habits, trying to establish what made me the character that I am today and why I persist in the belief and take public action to be the steward that helps to this produce this publication. The answer, of course, is that I believe in its mission, its purpose. I believe with all my heart, that it is inspired by all of the educators, colleagues, clinicians, patients, friends affected by diabetes, and the wealth of all of our experiences that make it success.

I believe this is also what made me live for, and work towards, making life better for those affected by diabetes. It has always been my destiny and who I am, yet today. It is no surprise to my colleagues that I already continue to participate in our beloved world of diabetes management and education. "Retirement" is just a word. Perhaps "revitalization" would be more descriptive. And may I quote my best friend who fondly says, "Look out world, Ms. Diabetes has even more time now!"

I am especially grateful to, and in awe of, our co-editors, Cindy and Susan, for their expertise and careful scrutiny of content, attention to detail, commitment of time, and tolerance for my demands. Importantly, I am deeply appreciative for the AADE staff, lead by Margaret, who devoted hours to making us "read better than we write," and sometimes "fussed" when our deadlines got away from us.

Finally, for the readers, this comes to the point where I now ask, "What is your destiny?" If you are reading this, I suspect you are as committed as I am. This, then, is the character we share—our mutual destiny.

So, carry on and make it so. . . .

> *When there's tough job to do,*
> *some run and hide.*
> *You stood up and did it,*
> *And I'm brimming with pride!*
>
> Dr. Seuss

Carolé Mensing, RN, MA, CDE, FAADE
Editor in Chief and Truly a "Character"

References

1. Wagner EH, Austin BT, Davis C, Hindmarsh M, Schaefer J, Bonomi A. Improving chronic illness care: translating evidence into action. *Health Aff* (Millwood). 2001;20:64-78.

2. Haas L, Maryniuk M, Beck J, Cox C, Duker P, et al. National Standards for Diabetes Self-Management Education and Support. *The Diabetes Educator* 2012;38:619-29. On the Internet at: http://www.diabeteseducator.org/export/sites/aade/_resources/pdf/general/2012NationalStandards.pdf (accessed 14 April 2014).

3. AADE Position Statements, 2008–2012. On the Internet at: http://www.diabeteseducator.org/ProfessionalResources/position/position_statements.html (accessed 14 April 2014).

4. Standards for Outcomes Measurement of Diabetes Self-Management Education. *The Diabetes Educator* 2003;(29)5:809. On the Internet at: http://www.diabeteseducator.org/export/sites/aade/_resources/pdf/PS-Outcomes.pdf (accessed 14 April 2014).

ACKNOWLEDGMENTS

Editor in Chief

Carolé Mensing, RN, MA, CDE, FAADE, was a manager for clinical and education programs and a CDE in the Strategic Initiatives department at the Joslin Diabetes Center in Boston. She is a nationally known speaker, published expert, and leader in the field of diabetes care and education. She was an invited lecturer for the first annual Harriet McKay Forum at Joslin's Center for Innovation in Diabetes Education.

Ms. Mensing has played an integral part in the establishment of a number of diabetes education programs throughout the country and chaired the task force that published the *National Standards for Diabetes Self-Management Education* (Washington, DC, May 2000). She is past coordinator of the recognized Diabetes Self-Management Program at the University of Connecticut, Farmington, and Health Partners in Minneapolis, Minnesota.

She has served on the AADE board of directors and is a past AADE chapter president and past officer. In 2012, Ms. Mensing received the Allene Von Son Distinguished Service Award in recognition of her outstanding contributions and services to AADE. She served as past president, Health Care and Education, of the American Diabetes Association.

Ms. Mensing served as the editor of the first and second editions of *The Art and Science of Diabetes Self-Management Education: A Desk Reference for Healthcare Professionals*, published in 2006 and 2011, respectively.

Associate Editor, Section One

Susan Cornell, BS, PharmD, CDE, FAPhA, FAADE, is the assistant director of experiential education and an associate professor in the department of pharmacy practice at Midwestern University Chicago College of Pharmacy in Downers Grove, Illinois. Dr. Cornell is also a clinical pharmacist consultant and certified diabetes educator, specializing in community and ambulatory care practice. She also serves as the Midwestern University American Pharmacists Association Academy of Student Pharmacists (APhA-ASP) faculty advisor and patient care project supervisor. She serves as the faculty advisor and supervisor of CHAT, an interprofessional team of students from the colleges of pharmacy, medicine, physician assistant, physical therapy, dental medicine, and biomedical sciences that provides diabetes self-management education and training to people in underserved areas and in free community clinics.

Dr. Cornell has served on the AADE board of directors and is a past president and a past chair of the board of directors of the Illinois Pharmacists Association. She has received numerous awards and recognitions, including the 2010 Teacher of the Year Award, the 2010 American Association of Colleges of Pharmacy Student Engaged Community Service Award, the 2008 AADE Fellow Award, the 2008 American Pharmacists Association Fellow award, and the 2005 Midwestern University Golden Apple Teaching Award.

Dr. Cornell has given numerous presentations to various healthcare professionals and community groups and has published and contributed to many peer-reviewed, professionally written, and online publications.

Associate Editor, Section Two

Cindy Halstenson, RD, LD, CDE, is a Clinical Program Consultant with Optum, a UnitedHealth Group company in Minnetonka, Minnesota. Ms. Halstenson has specialized in diabetes care and education over the past 20 years, including clinical care, population healthcare improvement, and clinical program management.

She has served as a past chair of the AADE Minnesota Network; the 2013 and 2014 chair, Professional Education, AADE Minnesota Network; the chair or president of the Minnesota area American Diabetes Association, the Minnesota Dietetic Association, the Diabetes Care and Education dietetic practice group of the Academy of Nutrition and Dietetics, and the board of directors of the National Certification Board for Diabetes Educators.

Ms. Halstenson currently serves on the editorial board for *AADE InPractice* magazine and served as a section editor of the second edition of *The Art and Science of Diabetes Self-Management Education: A Desk Reference for Healthcare Professionals*, published in 2011.

Reviewers

Susan Barlow, RD, CDE
National Medical Liaison
Field Medical Affairs
Valeritas, Inc.
Bridgewater, NJ

Joni Beck, PharmD, BC-ADM, CDE
Associate Professor and Clinical Programs Director
Pediatric Diabetes and Endocrinology
University of Oklahoma Health Sciences Center
College of Medicine
Edmond, OK

Gretchen Benson, RD, CDE
Manager, Healthcare Systems Integration
Minneapolis Heart Institute Foundation
Minneapolis, MN

Susan W. Butterworth, PhD, MS, CCP, RHC-III
Associate Professor
School of Medicine
Oregon Health Sciences University
Portland, OR

Amy Campbell, MS, RD, LDN, CDE
Education Program Manager
Joslin Diabetes Center Healthcare Services
Boston, MA

Michelle A. Dart, MSN, PNP, CDE
Dart Health Coaching & Consulting
Auburn, NY

Lea E. dela Pena, PharmD, BCPS
Associate Professor of Pharmacy Practice
Midwestern University Chicago
College of Pharmacy
Downers Grove, IL

Jane K. Dickinson, PhD, RN, CDE
Program Coordinator/Adjunct Associate Professor
Master of Science in Diabetes Education and
    Management Program
Teachers College, Columbia University
New York, NY

Alison B. Evert, MS, RD, CDE
Diabetes Educator
University of Washington
Endocrine and Diabetes Care Center
Seattle, WA

Deborah Fillman, MS, RD, LD, CDE
Public Health Director
Green River District Health Department
Owensboro, KY

Cindi Goldman-Patin, BA, BSN, RN, CDE
Principal
Integrative Diabetes Education Associates
Pittsfield, MA

Deborah Greenwood, PhD Candidate, MEd, CNS,
    RN, BC-ADM, CDE, FAADE
Diabetes Clinical Nurse Specialist
Sutter Medical Foundation
Granite Bay, CA

Carol J. Homko, PhD, RN, CDE
Temple University
Associate Professor, Department of Medicine,
    Section of Endocrinology, Metabolism, and
    Diabetes
Assistant Professor, Department of Obstetrics,
    Gynecology and Reproductive Sciences
Philadelphia, PA

Karen Kemmis, MS, PT, DPT, GCS, CDE
Physical Therapist/Diabetes Educator
Joslin Diabetes Center
Syracuse, NY

Jessica L. Kerr, PharmD, CDE
Associate Professor of Pharmacy Practice
Southern Illinois University
School of Pharmacy
Edwardsville, IL

Barbara Kocurek, PharmD, BCPS, CDE, FAADE
Diabetes Program Manager
Baylor Health Care System
Arlington, TX

Jodi Lavin-Tompkins, RN, BC-ADM, CDE
Diabetes Program Manager
Healthpartners
Minneapolis, MN

Susan McKenney, MSN, FNP-BC, ADM-BC, RN
Family and Advanced Diabetes Nurse Practitioner
Pardee Hospital/UNC Healthcare/Pardee Family
    Medical Associates
Hendersonville, NC

Lois Moss-Barnwell, MS, RD, LDN
Principal, Nutrition & Diabetes Consultant
Diet Rx, Ltd.
Highwood, IL

Cathy Mullooly, MS, RCEP, CDE
Medical Liaison
Novo Nordisk, Inc.
Waltham, MA

Patricia Moore, MSN, RN, CDE
Managing Partner
Clinical Solutions, LLC
Columbus, IN

Nathan A. Painter, PharmD, CDE
Associate Clinical Professor
University of California, San Diego
Skaggs School of Pharmacy and Pharmaceutical
    Sciences
La Jolla, CA

Katie Weinger, EdD, RN, FAADE
Investigator
Joslin Diabetes Center
Boston, MA

The editors of the third edition would like to acknowledge the contributions of the editors and the chapter authors of the first and second editions of *The Art and Science of Diabetes Self-Management Education Desk Reference*.

Anne J. Abbate, RN, CDE
Samuel L. Abbate, MD, CDE
Ann L. Albright, PhD, RD
Marilyn S. Arnold, MS, RD, LD, CDE
Rodolfo M. Banda, MD
Jackie L. Boucher, MS, RD, BC-ADM, CDE
Carol A. Brownson, MSPH
Dorothy Burns, PhD, RN
Laura D. Byham-Gray, PhD, RD, CNSD
Kiralee K. Camp, MS
Belinda P. Childs, MN, CNS, BC-ADM, CDE
Marjorie Cypress, MSN, C-CNP, CDE
Kim DeCoste, MSN, RN, CDE
Mary de Groot, PhD
Linda Delahanty, MS, RD, LD
Michael M. Engelgau, MD, MS
Edwin B. Fisher, PhD
Victor H. Gonzalez, MD
Felicia Hill-Briggs, PhD, ABPP
Deborah Hinnen, APRN, RN, BC-ADM, CDE,
    FAAN, FAADE
Tommy Johnson, PharmD, BC-ADM, CDE,
    FAADE
Edna G. Johnson-Gutierrez, MSN, ANP-BC, RN,
    CDE
Karmeen Kulkarni, MS, RD, BC-ADM, CDE
Daniel Lorber, MD, FACP, CDE

Gayle M. Lorenzi, RN, CDE
Sarah L. Lovegreen, MPH
Susan D. Martin, RD, LD, CDE
Lois Maurer, MS, RD, LDN, CDE
Susan McLaughlin, BS, RD, CDE
Gail D'Eramo Melkus, EdD, C-ANP, FAAN
Dara L. Murphy, MPH
K. M. Venkat Narayan, MD, MPH
James W. Pichert, PhD
Margaret A. Powers, PhD, RD, CDE
Robert E. Ratner, MD, FACP, FACE
Laurie Ruggiero, PhD
David G. Schlundt, PhD
Linda Siminerio, PhD, RN, CDE
Anne H. Skelly, PhD, ANP, RN, CS
Geralyn R. Spollet, MSN, ANP, CDE
Condit F. Steil, PharmD, FAPhA, CDE
Tricia S. Tang, PhD
Donna M. Tomky, MSN, C-ANP, RN, CDE
Ann Vannice, MSN, APRN, CDE
Jeffrey J. VanWormer, MS
Frank Vinicor, MD, MPH
Christopher J. Vito, PharmD
Julie Wagner, PhD
Elizabeth A. Walker, PhD, RN, CDE, FAADE
Judith Wylie-Rosett, EdD, RD

SECTION 1

The Art of Diabetes
Self-Management Education

Associate Editor
Susan Cornell, BS, PharmD, CDE, FAPhA, FAADE

> You cannot teach a person anything, you can only help them find it within themselves.
>
> Galileo Galilei

This proverb truly captures the importance of the *art* of diabetes education. Since most people with diabetes will spend less than 5% of their life with the healthcare professionals who care for them, it is essential that they be able to self-manage their disease so they can have a healthy, productive life without diabetes-related complications.

Diabetes self-management education (DSME), training, and support is the cornerstone of optimal care and outcomes. A patient-centered, team-based approach to diabetes care provides the essential components from key healthcare professionals, necessary for patients to receive, learn, comprehend, and implement the self-management education that is imperative to control their disease.

Healthcare professionals sometimes focus on their own agendas in providing education and care for patients. This has proven to be futile. People with diabetes have their own agenda—and often it does not match the healthcare professional's plan. Therefore, healthcare professionals should not be surprised that patients do not achieve the goals put in place for them or follow the instructions or advice they have

been given. Since people with diabetes live most of their life without input from healthcare professionals, it is imperative that the diabetes management plan include the patient's input. The goals set must be selected by the patient and fit into his or her daily life in order to succeed. Patients are experts in their own lives, and diabetes educators need to respect and work with them to meet their needs.

To this end, the focus of this section of the *Desk Reference* is on the educator. Information and skills are provided that diabetes educators can use to help patients solve their own problems to self-manage diabetes. Changes and additions have been made to section 1 to better equip the diabetes educator with the tools needed in the continually changing world of diabetes.

Chapter 1 discusses the impact of diabetes as a major public health concern associated with devastating social and economic burdens. The evolving role of the diabetes educator and changes in the practice of DSME and practice levels are discussed. Chapter 2 focuses on the changes that have occurred within the DSME process, and chapter 3 discusses how educators can individualize health behavior change to help people with diabetes improve their overall health. Chapters 4 through 10 address each of the AADE7 Self-Care Behaviors™, while providing practical tips and strategies to aid patients in attaining their health behavior and diabetes goals. Chapter 4 includes a discussion on the latest updates in nutrition. Chapter 7 has been revised to provide more extensive coverage of the various monitoring parameters enmeshed in diabetes management, in addition to glucose monitoring. Chapter 11 provides useful information for diabetes educators in regard to the business management of DSME programs. Finally, chapter 12 is a new addition to this book and focuses on aspects of transitional care for people with diabetes. This includes transitions of care from youth to adolescence to young adult, as well as transitions within residences, such as home, hospital, and rehabilitation and long-term care facilities.

In this section, chapter authors provide practical information and describe real-world application of effective diabetes education, also known as the *art* of DSME. Through the use of skills and techniques that focus on the patient's "agenda," the authors provide approaches that help patients "find it within themselves" to self-manage their diabetes successfully.

Finally, as associate editor for the third edition of the *Desk Reference*, I would like to thank the team of talented, creative, and dedicated authors and reviewers with whom I have had the privilege to work. These folks exemplify the true meaning of a diabetes educator and mentor. I would also like to thank the outstanding, passionate, and conscientious editorial team: Carole Mensing, editor-in-chief; Cindy Halstenson, associate editor; and Margaret Maloney, AADE publications manager. These folks truly demonstrate that hard work and dedication can make a difference and improve the lives and the quality of care for people with diabetes. They are inspirational and motivational role models for all diabetes educators. Lastly, I am grateful to my mom and all of the people with or at risk for diabetes who have taught me the purpose and true meaning of diabetes self-management.

Life is not merely being alive, but being well.
Marcus Valerius Martialis

Diabetes Self-Management Education: The Art and Science of Disease Management

Sandra Drozdz Burke, PhD, APN-BC, CDE, FAADE
Janet Thorlton, PhD, RN
Monica Hall, BSN, CDE, PhD candidate

Key Concepts

- ◈ Diabetes is a worldwide public health problem requiring a multilevel system response.

- ◈ The growing financial burden of diabetes management threatens the viability of healthcare systems around the world.

- ◈ Diabetes self-management education (DSME) has been shown to be valuable and effective in both lowering the use of preventive and acute care services and positively affecting behavior change in persons with prediabetes and diabetes.

- ◈ Diabetes educators are the key to the delivery of effective diabetes self-management education and support (DSME&S).

- ◈ A growing body of practice guidelines and documents supports the career path of the diabetes educator.

- ◈ Numerous barriers to providing equal access to DSME&S must be addressed.

Diabetes Education: Challenges and Opportunities

> *Learn from yesterday, live for today, hope for tomorrow.*
>
> Albert Einstein

Definitions of Terms

- ◈ **Epidemic:** A disease that affects a defined group of people in a specific geographic location simultaneously
- ◈ **Pandemic:** An extremely widespread or globally occurring disease that affects many populations simultaneously
- ◈ **Syndemic:** A combination of health or social conditions that interact to increase the disease burden to a community, further developing a public health concern

Diabetes mellitus is a leading public health concern that has been associated with harmful economic and social effects. No one can dispute the fact that diabetes has reached epidemic proportions in the United States. Worldwide, 1.3 million people died from diabetes in 2008, and the global prevalence was estimated to be 9%[1]; therefore, it can be argued that diabetes surpassed epidemic proportions to reach pandemic levels several years ago.[2] The development of type 2 diabetes is associated with a genetic predisposition compounded by the preventable risk factors of obesity, physical inactivity, and poor nutrition. Although type 1 diabetes cannot yet be prevented, clear evidence shows that the onset of type 2 diabetes can be delayed or prevented by disrupting the association of 1 or more risk factors.[3–6] For this reason, the case may be made that type 2 diabetes is also a *syndemic.*

The good news is that type 2 diabetes is preventable. And, once diabetes (type 1 or type 2) has been diagnosed, long-term complications associated with insufficient glucose control can be prevented or delayed with good glycemic control.[3–5] Diabetes control is achieved through effective disease management that includes education to facilitate a healthy lifestyle.

Global Impact of Diabetes

The global burden of diabetes continues to grow. In the United States, 1 in every 3 individuals born today will develop diabetes during his or her lifetime.[7] Currently, of the more than 25 million Americans believed to have diabetes, about 11% of those with type 2 diabetes are undiagnosed.[1,8] With an estimated prevalence of 25.8 million Americans in 2010 and nearly 1.9 million new adult diagnoses annually,[7] the United States ranks third in the world for the highest number of people with diabetes, behind only China and India.[2,9] In the United States, an additional 79 million people have prediabetes,[7] bringing the total number of Americans with or at risk for diabetes to over 100 million.[7] Therefore, about 1 in every 10 adults in the United States already has diabetes. This is sobering and very serious, but if current projections are accurate, by 2050 as many as 1 in 3 adults will have diabetes.[10] Looking at the problem from a world view, figures from the International Diabetes Federation (IDF) suggest that the number of people with diabetes will grow from the current level of 382 million to a projected 592 million people by 2035.[2] Throughout the world, the largest increases are expected to occur in developing countries where resources are most limited.[9] Moreover, the aging populations in all countries will be disproportionately affected.[11] Present healthcare systems remain unprepared to deal with the consequences associated with a pandemic of this magnitude. Experts believe that public health initiatives promoting an understanding of the multifactorial nature of diabetes and its complications may help reduce the spread and lessen the impact of this devastating disease. Indeed, in the United States, major prevention initiatives are already under way.[12]

Incidence vs. Prevalence

Health statistics often are expressed in terms of incidence and prevalence. The distinction between the two measurements is important when interpreting the data.

Incidence measures risk of the target population developing the disease or condition being tracked over a specific time period. *Prevalence* measures the portion of the target population that has the disease or condition being tracked.

Incidence is calculated by taking the number of new cases of a disease or condition within a specific time frame—usually a year—and dividing by the size of the population.

Prevalence is calculated by dividing the number of individuals with the disease or condition at a particular point in time by the number of individuals examined.

There are differences in the incidence and prevalence of the primary types of diabetes. Globally, nearly half a million children are living with diabetes, and more than 79,000 more children develop type 1 diabetes annually.[2] Compared with the number of people with type 2 diabetes, these figures may sound small, but the incidence of type 1 diabetes has been increasing at a rate of about 3.2% per year.[13] The reasons for this increase are unclear. Type 1 diabetes is commonly associated with childhood and youth, and the greatest increases in type 1 diabetes are predicted to occur in very young children.[13,14] Still, it would be wise for all clinicians to remember that the diagnosis of type 1 diabetes may occur at any point in the lifespan. And, once diagnosed, individuals with diabetes often live well into old age.

In the United States, non-Hispanic whites under 20 years of age have a relatively high incidence of type 1 diabetes at 23.6 per 100,000 person-years, compared with African-American (15.7 per 100,000), Hispanic (15 per 100,000), and Asian (7 per 100,000) youth.[14–18] Navajo youth have a relatively low incidence of type 1 diabetes, but by age 19 the incidence of type 2 diabetes in this group rises dramatically to 39.34 per 100,000 person-years.[14,19] Even though type 2 diabetes typically develops over many years and is more common in adults, the incidence of type 2 diabetes is increasing in children of Native American, Hispanic, African-American, and Pacific Islander ancestry, especially when the youth are overweight or obese.[16–19] Regardless of the type, acquiring diabetes at such early ages carries an increased lifetime risk of developing complications.

Worldwide, type 2 diabetes represents approximately 90% to 95% of all cases of diabetes.[2] There are no apparent gender differences in the prevalence of type 2 diabetes, but in the United States, diabetes is far more common in nonwhites and in older populations. Data from the National Health and Nutrition Examination Survey (NHANES) suggest that the prevalence of diabetes is 70% to 80% higher in non-Hispanic blacks and Mexican Americans compared with non-Hispanic whites.[20–22] As for the aging population, while 11.3% of the overall adult population has diabetes, when the data are broken down according to age, about 27% of people over age 60 are shown to have diabetes.[7] Cowie and colleagues[20] reported the sobering statistics that 3 out of every 4 older adults in the United States have diagnosed diabetes, undiagnosed diabetes, or prediabetes. In contrast, the greatest numbers of individuals with diabetes in developing countries are between 40 and 59 years of age.[9]

Financial Burden of Diabetes

The ever-increasing prevalence of diabetes is associated with substantial economic impact. Complications such as retinopathy, neuropathy, and nephropathy, which are commonly present at diagnosis of the disease in developing nations, make treatment very expensive.[23] In the United States, the economic impact of diabetes is staggering, as about $245 billion is spent annually on diagnosed diabetes. This represents a 41% escalation in cost over the previous 5 years.[24] Overall, persons with diabetes in the United States spend nearly 2½ times more dollars on medical costs than those without the disease.[7,24] Several years ago, the cost of caring for diabetes in the United States was expected to be 20% of the gross domestic product (GDP) by 2016.[25] As of 2013, this expectation was exceeded. Currently, more than 1 in every 5 dollars from the US economy is used to pay for costs linked to diabetes. These costs include substantial direct medical expenses for inpatient

care, outpatient care, emergency care, medications, and durable medical equipment, as well as indirect costs for absenteeism, reduced productivity at work, and lost productivity due to disability or premature death.[24,26] Individuals with diabetes are more likely to be absent from work (absenteeism) and at work, suffer from fatigue, or have reduced concentration; additionally, they may not be able to perform at a normal level (presenteeism). Nearly 11 million people with diabetes are Medicare eligible,[7] and this figure is expected to increase 34% to a level of 14.6 million by 2034.[27] The financial burden of diabetes is likely to continue to adversely affect the ability of developed countries to finance their national healthcare systems, and it will also have a considerable negative impact on the economic progress being made in developing countries. In a recent report forecasting the impact of diabetes over the next decade, Rowley and Bezold acknowledged the tremendous impact of preventing type 2 diabetes. They projected that effective management in just 50% of persons with existing diabetes would save over $50 billion in dialysis costs alone.[28]

At the individual level, great disparities exist in the economic resources available to persons with diabetes. The limited amount of personal disposable income available for expenses may complicate and possibly hinder desired practices related to diabetes. Recent economic trends have had a negative impact on personal disposable income. Whereas the median income in the United States was $52,029 in 2008, it dropped to $50,502 in 2011.[29] Income varies by age and by ethnic background. Historically, African-American, Pacific Islander, and Navajo youth have been most likely to reside in families with very low incomes (at or below $25,000 annually), whereas greater than 40% of Asian-American households report incomes in excess of $75,000.[16,18,19] Sixty percent of non-Hispanic whites with type 1 diabetes live in households with incomes reported greater than $50,000; however, Caucasians with type 2 diabetes were less likely to have similar income levels.[15] The US Census Bureau provides information on household income by race.[30] Older adult populations are also economically vulnerable. In 2008, the median income for Americans aged 65 and older was $41,851 (US Census Bureau, 2008[31]). Finally, according to the Henry J. Kaiser Family Foundation, 47 million Americans remained uninsured in

2013.[32] This number should decline as the Affordable Care Act continues to roll out; but at the time of this writing, the uninsured population continues to lack the resources for diabetes education and self-care.[33]

Because diabetes affects all segments of society, the impact of this disease is far reaching. In 2010, an estimated 4 million deaths were attributed to diabetes worldwide, with the proportionate number of deaths from diabetes in middle-aged women sometimes reaching nearly 25%.[34] By 2013, the annual death rate attributable to diabetes had exceeded 5 million worldwide.[35]

In the United States, diabetes is ranked as the seventh leading cause of death, and it is generally believed that estimates of mortality due to diabetes are greatly underestimated because the cause of death in persons with diabetes is often ascribed to other conditions.[7] Clearly, diabetes has major social, financial, and individual implications. Current evidence suggests the impact can be reduced by diabetes education, but what exactly *is* diabetes education?

Diabetes Education

A common impression is that diabetes education simply involves the transfer of information from a healthcare professional to a patient. This belief is rooted in the compliance/adherence model to guide care. Using this model, the healthcare provider serves as the expert and the patient as a passive recipient of information. The ultimate goal of diabetes education for many clinicians is improved glycemic control.

As it turns out, this is only partially correct. While improved glycemic control remains an important outcome of diabetes management, over the past 3 decades, it became clear that while knowledge is an essential prerequisite for self-care, knowledge alone is not enough to promote behavior change.[36–38] In response to a growing body of evidence, the process of diabetes education evolved from information delivery to a focus on techniques that promote effective self-management.[39–41] The process may begin with topical content, but to be effective the process of diabetes education must also include patient-directed goal setting and follow-up. Because the care of diabetes is primarily self-directed, self-management support is a key element in success and is now included in the National Standards for Diabetes Education.[42,43]

This important shift in focus led to DSME now being defined as "a collaborative process through which people with or at risk for diabetes gain the knowledge and skills needed to modify behavior and successfully self-manage the disease and its related conditions. It is an interactive, ongoing process involving the person with diabetes (or the caregiver or family) and a diabetes educator(s)."[44] The goal of DSME is no longer just about glycemic control; it now encompasses improved quality of life, self-care behaviors leading to improvements in a wide variety of clinical attributes, and decreased healthcare costs.[42,45,46] Ongoing support of and for diabetes self-management is recognized as a key strategy for success. National Standards for Diabetes Self-Management and Support (DSME&S) define diabetes self-management support as "activities that assist the person with prediabetes or diabetes in implementing and sustaining the behaviors needed to manage his or her condition on an ongoing basis beyond or outside of formal self-management training.[47] The type of support provided can be behavioral, educational, psychosocial, or clinical."[45]

Previous national standards used 5 evidence-based principles to guide the development and implementation of diabetes education.[41] These principles reflected the knowledge that current models of diabetes education improve clinical outcomes and that the approach and setting are important aspects for success. Patient-centered empowerment approaches to DSME have been very successful because they are based on principles of self-determination and support for autonomy.[38] Patients believe this approach acknowledges the value of the individual's voice in his or her own care, a fact that enables the well-informed patient to choose more effectively.[48] From the clinician's perspective, the essential outcomes of DSME include improved glycemic control and overall risk reduction. From the patient's perspective, the essential outcome of DSME is sufficient knowledge to perform necessary skills and make the lifestyle changes required to control diabetes and achieve a satisfactory quality of life. Effective diabetes education for self-management can lead to positive outcomes to satisfy both patients and clinicians. The addition of support to the framework of DSME acknowledges that education for self-management of this complex chronic disease cannot be a single or isolated process. Self-management is continuous and difficult, and it changes as the individual ages and the disease progresses. Ongoing education and support provide needed assistance for the patient and the family. Detailed information about various approaches to diabetes education can be found in chapter 3.

Evolution of the Term "Diabetes Self-Management Education/ Training" (DSME/T)

- ◆ The diabetes education process has been called diabetes self-management education (DSME).[46]
- ◆ DSME is the official term used in the National Standards for Diabetes Self-Management Education.[46] DSME&S represents the addition of support to DSME.
- ◆ Diabetes self-management training (DSMT) is the official terminology used by the Centers for Medicare and Medicaid Services (CMS).[46]
- ◆ In reality, diabetes educators provide more than training—they provide education. Because CMS and some other payers reimburse only for training and are unwilling to pay for education, AADE embraces both terms to reflect the accuracy of what is provided to the patient along with the pragmatism required by payer coverage and reimbursement policies.

Diabetes self-management support includes the activities that assist the person with prediabetes or diabetes in implementing and sustaining the behaviors needed to manage his or her condition on an ongoing basis beyond or outside of formal self-management training. The type of support provided can be behavioral, educational, psychosocial, or clinical.[43]

The process of diabetes education is clearly important, but process alone does not guarantee success. The AADE published an influential position statement in 2003 illustrating the importance of the outcome of DSME.[49] In this widely accepted and now classic position statement, the AADE established 5 standards for outcome measurement of DSME (see Table 1.1). In 2003, behavior change was identified as the unique outcome criterion for diabetes education

TABLE 1.1   Standards for Outcomes Measurement of DSME
1. Behavior change is the unique outcome measurement for DSME.
2. Seven diabetes self-care behavior measures determine the effectiveness of DSME at individual, participant, and population levels.
3. Diabetes self-care behaviors should be evaluated at baseline and then at regular intervals after the education program.
4. The continuum of outcomes, including learning, behavioral, clinical, and health status, should be assessed to demonstrate the interrelationship between DSME and behavior change in the care of individuals with diabetes.
5. Individual patient outcomes are used to guide the intervention and improve care for that patient. Aggregate population outcomes are used to guide programmatic services and for continuous quality improvement activities for the DSME and the population it serves.

Source: K Mulcahy, M Maryniuk, M Peeples, et al, "Position statement: standards for outcomes measurement of diabetes self-management education," *Diabetes Educ* 29, no. 5 (2003): 809.

for the first time. Seven specific self-care behaviors, now known as the AADE7™, were identified.

The position statement emphasized the need for baseline and periodic measurement of self-care behaviors that enable program staff to evaluate and use both individual and program data as guides for patient care and program improvement.[49] Diabetes education began moving from its position in health care as a ubiquitous term with questionable impact on a select group of patients to an established and legitimate intervention for a broad spectrum of patients.

AADE7 Self-Care Behaviors™

Healthy eating

Being active

Monitoring

Taking medication

Problem solving

Healthy coping

Reducing risks

Despite a growing body of literature supporting diabetes education, questions remained about the value and effectiveness of DSME. For well over a decade now, studies have demonstrated that structured (formal) DSME results in improved knowledge, along with improved fasting glucose, A1C, lipid, and blood pressure levels.[50–56] For example, a structured life coach program resulted in better A1C, lipid, and blood pressure goals for younger adult patients with type 1 diabetes or type 2 diabetes.[57] Diabetes disease management programs for the older adult can lead to better clinical outcomes including fewer hospitalizations and more effective use of medications and diagnostic testing.[58] More recently, diabetes education with follow-up support delivered by diabetes educators not only resulted in better self-management knowledge but also led to improved patient satisfaction and reductions in diabetes-related distress.[59] And, culturally appropriate diabetes education effectively improves knowledge, healthy lifestyles, and A1C levels in ethnic minority groups, at least in the short-term.[60] Engaging patients, providing self-management support along with comprehensive education, and using healthcare team members from a wide variety of disciplines are clearly effective.

The Chronic Care Model (CCM) identifies the essential elements of a healthcare system that encourage high-quality chronic disease care. These elements include the community, the health system, self-management support, delivery system design, decision support, and clinical information systems. The CCM fosters productive interactions between informed patients who take an active part in their care and providers with resources and expertise.

Source: Copyright 1996-2010 The MacColl Institute. The Improving Chronic Illness Care program is supported by The Robert Wood Johnson Foundation, with direction and technical assistance provided by Group Health's MacColl Institute for Healthcare Innovation.

Importantly, a cost-benefit analysis of the impact of DSME demonstrated that patients receiving formal diabetes education used preventive services more and acute care services less, often resulting in lower overall healthcare costs.[61] These patients were more likely

The CCM provides an ideal framework to support DSME because it provides a cogent basis on which to promote self-management based on the AADE7™ framework.

Source: LM Siminerio, SR Drab, RA Gabbay, "AADE position statement: diabetes educators: implementing the chronic care model," *Diabetes Educ* 34, no. 3 (2008): 455 (cited 2014 Mar 28). On the Internet at: http://www.diabeteseducator. org/export/sites/aade/_resources/pdf/PositionState ment_xChronicCareModelx_2008.pdf.

to have A1C levels tested, to get screening kidney and eye exams, and to show improvements in A1C levels. Diabetes self-management education is not just effective in treating people with diabetes. Because diabetes education leads to sustained behavior change, it is instrumental in preventing type 2 diabetes in people with prediabetes.[6,62,63] A follow-up cost-benefit analysis of diabetes education delivered by qualified diabetes educators not only demonstrated lower cost patterns but also demonstrated that patients educated in recognized or accredited programs were more likely to achieve self-management targets.[64] In short, it is now clear that DSME is valuable and effective, particularly when provided by a credentialed educator.[46,49,65,66] The importance of diabetes education is particularly relevant given that only 14.3% of all people with diabetes are successfully achieving target values in 3 key areas: glycemic control, blood pressure control, and lipid control.[67]

"Disease management is a system of coordinated health care interventions and communications for populations with conditions in which patient self-care efforts are significant."

Source: Population Health Alliance, "Definition of disease management," *Outcomes Guidelines Report*, vol. 5 (Washington, DC: Care Continuum Alliance, 2010; cited 2014 Mar 27). On the Internet at: http://populationhealthalliance.org/research/ phm-glossary/d.html.

Increasingly, third-party payers are recognizing the value of DSME and are willing to underwrite or reimburse for quality DSME. This willingness to support DSME&S will be a critical factor as healthcare delivery models are redesigned. Programs demonstrating quality in delivery and outcomes are expected to be highly sought after. One way to ensure quality is by achieving and maintaining accreditation or recognition status. The AADE and the American Diabetes Association (ADA) offer accreditation or recognition status to programs meeting established criteria. Additionally, The Joint Commission (formerly JCAHO) provides accreditation for inpatient diabetes management.

- ◆ AADE: Diabetes Education Accreditation Program (DEAP): http://www.diabeteseducator. org/ProfessionalResources/accred/
- ◆ ADA: Education Recognition Program (ERP): http://professional.diabetes.org/Home DiabetesEducationAndRecognition.aspx? hsid=4
- ◆ The Joint Commission: Inpatient Diabetes Certification: http://www.jointcommission. org/certification/inpatient_diabetes.aspx

Quality DSME&S programs are generally developed, managed, and led by qualified, experienced, and usually credentialed diabetes educators. Over the years, however, questions have emerged about the definition of the diabetes educator.

Diabetes Educators

According to the AADE, diabetes educators are healthcare professionals who focus on helping people with and at risk for diabetes and related conditions achieve behavior-change goals which, in turn, lead to better clinical outcomes and improved health status. Diabetes educators are clinicians who apply in-depth knowledge and skills in the biological and social sciences, communication, counseling, and education to provide self-management education, self-management training, and ongoing support to those affected by diabetes.[42]

The first educators were registered nurses and registered dietitians. Although more than 70% of today's diabetes educators still originate from these 2 professions, clinicians from a wide variety of other healthcare occupations, including pharmacy, social work, and exercise physiology, choose to specialize in diabetes education.[45,68,70] The newest group of diabetes educators are those individuals with a master certified health education specialist (MCHES) credential. Eligible for certification in 2014, this group of public health workers expands the pool of individuals qualified to engage in diabetes prevention and education. Depending on the setting and the educator's professional background and credentials, he or she may be active in providing DSME&S, medical nutrition therapy (MNT), clinical management, disease management, counseling, and/or health professional education and research.[45,69,71] Diabetes educators work in various settings including inpatient, outpatient, community, home care, retail outlets, industry, and academia. As well as growing numbers of diabetes educators in nontraditional settings, findings from the 2012 National Diabetes Education Practice Survey conducted by the AADE demonstrate growth in the number of both outpatient and hospital-based settings.[70] Some educators work in collaborative practice settings, others have established independent practices, and still others serve as consultants. Diabetes educators are involved in direct patient care, education of other healthcare professionals, research, social reform, and advocacy. Many diabetes educators obtain certification in the specialty and are credentialed as a certified diabetes educator (CDE) or board certified–advanced diabetes manager (BC-ADM) or, in some cases, both. An educational background in health care, considerable experience working with people with diabetes, and a comprehensive knowledge base enable a qualified healthcare professional to take a certification examination. It has long been the AADE's position that diabetes educators should work toward certification in the specialty. In the United States, the National Certification Board for Diabetes Educators sets the criteria for CDE certification, whereas the AADE establishes the criteria for the BC-ADM credential. Other countries often have their own standards, processes, and names for the credentialed educator. Of interest are results from recent surveys suggesting that while certification is valued by the educator, it may no longer be required for employment.[45,69] If this finding persists over time, it will become a trend suggesting that employers fail to understand the complexities of DSME&S and the critical role of the credentialed diabetes educator in the delivery of comprehensive care. Also troubling is the notion that primary care providers may not fully appreciate the contribution of diabetes educators in facilitating self-care management, a trend suggested by referral patterns.[42,46,68,72]

The practice of diabetes education has been guided by the Scope and Standards of Practice, Standards of Practice, and Standards of Professional Performance (Scope of Practice) for more than 2 decades. Revised several times since its inception, the Scope and Standards defines diabetes education and the role of the diabetes educator, providing a framework for practice and a guideline for excellence.[73–76] Historically, 3 practice options have been defined in the Scope and Standards: the diabetes educator, the CDE, and the BC-ADM. Six standards of practice provide a quality blueprint enabling diabetes educators to design, deliver, and evaluate programs and personnel. Moreover, people with diabetes, non–diabetes specialist providers, and other stakeholders can use these standards for quality assessment purposes.[77] Recognizing that many patients never have the opportunity to interface with a credentialed diabetes educator, the AADE takes the position that all healthcare providers should have sufficient diabetes knowledge to provide safe clinical care for people with diabetes. Healthcare providers with a strong foundation in diabetes knowledge are more likely to choose to partner with diabetes educators and possibly even choose a diabetes specialty career path.

At present, although some programs have emerged, few formal professional educational paths exist for diabetes educators, despite the considerable knowledge, skills, and abilities required for the job.[42,45,46,78,81] As stated in the Scope and Standards of Practice, "Mastery . . . is obtained through formal and continuing education, individual study and mentorship."[77,81] In 2009, the AADE published important companion documents to Scope of Practice, Standards of Practice and Standards of Professional Performance; Guidelines for the Practice of Diabetes Self-Management Education; and Competencies for Diabetes Educators.[42,46,76,78] Taken together, these materials were intended to support the specialty practice of diabetes education. One reason to develop and publish guidelines and competencies was to acknowledge the value of diabetes

education providers across a broad continuum, from the community health worker to the advanced-level diabetes care and education provider. People with diabetes obtain self-care information from a wide variety of sources, including physicians, pharmacists, hospital and/or clinic staff, and parish nurses, as well as from *promotoras* and other community health workers. While most of these individuals do not fit the traditional definition of a diabetes educator, these caregivers often serve as the patient's primary source of self-management information or support. Attempting to address this conundrum, the AADE defined 5 levels of practice.[82] The levels identified a spectrum of practice ranging from the community health worker to the expert practitioner of diabetes education and/or management. Although these initial guidelines outlined the key differences between the various levels of educator, a fundamental flaw in conceptualizing the levels existed. Specifically, the scope of practice is, first and foremost, defined by an individual's professional discipline of origin. Unless or until widespread state licensure is enacted for diabetes educators, registered nurses, licensed or registered dietitians, licensed pharmacists, and other licensed healthcare workers are legally bound by the limits set for their profession at the state level. The functions performed by healthcare workers falling outside the boundaries set by the various professions are limited to those which can be delegated to this level of health worker by licensed healthcare professionals. In accordance with state laws in some states, certain things, such as assessment, cannot be delegated to or conducted by a nonprofessional.

To address this weakness in the definition of functional levels of the diabetes educator, the AADE recently revised the levels of practice. Recognizing the important contributions of all care providers, including the nontraditional and/or non-licensed healthcare worker, the AADE developed a distinctly separate category, aptly termed the diabetes educator associate, with its own leveling process. The focus of the diabetes educator associate, who works under the direction of the diabetes educator, is to provide information and ongoing support to individuals.

The remaining 4 original levels of the diabetes educator were collapsed into 3 explicit levels. Each of these levels, which is aligned with specific competencies, defines the requisite professional background as well as the knowledge, skills, and behaviors expected of the diabetes educator. This type of practice-level model addresses the natural progression from novice to expert defined by Dreyfus[83] and then adapted to nursing by Benner[84] so many years ago. Collapsing the original 5 levels to 3 was designed to more explicitly define the career path needed for development of a workforce capable of providing high-quality, evidence-based diabetes care, education, and support. Importantly, the redefined levels are not only competency based but conceptualized according to the nature of the work of the educator. The percentage of time the educator engages in activities related to patient knowledge and skill development versus adaptation to self-management varies according to the experiential base of the educator. The latter term, "adaptation," recognizes that behavior change is the unique outcome of diabetes education. The term was selected because it can reflect all aspects required for self-management. This is further clarified in the following paragraphs.

Levels of practice are designed to help the individual clinician determine his or her appropriate entry point to the specialty practice of diabetes education and, importantly, to clarify the competencies required for advancement to the next level. Each level of practice builds on the previous one(s) and recognizes that clinical expertise within each level increases over time. The foundational concepts of diabetes education are covered in great detail in chapter 2. To be successful with diabetes self-management, the patient must know what to do (knowledge), how to do it (skill), and how to act on the results of the tasks of self-management (adaptation). Depending on the level of the educator, the focus of interaction with the patient will vary according to these elements. For example, at level 1, the educator's efforts are focused on transmission of knowledge and skills. As the diabetes educator becomes increasingly proficient, his or her time is more likely to be devoted to promoting behavior change at the patient level and, ultimately, higher level skills at the programmatic and systems levels. Over the course of time, each educator will move through the levels of proficiency, from novice to expert, and will be able to document development of an increasingly wider body of diabetes specialty knowledge and skills through achievement of competencies.

The revised levels of the diabetes educator are presented in Table 1.2. At level 1, educators are typically point-of-care healthcare professionals who have, at a minimum, completed the educational requirements for a specific health profession's degree. They are licensed to practice in their primary professional discipline or, in some cases, are members of a professional registry (eg, registered dietitians). Entry-level MCHESs would also fall into this category. Many level 1 educators have the basic background knowledge of diabetes inherent to academic training in health professions, but they have not developed a broad-based diabetes specialty practice knowledge base. People with diabetes commonly interface with level 1 educators in hospitals, clinics, home care, and pharmacy settings. It is critical that this level of provider have sufficient knowledge to provide safe care and accurate information to the individual with diabetes. Level 1 diabetes educators are at the novice or advanced beginner level on the Dreyfus continuum. The educator's focus at this level is on transmitting knowledge related to essential skills for safe self-management. Thinking about this level from the standpoint of the emphasis on Bloom's (revised) taxonomy, at level 1 the educator's focus is on the lowest-level objectives (eg, remembering, understanding, and applying). Petram provided an excellent and concise explanation of the revised taxonomy.[85] Clinicians at this level possess the teaching and learning skills learned in their professional program of origin. Most likely, level 1 educators incorporate information provided by preprocessed delivery models including online programs or existing programs such as the Stanford or other models. As an example, the newly diagnosed patient will need instructions about what to do before the first diabetes education appointment or class. The level 1 educator can instruct the patient on self-monitoring of blood glucose (SMBG), basic nutrition guidelines, record keeping, and the importance of attending DSME classes. Ideally, the level 1 educator follows up with the patient between diabetes education sessions to provide support.

According to the Dreyfus model, experience is gained over time, and an individual moves from the level of advanced beginner to competent and then to proficient professional. In diabetes education, level 2 includes those healthcare providers who have achieved an advanced body of core knowledge and

TABLE 1.2 Diabetes Educator Practice Levels

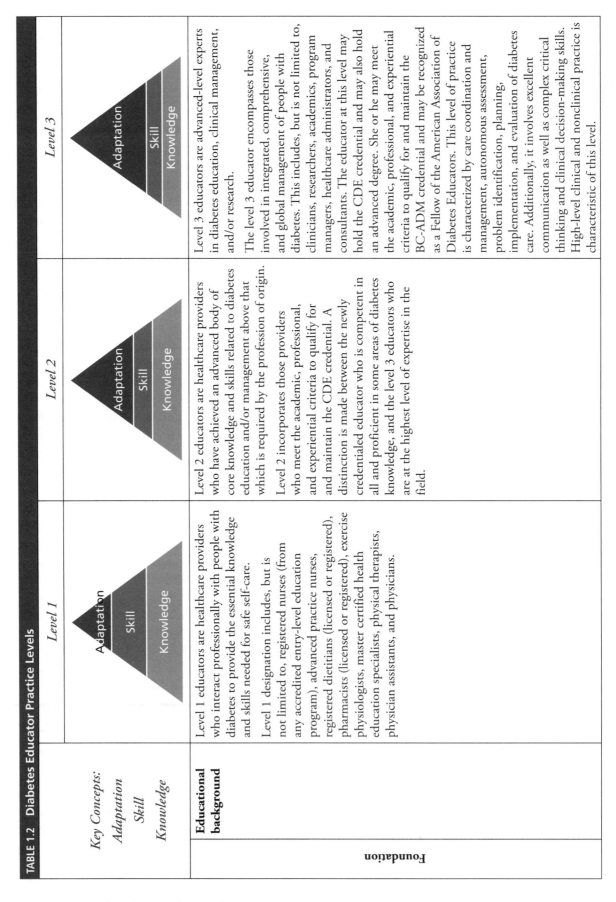

Key Concepts: *Adaptation* *Skill* *Knowledge*	*Level 1*	*Level 2*	*Level 3*
Educational background	Level 1 educators are healthcare providers who interact professionally with people with diabetes to provide the essential knowledge and skills needed for safe self-care. Level 1 designation includes, but is not limited to, registered nurses (from any accredited entry-level education program), advanced practice nurses, registered dietitians (licensed or registered), pharmacists (licensed or registered), exercise physiologists, master certified health education specialists, physical therapists, physician assistants, and physicians.	Level 2 educators are healthcare providers who have achieved an advanced body of core knowledge and skills related to diabetes education and/or management above that which is required by the profession of origin. Level 2 incorporates those providers who meet the academic, professional, and experiential criteria to qualify for and maintain the CDE credential. A distinction is made between the newly credentialed educator who is competent in all and proficient in some areas of diabetes knowledge, and the level 3 educators who are at the highest level of expertise in the field.	Level 3 educators are advanced-level experts in diabetes education, clinical management, and/or research. The level 3 educator encompasses those involved in integrated, comprehensive, and global management of people with diabetes. This includes, but is not limited to, clinicians, researchers, academics, program managers, healthcare administrators, and consultants. The educator at this level may hold the CDE credential and may also hold an advanced degree. She or he may meet the academic, professional, and experiential criteria to qualify for and maintain the BC-ADM credential and may be recognized as a Fellow of the American Association of Diabetes Educators. This level of practice is characterized by care coordination and management, autonomous assessment, problem identification, planning, implementation, and evaluation of diabetes care. Additionally, it involves excellent communication as well as complex critical thinking and clinical decision-making skills. High-level clinical and nonclinical practice is characteristic of this level.

Foundation

	Beginner/Advanced beginner Basic	Competent/Proficient Intermediate	Expert Advanced level
Educator/ Clinician level of practice	Beginner/Advanced beginner Basic	Competent/Proficient Intermediate	Expert Advanced level
Expected and domain-specific knowledge, skills, and abilities for delivery of diabetes education/ support (focus on the educator)	The educator's focus is on transmitting knowledge related to essential skills for safe self-management.	The educator/clinician's focus is on both knowledge and skills to create individualized self-management plans, coordinate care, interpret personal data, conduct focused and/or complete educational assessments and promote successful self-management through adaptation.	The clinician/educator's focus is on higher level counseling, regimen adjustment (as appropriate for scope of practice), therapeutic problem solving, and recognizing and prioritizing complex data. Focused and/or complete clinical and educational assessments are used to guide decision making. Develop management materials and policies
	See Scope of Practice, Standards of Practice, and Standards of Professional Performance for Diabetes Educators	See Scope of Practice, Standards of Practice, and Standards of Professional Performance for Diabetes Educators	See Scope of Practice, Standards of Practice, and Standards of Professional Performance for Diabetes Educators
Non-diabetes foundational skills for the delivery of diabetes education	Bloom's taxonomy: remembering, understanding, applying Teaching and learning skills: preprocessed delivery models	Bloom's taxonomy: applying, analyzing evaluating Teaching and learning skills: Individualized assessment & delivery Educator-facilitated group discussion. Differentiate teaching from learning objectives	Bloom's taxonomy: analyzing, evaluating, creating Teaching and learning skills: Creative, individualized teaching for self-management? Developing and evaluating new models of education
Novice to expert continuum (Dreyfus model) Expertise develops over time	Entry level	CDE	BC-ADM
Self-assessment based on competencies	TBD Pre-test	TBD Pre-test based on scenarios	TBD Pre-test based on scenarios

(Foundation)

skills related to diabetes education and/or management above that which is required by the profession of origin. The level 2 educator possesses the minimum competencies to qualify for licensure. Level 2 incorporates those providers who may meet the academic, professional, and experiential criteria to qualify for and maintain the CDE credential. Importantly, however, level 2 educators may or may not hold the CDE credential. A number of competent/proficient educators do not meet all criteria set by the certifying board or, for a variety of reasons, do not wish to sit for certification. These educators may be found in a variety of settings and may include home care nurses, pharmacists, hospital patient educators, public health professionals, and academics who have considerable experience working with people with diabetes but whose practice is not limited to diabetes. Thinking about Bloom's revised taxonomy, at this level, the educator's focus is on applying, analyzing, and evaluating. While these midlevel and higher level learning objectives still allow for transmission of knowledge and skill sets, there is an increased focus on facilitating healthy lifestyle behaviors. The level 2 educator has the knowledge, skill, and ability to provide individualized assessment of learning needs and deliver content specific to those needs. Teaching may be done individually or in groups. Instructional methodology (eg, facilitated discussion) is selected based on individual or group needs. Level 2 educators are skilled professionals in diabetes education. However, a distinction is made between the newly credentialed educator who is competent in all and proficient in some areas of diabetes education practice, and level 3 educators who are at the highest level of expertise in the field. Level 3 educators are advanced-level experts in diabetes education, clinical management, and/or research. On the Dreyfus continuum, this group constitutes the most expert diabetes educators (ie, those who have the greatest amount of experience and expertise in the field of diabetes education and management); thus, educators from this group are most likely to be inducted as Fellows of the American Association of Diabetes Educators (FAADE). Level 3 educator/clinicians are involved in integrated, comprehensive, and global management of people with diabetes. The educator at this level is likely to meet the academic, professional, and experiential criteria to qualify for and maintain the BC-ADM credential.

Like level 2 educators, those at level 3 may or may not hold voluntary credentialing in the specialty, but can demonstrate the competencies associated with the highest level of practice in diabetes education. This level of practice is characterized by care coordination and management, autonomous assessment, problem identification, planning, implementation, and evaluation of diabetes care. It involves excellent communication skills as well as complex critical thinking and clinical decision-making skills. An educator at level 3 typically has considerable experience and advanced skills in the delivery of DSME. This knowledge and experience enable the educator to work with even the most complex people with diabetes. Always guided by individual scope of practice, the clinician/educator's focus is on higher level counseling, regimen adjustment, therapeutic problem solving, and recognizing and prioritizing complex data. He or she engages in focused and/or complete clinical and educational assessments to guide clinical decision making and is a resource for the development of management materials and policies in a variety of settings, including public health. At the patient level, the level 3 educator maximizes teaching and learning skills to focus on the highest level of learning objectives: analyzing, evaluating, and creating. The level 3 educator may also be engaged in evaluation of existing models of education and development of new ones. And, at the systems level, this educator is often involved in program design and management. Between them, level 2 and level 3 educators demonstrate the composite array of competencies in the specialty that equip them to guide the self-management education trajectory of the person with diabetes.

With 100 million Americans already with or at risk for diabetes, educators from all levels are indispensable in the delivery of DSME and support of the person with diabetes. Recognizing the importance of non-licensed and/or supportive personnel, the AADE created a separate category of provider called the diabetes educator associate.

A document outlining the roles and responsibilities for the diabetes educator associate is in its initial stages of development. This document is intended to illustrate the important role of the wide variety of unlicensed health workers in the work associated with diabetes education and support. Whereas the diabetes educator associate is engaged in information transmission,[59,86] it is important to recognize the distinction between exchange of information and comprehensive learning assessment, targeted instruction and acquisition of knowledge. Level 3 educators should continue to assume key roles in designing and directing DSME practice, but should also focus on how best to educate, support, and mentor educators from all other levels of practice, including the diabetes educator associate.[86]

To assist with this, the AADE has a series of competencies for diabetes educators.[77] These competencies are intended to provide structure for the knowledge, skills, and abilities required for practice at each level across the continuum of diabetes care. The knowledge base needed to provide quality diabetes education is multifaceted, so the competencies are structured into 5 broad categories called domains (see Table 1.3). Domain I addresses the foundational knowledge of diabetes. It includes diabetes pathophysiology, epidemiology, and clinical guidelines. Domain II encompasses the competencies needed to provide culturally competent, supportive care across the lifespan. Domain III focuses on aspects of teaching and learning and behavior change. The competencies in this domain include a focus on healthy coping and problem solving, 2 of the behaviors identified in the AADE7™. Domain IV identifies the competencies

required to provide effective DSME. It incorporates the remaining 5 behaviors of the AADE7™. Domain V is focused on program and business management. Competencies in this domain enable the educator to create a climate that supports successful self-management of diabetes. Within each domain, the competency is defined by specific learner/user objectives. The objectives for level 1 provide basic background knowledge. Each subsequent level assumes proficiency with the competencies at the previous level. The competencies can be used by diabetes educators at all levels. They can serve as a framework to assist the educator in defining the knowledge, skills, and abilities needed to function effectively at his or her level and can also be used to identify the content needed for further professional development. When the competencies are updated and consistent with the revised levels of practice, the document will be available on the AADE Web site.

Revisions to the levels of practice were made to more explicitly define roles and responsibilities based on the educator's functional capacity, rather than on his or her professional background. Whereas the focus of education at level 1 is transmitting knowledge and skill, as the educator gains knowledge and experience, that focus shifts to increasingly less time with knowledge and skill development and more time

TABLE 1.3 **Competency Domains for Diabetes Educators**
Domain I: Pathophysiology, Epidemiology, and Clinical Guidelines of Diabetes
This domain addresses the competencies needed for individuals to demonstrate familiarity with pathophysiology, epidemiology, and clinical guidelines consistent with diabetes care provider level.
Domain II: Culturally Competent, Supportive Care Across the Lifespan
This domain addresses the competencies needed to provide diabetes support and care in a culturally competent manner across the lifespan.
Domain III: Teaching and Learning
This domain addresses the competencies needed to apply principles of teaching and learning and/or behavior change to facilitate self-management skills of individuals with diabetes.
Domain IV: Self-Management Education
This domain addresses the competencies needed to work with an interdisciplinary diabetes care team to tailor interventions to individual patient self-management education needs.
Domain V: Program and Business Management
This domain addresses the competencies needed to apply principles of program and/or business management to create a climate that supports successful self-management of diabetes.

Source: American Association of Diabetes Educators, *Competencies for Diabetes Educators* (Chicago: American Association of Diabetes Educators, 2009).

American Association of Diabetes Educators©

facilitating successful self-management. The levels are still based on the Dreyfus (novice to expert) model of practice, where clinicians move from the level of advanced beginner, to competence, to proficiency, and into expertise according to the amount of time they spend in the field of practice. There will always be some degree of overlap between the levels. This is because movement from level to level is competency driven. At any given level, educators may have more or less expertise in a particular competency. For example, level 2 educators who are RN CDEs will differ from RD/LD CDEs in their fundamental background knowledge of nutrition.

The Scope of Practice, Standards of Practice and Standards of Professional Performance for Diabetes Educators; the Competencies for Diabetes Educators; and the Guidelines for the Practice of Diabetes Education are designed to promote effective, quality DSME. They guide the diabetes educator's practice. An important issue to consider, however, is the availability of that practice within the community.

Barriers and Facilitators to Access

There is clear evidence that well-controlled diabetes is associated with fewer chronic complications and that DSME is associated with improved diabetes control.[3–5,66,87] Ideally, all people with diabetes would receive formal diabetes education from a qualified provider. Currently, only about 55% of people with diabetes in the United States receive DSME.[64] According to Healthy People 2010, the number of people receiving formal diabetes education did not reach the goal of 60%. Consequently, the proposed goal for Healthy People 2020 (HP 2020) remains the same, that is, "to increase the proportion of persons with diagnosed diabetes who receive formal diabetes education."[88] As well, healthy lifestyle behaviors for metabolic control and prevention of diabetes remain a 2020 goal. The initial goal to increase the number of people with diabetes who have their A1C level tested twice a year has already been met. However, while it is important that people with diabetes have A1C levels tested, it is more important that they achieve individualized glycemic targets. Nationwide,

an estimated 57% of people with diabetes had A1C levels at the target level (of under 7%) in 2004, but this fell to 52.5% from 2007 to 2010.[67] Data from NHANES and the Behavioral Risk Factor Surveillance System (BRFSS) continue to show significant disparities in control among minority populations, with non-Hispanic whites having the highest percentage of A1C at goal, followed by non-Hispanic blacks, then all Hispanics. And, as previously mentioned, very few individuals with diabetes achieve target levels in the 3 main areas of blood glucose, blood pressure, and blood lipid control.

Surveys have examined the profile of patients seen by the typical diabetes educator. According to Zrebiec,[69] the typical patient seen by a CDE is a Caucasian adult with type 2 diabetes taking oral agents alone or in combination with insulin. In a recent survey of practice settings, Martin and colleagues[68] found that while most diabetes educator practices were in the outpatient setting, the majority were in the most highly populous states. Similarly, demographic findings from the first AADE member salary survey showed that the majority (68%) of practices are outpatient based, with 75% in urban or suburban areas.[45] Children and older adults with diabetes represent particularly vulnerable populations. A key element in successful management for children is good control in the school setting, but school personnel are generally poorly prepared to support the needs of the child with diabetes.[89] The prevalence of type 2 diabetes among older adults is nearly twice that of young and middle adults, yet the frequency of diabetes education and the level of diabetes care in this population, particularly in the low-income elderly, are suboptimal.[69,90]

Findings from these studies reveal important barriers to access. First, geographic barriers limit access to qualified diabetes educators. Rural areas, particularly in the South, are underserved by diabetes educators. This is particularly troublesome because the so-called Diabetes Belt cuts a swath across the southern United States. This is where the highest concentration of adults with diabetes in the country can be found.[70] Next, there are demographic barriers influencing care management. Adults with type 2 diabetes make up the majority of patients seen by diabetes educators.[69]

Nearly 27% of adults age 65 or older have diabetes, yet the vast majority of these individuals fail to take advantage of diabetes education, an established Medicare benefit.[61,64] Most older adults live independently, but a particularly vulnerable group is those elders living in long-term care (LTC) settings. Neither the frail elder with diabetes in LTC nor his or her caregivers typically utilize the services or expertise of diabetes educators.[91] With respect to children, it is not surprising to see that they constitute smaller proportions of clinical practice, as people with type 1 diabetes represent only 5% to 10% of the diabetes population.[4] Even when parents and children with diabetes receive good clinical care, that care management knowledge rarely extends to personnel at school, where children spend nearly one-third of their lives. This lack of care management knowledge among teachers and school nurses is of even greater concern given the increasing prevalence of type 2 diabetes in children. Finally, there are cultural barriers. The majority of patients seen by diabetes educators are non-Hispanic whites, but the largest-growing populations of people with diabetes are from nonwhite cultures, races, and ethnicities. Clearly, meeting the goals of Healthy People 2020 will be difficult when some of the most vulnerable patients do not have access to quality diabetes education and/or support.

Some of the more common access barriers to DSME were identified in a 2009 national study of patients, educators, and physicians.[72,92] The results of this study showed that DSME is highly regarded among patients who have received it, and less so among those who did not. Patients and physicians alike want easier access to quality education programs. Patients value their doctor's opinions, so it was not surprising that primary care physicians were found to be essential to the referral process. Some physicians struggle with the referral process, and others report having limited access to local educators. Most physicians want patients to have more self-management support, but some disagree with the patient care recommendations provided by the educator. The natural tension caused by this paradox can be resolved with effective communication. Patients in this study valued traditional DSME sources and settings but also approved of some media-based education strategies.

It is important to note that the patient sample in this study was primarily white, well-educated, and insured.

Absence of communication about diabetes education between patients and physicians, conflict and misunderstandings between physicians and educators, and a number of patient-related factors may work together to create barriers to access. The diabetes educator is an essential component of the healthcare team, but one who must take the initiative to dispel myths and misconceptions, advocate with third-party payers for effective reimbursement, and create innovative strategies to deliver DSME&S.

Evolving Healthcare Systems in the United States

Few observers would dispute the fact that the healthcare system in the United States is fragmented and dysfunctional. Healthcare outcomes continue to be disappointing despite the allocation of nearly 18% of GDP to healthcare spending.[93,94] Although chronic diseases have supplanted acute illnesses as the primary reasons for seeking health care in the United States, the healthcare system continues to use an acute-care delivery model. Creative mechanisms are being explored in the hope of mitigating the impact of rising healthcare costs, and the fee-for-service model common to US health care is slowly being overtaken by alternative designs including the Patient Centered Medical Home (PCMH) and the Accountable Care Organization (ACO).

Diabetes Educators and the Affordable Care Act

It is clear that individuals with diabetes benefit from DSME&S. It is equally clear that in the current healthcare system, millions of people with diabetes have not had the advantage of working with a skilled diabetes educator. As healthcare delivery and payment structures in the United States are evolving, diabetes educators are wondering not only whether that pattern will change but also how the comprehensive changes to the healthcare system will affect them. An important aspect of the evolving healthcare system is the Patient Protection and Affordable Care Act.[95]

The Patient Protection and Affordable Care Act, originally known as the Affordable Care Act (ACA), is known colloquially as "Obamacare." The ACA became public law on March 23, 2010 (Pub. L. No. 111-148, 2010). Without question, the law will expand insurance coverage, consumer protections, and access to primary care services. The ACA contains several provisions of interest to persons with diabetes, policymakers, and healthcare providers—including diabetes educators. These provisions directly address gaps in diabetes prevention, screening, and care, and they create a comprehensive approach toward improved treatment.[96] Some provisions are intended to become effective in 2014, while others will be phased in gradually.[97] The Catalyst to Better Diabetes Care Act of 2009, built into the ACA, authorizes the Centers for Disease Control and Prevention (CDC) to enhance surveillance of the disease and to develop national quality standards for a national diabetes report card.[96] Additional diabetes-related provisions include wellness and prevention programs, Medicaid Health Homes for those with chronic conditions, the Medicaid Incentives to Prevent Chronic Disease Program, and the Medicare Independence at Home Demonstration Program.[96] The complete ACA contains 10 titles (or divisions), each addressing a particular aspect of reform, and can be found at the Department of Health and Human Services Web site: http://www.hhs.gov/healthcare/rights/law/index.html.

Because the entire law can be intimidating to the reader, this section describes the 10 titles and offers a consolidated summary of what is contained in the ACA, highlighting specific implications for the diabetes educator. The titles are summarized in Table 1.4. This brief summary is not intended to represent the entirety of this law. A PDF copy of the law can be downloaded from the US Department of Health and Human Services Web site: http://www.hhs.gov/healthcare/rights/law/index.html.

Title I: Quality, Affordable Health Care for All Americans

Through shared responsibility, the ACA will transform health insurance in the United States, employing individual and group market reforms designed to eliminate discriminatory practices. Preexisting condition exclusions based on health status are prohibited, and preventive health services, fair premiums, and guaranteed coverage with no lifetime or annual limits will be implemented. The ACA extends coverage for dependent children to age 26 and caps nonmedical administrative expenditures. Title I addresses individual and small-business tax credits, individual and employer responsibilities, and a variety of miscellaneous provisions. Consumers are offered affordable

TABLE 1.4 The Affordable Care Act: Titles and Sections Addressing Aspects of Reform		
Title	*Title Name*	*Sections of the ACA*
Title I	Quality, Affordable Health Care for All Americans	1001–2995
Title II	The Role of Public Programs	3001–3129
Title III	Improving the Quality and Efficiency of Health Care	3131–3602
Title IV	Prevention of Chronic Disease and Improving Public Health	4001–4402
Title V	Health Care Workforce	5001–5701
Title VI	Transparency and Program Integrity	6001–6801
Title VII	Improving Access to Innovative Medical Therapies	7001–7103
Title VIII	Community Living Assistance Services and Supports	8001–8002
Title IX	Revenue Provisions	9001–9023
Title X	Strengthening Quality, Affordable Health Care for All Americans	10101–10909

Source: Adapted from "An Act: The Patient Protection and Affordable Care Act." The Patient Protection and Affordable Care Act, Pub. L. No. 111-148, §2702, 124 Stat. 119, 318-319 (2010), US Government Printing Office, on the Internet at: http://www.govtrack.us/congress/bills/111/hr3590.

choices of health benefit plans; this permits individual state flexibility in the operation and enforcement of health insurance exchanges.

Health Insurance Exchanges

A health insurance exchange is an online store where consumers can compare and buy health insurance plans. Each US state had the option to run its own exchange, to work in partnership with the federal government to run an exchange, or to use a federal exchange. About half the states decided to use the federal exchange, and the rest selected either the state-run or partnership model.

Each exchange will do the following:

- Present benefit options in a standard format so it's easy for consumers to compare plans
- Operate a toll-free hotline where consumers can ask questions and get help
- Set up a navigator program to help consumers understand and purchase health insurance
- Certify the health plans that sell policies through the exchange and make sure health plans comply with regulatory standards and requirements
- Provide an online calculator so consumers can determine their costs; the calculator will factor in tax credits or subsidies available to the consumer
- Interact with other computer systems and databases to determine whether consumers are eligible for tax credits or subsidies on the exchange or if they qualify for Medicaid or the Children's Health Insurance Program (CHIP); this is called "no wrong door," and it will make it much easier for consumers to sign up for some kind of health coverage
- Certify which individuals are exempt from the individual mandate

Source: C Anderson, "What is a health insurance exchange? A closer look at what ACA's health insurance marketplace will do for you, starting October 1" (cited 2013 Oct 15), on the Internet at: http://www.healthinsurance.org/learn/what-is-a-health-insurance-exchange/.

The online marketplaces for state insurance exchanges are also known as the Obamacare Health Insurance Exchange Marketplace. Consumers can locate their marketplace through the State Health Insurance Exchange: State Run Exchanges Web site: http://obamacarefacts.com/state-health-insurance-exchange.php. Opened October 1, 2013, the Web site continues to be refined and improved. The Internet portal http://www.healthcare.gov has been established to assist Americans in identifying coverage options, obtaining answers to questions, and enrolling in Platinum, Gold, Silver, or Bronze marketplace insurance programs. These plans offer different coverage levels, which differ by cost-sharing requirements.[97] More than 7 million subscribers enrolled in programs before the first open enrollment period closed on March 31, 2014. Essential health benefits include at least the following general categories that apply to diabetes coverage and treatment: ambulatory care, emergency services, hospitalization, maternity and newborn care, mental health and substance use disorders, behavioral health treatment, prescription drugs, rehabilitative and habilitative services and devices, laboratory services, preventive/wellness chronic disease management, and pediatric services, including oral and vision care.[97]

Of Interest to the Diabetes Educator

Title I addresses provisions for health homes for enrollees with chronic conditions. The term "health home" is defined as a designated individual provider or a healthcare team selected by eligible individuals with chronic conditions. The term "chronic conditions" includes, but is not limited to, diabetes (Sec. 2703). Health home providers provide a cadre of services, including comprehensive care management, care coordination, and health promotion. Health services also encompass comprehensive transitional care (eg, follow-up from inpatient to other settings; patient and family support; referral to community and social support services, if relevant; and use of health information technology to link services, as feasible and appropriate). The ACA defines a "designated health provider" as a physician, clinical practice or clinical group practice, rural clinic, community health center, community mental health center, home health agency, or any other entity or provider (eg, pediatricians, gynecologists, obstetricians) that is determined by the state to be qualified to be a health home for eligible individuals with chronic conditions.

Title II: Role of Public Programs

The ACA improves access to Medicaid for the lowest-income populations, including coverage for former foster care children. Special adjustments will be considered for certain states recovering from a major disaster. Enhanced support is available for the CHIP, and between fiscal years 2014 and 2019, states will receive a 23 percentage point increase in the CHIP federal match rate, subject to a 100% cap. Subtitle F (Sec. 2510), Medicaid Prescription Drug Coverage, is of particular interest to the diabetes educator, as it addresses prescription drug rebates, the elimination of the exclusions of coverage for certain drugs, and provision of adequate pharmacy reimbursement. Improved coordination for individuals enrolled in Medicare and Medicaid, the so-called dual-eligible beneficiaries, will be addressed through a 5-year period of demonstration projects. In an effort to improve the quality of Medicaid for both patients and providers, Sections 2701 to 2707 address adult health quality measures, payment adjustment for healthcare-acquired conditions, provision of health homes for enrollees with chronic conditions, and 4 demonstration projects. The demonstration projects are the following: (1) evaluation of integrated care around a hospitalization, (2) the Medicaid Global Payment System Demonstration Project, (3) the Pediatric Accountable Care Organization Demonstration Project, and (4) the Medicaid Emergency Psychiatric Demonstration Project. Of special note, the ACA has incorporated protections for American Indians and Alaska Natives, containing special rules relating to Native Americans including the elimination of sunset for reimbursement for all Medicare Part B services furnished by certain Indian hospitals and clinics.

Of Interest to the Diabetes Educator
The Independence at Home Medical Practice Demonstration Program is amended from Title XVIII of the Social Security Act, inserted under Section 3023: National Pilot Program on Payment Bundling. Applicable beneficiaries is defined with respect to an individual who has 2 or more chronic illnesses, such as congestive heart failure, diabetes, chronic obstructive pulmonary disease, stroke, ischemic heart disease, Alzheimer's disease, neurodegenerative diseases, or other diseases and conditions that result in high costs under this title (Sec. 3023).

Title III: Improving the Quality and Efficiency of Health Care

The ACA will make substantial investments to improve quality and delivery of care, supporting research to inform consumers about outcomes resulting from differing approaches to treatment and care delivery, via new patient care models. Payments will be linked to quality outcomes under the Medicare program, with a national strategy designed to improve healthcare quality through quality measure development, measurement, data collection, and reporting. Diabetes-specific information will be available biennially through the Diabetes Report Card on the US Department of Health and Human Services, CDC Web site (http://www.cdc.gov/diabetes/pubs/pdf/DiabetesReportCard.pdf). Improvements in rural care and payment accuracy will occur, and the Medicare Part D prescription drug benefit will be expanded, with a reduction in the "donut hole."

Of Interest to the Diabetes Educator
Diabetes educators are focused on improving outcomes. Current evidence already suggests that although Medicare patients who receive diabetes education are more likely to receive preventive services, diabetes education is an underutilized service.[61,64] There is an opportunity for enterprising diabetes educators to partner with health home providers to address the diabetes-specific quality measures (ie, DSME, foot exams, eye exams, SMBG, A1C testing, and influenza vaccines).

Title IV: Prevention of Chronic Disease and Improving Public Health

Sections 4001 to 4402 of the ACA are designed to better position the nation's healthcare system toward disease prevention and health promotion. A variety of initiatives will provide the impetus and infrastructure through a new Prevention and Public Health Investment Fund. Education about preventive benefits for clinical and community services is addressed in this section. The ACA authorizes these benefits through school-based health clinics, Medicare annual wellness visits with personalized prevention plans, evidence-based coverage of preventive services in Medicare, and incentives for prevention of chronic diseases in Medicaid. Healthier communities will be created through community transformation grants and through healthy aging and living well programs. Nutrition labeling will be required for standard menu items at chain restaurants, and funding will be available for the Childhood Obesity Demonstration Project. An Institute of Medicine (IOM) conference on pain care will evaluate adequacy of pain assessment, treatment, and management, thereby raising awareness and advancing research and treatment for pain care management.

Of Interest to the Diabetes Educator

Section 4108 of the ACA specifies that states shall be awarded grants to carry out initiatives to provide incentives to Medicaid beneficiaries who successfully participate in a program, and upon completion of such participation, demonstrate changes in health risk and outcomes, including the adoption and maintenance of health behaviors by meeting established measurable standards and health status targets. The purpose of these initiatives is to test approaches that may encourage behavior modification and determine scalable solutions. In general, a "program" is comprehensive, evidence based, widely available, easily accessible, and designed and uniquely suited to address the needs of Medicare beneficiaries and has demonstrated success in helping individuals achieve 1 or more of the following from Section 4108:

- Cease use of tobacco products
- Control or reduce weight
- Lower cholesterol
- Lower blood pressure
- Avoid the onset of diabetes, or in the case of someone with diabetes, improve management of the existing condition

In general, grants shall be awarded to state or local health departments and Indian tribes to carry out 5-year pilot programs to provide public health community interventions, screenings, and, where necessary, clinical referrals for individuals who are between 55 and 64 years of age (Sec. 4202). In addition to community-wide public health interventions, a state or local health department will be mandated to use funding received in conducting ongoing health screening to identify risk factors for cardiovascular disease, cancer, stroke, and diabetes among individuals in both urban and rural areas who are between 55 and 64 years of age (Sec. 4202). Individuals who are found to have chronic disease risk factors through these screening activities will receive clinical referral/treatment for follow-up services to reduce risk. With respect to each individual with risk factors for or having heart disease, stroke, diabetes, or any other condition for which they were screened, grantees shall determine whether these individuals are covered under a public or private health insurance program. Insured individuals will be referred to an in-network provider, with respect to the program involved. Uninsured individuals can be assisted in determining eligibility for available public coverage options and identify other appropriate community healthcare resources and assistance programs (Sec. 4202).

There is an opportunity for diabetes educators to partner with state or local health departments as direct providers or as consultants. Community-based resources may need to be developed to serve the collective needs of individuals with or at risk for diabetes as they work to reduce risks and/or improve all aspects of control.

Title V: Health Care Workforce

The ACA will encourage innovations in healthcare workforce training, recruitment, and retention, and through a national healthcare workforce commission designed to support increasing the supply of healthcare workers. This will be supported through a variety of student loan and loan repayment programs and provision of nurse-managed health clinics. A commission on key national indicators is established under Improving Access to Health Care Services.

Of Interest to the Diabetes Educator

Section 399V-3 of the Public Health Service Act: National Diabetes Prevention Program has been amended under Sec. 5313. As a result, the CDC established the National Diabetes Prevention Program (NDPP), targeted to adults at high risk for diabetes, in order to eliminate the preventable burden of diabetes. The NDPP includes a grant program for community-based diabetes prevention program model sites, a program within the CDC to determine eligibility of entities to deliver community-based diabetes prevention services, a training and outreach program for lifestyle intervention instructions, and evaluation, monitoring, technical assistance, and applied research carried out by the CDC.

The subspecialty of diabetes education has long been populated primarily by nurses and dietitians. The former group is in a state of impending critical shortage. A workforce analysis commissioned by the AADE projected a significant increase in the demand for diabetes educators through 2025.[98] The analysis identified all healthcare professions, including nursing, as continued sources of diabetes educators. Therefore, having programs that support the education and training of nurses provides an ongoing source of trained professionals who can migrate into the field of diabetes education. To sustain and grow the specialty, current diabetes educators have an obligation to serve as models and mentors for new professionals entering the field.

Title VI: Transparency and Program Integrity

Transparency, in a social context, implies open communication and accountability, thereby operating in a way that allows others to easily see actions being performed. This title addresses physician ownership, nursing home transparency of information, improving staff training, and patient-centered outcomes research and its coordinating council for comparative effectiveness research. Medicare, Medicaid, and CHIP program integrity provisions are described in Sections 6301 to 6607 of the ACA. The Elder Justice Act will raise awareness for the prevention and elimination of elder abuse, neglect, and exploitation, particularly in LTC facilities.

Of Interest to the Diabetes Educator
According to the interpretation given by the Department of Health and Human Services, this section of the law is aimed, in part, at promoting more effective provider-patient relationships.[99] Consider this section in terms of the CCM.[100] Improved transparency and improved communication can be linked to the engaged, activated patient. Diabetes educators, with their expertise in chronic care management, are well positioned to serve as resources and consultants for agencies working to bring more transparency into their processes.

Title VII: Improving Access to Innovative Medical Therapies

The ACA makes a provision for biologics price competition and innovation under Sections 7001 to 7003, and allows more affordable medicines for children and underserved communities through the 340B program.

Of Interest to the Diabetes Educator
The intent of this section is to enhance access to medications by making them more affordable. Diabetes educators have long advocated, individually and in the aggregate, for underserved populations to have access to *all* diabetes medications and devices. Price competition brings with it a potential for compromised quality. Diabetes educators have an opportunity to serve as a watchdog group to ensure that as access to medications is improved, quality does not deteriorate.

Title VIII: Community Living Assistance Services and Supports

The ACA establishes a national voluntary insurance program, the Community Living Assistance Services and Supports (CLASS) Independence Benefit Plan, for the purchase of community living assistance services and support. The intent is to provide a mechanism for beneficiaries to live as independently as possible in their own homes or a residential facility of choice.

Of Interest to the Diabetes Educator
Title VIII is specific to development and enrollment issues rather than provider-linked services. However, diabetes educators who are actively engaged with the older adult population should be aware of Title VIII and its intent to ensure that beneficiaries have access to the equipment and services needed for independent living.

Title IX: Revenue Provisions

When fully enacted, the ACA is designed to, ultimately, reduce the federal deficit. Title IX outlines tax cuts to citizens as well as the consequences for insurance companies and plan administrators, and it specifies the taxes and fees imposed on agencies and industry.

Of Interest to the Diabetes Educator

Section 9003 is of specific interest to diabetes educators, in that it specifies distributions for medicine qualified only if it is for prescribed drugs or insulin. An annual fee can be imposed on manufacturers and importers of branded pharmaceuticals and on medical devices.

Title X: Strengthening Quality, Affordable Health Care for All Americans

Sections 10101 to 10909 address revisions, modifications, clarifications, expansions, and amendments made to the original ACA. Of interest to diabetes educators, Section 10407 addresses better diabetes care.

Of Interest to the Diabetes Educator

Section 10407 may be cited as the "Catalyst to Better Diabetes Care Act of 2009" and includes provisions for a national diabetes report card, prepared biennially in collaboration with the CDC. In general, each report card will include aggregate health outcomes related to individuals diagnosed with diabetes or prediabetes, including preventive care practices, quality of care, risk factors, and outcomes. Each report card will include trend analysis for the nation and, to the extent possible, for each state, for the purpose of tracking progress in meeting established national goals and objectives for improving diabetes care, costs, and prevalence and informing policy and program development. The report card is available to the public and is posted on the CDC's Web site: http://www.cdc.gov/diabetes/pubs/pdf/diabetes reportcard.pdf. Also under this section is a mandate for improvement of vital statistics collection, which promotes the education and training of physicians on the importance of birth and death certificate data and how to properly complete these documents, including the collection of such data for diabetes and other chronic diseases. In carrying out this subsection, improvements may be promoted for the collection of diabetes mortality data, including the addition of a question for the individual certifying the cause of death regarding whether the deceased had diabetes. The IOM and appropriate associations and councils will collaborate to conduct a study of the impact of diabetes on the practice of medicine in the United States, and the appropriate level of diabetes medical education that should be required prior to licensure, board certification, and recertification (Sec. 10407).

Also under Title X, Section 10401: Centers of Excellence for Depression is a provision specifying that each national center shall collaborate with other centers to carry out general activities that foster communication with other providers attending to co-occurring physical health conditions such as cardiovascular, diabetes, cancer, and substance abuse disorders.

Summary

As a result of the ACA, persons with diabetes will not be penalized for having a preexisting condition and can expect reduced healthcare expenses due to annual caps for out-of-pocket spending. Those with diabetes will be able to select a plan that is best suited to their needs, obtain coverage for preventive health screenings, and over time, experience fewer health disparities.

This section addressed provisions in the ACA that may be of particular interest to diabetes educators. These provisions include insurance components, diabetes prevention, chronic disease management, and improved standards and reporting mechanisms. Some of these provisions become effective in 2014. Others will be rolled out more slowly. The ACA is a comprehensive law that receives ongoing revision, modification, clarification, expansions, and amendments. To track the status of this law, readers are encouraged to query for updates on the Patient Protection and Affordable Care Act, Public Law 111-148 by visiting GovTrack at https://www.govtrack.us/.

A Changing Paradigm for the Diabetes Educator

Diabetes education is not only valuable, it is cost-effective. Regrettably, the limited numbers of diabetes educators who are in practice are not equally distributed geographically. Although there seems to be movement back to the inpatient arena, most diabetes education continues to occur in outpatient settings. Because the epidemic of diabetes continues to escalate, and because the populations with or at risk for diabetes are currently underserved, the diabetes educator needs to think about how to augment current programs in innovative ways. Traditional sources and settings for DSME&S continue to be important, but the significance of meeting people where they are while maintaining quality of programming should not be underestimated. Diabetes educators have been successfully embedded in primary care practices. Evidence supports using disease management strategies and the CCM to improve access to diabetes care and education as well as provide systematic self-management support.[100-106]

Research investigating the value of DSME&S in community-based settings has been occurring for decades.[107-110] Approaches to diabetes prevention based on the interventions used in the Diabetes Prevention Program are now being commonly employed in community settings using lifestyle coaches and peer supporters.[63] Given what is now known, it is reasonable to conclude that diabetes educators would be well suited to hold active roles as care coordinators in the PCMH. However, it will be essential to back up this assumption with additional research. Diabetes educators not only have access to a vast array of innovative approaches to DSME&S, many have the education and experience to determine the best model of care to serve the local community. Discovering innovative ways to partner with other members of the healthcare team using the levels of practice, guidelines, and competencies may well serve to improve access to DSME&S, help eliminate disparities, and achieve an overall goal of better diabetes care for all.

Focus on Education

Teaching Strategies

⤷ **Diabetes can be viewed as a syndemic, a combination of health or social conditions that interact to increase the disease burden to a community, further developing a public health concern.** A comprehensive approach to diabetes care is needed to minimize its negative social impact. Disease management strategies and the CCM might be used to improve access to diabetes care and education and provide systemic self-management support. Diabetes control is achieved through effective disease management that includes education to facilitate healthy lifestyle behaviors.

⤷ **One in every three individuals born today will develop diabetes during his or her lifetime.** The largest increases are expected in the developing countries where resources are limited. Children and older adults are particularly vulnerable when they develop diabetes. Type 2 diabetes is increasing in children of Native American, Hispanic, African-American, and Pacific Islander ancestry, especially in those who are overweight or obese. Type 2 diabetes represents 90% to 95% of all cases of diabetes worldwide. Currently more than 1 in every 5 dollars from the US economy is used to pay for the costs linked to diabetes.

⤷ **Diabetes self-management support is the activities that assist the person with prediabetes or diabetes in implementing and sustaining the behaviors needed to manage his or her condition on an ongoing basis beyond or outside of formal self-management training.**[47] The type of support provided can be behavioral, educational, psychosocial, or clinical.

↻ **Third-party payers recognize the value of DSME&S and in some cases underwrite or reimburse for quality DSME.** One way to ensure quality is by achieving program accreditation or recognition by the AADE or the ADA. The Joint Commission provides accreditation for inpatient diabetes management. Diabetes self-management education programs are typically developed, managed, and led by qualified diabetes educators.

↻ **Diabetes educators are the primary providers of DSME&S.** Diabetes educators are involved in direct patient care, public health, education of other healthcare professionals, research, social reform, and advocacy. Some educators obtain certification and are credentialed as a CDE, BC-ADM, or both. The Scope and Standards of Practice guides the practice of diabetes education. The Standards of Professional Performance defines diabetes education and the role of the diabetes educator, and provides a framework for practice and a guideline for excellence.

↻ **Healthy People 2020 targets related to diabetes remain essentially the same as the Healthy People 2010 target as the number of patients receiving formal diabetes education failed to reach the goal of 60%.** Barriers to access continue to be a primary challenge in providing diabetes education.

Messages for Patients

↻ **Diabetes self-management education and support is a collaborative process between you and your healthcare team.** With effective diabetes education, you will increase the knowledge and skills you need to make healthy choices and manage your diabetes. Diabetes education is an ongoing process that includes support. Diabetes educators will not only teach but also coach you as you work to put new knowledge into practice.

↻ **Diabetes educators can be lifelong partners and advocates, but you are responsible for 98% of your diabetes care.** You need a diabetes educator who will help you gain the knowledge and

skills necessary for successful self-care. Learning about healthy choices and how to include them in your daily life is a process. Choose educators with whom you feel comfortable and who will support your efforts and accept your limitations for self-care.

↻ **Everyone with diabetes needs structured diabetes education.** A Healthy People 2020 goal is to increase access to diabetes education by making sure that at least 6 out of every 10 people with diabetes receive diabetes education. Work with your diabetes care provider to locate a diabetes education program near you—and then call to make an appointment.

↻ **Many types of healthcare professionals are needed to help you care for your diabetes.** Be sure to communicate any challenges you are having in managing diabetes. When you have challenges, ask your diabetes care team for help. Be open to new ways and ideas. Don't expect to be perfect. Some days you won't succeed, but it's important to try again, using the same strategy or trying a new one. Diabetes is a lifelong condition with lifelong education opportunities. As your diabetes changes, so does diabetes education and its approaches.

Health Literacy

↻ **Health literacy is a multifactorial phenomenon that involves individuals, families, communities, and systems.** When addressing health literacy, consider access to care and resources; the knowledge, skills, and abilities of everyone involved; the culture of healthcare providers and public health systems; and demographics.

↻ **The Patient Protection and Affordable Care Act of 2010 addresses health literacy both directly within 4 provisions and indirectly in the following broad themes:**[111]
- *Coverage expansion:* Enrolling, reaching out to, and delivering care to health insurance coverage expansion populations in 2014 and beyond
- *Equity:* Ensuring equity in health and health care for all communities and populations

- *Workforce:* Training providers on cultural competency and diversifying the healthcare provider workforce
- *Patient information:* At appropriate reading levels in print and electronic media
- *Public health and wellness*
- *Quality improvement:* Innovation to create more effective and efficient models of care, particularly for individuals with chronic illnesses requiring extensive self-management.

(>) **The Hospital Consumer Assessment of Healthcare Providers and Systems Survey—also known as Hospital CAHPS®, developed by the CMS, along with the Agency for Healthcare Research and Quality (AHRQ)—addresses health literacy and numeracy issues through survey questions on doctor and nurse communication, communication about medicines, and discharge information.**[112]

Focus on Practice

(>) **Improve care and enhance quality by facilitating and critically considering feedback from all patients regarding coordination of their care.** People with diabetes choose where and how they want their DSME to be done. Continuous quality assurance will allow DSME program managers to evaluate the quality of patient-focused interventions provided.

(>) **Effectively communicate around all clinical care services.** Communicate with referring providers what DSME is and what is involved. Communicate the interventions, goals, expected outcomes, and support mechanisms needed to deliver DSME among all providers involved.

References

1. World Health Organization. Global Health Observatory. Deaths from CVD and diabetes (cited 2013 Jul 12). On the Internet at: http://www.who.int/gho/ncd/mortality_morbidity/cvd_text/en/.

2. International Diabetes Federation. IDF Diabetes Atlas. 5th ed. Brussels, Belgium: International Diabetes Federation; 2011.

3. The Diabetes Control and Complications Trial (DCCT) Research Group. The effect of intensive treatment of diabetes on the development and progression of long term complications in insulin-dependent diabetes mellitus. N Engl J Med. 1993;329:977-86.

4. The Diabetes Control and Complications Trial (DCCT)/ Epidemiology of Diabetes Interventions and Complications Research Group (EDIC). Retinopathy and nephropathy in patients with type 1 diabetes four years after a trial of intensive therapy. N Engl J Med. 2000;342(6):381-9.

5. UK Progressive Diabetes Study (UKPDS) Group. Intensive blood glucose control with sulfonylureas or insulin compared with conventional treatment and risk of complications in patients with type 2 diabetes (UKPDS 33). Lancet. 1998;352(9131):837-53.

6. Knowler WC, Barrett-Conner E, Fowler SE, et al. Reduction in the incidence of type 2 diabetes with lifestyle intervention or metformin. N Engl J Med. 2002;346: 393-403.

7. Centers for Disease Control and Prevention. National diabetes fact sheet: general information and national estimates on diabetes in the United States. Atlanta, Ga: Centers for Disease Control and Prevention; 2011 (cited 2014 Mar 27). On the Internet at: http://www.cdc.gov/diabetes/pubs/pdf/ndfs_2011.pdf.

8. Selvin E, Parrinello CM, Sacks DB, Coresh J. Trends in prevalence and control of diabetes in the United States, 1988-1994 and 1999-2010. Ann Int Med. 2014;160(8): 517-25.

9. Shaw J, Sicree R, Zimmet P. Global estimates of the prevalence of diabetes for 2010 and 2030. Diabetes Res Clin Pract. 2010;81(1):4-14.

10. Boyle JP, Thompson TJ, Gregg EW, Barker LE, Williamson DF. Projection of the year 2050 burden of diabetes in the US adult population: dynamic modeling of incidence, mortality, and prediabetes prevalence. Popul Health Metr. 2010;8(29):1-12.

11. Whiting DR, Guariguata L, Weil C, Shaw J. IDF Diabetes Atlas: Global estimates of the prevalence of diabetes for 2011 and 2030. Diabetes Res Clin Pract. 2011;94(3):311-21.

12. Centers for Disease Control and Prevention. National diabetes prevention program (last reviewed 2013 Oct 1). On the Internet at: http://www.cdc.gov/diabetes/prevention/index.htm.

13. Patterson CC, Dahlquist GG, Gyürüs E, et al. Incidence trends for childhood type 1 diabetes in Europe during 1989-2003 and predicted new cases 2005-20: a multicentre prospective registration study. Lancet. 2009;373(9680):2027-33.

14. The Writing Group for the SEARCH for Diabetes in Youth Study Group. Incidence of diabetes in youth in the United States. JAMA. 2007;297(24):2716-24.

15. Bell RA, Mayer-Davis EJ, Beyer JW, et al. Diabetes in non-Hispanic white youth: prevalence, incidence, and clinical characteristics: the SEARCH for Diabetes in Youth Study. Diabetes Care. 2009;32(2 Suppl 2):S102-11.

16. Mayer-Davis EJ, Beyer J, Bell RA, et al. Diabetes in African American youth: prevalence, incidence, and clinical characteristics: the SEARCH for Diabetes in Youth Study. Diabetes Care. 2009;32(2 Suppl 2):S112-22.

17. Lawrence JM, Mayer-Davis EJ, Reynolds K, et al. Diabetes in Hispanic American youth: prevalence, incidence, and clinical characteristics: the SEARCH for Diabetes in Youth Study. Diabetes Care. 2009;32(2 Suppl 2):S123-31.

18. Liu L, Yi JP, Beyer J, et al. Type 1 and type 2 diabetes in Asian and Pacific Islander U.S. youth: the SEARCH for Diabetes in Youth Study. Diabetes Care. 2009;32(2 Suppl 2):S133-9.

19. Dabelea D, DeGroat J, Sorrelman C, et al. Diabetes in Navajo youth. Diabetes Care. 2009;32(2 Suppl 2):S141-7.

20. Cowie CC, Rust KF, Ford ES, et al. Full accounting of diabetes and pre-diabetes in the US population in 1988-1994 and 2005-2006. Diabetes Care. 2009;32(2):287-94.

21. Mainous AG 3rd, Baker R, Koopman RJ, et al. Impact of the population at risk of diabetes on projections of diabetes burden in the United States: an epidemic on the way. Diabetologia. 2007 May;50(5):934-40.

22. Lin SX, Pi-Sunyer EX. Prevalence of the metabolic syndrome among US middle-aged and older adults with and without diabetes—a preliminary analysis of the NHANES 1999-2002 data. Ethn Dis. 2007;17(1):35-9.

23. Ringborg A, Cropet C, Jonsson B, et al. Resource use associated with type 2 diabetes in Asia, Latin America, the Middle East and Africa: results from the International Diabetes Management Practices Study. Int J Clin Pract. 2009;63(7):997-1007.

24. American Diabetes Association. Economic costs of diabetes in the U.S. in 2012. Diabetes Care. 2013;36(4):1033-46. doi: 10.2337/dc12-2625

25. Boren SA, Fitzner KA, Panhalkar PS, et al. Costs and benefits associated with diabetes education: a review of the literature. Diabetes Educ. 2009;35(1):72-96.

26. American Diabetes Association. Economic costs of diabetes in the US in 2007. Diabetes Care. 2008;31:1-20.

27. Huang ES, Basu A, O'Grady M, et al. Projecting the future diabetes population size and related costs for the US. Diabetes Care. 2009;32(12):2225-9.

28. Rowley WR, Bezold C. Creating public awareness: state 2025 diabetes forecasts. Popul Health Manag. 2012;15(4):194-200. doi: 10.1089/pop.2011.0053

29. United States Census Bureau. Household income for states: 2010 and 2011. American Community Survey Briefs, September 2012, Appendix Table 1, page 5.

30. United States Census Bureau. 2006-2010 American Community Survey. 2010.

31. Greenberg SA, ed. Profile of Older Americans. Washington, DC: US Department of Health and Human Services Administration on Aging; 2008 (cited 2010 Nov 1). On the Internet at: http://www.aoa.gov/AoAroot/Aging_Statistics/Profile/2008/docs/2008profile.pdf.

32. Henry J. Kaiser Family Foundation. Key facts about the uninsured population. 2013 Sep 26 (cited 2013 Oct 1). On the Internet at: http://kff.org/uninsured/fact-sheet/key-facts-about-the-uninsured-population/.

33. Denavas-Walt C, Proctor BD, Smith JC. Income, poverty, and health insurance coverage in the United States: 2011. Washington, DC: US Government Printing Office; 2012.

34. Roglic G, Unwin N. Mortality attributable to diabetes: estimates for the year 2010. Diabetes Res Clin Pract. 2010;87(1):15-9. Epub 2009 Nov 14.

35. International Diabetes Federation. IDF Diabetes Atlas. 6th ed. Brussels, Belgium: International Diabetes Federation; 2013.

36. Glasgow RE, Eakin KG. Issues in diabetes self management. In: Shumaker S, Schron E, Ockene J, McBee WL, eds. The Handbook of Health Behavior Change. New York: Springer; 1997.

37. Anderson RM, Funnell MM. Patient empowerment: reflections on the challenge of fostering the adoption of a new paradigm. Patient Educ Couns. 2005;57(2):153-7.

38. Coates VE, Boore JRP. Knowledge and diabetes self-management. Patient Educ Couns. 1996;(290):99-108.

39. Funnell MM, Tang TS, Anderson RM. From research to practice/DSME support. From DSME to DSMS: developing empowerment-based diabetes self-management support. Diabetes Spectr. 2007;20(4):221-6.

40. Mensing C, ed. The Art and Science of Diabetes Education. Chicago: American Association of Diabetes Educators; 2006.

41. Funnell MM, Brown TL, Childs BP, et al. National standards for diabetes self-management education. Diabetes Care. 2009;32 Suppl 1:S87-94.

42. American Association of Diabetes Educators. AADE guidelines for the practice of diabetes self-management education and training (DSME/T). Diabetes Educ. 2009;35 Suppl 3: 85S-107.

43. Haas L, Maryniuk M, Beck J, Cox CE, Duker P, Edwards L; Standards Revision Task Force. National standards for diabetes self-management education and support. Diabetes Care. 2013;36 Suppl 1:S100-8. doi: http://dx.doi.org/10.2337/dc13-S100

44. American Association of Diabetes Educators. What is diabetes education? On the Internet at: http://www.diabeteseducator.org/DiabetesEducation/Definitions.html.

45. Tobin CT. Highlights from the salary survey of diabetes educators—2008. Diabetes Educ. 2008;35(8):931-3.

46. American Association of Diabetes Educators. Guidelines for the Practice of Diabetes Self-Management Education. Chicago: American Association of Diabetes Educators; 2009 (cited 2010 Nov 2). On the Internet at: http://www.diabeteseducator.org/export/sites/aade/_resources/pdf/PracticeGuidelines2009.pdf.

47. Burke SD, Sherr D, Lipman RD. Partnering with diabetes educators to improve patient outcomes. Diabetes Metab Syndr Obes. 2014 Feb 12;7:45-53.

48. Weiss MA. Empowerment: a patient's perspective. Diabetes Spectr. 2006;19(2):116-8.

49. American Association of Diabetes Educators. Standards for outcomes measurement of diabetes self-management education. Diabetes Educ. 2003;29(5):804-16.

50. Brown SA, Garcia AA, Kouzekanani K, et al. Culturally competent diabetes self-management education for Mexican Americans. Diabetes Care. 2002 Feb;25(2):259-68.

51. Piatt GA, Orchard TJ, Emerson S, et al. Translating the chronic care model into the community. Diabetes Care. 2006 Apr;29(4):811-7.

52. Lorig KR, Ritter PL, Laurent DD, et al. Internet-based chronic disease self-management: a randomized trial. Med Care. 2006;44(11):964-71.

53. Mensing CR, Norris SL. Group education in diabetes: effectiveness and implementation. Diabetes Spectr. 2003; 16(2):96.

54. Norris SL, Engelgau MM, Narayan KMV. Effectiveness of self-management training in type 2 diabetes: a systematic review of randomized controlled trials. Diabetes Care. 2001;24(3):561-87.

55. Norris SL, Lau J, Smith SJ, et al. Self-management education for adults with type 2 diabetes: a meta-analysis of the effect on glycemic control. Diabetes Care. 2002;25(7): 1159-71.

56. Whittemore R. Strategies to facilitate lifestyle change associated with diabetes mellitus. J Nurs Scholarsh. 2000;32(3): 225-32.

57. Bray K, Turpin RS, Jungkind K, et al. Defining success in diabetes disease management: digging deeper in the data. Dis Manag. 2008;11(2):119-28.

58. Berg GD, Wadhwa S. Health services outcomes for a diabetes disease management program for the elderly. Dis Manag. 2007;10(4):226-34.

59. Siminerio L, Ruppert KM, Gabbay RA. Who can provide diabetes self-management support in primary care? Findings from a randomized controlled trial. Diabetes Educ. 2013;39(5):705-13. doi: 10.1177/0145721713492570

60. Hawthorne K, Robles Y, Cannings-John R, et al. Culturally appropriate health education for type 2 diabetes mellitus in ethnic minority groups. Cochrane Database Syst Rev. 2008(3):CD006424.

61. Duncan I, Birkmeyer C, Coughlin S, et al. Assessing the value of diabetes education. Diabetes Educ. 2009;35: 752-60.

62. The DPP Research Group. The Diabetes Prevention Program (DPP). Diabetes Care. 2002;25(12):2165-71.

63. Finch EA, Kelly MS, Marrero DG, et al. Training YMCA wellness instructors to deliver an adapted version of the diabetes prevention lifestyle intervention. Diabetes Educ. 2009;35(2):224-32.

64. Duncan I, Ahmed T, Li Q, et al. Assessing the value of the diabetes educator. Diabetes Educ. 2011;37(5):638-57. doi: 10.1177/0145721711416256

65. Coonrod BA, Betschart J, Harris MI. Frequency and determinants of diabetes patient education among adults in the U.S. population. Diabetes Care. 1994;17:852-8.

66. Zhang Y, Dall TM, Mann SE, et al. The economic costs of undiagnosed diabetes. Popul Health Manag. 2009;12(2): 95-101.

67. Ali MK, McKeever-Bullard K, Saaddine JB, Cowie C, Imperatore G, Gregg, EW. Achievement of goals in U.S. diabetes care, 1999-2010. N Engl J Med. 2013;368(17): 1613-24.

68. Martin AL, Lumber T, Compton T, et al. Insights and trends in diabetes education: results of the 2008 AADE National Diabetes Education Practice Survey. Diabetes Educ. 2008;34(6):970-86.

69. Zrebiec J. A national study of the diabetes educator: report on a practice analysis conducted by the National Certification Board for Diabetes Educators. Diabetes Educ. 2009; 35(4):657-63.

70. Martin AL, Warren JP, Lipman RD. The landscape for diabetes education: results of the 2012 AADE National Diabetes Education Practice Survey. Diabetes Educ. 2013;39(5):614-22. doi: 10.1177/0145721713499412

71. Funnell MM, Anderson RM, Nwankwo R, et al. A study of certified diabetes educators: influences and barriers. Diabetes Educ. 2006;32(3):359-62, 364-6, 368-72.

72. Peyrot M, Rubin RR, Funnell MM, et al. Access to diabetes self-management education: results of national surveys of patients, educators, and physicians. Diabetes Educ. 2009;35(2):246-63.

73. American Association of Diabetes Educators. The scope of practice for diabetes educators and the standards of practice for diabetes educators: developed under the aegis of a multidisciplinary task force of the American Association of Diabetes Educators. Diabetes Educ. 1992;18(1):52-6.

74. American Association of Diabetes Educators. The 1999 scope of practice for diabetes educators and the standards of practice for diabetes educators. Diabetes Educ. 2000;26(3):519-25.

75. American Association of Diabetes Educators. The scope of practice, standards of practice, and standards of professional performance for diabetes educators. Diabetes Educ. 2005;31(4):487-512.

76. American Association of Diabetes Educators. Scope of Practice, Standards of Practice and Standards of Professional Performance. Chicago: American Association of Diabetes Educators (cited 2010 Nov 2; site no longer available). On the Internet at: http://www.diabeteseducator.org/export/sites/aade/_resources/pdf/The_Scope_of_Practice_07_14_08_Update.pdf.

77. American Association of Diabetes Educators. The Scope of Practice, Standards of Practice, and Standards of Professional Performance for Diabetes Educators: 2011 update. On the Internet at: http://www.diabeteseducator.org/export/sites/aade/_resources/pdf/research/ScopeStandards_Final2_1_11.pdf.

78. American Association of Diabetes Educators. Competencies for Diabetes Educators. Chicago: American Association of Diabetes Educators; 2009 (cited 2010 Nov 2). On the Internet at: http://www.diabeteseducator.org/export/sites/aade/_resources/pdf/competencies.pdf.

79. The Diabetes Education and Management Program [home page]. New York: Teacher's College, Columbia University. On the Internet at: http://www.tc.columbia.edu/diabetes/.

80. Master of Science in Nursing, Diabetes Nursing Specialization [home page]. Minneapolis, Minn: Capella University. On the Internet at: http://www.capella.edu/online-degrees/masters-diabetes-nursing/.

81. American Association of Diabetes Educators. The 2008 Scope of Practice for Diabetes Educators, Standards of Practice and Standards of Professional Performance (cited 2010 Nov 2). On the Internet at: http://www.diabeteseducator.org/export/sites/aade/_resources/pdf/The_Scope_of_Practice_07_14_08_Update.pdf.

82. American Association of Diabetes Educators. AADE guidelines for the practice of diabetes self-management education and training (DSME/T). Diabetes Educ. 2009;35(3 Suppl):85S-107. doi: 10.1177/0145721709352436

83. Dreyfus HL. Mind Over Machine: The Power of Human Intuitive Expertise in the Era of the Computer. New York: Free Press; 1986.

84. Benner P. From Novice to Expert: Excellence and Power in Clinical Nursing Practice. Upper Saddle River, NJ: Prentice-Hall; 2001.

85. Petram K. Bloom's taxonomy: levels of understanding. 2010 Jun 15 (cited 2014 Mar 22). On the Internet at: http://www.psia-nw.org/newsletter-articles/blooms-taxonomy-levels-of-understanding/?doing_wp_cron=1395585640.8118510246276855468750.

86. Maryniuk M D, Mensing C, Imershein S, Gregory A, Jackson R. Enhancing the role of medical office staff in diabetes care and education. Clin Diabetes. 2013;31(3):116-22.

87. Norris SL, Engelgau MM, Venkat Narayan KM. Effectiveness of self-management training in type 2 diabetes. Diabetes Care. 2001 Mar;24(3):561-87.

88. US Department of Health & Human Services. Proposed Healthy People 2020 Objectives. Washington, DC: Office of Disease Prevention & Health Promotion; 2010.

89. Lewis DW, Powers PA, Goodenough MF, et al. Inadequacy of in-school support for diabetic children. Diabetes Technol Ther. 2003;5(1):45-56.

90. McCall DT, Sauaia A, Hamman RF, et al. Are low-income elderly patients at risk for poor diabetes care? Diabetes Care. 2004;27(5):1060-5.

91. Haas L, Burke SD, eds. Diabetes Management in Long-Term Settings: A Clinician's Guide to Optimal Elderly Care. Alexandria, Va: American Diabetes Association. In press.

92. Peyrot M, Rubin RR. Access to diabetes self-management education. Diabetes Educ. 2008;34(1):90-7.

93. Martin A, Lassman D, Whittle L, et al. Recession contributes to slowest annual rate of increase in health spending in five decades. Health Aff (Millwood). 2011;30(1):11-22. PMID: 21209433.

94. McGlynn EA, Asch SM, Adams J, et al. The quality of health care delivered to adults in the United States. N Engl J Med. 2003;348(26):2635-45. PMID: 12826639.

95. Patient Protection and Affordable Care Act. http://www.hhs.gov/healthcare/rights/law/index.html.

96. Centers for Disease Control and Prevention. Diabetes report card 2012. Atlanta, Ga: Centers for Disease Control and Prevention; 2012 (cited 2014 Jan 1). On the Internet at: http://www.cdc.gov/diabetes/pubs/pdf/diabetesreportcard.pdf.

97. Mason K. Federal health reform provisions related to diabetes. National Conference of State Legislatures. 2011 May (cited 2014 Jan 1). On the Internet at: http://www.ncsl.org/portals/1/documents/health/DiabetesinHR511.pdf.

98. Dobson A, DaVanzo JE, El-Gamil A, Freeman J. Diabetes Education in a New World of Healthcare Delivery System Innovation: A Workforce Analysis. Chicago: American Association of Diabetes Educators; 2011.

99. US Department of Health and Human Services. The Affordable Care Act, section by section (cited 2014 Mar 27). On the Internet at: http://www.hhs.gov/healthcare/rights/law/index.html.

100. Bodenheimer T, Wagner EH, Grumbach K. Improving primary care for patients with chronic illness. JAMA. 2002;288(14):1775-9. doi: 10.1001/jama.288.14.1775

101. Siminerio LM, Piatt G, Zgibor JC. Implementing the chronic care model for improvements in diabetes care and education in a rural primary care practice. Diabetes Educ. 2005;31(2):225-34.

102. Philis-Tsimikas A, Walker C. Improved care for diabetes in underserved populations. J Ambul Care Manage. 2001 Jan;24(1):39-43.

103. Steinman K, Steinman MA, Steinman TI. Disease management programs in the geriatric setting: practical considerations. Dis Manag Health Out. 2003;11(6):363-74.

104. Taub LM. Concordance of provider recommendations with American Diabetes Association's guidelines. J Am Acad Nurse Pract. 2006 Mar;18(3):124-33.

105. Glasgow RE, Orleans T, Wagner EH. Does the chronic care model serve also as a template for prevention? Milbank Q. 2001;79(4):579-612.

106. Bodenheimer T, Wagner EH, Grumbach K. Improving primary care for patients with chronic illness: the chronic care model, part 2. JAMA. 2002;288(15):1909-14.

107. Lorig KR, Hurwicz M, Sobel D, et al. A national dissemination of an evidence based self-management program: a process evaluation study. Patient Educ Couns. 2005;59:69-79.

108. Lorig KR, Sobel DS, Stewart AL, et al. Evidence suggesting that a chronic disease self-management program can improve health status while reducing hospitalization: a randomized trial. Med Care. 1999;37(1):5-14.

109. Norris SL, Nichols PJ, Caspersen CJ, et al. Increasing diabetes self-management education in community settings: a systematic review. Am J Prev Med. 2002.

110. Norris SL, Chowdhury FM, Van Le K, et al. Effectiveness of community health workers in the care of persons with diabetes. Diabet Med. 2006;23(5):544-56.

111. Somers S, Mahadevan R. Health literacy implications of the Affordable Care Act (ACA). Presentation to the Institute of Medicine's Roundtable on Health Literacy, Center for Health Care Strategies; November 10, 2010. On the Internet at: http://www.iom.edu/~/media/Files/Activity%20Files/PublicHealth/HealthLiteracy/2010-NOV-10/Somers.pdf.

112. Medicare.gov. Survey of patients' experiences (cited 2014 Jan 1). On the Internet at: http://www.medicare.gov/HospitalCompare/Data/Overview.html?AspxAutoDetectCookieSupport=1.

CHAPTER 2

The Diabetes Self-Management Education Process

Barb Schreiner, PhD, APRN, CPLP, CDE, BC-ADM

Key Concepts

- ◆ Successful management of diabetes requires collaboration between the person with diabetes, the healthcare providers, and others in the support system.

- ◆ Components of diabetes self-management education (DSME) include assessment, goal setting, planning, implementation, and evaluation/monitoring, all of which focus on the individualized needs and goals of the person with diabetes.

- ◆ Review alternatives of what to ask and how to ask for information to individualize management and intervention plans.

- ◆ The plan for DSME must be individualized and sequenced to address objectives outlined in the medical plan, and include the desired needs and capabilities of the person with diabetes.

- ◆ Effective plans differentiate between treatment, learning objectives, and lifestyle behavioral goals. All are essential.

- ◆ Diabetes self-management education is a dynamic plan and a lifelong process.

- ◆ Diabetes educator competencies include refined assessment and clinical skills based in critical thinking; knowledge about diabetes, the chronic disease model, and the learning process; effective use of teaching tools and a variety of delivery methods; application of empowerment strategies and facilitation skills.

- ◆ Documentation provides data for collaboration, tracking patient outcomes, and overall program evaluation.

Introduction

Diabetes self-management education and support (DSMES), also known as diabetes self-management training (DSMT), is defined as a collaborative process through which people with or at risk for diabetes gain the knowledge and skills needed to modify behavior and successfully self-manage the disease and its related conditions.[1] Diabetes self-management education and support is an interactive, ongoing process involving the person with diabetes (or the caregiver or family), a diabetes educator, and other members of the healthcare team.[1] The diabetes educator continues to be the recognized coordinator and

is most often the provider of the diabetes knowledge, skills, and adjustment support for this chronic disease and its demands.

Diabetes self-management education is the cornerstone for the management of diabetes. In recent years, there has been a paradigm shift from the didactic (lecture) teaching style of self-management skills to a patient-centered facilitation approach that encourages behavior change. It is critical that the person with diabetes has the knowledge, skills, and behaviors needed to successfully manage the disease. Measurable behavior change is the desired outcome of diabetes education.[2,3] Therefore, the intervention—the DSME process—aims to achieve optimal health status and better quality of life, and reduce the need for costly health care.

The overall objectives of DSME are to support the following[4]:

♦ Informed decision making
♦ Self-care behaviors
♦ Problem solving
♦ Active collaboration with the healthcare team to improve clinical outcomes, health status, and quality of life

In 2007, the task force working on the National Standards for Diabetes Self-Management Education identified overriding principles based on existing evidence that were used to guide the review and revision of the Standards. These principles were the following[5]:

1. Diabetes education is effective for improving clinical outcomes and quality of life, at least in the short term.
2. DSME has evolved from primarily didactic presentations to more theoretically-based empowerment models.
3. There is no one "best" education program or approach; however, programs incorporating behavioral and psychosocial strategies demonstrate improved outcomes. Additional studies show that culturally and age-appropriate programs improve outcomes and that group education is effective.
4. Ongoing support is critical to sustain progress made by participants during the DSME program.
5. Behavioral goal setting is an effective strategy to support self-management behaviors.

These overriding principles support the efficacy of DSME and guide the development of sound DSME programs.

In 2012, the task force expanded the National Standards to include support, underscoring the need for continued interaction with patients after formal educational sessions have ended. The other addition to the Standards was the inclusion of educating people with prediabetes, as this is an underserved population in need of content and support similar to that given to those with diabetes.[4]

This chapter describes the 5-step process of DSME as detailed in *The AADE Guidelines for the Practice of Diabetes Self-Management Education and Training*.[6]

The steps are as follows:

1. Assessment
2. Goal setting
3. Planning
4. Implementation
5. Evaluation/monitoring

Each step of this process is detailed in its own section. Skill builders, knowledge builders, tips on patient handouts, and documentation reminders are included at each step. The educational process chart (Figure 2.1) graphically displays this process. It is important to note that the DSME process is presented in this chapter in a linear fashion for ease of comprehension. In practice, the 5 steps are not necessarily sequential, and often the diabetes educator finds it necessary to return to an earlier step in the process to address the individual needs of the person with diabetes.

Assessment

Assessment is the first, and arguably the most important, step in the process of DSME and includes collection and interpretation of relevant patient information. The educator and the patient use these data to mutually identify goals and then progress to implementation of an individualized education plan. Assessment is ongoing and involves reassessment throughout the process. Reassessment occurs as goals and plans are updated to reflect changing priorities and to determine attainment of educational goals. Because of the chronic nature of diabetes, it is recognized that DSME is a lifelong process and that there may be life events that interrupt the learning process or cause the patient's goals to be changed or put on hold.[7]

Assessment sets the foundation for helping patients find their motivation to manage their diabetes and to adopt healthier lifestyle habits. The initial assessment is important for establishing rapport and developing trust between the educator and the patient. The objective of the assessment is to gather sufficient information, including the patient's expectations,

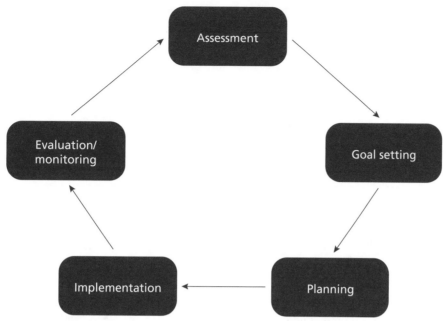

FIGURE 2.1 **The DSME Process**

perceptions, and fears, so that the patient, along with his or her healthcare team, may identify goals and develop an individual education plan. The educator determines both the *scope* and the *content* of the assessments and manages the flow to allow for sufficient time to gather information needed to engage in goal setting and education planning.[8]

Conducting an Effective Assessment

According to the Standards of Practice, the diabetes educator conducts a thorough, individualized assessment of the person with or at risk for diabetes.[7] The assessment process requires ongoing collection and interpretation of relevant data.[7] Assessment can be done by a variety of methods: face-to-face individual interview, group discussion, or a paper-based or electronic self-assessment tool. Detailed measurement criteria for assessment are included in the Standards of Practice[7] and are summarized in Table 2.1.

Beginning an Assessment

When preparing to work with people with diabetes, the effective diabetes educator conducts a careful self-assessment. Common questions to ask yourself include the following: What words do I use to describe a person with diabetes? Do I find myself saying "diabetic," "compliant," "should," "must," "can't," or "don't"? Do I use such phrases as "I want you to" or "You need to"? Other areas to explore are personal biases related to race, ethnicity, social status, education, body size, sexual orientation, and religion. By reflecting on personal biases and beliefs, the educator becomes more open to cultural sensitivity and more attune to and accepting of individual differences. This self-awareness translates to a trusting environment.

When starting an effective assessment, the diabetes educator examines the patient's expectations for the visit. In the initial meeting, the educator builds trust and rapport with the patient while creating an environment in which people feel comfortable talking about their needs, motivations, goals, problems, and feelings. One strategy for building rapport is to get to know the person by asking about his or her daily life and family, and what is most important in life. This builds a holistic assessment and demonstrates the educator's interest in both the person's diabetes and the nonmedical aspects of the person's life. Such an approach can also yield information about the person's affect and may uncover signs of emotional distress or depression. The diabetes educator uses a range of assessment strategies and interviewing

TABLE 2.1   Data Needed for Effective Assessment
Approach to Gathering Information
A systematic, organized, and holistic approach is called for, with data collected from the following sources: • Person with diabetes • Family members and members of the client's social support network, as appropriate • Existing medical records • Referring healthcare providers
Data to Be Collected
It is appropriate to gather information on the following topics: • Personal health history, family health history • Nutrition history and practices • Physical activity and exercise behaviors • Prescription and over-the-counter medications; use and practice of complementary and alternative therapies • Factors that influence learning, such as education and literacy levels, health beliefs, perceived learning needs, motivation to learn, preferred sources of information, and preferred learning style (eg, audio, visual, kinesthetic) • Diabetes self-management behaviors, including experience self-adjusting the treatment plan • Previous DSME, actual knowledge, and skills • Physical factors, including age, mobility, visual acuity, hearing, manual dexterity, alertness, attention span, and ability to concentrate; special needs or limitations requiring accommodations or adaptive support and use of alternative skills • Psychosocial concerns, factors, or issues, including family and social supports; experience with diabetes in friends or family; fears about diabetes • Current mental health status, including preferred stress management or coping strategies, history and treatment of eating disorders or depression • History of substance use, including alcohol, tobacco, and recreational drugs • Occupation; vocation; financial status; and social, cultural, and religious practices • Access to and use of healthcare resources
Data for Prediabetes Assessment
For an individual with prediabetes, the following information must be gathered in addition to the above information: • Knowledge of prediabetes and risks: Evaluate person's understanding of prediabetes and the risks associated with it • Weight loss and weight management: Evaluate the person's understanding of the role of weight loss and weight management through nutrition modification and healthy eating in the management of prediabetes • Physical activity: Determine the individual's habits and behaviors associated with physical activity and the individual's understanding of the role of physical activity in management of prediabetes • Motivation: Assess the individual's motivation skills for maintaining positive behavioral change

Source: JA Pichert, DG Schlundt, "Assessment: Gathering Information and Facilitating Engagement," in C Mensing, ed, *The Art and Science of Diabetes Self-Management Education: A Desk Reference for Healthcare Professionals* (Chicago: American Association of Diabetes Educators, 2006), 580.

skills to develop an understanding of clients and their specific problems.

The following outline provides an example of an effective opening:

1. Provide brief orientation. Introduce yourself and explain your role.
2. Share the objectives. Ask the patient what his or her goals are for the meeting. Share with the patient what you hope will happen in your time together.
3. Explain rationale. Help the patient understand why you are collecting this information and how his or her sharing will be of benefit.
4. Assess receptivity. Ask the patient's permission to move on with the assessment. Listen to the patient and observe the response. Does the patient find this acceptable, or does he or she express reluctance, dissatisfaction, or discomfort? Listen to what the patient says and observe nonverbal behaviors. Is the patient ready to engage in the assessment, or are more discussion and negotiation necessary?

Despite the fact that, ideally, an assessment is completed before an education plan is developed, the diabetes educator may encounter a patient for the first time in a group (class) environment with no prior information from medical records or a referral form. A basic needs assessment of all patients can be conducted efficiently by having each patient complete a short, written assessment tool and answer questions during group introductions. In addition to asking patients to share some basic diabetes information, such as duration of diabetes, type of diabetes medication being taken, current A1C, target goal, and previous diabetes education, the educator might also ask, "What one question do you hope to have answered in this next hour?"

In Practice: Tips for a Quick Assessment

Diabetes educators often are faced with groups of patients, late arrivals, and tight time schedules. Assessing health literacy can easily fall in the list of priorities. Following are a few key points on how to conduct a quick assessment of health literacy and safety:

1. Create an environment which recognizes health literacy challenges.[9] The following are key questions:
   ◈ How often do you need to have someone help you when you read instructions, pamphlets, or other written material from your doctor or pharmacist?
   ◈ What do you find most difficult in filling out medical forms by yourself?
   ◈ Reading and understanding health information can be difficult. Has that been your experience?
2. Ask the patient how he or she prefers to learn new information
3. Ask about what he or she would like to learn. "What part of living with diabetes is most difficult?"
4. Ask about his or her feelings about having diabetes. "How does (the situation described in the previous question) make you feel?"
5. Ask about changes he or she has already tried and past experiences. "How would this situation have to change for you to feel better about it?"
6. Ask about support. "Who in your family do you turn to for support with your diabetes?" or "Which friend helps support you with your diabetes?"

In summary, the educator is able to answer the following inquiries:

◈ Attitude: Do you understand enough about the person's needs and beliefs?
◈ Health: Do you have enough information about the person's physical and medical needs? What are the current medications and laboratory values?
◈ Psychosocial: Who supports the patient? What emotional needs does the person have? What cultural differences should be respected?
◈ Knowledge: Is the person ready to learn? What will support knowledge gain and behavioral change? What are the barriers to knowledge gain and behavioral change?

Due to time constraints related to group classes, have the patient complete a self-assessment prior to the initial face-to-face encounter. This may be done on paper or electronically. If there are literacy issues or if Internet access is not available, other arrangements can be made for completion. This self-assessment, combined with a short face-to-face assessment, assists the educator in understanding a patient's individual needs.

When conducting a brief group assessment, the educator must also focus on anything that may be a risk for the class. Pay close attention to physical signs and symptoms that a person may be exhibiting. For instance, watch for signs of hypoglycemia.

Characteristics of Effective Assessments

Effective assessments give the educator the information needed to create an individualized approach to education and support. Effective assessments must be merged with critical thinking, clinical reasoning, and professional experience to best address a patient's needs. The following are characteristic of effective assessments:

- They reveal lifestyle issues and factors.
- They are patient centered, elicit sufficient participation, and promote honest self-disclosure.
- They involve family members and caregivers when appropriate.
- They identify the needs of those in special populations, searching for factors that interfere with an individual's activities of daily living.
- They respectfully honor cultural differences to garner cooperation, information, and trust.
- They uncover high-priority problems to be solved.

These characteristics are discussed more fully below.

Lifestyle Issues

Effective assessments address lifestyle as well as diabetes-specific content. Most diabetes educators are aware of and very knowledgeable about the diabetes-specific elements of an assessment. However, it is important that diabetes educators employ strategies to learn about both the diabetes- and the lifestyle-related components of assessments. The following is a quick summary of some lifestyle-related aspects to be addressed with sample questions:

- Current behaviors in terms of nutrition, exercise, medication, and monitoring. What is the most challenging aspect of diabetes self-care for you?
- Current desired health outcomes and goals. How do you envision your health in the next 5 years?
- Resources and barriers to achieving health outcomes. What seems to get in the way of your achieving your health goals?
- Psychosocial and cultural contexts. How does your culture view people with diabetes or chronic diseases? What is the most important thing you would like for me to know about your cultural, religious, or spiritual beliefs?
- Attitudes or health beliefs. What was it like to find out you have diabetes? How did you get diabetes? What are one or two things you want more of in your life?
- Knowledge, past experiences, stress, emotions, and values. How have you dealt with stress or emotional problems in the past?
- Psychomotor skills. What physical limitations do you have?

Skill Builder: Appreciative Coaching

Appreciative inquiry or appreciative coaching[10] approaches assessment with an attitude of curiosity. If you are truly curious, you behave less like an expert and more like a trusted facilitator or coach. Kimsey-House et al[11] said it well:

"Asking questions for data will yield analysis, reasons, rationale, explanation. Asking questions out of curiosity will yield deeper—often more authentic—information about feelings and motivation" (p. 68).

Consider the different levels of responses from these questions:

- Why did you regain the weight? (asking for explanation)
- I am wondering what made it difficult to keep the weight off? (asking out of curiosity)

Family and Caregivers

Involving the patient's family or caregiver can create both challenges and opportunities for self-management. In general, directing questions to the person with diabetes is best. Family members may agree or disagree with, elaborate on, or interrupt the responses of the person with diabetes or take over answering all the questions. Every one of these actions provides insight into family dynamics or cultural standards. It is important to understand the patient's role in the family. This will often dictate who will participate with the patient during an interview. One approach is for the educator to explain the purpose of the interview and the importance of hearing from each family member, including the patient. What is important is reassuring each party that his or her input is valued.

Special Populations

Just as the education plan is individualized, the assessment takes into consideration unique or special needs. Assessment of a teenager, for instance, might include the HEEADSSS[12] list of questions, which focuses on the home environment, eating, education, activities, drugs, sexuality, suicide/depression, and safety. For older adults and the elderly, the SPICES list of questions would be appropriate.[13] This tool focuses on sleep, problems with eating, incontinence, confusion, evidence of falls, and skin breakdown. Assessment should address the special challenges often faced by members of a particular population or cultural group. For example, assessing religious practices with a Muslim or Jewish individual will increase the educator's understanding of the impact of fasting or food preferences on diabetes management or blood glucose levels.

Practice Setting

Gear assessments to the demands of the practice setting and the patient's previous history in that setting:

- ◆ Initial inpatient: Assessments conducted on inpatient units for immediate "survival" skills training and/or discharge planning focus on those elements germane to the immediate safety needs for a successful transition to home.
- ◆ Repeat hospitalization: A patient repeatedly hospitalized for diabetic ketoacidosis (DKA),

on the other hand, will require a more specific, targeted assessment focused on the causes of DKA and barriers to care.

- ◆ Outpatient: Assessments conducted in outpatient clinics with a high probability of continuous follow-up visits may be more comprehensive and may be conducted in segments over time.
- ◆ Consultant: Assessments conducted by consultants who refer persons with diabetes back to other professionals in "shared care" arrangements may focus on previously negotiated goals and management approaches.

Structure the nature and depth of the assessment to both the patient's needs and the boundaries and limitations imposed by the practice setting.

Activities of Daily Living

It is important to determine the individual's ability to safely and correctly perform self-care skills. Many patients tell their educator that maintaining their independence is very important and is the reason that making behavior changes is something they want to do. On the other hand, the educator may need to ask about their ability to continue to live independently. Some questions to ask are:

- ◆ Do you require help in shopping or preparing your food, personal hygiene, medication, monitoring, or being active?
- ◆ Do you need assistance with transportation to medical appointments, social activities, or other important activities?
- ◆ Is assistance available from family, friends, colleagues, community, or social groups?
- ◆ Do you have daily living skills, such as cooking and doing laundry?

The diabetes educator should also make the following assessments:

- ◆ Is the patient so anxious, disoriented, or depressed by the diagnosis of diabetes or the onset of a new complication that learning a new skill would be extremely difficult? If so, more time may be needed for learning or teaching diabetes skills.
- ◆ Does the patient have adequate cognitive ability to learn new skills?

◈ Has the individual experienced short-term memory loss? If so, does he or she have adequate memory to learn new ways of performing reliable diabetes self-care?

Cultural Considerations

Since studies[14] confirm that culture influences the effectiveness of health care, educators are encouraged to become familiar with the health-related cultural influences of the populations they serve. Culture is that constellation of values and beliefs, traditions and mores which define a group. Taking the broad view of culture, then, the educator may view even generations as having cultural differences. For instance, a baby boomer may have a very different learning style and preferences than a millennial.

For some ethnic cultures, the educator may want to consider incorporating community or lay health workers, also known as promotoras, as part of the assessment visit. Lay health workers are generally trusted and respected members of the community who act as a link between the healthcare system and the community.[15]

Effective educators also consider the culture of generations. The impact of diabetes spans generations, from the traditionalists to the baby boomers to generations X, Y, and Z. Just as in ethnic cultures, members of a generation share political and social influences, values, and characteristics. The impact of generation is addressed in detail later in this chapter.

Prioritizing Needs and Interventions

The assessment will likely reveal more than can possibly be covered in a single class or individual visit. The educator prioritizes the learning objectives into those that must be handled immediately for patient safety, such as hypoglycemia teaching or starting on insulin, and those that can wait. One technique to help engage a patient during the assessment in setting priorities is to suggest a list of possible topic questions and compromise on the assessment agenda.

Clinical judgment, knowledge of diabetes, and patient experience will provide the framework for successfully identifying the most pressing needs. Several resources, including the following Skill Builder, can help the educator hone these clinical decision-making skills.[16,17]

Skill Builder: Applying Critical Thinking to Patient Assessment

◈ Draw from your knowledge, experience, frame of reference, and intuition.
◈ Listen to the patient's story and consider a list of possible problems, making some reasoned assumptions to test out.
◈ Gather data by asking powerful questions which promote insight.
◈ Create an accurate representation of the problem.
◈ Fill in information gaps by asking more questions and seeking more data.
◈ Interpret the information and confirm with the patient what you believe or what you have heard.
◈ Use evidence-based concepts, models, and theories to support or explain the data collected.
◈ Develop conclusions and solutions.
◈ Be open-minded and curious, applying a healthy skepticism as needed.
◈ Learn from the experience through self-reflection.

Assessing Education Needs and Readiness to Change

While the education approach may be well matched to the person or population being served, if those on the receiving end are not ready to receive information or if the information is unimportant to them at the time, learning will likely be compromised.

Consider the following: An individual with type 2 diabetes has just been given a prescription for insulin. You are responsible for educating her. The information you have to share is important. Is the person agreeable, or is she angry and resistant to learning about insulin today? You are adamant that the information you have to share is important for the person to know and understand. However, the person you are trying to help may not agree with your assessment. You know that her history of glycemic control has been suboptimal for years; however, she reports feeling "just fine." What are the chances that the information you have to offer her will be heard today? Will this one-time education session achieve your goals or meet the patient's needs?

A key component of the assessment is determining not only the individual's education needs but also his or her willingness to learn and readiness to change. In situations where the education method and message are not aligned with learner readiness, the outcome will likely be less than desired.[18–21] Issues to consider when assessing educational needs and readiness to learn are summarized in Table 2.2.

TABLE 2.2 **Assessing Education Needs and Readiness to Change**		
Assessment	*Issues to Consider*	*Negative Impact if . . .*
Attitude, knowledge, psychomotor, and psychosocial background	• Attitude and health beliefs and feelings about diabetes: severity, susceptibility, costs, and benefits • Attitude toward participating in education program • Individual goals of treatment: A1C, blood pressure, weight, etc • Experience with diabetes to date • Presence of other confounding health conditions • Presence or absence of a support network	• Diabetes is viewed as unimportant, education is not desired, goals are different, diabetes is not a priority, prior negative experience with friend or family member, or support is lacking
Knowledge and practice of self-care or level of self-care	• Individual ability to perform complex tasks • Willingness to devote more time to management	• Individual not interested in being actively involved in self-management, attitude of "why bother"
Knowledge and preferred learning style	• Preferred method: read, listen, discuss • Usual method of acquiring new information: media, Internet, friends/family, etc • Preference for group vs. individual instruction	• Ability to learn depends on a method that is not available • Individual instruction is required but not available
Psychosocial status and level of stress	• Acute vs. chronic • Influence on ability to learn or make changes	• Stress is high enough to interfere with learning or prioritization of diabetes • Presence of depression may interfere with ability to learn
Psychosocial status and social, cultural, and religious preferences	• Influence on willingness to learn new behaviors • Potential for conflict between treatment recommendations and cultural beliefs	• Education message or methods or treatment recommendations conflict with belief system
Health literacy	• Years of formal education • Learning style and ability to tolerate complexity • Directive teaching may be beneficial • Previous experience with diabetes education or diabetes educators	• Assumptions are made solely on years of education • Literacy level of education method and materials is not appropriate
Readiness for change	• Extent that need for change is recognized • Create conditions that stimulate desire to change or capitalize on readiness to change	• Expressed desire to change does not reflect willingness to change • Readiness for change is not aligned with education goals • Assumptions are made that the individual will never change

Source: Adapted from RM Anderson, "Applied Principles of Teaching and Learning," in MJ Franz, ed, *A Core Curriculum for Diabetes Education and Program Management*, 4th ed (Chicago: American Association of Diabetes Educators, 2001), 7-8.

American Association of Diabetes Educators©

Assessment Skills: Knowing What to Ask

A variety of strategies may be used to systematically gather information[22-36]:

- Direct questions
- Regimen or daily review
- Deviation review
- Specific examples
- Hypothetical situations
- Common obstacles

Direct Questions

Sometimes the best way to get information is to ask for it directly. Decide what information is needed and then formulate a question that will get at that information directly. Open-ended questions allow for general, descriptive answers, while closed-ended questions permit more focused, narrow answers.

Regimen or Daily Review

A regimen review asks individuals to summarize or describe what they typically do to take care of themselves. For example, "Please tell me what you do to care for your diabetes in the morning when you get up" or "Please walk me through a typical day, including what you do for your diabetes."

Deviation Review

When asking people to describe their typical routines, ask them also to describe times when they deviate from their routines. The educator benefits from knowing about both usual routines and exceptions to them. For example, "What happens on the weekend that is different from the weekday?"

Specific Examples

People often find it easier to provide details about a general problem or a behavior if asked to describe a specific example. Ask the person to recall a recent incident or day, and have them describe each episode in detail. For instance, "Please tell me about a time when you were able to follow your meal plan exactly" or "Tell me about a time when you successfully lost weight."

Hypothetical Situations

The educator can sometimes learn a great deal and have hypotheses confirmed or denied by posing a hypothetical situation. Hypothetical situations ask the person to consider what he or she would say, think, or do if a certain situation were to occur. For example, the educator might ask the person to describe what he or she would do at a restaurant after suddenly realizing that insulin or blood glucose monitoring supplies were left at home. Hypothetical situations can provide a great deal of useful assessment information. The educator might pose what-if questions such as, "What if you accidentally left your meter in a hot car all day?"

Common Obstacles

Hypothesis testing offers diabetes educators opportunities to evaluate whether any common obstacles to regimen adherence may be interfering with a person's self-care.[37] When the person's blood glucose level is not consistently in the target range, the educator might ask what could be contributing to this problem. Thoughtful educators will ask questions designed to reveal problems in areas such as these:

- Lack of knowledge or skill
- Competing priorities (lack of time)
- Treatment costs (money, social sacrifices)
- Habit patterns
- Family or social support
- Stress
- Unhelpful thoughts or beliefs
- Language-learning difficulties
- Other aspects

The obstacles to adherence that are present or may arise often can be anticipated. When the educator sees potential trouble, assessing for its presence can minimize problems for the patient. The assessment sets the stage for the educator and the patient to develop both a plan for overcoming existing obstacles and plans for dealing with potential ones. The focus is on helping the person devise new and more effective ways of responding to situations that present adherence obstacles. The person may be encouraged to practice or rehearse the plan to ensure success. For more on problem solving, see chapter 8.

Assessment Strategies

Give Time to Answer

Conducting an assessment can be difficult when the patient is slow to respond or reticent. People have different response times, information processing rates, and social interaction styles. These factors vary widely from one culture to another. Trying to rush the discussion along may be perceived as disrespectful. Before moving on, be patient and provide enough time for inquiries to be answered.

Use Active Listening Skills

Most diabetes educators are aware of and employ one or more of 4 verbal and nonverbal behaviors generally referred to as active listening skills: clarifying, paraphrasing, reflecting feelings, and using minimal encouragers.

Clarifying   Asking for clarification helps the educator ensure he or she understands what the patient has said. The educator is checking the patient's understanding of a particular word, phrase, or idea that the patient has used. For instance, "When you said you had 'high blood' did you mean blood sugar or blood pressure?"

Paraphrasing   Paraphrasing tells the other person that he or she has been heard and understood. The educator restates what the patient has said in slightly different words that have the same meaning. Paraphrasing responds to the factual or informational content of what the patient is saying. Unlike clarification, paraphrasing does not involve asking a question. Instead, the educator confirms what was heard by restating it to the person. For example, "I think I heard you say that eating pizza really affects your blood glucose for hours after the meal."

Reflecting Feelings   Reflecting feelings involves giving feedback to the patient on the affective tone of what is being said. Thus, the emotion or feeling expressed in the patient's verbal or nonverbal behavior is made explicit by reflecting feeling. Paraphrasing, in contrast, involves giving feedback on factual information. When a person is expressing an emotional reaction, reflecting this emotion back to the person is often helpful. Sometimes, patients are not aware of their emotional reactions, so by reflecting feelings the educator is able to help them become more aware of how they appear to be reacting emotionally to a particular situation. Reflecting feelings can also be useful as a way for the educator to check whether he or she is accurately reading the patient's feelings about a particular event or situation. Reflecting another's

feelings might sound like, "You sound so sad when you describe what happened." Paraphrasing, on the other hand, sounds like, "What I hear you say is that checking your blood glucose is a hassle." Notice that both comments will encourage further dialogue, but reflecting feelings will foster further discussion at a deeper emotional level.

Using Minimal Encouragers   Minimal encouragers are the verbal and nonverbal behaviors people use to signal to another person that they are listening and the person speaking should continue. The best way for educators to learn how well they use minimal encouragers is to watch one of their interviews on videotape. Examples of minimal encouragers include eye contact while listening, nodding the head, and saying short phrases like "yes," "continue," "uh-huh," and "ok."

One caveat: Avoid minimal encouragers if and when individuals engage in any kind of "jousting," such as blaming other healthcare professionals or family members for their poor control, for creating barriers to regimen adherence, or for their complications. People may interpret minimal encouragers as agreement with their negative evaluations of others. In such cases, the diabetes educator must be especially attentive to listening carefully but studiously avoiding any appearance of agreeing. Otherwise, the educator may become an enabler or encourager of such behavior. The educator also may one day hear from colleagues or family members who were surprised to hear the educator had "accused" them of some wrongful behavior.

In conducting an individual or group assessment, a variety of practical strategies and skills can be used to gain a better understanding of a patient. A summary appears in Table 2.3.

Techniques for Closing the Assessment

Give Feedback   At the end of an assessment, or when a portion of the assessment has been completed, the educator gives feedback to the patient. Feedback involves not just a summary but an interpretation of what the educator learned in the assessment. Normalizing the patient's problem and providing ideas that have been tried by others is a useful strategy. The patient's learning that he or she is not alone may be reassuring. As described in the

TABLE 2.3   Effective Assessments at a Glance

Set the Tone
- Decrease background sounds, especially for those who may have hearing or attention deficits
- Avoid interruptions
- Include family members and caregivers
- When addressing an elderly adult, speak clearly and face-to-face
- Avoid patronizing titles ("dear," "hon"); use formal salutations ("Ms. Jackson," "Dr. Jones")

Open and Close Effectively

Opening
- Orientation
- Objectives
- Rationale
- Receptivity

Closing
- Summary
- Transitions

Build Trust and Encourage Honest Communication

Do:
- Build trust
- Encourage openness and honesty
- Form a collaborative relationship, including caregivers as appropriate
- Accept the person unconditionally
- Express empathy
- Be an active listener

Don't:
- Use fear or scare tactics
- Be judgmental
- Interrupt or hurry
- Ignore feelings and emotion
- Use jargon or unfamiliar terms
- Underestimate people's desire and ability to learn
- Appear distracted

Improve Skill in Information Gathering
- Use this checklist while reviewing videotaped assessments
- Watch and emulate expert colleagues
- Offer to teach these skills to others

Ask Good Questions
- Pause and think
- Be direct
- Ask for specifics
- Be persistent
- Ask follow-up questions
- Make mental notes
- Ask for examples

Identify Sensory and Cognitive Deficits

Assess for:
- Hearing deficits
- Visual impairment
- Literacy and language problems
- Cognitive impairment

Know What Type of Questions to Ask
- Direct questioning: What do you want to know?
- Regimen review: What do you usually do?
- Deviation review: Tell me about exceptions or special circumstances.
- Specific examples: Give me an example of when that happened.
- Hypothetical situations: What would you do if . . .

Encourage Patient Participation
- Allow time to answer, recognizing individual and cultural differences
- Use active listening skills
- Summarize
- Give feedback

Gather Information Using a Variety of Strategies
- Paper-and-pencil measures
- Physical and laboratory data
- Self-monitoring (blood glucose, meal plan, activity)
- Observe behavior (skills checks)
- Solicit information from client, family, caregivers

Acknowledge Client's Feelings and Frustrations
- Listen to how it is said
- Watch body language
- Give feedback
- Be sympathetic

Source: JA Pichert, DG Schlundt, "Assessment: Gathering Information and Facilitating Engagement," in C Mensing, ed, *The Art and Science of Diabetes Self-Management Education: A Desk Reference for Healthcare Professionals* (Chicago: American Association of Diabetes Educators, 2006), 592.

Knowledge Builder, a careful assessment can help the educator understand how the individual is normalizing the experience of having diabetes.

Knowledge Builder: Normalization and Chronic Disease

Kralik and colleagues discovered that while professionals view self-management as a form of structured education, patients see self-management as a way to create a new normal in their lives. To do this, individuals had to recognize the boundaries imposed by the disease, redirect resources to manage the disease, consider their new identity as a person with a chronic disease, and seek a new balance by planning and prioritizing their daily demands of the disease.[38]

Educators can use the work of Kralik et al to assess how their patients have normalized the experience of living with diabetes.

Summarize Summarizing is similar to paraphrasing in that the educator restates what the patient has just said. A summary allows the educator to see whether he or she has learned the gist of what the patient has been talking about. A summary gives the patient an opportunity to correct the educator's perception or to add information that has been omitted and also serves to create a smooth transition between topics. A large component of critical thinking involves interpreting the data and confirming with the patient what was discussed. Using a summary can help the educator be ready for goal setting.

Summary for Assessment

To complete a comprehensive diabetes education assessment efficiently, the educator utilizes his or her well-developed interviewing skills and critical thinking skills. Once the assessment is completed, the educator synthesizes the information and develops a sense of which topics and behavior targets need focus, while always remembering that DSME is patient-driven and that the goals and plan are developed in cooperation with the patient. The next step in the DSME process is goal setting.

Goal Setting

Goal setting is a critical component in successful DSME.[6] The process of developing goals is based on assessment and collaboration among the patient, the healthcare provider and other team members, and the patient's support system. Goals can later serve as a method to evaluate a patient's progress.

Goals are defined in measurable terms stated in behavioral objectives.[3] These goals are monitored and measured throughout the DSME process. As defined by AADE, the diabetes educator works with the person with or at risk for diabetes to identify patient-centric DSME outcomes.[3] The goals reflect information obtained through the assessment process and also serve as a tool to evaluate progress toward individual, program, institutional, or community-level goals. The delivery of the education to reach the goals is coordinated with the healthcare team members.

The Standards of Practice include criteria to be considered in goal setting, and this step in the process includes the following[7]:

- Write desired goals in measurable terms.
- Define specific behavioral objectives and actions in an educational setting.
- Develop goals that are consistent with diabetes practice guidelines and honor the patient's role.
- Incorporate consideration of risks and benefits of the proposed outcomes.
- Develop goals with consideration for resources available to that person to increase the likelihood that the suggested behavior change will be adopted.
- Define goals that are tailored and appropriate to a person's state of health.
- Redefine goals as needed to meet the needs of the person.

In addition to the AADE Scope of Practice (addressed later in this chapter), the National Standards for Diabetes Self-Management Education and Support include 2 directions for goal setting.[4] Standard 7 states that the assessment and education plan will be developed collaboratively by the participant and the instructor(s) to direct the selection of appropriate education interventions and self-management support strategies. This assessment and education plan and the intervention outcomes will be documented in the education record.[4] One of the indicators for meeting this standard is showing evidence of ongoing education planning and behavioral goal setting based on the assessed and/or reassessed needs of the person.

This standard reflects on the patient's selected behavioral objective and measurable learning objectives. The objectives are mutually determined, but most important is that the person is involved in the process of the development and final selection of his or her goals.

Standard 9 states that the provider(s) of DSME and DSMS will assess each participant's personal self-management goals and progress toward those goals.[4]

This standard addresses the individual achievement of goals while Standard 10 addresses the program assessment of targeted goal achievement for the population served and actual goal achievement. This information can be used to reflect on the effectiveness of the program. For more on program management, see chapter 11.

Goal-Setting Considerations

A person's goals are tailored to his or her attitude, knowledge, and behavioral skills. It is important to recognize where the patient is in the learning process and the individualized needs for patient safety. For example, a patient new to the disease may require basic information and "survival skills."

When working with the patient to develop goals, educators can do the following:

◆ Recognize that the goal belongs to the patient, not to the educator.
◆ Identify options for achieving a goal, including the desired overall outcome(s).
◆ Choose the best agreed-upon option to start. Include a person's needs, skills, and learning preferences.
◆ Demonstrate respect for cultural, lifestyle, and health beliefs.
◆ Develop specific implementation of goals addressing strengths and barriers and determine a person's commitment to his or her goals.

◆ Recognize goal setting as a lifelong process that evolves with changing needs, desires, and abilities of the person living with a chronic illness.
◆ Goal setting is iterative and dynamic. Expect goals to be refined, expanded, or even discarded as individuals form new behaviors and gain new knowledge.

During the assessment process, it is common for an educator to uncover several patient needs. Where to begin in setting goals can be daunting. A simple approach is to ask the patient, "Is there anything you would like to do this week to improve your health?"[39] This allows the patient a voice in the experience of goal setting and sets a level of interest and commitment.

Collaborating on Educational Goals

An important component in the process of program evaluation of outcomes is understanding the person's point of view, expectations, and desired outcomes as well as those of the referring provider. The educator may find that these don't always match. In addition, during the assessment an educator may discover additional behavioral and learning needs that should be included in the goals. A skilled educator will explore a variety of options for the person to select and to accomplish in a specific period of time.

Use the AADE7™ as a Guiding Tool to Goal Setting

The desired outcomes must be clearly defined and mutually agreed upon. Ideally, the educator has sufficient information from the person with diabetes, the family and others in the case of a child, and from the referring provider. The AADE7 Self-Care Behaviors™ provide a comprehensive framework for formulating goals. Because behavior change is a unique outcome measure for DSME, the outcomes may focus on knowledge, behavior, or clinical results. Goals should be quantifiable so that behavior change can be measured and documented.

Obtain Buy-in
A large part of the initial visit and assessment is to establish a rapport with the person while setting

up an agenda to include goals and follow-up plans, which can be in either a group or an individual setting. Essential to goal development is helping the patient explore his or her commitment.[40] Asking a patient to tell his or her story and share his or her perspective about diabetes helps the educator understand the individual's experience and get to the core of what that patient needs in terms of knowledge, skills, and a deeper understanding of his or her disease.

Understand and Respect Each Patient as an Individual

Each person comes for DSME with a unique set of experiences. The educator uses the person's initial information to further determine his or her level of conviction and confidence in goal setting. A person's conviction is his or her belief in how important it is to make a change. A conversation about the person's strengths and barriers can help the educator assess readiness to learn. A person's confidence is his or her belief in an ability to be successful and to overcome obstacles and is intimately linked to self-esteem, knowledge, and past experiences. For the educator, understanding a person's conviction and confidence offers a measure of the potential for successful behavior change and is a key factor in establishing appropriate, realistic behavior goals. A person's goals reflect his or her needs, skills, learning style, and preferences. The goals also respect a person's cultural, lifestyle, and health beliefs.

Keep the Patient's Agenda in Mind

Educators often feel that they know what their patients need to do to improve their health, but working under this assumption is often counterproductive. It is not uncommon for educators to suggest that a patient try something, only to receive a "Yes, but . . ." from the patient. This is what is called a "premature focus trap."[41] To be effective, goals need to be owned by the patient and supported by the educator.

Individualize the Goals

A key to successful goal setting is effective questioning. For example, if a patient goal is weight loss, some questions on the person's past experiences with weight loss can be beneficial: What were the

individual's most successful attempts and what were some barriers? What needs to be different this time to be successful? A simple tool used in motivational interviewing is the acronym DARN[42]:

Desire: "What do you want, or like, or wish, hope, etc?"
Ability: "What is possible?" or "What can or could you do?"
Reasons: "Why would you make this change?" or "What are the benefits and risks?"
Need: "How important is this change?" "How much do you need to do this?"

The more details generated by the patient, the more likely the chance for success. This helps not only the patient but also the educator see difficulties or barriers with achieving the goal. For example, if a patient's goal is meal planning, there may need to be a discussion around certain meals or snacks. It may turn out that the real issue is nighttime snacking, which narrows the goal and action plan.

Take a Step-by-Step Approach

The patient needs to identify the first step in reaching his or her goal. The patient may have a broad overall goal of reducing his or her A1C and a smaller goal to begin walking several times a week. The role of the educator is to help the patient generate strategies for success. For example, in terms of the walking goal, there may need to be a discussion about when, where, and how long the person will walk. Sharing information such as "Studies show that people who exercise in the morning tend to stay with their program longer" can be very useful. Encouraging the person to keep a record of his or her walking to demonstrate success is another strategy to share for achievement of a goal.

Focus on the Behavior, Not on the Outcome

Patients are more likely to achieve improved outcomes such as lowering A1C or losing weight by focusing on the behavior change. A behavior change is something a person can do that will influence the broader identified outcome.

Have a Written Agreement

Writing down a patient's ideas for short-term goals and making an agreement to try new behaviors in the next week can prove effective. Both the educator and the patient have a clear understanding of the plan.

A well-written agreement is goal-specific, measurable, achievable, and timely. Between the educator and the patient there may even be a discussion of a reward at the end of a specific timeframe. Rewards don't have to involve money; a reward could be the patient having time to pursue a hobby or a family member cooking dinner.[41]

Involve Family Members and Friends

Diabetes may affect the lives of everyone who loves, lives with, or cares about the person with this disease. Family and friends can support the patient in a number of ways. Having the educator learn about a patient's support system may be useful when goal setting is discussed. Perhaps a family member could volunteer to cook one meal a week and give the patient the night off from that responsibility. Ideas for rewards and psychological support can be encouraged during the goal-setting process.

Keep Cultural Considerations in Mind

A community health worker may be a valuable resource in helping to understand cultural preferences when selecting attainable goals. Other diabetes educators who work with ethnically diverse patients may also be a source of information and support. With social media outlets, access to educator colleagues is increasingly available.

A Word About Children

In the case of children, their readiness to learn can change considerably with age and maturation. Included in the goal-setting process with children are other significant people in a child's life, such as parents, siblings, grandparents, extended family members, and teachers. A child's support system is usually much broader than that of an adult, and these other people must be included in the goal-setting process. The educator must also take into consideration age-specific behavioral and learning objectives.

Strategies for Developing Goals

Behavior-change counseling may be used to elicit participation in goal setting. By helping the patient become motivated, the educator is also helping the patient make progress in identifying personal goals. The educator has to continue to spend time building rapport.[42] Strategies include the following:

◆ Begin with open-ended questions: "So you would like to . . ."

◆ Reassure patient of confidentiality: "This is just between us, talking out loud to try and come up with a plan."

◆ Show interest in what the patient has to say: "I am happy to hear that you . . ."

◆ Be accepting and nonjudgmental: "You have really given this some thought."

◆ Be very slow to interrupt. Listen; try to allow time for a quiet pause for the patient to think a little bit more and process information. Simply counting slowly (and silently) to 5 will show the educator's patience and encourage the patient to be the one to break the awkward silence.

◆ Continue to explore what is most important for the person and what is most reasonable to work on.

Trust and Rapport

Ideally, an environment has been created during the assessment process that supports honest self-disclosure. Just as in the assessment process, honest self-disclosure of personal goals occurs only when people trust each other. The educator's task is to maintain an atmosphere of trust and nonjudgmental acceptance.[41] This means listening, reflecting back what the patient says, and asking for clarification, as described in the previous section.

Assess Patient Skills to Plan Goals

The diabetes educator uses 4 critical skills to determine the patient's abilities for goal setting[43]:

1. **Interpret information gathering.** The educator uses data obtained from patients during the assessment phase, including their attitude, knowledge, and skills related to their abilities, to assist with goal setting.

2. **Facilitating engagement.** These are skills the diabetes educator uses to create a safe, trusting atmosphere in which the individual feels comfortable divulging details about personal

health, self-management, and possible lifestyle changes. These skills include the following[32]:

—Listening skills

—Empathy

—Making conversation easy and enjoyable

—Awareness of his or her own nonverbal behaviors that can discourage conversation and brainstorming (eg, crossing arms, pushing chair away from the patient, and repeatedly checking the time)

3. **Hypothesis testing.** The process of identifying and understanding a patient's ideas about problem solving is best accomplished via hypothesis testing. Effective and efficient interviewers develop hypotheses—educated guesses—about problems that are specific to a particular person. The educator asks questions designed to elicit information that will eliminate some hypotheses and confirm others. Using a hypothesis testing approach, the educator zeros in on a problem and develops an understanding of the issues in a relatively short period of time.

4. **Problem analysis.** Problem analysis refers to developing an understanding of the "whats and whys" of a patient's medical and self-management problems. Understanding the kinds of problems typically faced and the most common obstacles to behavior change helps the educator develop reasonable hypotheses. These can then be tested by asking pertinent questions, analyzing the answers, and thereby increasing the understanding of the issues for subsequent problem solving. Each item addresses a specific event or behavior and employs multiple-choice responses, so the alternatives cover the range of possible responses.

In Practice Tip: Using Past Experiences with Self-Monitoring to Assist in Goal Setting

Self-monitoring involves asking people to keep a diary or record of a specific behavior. For example, the person can be asked to self-monitor (ie, count) the number of cigarettes smoked each day. A diary's purpose is twofold:

1. It provides the person with immediate feedback on his or her success at meeting the treatment goal.
2. It provides the healthcare professional with an ongoing record of behavior that can be used to identify specific problems.

Be sure to discuss the purpose of the self-monitoring activity with the patient, as well as the specifics on how to report on the activity:

◆ **Rationale:** Give a clear rationale for keeping records. Explain how the data will be used and why a diary will be helpful. People who understand the importance of keeping good records are more likely to do so.

◆ **Willingness:** Make sure the person is willing to keep a diary.

◆ **Report:** The person should be instructed on where to keep the record and when to complete it.

◆ **Simplicity:** Make the record-keeping task as simple as possible. For some patients, using a smartphone app may be the best approach. Numerous apps are available that support diabetes behaviors.[44] For others, a handwritten log may be the best choice.

◆ **Understanding:** Ask the person to reiterate the instructions. For example: "Tell me in your own words what you are going to record." Educators may assume the person understands; in fact, they are often surprised that an assignment they thought was clear confused the client.

◆ **Receipt:** Make a note in the medical record to ask for the diary at the next meeting. When the person gives you a completed diary, give ample praise. Use the information in the teaching/counseling session. Help the person feel the effort was worthwhile.

Observe Behavior

Sometimes the educator has questions about a person's skills and abilities to do certain things.

Observing the person performing the skill is often preferable to asking about self-perceived capabilities. For example, to assess someone's skill in using a particular blood glucose meter, give the person the meter and ask him or her to perform a blood glucose check. Use role-playing techniques, too. For example, give the person a restaurant menu and say, "Pretend I am a waiter at the restaurant and you are a customer. Order a meal that fits the meal plan you have chosen to follow."

Collaboratively Establishing Goals

In collaboration with each patient, the diabetes educator establishes and documents specific goals and objectives. The aim is to set goals and write specific behavioral objectives that are important to the individual and that the individual feels confident about achieving. It is important that the educator and the patient are clear on what is meant by a goal, as well as the distinctions between a learning objective and a behavioral objective.

- **Goal:** This serves as a big-picture, directional guide; it is the focal point for the objectives and the end result of meeting the objectives.
- **Learning objective:** This is the objective the individual with diabetes plans to meet at the end of the educational intervention. Examples of learning objectives are the following:
  —"Identify 3 foods with carbohydrate"
  —"Discuss sick-day treatment guidelines"
- **Behavioral objective:** Also referred to as "a behavioral goal," this is a planned, measurable change in behavior that is likely to achieve a positive health outcome over a period of time once the initial intervention is completed. Examples of behavioral objectives are the following:
  —"Eat 3 to 4 carbohydrate choices per meal"
  —"Monitor blood glucose 4 times per day before meals"

Both learning objectives and behavioral objectives are written as measurable, observable statements so the participant and the educator can clearly determine whether objectives have been met.[45] Table 2.4 gives examples of each type of objective. Table 2.5 is an aid, based on Bloom's Taxonomy, for writing both types of objectives.[45]

TABLE 2.4   Differentiating Between Learning and Behavioral Objectives
Sample Learning Objectives
• Identify carbohydrate foods
• List 4 treatments for hypoglycemia
• Discuss differences between saturated and unsaturated fats
Sample Behavioral Objectives
• Record food intake and activity in a logbook 4 days per week for 1 month
• Eat 4 carbohydrate servings at lunch and dinner and 1 carbohydrate snack for 2 weeks
• Drink noncaloric beverages instead of sweetened ones until follow-up class

Source: JVC Hill, "Writing Behavioral Objectives: Tips From an Educator and Auditor," in MD Maryniuk, theme ed, *On the Cutting Edge* [DCE newsletter] 26, no. 2 (2005): 25-29.

Since learning cannot be witnessed directly, objectives provide a basis for making the best possible inferences about whether learning has occurred. Objectives clarify the purposes and intent of instruction, and they enable the person with diabetes to know what the plan is, which helps improve communications.

Behavioral Objectives: Characteristics
A behavioral objective should have the characteristics described below.

A simple acronym to guide educators in assessing the completeness of their objectives is to determine whether they are SMART: specific, measurable, achievable, realistic, and time-bound (ie, stated in terms of a specific time when they will happen).

SMART goal setting is defined as:

- **Specific:** What, why, and how? Encourage the patient to be specific and identify details.
- **Measurable:** If the goal can't be measured, it can't be managed. Accurate tracking and the ability to identify progress are necessary components of goal achievement.
- **Achievable:** Help the patient identify what is important to him or her. The goal requires commitment and should stretch the patient slightly, but it should not be too far out of reach. Success in goal achievement will help develop confidence and self-efficacy.

❖ **Realistic:** This doesn't mean easy, just doable. The educator can help the patient evaluate how realistic the chosen goal is in the given situation. Work with the patient to identify what he or she is or is not willing (or able) to do to meet the goal.

❖ **Time-bound:** Set a time frame for the goal. This gives a clear target to work toward. Setting very short-term goals such as "for the next week" gives an opportunity for more immediate feedback.

TABLE 2.5 Guide for Writing Learning and Behavioral Objectives		
Sample Verbs	*Learning Objective*	*Behavioral Objective*
1) REMEMBERING Learner recalls or recognizes information, ideas, and principles in the approximate form in which they were learned.		
List Identify Record Recall	List 3 treatments for hypoglycemia.	Record how I treat hypoglycemia in my log for the next 2 weeks.
2) UNDERSTANDING Learner translates, comprehends, or interprets information based on prior learning.		
Describe Summarize Explain Compare	Describe rationale for the 15-15 rule in hypoglycemia treatment.	Describe treatment for hypoglycemia to my husband and coworker within the next week.
3) APPLYING Learner selects, transfers, and uses data and principles to complete a problem or task with a minimum of direction.		
Demonstrate Choose Implement Complete	Choose food models of 15-g carbohydrate portion sizes.	Choose foods that match meal plan during the next month and discuss with registered dietitian at follow-up class.
4) ANALYZING Learner breaks material or ideas apart, determines how the parts relate to each other by organizing the material.		
Analyze Determine Summarize Organize	Determine carbohydrate foods that have a higher glycemic index based on case example information.	Analyze effect of different carbohydrate foods on blood glucose by keeping records for 1 month.
5) EVALUATING Learner originates, integrates, and combines ideas or parts into a whole idea, product, plan, or proposal that is new to him or her.		
Check Order Prepare Critique	Prepare a sample meal incorporating carbohydrate allowance and principles of healthy eating.	Prepare a set of sample menus for 1 week incorporating carbohydrate allowances and principles of healthy eating.
6) CREATING Learner puts elements together into a functional whole by reorganizing components in new ways.		
Generate Plan Produce	Create a meal from a list of preferred foods.	Create a week of breakfast meals each containing 45 g of carbohydate using a list of preferred foods.

Source: DR Krathwohl, "A revision of Bloom's Taxonomy: an overview," *Theory Pract* 41, no. 4 (2002): 212-8.

Common Mistakes The following 3 examples represent behavioral objectives that are not SMART goals:

◆ "I will eat healthier foods."

Rationale: This is not a specific objective. What is a "healthier food"? Guide the patient in making this more specific and measurable by asking, "What would this look like to you?" A more specific goal in this case might be, "I will eat 5 servings of fruits and vegetables each day for the next month and reevaluate the goal at my next clinic visit."

◆ "I will lose 5 pounds."

Rationale: This is not an objective but an outcome of practicing healthy behaviors (such as eating less or exercising more). An objective is something the person can actually do that will result in weight loss. Help the patient create an objective by asking, "How will you lose 5 pounds?" The answer will often be phrased as an objective such as, "I will limit my meat servings at lunch and dinner to 4 oz at least 5 evenings per week."

◆ "I will join a gym and go for 1 hour every day."

Rationale: Check with the person to see whether this is achievable. A daily, hour-long visit to the gym may be tough for even the most avid exercise enthusiast to meet. It is important to guide the person in setting small goals to ensure they can be met and to evaluate them after a short period to reward success.

Action Planning

Another form of goal setting is action planning. Action plans tend to use more informal goal setting. Behavioral goals are replaced with statements of intent, for example. Action planning has been found to be an effective component of health education programs.[46] Polonsky (written communication, January 2006) describes the critical elements of action planning to include the following:

◆ *Specificity:* The patient clearly understands exactly what he or she needs to do.

◆ *Reasonableness:* The patient believes the plan for action is achievable.

◆ *Patient-centered:* The patient perceives some sense of personal ownership of the plan and its development; it is not merely a set of instructions delivered by the educator.

◆ *Meaningfulness:* The patient perceives that accomplishing the plan will be of personal value.

An excellent example of how action planning that meets these criteria can produce positive outcomes is illustrated in a study assessing implementation intentions in the following Knowledge Builder.

Knowledge Builder: Action Plans at Work

Sheeran and Orbell[47] asked a sample of 114 women to make appointments for cervical cancer screening. Half of the sample served as controls, that is, they were given no further instructions, while the remaining half were asked to specify in writing their intention to implement this recommendation. They were asked to write down when, where, and how they would make the appointment. Of this latter group, 92% attended screenings. In contrast, only 69% of the control group attended screenings. These data lend further support to the importance of personalized, specific behavioral objectives or action planning. When people have detailed their own "implementable" plan for action, they are equipped with a plan that is likely to be specific, reasonable, and, of course, patient-centered. This enhances their intent to take action; therefore, behavior change is more likely to happen.

Preparing for Success The process of goal setting is fairly straightforward: Establish one or more SMART goals or an action plan and see what happens. Yet there are several considerations in predicting whether the goals are the most appropriate for the patient and the identified needs. Here are some questions to explore[46]:

◆ Does the patient:
  —Value the goal and perceive a need for it?
  —Understand the steps needed to change the behavior?

—Have conviction (ie, believe) that changing the behavior is important and will improve his or her health or quality of life?

—Have confidence (ie, believe) that he or she has the necessary resources and is likely to be successful in both changing the behavior and overcoming the obstacles to behavior change?

Simple behavioral rulers can help answer these questions. Further described in chapter 5, rulers help gauge the patient's conviction and confidence in launching new behavioral goals.

Summary for Goal Setting

The patient owns his or her goals. Supporting patients in their effort to establish goals that initiate and maintain healthy patterns of self-care is a major role of the diabetes educator. An educator is a facilitator in the change process, which also involves ongoing follow-up visits or communication. The patient's role is to make the change and communicate the results. The educator's skills are measured in the ability to ask the right questions and offer options rather than issue directives. The skilled educator has a firm understanding of the role the patient's view of diabetes, including health beliefs, locus of control, and self-efficacy, plays in motivating behavior change. Further, the effective educator understands how the patient's support system of family, coworkers, and community enhances and sustains the patient's successful change.

Self-care behaviors are assessed at baseline and at specific intervals during and after the education program.[3] Once the goals of the learning experience are established, the plan can be developed and implemented.

Planning

Planning is the third step in the DSME and training process. As described by AADE in The Scope of Practice, Standards of Practice, and Standards of Professional Performance for Diabetes Educators,[7] the diabetes educator develops the DSME plan to help the person with their desired health outcomes. The plan integrates evidence-based diabetes care practices

and established principles of teaching and learning. The plan is coordinated among the diabetes healthcare team members, the person with or at risk for diabetes, the person's family and other relevant support systems, and the referring provider. The plan for education must be individualized and appropriately paced and address not only the objectives outlined in the medical plan but also the needs and capabilities of the person with diabetes. Linked closely to the findings in the assessment, the most effective therapeutic plan is individualized and prioritizes the knowledge, skills, and behaviors required for desired behavior change and metabolic outcomes.

The planning process is thoroughly described in *The AADE Guidelines for the Practice of Diabetes Self-Management Education and Training*. Key components include the following[6]:

◆ Development of a detailed intervention plan to address both clinical and behavioral goals established in the goal-setting process

◆ A learning plan to address gaps in knowledge and plan strategies for addressing identified barriers and referrals as needed

Planning is also described in Standard 7 of the National Standards for Diabetes Self-Management Education and Support[4] as well as in a standard in The Scope of Practice, Standards of Practice, and Standards of Professional Performance for Diabetes Educators.[7] Given the time limits of most education sessions, planning may be the one step which is abbreviated. However, planning serves as a road map or guide for the delivery of education. Planning is dynamic, changing as the needs of the patient change and as further assessment dictates.

According to the AADE Standards of Practice,[7] the education plan includes the following:

◆ Specific outcomes
◆ Measurable, behaviorally focused terms
◆ Specific instructional strategies honoring the individual's cultural, lifestyle, and health beliefs
◆ Evaluation of the plan's effectiveness

In addition to guiding the service, an education plan is a required part of program accreditation/recognition. It must reflect collaboration and appropriate educational interventions and self-management support strategies.

American Association of Diabetes Educators©

The plan addresses issues identified in the multi-faceted assessment, including gaps in knowledge and information and/or skills needed to address identified behavioral goals.[4] Barriers identified during the assessment, such as lack of transportation, difficulty in paying for medications or supplies, and psychosocial problems, must be considered when developing the plan.[4] The education plan, along with the outcomes, is documented in the patient record.[4]

In developing a successful education plan, the diabetes educator uses a number of important skills:

◆ Synthesis of information
◆ Logical thinking
◆ Prioritizing interventions
◆ Developing objectives and targeting outcomes
◆ Maintaining engagement

It often can be challenging to analyze all the available assessment information and propose a realistic plan within the constraints of the individual or group visit. The educator prioritizes the learning objectives into those that must be handled immediately for patient safety and those that can wait, while keeping in mind adult learning theory and the importance of responding to the patient's priorities.

Components of the Education Plan

Elements of the plan include specific desired outcomes, instructional approaches, and evaluation ideas. A template is provided in Table 2.6, and a sample completed plan is offered in Table 2.7.

Specific Outcomes

An important part of assessment is clarifying the individual's expectations and desired outcomes, as well as those of the referring provider. These may or may not be the same. In addition, during the assessment, the needs that should be addressed in the education plan are identified, including those of family members who are part of the visit. The skilled educator identifies all areas to be covered for comprehensive education and works with the patient and the education team to develop an education plan that includes learning objectives for the group or individual visit. Typically, behavioral objectives are determined at the end of the

TABLE 2.6 Template: Diabetes Education Plan				
Patient:				
Self-management goal(s):				
Behavioral objectives to achieve goal:				
Evaluation of goal achievement:				
Topic:				
Learning Objective	**Content**	**Teaching Strategies**	**Evaluation**
Topic:				
Learning Objective	**Content**	**Teaching Strategies**	**Evaluation**
Topic:				
Learning Objective	**Content**	**Teaching Strategies**	**Evaluation**

TABLE 2.7   Sample Diabetes Education Plan

Self-management goal(s): Decrease A1C 1%

Behavioral objectives to achieve goal:

Walk 15 minutes after breakfast and lunch for 2 weeks.

Decrease sugary drinks from 3 per day to 1 or less for 2 weeks.

Evaluation of goal achievement:

Short-term: Patient activity and diet logs and self-report

Long-term: A1C decreases 1% in 3 months

Topic: Exercise

Learning Objective	Content	Teaching Strategies	Evaluation of learning
Verbalize benefits of exercise	Benefits and risk of exercise	Handout Discussion	Actively involved in discussion
List preferred activities	Types of activities: aerobic, anaerobic, flexibility, strength activities	3-minute YouTube video	Lists and prioritizes preferred activities
Discuss safety and exercise	Blood glucose safety Foot safety Using a pedometer Clothing selection	Pedometer practice Options for blood glucose equipment Options for treating hypoglycemia	Practices with a pedometer Lists one or two safety issues and how to address

Topic: Nutrition

Learning Objective	Content	Teaching Strategies	Evaluation
List favorite beverages and carbohydrate content	Hidden sources of sugar and carbohydrate	Handout Label reading examples	Reads label accurately
Select alternatives to sugary drinks	Fluid options Making non-sugary drinks flavorful	Web search for non-sugary drink alternatives	Describes a plan for locating other beverages

session. Learning and behavioral objectives are incorporated into the DSME follow-up and reassessment.

Measurable, Behaviorally Focused Goals

Measurable, behaviorally focused goals are part of the plan. The mutually agreed-upon goals give direction to the DSME plan. Utilizing the AADE7 Self-Care Behavior™ framework for DSME gives a behaviorally focused, action-oriented direction in the plan of care. See the section on goal setting for more information on creating measurable, behaviorally focused goals.

Content

Understanding what has gone awry in the body in the presence of diabetes is important. However,

understanding how to manage the disease on a daily basis is critical to the individual's short- and long-term health and quality of life. Beyond the "what" and "why," adequate attention must be paid to the "how."

The challenge for healthcare educators is to effectively provide the individual with sufficient information to facilitate translation of new information into positive behavior change. An individual's management of diabetes requires integration of several skill sets: specific self-care skills, self-management skills, and coping skills.[48] This content must be considered in the DSME plan.

Self-Care Skills

Essential self-care skills include making food choices, monitoring blood glucose, taking medications (orally or by injection), adjusting for food or activity variations, and managing hyperglycemia and hypoglycemia. These are commonly referred to as "survival skills"; however, many people with diabetes have "survived" knowing less than this amount of information. Many self-care skills are psychomotor in nature. In this case, discussing the content will not be enough. Interactive strategies will be critical.

Self-Management Skills

Mastery of the essential self-management skills requires incremental learning that incorporates information and personal experience. Diabetes education is an ongoing process, not a once-in-a-lifetime experience. Development of self-management skills requires that learning be pushed to the next level. For this to happen, an individual must incorporate previously acquired information into situational decision-making. Utilization of anticipatory planning and problem solving promotes the development of self-management skills. For example, adjusting the insulin dose to compensate for pizza and beer involves anticipatory planning. Evaluating the outcome of this adjustment using postmeal blood glucose data allows the individual to assess the effectiveness of the decision. In the DSME plan, the content should include didactic information as well as practical application and problem solving.

Coping Skills

Equally important to self-care is the identification and cultivation of appropriate coping skills. The presence of diabetes adds multiple stressors to the individual's life. The ability to manage the usual stressors (job, family, etc) will directly influence the individual's ability to manage the stressors associated with diabetes (inconvenience of daily care, potential for hypoglycemia, evolving complications, etc). Thus, helping the individual recognize and evaluate his or her usual coping strategies assists in the development of diabetes-specific coping behaviors. For example, if an individual typically responds to unplanned situations with frustration and agitation, helping him or her to anticipate and problem solve about delayed meals or unexpected schedule changes may decrease the frustration and agitation felt during these unplanned times. In this way, the event may be viewed as a learning opportunity rather than as a threat.

Finally, the person with diabetes needs to understand the goals and limitations of diabetes management. Maintenance of daily glycemic control is a potential challenge. If the learner has access to self-management information and that information is presented in an effective manner, diabetes can be managed. In the DSME plan, content related to coping and normalizing diabetes is important. This may be the perfect time to share stories of successfully living with diabetes.

Specific Instructional Strategies

Each individual has character traits, personality styles, and learning preferences that can affect the overall education intervention. Acknowledging that these differences exist is an important first step by the diabetes educator toward adapting and adjusting teaching styles.

Instructional strategies used in a DSME encounter reflect the needs, skills, learning style, and preferences of the person with diabetes. Though a number of instructional methodologies are available to meet the needs of different learners, most individuals learn best when they are actively engaged (eg, through discussion groups, practice, and teaching others) rather than passively involved in learning (eg, listening to a lecture).[49] Choosing the appropriate method of instruction is a critical determinant of effective education. While teaching and learning can occur informally, in person or remotely via phone or computer, more formal education requires planning to maximize success. Identification of content and skills to be learned, access to audiovisual materials, class size and composition, and time and available resources should all be considered when developing a teaching plan. Several teaching strategies can be considered, individually or collectively, to deliver information depending on the education needed for the expected outcome (see Table 2.8).

No single format is conducive for teaching all components of diabetes self-management to all persons with diabetes. Using a combination of various media, tools, and materials can enhance integration of the information and skills needed to effectively self-manage diabetes. Creativity and ongoing assessment of the methods used to impart information to the learner will prevent monotonous delivery of outdated or irrelevant content—and make the education

TABLE 2.8   Teaching Strategies and the Learning Experience

Teaching Format	*Goal*	*Learner's Experience*	*Attributes*	*Limitations*
Lecture	Present information	Passive—listens	Easy to implement and control content	Educator-centric; limited applicability of information to the individual
Discussion	Seek and acquire information	Active—asks questions, shares information and experiences	Patient-centric; active participation and learning; ability to learn from others	Less control over content and time; agenda may be influenced by outspoken few
Demonstration	Teach psychomotor or social skills	Active—if return demonstration included	Allows learner to observe, perform, and be evaluated	Takes more time; easier to do in small groups or one-to-one
Print materials	Provide and/or reinforce information	Passive—self-initiated	Augments in-person education and provides enduring resource	Does not replace in-person education; effectiveness influenced by congruence between materials and individual characteristics (literacy, language, readability, etc)
Audiovisual aids	Enhance presentation of information	Passive and active learning	Provides variety in presentation of information; assists those who are visual learners; adaptable to audience size and composition	Can decrease integration of information if used alone; complexity/simplicity needs to be balanced and targeted to audience
Computer-based or Web-based	Enhance self-directed education	Active learning—information resource with interactive potential	Provides opportunity for self-directed learning and problem-solving; 24-hour accessibility	Comfort with technology varies by age, socioeconomic status, and prior comfort and/or experience; questionable credibility and authority of some Web sites
Role-playing	Practice, express, explore, discuss, share	Active learning—facilitates sharing of information and exploration of what-if situations	Useful in individual or group setting	Requires cohesiveness of participants and instructor with good interpersonal skills; not palatable to some learners
Games	Enhance learning	Active learning—interactive	Can make learning more enjoyable or comfortable	Can detract from learning if not well planned or executed or if incongruent with content being taught
Case study or stories	Explore, discuss, share	Active, applied learning and problem solving	Ability to learn from others and apply concepts to "real life" experience; taps into the human preference for stories	Larger concepts may be lost in details of case studies; studies may have extraneous material
Conversation maps	Focus on health information most relevant to them	Active learning—interactive	Useful in individual or group settings; tool is colorful and engaging	Requires a skilled educator comfortable with content and with good interpersonal skills to keep the group engaged

(continued)

TABLE 2.8   Teaching Strategies and the Learning Experience (continued)

Teaching Format	Goal	Learner's Experience	Attributes	Limitations
Blended learning	Combination of a form of electronic learning and human interaction	Combination of the learning experiences listed above (computers, lecture, discussion)	Engages learners with a variety of learning styles; useful when resources or educators are limited	Requires a skilled educator comfortable with providing content in multiple technologies; lack of access to the technologies for both the patient and the educator

Source: Adapted from RM Anderson, "Applied Principles of Teaching and Learning," in MJ Franz, ed, *A Core Curriculum for Diabetes Education: Diabetes Education and Program Management*, 4th ed (Chicago: American Association of Diabetes Educators, 2001), 9-11.

experience more rewarding for the teacher and the learner. In selecting effective teaching strategies, it is critical for the educator to consider health literacy and culture.

Health Literacy

Health information can be very confusing, and the amount of information needed to effectively self-manage diabetes can be overwhelming. Health literacy is defined as the ability to read, understand, and act on health information.[50] Because it includes the word "literacy," people often assume it is concerned only with being unable to read. It includes the ability to not only read but also process numbers and navigate the healthcare system. The inability to understand and act on the health information can have a negative impact on health outcomes. Health information can be misunderstood for a number of reasons, including literacy, disability, age, language, culture, and emotion.[51] Though everyone is at risk for low health literacy, limited literacy skills are the strongest predictor of health status—stronger than age, income, employment status, education level, and racial or ethnic group.[52] There are several screening tools available for assessing health literacy. The Newest Vital Sign, a new screening tool based on a nutrition label from an ice cream container, can be administered in as little as 3 minutes. The healthcare provider asks the patient 6 questions about the nutrition label in order to assess the patient's health literacy level.[50] Understanding a patient's health literacy is useful when developing the plan for DSME, and clearly communicating the health information is imperative to the success of the intervention. The words used to deliver the message, give directions,

and present materials are all important. Identifying and incorporating health literacy into planning and implementation increases the possibility of influencing the person's actions and decisions. Osborne describes a working definition of health literacy as a shared responsibility in which patients and providers must communicate in ways the other can understand.[52]

When planning DSME, it is important to consider the literacy level of the patient. In addition, the readability, appropriate adaptation, culture, personal relevance, and language should all be reviewed. A common misconception is that translation of educational materials from English to another language is sufficient for educating non-English-speaking individuals. Direct translation of words without an appreciation of the context or interpretation can create confusion. Practical guidelines to consider when choosing or creating educational materials include the following[53]:

- ◆ Use active voice; write the way you talk.
- ◆ Use short, simple sentences and common words.
- ◆ Give examples or tell a story to explain difficult words or concepts.
- ◆ Include the opportunity for interaction and informational review.

A checklist for evaluating handouts is found in Table 2.9.

Plan to use educational materials that have personal relevance. Does the material motivate readers and encourage them to take action? When creating materials, it is not adequate to rely strictly on the reading grade-level formulas included in word processing programs. These often look at the length

TABLE 2.9 Checklist for Evaluating Handouts	Yes	No
The purpose of the handout is clear		
Key messages are included		
Content is consistent with the lesson or curriculum		
Font is readable for the intended audience		
White space is used effectively so handout is uncluttered		
Design strategies make important text stand out		
Information is organized (tables labeled, pages numbered)		
Spelling and grammar are correct		
Pictures/graphics are relevant and realistic		
There is no commercial bias		
Content and graphics are culturally respectful		

In Practice Tip: Assess, Don't Assume

Consider the following example: You are covering the inpatient diabetes service and are scheduled to meet with a 45-year-old man to provide basic diabetes education before discharge. You go armed with all the pamphlets and handouts you can find, knowing that your time with him is limited to 45 minutes. Early in the conversation, he shares that he "doesn't read much." However, his medical record indicated he has a very successful business, and thus you expect he will be able to understand the new information in the written materials with minimal difficulty. He must be literate; after all, he runs a successful business. Is your assumption accurate? Could it be that he is successful in business because he has surrounded himself with individuals who provide oral reports? While literacy is one stepping stone to success, it is not the only one.

of sentences and the number of syllables in words. Though they provide a start, other factors that are not assessed by these programs are important as well. Just because educational material is statistically readable doesn't mean it can be understood. Feedback from your patients may be the best judge of readability.[52]

Most individuals are able to learn despite their literacy level, so long as the method of instruction is designed to recognize and compensate for the literacy deficits.[53] Within health care, there is a mismatch between the general literacy level and the literacy demands of healthcare instructions; this disparity impacts healthcare costs. Those with lower levels of literacy are more apt to put off preventive care measures or delay seeking medical assistance than those with high literacy levels, contributing to higher healthcare costs.[54] The diabetes educator incorporates aspects of assessing health literacy into individual and group plans. Communicate in whatever way works, applying the principles of "plain language" to all forms of communication. Remember, the diabetes educator's role as a health communicator is to translate difficult health information into words and concepts that patients and their support persons can understand and use in self-management.[52]

Individual's Cultural, Lifestyle, and Health Beliefs

In addition to literacy, the educator considers cultural factors when developing the DSME plan. Each individual comes for DSME with a unique set of experiences. These experiences affect the individual's ability to learn and level of readiness to change behaviors. The individual's cultural, lifestyle, and health beliefs may be very different from those familiar to the health educator, and this needs to be acknowledged, honored, and respected. The impact of the steadily increasing diversity in the United States means that the diabetes educator must learn to manage differences in communication styles, attitudes, expectations, beliefs, and world views. Different approaches must be taken to remove barriers created by racial, ethnic, cultural, and linguistic differences. A large body of research underscores the existence of disparities in health care. The literature shows that US racial and ethnic minorities are less likely to receive routine medical procedures and more likely to experience a lower quality of health services compared with their counterparts in the white population. In addition, the Office of Minority Health and Health Disparities has identified other vulnerable populations, including those defined by socioeconomic status, geography, gender, age, and disability.[49] Addressing health disparities is a core goal of the National Diabetes Education Program (NDEP).[55] In response to this need, the NDEP and its minority work groups have developed and adapted materials to reach audiences at highest risk for developing diabetes and with the highest prevalence of the disease. These materials address cultural issues like food choices and health literacy needs and can be accessed from the NDEP.[4] See Table 2.10 for more on the levels of cultural

TABLE 2.10 Cultural Competence in the Delivery of Healthcare Services: Foundation of the Practice Model	
Level	*Strategies to Promote the Competency*
Cultural awareness	Recognize personal prejudices and biases toward other cultures
	Understand personal cultural/ethnic background
Cultural humility	Commit to ongoing self-evaluation and self-critique
	Be willing to address power imbalances in patient-provider relationship
	Develop mutually beneficial partnerships with communities/organizations on behalf of defined populations
Cultural knowledge	Develop an education foundation that incorporates various world views of different cultures
	Identify and integrate knowledge regarding biological variations, disease and health conditions, and variations in drug metabolism
Cultural skill	Collect culturally relevant data regarding the individual's presenting problem and health history
	Conduct culturally based physical assessments in a culturally sensitive manner
Cultural desire	Commit to engage in the process of cultural competence
	Demonstrate compassion, authenticity, humility, openness, availability, and flexibility
	Provide care, regardless of conflict

Source: Adapted from J Campinha-Bacote, "The process of cultural competence in the delivery of healthcare services: a model of care," *J Transcult Nurs* 13 (2002): 181-4.

competence and how an educator can further develop those competencies.

Knowledge Builder: Health Disparities Linked to Ethnicity and Socioeconomic Factors

One example of health disparity tied to ethnicity is an analysis of data from the 2001 Behavioral Risk Factor Surveillance System. This demonstrated that frequency distributions of selected diabetes management variables were widely variant across levels of race/ethnicity. Overall, those in the Hispanic population were significantly less likely to have positive self-management behaviors.[56] A qualitative study on knowledge and perceptions of diabetes in an Appalachian region observed that socioeconomic factors appear to be major influences on health-related decision making. Also noted was that what is sometimes labeled as "nonadherent behavior is often a common-sense adaptation for the patient from within his or her belief framework, cultural context, and outside influences" (p. 5).[57]

A culturally sensitive and informed healthcare professional understands and addresses the cultural beliefs and myths that may influence the patient's ability and willingness to follow directions, ask questions, or seek additional information. When the diabetes educator understands the cultural factors and beliefs that can contribute to these differences, a plan that reflects the needs of the individual can be developed and effective interventions can be designed.

Storytelling as a Teaching Strategy   One way to overcome some of the challenges of literacy and culture is to use stories. Stories address a variety of learning styles and engage the individual at both cognitive and emotional levels. They create bonds, connections, and relationships between the educator and the learner.[58] Stories can help patients make sense of their own journey with chronic disease.[59] Patients are already sharing stories informally through social media[60] and support groups. Storytelling can also be incorporated into the DSME plan. Most stories are a hero's quest: encountering an obstacle and overcoming the challenge. A simple outline for constructing an engaging story with a message includes the following[58]:

- ◆ Set the scene: Provide some background detail.
- ◆ Introduce the characters: Create a visual picture of the people involved in the story. What are their personalities, needs, and desires? Do you want the characters to share some of the characteristics of your learners?
- ◆ Begin the journey.
- ◆ Encounter the obstacle.
- ◆ Overcome the obstacle: Who helped in the journey?
- ◆ Resolve the story and reinforce the key message.
- ◆ Debrief the story and its meaning: Has this ever happened to you? What did you do?

Teaching Across the Lifespan

When developing and implementing the diabetes education plan, it is important to consider how people learn at different stages of life. It is important that principles of learning be considered when identifying the individual's motivation to learn, in designing the curriculum to be taught, and in creating the learning environment.

Children and Adolescents

Readiness to learn in childhood changes considerably with age and maturation. A wide array of caregivers, including parents, siblings, grandparents, other family members, the primary care provider, school personnel, coaches, and babysitters, are included as part of the healthcare team, and considerable planning must occur for all to be included in the education process at relevant times. When educating the parents of a newly diagnosed child with type 1 diabetes, it is important to remember that their ability to learn may be impacted by fear of the diagnosis. They must be reassessed regularly, along with the child, and the assessment information incorporated into the planning and implementation of DSME. In addition to imparting facts and teaching practical skills, diabetes education promotes desirable health beliefs and attitudes in the young person. This is often best accomplished in a setting where age-appropriate peer education can occur, such as in summer camps or on moderated Web site discussion boards. It is

important that the child be included in education that is age appropriate. A recommended approach for a child with diabetes is for the child and the parent to attend several single-topic-focused sessions scheduled for no longer than 30 minutes. This will also offer the opportunity for reinforcement, which is important in successful achievement of mutually defined self-management goals.[61]

Young children often learn best by example and simple explanation using words they are familiar with and incorporating play when possible. It is also important that at the appropriate stage in development, self-management responsibility begins to shift from the parent or caregiver to the individual with diabetes. This must be considered on an individual basis and will be guided by the child's developmental phase, intellect, ability, and willingness to assume responsibility. Understanding what the child is managing in his or her routine life can serve as a guide for encouraging increasing independence in diabetes management.[62,63]

Adults

In developing the plan for the adult learner, it is important to incorporate principles of learning.[64] These include the following:

- ◆ Adults are self-directed. They will decide for themselves what is important to be learned. The educator can only suggest and guide.
- ◆ Adults are task- or problem-oriented learners. The adult doesn't like to just sit back and listen. They prefer practical activities such as discussion, hands-on work, or a project related to a concept. Examples of this include interpreting a blood glucose log to identify patterns or using food models to build a plate with the appropriate amount of carbohydrates.
- ◆ Adults bring experience to the learning situation. This can be a rich resource for themselves and for others. This experience can be used effectively by connecting it to new learning.
- ◆ Adults are more likely to learn when learning has meaning for who they are and their social roles and responsibilities. This is sometimes described as WIIFM (What's in it for me). An adult's most teachable moment is when they believe they need to learn something new or different.[64]

Older Adults

There are special considerations when developing the individualized DSME plan for older adults. The plan incorporates assessment information related to the patient's functional, cognitive, and psychosocial status, recognizing that these change over time.[64] It is important to consider comorbidities and the impact of coexisting conditions on the functional capacity of the individual. Quality of life and life expectancy must be considered when prioritizing the topics and content for the older adult. Older adults may require more time to assimilate the information and may benefit from a slower-paced education session. It may be necessary to involve a care partner in DSME if the patient is unable to assume full responsibility for his or her self-care.[65]

Generational Differences in Learning

For the first time, adults in the United States come from 4 generations: veterans (born before 1946), baby boomers (born between 1946 and 1964), generation X (born between 1965 and 1980), and generation Y or millennials (born between 1981 and 1995). Imagine the world in which each generation was raised. The impact of the world and the early school experiences contribute to how each generation now approaches education and learning[66] (see Table 2.11).

Whether planning for group or individual education sessions, consider age as well as the individual's stage of life, as each presents unique issues and needs. Regardless of age or stage of life, the education process must accomplish the following:

⬥ Include information that is viewed as important to the individual
⬥ Recognize the individual's experiences and integrate them into the learning process
⬥ Foster the development of problem-solving skills
⬥ Promote active participation in one's self-care

The DSME/S Plan Is Dynamic

In addition to the recognition that each plan must be individualized is that the plan is fluid and must be adjusted and updated to reflect the changing needs of the patient. This indicates the need for ongoing assessment and evaluation of the plan's effectiveness.

The DSME/S Process Is Lifelong

Standard 8 of the National Standards for DSME and Support includes a collaboratively developed follow-up plan for ongoing DSMS.[4] It is recognized that to sustain behavior change at the level necessary to manage diabetes, most patients need ongoing self-management support. Diabetes self-management support is a process of receiving education and motivation beyond the visits with the patient's healthcare providers. The process of DSMS planning can begin within the framework of the assessment and may include discussion of complementary education experiences while in the DSME program or to start upon completion. The DSMS may occur within the DSME program, but a number of opportunities exist outside. Strategies may include support groups; disease management, case management, or care coordination programs; media or online support; medical nutrition therapy (MNT); and programs utilizing community health workers who work under the guidance of the diabetes educator.[6] Community initiatives can include health fairs, breakfast clubs, and social events for patients and their families promoting self-management opportunities. Very important is that follow-up and support provide individuals with choices that meet their individual needs and are readily available and convenient. Personal connection or consistent contact with someone who knows them is also important.[67]

Summary for Planning

Planning is the step in the DSME/S process that involves the selection of specific interventions and goals that are based on a multifaceted assessment of the individual. Planning requires collaboration among the person with diabetes, their family members (as appropriate), the diabetes educator, the referring provider, and other members of the healthcare team to develop a mutually agreed-upon individualized, realistic, and effective plan for DSME/S. The next step in the process is implementing the plan.

Implementation

The fourth step of the DSME process is implementation of the agreed-upon plan. Implementation involves interfacing with the patient and various care providers and linking the patient to community and professional resources and services. According to *The AADE Guidelines for the Practice of Diabetes Self-Management Education and Training*, implementation involves

TABLE 2.11 Generational Differences				
	Veterans (born before 1946)	*Baby Boomers (born between 1946 and 1964)*	*Generation X (born between 1965 and 1980)*	*Generation Y or Millennials (born between 1981 and 1995)*
World events	WWII Great Depression	Vietnam Sexual revolution	Gulf War Fall of Berlin Wall Challenger disaster End of Cold War High divorce rates AIDS	Terrorism: local and global 9/11
Technology	Radio Phones	Television Compact discs Handheld calculator Transistor radio Typewriter	Early computers	World Wide Web Cell phones Computers
Education	Rote memorization Classroom Lectures	Classroom Participation in class	Games Role playing PowerPoint® presentations Educational videos and TV	Wikis Blogs Social media On demand
Implications for diabetes education	Expect respect Formal relationship (Mr., Mrs.) Look to authority Prefer individual work, not groups	Want to be part of the solution Less impressed with authority figures	More informal Technologically able with devices Want relevant information delivered quickly	Sharing information is the norm Multitasking Social learning
Teaching techniques	Traditional approaches (lecture, reading) Stories and sharing experiences Use large font size	Visual tools Interactive May not like role playing	Expect slides or video Group activities Use bullet points Provide ample feedback	Internet sources Smartphone apps Group work

Source: Adapted from Baker College, *Teaching Across Generations*, 2004 (cited 2013 Jun 30), on the Internet at: http://www.mcc.edu/pdf/pdo/teaching_across_gen.pdf.

recommendation and execution of the plan; ensuring that the patient has the knowledge, skills, and resources necessary to follow through on the plan; and identification and assistance with removal of barriers identified throughout the process.[6]

The DSME Team

One question that often arises is who should deliver DSME to the person with diabetes. Although reports on the effectiveness of different disciplines are mixed, registered nurses, registered dietitians, and registered pharmacists most commonly make up the DSME team.[6] Standard 5 of the National Standards for DSME states that at least one of the instructors will be from one of these disciplines. Other health professionals (eg, behaviorist, exercise physiologist, and physicians) may be included as well.[4] The AADE supports the role of the community or lay health worker serving as a bridge between the healthcare system and the patients.[6]

Standards of Practice

Measurement criteria for implementation identified in The Scope of Practice, Standards of Practice, and Standards of Professional Performance for Diabetes Educators include the following[7]:

◆ Provides an accessible, safe, and appropriate environment for DSME

◆ Uses teaching materials appropriate to the learner's age, culture, learning style, and abilities

◆ Structures DSME to progress from basic safety and survival skills to advanced information for daily self-management and improved outcomes

◆ Addresses basic diabetes self-management skills, including safe medication use, meal planning, self-monitoring of blood glucose, and recognizing when and how to access professional services

◆ Provides increasingly advanced DSME, based on the client's needs and goals, on topics including preventing and managing chronic complications, psychosocial adjustment, developing problem-solving skills, managing physical activity, adjusting treatment regimens (including insulin and oral diabetes medications), stress management, travel situations, and pattern management

◆ Provides opportunities for peer support

◆ Integrates the DSME plan into the overall plan of care

◆ Shares the diabetes educational plan and progress with referring providers

◆ Establishes means for follow-up and continuity of DSME, including referrals to other providers

◆ May provide a format of group education for DSME, if desired, to foster the support, encouragement, and empowerment of clients; group education can lead to behavior change as participants share ideas and experiences

Curriculum Content

Standard 6 of the National Standards for DSME and Support addresses the importance of having a written curriculum with measurable learning goals.[4] A curriculum meeting the patient's needs will be maintained and updated to reflect current evidence and practice guidelines. Programs recognized by the Centers for Medicare and Medicaid Services (CMS), credentialed organizations (eg, the AADE Diabetes Education Accreditation Program [DEAP]), and the ADA (American Diabetes Association) Education Recognition Program (ERP) are advised to have a written set of lesson plans (curriculum) to guide instructors for information consistency.

Assessed needs of the individuals will determine the content to be provided. The content of the curriculum will include the principles and concepts of the AADE7 Self-Care Behavior™ framework. In addition, content about the diabetes disease process will be included. To increase the likelihood of success, the curriculum and educational materials used should take into account previously discussed concepts like health literacy, cultural beliefs and attitudes, and practices of the target population. The curriculum will use primarily interactive, collaborative, skill-based training methods.[4]

Mensing and Norris[68] suggest that new educators may find it useful to adapt an existing commercial curriculum to meet the standards, while more experienced educators may develop their own, focusing on unique delivery methods, creative alternatives, and a more interactive delivery style.

Strategies for Implementing DSME

A frequently asked question when the Diabetes Control and Complications Trial (DCCT) ended was, "How was it done?" Specifically, healthcare professionals and people with diabetes were curious: What strategy was used to treat the intensive treatment group that resulted in achievement of the desired outcome? The DCCT illustrated the need for patient education, the importance of multidisciplinary team care, the value of incorporating regimens that were most consistent with the individual's lifestyle, and the importance of ongoing support. Various education strategies and tactics that recognized and capitalized on the individual's needs, attributes, and limitations were used. However, no universal strategy or education approach could be identified. So, what does this tell us about how to best educate people with diabetes? If there is no "right" way to do it, what factors should be considered to improve effectiveness?[48]

Compliance and Empowerment Approaches to Education

While the compliance and empowerment approaches to education have specific attributes and limitations, they are not mutually exclusive, nor is one approach ideal for all individuals throughout the learning process. Consider the person recently diagnosed with diabetes. He will require basic information and instruction to prevent hospitalization and ensure safety. Adjusting insulin doses for eating out may not be relevant to him at this time. However, learning how and why he got diabetes, what has gone wrong in his body, how and when to take medication or give an injection, and why medication is needed every day are all vital pieces of information during these early weeks. Conversely, the individual who has had diabetes for several years may gain more from an interactive session about carbohydrate counting that allows opportunities to ask about adjustments that would be needed to cover her favorite foods or includes practice on making healthy choices at her favorite restaurant. Table 2.12 highlights distinct characteristics of the compliance and empowerment approaches to patient education.

The educator considers the order or sequence in which topics are to be presented. Are you planning to teach about diabetes the way you, as a healthcare professional, were taught, beginning with definitions, basics of diagnosis, pathophysiology, and treatment? Are psychosocial issues pushed to the very end? Consider switching the order around. In general, individuals are not interested in diabetes as an academic subject but in how it affects them in their day-to-day life. Funnell and Anderson have long described an empowerment model, making the experiences of the person with diabetes the basis for the curriculum.[69] Discussing the nature of a self-managed disease such as diabetes at the beginning of an education program helps participants

TABLE 2.12 Approaches to Patient Education		
	Compliance Approach	*Empowerment Approach*
Assumptions	Healthcare professionals are the experts	Patients are capable of making complex decisions
	Patients comply with recommendations	Patients have the right and responsibility to manage their diabetes
	Patient must follow instructions for success	Healthcare professionals provide guidance and support
Strategies	Healthcare professional identifies important aspects of care and provides education	Basic understanding of disease and management tools needed
	Instructions are directive and approach is often uniform over time	Healthcare professional provides guidance regarding specific aspects of management, directed by the patient
Goal	Patient complies with treatment recommendations	Recommendations often replace standardized instructions
		Education focuses on self-care, self-management, and coping skills
		Patient assumes primary responsibility for daily decision-making
Usefulness of approach to patient	Early in disease process, beyond survival skills	After individual has a good understanding of diabetes survival skills
	If unable to assume greater responsibility for personal healthcare decisions	If willing to actively participate in care decisions
	If unable to focus on specifics of self-care due to other life issues	If able to make informed decisions and recognize when to seek assistance

Source: Adapted from RM Anderson, "Applied Principles of Teaching and Learning," in MJ Franz, ed, *A Core Curriculum for Diabetes Education: Diabetes Education and Program Management,* 4th ed (Chicago: American Association of Diabetes Educators, 2001), 9-11.

understand why the interaction with the group and information presented are so important. Participants also then see that the role of the healthcare professional is to be a source of expertise, support, and inspiration rather than a teacher or caregiver. This approach recognizes that the person living with diabetes has as important a contribution to make to the session as the diabetes educator. This view redefines the purpose of diabetes education, taking it from providing information so individuals will know why their behaviors need to change to providing information so individuals can make informed decisions about their behaviors. This empowerment-based approach for DSME has also demonstrated effectiveness in marginalized populations.[70]

Problem-Based Learning

One challenge to education or training is whether the learner ever transfers the knowledge or skill to practice. Another issue is how to teach a general concept yet keep it meaningful for each learner in the group. Problem-based or problem-focused learning is a strategy to address these concerns. In problem-based learning (PBL), the educator relies on case studies, stories, and what-if questions. Problem-based learning has been effective in diverse populations.[71,72] The Skill Builder provides tips for integrating PBL into diabetes education sessions.

Skill Builder: Using PBL

It is quite easy to incorporate PBL techniques into diabetes education sessions. Following these steps will integrate the problem-solving aspects of PBL[72]:

- ◆ Invite a learner to share a problem or concern he or she is experiencing.
- ◆ As a group, generate solutions to the problem.
- ◆ Explore how easy or hard it would be to implement the possible solutions.
- ◆ Discuss how relevant the problem is for each learner.
- ◆ Create action plans based on the discussion.

Individual versus Group

Diabetes self-management education may be conducted in either group or individual counseling settings.

Mensing and Norris describe how the process of group education has evolved over time.[68] Not long ago, diabetes group education might have been described as a set of didactic classes, presented lecture style, where the teacher would impart knowledge. Now, group education meetings are more interactive sessions or gatherings where the facilitator elicits discussion based on the participants' interests and needs. The shift to group education puts more responsibility on the patient to complete the assessment and the goal-setting activities with assistance and review by the educator.

Not only is group education the method required in most instances for Medicare reimbursement, the group setting has been found to be effective from both a clinical and cost perspective.[73] One study comparing individual versus group insulin instruction found group education offered a greater level of treatment satisfaction at 1 year with similar glycemic control (Eskerine as cited in Mensing and Norris, 2003[68]). While many studies have demonstrated that group classes improve metabolic and behavioral measures,[74] other studies have found that individual classes are superior in achieving these goals.[75] Therefore, the educator must accurately determine which approach will best match the needs, preferences, and resources of the individual.

In Practice Tip: Exceptions to Medicare Requirement

Following are exceptions to the Medicare regulation requiring group instruction:

- ◆ No group session is available within 2 months of the date the education is ordered.
- ◆ The individual has severe vision, language, or hearing limitations.
- ◆ Other conditions are identified by the treating physician or nonphysician practitioner.
- ◆ If the education assessment indicates that individual instruction would better meet a person's needs, the diabetes educator should let the referring physician know this promptly so that the referring provider can document this request.

Since rules and regulations change, check CMS for the most current information.

Managing Education Session Challenges

As important as it is to have a plan, having a backup plan is also important. Diabetes educators are flexible and spontaneous, and maintain a calm ride even through what may feel like stormy seas. Listed below are a couple of scenarios that diabetes educators may face from time to time, with suggestions for how to quickly make the best of the situation.[48]

A Group of One?

You have spent time preparing for class. You have content maps, slides, and handouts and are ready for a 1-hour session, but when you arrive at the classroom, only 1 person is there. You are tempted to deliver the "class" you are accustomed to giving each week. Do not! Instead of delivering the class you had planned, treat the session as one-to-one counseling. Determine exactly what the person's needs are and individualize your messages to meet those needs directly. Although the person will not have the benefit of the group interaction, he or she will benefit from much more personal attention.

Attendance Exceeds Expectation

You enter the classroom expecting to encounter 8 individuals and instead you find 15. Acknowledging your surprise with the bigger group is fine, but avoid showing that you feel hassled or annoyed. Ask the group to assist you in making a few adjustments so that everyone with diabetes can be best accommodated. For example, guests who have accompanied class participants can be asked to sit in the outer circle behind their partners to give them priority at the table or inner circle. Ask participants to share materials and say that you will arrange to get everyone a set later. Use tools from effective group process such as setting the ground rules for the session. Smile. Show a sense of humor, and all will be fine.

Technical Difficulties

Access to technology means an increased chance for equipment failure. Are you prepared if the projector does not work or your handouts do not get delivered from the copy center? Unless you have unlimited financial resources, you do not need two of everything "just in case." Instead, think about how you might get by on your own. If you are accustomed to using overheads or slides, have a handout set for yourself so you can at least use them as prompts to know what topic comes next. Use a flipchart or white board on which to write key points that may need emphasis. In fact, teach some classes without any audiovisual aids from time to time. Avoid overreliance on technology and ensure room for individualization and flexibility based on group needs.

Teaching Materials and Audiovisual Materials

Teaching materials must be available to support the curriculum. Patients often find these materials very useful in their ongoing self-management and behavior-change efforts. The materials used should take into consideration previously discussed issues like health literacy and culture, attitudes, and health beliefs.

Audiovisuals such as PowerPoint® slides, electronic presentations, or videos are available alternatives. They may help support the educator in ensuring completeness of delivery of content. On the other hand, media can get in the way of learning. Software such as PowerPoint® packages an amazing array of graphical elements to enhance the visual appeal of slides. Dozens of fonts, animation options, and color palettes are available to the educator. It is easy to confuse attraction with education. Colorful slides with moving parts often overshadow the key message of the slide. This is one area where simpler truly is better (see Knowledge Builder for tips on cognitive overload).

Knowledge Builder: Cognitive Overload

Cognitive science reminds us that the human brain has 2 channels for taking information into working memory: an auditory channel and a visual channel.[76,77] Distractions from the visual channel (such as animated slides) can hinder the impact of information entering through the auditory channel. This is particularly true if the messages are incongruent. For instance, if the educator is discussing hypoglycemia and the slide has titles twirling and fireworks exploding, the learner's brain will expend unnecessary (and precious) cognitive energy trying to make sense of the messages. When an individual finds complex, animated, overly designed presentations distracting, cognitive overload is at work.

What all this means for the educator is important:

- Keep your messages simple.
- Use media which best deliver the message in a clean and clear way.
- When tapping both cognitive channels, keep the message and media congruent.
- Avoid distractions when delivering a message.
- Just because a media tool *can* do something doesn't mean the educator *should* use it.
- Be prepared for technology failures (eg, power failures, device malfunctions) with a low-tech alternative (eg, handouts, whiteboards, flipcharts, drawings).

Educational materials from pharmaceutical companies and even government programs can be a huge boon to education programs with limited budgets. That is the good news—these materials are plentiful, very often Web based, and easily accessible. The challenge is when the materials are not consistent with the program's curriculum. Nuances in terms and procedures can be confusing to patients. Does the program use "blood glucose checks" where the materials use "blood sugar tests"? Other differences may be more philosophical. Does the program advocate the use of alcohol to clean the skin before injection, whereas the pamphlet eliminates this step? Materials used from sources outside the education program must be carefully scrutinized with these goals:

- Decrease as much inconsistency as possible.
- Ensure readability and language are appropriate for the program's target audience.
- Ensure ethnicity and culture portrayed in the materials are acceptable to the target audience.

Consider creating your own materials when feasible. Creating your own educational materials is much like cooking your own meal versus buying a frozen dinner. You will know what went into the final product.

Applying Learning Theory

Malcolm Knowles,[64] often cited as the "father of adult learning theory," wrote, "The richest resources for learning reside in the adult learners themselves.

Hence, the greater emphasis in adult education on experiential techniques—techniques that tap into the experience of the learners, such as group discussion, simulation exercises, problem-solving activities, case method, and laboratory methods—over transmittal techniques" (p. 59). Adult learners come with a history, with experiences, with a need to know. These elements drive their readiness to learn.

Other learning theories such as Transformational Learning reinforce the importance of life experience as well as critical reflection on learning outcomes.[78] Effective educators tap into their patients' experiences and encourage their patients' self-reflection by keeping them involved in the learning. The following Skill Builder offers some examples of interactive learning strategies.

Skill Builder: Making Learning Active

Learning is most effective when the person is involved in making the content his or her own. The educator can use several strategies to make content informative and the learning interactive.

Topic menu: Create a list of topics (like a menu) for the class to choose from. Start with the first topic chosen and then move to another topic. You might keep all the topics within a certain category.

Interactive handouts: Create handouts that require filling in the blanks.

Each one teach one: Have partners teach each other the important concepts or a specific subject they have just learned.

Matching activities: Using flashcards, have participants match a concept to a definition, or a symptom to a condition, or a treatment to a condition.

Skill sequence: Make and print photos of the key steps in a particular skill. Mix up the photos and ask learners to put the photos in the correct order of the steps in the skill.

Create a meal: Using photos, food models, or information from nutrition Web sites, ask learners to create a meal of 30 g (or any number) of carbohydrate.

Applying Cognitive Science

Learning theory can support the curriculum and the type of teaching tools used. So can cognitive science. Part of the role of the diabetes educator is to build expertise in persons with diabetes. While experts have developed extensive knowledge, they are also able to organize information, remember details, and solve problems.[79] This means that diabetes education should incorporate plenty of opportunity to learn new information, remember and retrieve that information, and apply that knowledge in practical ways to solve problems.

Memory becomes an important cognitive concept for educators to understand. The human brain takes in information through sensory pathways. While all experiences are registered in the brain, many are not remembered. Memory depends on the meaning the experience has for the individual. If a person is taking oral medications, for instance, will a class on insulin therapy be remembered? Memories become linked to emotions as well. What do you remember of your first kiss, for example? Patients will often remember what their healthcare team said on the day of diagnosis.

Helping learning to stick is all about creating enduring memory. Here are some practical ways to help patients remember content[80]:

- Use a variety of approaches which engage the senses. Cooking classes are a great way to teach nutrition concepts.
- Encourage discussion about the emotional impact of the new information being presented.
- Repeat important concepts in varied ways. Repetition is a key way that the brain settles new information into long-term memory.
- Recognize that memory is enhanced when blood glucose levels are normal.
- Because content at the beginning and the end of a session is remembered best, keep sessions of content short, with adequate breaks, so there are many beginnings and endings.
- Ask patients to summarize what they have learned. For example, "What are the 3 things you will probably remember about today's session?" "What are 2 things that you still wonder about?"

- Allow patients to make mistakes and problem solve when they are learning a new skill. Balance self-discovery with careful coaching to avoid too much frustration (a memory killer).

Teaching Environment

Controlling and modifying the learning environment is another way to promote memory. Careful consideration of the teaching environment is a component of an educator's ability to effectively lead a group or individual education session.[48] In a group, when possible, create a room arrangement that encourages interaction and discussion. Alternatives to traditional classroom style should be considered. Will the educator be sitting in a circle with the class, standing in the front, or moving around, or will it be a blend of all three? Generally, a combination works best for most kinds of groups. In individual education sessions, patients often discuss very personal healthcare matters that can become emotional. The interaction can be more difficult in a setting that feels cold and impersonal or lacks adequate privacy. Whether providing a group or individual intervention, consider the lighting, color, sound, movement, artwork, and clutter; also make sure that the facilities are accessible for patients with disabilities.[40] The environment should be inviting and elicit curiosity while minimizing distractions.

Create an inviting space by posting a welcome message on the door or as the first slide. Elicit curiosity by posting your key message with some of the words missing. For example, the message might state: "The best way to lose weight is . . ." Patients will wonder what is missing and will stay engaged as they listen for the message to be completed. When teaching a class on foot care, place paper cutouts of footprints around the room, perhaps ending at a key message posted. Enlist the whole environment as a teaching tool.

The environment should support your teaching. Plan ahead so that handouts and materials to be distributed are well organized for easy referencing and accessibility. Be prepared. Before leading a group, you might consider practicing delivering a mini-presentation to colleagues to confirm that the use of audiovisual aids, lighting, sound, your voice projection, and other elements all work well in a particular room. Patient safety is a priority. Have supplies available to treat emergencies such as a hypoglycemic reaction.

Disabilities

The Standards of Care[4] suggest that it is incumbent on the provider to ensure that DSME is available for all people with diabetes. Diabetes educators can play a key role in the diabetes care of individuals with disabilities and diabetes by providing DSME in a way that enables them to achieve similar behavioral change goals as persons with no current disability.[62] Disabilities do not necessarily preclude effective diabetes self-management.

People who have disabilities and diabetes are usually capable of caring for themselves when they are provided with appropriate adaptive DSME tools and techniques. Physical factors identified in the assessment—mobility, visual acuity, hearing, manual dexterity, alertness, attention span, ability to concentrate, mental health status (including depression), and other special needs or limitations, either physical or psychological—must be considered when implementing DSME. The process and the content must be both accessible and meaningful for the patient with disabilities. The AADE supports application of universal design to DSME programs in general and to consumer medical products.[81]

In Practice Tip: Definition of Universal Design

The design of products, environments, and services to be effectively and efficiently used by persons with a wide range of abilities to the greatest extent possible, without adaptation or specialized design.[81]

In 1990, the Americans with Disabilities Act (ADA) was enacted to offer protection to those with disabilities in the workplace, healthcare setting, and general community.[82] Specifically, the act prohibits discrimination against those with disabilities and ensures they are afforded the same opportunities related to employment, services, commercial and public facilities, and transportation as those without disabilities. This act further defines the rights of those with disabilities:

- ◆ A right to reasonable accommodations to make goods, services, and facilities available
- ◆ Access to the goods, services, facilities, accommodations, privileges, and advantages available to those without disabilities, provided this is appropriate for the individual

The presence of a disability must be incorporated into the entire education process. Assessment of individual capability, planning that incorporates accommodations specific to the person, implementation of the plan that includes ongoing evaluation, and subsequent modification as needed are key components of an education intervention designed for success. Additionally, including others who assist in the care of the person with a disability can provide helpful insight about the person's capabilities and challenges, while also educating the person about appropriate diabetes management. Community and professional organizations that support the needs of those with disabilities can be excellent resources for materials, adaptive devices, and general information about the issues to be considered in dealing with a particular disability. In addition, several of these organizations offer support resources for both the person with diabetes and his or her support network.[48]

Working With a Special Population: Hearing Impaired

- ◆ Arrange the room in a way that does not block the view of the ASL (American Sign Language) interpreter. All participants must be able to view the interpreter whenever you and the interpreter are speaking.
- ◆ Write out medication names and other medical terms and keep them posted during the class so the interpreter can simply point to them rather than having to spelled out each name and term letter by letter.
- ◆ Be sure to address questions and answers to the participant and not to the interpreter.
- ◆ Visual tools are extremely important for this population. These include props, handouts, slides, freehand drawings, and well-written instructions for completing paperwork.

Identifying and Addressing Barriers

Barriers are factors that interfere with disease self-management, for example, stress, lack of social support, and environmental factors such as unavailability of grocery stores or parks in the neighborhood.

In Practice Tip: Addressing Barriers

A simple question, "What's standing in the way of your taking care of your diabetes?" is a great lead-in to help the patient identify barriers to achieving their goals.

Barriers to successful implementation of the DSME plan and achievement of identified goals may continue to become evident throughout each step of the process. A patient's lack of follow-through with a plan may be misinterpreted by a provider as noncompliance when it is actually related to a barrier to achieving DSME goals. One study demonstrated that 49% of patients interviewed didn't participate in regular self-monitoring of blood glucose because of high out-of-pocket expenses (Simmons as cited in Zgibor and Songer, 2001[83]). Barriers related to access to care, finances, limitations on number and frequency of visits, functional health literacy, comorbid conditions (ie, depression or chronic pain), acute illness or hospitalization, disability, social or cultural barriers, and many others have been identified. Issues related to access may be more prevalent in rural areas versus urban settings. There may also be more challenges related to transportation in rural settings.[83] Following the State of the Science Symposium in September 2006, *Barriers to Optimal Care for Patients With Diabetes and Strategies to Overcome Them* was published.[83] When implementing DSME it is important to work with the patient, the patient's support system, and outside resources and providers for assistance in removing the barriers. The following themes were identified at the Science Symposium[83]:

♦ Difficulty navigating the healthcare system
♦ Diagnosis of diabetes not automatically leading to DSME
♦ Limited time to see provider
♦ Episodic versus comprehensive focus
♦ Patient education is undervalued by the healthcare system and payers
♦ The complexity of diabetes education
♦ Low level of health literacy

Table 2.13 lists barriers and tips for addressing them.

TABLE 2.13 Addressing Barriers to DSME	
Barrier	*Tips for Addressing the Barrier*
Access to care: May include a lack of referral or availability of DSME, lack of transportation, financial issues	Outreach to providers about importance of DSME; link patient to community resources; support availability of diabetes education in provider's office. Include key messages in community campaigns (eg, NDEP's ABC message).
Finances	Link patient to community resources; several pharmaceutical companies and diabetes education supply companies have uninsured and underinsured patient assistance programs. Develop a plan with the patient that works within his or her means.
Comorbid conditions (depression, chronic pain)	Work collaboratively with primary care provider and other care providers related to the comorbidity. Individualize strategies related to the comorbidity.
Acute illness or hospitalization	Sessions should be short. Give small segments over several days. Prioritize content to what is necessary for the patient to learn to be safely discharged.
Health literacy	Assume low level of health literacy when choosing materials for DSME; simplify information; use additional strategies other than print; use clear and plain language
Cultural beliefs and attitudes	Individualized approach. Recognize and respect social and cultural barriers. Help patient develop an action plan for working within these cultural boundaries. For example, in some cultures not being willing to eat traditional foods may be a sign of disrespect. Help the patient develop and implement an action plan with this in mind.
Disabilities	Make programs accessible without needing special adaptations if possible; communicate among all healthcare team members, sharing the effects of the disability on DSME; help patient acquire assistive devices and/or appropriate self-management supplies if necessary

Being an Agile Educator

Imagine the following scenario: Four patients sit around the table listening to the diabetes educator discuss the possible complications from diabetes. Suddenly one patient begins to cry. The educator hands her patient a tissue and continues to flip through the slides recognizing that the session must cover this content to be able to move to the next lesson. There is also a curriculum checklist that must be completed.

Whose agenda was addressed? What would you have done? Is this an opportunity for additional education and support, or is it a distraction that is interfering with the planned lesson?

Educators frequently must find a balance between the volume of information and skills to be addressed and the constraints of time and patient needs. Being an agile educator means using highly refined assessment skills, even after the assessment stage. It also means reacting to situations and shifting priorities as needs change.

In this scenario, how different it would have been if the educator had stopped to explore the impact of the lesson on the patient. How powerful it would have been to take the chance to debrief what diabetes means, how to achieve a new normal, how fears might become barriers to care, and how to overcome those barriers. How much richer the learning experience might have been for the participants.

Being an agile educator means putting the patient's needs ahead of the planned lesson or curriculum. It means assessment skills continue throughout the education process.

Promoting Standards of Care and Follow-up Care

As part of DSME a personalized follow-up plan is developed by the patient and the diabetes educator[4] (Standard 8). In practice, in addition to educating patients on and promoting the importance of the Standards of Care and Clinical Practice Recommendations, the diabetes educator may be the one who helps facilitate access to important aspects of care like a dilated eye exam or flu shot or important risk reduction resources like smoking cessation or weight loss classes. As previously discussed, ongoing self-management support is necessary to sustain behavior change and is now an emphasis of the National Standards for Diabetes Self-Management Education and Support.[4] The type of support provided can include behavioral, psychosocial, or clinical. Access to diabetes support groups, camps, and other community resources may be facilitated by the diabetes educator. Communication back to the referring provider includes the patient's goals and the plan for ongoing self-management support. While the primary responsibility for DSME rests with the diabetes education team, it is very helpful to the patient to receive ongoing reinforcement and support for his or her evolving self-management plan from the entire healthcare team.[4]

One example of DSMS is the use of "Graduate School," a support group of people who have completed DSME classes. They choose topics based on their interests and needs. The group is interactive and offers opportunities for discussion and sharing. Celebrations are shared each month and are primarily tied to success in behavior change. This support group could take place face-to-face or through social media interest groups.[84,85]

Community approaches to diabetes awareness, prevention, and advocacy can be a successful approach to DSMS. Health fairs are excellent for reaching out into the community and providing basic diabetes information and awareness. Additionally, they serve as a link for the patient to diabetes education. Information about DSME programs and the importance of DSME for successful diabetes management is shared. School-based interventions are an opportunity to make an impact at an early age. Age-specific programs related to diabetes prevention and awareness can be presented to most any school-aged child.

Examples of Community Approaches

◆ School Walk for Diabetes, ADA: In addition to the fund-raising efforts for diabetes research, the children participate in interactive classes and a walk or physical activity highlighting the importance of physical activity in diabetes prevention. The ADA provides lesson plans and teaching materials in its School Walk campaign.[86]

◆ Workplace or faith-based community diabetes programs are offered as an employee benefit or as part of faith community health initiatives.

Diabetes educators are often called on to participate in advocacy related to diabetes prevention and awareness, and barriers to care or systems changes.[6] Examples include the following:

◆ Advocate for the removal of barriers that stand in the way of children self-administering insulin or checking blood glucose during the school day.

◆ Speak to the mayor of the patient's community about building sidewalks in neighborhoods so that persons with diabetes (and all community members) can successfully meet their behavior goal related to being active.

◆ Meet with legislators and ask them to include reimbursement for certified diabetes educators to improve access to care for the many Medicare recipients.

Such examples demonstrate how diabetes educators provide DSMS at an organizational level. These examples are also concrete ways that educators meet the competencies identified in the Diabetes Educator Practice Guidelines for Level 2–5 educators.[87]

Summary for Implementation

A key to effective implementation of DSME and DSMS is building relationships with the patient and his or her support persons, identifying and individualizing appropriate goals and a realistic time frame, and implementing the plan. This sets the stage for supporting the patient's quest to achieve goals established in the collaboratively developed plan, leading to improved care and evaluation of patient and program outcomes.

Evaluation/Monitoring

Evaluation/monitoring is the fifth step in the DSME process described in the *AADE Guidelines for the Practice of Diabetes Self-Management Education and Training*.[6] The assessment, goal setting, planning, and implementation of the DSME process have occurred with consistent documentation. Recording of this ongoing education process supports each step of the DSME process and provides data for individual and program evaluation. Standard 9 of the National Standards for Diabetes Self-Management Education

and Support states that "the provider(s) of DSME and DSMS will monitor whether participants are achieving their personal diabetes self-management goals and other outcome(s) as a way to evaluate the effectiveness of the educational intervention(s), using appropriate measurement techniques" (p. 624).[4] To facilitate evaluation, educators must document the individual's assessment, education plan, intervention, and follow-up status in the patient's permanent confidential education record.[88–90] The more complete the documentation, the more accurate the patient or program evaluation will be.

Evaluation should be considered in terms of time and population. Whether the educator is evaluating an individual's outcomes or the success of a program, the approaches and processes are similar.

Understanding What to Document

Clear documentation provides the necessary data to make decisions about patient and program outcomes. Quality documentation is relevant, accurate, and timely. Table 2.14 describes the information to be included at each step to ensure accurate, quality documentation throughout the DSME process.

Documentation might be organized around the AADE7 Self-Care Behaviors™.[3] These standards complement the National Standards for Diabetes Self-Management Education and Support by recognizing that behavior change is the unique outcome measurement for DSME. These measures can be used to determine the effectiveness of DSME at the individual, group, and population levels:

◆ Being active
◆ Healthy eating
◆ Monitoring
◆ Taking medication
◆ Problem solving
◆ Healthy coping
◆ Reducing risks

Diabetes self-care behaviors should be evaluated at baseline and then at regular intervals following the initial education program. The continuum of outcomes, including learning, behavioral, clinical, satisfaction, and health status, should be assessed to demonstrate the interrelationship between DSME and behavior change in the care of individuals with

TABLE 2.14 Documentation of the DSME Process

DSME Process	What to Document
Step 1: Assessment	• Date and time of assessment • Pertinent medical history from referring providers, person with diabetes, and family members/support persons • Comparison of data collected with standards • Patient's attitude, health beliefs, values, perceptions, and readiness to change • Knowledge or level of understanding, expectation of learning self-care behaviors, and pertinent clinical or functional outcomes • Psychosocial status • Psychomotor skills
Step 2: Goal setting	• Date and time • Specific treatment and behavioral goals and expected outcomes as identified as part of the assessment process
Step 3: Planning	• Date and time • Recommended interventions and instructional strategies to be used, and who on the care team will provide those interventions • Plans for follow-up and frequency of care and how the care will be evaluated
Step 4: Implementation	• Date and time interventions provided • Description of interventions provided, including educational materials used, and patient receptivity/understanding • Referrals made, resources used, and communication with referring provider (if appropriate) • Rationale for discharge/discontinuation of care, if appropriate
Step 5: Evaluation/ monitoring	• Date and time • Specific outcomes measured (ie, learning, behavioral, clinical, and health status) and results • Progress toward goals and/or barriers to achieving goals

Sources: American Association of Diabetes Educators, "The scope of practice, standards of practice, and standards of professional performance for diabetes educators," *Diabetes Educ* 31 (2005): 487-513; K Lacey, E Pritchett, "Nutrition care process and model: ADA adopts road map to quality care and outcomes management," *J Am Diet Assoc* 103, no. 8 (2003): 1061-72.

diabetes (see Figure 2.2). Individual patient outcomes are used to guide the intervention and improve care for that individual. The aggregate population outcomes are used to guide programmatic services and continuous quality improvement (CQI) activities for the DSME program and the population it serves.

Evaluation

Diabetes educators are in the position to promote healthy lifestyles. Integrating disease-state knowledge, educational theories, and health behavioral models allows educators to approach the shaping of patient health behaviors. The educator role includes behavior-change facilitator, goal-setting coach, organizer of the learning environment (space, sequence, and materials), and evaluator. As an evaluator, the educator ensures educational programs are accountable to the learner and his or her family and to consumers in the health service community. This accountability is ensured by evaluation in the form of patient objectives and health outcomes for DSME as step 5 of the educational process. Evaluation is a process that provides evidence that what is done makes a value-added difference in the service/care provided. Evaluation is defined as a systematic process by which the worth or value of something—in this case teaching, learning, and support—is judged.

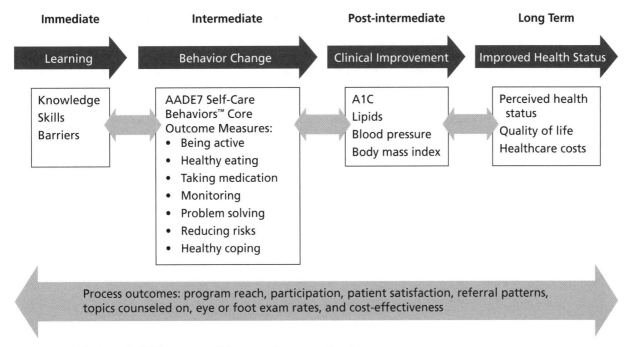

FIGURE 2.2   Diabetes Self-Management Education Outcomes Continuum

Sources: Adapted from the following: K Lacey, E Pritchett, "Nutrition care process and model: ADA adopts road map to quality care and outcomes management," *J Am Diet Assoc* 103, no. 8 (2003): 1061-72; American Association of Diabetes Educators, "Standards for outcomes measurement of diabetes self-management education," *Diabetes Educ* 29 (2003): 804-16.

The outcome of education for the learner must be measurably effective.

It is the diabetes educator's responsibility to ensure that the evaluation is based on objective assessment of collecting quantitative and qualitative data. The more the process is rooted in evaluation principles, the greater the confidence in the objectivity and meaningfulness of the evaluation. The timing of the evaluation determines the type of evaluation used. The 2 types are formative (or process) and summative (or outcomes) evaluation.

Formative Evaluation

The purpose of formative or process evaluation is to make adjustments in the educational process as they are needed. Process evaluation is integral to the education process and is an ongoing component of assessment, planning, and implementation. The scope is limited to a learning experience such as a class or workshop. Formative evaluation is used for patient experience as well as the program's outcomes. Sample questions for each are include in Table 2.15.

Summative Evaluation

The purpose of summative or outcomes evaluation is to determine the effects or outcomes of teaching or program efforts. Its intent is to sum what happened as a result of education or support. Some guiding questions in outcomes evaluation are listed in Table 2.15.

Both process and outcomes evaluation should be used for diabetes patient education.

It is worthwhile to note that while assessment and evaluation are interrelated and often used interchangeably, they are not synonymous. The process of assessment is to gather, summarize, interpret, and use data to determine a direction for action. The process of evaluation is to gather, summarize, and interpret data to determine the extent to which an action was successful. Evaluation is a value judgment that attaches meaning to the data obtained by measurement and gathered through assessment. It is guided by professional judgment and involves interpreting the accumulated information and how it can be used.

Formative and summative evaluations provide the educator with data to make decisions and to make

TABLE 2.15	Distinguishing Between Forms of Evaluation	
Type of Evaluation	*Patient Experience*	*Program Results*
Formative (or Process)	• Is there enough time for patients to ask questions? • Is the information in class consistent with information included in handouts? • Should additional opportunities be given for return demonstration? • Is the session honoring multiple learning preferences?	• How many patients were scheduled for the session and how many attended the session? • Are participants satisfied with the sessions?
Summative (or Outcomes)	• Did the individual(s) learn? • Were behavioral goals achieved? • Did the patient learn the skill taught and use it correctly?	• Was teaching appropriate? • What was the aggregate decrease in weight or A1C? • How many patients completed the program? • What was the cost to run the program?

needed changes in the curriculum. With systematic collection of information about the activities, characteristics, and outcomes of programs, judgments can be made about the program to improve its effectiveness and/or enable informed decision making for future program development.[91] While program evaluation is discussed in detail in chapter 11, this chapter will address evaluation as applied to the individual patient.

Individual Evaluation

Evaluation is the final step in the DSME process, before the process cycles again into reassessment, goal setting, planning, and implementation. At the individual patient level, assessment and evaluation examine processes and outcomes to determine whether an individual has achieved his or her behavior-change goals and health outcomes.[92] Together at each encounter the educator and the patient review the progress toward the patient's established goals. Patients receive feedback and support. Programs can then aggregate the outcome data to make decisions about program changes and upgrades. Aggregate patient data also contribute to requirements for maintaining program recognition or accreditation.

What Should Be Evaluated?

Guidelines for documentation and evaluation are outlined in Outcome Standards 9 and 10 of the National Standards.[4] These include a structured educational process based on the critical elements of diabetes care that address the critical self-care activities. Elements include educational, behavioral, and psychological elements which target lifestyle change and factors of self-efficacy and empowerment. Behavioral goal-setting is an effective strategy to support diabetes self-care.

Of course, goal setting is preliminary to behavior change and outcome evaluation. Goal setting helps the patient define what a current behavior is and what a desired behavior would be. Patients and educators can use individual outcome data to make comparisons against expected or desired results. They can then decide which interventions are most effective and which will need to be adjusted.

Setting goals and monitoring/evaluating progress provide both the educator and the person with diabetes with information on what is working and what is not. Evaluation is based on individual variables but allows others (such as accrediting bodies or program administrators) to see the bigger picture.

Evaluating learner or patient outcomes should consider 3 components: knowledge, skills, and satisfaction. Knowledge involves remembering and applying critical self-care information. Skills include mastering the necessary psychomotor tasks for diabetes self-care. Satisfaction involves the sense of fulfillment with attending the education session or program. Satisfaction can be a powerful motivator in self-care behavior.[93]

Use of forms or checklists can help the educator and the patient track different behaviors, assess progress toward goals, and see how achievement or lack of achievement of those goals impacts treatment outcomes. Forms can be used for both individual-level interventions and group classes. Lorig[94] cautions that in any evaluation it is important to ask yourself 2 questions: "What do you want to know?" and "What difference does it make?" Ask thoughtful evaluation questions that make sense with the goals. In essence, has the intervention changed knowledge, behaviors, attitudes, health status, or healthcare utilization?

One example of a tool for tracking knowledge and skills progress is the AADE7 Self-Care Behaviors™ Goal Sheet (Figure 2.3). This tool not only allows the educator to introduce the concept of the 7 critical self-care behaviors to patients, but allows the educator, care team, colleagues, and patients to track goals and goal achievement in a consistent manner.

Patient outcomes within the AADE7 Self-Care Behaviors™ may also be considered in terms of immediate or intermediate outcomes. Documentation should ultimately capture immediate, intermediate and post-intermediate, and long-term outcomes.[3]

- ◈ *Immediate outcomes* are those that can be measured at the time the intervention is delivered. Teaching and learning, for example, are immediate outcomes.
- ◈ *Intermediate and post-intermediate outcomes* result over time. Behavior change and clinical improvements are examples of intermediate outcomes.
- ◈ *Long-term outcomes* result from multiple variables over an extended period of time. Reduction in healthcare costs or complications, and improvements in quality of life are examples of possible long-term outcomes.
- ◈ Approaches to measuring immediate and intermediate outcomes are listed in Table 2.16.

In addition to measuring knowledge and skills, educators should ascertain whether patients are satisfied with their education. One method of determining satisfaction is to provide the patient with a brief satisfaction survey. Content includes items related to education and may use a Likert scale (in which information is ranked from 1 to 10). In setting up a satisfaction survey, consider what elements of the education session or program are important in pleasing a patient. Do you believe that the environment should be pleasant and conducive to learning? Do you want to learn whether the educator's style is facilitating learning? Some typical satisfaction questions are listed in Table 2.17.

The satisfaction survey may be in a paper-and-pencil format that is given at the end of the session or it may be an online survey. Online surveys are inexpensive (even free) and are easy to set up. Survey Monkey.com and Zoomerang.com are 2 examples.

Tools to Track Progress

In addition to tools for tracking satisfaction, there are a variety of means for collecting information about knowledge and skills outcomes. These are listed in Table 2.18.

Making Use of Patient Evaluation Data

Once evaluation information is collected, it is time to sift through the data and make follow-up decisions. First, the educator revisits the patient's goals. Then the educator asks a series of questions.[68]

What is the patient's assessment of the goal?

- ◈ Did the patient feel he or she achieved the goal?
- ◈ How would the patient rate his or her progress?

What is your collaborative assessment of the goal?

- ◈ Was the goal appropriate for the patient?
- ◈ Did the patient have adequate time to achieve the goal?
- ◈ Did the goal achieve the expected outcome?
- ◈ Did that outcome impact the diabetes treatment plan?
- ◈ If so, does therapy need to change?

What should the next steps be?

- ◈ Should the goal be changed or continued?
- ◈ Should additional goals be added or other goals changed?
- ◈ When will new goals be evaluated?
- ◈ What other changes in the diabetes treatment plan need to occur to support the goal(s)?

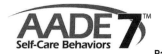

Patient Name _____

Goal Setting		Follow Up		Goal Review
Date	Goal	Date I Achievement		Documentation

Date	☐ **Healthy Eating**	Date	I Achieved	☐ Achieved ☐ Continued ☐ Modified
	☐ Make better food choices ☐ Reduce portion size ☐ Follow meal plan **Goal individualization:**_____ _____	☐ 1 mo. ☐ 3 mo. ☐ 6 mo. ☐ 12 mo.	Rate 0-10 _____	_____ _____ _____ _____ _____
Date	☐ **Being Active**	Date	I Achieved	☐ Achieved ☐ Continued ☐ Modified
	☐ Exercise longer ☐ Exercise more often ☐ Follow exercise plan **Goal individualization:**_____ _____	☐ 1 mo. ☐ 3 mo. ☐ 6 mo. ☐ 12 mo.	Rate 0-10 _____	_____ _____ _____ _____ _____
Date	☐ **Monitoring**	Date	I Achieved	☐ Achieved ☐ Continued ☐ Modified
	☐ Follow monitoring schedule ☐ Monitor more often ☐ Monitor health status **Goal individualization:**_____ _____	☐ 1 mo. ☐ 3 mo. ☐ 6 mo. ☐ 12 mo.	Rate 0-10 _____	_____ _____ _____ _____ _____
Date	☐ **Taking Medication**	Date	I Achieved	☐ Achieved ☐ Continued ☐ Modified
	☐ Increase taking medications on time ☐ Miss fewer medications ☐ Take medications as prescribed **Goal individualization:**_____ _____	☐ 1 mo. ☐ 3 mo. ☐ 6 mo. ☐ 12 mo.	Rate 0-10 _____	_____ _____ _____ _____ _____
Date	☐ **Problem Solving**	Date	I Achieved	☐ Achieved ☐ Continued ☐ Modified
	☐ Identify potential problems ☐ Plan problem situation treatment ☐ Prevent problem situations **Goal individualization:**_____ _____	☐ 1 mo. ☐ 3 mo. ☐ 6 mo. ☐ 12 mo.	Rate 0-10 _____	_____ _____ _____ _____ _____
Date	☐ **Healthy Coping**	Date	I Achieved	☐ Achieved ☐ Continued ☐ Modified
	☐ Cope with diagnosis of disease ☐ Adapt to lifestyle changes ☐ Get support from family/friends **Goal individualization:**_____ _____	☐ 1 mo. ☐ 3 mo. ☐ 6 mo. ☐ 12 mo.	Rate 0-10 _____	_____ _____ _____ _____ _____
Date	☐ **Reducing Risks**	Date	I Achieved	☐ Achieved ☐ Continued ☐ Modified
	☐ Stop smoking ☐ Get health checkups ☐ Perform daily self care activities **Goal individualization:**_____ _____	☐ 1 mo. ☐ 3 mo. ☐ 6 mo. ☐ 12 mo.	Rate 0-10 _____	_____ _____ _____ _____ _____

Diabetes Educator Name and Initial Index:
Name: _____ Initial: _____   Name: _____ Initial: _____

Name: _____ Initial: _____   Name: _____ Initial: _____

FIGURE 2.3   **AADE7 Self-Care Behaviors™ Goal Sheet**

Answers to open-ended questions provide detail and depth. For some of the questions, the educator might also use a rating scale. For example, the person can be asked to rate his or her progress on a Likert scale from 1 to 10 (1 = did not meet goal; 10 = achieved goal) or given word choices (eg, met goal most of the time, met goal some of the time, did not meet goal, or changed goal).

TABLE 2.16 Outcomes for the AADE7 Self-Care Behaviors™					
	*Immediate Outcome**			*Intermediate Outcome†*	
	Knowledge	*Skill*	*Barriers*	*Measures*	*Methods of Measurement*
Being Active physical activity, exercise	Type; duration; intensity; safety precautions.	Develops appropriate activity plan; balances food and medication with activity.	Physical limitations; time; environment; fear.	Type; frequency; duration; intensity.	Patient self-report; observation; use of tools such as a pedometer.
Healthy Eating	Effect of food on blood glucose; sources of carbohydrate; meal plan (what to eat, when to eat, how much to eat); resources to assist in food choices.	Meal planning; weighing and measuring food; carbohydrate counting; label reading.	Environmental triggers; emotional eating; cultural influences; financial issues.	Type of food choices; amount of food eaten; timing of meals; alcohol intake; effect of food on glucose; special situations and problem solving.	Patient self-report; observation; records of food and blood glucose; food recall (eg, 24-hour recall or food frequency questionnaires).
Taking Medication	Name, dose, frequency; medication action; action for missed dose; side effects, toxicity; action for side effect; storage, travel, safety; recognition of efficacy.	Preparation, technique, administration; safe handling, disposal of equipment; dose adjustment; recognition, treatment, prevention of low blood glucose.	Vision or dexterity; financial; fear of needles; cognitive, math skills; embarrassment.	Adherence to medication; dose accuracy.	Pill count; review of pharmacy refill; demonstration, patient self-report; records of blood glucose and medication; observation and role playing.
Monitoring of blood glucose	Schedule for checking; target values; proper disposal of sharps; interpretation, use of results.	Self-monitoring of blood glucose; records of blood glucose values; equipment use, care.	Physical; financial; cognitive; time; inconvenience; emotional.	Frequency of missed tests; frequency and schedule of monitoring (eg, times/day, days/week); planned, unplanned testing; review of pharmacy refill record.	Review of logbook; meter memory review or printout; patient self-report; demonstration of technique.

(continued)

TABLE 2.16 Outcomes for the AADE7 Self-Care Behaviors™ (continued)				
	Immediate Outcome*			Intermediate Outcome†	
	Knowledge	Skill	Barriers	Measures	Methods of Measurement
Problem Solving especially for blood glucose: high and low levels and sick days	Signs, symptoms, causes; treatment, guidelines, prevention strategies; sick-day rules; safety concerns (eg, driving, operating equipment).	Hypoglycemia treatment; glucagon administration (if applicable); use of blood glucose data to determine appropriate actions related to food, exercise, medication.	Cognitive; financial; coping strategies; emotional; physical.	Blood glucose checks; adjusting food, medication, activity; contact with healthcare provider for problem resolution; checking meter and strips for function; number of blood glucose checks per month that require assistance; number of times ketones are checked (when appropriate); missed days from work, school, or related activities.	Patient self-report; review of logbook; meter memory review or printout; medical chart review; frequency of medication adjustment.
Reducing Risks of diabetes complications	Standards of care; therapeutic goals; how to decrease risks (through preventive services).	Foot exam; blood pressure (self); self-monitoring of blood glucose; maintaining personal care record.	Financial; time; unaware of disease process or seriousness; lack of rapport with provider; travel; physical disabilities.	Smoking status; frequency of foot self-exam; aspirin therapy; eye exam; MD visit; diabetes educator visit; RD visit; lipids checked; blood pressure checked; flu vaccine, pneumonia vaccine; urine check for protein; prepregnancy counseling.	Patient self-report; chart or exam code audit for demonstration of self-care activities.
Healthy Coping living with diabetes (psychosocial adaptation)	Recognizing that everyone has problems; benefits of treatment and self-care; motivation is internal function.	Goal setting; problem solving; coping strategies; self-efficacy.	Lack of awareness; financial; lack of support; physical; psychosocial distress.	Depression score; stress; quality of life; functional measurement; treatment self-efficacy; patient empowerment; self-report.	SF-36/SF-12; PAID; Zung/Beck Depression Scale; D-SMART.

*Immediate outcomes are those that can be measured at the time of the intervention (eg, learning).

†Intermediate outcomes result over time (eg, behavior change) and require more than a single measurement.

Source: Adapted from K Mulcahy, M Maryniuk, M Peeples, et al, "Diabetes self-management education core outcomes measures," *Diabetes Educ* 29 (2003): 768-88.

TABLE 2.17	Sample Statements in a Satisfaction Survey
Environment	The classroom was comfortable.
	The registration process was easy.
	There was adequate parking.
Educators	The educator was effective in teaching me to use my pump.
	The educator provided enough time to practice the skill.
Education	As a result of the education, I am better able to take care of my diabetes.
	The handouts were easy to follow.
Value	I received good value for my money.
	I would recommend this program to other patients.

Once the analysis is complete, the educator and the patient establish the next goal and implement the next set of tactics to reach the goal. In doing this, the educator models for the patient one form of problem solving and how future decisions can be based on past experience.

Finally, the educator sends a summary of the patient outcomes and recommendations for future DSME and medical follow-up to the referring provider. The information can also be reviewed by the educational team, and summarized (without identifying details) and presented to the advising group, directors, or administrators for use in program reviews and program outcome studies.

TABLE 2.18   Data Collection Tools

Method	Examples of Outcomes Collected	Easy to Use?	Yields Reliable Data?	High Response Rate?
Survey Method used to question individuals in writing, face-to-face, by phone, or by mail	Learning; behavior change; quality of life; satisfaction	Yes; can be designed to be simple and easy to use	Yes; although respondents' interpretation of survey questions can vary; surveys more reliable if surveyor is not the diabetes educator	Depends; telephone or face-to-face surveys can have a high response rate
Chart/File Audit Review of closed, open, or computerized medical records to retrieve information	Lab data (A1C, lipids); process data (eye or foot exam)	Depends; paper chart review can be labor-intensive and time-intensive	Depends on skill of individuals doing the review	Yes
Checklist Data collection sheet for gathering concurrent information during a study	Behavior change; process and implementation tasks	Yes; can be designed to be simple and easy to use	Depends; all people who will be completing the checklist during the data collection must be trained on how to use the data collection instrument	Depends on the cooperation and availability of the personnel completing the forms
Time Study Concurrent information about time to complete a process such as turnaround time	Cycle time to schedule a patient for a visit	Usually very time-intensive and labor-intensive	Depends; all people who will be completing the time study during the data collection must be trained on how to use the instrument	Depends on the cooperation and availability of the personnel completing the study

Source: Adapted from K Mulcahy, "Management of Diabetes Education Programs," in MJ Franz, ed, *A Core Curriculum for Diabetes Educators*, 5th ed (Chicago: American Association of Diabetes Educators, 2003), 203.

American Association of Diabetes Educators©

Case: The DSME Process

LC, a 60-year-old man, was diagnosed with type 2 diabetes less than 1 year ago. Upon referral from his primary care provider (PCP), he was scheduled to meet with the diabetes educator. Information provided includes the following:

- A1C: 7.8%

- Metformin 500 mg twice a day

Assessment

At the initial visit, the educator began with an assessment of LC's learning needs, self-management behaviors (including current nutrition, physical activity, and medication-taking practices), and current treatment plan. The educator also assessed health literacy and physical and psychosocial factors impacting learning. LC indicated he was motivated to learn what he needed to know to prevent complications, because his mother had "bad diabetes." LC has not received previous diabetes education. He looked for information on a few Web sites but found it overwhelming. He has not had a dilated eye exam in over 4 years. He is willing to monitor but is a little unsure of how to use the equipment and when he should perform the blood glucose checks.

Goal Setting and Plan

At LC's initial DSME visit, the diabetes educator used the information provided by LC's PCP and gathered in his assessment to develop an education plan to meet his needs. It was mutually decided to begin with some basic diabetes information and a review of home monitoring. They also agreed on the importance of scheduling an eye exam.

His overall stated goal was to "decrease risks of complications."

Learning Goal

Monitoring of blood glucose including correct use of monitor and frequency and timing of testing.

Goals

AADE7 Self-Care Behavior™: Monitoring

- Monitor once a day at alternating times (fasting, before meals, 2 hours after meals, and before bed) for 2 weeks and write down results in a glucose logbook.

- Call diabetes educator to report blood glucose results in 2 weeks.

AADE7 Self-Care Behavior™: Reducing risks

- Within the next week, call to schedule an appointment for an eye exam.

Implementation

The educator shared basic information about diabetes, promoting a healthy lifestyle, and reducing risks of complications, including healthy checkups and recommended tests and exams. LC also was educated on the importance of monitoring, including guidelines for frequency, keeping records, and reporting results to his healthcare team. He demonstrated appropriate monitoring technique. Below is a sample of a piece of documentation from the education record.

For his DSMS plan, LC chose to subscribe to a popular diabetes magazine. To extend his learning, he was given a diabetes self-care workbook, which had additional references. LC agreed to the plan that he would call the educator with his blood glucose results in 2 weeks, and a return visit was scheduled in 1 month.

Assessment Summary Date: **5/22/14**	Behavioral Objectives	Instruction Given					Goal Reached
		Insert total time spent with patient					Date/Initial
		60 min					
		Date: **5/22/14**	Date:	Date:	Date:	Date:	
	Monitoring						
① 2 3 0	Demonstrates monitoring skills						**5/22/14 LM**
1 ② 3 0	Monitors BG according to plan						
1 2 3 ⓪	Uses results of monitoring						

1 = completed, 2 = review needed, 3 = full education needed, 0 = not applicable

Communication Back to the Referring PCP

Included a summary of the visit, patient goals, and the plan for ongoing self-management support.

Follow-Up Phone Call

LC phoned the diabetes educator 2 weeks after the initial visit with monitoring results as planned. During the phone call he reported his blood glucose records, and he also mentioned that he noticed some high numbers after a meal of spaghetti and meatballs. He learned that exercising on his treadmill lowered his blood glucose levels. He was pleased to report that his weight had dropped 2 pounds over the last 2 weeks. His educator agreed that he was doing well. He said that at the next visit, he would like to learn more tips that will help him avoid complications like his mother had. He would especially like more help with choosing what to eat and learning how his food affects his blood glucose. He also reported that he has not had a chance to schedule his eye exam.

Evaluation of Patient Goals

AADE7 Self-Care Behavior™: Monitoring

- Monitor once a day at alternating times (fasting, before meals, 2 hours after meals, and before bed) for 2 weeks and write down results in a glucose logbook.

- Call diabetes educator to report blood glucose results in 2 weeks.

AADE7 Self-Care Behavior™: Reducing Risks

- Within the next week, call to schedule an appointment for an eye exam.

Monitoring Behavior Evaluated

Blood glucose records shared with the educator showed that LC had checked his blood glucose at least once a day at different times of the day. He called to report the results as planned. His goal of monitoring once a day will continue, and he will bring his blood glucose log to the follow-up visit.

Reducing Risks Behavior Evaluated

LC did not schedule his eye exam within the week, so he and the educator adjusted his goals to state the following: Prior to next appointment with the diabetes educator, schedule an appointment for an eye exam.

Follow-up Visit

LC brought his blood glucose logbook to his follow-up visit. He and the educator reviewed the logbook together, and LC again mentioned that he noticed that certain foods affect his blood glucose more than others. He is interested in learning more about carbohydrate counting and getting help with his personal meal plan. The educator updated LC's assessment and provided him with some basic carbohydrate information. He was able to identify a list of foods containing carbohydrate. A referral to a registered dietitian (RD) for medical nutrition therapy (MNT) was arranged with his PCP's office. He would like to get additional DSME from a diabetes class since he enjoys participating in groups. A referral to a group class was made as well. LC wondered whether there were other things he should be tracking to decrease his risk of complications. The educator reviewed the impact of blood pressure and weight on long-term health and suggested that LC monitor these things routinely. The educator showed LC how to accurately check his blood pressure. LC decided to weigh himself every week and check his blood pressure each evening. In addition to communicating a summary of the visit to LC's PCP, information was shared with the RD and the diabetes education team leading the classes.

Learning Goal

LC's learning goal is to use carbohydrate counting in his meal planning.

AADE7 Self-Care Behavior™: Healthy Eating

- Practice carbohydrate counting for at least 1 meal a day by identifying and writing down foods that contain carbohydrate.

AADE7 Self-Care Behavior™: Reducing Risks

- Check weight weekly on Friday and record.

- Check blood pressure each evening and record.

Evaluation/Monitoring Summary

Documentation and evaluation are critical components of the DSME process. Both are considered "standards" of diabetes care.[4,5] The information is needed to evaluate both outcomes related to the individual and a DSME program's progress toward achieving its goals. Without such documentation, providing ongoing education that evolves to match the changing needs of the person with diabetes is difficult.

For individuals and programs to be successful, the following elements are required[3]:

- ◆ Outcomes measurement: Consistent measurement of specific indicators
- ◆ Outcomes monitoring: Measurement of those indicators at specified intervals
- ◆ Outcomes management: Use of those outcomes to drive educational and clinical decision making

Standardized tools and methods to track and report outcomes can help the educational process and improve the health of individuals and the quality of programs when the documentation is reviewed regularly.

Conclusion

Diabetes self-management education is a critical component of care for people with diabetes. It is not a singular event but an ongoing process of facilitating knowledge, skill, and ability necessary for self-care leading to improved health outcomes and quality of life. The process outlined in this chapter includes assessment, goal setting, planning, implementation, and evaluation/monitoring that is based on the DSME process outlined in the *AADE Guidelines for the Practice of Diabetes Self-Management Education and Training* and the National Standards for Diabetes Self-Management Education and Support.

The DSME process described in this chapter begins with assessing an individual with diabetes or prediabetes to determine understanding, knowledge, and experiences of the person. Assessment is the cornerstone of diabetes education and management and relies on critical thinking and clinical judgment.

Next, empowerment models are employed to explore the needs and goals of the individual and his or her family or caregivers to become self-managers of their diabetes. The process is dynamic and ongoing. A variety of healthcare professionals are responsible for assessing, planning, and implementing appropriate healthcare education that promotes longevity and productivity for the people served. Appropriate education incorporates information from a comprehensive curriculum of content areas that is tailored to the individual and delivered in a manner that both facilitates learning and honors learning styles and preferences. Those implementing the plan to provide diabetes education must then adapt teaching tactics, methods, and materials to be sensitive to the learning capability, readiness, needs, and cultural influences of the learner.

Diabetes self-management education incorporates educational, behavioral, and psychosocial strategies to implement the plan. For this reason, DSME is ideally delivered collaboratively by a multidisciplinary team with a comprehensive plan of care. Team members work toward collaborative objectives using expertise in clinical care of diabetes, MNT, learning and teaching strategies, and psychosocial and behavioral aspects of diabetes self-management.

The AADE Scope of Practice, Standards of Practice, and Standards of Professional Performance for Diabetes Educators addresses the process of assessment, goal setting, planning, implementation, and evaluation of DSME. The components and issues to consider when implementing an education plan have been addressed throughout this chapter. In summary, to implement diabetes education successfully, confirm the individual's readiness to learn, identify teaching methods appropriate for the person's literacy level, recognize the importance of cultural influences, and integrate these factors into the education process. Additionally, strive to motivate the people with diabetes you serve by understanding what is important to them and why, helping them identify barriers they may encounter, and working with them to address those barriers. Keep in mind that you cannot "make" someone learn, but inability or unwillingness to learn is not a permanent state.

Documentation and evaluation are critical components of the DSME process. Both are considered to be "standards" of diabetes care. To maintain continuity of care, it is important to document the patient's progress in attaining the mutually determined goals. Progress in achieving goals leads to effective reassessment or evaluation. Patient outcomes are the most important elements of DSME.

This chapter considered AADE Standards for Outcomes Measurement of Diabetes Self-Management Education, a tool which specifies self-management behaviors as the key outcomes for DSME, to be ideal for the evaluation. These self-care behaviors include physical activity, healthy eating, medication taking, monitoring blood glucose, diabetes self-care-related problem solving, reducing risks of acute and chronic complications, and psychosocial aspects of living with diabetes. Standardized tools such as the AADE7 Self-Care Behaviors™ Goal Sheet are useful for tracking and reporting outcomes.

Finally, this chapter emphasized the crucial role of the diabetes educator in applying a systematic process to providing diabetes education and support. Effective care of people with diabetes is dependent on a clinician or educator who continually assesses changes in the patient, the family, and the environment to make the best decisions about care and support.

Focus on Education

Teaching Strategies

→ **Foster an atmosphere of trust.** Maintaining a nonjudgmental attitude improves identification of other teaching opportunities.

→ **Prioritize.** A person's goals, interests, and needs guide what to cover and when. There are always more topics and more information to discuss than there is time. Focus on the patient's ability to make safe and informed decisions.

→ **Be flexible.** Plan to deliver information in several ways, adjusting the teaching plan to accommodate patient needs at that time. Avoid information overload. Be practical in collaborating on actionable behaviors. It will increase the likelihood of improved outcomes.

→ **Keep the pace.** Allow time to discuss goals, application, and next steps. Covering fewer topics and having a behavioral action plan is preferable to covering many topics with no discussion or implementation intentions.

→ **Use novel, engaging approaches to educate.** Use effective strategies, not just the latest technology. Low-tech options (drawings, handouts, etc) can be as effective as high-tech options and are an important tool in the educator's toolkit.

Messages for Patients

→ **Permission to ask as well as answer.** No question or answer is silly or dumb. Clarify what each person on the care team needs and ask for help so you have a clear path to progress.

→ **Education is ongoing.** Diabetes education is not just a one-time event. Take as much time as you need to understand the information and make choices.

→ **Rights and responsibilities.** You have the right and responsibility to ask questions, seek clarification, and make decisions and changes in managing your diabetes and overall health. You have a right to know all the choices, alternatives, and potential outcomes of your choices. You have the right to a second opinion, to ask your family or others for advice, and to take as much time as needed.

Health Literacy

→ **Learning principles.** Consider preferred learning styles, learner readiness, and special needs of the learner (vision, concentration, physical health, etc) when determining educational content and delivery. Health literacy is different from reading literacy or mental capacity.

⊘ **Educational content.**   Ensure that materials and methods are at the appropriate literacy level. Build on existing knowledge. Move in sequence from simple to more complex information. Materials should reflect sensitivity and awareness of cultural differences. Adjust teaching options to fit the person's style.

⊘ **Tune in to culture.**   Be sensitive to differences in cultural and ethnic backgrounds during assessment. Appropriate tone of voice, rate of questioning, and nonverbal cues are critical in establishing rapport and the success of future educational encounters.

Focus on Practice

⊘ **Documentation is critical and an ongoing process.**   Documentation chronicles past care and outcomes and serves as a road map for future encounters and expected outcomes. Create documentation that allows multiple team members to accumulate information and data to foster reinforcement of the self-management plan and to evaluate the program.

⊘ **Evaluation.**   Data can be captured, reviewed, and evaluated more easily when tools are consistent. Patient education and behavioral outcomes, along with program data, are used to update curriculum, educational materials, delivery methods, and instructors to enhance effectiveness of care in meeting program goals.

References

1. American Association of Diabetes Educators. Definition of diabetes education (cited 2013 Jun 10). On the Internet at: http://www.diabeteseducator.org/DiabetesEducation/Definitions.html.

2. American Association of Diabetes Educators. Measurable behavior change is the desired outcome of diabetes education (cited 2013 Jun 10). On the Internet at: http://www.diabeteseducator.org/ProfessionalResources/AADE7.

3. American Association of Diabetes Educators. Standards for outcomes measurement of diabetes self-management education. Diabetes Educ. 2003;29:804-16.

4. Haas L, Maryniuk M, Beck J, et al. National standards for diabetes self-management education and support. Diabetes Educ. 2012;38(5):619-29.

5. Funnell MM, Brown TL, Childs BP. National standards for diabetes self-management education and support. Diabetes Educ. 2007;33(4):599-614.

6. American Association of Diabetes Educators. The AADE Guidelines for the Practice of Diabetes Self-Management Education and Training (DSME/T). Chicago: American Association of Diabetes Educators; 2009:15-9.

7. Martin C, Daly A, McWhorter LS, Shwide-Slavin C, Kushion W; for the American Association of Diabetes Educators. The scope of practice, standards of practice, and standards of professional performance for diabetes educators. Diabetes Educ. 2005;31(4):487-512.

8. Pichert JA, Schlundt DG. Assessment: gathering information and facilitating engagement. In: Mensing C, ed. The Art and Science of Diabetes Self-Management Education: A Desk Reference for Healthcare Professionals. Chicago: American Association of Diabetes Educators; 2006:578-9.

9. Cornett S. Assessing and addressing health literacy. OJIN: The Online Journal of Issues in Nursing. 2009; 14(3, Manuscript 2). On the Internet at: www.nursingworld.org/MainMenuCategories/ANAMarketplace/ANAPeriodicals/OJIN/TableofContents/Vol142009/No3Sept09/Assessing-Health-Literacy-.html.

10. Orem SL, Binkert J, Clancy AL. Appreciative Coaching: A Positive Process for Change. San Francisco: Jossey-Bass; 2007.

11. Kimsey-House H, Kimsey-House K, Sandahl P. Co-Active Coaching. 3rd ed. Boston: Nicholas Brealey Publishing; 2011.

12. Goldenring JM, Rosen DS. Getting into adolescent heads: An essential update. Contemp Pediatr. 2004;21:64.

13. Fulmer T. How to try this: Fulmer SPICES. Am J Nurs. 2007;107(10):40-8.

14. Zeh P, Sandhu HK, Cannaby AM, Sturt JA. The impact of culturally competent diabetes care interventions for improving diabetes-related outcomes in ethnic minority groups: A systematic review. Diabet Med. 2012;29(10):1237-52. doi: 10.1111/j.1464-5491.2012.03701.x.

15. American Association of Diabetes Educators. Community health workers in diabetes management and prevention (position statement). Diabetes Educ. 2009;35 Suppl 3: 48S-52.

16. Benner P, Hughes RG, Sutphen M. Clinical reasoning, decision-making, and action: thinking critically and clinically. In: Hughes RG, ed. Patient Safety and Quality: An Evidence Based Handbook for Nurses. Rockville, Md: Agency for Healthcare Research and Quality; 2008(cited 2013 Jun 30):1:87-109. On the Internet at: http://www.ncbi.nlm.nih.gov/books/NBK2643/.

17. Bowen JL. Educational strategies to promote clinical diagnostic reasoning. N Engl J Med. 2006;355:2217-25.

18. Anderson RM. Applied principles of teaching and learning. In: Franz MJ, ed. A Core Curriculum for Diabetes Education: Diabetes Education and Program Management. 4th ed. Chicago: American Association of Diabetes Educators; 2001:3-18.

19. Rubin RR, Napora JP. Behavior change. In: Franz MJ, ed. A Core Curriculum for Diabetes Education: Diabetes Education and Program Management. 4th ed. Chicago: American Association of Diabetes Educators; 2001:72-92.

20. Weinger K, McMurrich SJ. Behavioral strategies for improving self-management. In: Childs B, Cypress M, Spollet G, eds. Complete Nurse's Guide to Diabetes Care. Alexandria, Va: American Diabetes Association; 2005:199-206.

21. American Association of Diabetes Educators. Standards for outcome measurement of diabetes self-management education (position statement). Diabetes Educ. 2003; 29(5):804-15.

22. Lipkin M Jr, Putnam SM, Lazare A. The Medical Interview, Clinical Care, Education and Research. New York: Springer-Verlag; 1995:71-2.

23. Tresolini CP; and the Pew-Fetzer Task Force. Health Professions Education and Relationship-Centered Care. San Francisco: Pew Health Professions Commission; 1994.

24. Lewin SA, Skea ZC, Entwistle V, Zwarenstein M, Dick J. Interventions for providers to promote a patient-centered approach in clinical consultations. Cochrane Database Syst Rev. 2001;(4):CD003267.

25. Greenfield S, Kaplan S, Ware JE. Expanding patient involvement in care—effects on patient outcomes. Ann Intern Med. 1985;102:520-8.

26. Orth JE, Stiles WB, Scherwitz L, et al. Interviews and hypertensive patients' blood pressure control. Health Psychol. 1987;6:29-42.

27. Smith RC. Patient-Centered Interviewing: An Evidence-Based Method. 2nd ed. Philadelphia: Lippincott Williams & Wilkins; 2002.

28. Lipkin M Jr, Frankel RM, Beckman HB, et al. Performing the interview. In: Lipkin M Jr, Putnam SM, Lazare A, eds. The Medical Interview: Clinical Care, Education, and Research. New York: Springer-Verlag; 1995:75-6.

29. Stewart M, Brown JB, Donner A, et al. The impact of patient-centered care on outcomes. J Fam Pract. 2000;49: 796-804.

30. Swenson SL, Buell S, Zettler P, White M, Ruston DC, Lo B. Patient-centered communication: do patients really prefer it? J Gen Intern Med. 2004;19:1069-79.

31. Schlundt DG, Pichert JW, Gregory B, Davis D. Eating and diabetes: a patient-centered approach. In: Anderson BJ, Rubin RR, eds. Practical Psychology for Diabetes Clinicians: How to Deal With the Key Behavioral Issues Faced by Patients and Health Care Teams. Alexandria, Va: American Diabetes Association; 1996.

32. Funnell MM, Hunt C, Kulkarni K, Rubin R, eds. A Core Curriculum for Diabetes Education. 3rd ed. Chicago: American Association of Diabetes Educators; 1998.

33. Franz MJ, ed. A Core Curriculum for Diabetes Education: Diabetes Education and Program Management. 4th ed. Chicago: American Association of Diabetes Educators; 2001.

34. Roter D, Hall JA, Kern DE, et al. Improving physicians' interviewing skills and reducing patients' emotional distress: a randomized clinical trial. Arch Intern Med. 1995;155:1877-84.

35. Roter DL, Hall JA. Physicians' interviewing style and medical information obtained from patients. J Gen Intern Med. 1987;2:325-9.

36. Schlundt DG, Rea MR, Kline SS, Pichert JW. Situational obstacles to dietary adherence for adults with diabetes. J Am Diet Assoc. 1994;94:874-6.

37. Anderson BJ, Rubin RR, eds. Practical Psychology for Diabetes Clinicians: How to Deal With the Key Behavioral Issues Faced by Patients and Health Care Teams. Alexandria, Va: American Diabetes Association; 1996.

38. Kralik D, Koch T, Price K, Howard N. Chronic illness self-management: Taking action to create order. J Clin Nurs. 2004;13(2):259-67.

39. Bodenheimer T, Davis C, Holman H. Helping patients adopt healthier behaviors. Clin Diabetes. 2007;25(2): 66-70.

40. Rollnick S, Miller WR, Butler CC. Motivational Interviewing in Health Care: Helping Patients Change Behavior. New York: Guilford Press; 2008.

41. Maryniuk MD. Developing the plan for education. In: Mensing C, ed. The Art and Science of Diabetes

Self-Management Education: A Desk Reference for Health-care Providers. Chicago: American Association of Diabetes Educators; 2006.

42. Cohen-Cole SA, Bird J. Function 2: building rapport and responding to patient's emotions (relationship skills). In: Cohen-Cole SA, ed. The Medical Interview: The Three Function Approach. St. Louis, Mo: Mosby Year Book; 1991:21-6.

43. Schlundt DG, Pichert JW, Gregory B, Davis D. Eating and diabetes: a patient-centered approach. In: Anderson BJ, Rubin RR, eds. Practical Psychology for Diabetes Clinicians: How to Deal with the Key Behavioral Issues Faced by Patients and Health Care Teams. Alexandria, Va: American Diabetes Association; 1996.

44. Chomutare T, Fernandez-Luque L, Arsand E, Hartyigsen G. Features of mobile diabetes applications: review of the literature and analysis of current applications compared against evidence-based guidelines. J Med Internet Res. 2011;13(3):e65.

45. Krathwohl DR. A Revision of Bloom's Taxonomy: An Overview. Theory Pract. 2002;41(4):212-8.

46. Gibson PG, Powell H, Coughlan J, et al. Self-management education and regular practitioner review for adults with asthma. Cochrane Database Syst Rev. 2003;(1):CD001117.

47. Sheeran P, Orbell S. Using implementation intentions to increase attendance for cervical cancer screening. Health Psychol. 2000;19(3):283-9.

48. Lorenzi GM. Implementation of diabetes education. In: Mensing C, ed. The Art and Science of Diabetes Self-Management Education: A Desk Reference for Healthcare Providers. Chicago: American Association of Diabetes Educators; 2006.

49. Office of Minority Health and Health Disparities. Eliminating racial and ethnic health disparities (cited 2013 Jun 30). On the Internet at: http://www.cdc.gov/omhd/About/disparities.htm.

50. Pfizer. The Newest Vital Sign: a health literacy assessment tool for patient care and research (cited 2013 Jun 30). On the Internet at: http://www.pfizerhealthliteracy.com/public-policy-researchers/NewestVitalSign.aspx.

51. Ad Hoc Committee on Health Literacy for the Council on Scientific Affairs, American Medical Association. Health literacy: Report of the Council on Scientific Affairs. JAMA. 1999;281(6):552-7.

52. Osborne H. Health Literacy from A to Z: Practical Ways to Communicate Your Health Message. Sudbury, Ma: Jones and Bartlett; 2005.

53. Doak CC, Doak LG, Root JH. Teaching Patients With Low Literacy Skills. Philadelphia, Pa: JB Lippincott Co; 1996 (cited 2013 Jun 30). On the Internet at: http://www.hsph.harvard.edu/healthliteracy/resources/teaching-patients-with-low-literacy-skills/.

54. Weiss BD, Blanchard JS, McGee DL, et al. Illiteracy among Medicaid recipients and its relationship to health care costs. J Health Care Poor Underserved. 1994;5(20):99-111.

55. National Diabetes Education Program. Changing the way diabetes is treated. 2012 (cited 2014 Apr 17). On the Internet at: http://ndep.nih.gov/media/NDEP_15th_year_508.pdf.

56. Thackeray R, Merrill RM, Neiger BL. Disparities in diabetes management practice between racial and ethnic groups in the United States. Diabetes Educ. 2004;30:665-75.

57. Tessaro I, Smith S, Rye S. Knowledge and perceptions of diabetes in an Appalachian population. Prev Chronic Dis. 2005;2(2):1-9.

58. Stevenson D. Story Theatre Method. Colorado Springs, Co: Cornelia Press; 2008.

59. Haigh C, Hardy P. Tell me a story—a conceptual exploration of storytelling in healthcare education. Nurse Educ Today. 2011;31(4):408-11.

60. Greene JA, Choudhry NK, Kilabuk E, Shrank WH. Online social networking by patients with diabetes: A qualitative evaluation of communication with Facebook. J Gen Intern Med. 2011;26(3):287-92.

61. Atkinson A, Radjenovic D. Meeting quality standards for self-management education in pediatric type 2 diabetes. Diabetes Spectr. 2007;20(1):40-6.

62. Redman BK. The Practice of Patient Education. 9th ed. St Louis, Mo: Mosby; 2001.

63. Grey M, Boland ED, Davidson M, et al. Coping skills training for youth with diabetes mellitus has long-lasting effects on metabolic control and quality of life. J Pediatr. 2000;137:107-13.

64. Knowles M. Adult Learner: A Neglected Species. Houston, TX: Gulf Publishing Co; 1990.

65. Suhl E, Bonsignor P. Diabetes self-management education for older adults: general principles and practical application. Diabetes Spectr. 2006;19:234-40.

66. Baker College. Teaching across generations. 2004 (cited 2013 Jun 14). On the Internet at: http://www.mcc.edu/pdf/pdo/teaching_across_gen.pdf.

67. Fisher EB, Brownson CA, O'Toole ML, et al. Ongoing follow-up and support for chronic disease management in the Robert Wood Johnson Foundation Diabetes Initiative. Diabetes Educ. 2007;33(6):201S-7.

68. Mensing CR, Norris SL. Group education in diabetes: effectiveness and implementation. Diabetes Spectr. 2003;16:96-103.

69. Funnell MM, Anderson RM. Empowerment and self-management of diabetes. Clin Diabetes. 2004;22(3):123-7.

70. Glazier R, Bajcar J, Kennie N, et al. A systematic review of interventions to improve diabetes care in socially disadvantaged populations. Diabetes Care. 2006;29:1675-88.

71. Hill-Briggs F, Lazo M, Peyrot M, et al. Effect of problem-solving-based diabetes self-management training on diabetes control in a low income patient sample. J Gen Intern Med. 2011;26(9):972-8. doi: 10.1007/s11606-011-1689-6

72. Funnell MM, Tang TS, Anderson RM. Empowerment-based diabetes self-management support. Diabetes Spectr. 2007;20(4):221-6.

73. Rickheim P, Weaver T, Flader J, Kendall D. Assessment of group versus individual diabetes education. Diabetes Care. 2002;25:269-74.

74. Steinsbekk A, Rygg L, Lisulo M, et al. Group based diabetes self-management education compared to routine treatment for people with type 2 diabetes mellitus. A systematic review with meta-analysis. BMC Health Serv Res. 2012;12:213. doi: 10.1186/1472-6963-12-213

75. Sperl-Hillen J, Beaton S, Fernandes O, et al. Comparative effectiveness of patient education methods for type 2 diabetes: A randomized controlled trial. Arch Intern Med. 2011;171(22):2001-10.

76. Clark R, Nguyen F, Sweller J. Efficiency in Learning: Evidence-based Guidelines to Manage Cognitive Load. San Francisco: Wiley; 2006.

77. Medina J. Brain Rules. Seattle, Wash: Pearl Press; 2008.

78. Merriam SG, Caffarella RS. Learning in Adulthood: A Comprehensive Guide. 2nd ed. San Francisco: Jossey-Bass; 1999.

79. Bransford JD, Brown AL, Cocking RR, eds. How People Learn: Brain, Mind, Experience, and School. Washington, DC: National Academy Press; 2000 (cited 2013 Jun 30). On the Internet at: http://www.nap.edu/catalog.php?record_id=9853.

80. Jensen E. Brain-based Learning: The New Paradigm of Teaching. 2nd ed. Thousand Oaks, Calif: Corwin Press; 2008.

81. American Association of Diabetes Educators. Diabetes education for people with disabilities (position statement). Diabetes Educ. 2002;28(6):916-21.

82. Americans with Disabilities Act of 1990: Public Law 101-336, 101st Congress. Washington, DC: US Government Printing Office; 1990.

83. Zgibor J, Songer T. External barriers to diabetes care: Addressing personal and health systems issues. Diabetes Spectr. 2001;14(1):23-8.

84. Zrebiec JF, Jacobson AM. What attracts patients with diabetes to an internet support group? A 21-month longitudinal website study. Diabet Med. 2001;18(2):154-8.

85. Barak A, Boneil-Nissim M, Suler J. Fostering empowerment in online support groups. Comput Human Behav. 2008;24(5):1867-83.

86. American Diabetes Association. School walk for diabetes (cited 2013 Jun 16). On the Internet at: http://schoolwalk.diabetes.org/site/PageServer?pagename=SW_teach.

87. American Association of Diabetes Educators. Competencies for Diabetes Educators: A Companion Document to the Guidelines for the Practice of Diabetes Educators. 2009 (cited 2013 Jun 16). On the Internet at: www.diabeteseducator.org/competencies.

88. Seley J, Weinger K. Barriers to optimal care for patients with diabetes and strategies to overcome them. AJN. 2007; 107(6 suppl):4-5.

89. Mensing C, Boucher J, Cypress M, et al. National standards for diabetes self-management education. Task force to review and revise the National Standards for Diabetes Self-Management Education Programs. Diabetes Care. 2000;23:682-9.

90. Report of the task force on the delivery of diabetes self-management education and medical nutrition therapy. Diabetes Spectr. 1999;12:44-7.

91. Mulcahy K. Management of diabetes education programs. In: Franz MJ, ed. A Core Curriculum for Diabetes Educators: Diabetes Education and Program Management. 5th ed. Chicago: American Association of Diabetes Educators; 2003:181-218.

92. Lacey K, Pritchett E. Nutrition care process and model: ADA adopts road map to quality care and outcomes management. J Am Diet Assoc. 2003;103(8):1061-72.

93. Hagger MS, Chatzisarantis NLD, Harris J. From Psychological Need Satisfaction to Intentional Behavior: Testing a Motivational Sequence in Two Behavioral Contexts. Pers Soc Psychol Bull. 2006;32(2):131-48.

94. Lorig K. Patient Education: A Practical Approach. 3rd ed. Thousand Oaks, Calif: Sage Publications, 2001.

CHAPTER 3

Theoretical and Behavioral Approaches to the Self-Management of Health

Martha M. Funnell, MS, RN, CDE
Gretchen A. Piatt, MPH, PhD
Bob Anderson, EdD

Key Concepts

◈ Be familiar with behavioral and educational theories, models, and approaches that support self-management of health. These include the Health Belief Model, Social Cognitive Theory, the Theory of Reasoned Action and Theory of Planned Behavior, and the Transtheoretical Model, with its construct of stages of change.

◈ Be aware that some models and approaches go beyond theories that address the behavior of patients. Patient empowerment and motivational interviewing describe the skills, expertise, and values needed by educators to effectively engage in patient-centered, collaborative diabetes care, education, and ongoing support.

◈ Learn to assess whether a theory will assist in understanding the intended goals and purpose if applied in the specific situation, for example, in program design or individual practice. Will the theory describe, explain, predict, or influence outcomes as desired?

◈ Think critically about the appropriateness of a theory if it is applied to program design or individual practice: Does the theory resonate within this context? Does it extend thinking? Is the approach useful in this situation? Can its main attributes be measured if applied in this situation?

◈ Think critically about depending solely on models that focus only on patient behavior versus including one of the models that address the skills, expertise, and values necessary to effectively engage in patient-centered, collaborative diabetes care and education.

◈ Be able to choose an approach that includes behavior change as well as addresses the emotional, psychosocial, cultural, and health literacy issues that significantly influence self-management behaviors and quality of life.

Introduction

The mission of diabetes self-management education and support (DSME/S) is to help individuals with diabetes acquire the knowledge, skills, attitudes, and behaviors needed to optimize both self-management of their diabetes and their quality of life. The field of diabetes education has advanced substantially over the past 30 years. Originally, diabetes education focused on acquiring knowledge and skills. More recently, diabetes education focused on behavior change as both a strategy and an outcome. However, it has become clear that neither of these approaches to DSME/S is adequate to accomplish this mission. Knowledge and behavior-change strategies are necessary components of DSME/S, but they are not enough to ensure that patients and their families are adequately prepared to live well with a lifelong chronic illness. Because diabetes-related distress and other psychosocial issues profoundly affect self-management behaviors, these issues also must be addressed as part of the educational process.[1]

Ideally, modern diabetes education programs focus on helping people with diabetes identify and adopt the behaviors and coping strategies that will optimize their diabetes self-management and overall well-being. These education programs address knowledge and skill acquisition, but they include much more. For example, they both teach and help patients learn how to solve problems and set goals, they address the psychosocial aspects of diabetes along with the clinical aspects, they help the person with diabetes define and acquire social support, and they provide the knowledge and skills necessary for effective coping and managing diabetes in challenging social situations and personal relationships.

The role of the diabetes educator has evolved as well. To be effective, the modern diabetes educator needs to have the interpersonal skills, expertise, and values necessary to effectively engage in patient-centered, collaborative diabetes care and education. Because of the need for ongoing support throughout a lifetime of diabetes, providing ongoing diabetes self-management support (DSMS) programs as follow-up to initial DSME is now a prominent component of the National Standards for DSME/S.[2] Diabetes educators also need the skills to provide DSMS, which can include psychosocial, behavioral, educational, and clinical support.[2,3]

The purpose of this introduction is not to list all the attributes of modern DSME/S or to address all of the variables that influence behavior, but to illustrate how complex and sophisticated this specialty has become. In addition to having clinical and teaching skills, today's diabetes educator needs to understand and be able to apply theoretical approaches to facilitating healthy coping and self-directed behavior change. Moreover, those involved in this educational effort need to be able to distinguish and combine evidence-based theories with sophisticated approaches to behavior change that have proved efficacious in DSME. The purpose of this chapter is

to help educators gain the knowledge necessary to develop and apply a sound theory-based approach to DSME and ongoing DSMS.

Before presenting several major theoretical approaches related to self-management behavior of those with diabetes, this chapter outlines considerations pertinent to choosing theories appropriately for application in diabetes education. After discussing how to choose theories to apply to a program or individual practice, the chapter describes 4 theories that are of value in understanding an individual's health behavior. The chapter ends with a description of 2 approaches shown to be effective in facilitating self-directed behavior change to illustrate how to put a theory into practice. Each approach is summarized and the body of evidence regarding its use in diabetes education is reviewed. It should be noted that many theories, models, and approaches from the fields of nursing, education, and psychology are relevant for diabetes educators. The theoretical approaches chosen for this chapter were selected because of their frequent use by diabetes educators and the amount of available evidence. They also serve as examples of how to choose a theory or model and then use an approach (eg, patient empowerment, motivational interviewing) that is consistent with the theory or model in practice. This chapter is meant to be illustrative rather than definitive and will address the following:

◆ Health Belief Model
◆ Social Cognitive Theory
◆ Theory of Reasoned Action and Theory of Planned Behavior
◆ Transtheoretical Model, specifically the construct of stages of change
◆ Patient empowerment
◆ Motivational interviewing

Applying Theory in Diabetes Education

The words "theory," "model," and "approach" were used several times in the introduction. Although these words are often used interchangeably, they are somewhat different. A *theory* is a set of assumptions or facts that attempt to provide an explanation or link for an observed phenomenon. A *model* is a representation of a phenomenon and is sometimes used to explain or apply a theory. This chapter includes *theoretical approaches* to behavior change, which are ways to put into practice a theory or philosophy.

Before an educator selects specific theories, models, and/or approaches to apply in program design or individual practice, he or she needs to think about the usefulness of theories and approaches in producing the desired outcomes. To be effective, educators need to carefully choose the theories and approaches to behavior and education they will apply—both for individual practice and in the design, conduct, and evaluation of education programs.[4] Chosen wisely, the theories help members of the diabetes care team understand the behavior of the individuals with diabetes whom they serve and subsequently teach them effective strategies for making self-directed behavioral changes. With a clear conception of what theories and approaches to behavior change are and how they can be used, educators are then prepared to compare the relative merits of each and choose those most suitable to their situation.

Matching Theory With Purpose

Behavioral and educational theories are usually selected for use in educational program design and individual practice based on how well they meet 1 or more of the following 4 purposes: describing, explaining, predicting, and controlling/influencing health behavior.[5–7]

Describing

The first purpose of a theory is describing the phenomena of interest. The theory tells us the way things are, but not why they are the way they are or how they are likely to change. The value of descriptive theory is largely dependent on how coherent and thorough it is. For example, suppose you noticed that patients graduating from the diabetes education program on the east side of town got consistently higher scores on the same knowledge test than patients graduating from another program on the west side of town. You could begin theory building by developing a thorough description about what you have observed. How many observations were involved? Were the differences in test scores always in the same direction and similar in magnitude? Were the patients in both programs similar (eg, age, gender, socioeconomic status)? Were

the educators in both programs Certified Diabetes Educators? Do both educational programs meet the National Standards for DSME/S? Do both programs provide DSMS? Are families included in the education program? The answers to these and similar questions would constitute your descriptive theory.

Explaining

The second purpose of a theory is explanation. Your descriptive theory has answered the question "What is happening?" Now attention turns to the question "Why is it happening?" You want to know what is causing the differences in the knowledge test scores. You could carefully examine the descriptions of the 2 programs you observed to determine whether you could enhance your theory by incorporating an explanation of what you observed. If the only significant difference you found between the 2 programs was that the east-side program provided 60% more instructional time than the other, you might theorize that increasing the amount of time spent on instruction accounted for the better test results.

Predicting

The third purpose of a theory is prediction. Using the example above, your new educational theory would be considered robust if it proved to be true in other settings (ie, other diabetes programs). Consistent correlations, in the expected direction between instructional time and educational achievement, derived from data found in other studies would support a prediction of similar results based on these factors.

Controlling or Influencing

Your new educational theory would be viewed as even more robust and useful if you conducted experiments that demonstrated that you could increase instructional time to produce better educational outcomes. The ability of your theory to influence educational achievement in this example could be contrasted with a theory that is less useful (eg, a theory about IQ and learning) because it cannot be manipulated to produce better outcomes.

Choosing a Theory That Fits

When choosing a theory and/or approach to apply to a program design or for working with individual patients, 3 areas of inquiry are important to consider:

how well the theory resonates with you, how the theory extends your thinking, and how useful the theory appears to be.

Does It Resonate?

The first area of inquiry addresses the compatibility between the theory and your sense of how people learn and behave. Questions to ask are, Does this theory fit with my experiences of how I learn and change? and Does this theory resonate with how I view my patients and my approach to them? Does it fit with how I define success when I provide diabetes education? Those working in diabetes education are unlikely to make effective use of a theory unless they feel an affinity for the vision or world view embedded in it.

Does It Extend Thinking?

The second area of inquiry considers whether the theory helps organize and expand your ideas and observations into a coherent pattern. Questions to ask are, Does this theory provide a thorough description of the phenomena of interest? Does this theory offer a plausible explanation for why things happen the way they do? Does this theory help me to better understand and relate to my patients? Does the theory challenge me to reflect on aspects of my practice or program design that I may not have considered fully? In other words, is the theory consistent with your perspective on learning and behaving, and does it help enhance and expand your perspective and practice?

Is This Approach Useful?

The third area of inquiry should address the utility of the theory. Questions to ask are, Can this theory be translated into specific practice behaviors or strategies (approach) that will help me become a more effective educator? Does this theory help me design and evaluate my education program? Will my patients benefit from this approach?

Choosing an Approach That Can Be Measured

A theory's usefulness is very much related to the user's ability to measure its main attributes. The user will need to answer the following questions: What measures/instruments exist to evaluate this theory? Have these measures/instruments been shown to be valid and reliable in similar populations? Are they sensitive to change? Have the measures been used successfully in previous diabetes education and support studies?

Ensure the theory is appropriate to the specific practice or program:

- Is there a convincing evidence base indicating that this theory can be used to facilitate learning and behavior change, and impact quality of life effectively?
- Is it a good fit with the kind of diabetes care and education I provide?
- Can this theory help guide my interactions with patients and program design in one or more of these ways: Can I visualize how I would apply this theory in one-to-one interactions with patients? Can I visualize how I would apply this theory when group teaching? Can I incorporate this theory into the design of my program?
- After conducting some sessions or programs, will it be apparent whether this theory has improved my practice or programs?
- After conducting some sessions or programs, will it be apparent whether this theory is viewed positively by my patients?
- Do I possess the knowledge, skills, and experience to use this theoretical approach to practice patient-centered, collaborative DSME and/or DSMS?

Combining Theories and Approaches to Behavior Change

Educators can and often do use more than 1 theory or combine a theory with an approach to behavior change in individual practice and in developing education and ongoing support programs. When using a combination of theories, compatibility is important; the theories must embody the same world view. Also, each theory or approach must independently contribute to the user's effectiveness. For example:

⬧ *The patient empowerment approach posits this:* Individuals will carry out self-management tasks more consistently and over a longer period of time if those tasks were freely chosen by patients to help them reach their own goals.[8]

⬧ *The Health Belief Model posits this:* The health-related choices people make are a function of their beliefs about their susceptibility to the disease (diabetes, in this instance) and its complications, the severity of diabetes and its complications, the efficacy of available treatments, and the ability to carry out those treatment options.[9]

⬧ *In combination:* These 2 frameworks could be combined and incorporated into the design of a DSME and/or a DSMS program. Patient empowerment could be used as the program's overall approach to facilitating self-directed behavior change and healthy coping, and the Health Belief Model could be used to order and sequence the educational content of the program.

At both the individual practitioner and program levels, theories and approaches to behavior change can be important tools for the design, understanding, and conduct of DSME and DSMS. Theory-based practice and evaluation add to professionals' understanding of how to be effective educators, and enhance the credibility of the profession.

Theoretical Approaches to Behavior Change

Four current and well-developed approaches to influencing the health behavior of persons with diabetes are described in this section:

⬧ Health Belief Model
⬧ Social Cognitive Theory
⬧ Theory of Reasoned Action and Theory of Planned Behavior
⬧ Transtheoretical Model

In addition, this section describes 2 well-developed approaches to facilitating self-directed behavior change

that are effective at improving diabetes self-management and quality of life:

⬧ Patient empowerment
⬧ Motivational interviewing

This chapter describes each theory and approach and its primary components, applies the theory/approach to diabetes-related behavior, and summarizes the research to date that has been used to evaluate the theory in understanding and promoting diabetes self-management. The case shows how the principles embedded in each approach can be applied to a diabetes-specific patient example. Tables throughout the chapter summarize information on each approach and then address issues pertinent to the case so readers can see the differences and similarities among the components of each model.

Health Belief Model

The Health Belief Model (HBM) has been widely used as a theoretical framework to understand health behavior change and maintenance.[9,10] The model was first introduced in the 1950s when behavioral scientists at the US Public Health Service sought to understand the low participation rates in government-sponsored, cost-free, and easily accessible screening, detection, and immunization programs.[9,11] As the model matured, the nature of events underlying beliefs about health problems was extended to include diagnosed conditions, such as diabetes.[12] The HBM underscores the importance of individuals' perceived risk and perceived seriousness as part of their health beliefs and determines the likelihood of adopting preventive health behaviors.[13] The more an individual perceives himself or herself to be at a particular health risk and considers this risk to be serious and important, the more likely it is that he or she will make the necessary changes to prevent health problems from occurring.

Under this model, a patient's decision to perform a "target" health behavior is influenced by the following factors[9]:

⬧ Level of personal vulnerability the patient feels about developing the illness
⬧ How serious the patient believes the illness is or has the potential to be

◈ Efficacy of the behavior, in the patient's view, in preventing the development or minimizing the consequences of the illness

◈ Costs or deterrents associated with performing the behavior relative to the benefits achieved as a result

When it was determined that self-efficacy fit conceptually within the HBM framework and was a strong predictor of health behaviors, an expanded HBM that incorporates readiness and self-efficacy was developed to provide a more powerful approach to understanding health-related behavior.[9,14] The Expanded Health Belief Model (EHBM) has become the most frequently used theoretical model to predict health behaviors.[15] The 2 additional constructs are the following[9]:

◈ Cues to action
◈ Self-efficacy

Table 3.1 provides definitions of the expanded model's constructs and examples of these constructs in relation to diabetes self-management. Of these, beliefs about treatment effectiveness and seriousness are most important in diabetes self-management,

although the emotional response to diabetes may influence the relationship between beliefs and behaviors.[10]

Evidence Base

A large body of research has utilized the HBM in explaining diabetes self-care behaviors.[13–26] Among a sample of 31 African-American women diagnosed with type 2 diabetes, Koch investigated differences between women who engaged in regular physical activity and those who did not.[16] He found significant group differences in the perceived benefits and perceived barriers: The physical activity group reported greater perceived benefits and fewer perceived barriers than their counterparts. Another study conducted by Aljasem and colleagues examined the role of barriers and self-efficacy in self-management behaviors in 309 individuals diagnosed with type 2 diabetes.[17] The data revealed that the more barriers patients perceived to performing self-care behaviors, the less likely they were to follow a healthy diet or engage in physical activity. Additionally, patients who reported a greater level of self-efficacy were more likely to test their blood glucose frequently and less likely to forget to take

TABLE 3.1 Health Belief Model: Constructs and Application to Diabetes Self-Management		
Construct	*Definition*	*Case*
Perceived susceptibility	Estimate of personal vulnerability of developing an illness	MG's A1C levels have been high for 5 years, and her father had gone blind as a result of diabetes. Therefore, she believes her risk level for developing diabetes-related complications is high.
Perceived severity	Perception of how serious an illness is and can be if diagnosed	MG thinks that if she does not keep her blood glucose closer to normal she will go blind or lose a leg because of her diabetes.
Perceived benefits	Perception of how a specific action will lead to a positive outcome	MG believes that checking her blood glucose frequently and taking her diabetes medication as prescribed will substantially minimize the long-term chances of her going blind or having her leg amputated.
Perceived barriers	Perception of the deterrents to engaging in a behavior or the costs associated with a behavior	MG feels that checking her blood glucose several times a day is a burden. She also does not want her coworkers to find out she has diabetes because she is worried they will start monitoring what she eats throughout the day.
Self-efficacy	Level of confidence one has in engaging in the identified health behavior	MG feels fairly confident that she can find a private place to check her blood glucose during the workday.
Cues to action	External stimulus used to activate health behavior	MG sees TV commercials about the latest blood glucose monitors and remembers to check her own blood glucose.

their medication or engage in binge-eating behavior. In the same vein, Cerkoney and Hart demonstrated that, in a group of people taking insulin for their diabetes, there was a positive correlation between the patient's adherence to guidelines and his or her belief model score.[23] A recent study was conducted to develop a behavioral model to better understand the mechanisms for the effectiveness of text-message-based DSME for African Americans with type 2 diabetes.[24] Surveys conducted with participants at the end of the program revealed that their self-management was influenced through multiple behavioral constructs, including health beliefs, self-efficacy, and social support. This information will be used to create a framework for future programs that use this technology. The HBM has also been used as the framework for conducting focus groups to develop educational materials for weight management for African-American women[25] and for the Diabetes and Healthy Eyes Toolkit.[26]

Although all of the aforementioned findings are important, to date, there has not been a substantial amount of literature on using the HBM as a basis for DSME interventions in people with type 2 diabetes. Indeed, substantially more research has been conducted on the use of the HBM in individuals with type 1 diabetes, where adherence to a treatment plan (ie, insulin use) is of critical importance. Charron-Prochownik and colleagues examined the use of the HBM in terms of understanding young children's health beliefs and diabetes regimen adherence.[14] They found that, overall, both children and their parents reported moderate to very strong health beliefs (eg, diabetes is severe), while barriers to management were perceived as low to moderate as predicted by the HBM. Also, both children and parents reported high degrees of self-efficacy, as they felt very confident in being able to assist in performing diabetes self-care behaviors and carrying out the diabetes treatment plan. Children's perception of the severity of their illness, barriers to treatment, and self-efficacy were found to be significantly correlated with observable adherence or metabolic control. In a second study conducted by Charron-Prochownik and colleagues, the objective was to identify significant correlates among constructs of the EHBM with reproductive behaviors and metabolic control in teens with type 1 diabetes.[15] It was found that being

told by a healthcare professional to seek out preconception counseling was a motivational cue that triggered an action step. Several major constructs of the EHBM were significantly correlated with beneficial reproductive health behaviors and metabolic control.

The HBM has also been applied to diabetes self-management research conducted outside the United States.[27–29] In a sample of 128 Chinese men and women diagnosed with type 2 diabetes, Tan reported that subjects who felt a greater vulnerability of developing diabetes-related complications, who believed diabetes to be a very serious condition, and who reported fewer deterrents to engaging in self-care behaviors were more likely to engage in diabetes-related preventive care behaviors.[27] Similarly, a study conducted with 34 aboriginal subjects with type 2 diabetes living in British Columbia found perceived severity and perceived barriers to be predictors of A1C improvement over a period of 18 months.[28] Moreover, subjects who believed diabetes to be a serious condition and reported fewer barriers to self-management at 18 months were more likely to have reduced their A1C between baseline and an 18-month follow-up.

Given the research supporting the HBM in explaining and predicting diabetes self-management behaviors, it is not surprising that many researchers have used it as the framework in designing self-management interventions. For instance, using this model as a framework, Wdowik et al conducted focus groups and interviews with college students diagnosed with type 1 diabetes to explore factors associated with diabetes self-management practices.[30] The results identified prominent barriers to self-care in this group, including such things as economic constraints, stress, fear of hypoglycemic events, and dietary restrictions. Findings from this qualitative study were used to design an intervention called "Control on Campus." The researchers found that students assigned to the intervention group demonstrated greater improvements in diabetes-related knowledge, attitudes, and behaviors than the control group. Specifically, they found at the end of the study that the intervention students reported reduced anxiety around glucose testing, greater frequency of glucose testing, and greater likelihood of glucose testing when experiencing symptoms.

Following the constructs of the HBM, Scollan-Koliopoulos developed and implemented a church-based educational intervention aimed at improving foot care among African Americans diagnosed with type 2 diabetes.[31] Prior to the intervention, participants completed self-report surveys assessing their perceived risk for diabetes-related amputation as well as beliefs and behaviors related to amputation. The intervention consisted of 3 parts: viewing a video on how to perform foot care, observing a foot care demonstration by a healthcare provider, and developing the skills to use a monofilament. In addition, participants were given educational materials on diabetes and foot care. Following this intervention, several participants served as outreach educators and disseminated information to 27 other African Americans, distributed 36 pamphlets, and demonstrated foot care to 12 others.

Wang et al compared the strength of 3 theories (HBM, Theory of Reasoned Action, and Social Cognitive Therapy) in predicting reproductive health behavioral intention among 87 adolescent women with type 1 diabetes. The HBM was the strongest predictor of pre-conception planning, with perceived barriers, cues to action, and self-efficacy (from Social Cognitive Theory) as the constructs that significantly affected intention.[32]

Social Cognitive Theory

Social Cognitive Theory (SCT) evolved from Bandura's Social Learning Theory (SLT), which states that individuals learn not only from their own personal experiences but also from observing the behaviors and behavioral consequences of others.[33] Adding further complexity, SCT examines health behavior as a constantly changing and evolving interaction between the individual and his or her environment. Social Cognitive Theory contains multiple constructs that can be used to understand health behavior change. This section describes the major constructs and applies them to diabetes self-management. Social Cognitive Theory addresses 2 areas[9]:

- Psychosocial factors that influence health behavior
- Methods of stimulating behavior change

Table 3.2 presents and defines the concepts of SCT and applies them to an example of diabetes self-management.

Evidence Base

Social Cognitive Theory has been widely used in understanding diabetes care practices and designing diabetes intervention programs. The theory has been applied to people with type 1 diabetes or type 2 diabetes and used across different age groups, including adolescents and adults.[33-42] Self-management interventions have focused on the following:

- Increasing physical activity
- Improving dietary choices and patterns
- Promoting frequent blood glucose testing

A literature review conducted by Allen examined the research, from 1985 to 2002, on the role of SCT, specifically the construct of self-efficacy, in explaining and predicting physical activity and the long-term maintenance of activity among people with diabetes.[33] Of the 13 studies reviewed that met preestablished criteria, all studies with a correlational design found a significant positive association between self-efficacy and physical activity, and all studies with a predictive design found self-efficacy to be a significant predictor for physical activity. The studies that specifically examined physical activity maintenance found that self-efficacy predicted patient ability to sustain physical activity over the study follow-up period.

Other self-management studies using SCT as a framework have focused exclusively on improving dietary habits. For instance, Miller et al applied the SCT principles of expectations and self-efficacy in developing a 10-week intervention aimed at increasing food label knowledge and skills among 93 older individuals recently diagnosed with type 2 diabetes.[35] Compared with the control group, subjects in the experimental group demonstrated a greater knowledge of food labels and a greater number of positive outcome expectations. The experimental group also reported greater confidence for engaging in behaviors that facilitated self-management and avoiding behaviors that deterred self-management.

Glasgow et al created a brief computer-assisted intervention focused on healthy eating and weight loss for type 2 diabetes patients and compared the effects with a computer-aided enhanced usual care group in a randomized controlled trial among primary care patients.[37] The intervention was based on SCT and included computer-based self-management assessment and feedback, tailored goal-setting, barrier

TABLE 3.2 Social Cognitive Theory: Concepts, Definitions, and Application to Diabetes Self-Management

Concept	Definition	Case
Reciprocal determinism	The constant interaction of the individual, behavior, and environment	MG wants to take better care of her diabetes, so she cooks lower fat dinners. Her family complains that the meals do not taste good. Additionally, fresh produce is very costly at the local grocery. Given these issues, after 2 weeks MG returns to her previous style of cooking.
Environment	The external factors and surroundings of an individual	The climate and atmosphere of MG's home/family, work, community, neighborhood, social circle, etc.
Behavioral capability	The knowledge and skills required to perform a specific behavior	MG recently attended a DSME/S program in which she learned how to check her blood glucose in a way that does not invite attention or disrupt her workday. As a result, her capability in performing this behavior is high.
Expectations	The outcome that an individual anticipates as a result of performing a specific behavior	MG believes that if she starts exercising and playing tennis regularly, her A1C will probably be lower at the next physician visit.
Observational learning	Utilizing the experiences of others' performance of a behavior as a way to acquire that specific behavior	MG has seen her father's health deteriorate as a result of not taking care of his diabetes. He also did not receive annual retinopathy screenings. At the age of 64, her father went blind. Due to this experience, MG has received annual eye exams.
Reinforcements	The responses an individual receives that facilitate or deter the future performance of a specific behavior	Three weeks after starting tennis, MG noticed her clothes were fitting better. This weight loss served as a positive reinforcement for her to continue playing tennis 3 times per week.
Self-efficacy	The level of confidence an individual has with regard to performing a behavior successfully	Given that MG enjoys playing tennis and uses it as a time to socialize with her friends, she has a high level of confidence that this will remain a permanent part of her lifestyle.

identification, and problem solving, followed by a health counselor interaction and follow-up calls. The participants assigned to the SCT computer-aided group reduced their dietary fat and weight significantly more than patients in the enhanced usual care group at the end of the 2-month intervention.

Some studies have developed SCT-guided interventions to improve multiple diabetes care–related behaviors. Toobert and colleagues utilized SCT principles in developing the Mediterranean Lifestyle Trial, an intervention aimed at preventing coronary heart disease among high-risk women diagnosed with type 2 diabetes.[38] These authors hypothesize that self-efficacy, along with other concepts, is a key mechanism in improving and maintaining self-care behaviors such as healthy nutritional choices, physical activity, and emotional coping.

Finally, a more recent study used SCT to implement a culturally adapted, brief DSME program for Native Hawaiians and Pacific People—Partners in Care.[39] Emphasis was placed on the SCT constructs of behavioral capability, self-control, emotional response, and self-efficacy. In the short term, participants in the program experienced significant improvements in A1C and in understanding and performing diabetes self-management. The authors hypothesize that combining the theoretical framework with community-based peer education, cultural adaptation, and use of focus groups in program development increased the effectiveness of the program.

Self-efficacy, as one component of SCT, was used as the basis for the development and implementation of a standardized peer-based program in diabetes: the Stanford Diabetes Self-Management Program (DSMP), offered in-person[40] or online[41] and adapted into Spanish.[42] This program was an adaption of an evidence-based chronic disease self-management program.[43]

The online DSMP program showed improvements in activation and self-efficacy, which were sustained at 18 months.[41] In the English-speaking community-based program, participants showed initial improvements in depression, symptoms of hypoglycemia, communication with physicians, healthy eating, reading food labels, patient activation, and self-efficacy. At 12 months, improvements were sustained for depression, communication with physicians, healthy eating, patient activation, and self-efficacy.[40] In the Spanish-speaking community-based program, health distress, symptoms of hypo- and hyperglycemia, and self-efficacy significantly improved and were sustained at 18 months.[42] In addition, further improvements were found at 18 months for self-rated health, communication with physicians, and fewer emergency room visits. Both the online and the Spanish-speaking programs demonstrated statistically significant improvements in A1C; however, the in-person program did not.

Theory of Reasoned Action and Theory of Planned Behavior

The Theory of Reasoned Action (TRA), developed by Fishbein, is extended by Azjen in the Theory of Planned Behavior (TPB).[44,45] This combined model (TRA-TPB) of behavior change operates through 3 major constructs:

- Attitude and beliefs the individual has toward the target health behavior
- How the individual thinks others in the general public or community view the health behavior (subjective norm)
- Extent to which the individual is equipped with the knowledge and skills to perform the behavior (perceived behavioral control)

These 3 constructs work together to determine how strong an individual's intention is related to performing the health behavior, which, consequently, leads to the likelihood that the individual will demonstrate the health behavior.[9] Table 3.3 lists the elements of the TRA-TPB model and applies them to a diabetes-specific example.

Evidence Base

A study conducted by Syrajala and colleagues utilized the TRA-TPB to examine the relationship between dental care practices and diabetes self-management among people diagnosed with type 1 diabetes.[46] In a sample of 149 patients ages 16 to 72 attending a

TABLE 3.3   Theory of Reasoned Action and Theory of Planned Behavior—Concepts and Application to Diabetes Self-Management

Concept	Case
Attitude and beliefs about behavior	MG believes that physical activity is an effective method of managing her blood glucose levels.
Subjective norm	MG values the opinion of her healthcare team (physician, nurse educator, and dietitian), who have all recommended that engaging in some type of physical activity will help manage her diabetes.
Perceived behavioral control	MG would like to play tennis as her physical activity. She took tennis lessons in the past, knows there are tennis courts near her house, and has 2 friends who have offered to play with her.
Behavioral intention	Based on the factors above, MG's intention to start playing tennis as one way of managing her diabetes is fairly strong.
Behavior	MG incorporates physical activity into her schedule 3 times a week for 60 minutes.

diabetes clinic affiliated with a teaching institution in Finland, these researchers found a significant positive relationship between attitudes toward and normative beliefs related to toothbrushing and toothbrushing intentions and behavior. Additionally, individuals who expressed a greater intention to brush their teeth were more likely to report more frequent brushing behavior. Finally, individuals with better attitudes and greater intentions to brush demonstrated better diabetes self-management and had lower A1C levels, respectively.

Components of the TRA-TPB have been integrated into a proposed prevention program targeting minority children at risk for developing type 2 diabetes. Specifically, Burnet et al outlined the TRA-TPB–related constructs, including beliefs and knowledge, attitudes, normative beliefs, and behavioral intention, as critical aspects of prevention behavior.[47] Burnet et al theorize that a child's beliefs and knowledge about an illness or associated health behaviors influence the child's attitudes about the health behavior. In turn, attitudes in combination with a child's belief about the public perception of the health behavior (normative beliefs) factor into the child's intention to perform the behavior. Finally, a child's level of intention to take action will ultimately determine the actual occurrence of the health behavior.

Transtheoretical Model

The Transtheoretical Model (TTM) was first introduced by Prochaska et al as a framework for understanding smoking cessation behavior.[48] Although the model includes decisional balance (ie, weighing the pros and cons), self-efficacy, and 10 identified processes of change, the major construct used in diabetes education research and practice is stages of change. Within this construct, the behavior-change process is marked by 6 distinct stages that are defined in terms of a person's past behavior and plans for future action[48]:

- ◈ Precontemplation
- ◈ Contemplation
- ◈ Preparation
- ◈ Action
- ◈ Maintenance
- ◈ Termination

The model focuses on an individual's "readiness" to make a behavior change. Behavior change, viewed in a temporal perspective, is seen as an ongoing process rather than as a specific outcome. During the process, an individual has different levels of motivation to change a behavior. Relapsing or "recycling" is considered a natural part of the change process and not a failure, as movement through the stages is not necessarily a linear process.

Table 3.4 lists and defines the stages of change in the TTM and applies them to a diabetes-specific example. The final, ongoing stage—termination—occurs when the change is a permanent part of the patient's lifestyle.

Evidence Base

The TTM has been used for the following in diabetes management:

- ◈ To understand diabetes self-management behaviors

- ◈ To customize self-care interventions aimed at promoting physical activity,[49–54] healthy dietary habits,[55,56] and blood glucose testing[57] (see chapter 5, Being Active)

Researchers have examined the stages of change in relation to metabolic control after a DSME intervention was delivered.[58,59] Kavookjian[58] found that although a patient may become ready for action toward self-care, a decrease in A1C levels might change more slowly. Peterson and Hughes[59] found that patients in the preparation and action stages achieved a significantly larger reduction in A1C levels in a shorter time than patients in the precontemplation and contemplation stages. The authors concluded that stages of change were significantly associated with clinical improvement in A1C levels at 3 months after an educational intervention, and these significant differences in clinical improvement between groups were sustained for at least 12 months. However, it should be noted that although study patients had significant reductions in A1C levels, none achieved an A1C level of ≤8%.[59]

Kirk and colleagues conducted a randomized controlled trial of 70 individuals with type 2 diabetes comparing usual exercise information plus an exercise consultation with usual exercise information.[49] Guided by the TTM, the exercise consultation was tailored to the stage of physical activity readiness in which subjects were classified. The intervention group received the stage-matched consultation at the start of the study and 6 months later. Follow-up telephone consultations were also conducted at 1 month and 3 months post-intervention. The intervention group members significantly increased the number of minutes of moderate activity per week and the number of times per week they engaged in physical activity, while the control group showed no changes in either indicator. A greater number of participants from the intervention group advanced across a stage of change. Similar to the study of Kirk et al,[49] Kim and colleagues developed a stage-matched intervention to promote physical activity among Korean individuals with type 2 diabetes.[52] The intervention consisted of 3 components: a counseling technique based on TTM-related constructs, physical activity training customized to the participant, and telephone counseling. Following the 12-week intervention, compared with the control group, the intervention group

TABLE 3.4   Transtheoretical Model: Stages of Change and Application to Diabetes Self-Management

Stage	Definition	Case
Precontemplation	Individual is not aware of the problem and has no intentions of changing his or her health behavior	MG was diagnosed with type 2 diabetes 5 years ago. At that time, she was not aware of the long-term health-related complications and, therefore, did nothing to lower her blood glucose.
Contemplation	Individual is aware of the problem and intends to change the behavior; knows the benefits associated with the health behavior change but also is acutely aware of the drawbacks; can be in a state of ambivalence	Last year, MG started to understand that if she did not take care of her diabetes, she could eventually develop kidney or eye problems. She also knew that self-management involved a set of responsibilities including regularly checking her blood glucose.
Preparation	Individual makes plans that will facilitate the health behavior change	Three months ago, MG started looking for diabetes education and support groups. She also looked into joining a tennis club so that she could actively start playing tennis.
Action	Individual actively engages in the behavior change	MG checks her blood glucose before and 2 hours after every meal. She also plays tennis 3 times a week.
Maintenance	Individual demonstrates the ability to sustain the behavior change	MG continues to check her blood glucose prior to and following meals and continues to play tennis 3 times per week.

progressed to a more advanced change stage, increased physical activity levels, decreased fasting blood glucose levels, and decreased A1C. Dutton et al used this model to create tailored print materials based on the assessed stage of readiness to promote physical activity among people with type 2 diabetes.[54] At the end of 4 weeks, intervention participants were more likely to progress to another stage than those receiving usual care. The amount of weekly activity also improved in this group, but not significantly. Studies evaluating the usefulness of the TTM for understanding readiness to change dietary behaviors have been mixed, although reviews have been hampered by the lack of high-quality studies.[60,61] In a sample of 768 overweight patients enrolled in a diabetes self-management trial, Vallis et al identified patient-specific factors associated with different stages of changing dietary behavior.[56] Among those subjects diagnosed with type 2 diabetes, the subjects classified in the action stage were significantly more likely to be female, report a higher quality of life, and engage in healthy dietary habits than those in other stages. Limited literacy does not appear to negatively affect readiness to change.[62]

A study conducted by Jones and colleagues compared a TTM-based intervention (Pathways to Change) with usual care in improving 3 self-care behaviors: blood glucose testing, dietary habits, and smoking cessation.[57] The intervention was delivered via mail and telephone counseling over a 12-month period. Distinct components of the intervention targeted readiness to change for the 3 self-management behaviors. Compared with the usual care group, the intervention group demonstrated significant improvements in frequency of blood glucose testing, percentage of calorie intake from fat, and fruit and vegetable consumption per day. With regard to smoking cessation behavior, a greater proportion of the intervention group than the control group advanced to the action-oriented stage.

The TTM was the basis for the development and implementation of the interventions for providing resources and supports for self-management by the 14 sites participating in the Robert Wood Johnson Foundation diabetes initiative.[63] The use of TTM strategies to identify processes appropriate for the stage of readiness was shown to enhance at least 3 of these constructs (individualized assessment, collaborative goal setting, and skill building) and also provides support for the use of this theory in developing self-management support interventions.

Systematic Approaches to Facilitating Self-Directed Behavior Change

Patient Empowerment and Behavior-Change Theories

The differences between patient empowerment and the theories discussed above are crucial and have the potential to have a significant impact on the practice of diabetes education. These differences and their significance are discussed below.

Effective diabetes education involves a combination of art and science. The designs of DSME and DSMS programs should be based on scientifically derived evidence and standards of education and care. However, communicating effectively with patients in the context of a positive human relationship is an art. Central to empowerment is the development of a less hierarchical relationship and a collaborative approach to DSME/S and behavior change.[3] Diabetes educators have interpersonal skills, personal values, and character traits that play an important role in their practices. They can feel and express compassion, empathy, and warmth. They can establish relationships with patients that are characterized by trust, respect, and acceptance. Such relationships create an environment of psychological safety and caring that nurtures patients. Furthermore, such relationships facilitate high levels of patient candor and self-disclosure, laying the groundwork for growth and behavior change.[64,65]

Counseling psychology defines this relationship as a therapeutic alliance. Establishing a therapeutic alliance is an art. It's an art because it is dynamic and fluid and cannot be reduced to a set of algorithms. It involves the creativity, values, and personalities of diabetes educators as well as their ability and willingness to respond to the unique needs and personality of each of their patients.[45] Although scientific research has demonstrated the effectiveness of the empowerment approach, the art of diabetes patient education has always been a fundamental component of the empowerment approach.[8,64–66] The art and science of diabetes education are brought together in the person of the diabetes educator.

Although the empowerment approach to diabetes education contains fundamental elements of a behavior-change theory,[8,64,66–69] it is thought of as an approach, a philosophy, a vision, or a paradigm.[7,45,70]

Although evidence-based behavior-change theories are necessary, they are not sufficient to ensure that DSME and DSMS programs are effective, especially if educators aspire to heal as well as teach. Just as important are knowledgeable, compassionate educators, skilled in the art of diabetes education.[65] Diabetes educators are responsible for translating abstract behavioral concepts and theories into concrete programs and systematic approaches in order to meet the needs of different types of patients and their families in both group and one-to-one settings. The most carefully designed, theory-based DSME and DSMS programs are only as effective as their least effective educator.

Patient Empowerment and Diabetes Education

Patient empowerment was introduced in the diabetes literature[66] and has been incorporated into a variety of DSME and DSMS programs.[71–89] Empowerment grew out of the traditions of community psychology, adult education, and counseling psychology. Empowerment is defined "as helping patients discover and develop their inherent capacity to be responsible for their own lives and gain mastery over their diabetes" (p. 38).[66] The empowerment approach is based on 3 characteristics of diabetes that differentiate this disease from an acute illness[3,8]:

1. The choices that have the greatest effect on metabolic and other outcomes are made by patients, not health professionals.
2. Patients are in control of their self-management.
3. The consequences of self-management decisions accrue first and foremost to patients; thus, it is both their right and their responsibility to be the primary decision-makers.

Unlike the theories described above, the empowerment approach addresses in considerable detail the importance of the educators' interpersonal skills, expertise, values, and experience.[7] Table 3.5 outlines the differences between empowerment-based DSME and DSMS and traditional diabetes education.[69]

TABLE 3.5 Comparison of Traditional and Empowerment-Based DSME and DSMS	
Traditional DSME and DSMS	*Empowerment-Based DSME and DSMS*
Diabetes is a physical illness.	Diabetes is a biopsychosocial illness.
Professional is viewed as teacher and problem solver, and responsible for outcomes.	Patient is viewed as problem solver and self-manager; professional acts as a resource and shares responsibility for outcomes.
Learning needs are usually identified by professional.	Problems and learning needs are identified by patient.
Education is curriculum-driven.	Education is patient-centered and consistent with adult learning principles.
Education is primarily didactic.	Patient experiences are used as learning opportunities for problem solving and serve as the core for the curriculum.
Emotional issues are a separate component of the curriculum.	Emotional issues are integrated with clinical content.
Behavioral strategies are used to increase compliance with recommended treatment.	Behavioral strategies are integrated with clinical content and taught to patients to help them change behaviors of their choosing.
Goal of education is compliance/adherence with recommendations.	Goal is to enable patients to make informed choices.
A lack of goal attainment is viewed as a failure by both the patient and the educator.	A lack of goal attainment is viewed as feedback and used to modify goals and action plans.
Behavior changes are externally motivated.	Behavior changes are internally motivated.
Patient is relatively powerless, professional is powerful.	Patient and professional are equally powerful.

Source: Adapted from MM Funnell, RM Anderson, "Patient empowerment: from revolution to evolution," *Treat Strategies Diabetes* 3 (2011): 98-105.

Empowerment-Based Behavior-Change Protocol

The following protocol includes a series of questions to help patients identify and commit to a behavior-change plan. The questions follow a logical sequence of identifying problems, addressing emotions influencing the problem, moving toward their solution, and evaluating the outcome. However, because empowerment is an overall approach to care and not a technique, the questions should not be used as a rigid sequence for interacting with patients. There are many situations in which the natural flow of the interaction would result in a discussion of the questions in a different order and/or the addition or deletion of some questions.[8,90]

This protocol is meant to provide guidance in helping patients consider how they can make changes in how they care for their diabetes. There may be instances when the health professional needs to provide information about diabetes care during the discussion. With some patients, the behavior-change plan may focus on short-term behavioral goals so that patients can experience the change process and become familiar with an incremental approach to behavior change. With other patients, the focus may be on acquiring the information and skills necessary to make informed choices or on addressing the emotions or barriers hindering their ability to reach their goal. These questions are meant to help support a process of patient-centered decision making. No matter how much or how little patients know about diabetes, they are capable of making changes as long as they have some insight into their own behavior.

This protocol is equally effective in an individual or group situation. In a group situation, you can ask patients to think about or write down a response as you read each question to the group. You can also ask participants to volunteer a common problem (eg, handling an upcoming holiday, stress) or ask if one

Case: Applying Behavioral Approaches in Diabetes Care and Education

MG is a 48-year-old woman who was diagnosed with type 2 diabetes 5 years ago. She is a mother of 2 children, ages 13 and 16. For the past 12 months, MG has been working as a receptionist at the internal medicine outpatient clinic affiliated with a teaching hospital in the greater Detroit area. Prior to this position, she worked as an office assistant at a small advertising agency. Her current job provides healthcare benefits, whereas her previous position did not.

- MG does not check her blood glucose regularly during her workday because she feels self-conscious about coworkers discovering she has diabetes.

- She encounters difficulty when making food choices because her husband and children prefer high-fat and high-sugar foods.

- Until several months ago, she had not been exercising regularly.

Within the empowerment approach, the purpose of education is to enable participants to gain more power over their lives, increase the number of choices available to them, and enhance their ability to influence the individuals and organizations around them.[8] A 5-step behavior-change model was developed as a fundamental component of this approach and a systematic method to use when working with people who have diabetes, both one-to-one and in groups.[8,90] Each step is important; however, defining the problem and identifying emotions are the most critical to the process. Once the problem is fully explored, it will be easier for patients to identify a solution and establish meaningful and relevant goals. The 5 steps are as follows:

1. Define the problem

2. Identify feelings

3. Identify long-term goals

4. Identify a short-term behavior-change experiment (I-SMART)

5. Experiment with and evaluate the short-term behavior-change plan

The purpose of the 5-step model is to assist patients in identifying behaviors they wish to address, and then create a self-directed behavior-change plan. The role of the diabetes educator is to ask questions and actively listen to the patients' responses so that patients learn through hearing themselves and through reflection prompted by the educator's questions. The patient uses this information to create both a long-term goal and a short-term behavioral experiment as a first step toward achieving this goal. Table 3.6 elucidates the steps in the protocol, and Table 3.7 illustrates the use of this protocol with a patient.

participant would be willing to identify a real problem and discuss it in the group. The patient then works through the process with the educator and the other participants to create an action plan as part of the group session.[88,90]

In traditional care, health professionals evaluate patient behaviors and offer positive or negative feedback based on their judgment of the patient's success or failure. When using the empowerment approach, it is essential that the patient rather than the professional evaluate the outcome. This reinforces the concepts that patients are responsible for their own efforts and decisions and that the health professional is not the judge of their efforts or behaviors.

Evidence Base

Patient empowerment has been used as the theoretical basis for DSME and DSMS provided to both individuals[49,61,72,73,89] and groups of patients.[71–88,91–93] A randomized controlled trial conducted to evaluate an empowerment-based education intervention designed specifically to enhance psychosocial self-efficacy resulted in significant improvements in self-efficacy and metabolic outcomes, although diabetes clinical content was not part of the program.[85,86]

In another randomized controlled trial with African Americans, the empowerment approach was used to develop a problem-based, culturally tailored diabetes self-management group education program offered at a variety of community-based settings in a large urban area.[87] Using a wait-listed control group design, the intervention was provided over 6 weeks for a total of 10 hours of education. A nurse and dietitian, both of whom were Certified Diabetes Educators, led the sessions. The mean number of sessions

TABLE 3.6   Behavior-Change Protocol
What part of living with diabetes is the most difficult or unsatisfying for you?
(Would you tell me more about that? Would you give me some specific examples? Would you paint a picture of the situation for me?)
The purpose of this question is to focus the discussion on the patient's concerns about living with and caring for diabetes. Educators and patients often have different priorities about the most important issues related to diabetes care. Patients are most likely to make changes that will solve problems that are personally meaningful and relevant to them.
How does that (the situation described above) make you feel?
(What are your thoughts about this issue? Are you feeling [insert the feeling, eg, angry, sad, confused, etc]? Are you feeling [insert the feeling] because [insert the reason]?)
As mentioned earlier, patients seldom make and sustain changes in situations unless they care deeply about solving the problem or improving the situation. It is very common for people to repress uncomfortable emotions, and repressed emotions reduce the energy and clarity necessary for effective problem solving. Discussing the feelings associated with a particular diabetes care situation can energize patients. When patients experience the depth of their anger, sadness, or dissatisfaction by talking about their feelings, they are much more likely to take action.
How would this situation have to change for you to feel better about it? What do you think will happen if you don't make any changes?
(Where would you like to be regarding this situation in [insert specific time, eg, a month, 3 months]?)
The purpose of this question is to help patients concretely identify how the situation would appear if it were improved. This means imagining the particulars of the situation if it were to be changed and imagining how patients would feel if the situation improved. It is also useful to help patients imagine how they would feel if things did not improve. This question helps patients focus on tangible elements in the situation that must change for them to feel better.
What are some steps that you could take to bring you closer to where you want to be?
(What could you do to help solve this problem? Are there any barriers you would have to overcome? Are there other people who could help you?)
This question helps patients develop a specific plan that will operationalize their commitment to change. It is useful to consider the various actions that could be taken, barriers to those actions, and potential resources, personal and otherwise, that patients could employ to help themselves.
Is there one thing that you will do when you leave here to improve things for yourself?
This question helps patients to focus on the first thing they will do to begin to improve the situation. It is useful to end the session by having identified at least one immediate step the patient will take to begin the behavior-change process. Creating an I-SMART plan—one that is important and inspiring, specific, measurable, achievable, relevant to their long-term goals, and time-specific—is one approach that can help patients learn the behavior-change process.. Writing down the action serves as a reminder for subsequent visits to begin with a discussion of how the problem-solving process proceeded. Patients may wish to take a written copy of their commitment home with them. Participants in a group class can tell others in the group what they will do. Commitments tend to be more binding when they are expressed publicly and/or documented.
How did the plan we discussed at your last visit work out?
(What happened when you tried the behavior? Why do you think that it worked (or didn't work)? What did you learn? Would you do anything differently next time? Based on this experience, what action would you like to take or what goal would you like to set for next time?)
The purpose of this question is to help patients view the behavior and the behavior-change efforts as experiments. The purpose of experiments is to try something new and to learn from the experience. Whether the effort is successful or not, learning can still occur. In fact, some of our best lessons come from experiments that did not accomplish what we had planned.

TABLE 3.7   Empowerment-Based, Self-Directed Behavior-Change Model

Step	Questions	Case
Define problem	What part of diabetes is the most difficult or unsatisfying? What is hardest for you? What is causing you the most distress?	MG has struggled with losing weight and making changes in her eating habits since her diabetes was diagnosed. She identifies the "real" issue as her family and their lack of support for her efforts.
Identify feelings	How do you feel about this situation?	MG is very afraid that if she does not lower her blood glucose levels she will go blind or lose a leg. She also feels angry at her family that they do not seem concerned about her future health. She does not feel she can be open about her diabetes at work because she has heard other staff members make negative comments about noncompliant patients seen in the practice. She is worried the other staff members will judge her food and other choices just as harshly. During the discussion, she comes to realize that feeling alone in managing diabetes is the hardest thing for her.
Identify long-term goal	How would this situation have to change for you to feel better about it? What barriers will you face? How important is it for you to address this issue? What are the costs and benefits of addressing this problem? Of not addressing this problem?	MG believes that to truly take charge of her diabetes she needs to gain support for her efforts, primarily from her family.
Identify short-term behavior-change experiment	What are some steps that you could take to bring you closer to where you want to be? Is there one thing that you will do when you leave here to improve things for yourself?	MG feels that the first step is to write down exactly how she feels and what she wants so that she can do a better job of asking her family for their help. She will complete this during the next week.
Implement and evaluate plan	How did the plan we discussed at your last visit work out? What did you learn? What would you do differently next time? What will you do when you leave here today?	Upon reviewing what she had written, MG recognizes that while she cannot force her family to change, she also has not asked for their support or told them what she needs. She decides to speak with her husband privately next week. In addition, she will attend a weight-loss support group with a friend and see whether it is helpful.

American Association of Diabetes Educators©

attended was 5.2, and all participants showed a broad array of modest positive metabolic, psychosocial, and other changes that were maintained or improved during the 1-year follow-up period.[87]

Strategies implemented in this empowerment approach program included the following[88,90]:

- Affirming that the person with diabetes is responsible for and in control of daily self-management of diabetes
- Educating patients to promote informed decision making rather than adherence/compliance
- Teaching how to set goals and providing weekly experience in setting, implementing, and evaluating action plans
- Integrating clinical, psychosocial, and behavioral aspects of diabetes into education
- Affirming participants as experts in their own learning needs
- Affirming the ability of participants to determine an approach to diabetes self-management that will work for them
- Affirming the innate capacity of patients to identify and learn to solve their own problems
- Creating opportunities for social support
- Providing ongoing self-management support following diabetes self-management education

More recently, the efficacy of the empowerment approach was evaluated in a 2-year randomized controlled trial of a telephone-based intervention.[91] The intervention consisted of an annual meeting with patients, their physician, and the diabetes educator, usually as part of a regular medical visit. The focus of these 3-person meetings was the self-management concerns and goals of the patient. In addition, the educator called each patient monthly (more often if necessary) to review his or her self-management concerns and goals. These calls often included collaborative problem solving and goal setting using the empowerment-based 5-step model. The study resulted in improvements in diabetes quality of life, A1C, empowerment, perceived understanding of diabetes, and satisfaction with care.[91]

The empowerment approach has also been used in studies that have implemented the Chronic Care Model for improvements in diabetes care and outcomes in primary care settings.[74–78] Based on the

work done by Piatt, Zgibor, and Siminerio et al in Pittsburgh, Pennsylvania, a large US health system adopted the empowerment approach as its approach to DSME/S among all of its diabetes educators.

The empowerment approach has been used as the basis for studies in Europe as well. X-PERT was a patient-centered, group-based diabetes self-management program[79,80] in the UK. Participants in the X-PERT arm of the study were given six 2-hour weekly group sessions in a community setting designed to develop skills, build confidence, and enable patients to make informed decisions. After 14 months, the X-PERT group showed significant improvements in mean A1C as well as in body weight, body mass index (BMI), waist circumference, total cholesterol, empowerment, diabetes knowledge, physical activity levels, foot care, fruit and vegetable intake, enjoyment of food, and treatment satisfaction. Diabetes medications were also reduced.

The efficacy of 3 education programs for individuals with type 2 diabetes was tested in a randomized trial in Germany.[81] A traditional didactic education program was compared with an empowerment-based group program, which was then further compared with an empowerment-based individual program. The empowerment-based courses focused on the emotional, cognitive, and motivational processes of behavior change. There was no change in A1C for the traditional education group compared with the self-management group. The self-management group participants showed a significant improvement in A1C that was maintained for 15 months post-intervention. The participants in the individual program had a significant decrease in A1C at 3 months, but this was not sustained at 15 months. In addition, when compared with traditional education, the self-management group participants experienced further clinical (BMI and fasting blood glucose), psychological (control, irritability, hunger dependency of eating behavior, and trait anxiety), and behavioral (exercise) benefits. There were no significant benefits of the more individualized program compared with the group program.

The empowerment approach has also been recommended for the provision of DSMS, designed to sustain changes resulting from DSME.[91] A study providing weekly DSMS groups for African Americans demonstrated significant improvements in diabetes-specific quality of life and in following a healthy diet, spacing carbohydrates throughout the day, and using insulin as recommended.[92] One year after the conclusion of the program, participants not only had sustained the behavioral improvements but demonstrated significant improvements in glycemic control, serum cholesterol, and LDL levels.[93] Although the sessions were offered weekly for 24 months, participants were encouraged to attend only as often as they felt the need for group support. Twenty-one percent of the participants attended at least half of the sessions, with about one third of the participants attending each week. Although the sessions were guided by participants' self-management questions and emphasized experiential learning, coping, goal setting, and problem solving, the process for each session consisted of 5 key components:

1. **Reflecting** on diabetes self-management experiments: Sessions began with a discussion of participants' experiences over the past week.
2. **Discussing** the emotional impact of living with diabetes: Discussion of psychosocial aspects of diabetes was integrated with clinical content and behavior-change discussions.
3. **Solving problems** systematically in the group: Primary focus of program was participant-driven, based on their problems and concerns.
4. **Responding** to diabetes self-management questions: Clinical content typically provided by lecture was instead given in response to questions raised by participants.
5. **Choosing** a diabetes self-management experiment: Participants were encouraged to create an action plan working toward a long-term goal as a behavioral experiment for the next week.

Current research efforts in empowerment are designed to provide peer-based DSMS in community settings. A curriculum[94] was recently developed and tested in a pilot study to determine whether it was effective for training African-American adults to provide group-based peer support. The training program was found to be effective for providing potential peer leaders with the necessary communication, group facilitation, and behavior-change skills needed to provide effective DSMS.[95]

Motivational Interviewing

Motivational interviewing (MI) is a "collaborative, goal-oriented style of communication with particular attention to the language of change. It is designed to strengthen personal motivation for and commitment to a specific goal by eliciting and exploring the person's own reason for change within an atmosphere of acceptance and compassion." In terms of practice, it is defined as a "person-centered counseling style for addressing the common problem of ambivalence about change" (p. 29).[96]

Motivational interviewing can also be defined as a conversation about change.[96] A major focus and distinguishing feature of MI is eliciting change talk to assist individuals in working through their ambivalence about behavior change and resolve discrepancies between behaviors and their goals.[3] The tone of MI is nonjudgmental, empathetic, and encouraging, using a guiding style.[96] Counselors establish a nonconfrontational and supportive climate in which clients feel comfortable expressing both positive and negative aspects of their current behavior. Motivational interviewing also employs other more common communication techniques and strategies, such as reflective listening and shared decision making.[97]

An MI counselor does not attempt to convince, cajole, persuade, motivate, or impose change. Instead, the counselor helps clients think about and verbally express their own reasons for and against change and explore how their current behavior or health status may impact their ability to achieve their life goals or fulfill their core values. The MI approach encourages clients to make fully informed and deeply contemplated life choices, even if the decision is not to change.[98,99] Any appropriately trained health professional can successfully use MI.[100] However, learning about MI through self-study or in short 1- or 2-hour workshops is generally not adequate to master the necessary skills.[96–99] Although it appears simple, most health professionals need repeated practice with feedback and encouragement from knowledgeable guides to facilitate both skills and comfort.

Motivational Interviewing: Guiding Principles

The MI approach to behavior change rests on 4 guiding principles, which have been recently revised to better express the spirit of MI[96]:

- Collaboration with the patient
- Acceptance which includes recognition of the patient's absolute worth, accurate empathy or understanding of the patient's perspective, autonomy support, and affirmation or acknowledgement of the patient's strengths and efforts
- Evocation or calling forth the patient's strengths, resources, and motivation
- Compassion to actively promote the patient's welfare and give priority to his or her needs

Motivational interviewing has 4 key processes[96]:

- Engaging or establishing a working relationship
- Focusing on or developing and maintaining a specific direction of the conversation
- Evoking or eliciting the patient's motivations for change
- Planning involves developing both a commitment to change and a concrete plan

The 4 core communication skills used throughout MI are known as OARS: asking open-ended questions, affirming, reflecting, and summarizing and providing information and advice with permission.

Motivational interviewing emphasizes active listening as well as creating a safe and accepting environment in which the patient can express personal thoughts, feelings, and experiences. The counselor's primary role is to identify ambivalence, areas of discord in behavior, values, and aspirations; provide support; and relay facts. Giving advice without permission and direct teaching are avoided. The patient, not the counselor, determines the pace and direction of the conversation and makes the decision to embark on behavior change.

Five questions have been identified to facilitate the process of MI[96]:

1. Why would you want to make this change?
2. How might you go about it in order to succeed?
3. What are the three best reasons for you to do it?
4. How important is it for you to make this change and why?
5. So, what do you think you will do?

Developing discrepancies and reinforcing change talk involves identifying the core values of the patient and what the patient deems important in life, and whether the patient's current behavior is consistent with or runs counter to those values. The counselor attempts to uncover and reveal discrepancies among the patient's current behavior, values, and future aspirations. The counselor assists the patient in exploring the negative outcomes related to current behavior, experiencing a sense of discontent and discomfort, which ideally fosters an increasing internal motivation to change. The counselor provides any relevant factual information and highlights inconsistencies between goals and current health behavior. The patient serves as the active agent of change and is responsible for integrating the facts, resolving discrepancies, and building the necessary motivation to take action.

Supporting self-efficacy reinforces the patient's confidence in taking action and making behavior changes. The counselor promotes an atmosphere of optimism that helps solidify patients' beliefs that they can perform the specific tasks they set out to accomplish.

Table 3.8 gives examples of how MI principles and the 4 core communication skills can be applied in diabetes care.

Evidence Base

Motivational interviewing has gained increasing attention as a counseling technique useful for diabetes self-management interventions.[100–111] Smith et al investigated the unique benefit that MI might add to standard behavioral intervention aimed at improving self-care practices and promoting weight loss.[107] Twenty-two women over the age of 50 with type 2 diabetes were randomly assigned to either a standard 16-week group weight-control program (instruction in diet, exercise, and behavior modification) or the standard program plus 3 personal MI sessions. Compared with the control group, the MI group performed significantly better with regard

TABLE 3.8   Motivational Interviewing—Principles and Application to Diabetes Care and Education

Step	Case	Response From Educator
Engaging	"As much as I want to eat better, following my meal plan is hard because my husband and kids usually want pizza, fast food, or macaroni and cheese for dinner."	"It sounds as if it is important to you to eat better, but you are finding it tough to do that and to please your family by making them foods they like. On a scale of 1 to 10, with 1 not important at all and 10 very important, how important is it for you to make a change in how you are eating?"
Focusing	"It's about an 8, but I'm not sure what to do or if I can do this. Pleasing my family is very important to me."	"An 8 is a high number, so it is pretty important to you to eat better even though you are wondering how you are going to balance your needs and those of your family. You're not sure how to go about it."
Evoking	"Yes, I tried cooking different food for myself but that was too much trouble."	"Would you be interested in hearing some ideas that have worked for other people who struggled with a similar problem?"
Planning	"I like the idea you suggested of limiting fast food to weekends. That would make it more of a treat for everyone."	"What is something you might do in the next few days to get started on this?"

to maintaining food diaries and documenting blood glucose. While there were no differences in the amount of weight lost between the 2 groups, the mean A1C for the MI group was significantly lower than for their counterparts.

There have also been studies involving MI provided by specific groups of trained health professionals working with type 2 diabetes patients.[110–111] Welch et al found that MI delivered by diabetes educators was less effective than DSME alone for reducing A1C among adults with poorly controlled type 2 diabetes.[110] In a study of MI provided by nurse case managers working with high-risk type 2 diabetes, Gabbay et al found improvements in systolic blood pressure and complications screening for the case manager group compared with a usual care control group. Both the case management and the usual care participants demonstrated reduced A1C levels (1.0% vs. 1.1%), which were therefore not statistically different.[111]

The MI method has also been used in programs targeting adolescents with diabetes. In a group of 22 patients ages 14 to 18 years, Channon and colleagues examined the health impact of an MI-based counseling intervention on blood glucose control, quality of life, and psychological functioning.[109] Pre- and post-intervention results revealed a significant reduction in A1C, fear of hypoglycemia, and perceived difficulty of living with diabetes.

A meta-analysis[100] evaluated the effectiveness of using MI with patients who had various diseases and found that MI resulted in better outcomes than usual care in about 80% of studies. In addition, MI produced significant effects in some areas (BMI, total blood cholesterol, systolic blood pressure) but not in others (cigarettes per day and A1C levels). A more recent review examined the effectiveness of MI interventions on diet, exercise, diabetes, and oral health and found MI to be effective for each of these areas.[112] While data have been mixed among studies in diabetes, MI was found to be effective in helping patients control glucose levels, decrease weight, and make dietary changes and may have contributed to additional benefits such as greater self-efficacy and increased sense of control over diabetes.

Motivational interviewing can be effective in brief encounters of 15 minutes or less; however, it is assumed that more time spent increases the likelihood of favorable outcomes.[98] In addition, longer term studies are needed to determine whether gains made during the intervention are sustained over time.

Motivational Interviewing and Patient Empowerment

Motivational interviewing and patient empowerment share the same vision and values. However, there are both similarities and differences in these approaches

TABLE 3.9 Similarities Between Patient Empowerment and Motivational Interviewing	
Concept	*Vision and Values*
Spirit	Acknowledge and respect the right of patients to freely make decisions about how to manage their diabetes, ie, truly patient centered
Theory	Are compatible with Self-Determination Theory, especially Autonomy Support
Persuasion	View persuasion and cajoling as inappropriate and counterproductive
Empathy	Place a high value on the role of empathy in establishing an effective therapeutic relationship
Nonhierarchical	View the helping process as collaboration between equals with a goal of shared decision making
Communication Strategies	Use many of the same communication strategies, eg, reflective (active) listening, summarizing, decisional balance, identifying discrepancies, expressing empathy, resolving ambivalence
Skills	Require ongoing training and practice in interpersonal skills and communication strategies
Knowledge	Require thorough knowledge of the particular approach

TABLE 3.10 Differences Between Patient Empowerment and Motivational Interviewing		
Concept	*Patient Empowerment*	*Motivational Interviewing*
Outcomes	Goals and behavioral changes are viewed as steps on the way to achieving the fundamental purpose, ie, mastery over their diabetes and improved quality of life.	Goals are focused on specific behavior changes that are usually viewed as ends in themselves.
Scope	A comprehensive (eg, patient issues, educator issues, health system issues) approach to promoting patient-centered diabetes care; developed specifically for diabetes care and education but as yet not widely adapted to other chronic diseases. An appropriate metaphor would be to say that empowerment is deep while MI is wide.	A patient-centered approach to helping patients achieve specific goals used in a wide variety of areas, eg, chronic disease, addiction therapy, health promotion; initially developed for work in addiction and adapted to diabetes.
Focus	The focus is on helping patients achieve mastery over their diabetes, eg, self-confidence, acceptance, expertise, improved quality of life, perceived emotional and physical well-being, and behavior-change expertise.	The focus is on behavior change and goal attainment; it is assumed that if goals are achieved, mental and physical well-being will naturally follow.

to facilitating behavior change. An in-depth discussion of those differences is beyond the scope of this chapter. Tables 3.9 and 3.10 summarize some of the major ways that they are both similar and different.

Summary

Self-management of diabetes is a primary determinant of diabetes-related health outcomes, in the short and long term. With each passing year and the development of new technologies and therapies, diabetes self-management is becoming more complex. In response to the combination of this increasing complexity and the growing body of knowledge about diabetes distress and its impact on outcomes, health-related behavior change, DSME, and DSMS must become increasingly sophisticated to be effective. These programs are only as effective as the diabetes educators who design and conduct them. This chapter outlined the resources necessary to help educators develop the skills to incorporate evidence-based approaches to facilitating self-directed behavior change into their programs and practices and thus to ultimately improve the quality of life for people with diabetes.

Focus on Education

Teaching Strategies

⊙ **Select and employ theories that will effectively guide practice.** Establish a framework, define an approach and purpose, and provide a common language for the healthcare team and patients. This philosophy is then reflected in the program design and implementation.

⊙ **Base outcomes on evidence.** Use valid and reliable measures of self-management behavior, metabolic status, and diabetes-related distress and quality of life, and then compare and contrast the results with expectations.

⊙ **Match the content and educational materials to the particular characteristics of your audience.** Of particular importance are different cultures, ethnicities, ages, and levels of health literacy.

⊙ **Know yourself and play to your strengths.** Some educators are comfortable with patient-driven discussions that move from topic to topic. Some educators need a more structured approach to patient education. Take the time to reflect on your educational efforts and interactions with individual patients. Do they reflect your values and your philosophy of patient education?

⊙ **It is easy to underestimate the power of listening.** There are many situations where it would be more effective for the educator to listen than to talk. Experiment with reducing the time you spend talking and increasing the time you spend listening.

⊙ **Recognize that changing how you communicate with and relate to patients can be challenging.** It takes training, practice, and reflection.

Messages for Patients

⊙ **Make decisions.** Gather as much information as is available. Learn the skills necessary to make decisions and create and implement effective behavior-change plans. Identify options and discuss them with the healthcare team, family, and educators to create a plan that will be most effective in helping you reach your goals.

⊙ **Learn about yourself.** Recognize that your emotional responses to diabetes, your culture, your family, your sources of support, your other priorities, and your values all influence your self-management and behavior-change efforts. While knowing about diabetes in general is helpful, it is more important to understand your own diabetes within the context of your life.

⊙ **Be involved in planning your care.** Be clear on what you plan to do and the criteria upon which you will judge your own success. Know that the plan can be altered and that every step forward is a step in the right direction.

⊙ **Involve family members, as they have a very specific and important role to play.** They share the burden of diabetes and provide the support needed to manage this complex disease that greatly impacts your day-to-day life as well as theirs. Invite them to attend diabetes education and support sessions with you. If they are struggling with how to be supportive, tell them specifically how they can help you. In return, ask what you can do to ease their burden.

⊙ **Realize how much impact your self-management has on your current and future health and well-being.** It is true that you are responsible for your own self-management. But remember that the other side of the responsibility coin is freedom. You have the freedom to adapt your self-management to the unique characteristics and needs of your life. Yes, you are responsible, but you can also take charge and take control over your own decisions.

Focus on Practice

→ **Be part of an organization's stewardship and acculturation of patient-centered communications.** The culture in which diabetes educators practice is reflective of the professional credibility and theoretical and behavioral approaches that are employed. Diabetes educators model the interpersonal skills, expertise, and confidence that are needed by patients in directing their own learning.

→ **Create patient-focused services with clear communications in interactions—from the reception desk to discharge planning.** Provide in-services on health literacy and what it takes to help patients change behaviors. Modify behavioral and psychosocial strategies to accommodate patients with special literacy and learning needs.

→ **Reflect on growth and development in delivering patient-centered education.** No matter which theoretical and behavioral approaches you learn, in order to facilitate change among patients, diabetes educators need to put theory into practice. Try modifying what is said to a patient and how it is said. Teaching skills are as important as clinical skills. It takes time to develop proficient skills as an educator, just as it takes time to study to become a nurse, dietitian, pharmacist, or other healthcare professional.

References

1. Skovlund SE, Peyrot M; on behalf of the DAWN International Advisory Panel. The Diabetes Attitudes, Wishes, and Needs (DAWN) program: a new approach to improving outcomes of diabetes care. Diabetes Spectr. 2005;18:136-42.

2. Haas L, Maryniuk M, Beck J, et al. National standards for diabetes self-management education and support. Diabetes Care. 2013;36 Suppl 1:S100-8.

3. Marrero DG, Ard J, Delamater AM, et al. Twenty-first century behavioral medicine: a context for empowering clinicians and patients with diabetes: a consensus report. Diabetes Care. 2013;36:463-70.

4. Fain J, Nettles A, Funnell MM, Charron-Prochownik D. Diabetes patient education research: an integrative literature review. Diabetes Educ. 1999;25 Suppl 6:7-15.

5. Meleis A. Theoretical Nursing: Development and Progress. 5th ed. Philadelphia: Lippincott; 2007.

6. Fawcett J. Criteria for evaluation of a theory. Nurs Sci Q. 2005;18:131-5.

7. Polit DF, Beck CT, Hungler BP. Essentials of Nursing Research: Appraising Evidence for Nursing Practice. 8th ed. Philadelphia: Lippincott; 2013.

8. Anderson RM, Funnell MM. The Art of Empowerment: Stories and Strategies for Diabetes Educators. 2nd ed. Alexandria, Va: American Diabetes Association; 2005.

9. Glanz K, Rimer BK, Marcus Lewis F, eds. Health Behavior & Health Education: Theory, Research & Practice. 4th ed. San Francisco: Jossey-Bass; 2008.

10. Harvey JN, Lawson VL. The importance of health belief models in determining self-care behaviour in diabetes. Diabet Med. 2009;26:5-13.

11. Rosenstock IM. Historical origins of the health belief model. Health Educ Monogr. 1974;2:328-35.

12. Kirscht J. The health belief model and predictions of health actions. In: Gochman D, ed. Health Behavior: Emerging Research Perspectives. New York: Plenum Press; 1988:27-41.

13. Bond GG, Aiken LS, Somerville SC. The health belief model and adolescents with insulin-dependent diabetes mellitus. Health Psychol. 1992;11:190-8.

14. Charron-Prochownik D, Becker MH, Brown MB, Liang WM, Bennett S. Understanding young children's health beliefs and diabetes regimen adherence. Diabetes Educ. 1993;19:409-18.

15. Charron-Prochownik D, Sereika SM, Becker D, et al. Reproductive health beliefs and behaviors in teens with diabetes: application of the expanded health belief model. Pediatr Diabetes. 2001;2:30-9.

16. Koch J. The role of exercise in the African-American woman with type 2 diabetes mellitus: application of the health belief model. J Am Acad Nurse Pract. 2002;14:126-9.

17. Aljasem LI, Peyrot M, Wissow L, Rubin RR. The impact of barriers and self-efficacy on self-care behaviors in type 2 diabetes. Diabetes Educ. 2001;27:393-404.

18. Wdowik MJ, Kendall PA, Harris MA, Auld G. Expanded health belief model predicts diabetes self-management in college students. J Nutr Educ. 2001;33:17-23.

19. Pham DT, Fortin F, Thibaudeau MF. The role of the health belief model in amputees' self-evaluation of adherence to diabetes self-care behaviors. Diabetes Educ. 1996;22:126-32.

20. Swift CS, Armstrong JE, Beerman KA, Campbell RK, Pond-Smith D. Attitudes and beliefs about exercise among persons with non-insulin-dependent diabetes. Diabetes Educ. 1995;21:533-40.

21. Polly RK. Diabetes health beliefs, self-care behaviors, and glycemic control among older adults with non-insulin-dependent diabetes mellitus. Diabetes Educ. 1992;18:321-7.

22. Kurtz SMS. Adherence to diabetes regimens: empirical status and clinical applications. Diabetes Educ. 1990;16:50-9.

23. Cerkoney KA, Hart LK. The relationship between the health belief model and compliance of persons with diabetes mellitus. Diabetes Care. 1980;3:594-8.

24. Nundy S, Dick JJ, Solomon MC, Peek ME. Developing a behavioral model for mobile phone-based diabetes interventions. Patient Educ Couns. 2013;90:125-32.

25. James DCS, Pobee JW, Oxidine D, Brown L, Joshi G. Using the health belief model to develop culturally appropriate weight-management materials for African-American women. J Acad Nutr Diet. 2012;112:664-70.

26. Ammary-Risch NJ, Aguilar M, Goodman LS, Quiroz L. Diabetes and Healthy Eyes Toolkit: a community health worker program to prevent vision loss and blindness among people with diabetes. Fam Community Health. 2012;35:103-10.

27. Tan MY. The relationship of health beliefs and complication prevention behaviors of Chinese individuals with type 2 diabetes mellitus. Diabetes Res Clin Pract. 2004;66:71-7.

28. Daniel M, Messer LC. Perceptions of disease severity and barriers to self-care predict glycemic control in aboriginal persons with type 2 diabetes mellitus. Chronic Dis Can. 2002;23:130-8.

29. Spikmans FJ, Brug J, Doven MM, Kruizenga HM, Hofsteenge GH, van Bokhorst-van der Schueren MA. Why do diabetic patients not attend appointments with their dietitians? J Hum Nutr Diet. 2003;16:151-8.

30. Wdowik MJ, Kendall PA, Harris MA, Keim KS. Development and evaluation of an intervention program: "Control on Campus." Diabetes Educ. 2000;26:95-104.

31. Scollan-Koliopoulos M. Theory-guided intervention for preventing diabetes-related amputations in African Americans. J Vasc Nurs. 2004;22:126-33.

32. Wang S-L, Charron-Prochownik C, Sereika SM, Siminerio L, Kim Y. Comparing three theories in predicting reproductive health behavioral intention in adolescent women with diabetes. Pediatr Diabetes. 2006;7:108-15.

33. Allen NA. Social cognitive theory in diabetes exercise research: an integrative literature review. Diabetes Educ. 2004;30:805-19.

34. Hays LM, Clark DO. Correlates of physical activity in a sample of older adults with type 2 diabetes. Diabetes Care. 1999;22:706-12.

35. Miller CK, Edwards L, Kissling G, Sanville L. Evaluation of a theory-based nutrition intervention for older adults with diabetes mellitus. J Am Diet Assoc. 2002;102:1069-81.

36. Miller CK, Edwards L, Kissling G, Sanville L. Nutrition education improves metabolic outcomes among older adults with diabetes mellitus: results from a randomized controlled trial. Prev Med. 2002;34:252-9.

37. Glasgow RE, Nutting PA, Toobert JD, et al. Effects of a brief computer-assisted diabetes self-management intervention on dietary, biological and quality of life outcomes. Chronic Illn. 2006;2:27-38.

38. Toobert DJ, Strycker LA, Glasgow RE, Barrera M, Bagdade JD. Enhancing support for health behavior change among women at risk for heart disease: the Mediterranean lifestyle trial. Health Educ Res. 2002;17:574-85.

39. Sinclair KA, Makahi EK, Shea-Soltorio C, Yoshimura SR, Townsend CKM, Kaholokula K. Outcomes from a diabetes self-management intervention for Native Hawaiians and Pacific People: Partners in Care. Ann Behav Med. 2013;45:24-32.

40. Lorig K, Ritter PL, Villa FJ, Armas J. Community-based peer-led diabetes self-management: a randomized trial. Diabetes Educ. 2009;35:641-51.

41. Lorig K, Ritter PL, Laurent DD, et al. Online diabetes self-management program: a randomized study. Diabetes Care. 2010;33:1275-81.

42. Lorig K, Ritter PL, Villa F, Piette JD. Spanish diabetes self-management with and without automated telephone reinforcement. Diabetes Care. 2008;31:408-14.

43. Holman H, Lorig K. Advances in managing chronic disease. BMJ. 2000;320:525-6.

44. Ajzen I, Fishbein M. Understanding Attitudes and Predicting Social Behavior. Englewood Cliffs, NJ: Prentice Hall; 1980.

45. Madden TJ, Ellen PS, Azjen I. A comparison of the theory of planned behavior and the theory of reasoned action. Soc Psychol Bull. 1992;18:3-9.

46. Syrajala AH, Niskanen MC, Knuuttila ML. The theory of reasoned action in describing tooth brushing, dental caries and diabetes adherence among diabetic patients. J Clin Periodontol. 2002;29:427-32.

47. Burnet D, Plaut A, Courtney R, Chin MH. A practical model for preventing type 2 diabetes in minority youth. Diabetes Educ. 2002;28:779-95.

48. Prochaska JO, Norcross JC, DiClemente CC. Changing for Good: The Revolutionary Program That Explains the Six Stages of Change and Teaches You How to Free Yourself From Bad Habits. New York: W. Morrow; 1994.

49. Kirk AF, Higgins LA, Hughes AR, et al. A randomized, controlled trial to study the effect of exercise consultation on the promotion of physical activity in people with type 2 diabetes: a pilot study. Diabet Med. 2001;18:877-82.

50. Kirk A, Mutrie N, MacIntyre P, Fisher M. Increasing physical activity in people with type 2 diabetes. Diabetes Care. 2003;26:1186-92.

51. Kirk AF, Mutrie N, MacIntyre PD, Fisher MB. Promoting and maintaining physical activity in people with type 2 diabetes. Am J Prev Med. 2004;27:289-96.

52. Kim CJ, Hwang AR, Yoo JS. The impact of a stage-matched intervention to promote exercise behavior in participants with type 2 diabetes. Int J Nurs Stud. 2004;41:833-41.

53. Yoo JS, Hwang AR, Lee HC, Kim CJ. Development and validation of a computerized exercise intervention program for patients with type 2 diabetes mellitus in Korea. Yonsei Med J. 2003;44:892-904.

54. Dutton GT, Provost BC, Tan F, Smith D. A tailored print-based physical activity intervention for patients with type 2 diabetes. Prev Med. 2008;4:409-11.

55. Kasila K, Poskiparta M, Karhila P, Kettunen T. Patients' readiness for dietary change at the beginning of counseling: a transtheoretical model-based assessment. J Hum Nutr Diet. 2003;16:159-66.

56. Vallis M, Ruggiero L, Greene G, et al. Stages of change for healthy eating in diabetes: relation to demographic, eating-related, health care utilization, and psychosocial factors. Diabetes Care. 2003;26:1468-74.

57. Jones H, Edwards L, Vallis TM, et al. Changes in diabetes self-care behaviors make a difference in glycemic control: the diabetes stages of change (DiSC) study. Diabetes Care. 2003;26:732-7.

58. Kavookjian J. Does readiness for self-care behaviors predict glycemic control? Diabetes. 2002;51:A437.

59. Peterson KA, Hughes M. Readiness to change and clinical success in a diabetes educational program. J Am Board Fam Pract. 2002;15:266-71.

60. Riemsma RP, Pattenden J, Bridle C, et al. A systematic review of the effectiveness of interventions based on a stages-of-change approach to promote individual behavior change. Health Technol Assess. 2002;6:1-242.

61. Salmela S, Poskiparta M, Kasila K, Vahasarja K, Vanhala M. Transtheoretical model-based dietary interventions in primary care: a review of the evidence in diabetes. Health Educ Res. 2009;24:237-52.

62. Powell CK, Hill EG, Clancy DE. The relationship between health literacy and diabetes knowledge and readiness to take health actions. Diabetes Educ. 2007;33:144-51.

63. Highstein GR, O'Toole ML, Shetty G, Brownson CA, Fisher EB. Use of the transtheoretical model to enhance resources and supports for diabetes self management: lessons from the Robert Wood Johnson Foundation Diabetes Initiative. Diabetes Educ. 2007;33 Suppl 6:193S-200.

64. Anderson RM, Funnell MM. The art and science of diabetes education. Diabetes Educ. 2008;34:109-17.

65. Funnell MM, Anderson RM. Empowerment and diabetes: why bother? J Diabetes Nurs. 2012;16 Suppl 1:2.

66. Funnell MM, Anderson RM, Arnold MS, et al. Empowerment: an idea whose time has come in diabetes education. Diabetes Educ. 1991;17:37-41.

67. Anderson RM, Funnell MM. Patient empowerment: myths & misunderstandings. Patient Educ Couns. 2010;79:277-82.

68. Anderson RM, Funnell MM. Ten things patient empowerment is not. Published in line with the EASD Congress, September 2010. Treat Strategies Diabetes. 2010;2(1):185-92.

69. Funnell MM, Anderson RM. Patient empowerment: from revolution to evolution. Treat Strategies Diabetes. 2011;3:98-105.

70. Funnell MM, Anderson RM. Patient empowerment: a look back, a look ahead. Diabetes Educ. 2003;9:454-64.

71. Norris SL, Lau J, Smith SJ, Schmid CH, Engelgau MM. Self-management education for adults with type 2 diabetes: a meta-analysis on the effect on glycemic control. Diabetes Care. 2002;25:1159-71.

72. Davis ED, Vander Meer JM, Yarborough PC, Roth SM. Using solution-focused therapy strategies in empowerment-based education. Diabetes Educ. 1999;25:249-57.

73. Dijkstra R, Braspenning J, Grol R. Empowering patients: how to implement a diabetes passport in hospital care. Patient Educ Couns. 2002;47:173-7.

74. Piatt G, Orchard T, Emerson S, et al. Translating the chronic care model into the community: a randomized controlled trial of a multifaceted diabetes education intervention. Diabetes Care. 2006;29:811-7.

75. Siminerio L, Piatt G, Emerson S, et al. Deploying the chronic care model to implement and sustain diabetes self-management training programs. Diabetes Educ. 2006;30:253-60.

76. Siminerio L, Piatt G, Zgibor J. Implementing the chronic care model for improvements in diabetes care and education in a rural primary care practice. Diabetes Educ. 2005;31:225-34.

77. Siminerio L, Ruppert K, Emerson S, Solano F, Piatt G. Delivering diabetes self-management education (DSME) in primary care. Dis Manage Health Outcomes. 2008;16: 267-72.

78. Piatt G, Anderson R, Brooks M, Zgibor J. Three year follow-up of clinical and behavioral improvements following a multi-faceted diabetes care intervention: results of a randomized controlled trial. Diabetes Educ. 2010;36:301-9.

79. Deakin TA, Cade JE, Williams R, Greenwood DC. Structured patient education: the X-PERT Programme makes a difference. Diabet Med. 2006;23:944-54.

80. Deakin T, Whitham C. Structured patient education: the X-PERT Programme. Br J Community Nurs. 2009;14: 398-404.

81. Kulzer B, Hermanns N, Reinecker H, Haak T. Effects of self-management training in type 2 diabetes: a randomized, prospective trial. Diabet Med. 2007;24:415-23.

82. Gillard ML, Nwankwo R, Fitzgerald JT, et al. Informal diabetes education: impact on self-management and blood glucose control. Diabetes Educ. 2004;30:136-42.

83. Pibernik-Okanovic M, Prasek M, Poljicanin-Filipovic T, Pavlic-Renar I, Metelko Z. Effects of an empowerment-based psychosocial intervention on quality of life and metabolic control in type 2 diabetic patients. Patient Educ Couns. 2004;52:193-9.

84. Skinner TC, Cradock S, Arundel F, Graham W. Lifestyle and behavior: four theories and a philosophy: self-management education for individuals newly diagnosed with type 2 diabetes. Diabetes Spectr. 2003;16:75-80.

85. Anderson RM, Funnell MM, Butler PM, Arnold MS, Feste CC. Patient empowerment: results of a randomized controlled trial. Diabetes Care. 1995;18:943-9.

86. Arnold MS, Butler PM, Anderson RM, Funnell MM, Feste C. Guidelines for facilitating a patient empowerment program. Diabetes Educ. 1995;21:308-12.

87. Anderson RM, Funnell MM, Nwankwo R, Gillard ML, Oh MS, Fitzgerald JT. Evaluation of a problem-based empowerment program for African Americans with diabetes. Results of a randomized controlled trial. Ethn Dis. 2005;15:671-8.

88. Funnell MM, Nwankwo R, Gillard ML, Anderson RM, Tang TS. Implementing an empowerment-based diabetes self-management education program. Diabetes Educ. 2005;31:53-61.

89. Anderson RM, Funnell MM, Aikens JE, et al. Evaluating the efficacy of an empowerment-based self-management

consultant intervention: results of a two-year randomized controlled trial. Ther Patient Educ. 2009;1:3-11.

90. Funnell MM, Anderson RM. Empowerment and self-management education. Clin Diabetes. 2004;22:123-7.

91. Funnell MM, Tang TS, Anderson RM. From DSME to DSMS: developing empowerment based self-management support. Diabetes Spectr. 2007;20:221-6.

92. Tang TS, Funnell MM, Noorulla S, Oh M, Brown MB. Sustaining short-term improvements over the long-term: results from a 2-year diabetes self-management support (DSMS) intervention. Diabetes Res Clin Pract. 2012;95:85-92.

93. Tang TS, Funnell MM, Oh M. Lasting effects of a 2-year diabetes self-management support intervention: outcomes at 1 year follow-up. Prev Chronic Dis. 2012;9:E109.

94. Tang TS, Funnell MM, Gillard M, Nwankwo R, Heisler M. The development of a pilot training program for peer leaders in diabetes. Diabetes Educ. 2011;37:67-77.

95. Tang TS, Funnell MM. Peer Leader Training Manual. Brussels, Belgium: International Diabetes Federation; 2011.

96. Miller WR, Rollnick S. Motivational Interviewing: Helping People Change. 3rd ed. New York: The Guilford Press; 2013:29.

97. Glynn LH, Moyers TB. Chasing change talk: The clinician's role in evoking client language about change. J Subst Abuse Treat. 2010;39:65-7.

98. Miller WR, Rose GS. Toward a theory of motivational interviewing. Am Psychol. 2009;64:527-37.

99. Miller WR, Rollnick S. Ten things that motivational interviewing is not. Behav Cogn Psychother. 2009;37:129-40.

100. Rubak S, Sandbaek A, Lauritzen T, Christensen B. Motivational interviewing: a systematic review and meta-analysis. Br J Gen Pract. 2005;55:305-12.

101. Carino JL, Coke L, Gulanick M. Using motivational interviewing to reduce diabetes risk. Prog Cardiovasc Nurs. 2004;19:149-54.

102. VanWormer JJ, Boucher JL. Motivational interviewing and diet modification: a review of the evidence. Diabetes Educ. 2004;30:404-6, 408-10, 414-6.

103. Doherty Y, Hall D, James PT, Roberts SH, Simpson J. Change counselling in diabetes: the development of a training programme for the diabetes team. Patient Educ Couns. 2000;40:263-78.

104. Trigwell P, Grant PJ, House A. Motivation and glycemic control in diabetes mellitus. J Psychosom Res. 1997;43:307-15.

105. Stott NC, Rees M, Rollnick S, Pill RM, Hackett P. Professional responses to innovation in clinical method: diabetes care and negotiating skills. Patient Educ Couns. 1996;29:67-73.

106. Stott NC, Rollnick S, Rees MR, Pill RM. Innovation in clinical method: diabetes care and negotiating skills. Fam Pract. 1995;12:413-8.

107. Smith DE, Heckemeyer CM, Kratt PP, Mason DA. Motivational interviewing to improve adherence to a behavior weight-control program for older obese women in NIDDM. A pilot study. Diabetes Care. 1997;20:52-4.

108. Clark M, Hampson SE. Implementing a psychological intervention to improve lifestyle self-management in patients with type 2 diabetes. Patient Educ Couns. 2001;42:247-56.

109. Channon S, Smith VJ, Gregory JW. A pilot study of motivational interviewing in adolescents with diabetes. Arch Dis Child. 2003;88:680-3.

110. Welch G, Zagarins SE, Feinberg RG, Garb JL. Motivational interviewing delivered by diabetes educators: does it improve blood glucose control among poorly controlled type 2 diabetes patients? Diabetes Res Clin Pract 2011;91:54-60.

111. Gabbay RA, Añel-Tiangco RM, Dellasega C, Mauger DT, Adelman A, Horn DH. Diabetes Nurse Case Management and Motivational Interviewing for Change (DYNAMIC): results of a 2-year randomized controlled pragmatic trial. J Diabetes. 2013;5:349-57.

112. Martins RK, McNeil DW. Review of motivational interviewing in promoting health behaviors. Clin Psychol Rev. 2009;29:283-93.

CHAPTER 4

Healthy Eating

Patti B. Geil, MS, RD/RDN, FAND, CDE

Key Concepts

- Healthy eating is an effective, but challenging, self-care behavior that improves metabolic control and quality of life in persons with or at risk for diabetes.

- The diabetes educator should support healthy eating behaviors that are grounded in evidence-based research, such as the American Diabetes Association Clinical Practice Recommendations. Clinical recommendations can be translated into self-management education guided by the AADE Guidelines for the Practice of Diabetes Self-Management Education and Training (DSME/T).

- Providers of DSME/T at every level of practice should work with an interdisciplinary diabetes care team to tailor interventions to individual patient self-management education needs as well as to the stage of readiness to change behavior.

- To facilitate healthy eating, the DSME/T provider assists the person with or at risk for diabetes in acquiring specific knowledge and skills by choosing the most appropriate meal-planning resource from the variety of approaches available. Key issues to address include, but are not limited to, portion sizes; food labels; meal planning, shopping, and cooking; modifying recipes; eating out; snacking; and special situations such as travel, alcohol, and parties/holidays.

Introduction

Healthy eating has a significant effect on the metabolic control of diabetes, including improvement in glycemic control and lipid profiles, maintenance of blood pressure in the target range, and weight loss or maintenance.[1] Many diabetes educators and clinicians consider healthy eating to be the most challenging of the AADE7 Self-Care Behaviors™ to implement successfully.[2] Healthy eating involves basic behaviors and decisions such as when to eat, what to eat, and how much to eat. Influencing these decisions are complex factors such as habits, emotions, food preferences, food availability, and family and cultural eating patterns. An American Association of Diabetes Educators (AADE) systematic review of the literature on incorporating nutritional management into lifestyle highlights the complex challenge of establishing healthy eating behaviors.[3] To help individuals with diabetes achieve effective behavior change to promote healthy eating, the diabetes educator's role encompasses the following:

- Providing the person with or at risk for diabetes with knowledge and skills training focused on healthy eating approaches grounded in evidence-based research
- Translating clinical recommendations into effective self-management education

◆ Facilitating successful behavior change by tailoring interventions to the individual's stage of readiness to embrace new behaviors

◆ Sharing practical information regarding meal-planning skills

Achieving successful self-management behaviors that are focused on making healthy food choices requires knowledge and skill on the part of the learner. This chapter focuses on the art of diabetes self-management education and training (DSME/T) and the areas that are important for the diabetes educator to teach, support, and promote to guide behavior change for healthy eating.

Promoting Healthy Eating: The Role of Medical Nutrition Therapy

Diabetes medical nutrition therapy (MNT) is the term for the specific nutrition diagnostic, therapy, and counseling services for the purpose of disease management furnished by a registered dietitian (RD)/registered dietitian nutritionist (RDN) or similarly qualified nutrition professional.[4] Successful MNT is grounded in evidence-based principles of nutrition for diabetes which are then translated into self-management education for healthy eating behaviors. Although diabetes

---

Case: Healthy Eating Through DSME/T

SM is a 30-year-old Caucasian female who has had type 1 diabetes since age 17. She is interested in preconception planning for her first pregnancy.

Assessment Data

- Height: 65 in (165 cm)
- Weight: 130 lb (58.5 kg)
- Body mass index (BMI): 21
- Blood pressure: 128/77 mm Hg

Most Recent Lab Values

- A1C: 8.5%
- Fasting blood glucose: 145 mg/dL (8.05 mmol/L)
- Total cholesterol: 226 mg/dL (5.85 mmol/L)
- Triglycerides: 128 mg/dL (1.45 mmol/L)
- HDL-C: 42 mg/dL (1.09 mmol/L)
- LDL-C: 113 mg/dL (2.93 mmol/L)

SM lives with her husband and travels frequently for her pharmaceutical sales job. She has been instructed on an 1800-calorie exchange diet, but she is not consistent with her intake. She often eats sporadically due to her hectic travel schedule. Breakfast during the workweek is typically a large bagel with low-fat cream cheese, a piece of fruit, and black coffee; on weekends at home she sleeps late and enjoys making a brunch of bacon, eggs, and fruit salad. On most days, lunch is a chef salad with low-fat ranch salad dressing, 2 packages of crackers, and a diet drink.

SM often goes out for a late dinner with friends, choosing items such as pasta with tomato sauce or grilled chicken with salad and bread, and an occasional alcoholic beverage.

SM currently takes 10 units of a rapid-acting insulin analog with meals and 20 units of glargine (Lantus®, sanofi-aventis) at bedtime. She is not adjusting her mealtime insulin doses. She is interested in using an insulin pump. SM checks her fasting blood glucose daily and tries to check her blood glucose at least one more time each day. SM is taking cinnamon capsules because her hairdresser told her it was "good for blood sugar." She denies taking other medications.

Her physical activity program consists of running 3 miles per day on the weekends. Her activity level during the week is much less intense, although she tries to attend a step aerobics class twice a week. Otherwise, her activity level is rather sedentary, as she spends much of her day in the car, driving between physicians' clinics in her sales territory.

Questions to Consider

1. What are the key healthy eating issues you might address at this visit?

2. How can you use the steps of the Nutrition Care Process and Model (NCPM) during SM's visit? (The NCPM is discussed later in this chapter.)

3. What are 2 behavior-change goals that focus on healthy eating that you might encourage SM to set?

4. List 3 skills related to healthy eating that you will review with SM during this visit.

educators at every level of practice must be able to apply the principles of MNT and use the same core set of behaviors to measure outcomes (see Table 4.1), the RD/RDN is the health professional with the greatest expertise in providing MNT. The RD/RDN's effectiveness has been documented in research studies that have achieved positive outcomes. The Nutrition Therapy Recommendations for the Management of Adults with Diabetes[5] highlights a comprehensive review of the evidence for the effectiveness of MNT and healthy eating in diabetes management. The authors cite randomized controlled trials in which MNT was either implemented independently or delivered as part of an overall diabetes self-management training (DSMT) program. The studies demonstrated the following:

◆ Decreases in A1C: –0.3% to –1% in type 1 diabetes and –0.5% to –2% in type 2 diabetes, reductions that are similar to or greater than reductions that would be expected with the use of currently available pharmacologic treatments for diabetes.

◆ Reductions in the various markers of cardiovascular and hypertension risk factors in the general population with an abnormal lipid profile: –5% to –8% daily fat intake, –2% to –4% daily saturated fat intake, and –232 to –710 daily energy intake. In addition, triglycerides were lowered –11% to –31%, LDL cholesterol –7% to –22%, and total cholesterol –7% to –21%.

◆ Reductions in diabetes comorbidities and decreased use of medications led to a reduction in the use of health services and costs, indicating that MNT is also cost-effective.

Strong evidence also suggests that interventions such as intensive lifestyle modifications based on healthy eating habits and physical activity are effective in delaying or preventing the onset of type 2 diabetes by 58% to 71%.[6]

TABLE 4.1 Healthy Eating Core Competencies for Diabetes Educators	
Provider Level	*Healthy Eating Competencies*
Level 1 Diabetes Educator Level 1 educators are healthcare providers who interact professionally with diabetes patients to provide the essential knowledge and skills needed for safe self-care. Level 1 designation includes but is not limited to registered nurses (from any accredited entry level education program), advanced practice nurses, registered dietitians (licensed or registered), pharmacists (licensed or registered), exercise physiologists, master certified health education specialists, physical therapists, physicians assistants, and physicians.	• Assesses meal plan and nutritional components of patient's lifestyle • Introduces patient to principles of healthy eating • Instructs patient about elements of the diabetes meal plan • Provides instruction on hypoglycemia prevention, identification, and treatment
Level 2 Diabetes Educator Level 2 educators are healthcare providers who have achieved an advanced body of core knowledge and skills related to diabetes education and/or management above that which is required by the profession of origin. Level 2 incorporates those providers who meet the academic, professional, and experiential criteria to qualify for and maintain the certified diabetes educator (CDE) credential. A distinction is made between the newly credentialed educator who is competent in all and proficient in some areas of diabetes knowledge, and the level 3 educators who are at the highest level of expertise in the field.	• Provides instruction about nutrition as a framework to guide patient toward successful management of personal meal plans • Assesses patient's ability to follow complex meal plan • Provides instruction on completing a food record • Introduces fundamental concepts of carbohydrate counting and meal-based insulin dosing • Explains the relationship between food, activity, and medication in preventing hypoglycemia • Explains interaction of food, activity, and medication

(continued)

TABLE 4.1 Healthy Eating Core Competencies for Diabetes Educators (continued)	
Provider Level	*Healthy Eating Competencies*
Level 3 Diabetes Educator Level 3 educators are advanced level experts in diabetes education, clinical management, and/or research. The level 3 educator encompasses those involved in integrated, comprehensive, and global management of people with diabetes. This includes, but is not limited to clinicians, researchers, academics, program managers, healthcare administrators, and consultants. The educator at this level may hold the CDE credential, meets the academic, professional, and experiential criteria to qualify for and maintain the board certified–advanced diabetes management (BC-ADM) credential, and may be recognized as a Fellow of the American Association of Diabetes Educators. This level of practice is characterized by care coordination and management, autonomous assessment, problem identification, planning, implementation, and evaluation of diabetes care. Additionally, it involves excellent communication as well as complex critical thinking and clinical decision-making skills. High level clinical and nonclinical practice is characteristic of this level.	• Uses comprehensive knowledge of nutrition and diabetes meal planning to provide (or support) MNT to a patient with complex needs • Assesses insulin-to-carbohydrate ratio (ie, must know if food portions are accurate) • Assesses for psychosocial adjustment, including coping strategies and eating disorders • Performs physical assessment, including signs of malnutrition and anthropometrics • Performs clinical assessment, including relevant lab values • Assesses for food/drug interactions • Reviews food intake in detail to assess accuracy of portions and specific carbohydrate intake or to refer to a registered dietitian (RD/RDN)

Note: It is assumed that competency requirements are cumulative throughout the levels.

Source: Adapted from American Association of Diabetes Educators, *The Diabetes Educator Career Path: Revised Levels of Practice,* 2014.

Registered Dietitian (RD)/ Registered Dietitian Nutritionist (RDN)

The team member with the most academic preparation, training, skills, and demonstrated effectiveness in fostering healthy eating for diabetes is the RD/RDN. The initials RD or RDN after a dietitian's name ensure that he or she has met and maintains the standards of the Academy of Nutrition and Dietetics.

Goals of MNT for Prediabetes and Diabetes

The American Diabetes Association (ADA) outlines the following goals of MNT for prediabetes and diabetes:

◆ For individuals with prediabetes, the goal of MNT is to decrease the risk of diabetes and cardiovascular disease (CVD) by intensive lifestyle modification, specifically healthy food choices and increased physical activity leading to moderate weight loss that is maintained.[7]

◆ For individuals with diabetes, the goals of MNT are the following:

—To promote and support healthful eating patterns, emphasizing a variety of nutrient-dense foods in appropriate portion sizes in order to improve overall health and specifically to

   ◆ Attain individualized glycemic, blood pressure, and lipid goals. General recommended goals from the ADA for these markers are as follows:

   • A1C <7%

   • Blood pressure <140/80 mm Hg

   • LDL cholesterol <100 mg/dL (2.95 mmol/L) in individuals without overt CVD, triglycerides <150 mg/dL (1.69 mmol/L), and HDL cholesterol >40 mg/dL (1.04 mmol/L) for men and >50 mg/dL (1.30 mmol/L) for women

◆ Achieve and maintain body weight goals

◆ Delay or prevent complications of diabetes

—To address individual nutrition needs based on personal and cultural preferences, health literacy and numeracy, access to healthful food choices, and willingness and ability to make behavioral changes, as well as barriers to change

—To maintain the pleasure of eating by providing positive messages about food choices while limiting food choices only when indicated by scientific evidence

—To provide the individual with diabetes with practical tools for day-to-day meal planning rather than focusing on individual macronutrients, micronutrients, or single foods[5]

Further information on the evidence-based research that supports these recommendations is provided in chapter 16, Nutrition Therapy.

MNT Considerations

Successful self-management for healthy eating requires DSME/T that focuses on concerns that are specific to the person's medical condition. One size does not fit all when educating an individual. Focus areas for healthy eating for type 1 diabetes are quite different from those for gestational diabetes, for example. Below are highlights of specialized issues that must be considered during DSME/T; more detailed information for each area can be found in chapter 16, Nutrition Therapy.

Nutrition Recommendations and Interventions for the Prevention of Diabetes

The prevalence of obesity continues to be high; more than one third of adults in the United States are obese.[8] Given that family history and overweight are strong risk factors for type 2 diabetes, healthy eating is a critical factor in diabetes prevention. Results from the Diabetes Prevention Program (DPP) confirm that lifestyle modification was nearly twice as effective as medication in preventing diabetes (58% versus 31% relative reductions, respectively).[6] The greater benefit of weight loss and physical activity strongly suggests that lifestyle modification should be the first choice

to prevent or delay diabetes. The following are recommended goals for diabetes prevention[7]:

◆ *Weight loss* of 7% of body weight

◆ *Increasing physical activity* to at least 150 minutes per week of moderate-intensity aerobic activity such as walking

Because this intervention not only has been shown to prevent or delay diabetes, but also has a variety of other benefits, healthcare providers should urge all overweight, obese, and sedentary individuals to adopt these lifestyle changes, and such recommendations should be made at every opportunity.

Healthy eating and physical activity strategies implemented in a community-based program can complement clinical preventive and treatment programs for those who are already obese. A review of DPP-based community interventions[9] concluded that prevention programs delivered in venues such as the YMCA showed promising results for long-term sustainability, making the goal of healthy eating more attainable for those working to prevent or delay the development of diabetes.

Nutrition Recommendations for the Management of Diabetes

The Nutrition Therapy Recommendations for the Management of Adults with Diabetes[5] state that nutrition therapy is recommended for all people with type 1 diabetes or type 2 diabetes as an effective component of the overall treatment plan. There is no ideal percentage of calories from carbohydrate, protein, and fat for all people with diabetes, so the choice of a healthy eating approach should be based on an individualized assessment of current eating patterns, preferences, and metabolic goals. Nutrition therapy goals should be created in collaboration with the individual with diabetes; the nutrition counselor's role is to share strategies to support the behavior changes necessary to achieve those goals.

Type 1 Diabetes Individuals with type 1 diabetes require exogenous insulin, so their primary nutrition goal is to integrate insulin therapy into their preferred eating routine and physical activity pattern. The total and type of carbohydrate in meals and snacks directly affects blood glucose levels, so this is a main area of focus. Those individuals on a fixed insulin regimen should strive for consistency in the timing and amount of their carbohydrate intake. Those using a multiple daily injection plan or insulin pump should adjust their insulin based on the carbohydrate content of their meals and snacks and may benefit from using the carbohydrate-counting meal-planning approach. For those on fixed daily insulin doses, consistent carbohydrate intake can result in improved glycemic control and reduced risk for hypoglycemia. Because hypoglycemia occurs more frequently in individuals with type 1 diabetes, reviewing the basics of hypoglycemia prevention and treatment is important. Because of the blood glucose–lowering effect of physical activity, the educator should share strategies such as adjusting insulin dosage for planned exercise to prevent hypoglycemia and also carrying a source of carbohydrate to treat hypoglycemia if needed. Additional information on this topic can be found in chapter 17, which deals with physical activity.

Type 2 Diabetes   Because most individuals with type 2 diabetes are overweight and insulin resistant, the educator should emphasize healthy eating behaviors that result in a reduction of energy, saturated and *trans* fat, and cholesterol and sodium, and an increase in physical activity in an effort to improve glycemia, dyslipidemia, and blood pressure. As in type 1 diabetes, individuals on fixed daily insulin doses may benefit from consistent carbohydrate intake to improve glycemic control and reduce risk for hypoglycemia.

  ❖ *Weight loss*—A single weight loss plan that is successful for all individuals with diabetes has yet to be created. Reducing energy intake while maintaining a healthful eating pattern is recommended to promote weight loss.
  ❖ *Physical activity*—Initial physical activity recommendations should be modest and based on the person's willingness and ability to change. Adults with diabetes should be advised to perform at least 150 minutes a week of moderate-intensity aerobic physical activity (50%-70% of maximum heart rate), spread over at least 3 days a week with no more than 2 consecutive days without exercise.

In the absence of contraindications, adults with type 2 diabetes should be encouraged to perform resistance training at least twice per week.[7]

  ❖ *Behavior change*—Patients who achieve behavior-change goals for weight loss will have better clinical outcomes and improved health status. Successful behavior-change strategies associated with weight loss and weight loss maintenance in addition to a reduced-calorie, low-fat diet include self-monitoring of weight and food intake; regular consumption of breakfast; increased, sustained levels of physical activity; and maintaining a consistent eating pattern across weekdays and weekends. Encouragingly, research has also shown that weight loss maintenance for an individual may become easier over time.[10]

Pregnancy and Lactation   Data from the Hyperglycemia and Adverse Pregnancy Outcome (HAPO) study have led to changes in the recommended criteria for the diagnosis and classification of hyperglycemia in pregnancy.[7] However, the MNT goals for pregnancy with diabetes continue to focus on minimizing blood glucose excursions and maintaining glucose values within target goal ranges before and after meals; providing a calorie intake that is neither inadequate nor excessive and will achieve an appropriate gestational weight gain without maternal ketosis; and ensuring adequate, safe nutrients for maternal and fetal health.[11] Breastfeeding is encouraged in all women with diabetes, with an emphasis on education for the prevention and treatment of hypoglycemia for women who require insulin. Specific nutrition issues with preexisting diabetes and gestational diabetes mellitus are noted below.

  ❖ *Preexisting diabetes:* Whether type 1 or type 2 preexisting diabetes, a major goal is "control before conception" because the risk of fetal anomalies is greater when blood glucose control is poor during fetal organogenesis, which occurs early in pregnancy.[12] Pregnancy for a woman with *type 1 diabetes* is often a time for intensive diabetes management involving an insulin pump or multiple daily injections of insulin. Concepts such as insulin-to-carbohydrate ratio must be mastered. The educator should also emphasize issues relating to food and the response of blood glucose during pregnancy. Hypoglycemia occurs more commonly in the first trimester because insulin requirements decrease and morning sickness leads to decreased food intake. As the pregnancy progresses, insulin resistance increases due to weight gain and increased placental hormones, necessitating increased insulin dosages to maintain optimal blood glucose control. Women with *type 2 diabetes* who become pregnant require much of the same information as women with type 1 diabetes. Often, a woman with type 2 diabetes is overweight or obese when she becomes pregnant. The educator should consider the pregravid BMI when setting gestational goals for weight gain, energy intake, and physical activity level. Additional information can be found in chapter 24, Pregnancy With Diabetes.

◆ *Gestational diabetes mellitus (GDM):* A healthy eating plan is the primary therapeutic strategy for managing GDM. Emphasis should be placed on maintaining normal blood glucose while consuming enough calories and carbohydrate to promote appropriate weight gain yet avoid maternal starvation ketosis. Dietary reference intakes (DRIs) are used to determine the estimated energy requirements in pregnancy. Because carbohydrate consumed affects postprandial blood glucose levels, the individualized eating plan for GDM focuses on total amount, type, and distribution of carbohydrate.[11] Women who develop GDM should be made aware of the lifestyle changes they will need to adopt to delay or prevent their increased risk for developing type 2 diabetes later in life. Additionally, children who were born to mothers who had GDM may also be at increased risk for obesity and type 2 diabetes throughout their lives. Additional information on GDM can be found in chapter 24, Pregnancy With Diabetes.

Children and Adolescents With Diabetes Nutrition education to promote healthy eating for children and adolescents with diabetes should involve the entire family as well as caretakers and should be geared toward the appropriate developmental stage of the child.[13] Food plans must be developed with both treatment goals and realistic lifestyle choices in mind. Consider these points for children with diabetes or at risk for type 2 diabetes when creating the healthy eating plan:

◆ Adjust the food plan to meet energy requirements for growth and activity.

◆ Focus on an intake of nutrient-dense foods (ie, fruits, vegetables, whole grains, and calcium-rich foods) versus nutrient-sparse foods (ie, excessive amounts of sweets or large amounts of juice and fruit drinks).

◆ Use the term "food plan" or "meal plan," rather than "diet," to avoid furthering negative connotations regarding healthy eating.

◆ Engage the child or adolescent in development of the food plan as well as in shopping for and preparing healthy foods for the entire family.

Type 1 Diabetes In addition to the points mentioned above, nutrition education for children with type 1 diabetes revolves around achieving blood glucose goals without excessive hypoglycemia while promoting normal growth and development. The key concepts discussed earlier about type 1 diabetes in adults also apply to children with type 1 diabetes. Discussions of DSME/T should address the following:

◆ Nutrition issues for school and day care, irregular schedules, sports activities, peer influences, and level of acceptance

◆ Effects of growth and hormonal changes on blood glucose

◆ Additional adjustments to be made in insulin administered at mealtime, for "picky" eaters

Type 2 Diabetes An estimated 1 out of 3 children born in the United States in the year 2000 will have diabetes in their lifetime.[14] This is due, in part, to the increasing number of children who are medically classified as "pediatric overweight." In addition to the previously mentioned points, lifestyle considerations for children at risk for or diagnosed with type 2 diabetes should include the following:

- Controlling portions by encouraging children to "eat to appetite" rather than "cleaning their plates" filled with adult-sized portions
- Slowing their rate of eating
- Striving for regular mealtimes and limiting distractions, such as eating while watching TV, working on the computer, or using a smartphone
- Promoting moderate physical activity of at least 60 minutes daily
- Limiting the amount of nonacademic "screen time" (TV watching, video games, or Internet or social media use) to less than 2 hours daily

Because of the strong genetic component of type 2 diabetes, the entire family often benefits from being involved in the lifestyle change program. Successful lifestyle change outcomes for children with type 2 diabetes are defined as follows[15]:

- Cessation of excessive weight gain with near-normal linear growth
- Near-normal fasting blood glucose and A1C values

The American Academy of Pediatrics suggests that clinicians incorporate the Academy of Nutrition and Dietetics' *Pediatric Weight Management Evidence-Based Nutrition Practice Guidelines*[16] into their nutrition counseling of children with type 2 diabetes at the time of diagnosis and as part of ongoing management. Additional information on nutrition therapy for children and adolescents with diabetes can be found in chapter 16.

Older Adults With Diabetes   Recommendations for making healthy food choices should be individualized regardless of a person's age, but the need for this is even more apparent when the numerous factors affecting the older adult are considered.

Older Adults

One-on-one sessions often eliminate visual and auditory barriers to learning. Family and caregivers can attend to offer additional support.

Older adults with diabetes vary widely in their physical and cognitive status; in the presence or absence of underlying chronic conditions and comorbidities; and in their cultural backgrounds, traditions, and beliefs. An older individual who is able and willing to undertake the responsibility for diabetes self-management should be encouraged to do so and should be treated using the previously stated metabolic goals for adults; for other older adults, glycemic goals may be reasonably relaxed.[17] The educator should provide meal-planning guidelines that incorporate cultural food favorites and meet calorie and nutrient needs while promoting glycemic control. Physical activity should also be encouraged as a regular part of the individual's daily routine. With the individual's permission, family and caregivers should be encouraged to attend the teaching sessions; one-to-one sessions may be preferable to group classes, in which visual and auditory barriers could arise. Healthy eating issues such as taste preferences, lifelong eating habits, finances, and food preparation ability are also important.[18] Additional information on nutrition therapy for older adults with diabetes can be found in chapter 16.

Eating Problems and Diabetes   Eating problems (both disordered eating behavior and eating disorders) are more common in adolescents with type 1 diabetes compared with their peers without type 1 diabetes, and both eating problems and diabetes are associated with poorer glycemic control.[19] Evidence also suggests an increasing trend in eating disorders for middle-aged women, as well as the trend of orthorexia nervosa, an unhealthful fixation about eating so-called healthful foods.[20] Types of eating disorders include the following:

- *Anorexia nervosa*, which centers on restricted energy intake relative to requirements, leading to a markedly low body weight; intense fear of gaining weight or becoming fat or persistent behavior to avoid weight gain, even though at a markedly low weight; disturbance in the way in which one's body weight or shape is experienced.
- *Bulimia nervosa*, which is characterized by recurrent episodes of binge eating with a sense of lack of control and inappropriate compensatory behavior; self-evaluation unduly

influenced by body shape and weight; and not occurring exclusively during episodes of anorexia nervosa. Purging may occur with self-induced vomiting, laxatives, diuretics, insulin omission or reduction, fasting, severe diets, or vigorous exercise.

⬥ *Binge eating disorder* is described as repeated episodes of overconsumption of food with a sense of a lack of control. While there may be no purging, there may be sporadic fasts or repetitive diets and often feelings of shame or distress after a binge.

Disturbed eating can have a potentially life-threatening impact on individuals with diabetes. Although early recognition of risk for an eating disorder may help with prevention, there are no validated screening tools to help identify those in need of intervention. Diabetes educators should be alert to warning signs that may suggest the presence of an eating disorder, such as deterioration in psychosocial function, neglect of diabetes management (particularly insulin omission), erratic clinic attendance, significant weight gain/loss, poor body image/low self-esteem, and recurrent/frequent diabetic ketoacidosis. Because eating disorders may be well hidden, it's important for the educator to use sensitive, open-ended questions to encourage discussion about body weight and shape. If an eating disorder is suspected, early referral to a mental health professional with experience working with individuals with eating disorders is indicated.

A multidisciplinary team approach to treatment is considered the standard of care for both eating disorders and diabetes. Initially, treatment of an eating disorder involves establishing medical safety, while members of the treatment team work to establish a positive rapport with the patient. Cognitive behavioral therapy has proven successful in the treatment of binge eating behaviors, but its use in anorexia nervosa is challenging because disruptions in neurotransmitter secretions and functions limit a patient's response to treatment.[20] A focus on carbohydrate or calorie intake can lead to over-restrictive eating in an individual with diabetes, so the nutrition treatment plan for the eating disorder should emphasize flexible and nondepriving approaches to eating that can be adopted by the patient's entire

family for overall health and wellness.[21] The total diet approach to healthy eating, which focuses on variety, moderation, and proportionality in the context of a healthy lifestyle, rather than targeting specific nutrients or foods,[22] may prove successful in the treatment of eating problems in individuals with diabetes.

Diabetes and the Gastrointestinal Tract *Celiac disease* and *gastroparesis* are 2 areas of concern relative to healthy eating, diabetes, and the gastrointestinal tract.

Celiac Disease Celiac disease (also known as gluten-sensitive enteropathy [GSE]) is an immune-mediated disorder that occurs with increased frequency in patients with type 1 diabetes (1%-16% of individuals compared with 0.3%-1% in the general population).[7] Individuals with celiac disease sustain damage to their intestinal epithelium after ingestion of foods made from the gliadin fraction of wheat gluten and similar molecules from barley, rye, and possibly oats, most commonly causing abdominal pain, diarrhea, malabsorption, and failure to thrive. While many patients with celiac disease are asymptomatic, current practice recommends that healthcare providers consider screening children with type 1 diabetes for celiac disease soon after the diagnosis of diabetes. If the diagnosis of celiac disease is confirmed, they should consult with an RD/RDN and begin a gluten-free eating plan to coordinate with their nutrition plan for diabetes management. In addition to strictly eliminating gluten-containing grains such as barley, bran, hydrolyzed wheat protein, oats, rye, wheat, wheat bran, wheat germ, and white, whole wheat, and graham flour, patients may require a multivitamin supplement daily to prevent deficiencies resulting from malabsorption.[23] Intensive education in label reading and identification of hidden sources of gluten is necessary. Sources are available to provide patients with celiac disease with pamphlets, books, and recipes,[24,25] although there is a need for more educational materials that address healthy eating for both celiac disease and diabetes.

Gastroparesis Gastroparesis is a form of autonomic neuropathy that delays the emptying of the stomach. Clinically, patients with diabetes and gastroparesis are at risk for erratic glycemic control as a consequence of unpredictable nutrient delivery of food into the upper gut, where it is absorbed. Hypoglycemia has resulted when insulin has been administered and gastric emptying of nutrients did not follow. Currently, there are no clinical trial results to determine the success of any particular nutrition intervention, and dietary suggestions are based largely on clinical experience. While therapies such as anti-emetic and prokinetic medications, as well as the emerging option of gastric electrical stimulation, are the main treatments of gastroparesis, some general healthy eating recommendations for patients with gastroparesis include the following[26]:

- Decrease volume of meals/eat smaller, more frequent meals throughout the day.
- Use more liquid calories—may need to switch to liquid calories over the course of the day as fullness worsens; if solids are not tolerated, consider a trial of a pureed/liquid diet.
- Chew foods well.
- Sit up for 1 to 2 hours after a meal.
- Decrease fiber in the diet, as it may delay gastric emptying and lead to bezoar formation.
- Evaluate fat intake—fat in liquid form is often tolerated; fat is a good source of calories and should only be limited after other measures have been exhausted or if intake of solid fat is excessive.
- Consider taking a daily multivitamin/mineral supplement if dietary intake is inadequate.

Because poor glycemic control and wide swings in blood glucose levels can exacerbate gastroparesis, it's important for people with diabetes to work toward improved blood glucose management. A basal/bolus insulin regimen before meals and snacks is recommended to match insulin needs to carbohydrate intake and promote optimal glucose control. Frequent blood glucose monitoring is necessary to achieve improved glycemic control.

In Summary: Which Approach to Healthy Eating for Diabetes Is the Most Effective?

Healthy eating for diabetes is a complex issue. At this time, no single, ideal approach to the amount of protein, fat, and carbohydrate in a diabetes meal plan has been established. An individualized assessment of a patient's current eating patterns, preferences, and metabolic goals can help determine macronutrient distribution. Emphasis should not be placed on individual micro- and macronutrients, but rather on eating patterns, a term used to describe combinations of different foods or food groups that characterize relationships between nutrition and health promotion and disease prevention. Framing nutrition recommendations in terms of eating patterns is consistent with the total diet approach suggested by the 2010 Dietary Guidelines for Americans, which consider the combinations of foods and beverages that provide energy and nutrients and constitute an individual's complete dietary intake, on average, over time.[22] The Nutrition Therapy Recommendations for the Management of Adults with Diabetes[5] review the evidence base in support of several eating patterns to evaluate their impact on diabetes nutrition goals for type 1 diabetes or type 2 diabetes:

- The *Mediterranean-style* eating pattern leads to improved CVD risk factors in individuals with diabetes. When supplemented with mixed nuts or olive oil, the Mediterranean eating pattern lowered combined end points for cardiovascular events and stroke. Individuals following an energy-restricted Mediterranean-style eating pattern also achieved improvements in glycemic goals.
- *Vegetarian and low-fat vegan* eating patterns did not consistently improve glycemic control or CVD risk in individuals with type 2 diabetes, except when energy intake was restricted and weight was lost.
- The *low-fat* eating pattern with reduced calories achieved moderate success for weight loss in the Look AHEAD trial, but in other cited research studies, lowering total fat intake didn't consistently improve glycemic control or CVD risk factors. The benefit from a low-fat eating pattern is more likely when energy intake is also reduced and weight loss occurs.
- Research on *low-carbohydrate* eating patterns is inconclusive when evaluating the effect of differing percentages of carbohydrate in

people with diabetes. However, monitoring the amount and type of carbohydrate consumed is a useful strategy for improving postprandial glucose control; the total amount of carbohydrate eaten is the primary predictor of glycemic response. Evidence is insufficient to support one specific amount of carbohydrate intake for all people with diabetes.

◆ The *DASH (Dietary Approaches to Stop Hypertension)* eating pattern has been shown to control blood pressure and lower risk for CVD in people without diabetes. Limited evidence exists on the effects of the DASH eating plan in individuals with diabetes, but one would expect similar results to other studies using the DASH eating plan.

Table 4.2 describes the key elements of each of these eating patterns and includes meal ideas to help translate these recommendations into a day's meals.

Glycemic Index

Monitoring carbohydrate intake remains a key strategy in achieving glycemic control. The *glycemic index* (GI) estimates the acute postprandial glycemic impact of a carbohydrate-containing food and ranks carbohydrates on a scale from 0 to 100 according to the extent to which they raise blood glucose levels after eating. Proponents of this often-controversial meal-planning approach explain GI by noting that foods with a high GI are those which are rapidly digested and absorbed and result in marked fluctuations in blood glucose levels; low-GI foods, by virtue of their slow digestion and absorption, produce gradual rises in blood glucose and insulin levels.[27] The Human Nutrition Unit, School of Molecular Biosciences, University of Sydney Australia maintains a comprehensive database of foods that have been tested for the GI and glycemic load.[28] Research on the effects of using a GI meal-planning approach on glycemic control and CVD risks factors is mixed; however, substituting low–glycemic load foods for high–glycemic load foods may modestly improve glycemic control.[5] Implementing a GI meal-planning approach can be complex, but individuals with diabetes who choose to use the GI can begin by incorporating one lower GI food in each meal and snack and making simple changes such as substituting a grainy or sourdough bread for white bread, natural muesli for puffed grain cereal, lentils or beans for potatoes, and nuts for snacks such as pretzels.

Because the literature suggests that several approaches to healthy eating for diabetes may be effective in improving glycemic and/or CVD risk factors, the educator should offer a choice of eating patterns based on the individual's health goals, personal and cultural preferences, health literacy and numeracy, access to healthful choices, and readiness, willingness, and ability to change.[5] For a more in-depth discussion on the evidence base supporting healthy eating, see chapter 16, Nutrition Therapy.

TABLE 4.2 Eating Patterns for Diabetes: Descriptions and Meal Ideas		
Eating Pattern	*Description*	*Meal Ideas*
Mediterranean style	Includes abundant plant food (fruits, vegetables, grains [mostly whole], beans, nuts, and seeds); minimally processed, seasonally fresh, and locally grown foods; fresh fruits as the typical daily dessert, and concentrated sugars or honey consumed only for special occasions; olive oil as the principal source of dietary lipids; dairy products (mainly cheese and yogurt) consumed in low to moderate amounts; fewer than 4 eggs per week; red meat consumed in low frequency and amounts; and wine consumption in low to moderate amounts, generally with meals	Breakfast—Greek yogurt topped with berries and walnuts, cubed cantaloupe Lunch—White bean soup, hummus and vegetables in a whole wheat pita Dinner—Grilled salmon stuffed with spinach and feta cheese, wheat berry salad (olive oil, vinaigrette, feta, parsley, and tomatoes), baked apples with cherries and almonds, glass of red wine Snacks—Nuts, whole grain crackers and cheese

(continued)

TABLE 4.2   Eating Patterns for Diabetes: Descriptions and Meal Ideas (continued)

Eating Pattern	Description	Meal Ideas
Vegetarian and vegan	Vegan meal plans are devoid of all flesh foods and animal-derived products; vegetarian meal plans are devoid of all flesh foods but include egg (ovo) and/or dairy (lacto) products. These meal plans feature lower intakes of saturated fat and cholesterol and higher intakes of fruits, vegetables, whole grains, nuts, soy products, fiber, and phytochemicals.	Vegan Meals: Breakfast—Whole grain cereal with soy milk, banana Lunch—Grilled vegetable sandwich (tomatoes, zucchini, peppers, onion, garlic, and beans), green spinach salad with vinaigrette dressing Dinner—Tofu stir-fry with sautéed vegetables such as broccoli, snow peas, baby corn, and water chestnuts, soy yogurt parfait Snacks—Fresh fruits and vegetables, soy almond milk fruit smoothie Vegetarian meals may include eggs and dairy products
Low fat	Emphasizes vegetables, fruits, starches (breads/crackers, pasta, whole grains, starchy vegetables), lean protein, and low-fat dairy products. Defined as total fat intake <30% or total energy intake and saturated fat intake <10%	Breakfast—Whole grain English muffin with fat-free cream cheese, blueberries, skim milk Lunch—Chicken noodle soup, green salad with chicken and fat-free French salad dressing, fresh pineapple Dinner—Grilled shrimp skewers on brown rice, tossed salad with fat-free Caesar salad dressing, watermelon Snacks—Nonfat yogurt, low-fat cheese with whole wheat crackers
Low carbohydrate	Focuses on foods higher in protein (meat, poultry, fish, shellfish, eggs, cheese, nuts, and seeds), fats (oils, butter, olives, avocado), and vegetables low in carbohydrate (salad greens, cucumbers, broccoli, summer squash). Amount of carbohydrate varies with most plans, allowing fruit and higher carbohydrate vegetables; however, sugar-containing foods and grain products such as pasta, rice, and bread are generally avoided. No consistent definition of "low" carbohydrate but may range from very low-carbohydrate (21-70 g per day of carbohydrate) to moderately low-carbohydrate (30 to <40% of calories from carbohydrates)	Breakfast—Eggs cooked in butter, Canadian bacon, fresh grapefruit Lunch—Sliced grilled chicken wrapped in lettuce with tomatoes and mayonnaise, Romaine lettuce salad with avocado slices and vinaigrette salad dressing Dinner—London Broil, mushrooms sautéed in oil, spinach salad with pecans and blue cheese dressing, sugar-free gelatin Snacks—Whole almonds, string cheese
DASH	Emphasizes fruits, vegetables, and low-fat dairy products, including whole grains, poultry, fish, and nuts; reduced in saturated fat, red meat, sweets, and sugar-containing beverages. The most effective DASH meal plan is also reduced in sodium.	Breakfast—Cooked oatmeal with low-fat milk, low-sodium vegetable juice, banana Lunch—Unsalted chicken salad on whole wheat bread with Dijon mustard, apple, low-fat milk Dinner—Baked turkey, broccoli, whole wheat roll with unsalted soft margarine, nonfat yogurt Snacks—Unsalted almonds or pretzels, fresh fruits and vegetables

Source: Adapted from AB Evert, JL Boucher, M Cypress, et al; American Diabetes Association. "Nutrition therapy recommendations for the management of adults with diabetes: a position statement of the American Diabetes Association," *Diabetes Care* 36 (2013): 3821-42.

American Association of Diabetes Educators©

Promoting Healthy Eating: The Role of DSME/T

Diabetes education, also known as diabetes self-management training (DSMT) or diabetes self-management education (DSME), is a collaborative process through which people with or at risk for diabetes gain the knowledge and skills needed to modify behavior and successfully self-manage the disease and its related conditions.[1] Using evidence-based clinical practice recommendations and taking into account the expected outcomes from MNT, diabetes educators translate clinical recommendations into self-management education. Registered dietitians/registered dietitian nutritionists are guided in this effort by 2 recommended tools, the Nutrition Care Process and Model and the Nutrition Practice Guidelines, both developed by the Academy of Nutrition and Dietetics.

The Nutrition Care Process and Model

The Nutrition Care Process and Model (NCPM)[29] outlines the consistent and specific steps to be used when delivering MNT and moves professionals beyond experience-based practice to evidence-based practice. Although the NCPM is intended for dietetics professionals, other healthcare professionals may find the process useful in providing quality care. Central to the effective provision of MNT is the relationship between the individual seeking care and the healthcare professional.

Four Steps in the NCPM

1. Assessment
2. Diagnosis
3. Intervention
4. Monitoring and evaluation

Step 1: Nutrition Assessment

An RD/RDN who provides MNT and education on healthy eating should follow a systematic process that begins with a nutrition assessment. Nutrition assessment is a systematic approach to collect, record, and interpret relevant data from patients, clients, family members, caregivers, and other individuals and groups. Nutrition assessment is an ongoing, dynamic process that involves initial data collection as well as continual reassessment and analysis of the patient's/client's status compared with specific criteria.[29] Other members of the diabetes healthcare team often provide information which makes the assessment more valuable. Types of data collected include the following:

- Food- and nutrition-related history
- Anthropometric measurements
- Biochemical data, medical tests, and procedures
- Nutrition-focused physical examination findings
- Client history

Conducting the assessment establishes rapport, which is particularly helpful as the process of DSME/T continues. The educator must learn the following about the individual: level of knowledge and skills, attitude and motivation, and readiness to learn new behaviors and interest in changing old ones, if appropriate, as well as preferred ways of learning.

During the assessment phase, the educator can determine the individual's preference for learning. This enables the educator to present information in a style tailored to promote success. Some people prefer to learn by reading, others by listening, others by watching, and still others by a hands-on approach; at times, an individual may combine learning styles. Health literacy is particularly relevant for diabetes education. The assessment phase yields information related to the individualization of self-management education which promotes consideration of each participant's educational concerns and priorities, recognizes the expertise and unique perspectives that each participant brings to the process of self-management education, incorporates psychosocial and behavioral aspects, and helps create collaborative partnerships between participants and diabetes educators that promote and sustain ongoing diabetes self-management.[30]

Health beliefs must be considered during the assessment. Food choices and why a person eats as he or she does are deeply embedded in the psyche and may be a result of strong cultural or ethnic traditions. The supportiveness of family members may not be obvious; further probing may be required. Visual status, disabilities, barriers to learning, and socioeconomic status are all important factors to determine in the assessment.

The Role of Ethnicity and Culture   Because ethnic diversity continues to increase, and because the prevalence of diabetes in minority groups throughout the United States is extremely high, the diabetes educator must be prepared to tailor DSME/T for healthy eating to fit a variety of cultural practices. The most effective diabetes educators are those who have a deep commitment to cultural sensitivity for the populations they serve.[31] Cultural competency is the ability to work effectively with people of different cultural backgrounds. Successful diabetes prevention and treatment in diverse ethnic populations requires sensitivity to cultural differences in health beliefs and eating habits.

A 4-Step Process to Improve Cross-Cultural Counseling

Eating is a personal matter that can carry great cultural significance. Health professionals can use a 4-step process to improve cross-cultural counseling.[32]

1. Self-evaluation of the educator's own cultural heritage
2. Preinterview research on the cultural background of each individual
3. In-depth, cross-cultural interview to establish individual's personal preferences and cultural background and eating habit adaptations made in the United States
4. Unbiased analysis of the data

In cross-cultural counseling, as in other situations, the person who came for assistance should be involved in problem solving and in developing strategies for behavior change. Include family members who are involved in food preparation. Establish respect and trust by having a nonjudgmental attitude and accepting cultural differences. Include as many familiar foods as possible in the healthy eating plan and explore the person's uses of special foods, beverages, or herbal therapies as folk remedies. Refer to chapter 20, on biological complementary therapies, for more information and a list of resources.

A variety of resources are available for learning more about a specific culture and are useful when providing MNT.[33,34] Existing educational materials may also be adapted to be culturally specific. Invite the individual with diabetes to teach the educator about the ingredients in and preparation of cultural and ethnic foods. Combining an individual's cultural expertise with the diabetes and nutrition knowledge of the educator allows for a true exchange of information that benefits both parties.

A comprehensive assessment is a crucial step in providing individualized diabetes nutrition therapy. The assessment requires adequate time to be performed thoroughly, but provides a wealth of information that allows the professional to tailor the intervention and the diabetes nutrition therapy to the individual. The RD/RDN cannot begin to develop a nutrition diagnosis or design a nutrition intervention without the sound basis of an assessment. A high-level assessment involves obtaining appropriate data as well as analyzing and interpreting the data in light of evidence-based standards.

Step 2: Nutrition Diagnosis
The nutrition diagnosis is the RD/RDN's identification and labeling of an existing nutrition problem that he or she is responsible for treating independently.[29] It determines the specific healthy eating behaviors that need to be modified. The nutrition diagnosis is not the same as the medical diagnosis, which is diabetes mellitus. Components of the nutrition diagnosis include a description of alterations in a patient's status, etiology of the problem, and signs/symptoms of the problem. While the patient may have a medical diagnosis of type 1 diabetes, after completing a nutrition assessment the RD/RDN establishes the nutrition diagnosis. A well-written nutrition diagnostic statement should be clear and concise, specific to a patient/client, limited to a single client problem, accurately related to one etiology, and based on signs/symptoms from the assessment data.[29] The following are examples of a nutrition diagnostic statement:

"Inconsistent carbohydrate intake"
"Overly large portion sizes"
"Excessive fat intake"

Determining a nutrition diagnosis will guide the educator and the person with or at risk for diabetes toward the appropriate selection of goals for behavior change and their desired outcomes.

Step 3: Nutrition Intervention
The third step of the NCPM, nutrition intervention, involves planning and implementing the activities

that specifically facilitate or support the individual's healthy eating behavior. It consists of 2 interrelated components: planning and implementation. Steps in planning include prioritizing diagnoses, writing a nutrition prescription, collaborating with the patient to identify goals, selecting specific intervention strategies, and defining time/frequency of care, including intensity, duration, and follow-up. Implementing the plan involves collaborating with the patient to carry out the plan, communicating the plan, modifying the plan as needed, following up and verifying that the plan is being implemented, and revising strategies based on changes in condition or response to the intervention.[29]

Education, the process of providing accurate and timely information to the individual who has or is at risk for diabetes, is key at this step. However, the role of the educator goes beyond merely supplying facts. The educator is a counselor and a coach, whose role is to help the person understand the disease and cope with its implications. The educator is a partner in disease management, assisting individuals in making their own decisions about self-care and healthy eating while helping them discover how they may be motivated to change their behavior.

After the nutrition diagnosis is made and behavior goals and desired outcomes are established, the nutrition intervention begins and healthy eating skills can be taught. A number of healthy eating resources are available; several are described later in this chapter. No single meal-planning approach works for every individual. The initial meal-planning approach is chosen with the understanding that it may change as the person's understanding of the disease and motivation to self-manage evolve.

Step 4: Nutrition Monitoring and Evaluation

Nutrition monitoring and evaluation identifies the amount of progress made and whether goals are being met. This step includes 3 distinct and interrelated processes: monitor progress, measure outcomes, and evaluate outcomes.[29] Successful MNT involves the process of problem solving, adjustment, and readjustment. Food diaries and records, such as blood glucose readings, are reviewed, evaluated, and reassessed. Measurable goals help make evaluation a straightforward task. Helping the person with

diabetes think in terms of a course correction, rather than a goal evaluation, makes this discussion less threatening. If initial goals are not met, they may need to be changed or renegotiated. If they have been met, new reasonable, attainable, and measurable goals should be designed.

Documentation is necessary at each stage of the NCPM. Documentation in the medical record aids in communication with other members of the healthcare team. Written documentation can be shared with the patient to demonstrate his or her progress and encourage further efforts.

Outline for a Well-Designed Diabetes Nutrition Education Encounter

- *Focus on the individual*—The encounter begins with the educator asking the individual what questions and concerns he or she has regarding healthy eating.
- *Assess, diagnose, plan*—The educator then completes the nutrition assessment, establishes a nutrition diagnosis, and works with the individual to set behavior-change goals and plan a nutrition intervention using an individualized healthy eating approach.
- *Wrap up for the individual's benefit*—The session ends with the educator answering remaining questions, asking the patient to summarize key points, and making a follow-up plan for the future.

The Nutrition Practice Guidelines

The Nutrition Practice Guidelines (NPGs) for type 1 diabetes and type 2 diabetes[35] and for GDM[11] have been developed to delineate the structure by which optimal care is provided. The NPGs are evidence-based protocols that, when used to deliver MNT, result in positive health outcomes. These guidelines outline both clinical outcomes and necessary lifestyle changes and suggest the frequency and length of contact with the RD/RDN as well as the amount of time between encounters, based on the specific situation of the person. For example, due to the time-sensitive nature of GDM, more frequent contact in a shorter period of time is generally required as compared with routine follow-up for an individual with long-standing type 2 diabetes. Together, the NCPM and NPGs form the framework for well-designed self-management education regarding healthy eating.

Promoting Healthy Eating: The Role of Behavior Change

Behavior change is the unique outcome measurement for DSME. For the individual who participates in self-management education focused on healthy eating, the goal is to improve overall health status by empowering him or her to do the following:

- ◆ Acquire knowledge (what to do)
- ◆ Acquire skills (how to do it)
- ◆ Develop confidence and motivation to perform the appropriate self-care behaviors (want to do it)
- ◆ Develop problem-solving and coping skills to overcome any barriers to self-care behavior (can do it)[36]

Outcomes

Measuring outcomes demonstrates the effectiveness of the diabetes educator and the unique contribution that he or she can make. For each of the AADE7 Self-Care Behaviors™, a continuum of outcomes related to diabetes education is expected:

- ◆ *Immediate outcomes:* Learning, knowledge, skill acquisition
- ◆ *Intermediate outcomes:* Behavior change
- ◆ *Post-intermediate outcomes:* Improved clinical indicators
- ◆ *Long-term outcomes:* Improved health status

Immediate Outcomes

Learning is the immediate outcome sought. After teaching a healthy eating behavior such as label reading, the diabetes educator can immediately ask the learner to demonstrate the new skill. The educator asks the learner, for example, to read a sample label for critical information, such as portion size or carbohydrate content. This enables the educator to determine whether the person learned the material that was taught.

Intermediate Outcomes

Behavior change, the intermediate outcome sought, is the unique outcome measurement for DSME/T. Although the learner may have acquired important information regarding label reading, the desired outcome is that this person uses the information to change his or her behavior and make healthier food choices. Behaviors such as choosing the proper type and amount of food or dealing with special situations such as illness or travel can be measured by observation, self-report of food intake, and review of records of blood glucose readings. Feeling empowered about making positive, sustainable behavior changes leads to increased energy levels and improved monitoring results.

Post-intermediate Outcomes

Improved clinical indicators, the desired post-intermediate outcome, can be measured via laboratory tests and clinical measurements such as A1C, blood pressure, and lipid levels.

Long-Term Outcomes

At the end of the continuum of outcomes are long-term outcomes such as improved health status. Long-term outcomes can be measured as improvement in quality of life, economic benefits from reduced healthcare costs, and increased productivity.

Behavior Change

Behavior-change theories and strategies are useful in planning effective counseling sessions on the topic of healthy eating. Using the Transtheoretical Model of Behavior Change,[37] the diabetes educator can match the nutrition intervention to the individual's stage of readiness to embrace new behaviors. In developing this model, Prochaska et al outlined the 5 stages of behavior change: precontemplation, contemplation, preparation, action, and maintenance. The stages are useful to consider when planning and implementing nutrition care. In making changes, people progress through these 5 stages, although not necessarily in a systematic manner. Being aware of the nature of this process can help the educator better understand and help the individual progress toward behavior changes that result in healthy eating. Recognizing that behavior change is a multistep process helps minimize unrealistic expectations. Table 4.3 illustrates the process.

The individual with diabetes and the educator work together to formulate goals and determine a plan of action. When establishing goals, the diabetes educator should distinguish not only between short-term goals for behavior change and long-term goals, but also between behavior-change outcomes that are the goals of the person seeking assistance and those that are the goals of the healthcare provider. Goals for both parties should be specific, reasonable, attainable, and measurable.[38] Examples of behavior-change goals for healthy eating are shown in Table 4.4. If the educator has established a good rapport with the person, negotiating attainable goals is easier. Healthy eating goals evolve over time and need to be evaluated and renegotiated as circumstances change.

A brief counseling approach that can be integrated with other diabetes nutrition education and counseling resources is the 5As (Assess, Advise, Agree, Assist, Arrange), which has proven helpful in counseling for smoking cessation. Research has shown that when clinicians spend as little as 3 minutes talking about a new behavior, patients will consider and even adopt a behavior change.[39]

Additional information about outcomes, goal setting, and behavior change can be found in chapters 2 and 3.

TABLE 4.4 Sample Behavior-Change Goals for Healthy Eating

I will measure my food and beverage intake for 3 days, record the amounts, and bring the records to my next clinic appointment.

I will substitute diet soda or water for sweetened soda at lunchtime at least 3 days per week.

I will check and record my blood glucose levels 2 hours after each meal every day.

I will modify 3 favorite recipes into lower fat and lower carbohydrate versions before my next clinic appointment.

I will limit my carbohydrate intake to 60 g of carbohydrate at each of my 3 meals and 15 g of carbohydrate at each of my 2 snacks at least 5 days per week.

Source: P Geil, T Ross, *What Do I Eat Now? A Step-by-Step Guide for Eating Right With Type 2 Diabetes* (Alexandria, Va: American Diabetes Association, 2009).

Promoting Healthy Eating: Theory Into Practice

No single meal-planning approach works for every individual, and no single approach has been proven to be more effective than another. Positive behavior change for healthy eating depends greatly on readiness to learn and the individualized needs of the person with diabetes. For each phase of education,

TABLE 4.3 The Process of Behavior Change: Healthy Eating for Weight Loss

Stage of Change	*Characteristics*	*Typical Patient Comments*
Precontemplation	Unaware that change is needed or having no intention of changing	"I feel fine, even though I might be a few pounds overweight."
Contemplation	Intends to change in the next 6 months; aware of the benefits and costs of change	"I will try to lose some weight. It will help improve my blood glucose, but I don't know if I can give up my wife's down-home cooking."
Preparation	Ready to change in the next 30 days; taking steps to begin making a change	"I've looked at all the diets out there. I think I'll stick with the meal plan I learned about at my last diabetes clinic visit."
Action	Has been making changes over the past 6 months	"I've been following my meal plan and weighing myself every week for the past month."
Maintenance	Has successfully made a change for more than 6 months; making efforts to avoid slipping into past behaviors	"Since the holidays are coming up, I need to plan on sticking with my current strategies so I won't gain weight again this year."

Source: P Geil, T Ross, *What Do I Eat Now? A Step-by-Step Guide for Eating Right With Type 2 Diabetes* (Alexandria, Va: American Diabetes Association, 2009).

different educational resources may be needed. Key topics for nutrition education, including coordinating food with diabetes medications, are available in the Nutrition Therapy Recommendations for the Management of Adults With Diabetes.[5]

Initial Education

Basic nutrition interventions are needed for beginning or "survival" education, while more in-depth tools may be needed as the counseling process continues. Basic or initial education provides the information needed at the time of diagnosis, when the treatment plan or person's lifestyle changes, or at the time of initial contact with a diabetes educator. Initial skill topics include the following:

◆ Information about basic nutrition guidelines
◆ Instruction on sources of carbohydrate, amount of carbohydrate to consume, portion sizes, and the need to space carbohydrates throughout the day to control blood glucose
◆ Symptoms and treatment of hypoglycemia, if appropriate

More Advanced Topics

Continuing self-management training provides more advanced education and includes both management and lifestyle skills. Topics to cover are chosen based on the individual's situation, level of nutrition knowledge, and experience in planning, purchasing, and preparing food. Individuals with diabetes can be taught more in-depth topics such as making adjustments in food and medication for sick days, physical activity, travel, and eating away from home.

Meal-Planning Resources

A healthy eating plan for diabetes is individualized and should emphasize a variety of minimally processed nutrient-dense foods in appropriate portion sizes.[5] The following meal-planning resources are helpful in translating the evidence-based science behind current diabetes nutrition recommendations into a healthy meal plan for everyday use.

Because healthy eating for diabetes is not "one size fits all," preprinted diet sheets are ineffective and should not be used. A number of meal-planning approaches are available to teach basic diabetes nutrition guidelines

as well as more in-depth nutrition interventions. The person with diabetes and the educator may begin with one meal-planning approach and then try other resources as the counseling process continues.

Dietary Guidelines for Americans, 2010[40] and the USDA Choose My Plate[41] (see Figure 4.1) can be used as an introduction to basic nutrition and to begin the process of changing eating behaviors. However, these resources do not address issues specific to diabetes; therefore, a diabetes-based resource such as the ADA's Create Your Plate[42] might prove more effective. These meal-planning approaches are especially useful for visual learners, those who do not speak English, persons with poor reading or math skills, and individuals with cognitive limitations.

Healthy Food Choices (English and Spanish)[43] is a pamphlet that illustrates the basics of good nutrition and includes food lists. It opens into a small poster that provides a general overview of what to eat and when. Space is provided to write in a detailed meal plan in any "meal-planning language" (ie, carbohydrate servings, food choice groups, or actual menu items).

Individualized menus can be developed by the RD/RDN to provide a written description of exactly what and when to eat. Individualized, preplanned menus help people with diabetes achieve healthy eating by specifying the foods and amounts to be consumed for meals and snacks each day. Menu resources often include simple recipes to help people with diabetes prepare their food. Menus are useful for initial or simplified diabetes meal planning; for those who have little experience or interest in meal

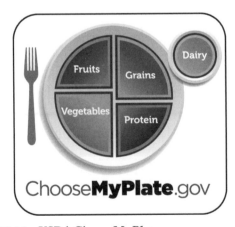

FIGURE 4.1   USDA Choose My Plate

Source: United States Department of Agriculture (USDA), "Choose my plate" (cited 2013 Nov 2), on the Internet at: http://www.choosemyplate.com.

planning; and for individuals with poor reading and math skills, cognitive limitations, or difficulty using more structured approaches. The ADA has developed healthy menus which are available in the *Month of Meals™ Diabetes Meal Planner* book.[44]

Eating Healthy With Diabetes: Easy Reading Guide[45] is intended for persons with diabetes who have limited reading skills or impaired vision. The guide offers a large-print format, numerous photos, and very little text. Food lists are presented in the context of breakfast, lunch, dinner, and snack choices.

Choose Your Foods: Food Lists for Diabetes[46] (English and Spanish) lists groups of measured foods of approximately the same nutritional value. Foods in each list can be substituted or exchanged for other foods in the same list. This continues to be the most complete set of food lists on which all other diabetes nutrition resources are based. The food lists are used with an individualized meal plan that specifies when and how many choices from each group are to be eaten for meals and/or snacks.

Choose Your Foods: Plan Your Meals[47] (English and Spanish) is a colorful trifold poster that introduces meal planning for people newly diagnosed with diabetes. It includes tips for using a plate to plan breakfasts, lunches, dinners, and snacks and features a meal planner that can be personalized.

Carbohydrate Counting

Carbohydrate affects blood glucose more directly than protein or fat, the other 2 sources of energy/calories. Both the amount (grams) and the type of carbohydrate in a food influence the blood glucose level. Monitoring total grams of carbohydrate remains a key strategy in achieving glycemic control. Using the carbohydrate-counting method, the person with diabetes counts the exact number of grams of carbohydrate in the foods eaten. Alternatively, each serving of starch, fruit, or milk and milk substitutes can be counted as 1 carbohydrate serving. Each carbohydrate serving has about 15 g of carbohydrate. An RD/RDN can help the person with diabetes determine the optimal number of carbohydrate servings or grams of carbohydrate to eat each day; the individual then follows this recommendation in planning meals. Food records and self-monitoring of blood glucose can be used to determine whether the amount of carbohydrate prescribed is appropriate. Carbohydrate counting can

be effective for individuals with all types of diabetes. Meal-planning resources for carbohydrate counting are divided into 2 levels of instruction:

- *Count Your Carbs: Getting Started*[48] is a booklet that introduces basic concepts of carbohydrate counting and blood glucose management. It provides guidance on how much carbohydrate to eat, record keeping, and where to find carbohydrate information.
- *Advanced Carbohydrate Counting*[49] is a booklet that is designed to teach blood glucose and pattern management and how to use insulin-to-carbohydrate ratios. An advanced carbohydrate-counting vocabulary list, a list of needed skills, practice exercises, and questions and answers are included. This booklet is intended to be used in conjunction with the *Choose Your Foods: Food Lists for Diabetes* or other carbohydrate-counting nutrition references, as food lists are not included.

Meal-Planning Skills

In addition to mastering the basic concepts described in a selected meal-planning resource, individuals with diabetes need to learn practical healthy eating skills to apply in a variety of real-life situations. The individual's specific needs and learning priorities should guide the diabetes educator in teaching topics such as portion sizes; food label reading; planning, shopping, and cooking; eating out; and special situations.

Portion Sizes

Portion sizes served are often in excess of what's needed to satisfy hunger and meet carbohydrate goals for meals and snacks. Many individuals don't realize that portion size might vary from the standard serving size listed on food labels. The diabetes educator can advise the person with diabetes to take advantage of the "tools of the trade":

- Use a measuring cup to serve foods such as soup, casseroles, cereal, rice, or cut-up fruit.
- Use measuring spoons for salad dressing, margarine, or peanut butter to get a visual of food portions.
- When possible, measure out appropriate individual portions of food and try to remember how the portion looks for the next time.

◆ Portions for meats, poultry, and fish are based on cooked weight, so allow shrinkage from raw.

◆ Measure your drinking cups so you'll know how much you drink when you use that cup, and measure your bowls so you'll know how much cereal or soup you're eating.

Visualize Portion Size[38]

Knowing portion sizes is crucial to successful diabetes control. Use plastic food models to demonstrate portion sizes and foods that contain carbohydrate. Compare small portions of common foods such as a cookie, frozen yogurt, or ice milk with the amount of sucrose in a 12-oz can of regular soft drink, gelatin, fruited yogurt, and other foods. Have the individual weigh and measure foods at home occasionally to improve portion-estimating abilities when eating away from home. Teach the following convenient guides to portion sizes:

◆ Thumb tip = 1 tsp
◆ Thumb = 2 Tb or 1 oz
◆ Fist = 1 c
◆ Palm = 3 oz of meat
◆ Handful = 1 to 2 oz of snack food

Food Label Reading

Food labels provide valuable information for healthy eating, but individuals with diabetes may feel overwhelmed by the wealth of facts and figures, making them uncertain about which numbers are most important. Some tips to share with patients about making the most of food label information are the following:

◆ *Take it from the top—size up the servings.* Compare the serving size recommended in diabetes meal-planning tools with the serving size listed on the food label and adjust the portion on your plate as needed.

◆ *How many servings are in there?* A quick check of the number of servings in the container is an easy portion tool.

◆ *Know your numbers—what's inside?* A quick way to determine whether the amount of a particu-

lar nutrient is high or low in a serving of food is to use the percent daily value data on the label: 5% or less is low, 20% or more is high.

◆ *Make a smart choice—it's all about you!* The RD/RDN can provide additional individualized guidance if nutrients such as fat or sodium are of concern.

If an individual with diabetes is still overwhelmed by label reading, he or she should be advised to go back to the basics and focus first on serving size and the amount of carbohydrate in the foods most commonly eaten.

Planning, Shopping, and Cooking

The heart of healthy eating is enjoying good food. With today's time crunch, cooking has become a lost art for many people. Encourage individuals with diabetes to take the time to plan meal and snack choices, shop economically, and begin cooking at home to improve their health and budget. Top tips include the following:

◆ Take the time to plan ahead for meals and snacks. Advance planning means healthier food choices, and using a list in the grocery store saves time and money.[50]

◆ Batch cooking (cooking once and serving twice) and planned-overs (key ingredients saved after a meal to use as part of another meal) help make the most of time in the kitchen.

◆ There's no need to give up favorite family recipes in order to eat healthfully for diabetes. Rethink recipes with an eye to reducing fat, sugar, and salt and increasing the fiber and flavor.

Eating Out

Individuals with diabetes often eat away from home. While dining out can make healthy eating a challenge, tips to share include the following:

◆ In a fast-food restaurant, keep it simple by sticking with foods in their simplest forms, such as a grilled chicken sandwich rather than processed chicken nuggets.

◆ When dining in a restaurant, plan ahead. Think about when you'll eat in order to time your medication correctly. Do some research on the menu prior to eating out, and identify choices at different restaurants that fit healthy eating needs so that ordering is simple.

◆ Don't hesitate to ask what's in a dish or to make special requests.

◆ Ask if calorie or other nutrition information is available, or check the restaurant's Web site ahead of time. Most chain restaurants provide this information.

Smart Snacking

Snacks fuel the body, curb the appetite, head off hypoglycemia, and boost calorie intake. Not everyone with diabetes needs snacks, so the individual with diabetes should discuss his or her specific situation with the diabetes educator to determine whether snacks are necessary to keep blood glucose and weight on target. While portion sizes for snacks are dependent on carbohydrate goals, some smart snack ideas include the following:

◆ Fresh fruit such as a medium-sized apple
◆ Frozen 100% fruit juice bars
◆ Air-popped or light microwave popcorn
◆ Fresh vegetable slices with salsa
◆ Lean turkey on whole grain crackers
◆ Celery sticks filled with peanut butter

Special Situations: Travel, Alcohol, Parties

Special situations are part of life. Individuals with diabetes need strategies for fitting them into their diabetes picture.

◆ Travel—Try to stay as close to your usual food and medication schedule as possible. Keep plenty of portable, ready-to-eat snacks on hand such as fresh fruit, small bags of high-fiber cereal, or individually wrapped reduced-fat cheese in case of delays or when food is not available.

◆ Alcohol—If drinking alcohol is part of your social life, keep in mind that the ADA recommends no more than 1 alcoholic drink per day for women and no more than 2 per day for men.[7] Alcohol can have unpredictable effects on blood glucose. Always eat something with carbohydrate when drinking alcohol, and use a carbohydrate-free mixer such as diet soda, diet tonic water, or club soda if you prefer mixed drinks.

◆ Parties—Focus on fun and fellowship rather than food. Eat a small snack before you leave home to curb your appetite. Take a look at the entire buffet table before filling your plate so you can make smart choices and plan the portions that best fit your carbohydrate goals.

Case: Wrap-Up

1. What are the key healthy eating issues you might address at this visit?

- Improving glycemic control prior to conception
- Matching insulin to carbohydrate intake
- Improving consistency of carbohydrate intake
- Addressing the use of complementary therapy

2. How can you use the steps of the NCPM during SM's visit?

- *Assessment*—Gather data, identify SM's goals and preferred learning style, establish rapport
- *Diagnosis*—Inconsistent carbohydrate intake
- *Intervention*—Choose the appropriate meal-planning resources. Begin with *Count Your Carbs: Getting Started* until SM achieves consistent carbohydrate intake and improved glycemic control. Move to *Advanced Carbohydrate Counting* when she is ready to learn more about insulin-to-carbohydrate ratio

- *Monitoring and evaluation*—Review, evaluate, and reassess food and blood glucose records via telephone or on a return visit

3. What are 2 behavior-change goals that focus on healthy eating that you might encourage SM to set?

- "I will measure my food and beverage intake for 3 days, record the amounts, and bring the records to my next clinic appointment."
- "I will keep my carbohydrate intake consistent by having 60 g of carbohydrate at each of my 3 meals and 15 g of carbohydrate at each of my 2 snacks at least 5 days per week."

4. List 3 skill areas related to healthy eating that you will review with SM during this visit.

- Portion control
- Eating out
- Special situations—travel, alcohol, parties

Summary

The epidemic of diabetes will continue to affect healthy eating and the delivery of DSME/T in a variety of ways. In the future, there will be a continued emphasis on prevention of diabetes and its complications. Individualized approaches to meal planning will require more in-depth assessment of an individual's health goals, personal and cultural preferences, and readiness to change. Methods of delivering education will rely more on electronic, online, and telemedicine approaches. Community-based programs will be used to deliver education alongside the traditional clinic-based programs.

Diabetes educators must be prepared to address healthy eating not only for diabetes itself but also for the many comorbidities that occur in individuals with diabetes. Behavior change, rather than content mastery, will continue to be the gold standard for outcomes of effective DSME/T for healthy eating. Educators at each level of practice can contribute to conquering the challenge of healthy eating for individuals with diabetes by translating evidence-based research into effective self-management education and training.

Focus on Education

Teaching Strategies

⟳ **Let the patient take the lead.** Encourage the patient to select a topic of interest. Start DSME/T sessions by asking the individual an open-ended question such as, "What would you like to work on today?" or display a list of nutrition-related topics and let the individual choose what seems most beneficial to learn. This technique encourages patient empowerment and relieves the educator of the unrealistic burden of trying to teach everything in a single session.

⟳ **Engage the learner.** Use menus from local restaurants or fast-food chains to help individuals plan a meal according to their healthy eating plan. Role-play so individuals can practice assertiveness skills by asking their "waiter" questions about ingredients, preparation, and presentation of food.

⟳ **Recognize cultural, ethnic, and family traditions.** Work to incorporate preferences or adapt recipes to include favorite foods and family traditions into meal planning to promote good health for the family.

⟳ **Stay current.** Nutrition is ever-evolving. The knowledge that "sugar is not a poison" is just one example of how evidence-based research on dietary carbohydrate has guided the remarkable changes that have occurred in clinical practice recommendations for healthy eating in recent years.

⟳ **Become familiar with diabetes apps.** For those individuals with diabetes who appreciate new ways to manage their condition on the go, apps (self-contained programs or pieces of software) that track food intake, physical activity, and blood glucose levels are available for smartphones and tablets. Information on health apps, many of which are free, can be found on reliable diabetes Web sites such as those of the ADA (http://www.diabetes.org) and the Academy of Nutrition and Dietetics (http://www.eatright.org).

Messages for Patients

⟳ **Be open to new information.** Recognize that learning about making healthier food choices takes time, but the extra effort will help achieve goals for improved diabetes management and overall health. Also, remember that recommendations for diabetes nutrition change and evolve as more is learned. Learning about the most current guidelines is worthwhile.

⟳ **Healthy eating is individualized.** What works for your friend or neighbor may not be appropriate for you. For example, whether a person with diabetes includes snacks in his or her meal plan depends on that person's medication, activity level, blood glucose levels, and nutrient needs.

Children with type 1 diabetes may require frequent snacks to maintain normal blood glucose levels, whereas adults with type 2 diabetes that is managed by lifestyle changes alone may not need the extra calories that snacks provide. A meal plan can be designed to meet your needs and work as part of your management plan.

Health Literacy

⟳ **Individuals with low health literacy and numeracy may have difficulty translating information from traditional diabetes nutrition education programs and materials into effective self-management.** The content of the material and its formatting should be designed to improve ease of use by adhering to a lower text-reading level, using illustrations for key concepts, and using color-coding and other modifications to guide patients through instructions for healthy eating. *Eating Healthy With Diabetes: Easy Reading Guide*[45] is an example of a meal-planning resource that is effective when health literacy is of concern.

⟳ **Consult additional resources on health literacy.** The National Network of Libraries of Medicine provides an extensive resource on health literacy.[51]

⟳ **Allow people with diabetes to experience healthy eating.** Do food preparation demonstrations, supermarket tours, restaurant menu selections, and restaurant/dining clubs for people with diabetes. This provides people with hands-on skills in food preparation and healthy eating experiences which include social interaction.

⟳ **Focus on what people can eat instead of what they can't eat.** Examine what people eat for breakfast, lunch, dinner, and snacks, in response to stress or special circumstances. Get an agreement from a patient on the alternative options, and write them down for the patient for easy reference.

⟳ **Health literacy plays an important role in the adoption of healthy eating.** Communication with the patient needs to focus on informed decision making within a typical environment and social economic circumstances. Each patient or specific population can be very different in seeking, interpreting, critically analyzing, and using information to make informed healthy eating decisions. Some patients might interpret "An apple a day keeps the disease away" literally and think that the only healthy fruit is an apple. Others might exclude favorite foods like bananas and carrots from their diet with the assumption that "they have too much sugar."

⟳ **Allow your patients to teach you about their healthy eating.** Most people with diabetes know that they need to eat healthfully, but they might not be very good about it or do not really know what it means. Ask your patients to tell you what they think they need to eat in order to be healthy or achieve better blood glucose management. This will allow you to identify their misconceptions and adjust accordingly.

⟳ **Focus on one meal at a time.** People with low health literacy will find it more manageable to understand one behavior change at a time. Add a meal or a snack with the additional visits. Ask your patient to summarize the strategy for that meal; that way you can evaluate whether he or she recalls it accurately.

Focus on Practice

⟳ **Invest in your physical environment.** In your waiting room, use colorful displays of charts or test tubes showing the amounts of sugar or fat in common foods to stimulate discussions of healthy eating.

⟳ **Make teaching creative and fun.** Ask patients to bring food labels from home to teach carbohydrate awareness. Use the Nutrition Facts to point out the grams of carbohydrate, protein, fat, and number of calories per serving. Use the label to illustrate that the serving size may differ from the food list value; for example, a label for brown rice lists a serving size of 1 cup while its serving size from the starch list is one-third cup.

⤴ **Consider the financial implications.** Diabetes self-management education and training for healthy eating should be part of the care plan of every individual with diabetes, regardless of his or her medication regimen. It is also part of diabetes prevention. Unfortunately, a large percentage of people with diabetes do not receive any structured diabetes education and/or nutrition therapy and may not be aware that these services are available to them. It is possible in this time of healthcare reform that DSME/T and MNT coverage will become more comprehensive and more accessible, given that healthy eating for diabetes helps improve quality of life and reduces healthcare costs.

References

1. American Association of Diabetes Educators. Guidelines for the practice of diabetes self-management education and training (DSME/T). 2011 (cited 2013 Aug 28). On the Internet at: http://www.diabeteseducator.org/export/sites/aade/_resources/pdf/general/PracticeGuidelines2011.pdf.

2. American Association of Diabetes Educators. AADE 7™ self-care behaviors. 2011 (cited 2013 Aug 28). On the Internet at: http://www.diabeteseducator.org/export/sites/aade/_resources/pdf/research/AADE7_Position_Statement_2011.pdf.

3. American Association of Diabetes Educators Position Statement. Healthy eating: incorporating nutritional management into lifestyle. Diabetes Educ. 2012;38:124-8.

4. Institute of Medicine. The Role of Nutrition in Maintaining Health in the Nation's Elderly: Evaluating Coverage of Nutrition Services for the Medicare Population. Washington, DC: National Academies Press; 2000.

5. Evert AB, Boucher JL, Cypress M, et al; American Diabetes Association. Nutrition therapy recommendations for the management of adults with diabetes: a position statement of the American Diabetes Association. Diabetes Care. 2013;36:3821-42.

6. Diabetes Prevention Program Research Group. Reduction in the incidence of type 2 diabetes with lifestyle intervention or metformin. N Engl J Med. 2002;346:393-403.

7. American Diabetes Association. Standards of medical care in diabetes—2014. Diabetes Care. 2014;37 Suppl 1:S14-80.

8. Centers for Disease Control and Prevention. NCHS data brief. Prevalence of obesity among adults: United States, 2011-2012. 2013 (cited 2013 Oct 14). On the Internet at: http://www.cdc.gov/nchs/data/databriefs/db131.htm.

9. Jackson L. Translating the diabetes prevention program into practice: a review of community interventions. Diabetes Educ. 2009;35:309-20.

10. Wing RR, Phelan S. Long-term weight loss maintenance. Am J Clin Nutr. 2005;82(1 Suppl): 222S-5.

11. Academy of Nutrition and Dietetics. Academy gestational diabetes evidence-based nutrition practice guideline. 2008 (cited 2013 Aug 22). On the Internet at: http://andevidence library.com/topic.cfm?cat=1399.

12. Kitzmiller JL, Block JM, Brown FM, et al. Managing preexisting diabetes for pregnancy. Diabetes Care. 2008;31:1060-79.

13. Silverstein J, Klingensmith G, Copeland KC, et al; American Diabetes Association. Care of children and adolescents with type 1 diabetes: a statement of the American Diabetes Association. Diabetes Care. 2005;28:186-212.

14. Narayan KM, Boyle JP, Thompson TJ, et al. Lifetime risk for diabetes mellitus in the United States. JAMA. 2003; 290:1884-90.

15. American Diabetes Association. ADA consensus statement: type 2 diabetes in children and adolescents. Diabetes Care. 2000;23:381-9.

16. Academy of Nutrition and Dietetics. Pediatric weight management evidence-based nutrition practice guideline. 2010 (cited 2013 Aug 22). On the Internet at: http://andevidencelibrary.com/topic.cfm?cat=2721.

17. Kirkman M, Briscoe VJ, Clark N, et al. Diabetes in older adults. Diabetes Care. 2012;35:2650-64.

18. Stanley K. Nutrition therapy for older adults with diabetes. In: Franz MJ, Evert AB, eds. American Diabetes Association Guide to Nutrition Therapy for Diabetes. Alexandria, Va: American Diabetes Association; 2012:169-80.

19. Young V, Eiser C, Johnson B, et al. Eating disorders in adolescents with type 1 diabetes: a systematic review with meta-analysis. Diabet Med. 2013;30:189-98.

20. American Dietetic Association. Position of the American Dietetic Association: nutrition intervention in the treatment of eating disorders. J Am Diet Assoc. 2011;111: 1236-41.

21. Goebel-Fabbri A, Uplinger N, Gerken S, et al. Outpatient management of eating disorders in type 1 diabetes. Diabetes Spectr. 2009;22:147-52.

22. Academy of Nutrition and Dietetics. Position of the Academy of Nutrition and Dietetics: total diet approach to healthy eating. J Acad Nutr Diet. 2013;113:307-17.

23. Schwarzenberg SJ, Bruzell C. Type 1 diabetes and celiac disease: overview and medical nutrition therapy. Diabetes Spectr. 2002;15:197-201.

24. American Diabetes Association. Gluten-free diets. 2013 (cited 2013 Aug 22). On the Internet at: http://www.diabetes.org/food-and-fitness/food/planning-meals/gluten-free-diets/.

25. Academy of Nutrition and Dietetics. Understanding celiac disease. 2012 (cited 2013 Aug 22). On the Internet at: http://www.eatright.org/Public/content.aspx?id=5542.

26. Parrish CR, McCray S. Gastroparesis and nutrition: the art. 2011 (cited 2013 Aug 23). On the Internet at: http://www.medicine.virginia.edu/clinical/departments/medicine/divisions/digestive-health/nutrition-support-team/nutrition-articles/ParrishGastroparesisArticle.pdf.

27. The University of Sydney. About glycemic index. 2013 (cited 2013 Aug 23). On the Internet at: http://www.glycemicindex.com/about.php.

28. The University of Sydney. Search for the glycemic index. 2013 (cited 2013 Aug 23). On the Internet at: http://www.glycemicindex.com/foodSearch.php.

29. American Dietetic Association. Nutrition care process and model part I: The 2008 update. J Am Diet Assoc. 2008;108:1113-7.

30. American Association of Diabetes Educators Position Statement. Individualization of diabetes self-management education. Diabetes Educ. 2007;33:45-9.

31. American Association of Diabetes Educators Position Statement. Cultural sensitivity and diabetes education. Diabetes Educ. 2012;38:137-41.

32. Kittler PG, Sucher KP. Diet counseling in a multicultural society. Diabetes Educ. 1990;16:127-34.

33. Goody CM, Drago L, eds; Diabetes Care and Education Dietetic Practice Group. Cultural Food Practices. Chicago: American Dietetic Association; 2009.

34. National Diabetes Education Program. Build cultural competency. 2013 (cited 2013 Sep 11). On the Internet at: http://ndep.nih.gov/hcp-businesses-and-schools/practice-transformation/patient-centered-interactions/cultural-competency.aspx.

35. Academy of Nutrition and Dietetics. Academy diabetes evidence-based nutrition practice guideline. 2008 (cited 2013 Aug 22). On the Internet at: http://andevidencelibrary.com/topic.cfm?cat=1615.

36. American Association of Diabetes Educators Technical Review. Diabetes self-management education and training outcomes measures. 2011 (cited 2013 Sep 9). On the Internet at: http://www.diabeteseducator.org/export/sites/aade/_resources/pdf/research/Outcomes_Technical_Review_2011.pdf.

37. Prochaska J, Redding C, Evers K. The Transtheoretical Model and Stages of Change. 2nd ed. San Francisco: Jossey-Bass; 1997:60-84.

38. Geil P, Ross T. What Do I Eat Now? A Step-by-Step Guide for Eating Right With Type 2 Diabetes. Alexandria, Va: American Diabetes Association; 2009.

39. Boucher J. Effective nutrition education and counseling. In: Franz MJ, Evert AB, eds. American Diabetes Association Guide to Nutrition Therapy for Diabetes. Alexandria, Va: American Diabetes Association; 2012:425-39.

40. US Department of Health and Human Services. Dietary guidelines for Americans, 2010 (cited 2013 Oct 24). On the Internet at: http://www.health.gov/dietaryguidelines/2010.asp.

41. US Department of Agriculture. Choose my plate. 2013 (cited 2013 Oct 24). On the Internet at: http://www.choosemyplate.gov/.

42. American Diabetes Association. Create your plate. 2013 (cited 2013 Aug 28). On the Internet at: http://www.diabetes.org/food-and-fitness/food/planning-meals/create-your-plate/.

43. American Diabetes Association and Academy of Dietetics and Nutrition. Healthy Food Choices. Alexandria, Va, and Chicago: American Diabetes Association and Academy of Dietetics and Nutrition; in press.

44. American Diabetes Association. Month of Meals™ Diabetes Meal Planner. Alexandria, Va: American Diabetes Association; 2010.

45. American Diabetes Association and Academy of Dietetics and Nutrition. Eating Healthy With Diabetes: Easy Reading Guide. Alexandria, Va, and Chicago: American Diabetes Association and Academy of Dietetics and Nutrition; in press.

46. American Diabetes Association and Academy of Dietetics and Nutrition. Choose Your Foods: Food Lists for Diabetes. Alexandria, Va, and Chicago: American Diabetes Association and Academy of Dietetics and Nutrition; in press.

47. American Diabetes Association and Academy of Dietetics and Nutrition. Choose Your Foods: Plan Your Meals. Alexandria, Va, and Chicago: American Diabetes Association and Academy of Dietetics and Nutrition; in press.

48. American Diabetes Association and Academy of Dietetics and Nutrition. Count Your Carbs: Getting Started. Alexandria, Va, and Chicago: American Diabetes Association and Academy of Dietetics and Nutrition; in press.

49. American Diabetes Association and Academy of Dietetics and Nutrition. Advanced Carbohydrate Counting. Alexandria, Va, and Chicago: American Diabetes Association and Academy of Dietetics and Nutrition; in press.

50. Geil P, Ross T. Diabetes Meals on $7 a Day—or Less! Alexandria, Va: American Diabetes Association; 2007.

51. National Network of Libraries of Medicine. Health literacy. 2013 (cited 2013 Oct 24). On the Internet at: http://nnlm.gov/outreach/consumer/hlthlit.html.

CHAPTER 5

Being Active

Sheri R. Colberg, PhD, FACSM

Key Concepts

◆ Support public health recommendations for physical activity and exercise by identifying lifestyle interventions.

◆ Understand the current recommendations for aerobic, resistance, and other structured exercise and physical activity for individuals with diabetes, along with daily lifestyle activity.

◆ Learn exercise modifications required by the presence of diabetes-related health complications to promote safe and effective practices.

◆ Understand behavior-change strategies that are effective in promoting self-care behaviors related to being physically active.

◆ Use evidence-based strategies for goal setting, including SMART strategies.

◆ Use motivational interviewing to foster the individual's readiness to make positive behavior changes in physical activity.

Introduction

Although many Americans do not meet the recommended guidelines for physical activity, just 39% of adults with diabetes are physically active (defined as engaging in moderate or vigorous activity for at least 30 minutes, 3 times per week), compared to 58% of other adults.[1,2] For most people with any type of diabetes, exercise can be undertaken safely and blood glucose levels managed effectively. Diabetes educators, therefore, have an important and challenging role in helping individuals with diabetes or prediabetes become more physically active. Effective behavior-change strategies, coupled with a solid understanding of current recommendations for physical activity and exercise, can be powerful tools for helping individuals incorporate regular physical activity into their diabetes management program.

Physical activity and exercise are important in both the prevention and the treatment of type 2 diabetes in particular. Regular physical activity can prevent or delay the onset of type 2 diabetes and its complications.[3–9] The Diabetes Prevention Program (DPP)[4,5] was a landmark randomized clinical trial of 3234 overweight individuals with prediabetes in the United States. The DPP found lifestyle intervention to be more effective than metformin in preventing type 2 diabetes. The trial reported that intensive lifestyle intervention decreased the incidence of type 2 diabetes by 58%, compared with 31% in the group taking metformin.[4] The lifestyle intervention included goals of engaging in moderate-intensity physical activity, such as brisk walking, for 150 minutes per week and consuming a healthy low-calorie, low-fat diet. Another goal for participants in this group was to lose 7% of their initial body weight and maintain that loss. Increased physical activity was shown to be important to sustain weight loss. Also, among 495 participants who did not meet the weight loss goal at the end of the first year, those who achieved the physical activity goal had a 44% lower incidence of diabetes.[9] This lifestyle intervention is similar to current public health recommendations for physical activity and exercise.

The mechanisms by which physical activity helps prevent type 2 diabetes continue to be investigated. Current evidence suggests physical activity improves insulin action, lowers blood glucose levels, improves body mass index (BMI), and reduces several risk factors for cardiovascular disease.[3,8] These important metabolic changes demonstrate the significant role that physical activity and exercise have in the prevention and management of type 2 diabetes. Improved insulin sensitivity may be related to the total exercise dose (expressed as average kilocalories expended per week) in a graded dose-response relationship, with exercise intensity being relatively more important than frequency.[10] More recently, others have suggested that higher volumes of sedentary time alone may be associated with the onset of type 2 diabetes and overall chronic disease, independent of physical activity and other factors,[11-13] and that simply breaking up sedentary time with any activity may lower postprandial glucose and insulin levels in individuals without diabetes.[14] In a recent meta-analysis, sedentary time was found to be associated not only with an increased risk of diabetes but also with cardiovascular disease and cardiovascular and all-cause mortality.[13]

Blood glucose management with physical activity as an added variable in type 1 diabetes can be more challenging, but most of the same metabolic benefits are possible for these individuals as well. In fact, regular participation in physical activity can prevent an increase in insulin resistance that can lead to "double diabetes" and greater exogenous insulin requirements if not managed effectively.[15]

Physical activity and exercise can be defined separately; however, these terms will be used interchangeably throughout this chapter for simplicity. Physical activity is defined as any bodily movement produced by skeletal muscle that requires energy expenditure in excess of resting energy expenditure.[16,17] Exercise is defined as planned, structured, and repetitive bodily movement done to improve or maintain one or more components of physical fitness.[16,17] Exercise training programs for individuals with diabetes typically include activities to enhance cardiovascular capacity (aerobic fitness) and muscular fitness and strength in individuals of all ages, as well as flexibility and balance in older individuals.

This chapter provides diabetes educators with tools and strategies for helping individuals with or at risk for diabetes make positive and lasting changes in physical activity and exercise habits.

Case: Weight, Blood Pressure, and Type 2 Diabetes

MT, a 48-year-old woman diagnosed with type 2 diabetes 7 years earlier, was having trouble controlling her weight and blood pressure. To address these issues and improve her overall health and diabetes management, she was referred to a diabetes educator by her physician to discuss safe and appropriate ways to be more physically active.

She received medical clearance to start increasing her activity level with no specific restrictions. Her medications include a sulfonylurea and an antihypertensive agent. MT reported testing her blood glucose fairly regularly (ie, at least once a day). She is not currently doing any structured physical activity and has not done any regular physical activity in the past. She stated that she is motivated to be more active, mainly because of her physician's recommendation and her unhappiness with her weight gain.

Vitals

- Height: 64 in
- Weight: 190 lb
- BMI: 33 kg/m^2

- Resting heart rate: 85 beats per minute
- Blood pressure: 138/86 mm Hg (medicated)

Lab Data

- Fasting plasma glucose: 158 mg/dL (8.8 mmol/L)
- A1C: 7.2%
- Total cholesterol: 190 mg/dL (4.91 mmol/L)
- Triglycerides: 200 mg/dL (2.26 mmol/L)
- HDL-C: 38 mg/dL (0.98 mmol/L)
- LDL-C: 132 mg/dL (3.41 mmol/L)

Questions to Consider

1. What recommendations would you give MT for increasing her activity level?
2. What precautions would you suggest?
3. What strategies might you suggest to help motivate and support her efforts to establish regular physical activity as a lifelong habit?

Preparing Individuals for Being Active

Medical Evaluation

Safe exercise participation can be complicated by the presence of diabetes-related health issues, such as cardiovascular disease, hypertension, neuropathy, or microvascular changes. For individuals who wish to participate in low-intensity activities like walking, healthcare providers should use clinical judgment in deciding whether to recommend pre-exercise testing.[18] Conducting exercise stress testing prior to starting a walking program is controversial, as no evidence suggests that it is routinely necessary as a diagnostic tool for cardiovascular disease, and requiring it may create barriers to participation.

For exercise that is more vigorous than brisk walking or that exceeds the demands of everyday living, sedentary and older individuals with diabetes will likely benefit from being assessed for conditions potentially associated with the risk of cardiovascular disease or that might contraindicate certain types of exercise or predispose them to injuries, such as severe peripheral neuropathy, severe autonomic neuropathy, or preproliferative or proliferative retinopathy.[19,20] Before undertaking higher intensity physical activity, they are advised to undergo a detailed medical evaluation and screening for blood glucose control, physical limitations, medications, and macrovascular and microvascular complications associated with the heart, blood vessels, eyes, kidneys, feet, and nervous system.[18]

Current guidelines attempt to avoid automatic inclusion of lower risk individuals, in whom the risk of a false positive test is higher and may outweigh the benefits of detection of cardiovascular abnormalities. Such testing is currently advised primarily for *previously sedentary* people with diabetes who want to undertake activity that is *more intense than brisk walking*.[19,20] Use of these criteria does not exclude the possibility of conducting electrocardiogram (ECG) stress testing on individuals with a low risk of coronary artery disease (CAD) or those planning to engage in less intense exercise. In the absence of contraindications to maximal stress testing, it can still be considered for anyone with diabetes. The potential benefits should be weighed against the risks for each individual.

A graded exercise stress test with ECG may be indicated for individuals based on the following criteria[19,20]:

- Age >40 years, with or without cardiovascular risk factors other than diabetes
- Age >30 years and
  —Type 1 diabetes or type 2 diabetes of >10 years' duration
  —Hypertension
  —Cigarette smoking
  —Dyslipidemia
  —Proliferative or preproliferative retinopathy
  —Nephropathy, including microalbuminuria
- Any of the following, regardless of age:
  —Known or suspected CAD, cerebrovascular disease, and/or peripheral artery disease
  —Autonomic neuropathy
  —Peripheral vascular disease

Individuals who exhibit nonspecific ECG changes in response to exercise or who have nonspecific ST and T wave changes on resting ECG may need follow-up testing. However, the cost-effectiveness and diagnostic value of more intensive testing remain in question.[18–20]

Other Program-Design Considerations

Clinical status and health needs, as well as the individual's personal interests and past and present activity patterns, should be considered in program planning. Specific goals identified by the individual are the ultimate target. All exercise programs need to be designed to address intensity (how difficult), duration (how long), frequency (how often), and mode (type of activity), as well as appropriate progression. Rates of progression depend on an individual's functional capacity, medical and health status, age, activity preferences and goals, and tolerance to the current level of activity.[18]

- *Type 1 diabetes:* For individuals with type 1 diabetes without complications, exercise recommendations are similar to those for individuals with no known health problems.
- *Type 2 diabetes:* Recommendations for individuals with type 2 diabetes closely align with guidelines for sedentary adults and older adults[21–23] but also focus on duration to achieve expected levels of calorie expenditure.[20]

Developing a Structured Physical Activity Program

Exercise Session Format

Structured exercise sessions generally have 3 parts:

- Warm-up
- Conditioning
- Cool-down

Warm-up

The warm-up phase includes doing 5 to 10 minutes of an activity at a slower speed or lower intensity. Warming up before moderate- or vigorous-intensity aerobic activity allows a gradual increase in heart rate and breathing at the start of the episode of activity.[24] It may also help reduce muscle injury and facilitate a safe transition from rest to exercise by stretching postural muscles, increasing blood flow, elevating body temperature, and increasing oxygen availability and metabolic rate. Warming up for a muscle-strengthening activity commonly involves doing exercises with lighter weights to start.

Conditioning

The conditioning phase includes activities to enhance cardiorespiratory fitness, muscle strength and endurance, or flexibility. Time spent warming up and cooling down may count toward meeting aerobic activity guidelines, but only if the activity is at least of moderate intensity (for example, walking briskly as a warm-up before jogging).[24]

Cool-down

The cool-down includes at least 3 to 5 minutes of a lower intensity activity to help the body gradually recover from the conditioning phase and safely transition back to a resting state. Doing so helps prevent blood from pooling in the arms and legs and removes metabolic by-products immediately after exercise.

Aerobic Exercise

Cardiorespiratory or aerobic exercise is defined as continuous, dynamic exercise that uses large muscle groups and requires aerobic metabolic pathways to sustain the activity.[16,21,23,24] Examples include walking, jogging, biking, swimming, water aerobics, cycling, rollerblading, and cross-country skiing. Aerobic exercise

has been the mode traditionally prescribed for diabetes management and prevention. Most of its benefits related to blood glucose control are realized through acute and chronic improvements in insulin action. The acute effects of a recent bout of exercise account for most of the improvements in insulin action, but are short-lived, while regular exercise training generally results in a more lasting effect.[25,26] Table 5.1 summarizes recommendations for aerobic exercise for individuals with diabetes.

Mode of Activity

The recommended types, or modes, of aerobic activity for diabetes are highly dependent on the individual's preferences and skill level. Health-related benefits of improved physical fitness do not appear to depend on the type of aerobic exercise done. Identifying activities that can safely and effectively improve cardiovascular endurance and maximize caloric expenditure is important.[20–22,24] Walking is the most common type of physical activity done by individuals with diabetes and often the most convenient. However, other low-impact or non-weight-bearing types of activity, such as bicycling, swimming, and aquatic or chair exercises, may be more appropriate for those with complications or coexisting conditions like peripheral or autonomic neuropathy.[20]

Intensity of Activity

Moderate- to vigorous-intensity physical activity is generally recommended to achieve aerobic and metabolic improvements.[16–20] Lower intensity activities will expend calories and help with weight maintenance, but they may have a lesser acute impact on blood glucose levels.

Estimating Intensity The intensity of aerobic activity can be easily based on measured or estimated maximal heart rate (HR). The American College of Sports Medicine (ACSM) recommends the following[16]:

- Exercise intensity of 40% to 89% of heart rate reserve (HRR)

The recommended intensity range is broad since deconditioned individuals can improve their cardiorespiratory fitness at lower intensities, while individuals with greater fitness typically require a higher minimal threshold.[16] The prescribed intensity range

TABLE 5.1   Summary of Aerobic Exercise Recommendations for Individuals With Diabetes

Screening

Diagnostic exercise stress testing for asymptomatic persons at low risk of CAD is not recommended. For individuals intending on participating in moderate- to high-intensity physical activity, an exercise stress test may be helpful based on the following criteria[1,2]:

- Age >40 years, with or without cardiovascular risk factors other than diabetes
- Age >30 years and
  - Type 1 diabetes or type 2 diabetes of >10 years' duration
  - Hypertension
  - Cigarette smoking
  - Dyslipidemia
  - Proliferative or preproliferative retinopathy
  - Nephropathy, including microalbuminuria
- Any of the following, regardless of age
  - Known or suspected CAD, cerebrovascular disease, and/or peripheral artery disease
  - Autonomic neuropathy
  - Peripheral vascular disease

Exercise Prescription, Type 2 Diabetes[2]

Intensity: moderate to vigorous (ie, 40%–89% of heart rate reserve, or rating of perceived exertion of 12–16)

Duration: a minimum of 150 minutes a week (with no less than 10 minutes per exercise session, with a goal of 30 minutes or more)

Frequency: spread over minimum of 3 nonconsecutive days per week, with no more than 2 consecutive days of inactivity; 5 days a week may be more effective

Exercise Prescription, Type 1 Diabetes

Intensity: moderate to vigorous (ie, 40%–89% of heart rate reserve, or rating of perceived exertion of 12–16)

Duration: a minimum of 150 minutes a week (minimum of 10-minute sessions), although individuals with higher aerobic capacities may exercise at a higher absolute intensity (ie, vigorously) for less total time and likely achieve the same benefits

Frequency: spread over minimum of 3 nonconsecutive days per week, with no more than 2 consecutive days of inactivity; consistency makes blood glucose control and regimen management easier

Safety Precautions

Warm-up and cool-down

Careful selection and progression of exercise program

Patient education

Monitor blood glucose pre- and postexercise, as well as during prolonged activities

Adjust medications and food intake to prevent hypoglycemia

Consult with healthcare personnel about regimen changes

Sources:

1. American Diabetes Association. Physical activity/exercise and diabetes. Diabetes Care. 2004;27:S58-S62.
2. Colberg SR, Albright A, Blissmer B, et al, for the American College of Sports Medicine and American Diabetes Association. Exercise and type 2 diabetes: position stand. Med Sci Sports Exerc. 2010;42(12):2282-303.

American Association of Diabetes Educators©

should be based on one's fitness level, duration of diabetes, degree of complications, and individual goals.

Exercise performed at low levels (<40% HRR) has less effect on glucose disposal than exercise performed at higher intensities. Glucose disposal during exercise is roughly proportional to the total work performed (time × intensity). It is likely that the total energy expenditure is more important than the exercise intensity for overall glycemic balance, however. For instance, when matched for energy cost, low- to moderate-intensity aerobic training has been shown to be as effective as moderate- to high-intensity training in lowering A1C levels and increasing whole body and skeletal muscle oxidative capacity in obese individuals with type 2 diabetes.[27] Even a single bout of low-intensity, as opposed to high-intensity, exercise substantially reduces the prevalence of hyperglycemia throughout the subsequent 24-hour postexercise period.[28] On the other hand, low-volume, high-intensity training has also been demonstrated to rapidly improve glucose control and induce adaptations in skeletal muscle that are linked to improved metabolic health in those with type 2 diabetes.[29] A note of caution is that vigorous exercise (>60% of HRR) may result in transient hyperglycemia and cause an excessive rise in systolic blood pressure.[20]

Exercise Intensity Defined by HRR and Perceived Exertion[16]

- HRR = Maximum HR – Resting HR
- % HRR = HRR × Percent intensity
- *Low intensity:* 30% to 39% HRR, or "light" (rating of perceived exertion [RPE] 10-11)
- *Moderate intensity:* 40% to 59% HRR, or "somewhat hard" (RPE 12-14)
- *Vigorous intensity:* 60% to 89% HRR, or "hard" (RPE 15-16)

Determining HR   Exercise intensity can be calculated more accurately using the results of an exercise stress test. Based on the individual's maximum HR response to the exercise stress test, the following HRR formula, also known as the Karvonen formula, is the commonly accepted method to calculate target HR or HR range in beats per minute (bpm)[16]:

$$\text{Target HR} = [(\text{HRmax} - \text{HRrest}) \times \text{Desired percent intensity}] + \text{HRrest}$$

Using HRR Formula to Determine Target Heart Rate Range

Example: Calculate the target HR range (40%–89% of HRR) for a 50-year-old man with a resting HR of 70 bpm and a maximum HR of 170 bpm.

Lower estimated range (40%)	$= [(170 - 70) \times 0.40] + 70$
	$= [100 \times 0.40] + 70$
	$= 40 + 70$
	$= 110$ bpm
Higher estimated range (89%)	$= [(170 - 70) \times 0.89] + 70$
	$= [100 \times 0.89] + 70$
	$= 89 + 70$
	$= 159$ bpm
Target HR range (40%–89%)	**= 110 to 159 bpm**

If the actual maximal HR is not known, the target HR range can be estimated using the following equation, although caution is required:

$$\text{Estimated HRmax} = 220 - \text{Age}$$

This equation should be used with caution due to the large standard deviation, which can cause the HR estimation to be off by 12 to 15 bpm.[16] This procedure may also overestimate the maximal HR of some individuals with type 2 diabetes, particularly those with autonomic neuropathy.[8,17,20] When cardiac autonomic neuropathy (CAN) is present, exercise intensity is better prescribed using the HRR method to approximate oxygen consumption during submaximal exercise with maximal HR directly measured, rather than estimated, for better accuracy.[30]

Due to the high prevalence of occult cardiovascular disease, caution should be used when applying standard HR formulas to an individual with diabetes. An alternate equation that utilizes 70% of age rather than full age may be more accurate for estimating maximal HR in an older population[16]:

$$\text{Estimated HRmax} = 208 - (0.7 \times \text{Age})$$

Rating of Perceived Exertion   The RPE is another useful guide for estimating exercise intensity (see Table 5.2). This is a subjective rating based on general fatigue and can be used along with target HR estimations or as a substitute to guide the intensity of activity.[19] There are 2 RPE scales appropriate to use with adults, including those with diabetes:

◈ Original RPE scale, which rates intensity from 6 to 20
◈ Category-Ratio scale, which rates intensity from 0 to 10+

When RPE scales are used, the individual is instructed to focus on full-body feelings of exertion and general fatigue. While performing the activity within his or her target exercise intensity, the individual is asked to identify feelings of exertion and fatigue. This elicits the recommended RPE range. Generally, a moderate-to-vigorous exercise intensity that corresponds to an RPE range of 12 to 16 ("somewhat hard" to "hard" using the 6-20 scale) or 3 to 7 (using the 0-10 scale) is recommended.[16]

Use of the "Talk Test"   For individuals who cannot or prefer not to measure HRs or use subjective ratings, another option is to gauge the upper limit of exercise intensity: the "talk test." This simply means that an individual should be able to carry on a conversation during aerobic activity without struggling to breathe while doing so. If an individual is breathing too heavily to talk, he or she is working above the ventilatory threshold and at an intensity that exceeds a moderate workload. Use of this test cannot discern when exercise intensity is lower than desired, however.

Duration of Activity

The duration of exercise is directly related to caloric expenditure requirements and inversely related to the intensity of exercise required to achieve the same results. To gain maximum caloric and glycemic benefits, lower intensity exercise needs to be performed for longer periods of time compared to higher intensity exercise. The exercise duration required to meet the recommended weekly energy expenditure differs by which current guidelines are consulted.

The 2007 joint guidelines from the ACSM and the American Heart Association for adults and older adults[21,22] recommended 150 minutes of moderate activity (30 minutes, 5 days per week) or 60 minutes of vigorous physical activity (20 minutes on 3 days) for all adults, while 2008 US federal guidelines[24] recommended 150 minutes of moderate or 75 minutes of vigorous activity, or an equivalent combination, spread throughout the week. The federal guidelines[24] suggest that an exercise volume of 500 to 1000 metabolic equivalent (MET) minutes per week (MET equivalent of physical activity × number of minutes) is optimal and can be achieved, for example, with 150 minutes per week of walking at 6.4 km/hour (4 mph; intensity of 5 METs) or 75 minutes of jogging at 9.6 km/hour (6 mph; 10 METs).

Unfortunately, most individuals with type 2 diabetes do not have sufficient aerobic capacity to jog for that duration, and they may have orthopedic or other limitations that would preclude them from doing so. The mean maximal aerobic capacity in individuals with diabetes was only 22.4 ml/kg/min, or 6.4 METs, in a 2003 meta-analysis.[31] Accordingly, 4.8 METs (~75% of maximal) is likely the highest sustainable intensity.

TABLE 5.2 Rating of Perceived Exertion		
Category Scale	*Category-Ratio Scale*	*Perceived Exertion*
6	0 Nothing at all	No intensity
7 Extremely light	0.3–0.5 Extremely weak	Just noticeable
8	1 Very weak	
9 Very light	1.5	
10	2 Weak	Light
11 Light	2.5 Moderate	
12	3	
13 Somewhat hard	4	
14	5 Strong	Heavy
15 Hard (heavy)	6	
16	7 Very strong	
17 Very hard	8	
18	9	
19 Extremely hard	10 Extremely strong	Maximal intensity
20 Maximal exertion	11	
	Absolute maximum	Highest possible

Source: Adapted with permission from G Borg, *Borg's Perceived Exertion and Pain Scales* (Champaign, Ill: Human Kinetics, 1998).

Thus, most individuals with type 2 diabetes require at least 150 minutes of moderate to vigorous aerobic exercise per week to achieve optimal cardiovascular risk reduction, as recommended in the joint position stand on exercise and type 2 diabetes by the ACSM and the American Diabetes Association (ADA).[20] Some cardiovascular and glycemic benefits may be gained from lower exercise volumes (although a minimum dose has not been established), whereas additional benefits likely result from engaging in durations beyond recommended amounts. Individuals with higher aerobic capacities (>10 METs), such as many younger individuals with type 1 diabetes, may exercise at a higher absolute intensity for less time to achieve the same benefits.

Physical activity may be broken down into a minimum of 10-minute sessions done throughout the day. Studies have shown that similar cardiorespiratory gains occur when physical activity is accumulated throughout the day in shorter bouts (3 bouts of 10 minutes) compared to a single prolonged activity session of similar duration and intensity (a 30-minute bout),[21,24] and glycemic benefits may be greater from the more frequent, shorter bouts of activity.[32] Structured exercise training of more than 150 minutes per week is associated with greater A1C declines than that of 150 minutes or less per week.[33] However, closer to 60 minutes of daily exercise appears to be required for significant weight loss in adults.[34,35] Severely deconditioned individuals may need to exercise in multiple sessions of short duration (5-10 minutes), begin at very low levels (30%-39% HRR) with brief rest intervals, and progress weekly to be able to sustain higher intensity exercise.[19] Initially, sessions can be done for 10 to 15 minutes, increasing progressively over time to a minimum of 30 to 60 minutes.[16]

Frequency of Activity

Individuals with diabetes should undertake physical activity at least 3 nonconsecutive days per week, but 5 or more weekly sessions of moderate activity will likely be even more beneficial to improving glycemic control and cardiorespiratory endurance and achieving target caloric expenditure.[8,18–20] Exercise that is limited to 2 days per week generally does not result in significant improvements in cardiorespiratory endurance. Since the duration of glycemic improvement after an exercise session is usually greater than 2 hours but less than 72 hours, regular physical activity is needed to lower blood glucose.[20,36,37] For individuals taking insulin, being active on a daily basis may help balance caloric needs with insulin dosages, as well as maintain higher levels of insulin sensitivity to allow for reduced insulin dosing.[18] Obese individuals may need to be active more frequently (5-7 days per week) at lower intensities to optimize weight loss and maintenance.[34,35] In addition, to achieve sustained major weight loss, the optimal level of activity needed is typically greater than that needed to improve glycemic control.

Energy expenditure can also be used to guide exercise programming. The ACSM recommends a target range of 150 to 400 calories per day expended via physical activity.[16] This represents a minimum threshold of 1000 calories a week, which is associated with a reduction in all-cause mortality risk. For previously sedentary individuals, recommend the minimum threshold as the initial goal, but encourage progress toward the upper target range of expending 300 to 400 calories per day, or 2000 calories per week, in physical activity to achieve maximal health benefits and weight loss. Energy expenditure in excess of 2000 calories per week in physical activity has been associated with successful short- and long-term weight loss.[16]

Progressing Toward Goals

Recommend appropriate rates of progression to help individuals effectively and safely achieve aerobic exercise goals. Initially, focus on increasing frequency and duration of the exercise, rather than its intensity. This provides a safe level of activity that can be done with little effort and increases the likelihood of creating and sustaining an activity habit.[16] See also the discussion that follows on putting the activity program into action, and chapter 17 for more information on maintaining a physical activity program.

Aerobic Exercise Summary

- *Frequency:* a minimum of 3 nonconsecutive days per week, with additional benefits likely from 5 or more days, and no more than 2 consecutive days without aerobic activity
- *Duration:* a minimum of 150 minutes spread throughout the week (minimum of 10 minutes per session, with 30 minutes or more as a goal), possibly a lower total time if done more intensely
- *Intensity:* moderate to vigorous (40%-89% of HRR)

Resistance (Strength) Training

Resistance exercise or strength training has been shown to improve musculoskeletal health, maintain independence in performing daily activities, and reduce the possibility of injury.[21–24] Properly designed resistance programs may improve indices of cardiovascular function, glucose tolerance, strength, and body composition.[38–41]

The term "muscular fitness" refers to both muscular strength and muscular endurance. Muscle strength is the ability of the muscle to exert force, while muscle endurance is the ability of the muscle to continue to perform without fatigue.[16] Resistance exercises are used to improve muscular fitness. Examples include the following:

◆ Weight lifting with free weights (dumbbells and barbells)
◆ Weight or resistance machines
◆ Resistance bands
◆ Isometric exercises
◆ Calisthenics using body weight as resistance (eg, push-ups)

Guidelines

Consider the following when helping individuals develop a resistance training program.

Exercise Selection Select at least 5 to 10 exercises that cover all of the major muscle groups in the upper body, lower body, and core, which include the back, legs, hips, chest, shoulders, arms, and abdomen.[24] Exercise selection should be based on individual goals, preferences, and skill. Specific muscle groups may also be targeted to enhance other components of the activity program, such as biking or swimming.

Sequence Exercise large muscle groups before small muscle groups, doing chest and back exercises before specific arm exercises, for example. In addition, recommend performing exercises involving multiple joints before those for single joints, for example, doing leg presses before leg extensions or leg curls. Doing exercises in this sequence helps ensure that adequate energy is available to effectively perform all exercises within a training session and lowers the potential for injury. Abdominal and core muscle exercises should always be performed at the end of the training session.

Amount of Resistance The resistance used is determined by the individual's 1-repetition maximum (1-RM), defined as the maximal amount of weight that an individual can successfully lift 1 time. Recommending training that is either moderate (50%-60% of 1-RM) or vigorous (75%-80% of 1-RM) in intensity allows for optimal gains in strength and insulin action.[20,24,41] No specific amount of time is recommended for muscle strengthening, but exercises should be performed to the point at which it would be difficult to do another repetition without help. Home-based resistance training is adequate for maintaining muscle mass and strength, but less effective than supervised, gym-based training for maintaining blood glucose control, as heavier weights or resistance may be needed to optimize insulin action.[42,43]

Frequency Recommend doing strength training exercises at least 2 times a week with a minimum of 48 hours of rest between sessions, but more ideally 3 nonconsecutive days per week, along with regular aerobic activities.

Progression Each training session should involve completion of 10 to 15 repetitions to near fatigue per set on every exercise early in training, progressing over time to using heavier weights or resistance that allows for completion of only 8 to 10 repetitions.[19–22,24] Recommend doing a minimum of 1 set of repetitions to near fatigue to start, with a later goal of completing as many as 3 to 4 sets. To avoid injury, progression of training should occur slowly. To be most effective, recommend first undertaking increases in weight or resistance, and only when the target number of repetitions per set can consistently be exceeded, followed by a greater number of sets, and lastly by increased training frequency. Progression over 6 months or more to thrice-weekly sessions of 3 sets of 8 to 10 repetitions done at 75% to 80% of 1-RM on 8 to 10 exercises is an optimal goal for most individuals with diabetes.[20,39]

Modifications For individuals who need to maintain a lower resistance program due to joint limitations or other health complications, recommend doing 1 set of exercises for all major muscle groups, starting with 10 to 15 repetitions and progressing to 15 to 20 repetitions before adding additional sets.[16]

Rest Adequate rest periods between sets are needed to successfully complete all sets on each exercise.

Typically, lower intensity training requires 15 seconds to 1 minute of rest, while higher intensity training may necessitate up to 2 to 3 minutes of rest between sets.[16] In addition, allow at least 48 hours between training sessions for optimal musculoskeletal recovery.

Resistance Training Summary

- *Activity:* 5 to 10 exercises that cover all the major muscle groups
- *Frequency:* 2 to 3 days per week
- *Duration:* 1 to 3 sets of 8 to 15 repetitions (eg, 1 set of 10-15 repetitions to fatigue initially, progressing to 8-10 harder repetitions, and finally to 3 sets of 8-10 repetitions)
- *Intensity:* moderate to vigorous; 50% to 80% of 1-RM

Considerations With Cardiovascular Disease

When working with individuals with cardiovascular disease, focus particular attention on blood pressure and HR responses to training. Advise these individuals to start resistance training with lighter resistances to help decrease the myocardial oxygen demand on the heart.[44] Heart rate and blood pressure need to be monitored during training and remain within the limits established by an exercise stress test, keeping in mind that myocardial perfusion will be similar or enhanced during resistance training at HR limits established during aerobic exercise testing. While cardiovascular disease is not a contraindication to any form of exercise, anyone with angina classified as moderate or high risk should preferably exercise in a supervised cardiac rehabilitation program, at least initially, and HR should be kept at least 10 bpm below the onset of exercise-induced angina (if present).[44]

Instruction and Supervision

Before starting a resistance exercise program, individuals must be instructed on proper weight lifting techniques to ensure that all exercises are performed safely and correctly. Recommend that a qualified exercise professional supervise the initial stages of the training program. Instruct individuals on the following guidelines[16]:

- Breathe continually and avoid breath-holding during movements.
- Exhale during the exertion or lifting phase, and inhale while returning to starting position.

- Avoid sustained, tight gripping and static lifts that may cause hypertensive responses.
- Lift weights with slow, controlled movements.
- Emphasize using a complete range of motion around each joint.
- Maintain good form and keep the body properly aligned throughout the lift, especially when using free weights or resistance bands.
- Adjust the resistance equipment to fit the body frame.
- Stop exercising if warning signs or symptoms occur, such as dizziness, unusual shortness of breath, or chest pain.

Resistance Training Precautions

- Individuals with microvascular or macrovascular complications require program modifications to decrease strain on their cardiovascular system.
- Advise those with unstable proliferative retinopathy or severe nephropathy against doing resistance training due to increased risk of an excessive systolic blood pressure response.[20]
- Before starting resistance training, individuals with diabetes and cardiovascular disease need to have an ejection fraction >45% and a cardiorespiratory fitness level of 7 METs, without ischemic ST segment depression hypotensive or hypertensive responses, serious ventricular arrhythmias, or symptoms of cardiovascular insufficiency.[44]
- Individuals with any complications that may be worsened by resistance training need to receive approval from their physician before starting a resistance program.

Flexibility and Stretching Exercises

Flexibility is defined as the ability to move a joint through its complete range of motion and is considered an important part of physical fitness.[21,22,24] Some types of physical activity require more flexibility than others. Both dynamic and static stretching exercises are effective in increasing flexibility and thereby can allow individuals to more easily do activities that require greater movement around joints. For this reason, flexibility activities are an appropriate part of a physical activity program, even though they have no known health benefits and it is unclear whether they reduce risk of injury. Flexibility exercises can be included as part of the warm-up or cool-down, but by themselves they are not counted toward meeting the aerobic or muscle-strengthening guidelines.[21,22,24]

Flexibility exercise, combined with resistance training, has been shown to increase joint range of motion in individuals with type 2 diabetes[45] and allow them to more easily engage in activities that require greater flexibility. For this reason, flexibility training may be included as part of a physical activity program, although it should not substitute for other training. Older adults are advised to undertake exercises that maintain or improve balance to prevent falls,[22,24,46] which may include flexibility training especially for many older individuals with type 2 diabetes or peripheral neuropathy who have a higher risk of falling.

The ADA's current position on flexibility exercises is that there is insufficient evidence to recommend for or against them as a routine part of the exercise prescription.[17,20] Therefore, flexibility exercise recommendations should be based primarily on the individual's specific needs and interests.

Combined and Other Forms of Training

Including both aerobic and resistance exercise in a weekly exercise program is recommended. Combined aerobic and resistance training done thrice weekly in individuals with type 2 diabetes may be of greater benefit to blood glucose control than either aerobic or resistance exercise alone.[47,48] However, in most studies, the total duration of exercise and caloric expenditure were greatest with combined training, and both were done on the same days during a single training session. One study that controlled for caloric expenditure reported that a group that performed a combination of aerobic and resistance training improved A1C levels in adults with type 2 diabetes compared with the nonexercise control group; this was not achieved by aerobic or resistance training alone.[49] No studies have yet investigated whether daily, but alternating, training would be more effective.

For individuals with type 1 diabetes, the order of the 2 activities undertaken during the same exercise session affects glycemic balance both during and following the combined activity. For example, in one study, performing resistance exercise before aerobic exercise improved glycemic stability throughout exercise and reduced the duration and severity of immediate postexercise hypoglycemia.[50] Although resistance exercise causes less initial decline in blood glucose during the activity, it is associated with more prolonged reductions in postexercise glycemia than aerobic exercise.[51]

Unconventional forms of physical activity, like yoga and tai chi, may benefit control of blood glucose, oxidative stress, flexibility, strength, balance, and more, but the results of studies investigating glycemic benefits have been mixed, and the inclusion of those activities as part of a weekly exercise program is not conclusively supported at this time.[41,52,53] Such exercises can be included according to individual preferences to increase flexibility, muscular strength, and balance, but their effects on aerobic fitness are likely minimal.

Safety Considerations

- ◆ Teach all individuals with diabetes who are treated with insulin, sulfonylureas, or meglitinides to carry rapidly absorbed carbohydrates (eg, glucose tablets or gels) with them while performing physical activity so that they can treat hypoglycemia quickly.
- ◆ Teach individuals to monitor blood glucose, both before and after activity, to promote safety and understanding of the glycemic effects of exercise.
- ◆ Advise individuals to wear some form of diabetes and personal identification.
- ◆ Advise individuals to avoid vigorous physical activity in extremely hot, humid, smoggy, or cold environments.
- ◆ Encourage individuals to wear clothing and shoes appropriate for the activity to reduce chance of injury.
- ◆ Be aware that certain medications can impair exercise tolerance; for example, beta-adrenergic blocking agents lower the HR response to physical activity, as well as mask hypoglycemic symptoms and lessen counterregulatory responses.
- ◆ Advise individuals to stop the activity if symptoms like pain, lightheadedness, or shortness of breath occur.
- ◆ Since seasonal changes in A1C have been related to environmental temperature,[54] encourage individuals to find places to be active indoors when the weather is cold.

Modifications for Diabetes Complications

Individuals with chronic complications of diabetes often do not undertake regular physical activity. Yet, increasing physical activity levels is especially useful for this group to improve or maintain functional capacity, strength, balance, and flexibility. Their participation can be undertaken safely and effectively as long as certain precautions are taken.

Cardiovascular Disease

Since individuals with diabetes have an increased risk of cardiovascular disease, a comprehensive assessment is recommended for those meeting the pre-exercise screening criteria to determine the most appropriate physical activity options.

- For all individuals, assess risk with a physical activity history and/or an exercise test, to guide prescription.
- Recommend that high-risk individuals with established cardiovascular disease (eg, recent acute coronary syndrome or revascularization, heart failure) be supervised in a cardiac rehabilitation or other medically supervised program during exercise.
- Encourage 30 to 60 minutes of moderate-intensity aerobic activity, such as brisk walking, on most, preferably all, days of the week, supplemented by an increase in daily lifestyle activities (eg, walking breaks at work, gardening, household work).[44]
- Recommend resistance training exercises at least 2 days per week.[44]
- Advise individuals to avoid activities that cause a hypertensive response (systolic blood pressure >260 mm Hg, diastolic blood pressure >125 mm Hg), including those that involve heavy lifting, straining, and Valsalva-like maneuvers.

Peripheral Artery Disease

Individuals with peripheral artery disease will experience ischemic pain during physical activity as a result of an insufficient oxygen supply and demand for the active muscles. A low-intensity walking program for intermittent claudication may improve collateral circulation and muscle metabolism and, in turn, decrease pain.[55] A training program using intervals of walk and rest periods may result in improved tolerance for exercise, which was previously limited due to pain, and even upper body (arm crank) training appears to improve pain tolerance and exercise capacity.[56]

- Advise individuals that daily physical activity sessions will maximize pain tolerance during movement.
- Help individuals determine the distance and duration for walking by a pain-limited threshold.
- Advise individuals to keep the intensity low, as higher intensity demands a greater blood supply and will likely cause claudication pain.[55]
- Encourage individuals to use conversation, music, and other elements to divert attention from the discomfort and pain.
- Stop activity when the discomfort or pain increases from moderate to intense and attention cannot be diverted from the pain.
- Recommend weight-bearing activities, although non-weight-bearing activities may be used if longer duration and higher intensity workouts are the goal.

Retinopathy

The level of retinopathy determines which activities are appropriate and which activities are to be avoided (see Table 17.13 in chapter 17, on exercise prescription). While background or preproliferative retinopathy requires no precautions, individuals with advanced proliferative retinopathy will have significant restrictions in their level of physical exertion and activity options.

- Provide physical activity recommendations based on the severity and stage of diabetic retinopathy.
- Advise individuals with unstable proliferative diabetic retinopathy that they must receive clearance for exercise from their ophthalmologist due to risk of vitreous hemorrhage or traction retinal detachment.
- Advise individuals with unstable, advanced proliferative disease that activities producing large increases in blood pressure are not advised, such as high-intensity aerobic exercise, heavy resistance training, jumping or jarring activities, or exercises in a head-down position.[20]

Visual Impairment

Visual impairment resulting from diabetes-related or other eye disease should not be considered a contraindication to exercise. Only in cases of unstable proliferative disease or high risk of retinal detachment would certain forms of exercise not be recommended (eg, high-intensity aerobic exercises, resistance training, or jarring activities).

- ◆ Recommend appropriate options for physical activity, such as swimming using lane guides, stationary cycling, treadmill walking, tandem cycling, and dancing, using a sighted person as a guide when appropriate.

Chronic Kidney Disease

Individuals with chronic kidney disease usually have low functional and aerobic capacity. Aerobic activities are preferred, but the individual's degree of kidney impairment dictates his or her ability to perform aerobic activity. Individuals who are weak can benefit from strength training interventions. Resistance and aerobic exercise programs should be initiated at relatively low intensity and progressed slowly as tolerated in order to avoid injury and discontinuation of exercise.

- ◆ Recommend that individuals begin aerobic activity at a low level, perhaps using interval work, followed by gradual increases in their activity plan.[57]
- ◆ Recommend progressing over time to brisk walking, swimming, and cycling activities, as well as resistance training to improve strength.
- ◆ Recommend that individuals on hemodialysis incorporate exercise into the dialysis session to increase participation and tolerance.[57,58]

Peripheral Neuropathy

Physical activity cannot fully reverse the symptoms of peripheral neuropathy, but it can prevent further loss of muscle strength and flexibility commonly seen in individuals with sensory polyneuropathy. Prior recommendations stated that individuals with severe peripheral neuropathy should avoid weight-bearing activities to lower their risk of foot ulcerations; however, recent studies show that moderate-intensity walking does not increase risk of foot ulcers or re-ulceration in those with peripheral neuropathy.[59,60] Moreover, mild to moderate exercise can actually prevent the onset of peripheral neuropathy itself.[61] Thus, individuals without acute foot ulcers can and likely should perform moderate weight-bearing exercise, although anyone with a foot injury or open sore should be restricted to non-weight-bearing activities. All individuals should closely examine their feet on a daily basis to detect sores or ulcers early.

- ◆ Recommend daily range-of-motion exercises to help minimize shortening of connective tissue.
- ◆ Advise individuals without acute foot ulcers to engage in mild or moderate weight-bearing exercise, although low-impact activities like cycling, swimming, and aquatic and chair exercise are viable options as well.
- ◆ Recommend that individuals with a foot injury or open sore avoid weight-bearing activities because of an increased chance of soft tissue and joint injury.
- ◆ Encourage individuals to wear proper footwear and inspect their feet after physical activity to prevent blisters and detect injuries.
- ◆ Advise individuals to avoid jogging, as it places a threefold increase in pressure on the foot compared with walking.
- ◆ Suggest chair exercises for individuals with limited mobility to improve flexibility and strength.

Autonomic Neuropathy

For individuals with autonomic neuropathy, increases in physical activity levels must be approached with caution because of the role of the autonomic nervous system in hormonal and cardiovascular regulation during exercise. The presence of CAN doubles the risk of mortality and is associated with more frequent silent myocardial ischemia, orthostatic hypotension, and resting elevations in HR, leading to impaired exercise tolerance and low maximal HRs and slower HR recovery.[62] Moderate-intensity aerobic training can improve autonomic function in individuals with and without CAN.[63] Individuals with CAN should have an exercise stress test and physician approval before commencing exercise. Exercise intensity may be accurately prescribed using the HRR method with maximal HR directly measured, rather than estimated, for better accuracy.[30]

- Advise individuals with autonomic neuropathy (particularly CAN) to avoid high-intensity physical activities unless they have been cleared by a physician to participate.
- Encourage individuals to avoid physical exertion in hot or cold environments since dehydration may be a risk for those who have difficulty with thermoregulation.
- Caution individuals that hypotension or hypertension may occur after vigorous activities.
- Recommend recumbent cycling or water aerobics for individuals with orthostatic hypotension.
- For better accuracy, advise individuals to monitor exercise intensity using the HRR method, using a measured maximal HR if possible.

Modifications for Obesity

Combined programs of physical activity, meal planning, and behavior change are effective for obese individuals. Physical activity combined with meal planning has been shown to be more effective for long-term weight loss than either done alone. Approaches that emphasize physical activity offer enhanced calorie expenditure and provide the benefits of improved fitness related to influencing blood lipids, blood glucose control, blood pressure, mood, and attitude.[16] Regular physical activity also helps maintain muscle mass while promoting fat loss during weight loss.[64]

The optimal volume of exercise needed to achieve sustained major weight loss is likely much larger than that needed to achieve improved blood glucose control and cardiovascular health. Individuals who successfully maintain large weight loss over at least a year typically engage in about 7 hours per week of moderate- to vigorous-intensity exercise,[65] although greater exercise volumes (2000 and 2500 calories per week) produce greater and more sustained weight loss than smaller exercise volumes (1000 calories per week).[66] When working with obese individuals, use the following guidelines to increase their physical activity level:

- Recommend an initial goal of simply increasing the amount of daily physical movement from an inactive level.

- Recommend moderate aerobic exercise that uses large muscle groups, with emphasis on increasing duration and frequency.
- Recommend walking as an effective choice for continuous aerobic exercise; alternative types of exercise include cycling and chair and water exercise.
- Recommend non-weight-bearing activities to reduce the risk of orthopedic injury; higher intensity weight-bearing activities like running and jogging are not recommended until body weight is reduced.
- Recommend aiming for 45 to 60 minutes of activity 5 to 7 days per week.
- Recommend a target range of 300 to 400 calories of energy expenditure per day, or 2000 calories per week in physical activity.
- Advise individuals to undertake recommended amounts of resistance training to build muscle strength and mass.

Modifications for Pregnancy

While most forms of exercise are safe during pregnancy, those that involve positions and movements that may be uncomfortable, tiring, or harmful should be avoided. After the first trimester of pregnancy, women should not do exercises that require them to lie flat on their back. Standing still for long periods of time should also be avoided. Engaging in 30 minutes of moderate-intensity exercise (eg, brisk walking) during most days of the week (eg, 2.5 hours per week), however, has been adopted as a recommendation for pregnant women without medical or obstetrical complications.[67] Women diagnosed with gestational diabetes mellitus (GDM) are at substantially increased risk of developing type 2 diabetes later in life, and physical activity of all intensities may be considered a tool to prevent both GDM and possibly diabetes onset at a later date.[68] Women with GDM who exercise have better blood glucose control, lower fasting and postprandial glucose concentrations, and improved cardiorespiratory fitness.[69]

- Recommend engaging in 30 minutes of moderate exercise most days of the week, aiming for a total of 150 minutes; individuals who were sedentary prepregnancy should start out slowly.[69]

- Advise individuals to avoid doing any exercise lying flat on their back after the first trimester of pregnancy.
- Recommend wearing comfortable clothing that will help individuals remain cool, along with a bra that fits well and gives adequate support.
- Encourage pregnant exercisers to drink plenty of water to help keep from overheating and dehydrating.
- Recommend consuming enough daily calories to replace those used during exercise.
- Recommend avoiding exercise done in hot, humid weather or with a fever.
- Running, certain racquet sports, and vigorous resistance training can be continued by women doing these activities before becoming pregnant, but do not advise beginning them during pregnancy.
- Advise pregnant women to avoid contact sports, downhill skiing, scuba diving, and sports requiring quick directional changes.
- All pregnant women may safely engage in light to moderate resistance training throughout pregnancy.[68]
- Advise pregnant women to stop exercising and call their physician if they develop symptoms during activity, including vaginal bleeding, dizziness, increased shortness of breath, chest pain, headache, muscle weakness, calf pain or swelling, uterine contractions, decreased fetal movement, or fluid leaking from the vagina.

Modifications for Older Adults

When working with older adults, give special consideration to changes in body composition that may have occurred over the years (eg, declines in muscle mass and muscle strength, with resultant decreases in basal metabolic rate, activity level, and energy expenditure). Guidelines for adults with and without diabetes also apply to older adults (ages 65 and older).[20,22,24] Brisk walking, gardening, yard work, and housework are good examples of recommended moderate-intensity activities. Simply decreasing total sitting time and having active breaks during sedentary activities may also be a useful goal for all older adults.[12]

Results from the DPP demonstrate that it is never too late to begin an exercise program. In that study, the older adults who met the activity goal of 150 minutes per week were found to have derived the greatest benefit from exercise in warding off type 2 diabetes when compared with their younger counterparts.[4] Table 5.3 summarizes the guidelines for aerobic exercise in older adults. As stated, guidelines for adults ages 18 to 64 for aerobic exercise, resistance training, and flexibility also apply to older individuals; however, special considerations may be needed.

Aerobic Activity: Older Adults

- Highly recommend that adults have a thorough medical exam before starting an exercise program of moderate or higher intensity.
- Recommend that older adults do at least 150 minutes a week of moderate- to vigorous-intensity aerobic exercise, performed in episodes of at least 10 minutes, and preferably spread throughout the week.

TABLE 5.3 Summary of Guidelines for Aerobic Exercise in Older Adults	
Activity	Cycling, brisk walking, swimming, dancing, rowing
Duration	A minimum of 150 minutes a week (with no less than 10 minutes per exercise session); intersperse initial activity sessions with brief rest periods until an activity can be performed for 10 minutes at a time, and add 2–5 minutes per week until desired goal is met
Frequency	At least 3 nonconsecutive days per week, but ideally spread out over 5 or more days per week
Intensity	Base initial training intensity on the individual's graded exercise test, risk factors, and medical history: moderate to vigorous (ie, 40%–89% HRR), but starting at a lower level if sedentary and progressing slowly to a recommended intensity
Assess progress and reevaluate the individual's fitness plan every 4–6 weeks until minimal recommendations are met	

- Instruct individuals to increase exercise duration and frequency before intensity.
- Recommend a conservative approach when increasing exercise intensity, avoiding vigorous aerobic activity at first (except for possibly shorter intervals interspersed throughout a lower intensity activity).
- Advise previously sedentary individuals to start at lower levels and gradually increase the duration and frequency to reach the desired fitness level.
- Advise older adults that if they cannot do 150 minutes of moderate-intensity aerobic activity a week because of chronic conditions, they should be as physically active as their abilities and conditions allow.
- Recommend aquatic or chair exercises and stationary cycling for individuals with less tolerance for weight-bearing activities, such as those with severe degenerative joint disease or osteoarthritis.
- Advise that no matter what its purpose—gardening, walking the dog, taking a dance or exercise class, or bicycling to the store—aerobic activity of all types counts toward meeting recommended levels of physical activity.
- Recommend that all older adults break up sedentary time with frequent movement and avoid prolonged periods of uninterrupted sitting.

Resistance Training: Older Adults

- Recommend a minimum of 1 set of 8 to 10 exercises for each major muscle group 2 to 3 times a week, progressing up to 2 to 3 sets per exercise session.
- Recommend doing 10 to 15 repetitions that are "somewhat hard" on the RPE scale (12-14), progressing slowly over time to 8 to 12 repetitions at a harder intensity.
- Recommend lower resistance for the first 8 weeks to accommodate changes in connective tissue and to prevent injury.
- Suggest using all means of muscle strengthening, including exercises using exercise bands, weight machines, and hand-held weights; calisthenic exercises (using body weight provides resistance to movement); digging, lifting, and

carrying as part of gardening; carrying groceries; some yoga exercises; and some tai chi exercises.
- Advise individuals with degenerative joint disease or osteoarthritis to avoid resistance training during active periods of joint inflammation or pain.

Flexibility and Balance Exercises: Older Adults

- Recommend a well-rounded stretching program to counteract decreases in flexibility and improve balance and agility.
- Advise older adults to do exercises that maintain or improve balance (such as backward walking, sideways walking, heel walking, toe walking, and standing from a sitting position) 3 or more times a week, particularly if they are at risk of falling, as long as they are done safely.
- Let individuals know that doing any type of lower body and core resistance training also counts as balance training.
- For deconditioned individuals who are just beginning to be more active, recommend devoting a significant portion of the exercise session to improving flexibility.

Considerations for Children and Adolescents

Type 2 diabetes is being diagnosed in children at an ever-increasing and alarming rate. While the causes for this looming epidemic are multiple, the decline in physical activity levels for children in the United States is partially responsible. Updated guidelines recommend that children and adolescents participate in at least 60 minutes of moderate-intensity physical activity most days of the week, preferably daily.[24] When working with children and adolescents, focus activity recommendations on enjoyable playtime activities, rather than structured exercise bouts. Encourage participation in school physical education classes, recreation leagues, school sports, and active family outings, as well as parental involvement in the planning and development of physical activity programs for children and adolescents.

For children with type 1 diabetes and those with type 2 diabetes taking insulin, careful review of insulin dosages, insulin peaks and durations of action, and timing of meals and snacks is critical if problems with widely variant blood glucose levels, related to physical activity, are to be avoided. Frequent self-monitoring of blood glucose (ie, before, during, and after exercise) will assist in guiding adjustments in insulin dosing that will help avoid the extremes of glycemic control. Due to an increased uptake of glucose into skeletal muscle during exercise, children who have not had a regular pattern of activity or conditioning may be particularly susceptible to hypoglycemic episodes near the time of the exercise or hours later. To avoid problems, a decrease in "insulin on board" during active periods and modifications in food intake may be needed.

A full discussion of insulin changes by regimen and activity is beyond the scope of this chapter. For comprehensive coverage of insulin, food, and exercise regimen changes for youth (and for adults with type 1 diabetes and other insulin users with type 2 diabetes), educators are referred to *Diabetic Athlete's Handbook: Your Guide to Peak Performance* (Human Kinetics, 2009).

Cultural Considerations

When assisting individuals in planning and preparing for physical activity, consideration must be given to their cultural practices and beliefs and how these may influence the adoption of physical activity behaviors.[70,71] Understanding and being sensitive to beliefs and perceptions regarding physical activity is crucial for successful planning of physical activity goals. Promote activities that do not offend or ignore the individual's cultural beliefs.[72] Elicit information from individuals and provide culturally appropriate suggestions to help tailor suitable physical activity recommendations for their particular group.

Dance and music are a vital part of tradition and celebration for many ethnically diverse groups, including Native, Hispanic, and African Americans. Asian and Middle Eastern groups may have other cultural traditions that can be brought into the fitness routine, such as yoga and tai chi. By reinforcing the regular inclusion of dance or other cultural physical activities as a healthy lifestyle choice, the diabetes educator can help individuals with diabetes (and their high-risk family members) make

increased activity a regular part of the family routine. The activity helps strengthen families as well.

Putting the Activity Program Into Action

Most diabetes educators are adept in interpreting and promoting recommendations for physical activity and exercise to individuals with diabetes. Educators who are skilled in behavior-change strategies and able to effectively tailor exercise programs to an individual's goals, needs, and interests are better equipped to help individuals become and stay more active. Physical activity programs that are designed primarily by the individual are more likely to be sustained. An individual who chooses enjoyable and convenient activities is more likely to participate regularly.

Adoption and Maintenance of Exercise by Persons With Diabetes

The following are central determining factors influencing activity across the life span in all individuals, with and without diabetes:

- Self-efficacy (ie, having confidence in one's ability to be active)
- Enjoyment of physical activity
- Lack of perceived barriers to being physically active
- Positive beliefs concerning the benefits of physical activity
- Support from others to continue exercising

Greater effort needs to be focused on the promotion of regular exercise among individuals with or at risk for developing type 2 diabetes in particular since lifestyle choices largely influence the onset of this condition. One of the most consistent predictors of greater levels of activity has been higher levels of self-efficacy[73,74] which reflect confidence in the ability to exercise.[75] In individuals with type 2 diabetes in particular, interventions should focus on enhancing self-efficacy, problem solving, and social-environmental support to improve self-management (which includes exercise, dietary, and medication behaviors).[76]

Enhancing Self-Efficacy

Beliefs about self-efficacy influence health behaviors. Individuals tend to pursue tasks they feel competent to perform and avoid those in which they feel incompetent. Diabetes educators can help individuals enhance self-efficacy in the following ways:

- Help the individual develop realistic activity goals.[77]
- Plan a gradual program with the individual, using small, incremental steps.[77-79]
- Encourage setting goals that the individual is likely to attain, to promote feelings of mastery.
- Provide suggestions or opportunities to observe others succeeding at being physically active, such as watching a video or exercise class.[16]
- Rehearse or practice the intended exercise behavior with the individual.[77]
- Provide regular, supportive feedback.

Problem Solving and Goal Setting

When planning to increase physical activity levels by overcoming potential obstacles or problems, individuals should be encouraged to develop realistic and practical goals. Goals that are too vague, too ambitious, or too distant do not provide enough self-motivation to maintain long-term interest. Encourage individuals to write down and track their goals to help see their progress and identify barriers. The acronym SMART may be used to help individuals set appropriate physical activity goals. SMART stands for specific, measurable, attainable, realistic, and time-frame specific, as explained below[16]:

- *Specific:* Encourage the individual to be as precise as possible when identifying details of frequency, duration, intensity, and type of activity.
- *Measurable:* Teach the person how to make goals that can be quantified so he or she can accurately track, measure, and identify progress.
- *Attainable:* Help the individual set goals that are challenging but reachable to increase confidence and the likelihood of setting even more challenging goals in the future.

- *Realistic:* Help the individual evaluate how likely he or she is to attain his or her chosen goals in a given situation.
- *Time-frame specific:* Encourage the individual to set short-term goals that provide more immediate feedback, such as setting goals for just the next week.

Social-Environmental Support

Social support is associated with greater levels of physical activity, supporting the role of social networks in modifying behavior patterns.[80] Fortunately, the same social dynamics may be exploited to increase the effects of interventions beyond the target individual and can potentially help spread exercise behavior.

Likewise, counseling delivered by healthcare professionals may also be a meaningful source of support and an effective source for delivery.[81] Physicians vary in counseling their patients to exercise: on average, advice or referral related to exercise occurred at 18% of office visits among diabetic patients, and 73% of patients reported receiving advice at some point to exercise more. The built environment (eg, availability of facilities, pleasant places to walk) may also be an important predictor of regular physical activity.

Similarly, exercise intervention studies showing the greatest impact on blood glucose control have all involved supervision of exercise sessions by qualified exercise trainers. In the 1-year Italian Diabetes and Exercise Study, for example, all participants with type 2 diabetes (intervention and control) received high-quality exercise counseling that increased self-reported physical activity substantially.[82] The intervention group also received supervised, facility-based combined aerobic and resistance exercise training twice weekly, resulting in greater improvements in overall blood glucose control, blood pressure, and body composition. A review of 20 resistance training studies on type 2 diabetes[41] also found that supervised training of varying volume, frequency, and intensity improved blood glucose control and insulin sensitivity, but that when supervision was removed, both compliance and glycemic control decreased. Thus, individuals with diabetes engaging in supervised training gain benefits that exceed those of exercise counseling and increased physical activity undertaken alone.

Effective Use of Step Counters (Pedometers)

Here are some points to consider when advising patients to use a pedometer to promote and record daily physical activity:

◆ Pedometers record ambulatory activity, such as walking, jogging, or running. They will not count steps during cycling, rowing, upper body exercise, swimming, or other activities.

However, steps can be estimated using the equivalent values listed in Table 5.4.

◆ To be considered a physically active adult, the patient will need to accumulate the equivalent of 10,000 steps per day.

◆ For most adults, 2000 steps is the equivalent of about 1 mile of walking.

◆ The most essential feature of any pedometer is the step count. Pedometers are most accurate in counting steps, less accurate in calculating

TABLE 5.4   Equivalent Steps of Physical Activities for Adults

Activity	Minute Step Count	15-Minute Step Count	30-Minute Step Count
Aerobic dance	197	2955	5910
Ballroom dancing, slow to fast	91–167	1365–2505	2730–5010
Bowling	91	1365	2730
Canoeing	106	1590	3180
Circuit training	242	3630	7260
Climbing, rock or mountain	273	4095	8190
Gardening	121	1815	3630
Golf	136	2040	4080
Gymnastics	121	1815	3630
Health club exercise, general	167	2505	5010
Hiking	182	2730	5460
Jogging	212	3180	6360
Jogging on mini-trampoline	136	2040	4080
Martial arts	303	4545	9090
Running, 5–8 mph	242–409	3630–6135	7260–12,270
Shopping	70	1050	2100
Stationary cycling, moderate to vigorous	212–318	3180–4770	6360–9540
Step aerobics	273	4095	8190
Swimming laps, moderate to vigorous	212–303	3180–4545	6360–9090
Swimming leisurely	182	2730	5460
Water aerobics	121	1815	3630
Water jogging	242	3630	7260
Weight lifting, moderate to vigorous	121–182	1815–2730	3630–5460
Yoga and stretching	76	1140	2280

Based on metabolic equivalents (METs) of various physical activities.

Source: BE Ainsworth, WL Haskell, MC Whitt, et al, "2011 Compendium of physical activities: a second update of codes and MET values," *Med Sci Sports Exerc* 43 (2011): 1575-81.

(continued)

American Association of Diabetes Educators©

distance walked, and even less accurate at estimating caloric expenditure.

❖ A variety of factors can affect step-counting accuracy, such as walking speed, waistband type, and abdominal size. In general, most pedometers are fairly accurate step counters at speeds of 2.5 mph and above.

❖ Pedometers are more accurate at counting steps when attached to a firm waistband in an upright position; pedometers attached to loose waistbands typically underestimate steps.

❖ Abdominal girth can also affect step-counting accuracy. For persons with large abdomens, consider placing the pedometer at the small of the back, or use one that can be placed in a pocket or other location (like around the knee).

❖ Recommended brands of pedometers include most Accusplit®, Yamax®, and Omron® models. Go for a simple but accurate model.

❖ To test a pedometer's accuracy, have the patient position the device on his or her belt or waistband in line with the knee on either side of the body and reset the pedometer's count to zero. Have the patient take 20 steps at a typical walking pace. If it records between 18 and 22 steps, it is reasonably accurate. If not, reposition it and try again. If it repeatedly fails this test, consider buying another type.

❖ A number of free online step-tracking programs are available, such as the one found on the America on the Move site (https://aom3. americaonthemove.org).

When prescribing physical activity for the prevention or control of type 2 diabetes, the effects of the dose of the prescription on adherence are small.[83] Therefore, educators are encouraged to focus more on factors like choice and enjoyment in helping determine specifically how an individual would meet recommended participation. Affective responses to exercise may be important predictors of its adoption and maintenance, and encouraging activity at intensities below the ventilatory threshold may be most beneficial.[84] Many individuals with prediabetes or diabetes prefer walking as an aerobic activity, and pedometer- or accelerometer-based interventions can be effective for increasing aerobic activity (see Table 5.4 for step equivalents per minute of activity undertaken with a pedometer).[85–88] Finally, based on what is now known about sedentary behaviors, interventions may also benefit from simply attempting to decrease sitting time and periods of extended sedentary activity and promote more lifestyle physical activity.

Promoting Lifestyle Physical Activity

For individuals with diabetes, who are frequently deconditioned and sedentary, the first major challenge is to help them incorporate more physical activity into daily living.[8] Significant health benefits, such as a reduction in coronary risk factors, can be obtained by incorporating frequent bouts of moderate-intensity activities on most, if not all, days of the week. In particular, older adults may benefit from simply reducing their total sedentary time and avoiding prolonged periods of sitting by increasing the number of breaks during sedentary time.[12] While lifestyle physical activity does not entirely take the place of a traditionally structured exercise program, it can be highly effective in helping individuals increase their daily activity level, build a fitness base, and possibly improve glycemic management.[14] In addition, those who have successfully implemented more physical activity into their daily lifestyle may feel more confident and ready, as well as able, to initiate more structured forms of activity.

Activity Pyramid

The Activity Pyramid is a useful tool to help individuals be more active (see Figure 5.1). It shows a variety of ways that physical activity, both structured and unstructured, can be included in daily life. Diabetes educators can use the Activity Pyramid to help individuals identify, plan, and progressively

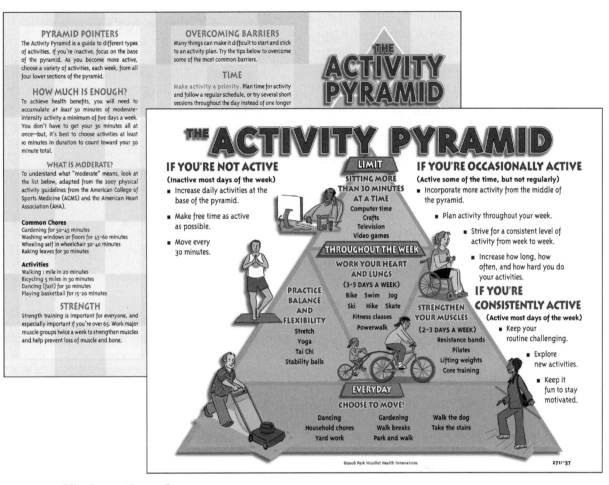

FIGURE 5.1   The Activity Pyramid

Source: From Type 2 Diabetes BASICS © 2010 International Diabetes Center. Adapted with permission from The Activity Pyramid © 2008 Park Nicollet HealthSource, Minneapolis, Minn.

increase regular physical activity, including lifestyle components.

- ◈ Suggest individuals begin by focusing on undertaking more daily activities from the base of the pyramid.
- ◈ Once the individual has established a solid base, encourage him or her to consider activities from other areas of the pyramid, starting and progressing slowly.
- ◈ Specific fitness areas can be enhanced by doing activities from a specific level of the pyramid:
  - —Activities from the base enhance overall health and well-being
  - —Activities from the middle level focus on improving aerobic fitness, muscular strength and endurance, and balance and flexibility
  - —The tip of the pyramid suggests ways to decrease sedentary activities
- ◈ Encourage individuals to move more and sit less by eventually incorporating activities from all areas of the pyramid.

Pedometers and Accelerometers

Both pedometers (small monitors that record the number of steps taken) and accelerometers (monitors that record all movement, including variations in exercise intensity) can be useful tools for increasing lifestyle physical activity. As they are inexpensive and easy to use, pedometers may be helpful to individuals in self-monitoring physical activity by providing immediate feedback, building confidence, and enhancing enjoyment. However, pedometers detect only walking-based activities and cannot detect changes in type, intensity, or pattern of activity, whereas accelerometers can. The main shortcomings of accelerometers are their low sensitivity to sedentary activities and their inability to register static exercise.[88] A recent meta-analysis found that pedometer users increased their overall physical activity by 26.9% over baseline in studies having an average intervention of 18 weeks, and an important predictor of increased levels was the use of a goal, such as to take 10,000 steps per day.[85] Assist individuals in using a pedometer effectively:

- Wear the pedometer correctly (usually attached to waistband of pants and centered above kneecap, or can be placed on small of back for persons with a large abdomen).
- Establish a baseline by tracking steps for a few days without intentionally increasing physical activity level.
- Set appropriate step goals by progressively increasing steps from baseline using small increases to start, such as taking an extra 500 to 1000 steps a day.
- Estimate step counts of time spent doing activities not recorded by the pedometer (refer to Table 5.4).
- Alternately, use accelerometers to track both total movement and intensity of activity for extended periods of time.

Using Stage-Matched Interventions

The Transtheoretical Model of behavior change, which uses progressive stages of readiness for behavior change, can be used to tailor exercise interventions.[89,90] Stage-matched interventions are widely accepted by healthcare practitioners in helping individuals make permanent lifestyle changes, including regular exercise.[16,79,91–93] The following stage-matched strategies can be used to help individuals overcome physical activity and exercise barriers.[5,16,79,89,94]

Stages of Change for Exercise Behavior[1,16,93]

1. *Precontemplation:* Not regularly active and has no intention of being active in the next 6 months
2. *Contemplation:* Not regularly active but thinking about starting in the next 6 months
3. *Preparation:* Doing some activity but not enough to meet current guidelines for regular physical activity
4. *Action:* Has become regularly physically active within the last 6 months
5. *Maintenance:* Has maintained regular physical activity for 6 months or more

Precontemplation

The goal at the precontemplation stage is for individuals to begin thinking about participating in more physical activity.

- Build trust with the individual and provide information as needed.
- Emphasize the individual's autonomy in decisions to be more active.
- Discuss pros and cons of physical activity.
- Encourage the individual to think about personally relevant benefits.
- Address the individual's specific barriers and encourage the individual to come up with possible solutions to these barriers.
- Use appropriate goal-setting activities focused on getting the individual to think about being more active, such as reading a pamphlet on the benefits of exercise.
- Suggest that the individual write down benefits of exercise, barriers to exercising, reasons to be active, and reasons not to be active.

Contemplation

The goal at the contemplation stage is for individuals to begin taking steps to be more active and to think about setting physical activity goals.

- Continue to use strategies from the precontemplation stage.
- Provide support and validation to the individual.

- Offer information on physical activity and exercise, emphasizing social, psychological, and general health benefits.
- Discuss the individual's personal preferences for physical activity.
- Encourage the individual to think about what has been successful in the past regarding physical activity or examples of family and friends who have been successful.
- Suggest that the individual use a reinforcement program that provides positive rewards when goals are achieved.
- Encourage the individual to identify other people to use for support.

Preparation

The goal at the preparation stage is for individuals to increase physical activity to recommended levels.

- Praise preparation taken to increase physical activity.
- Continue to use strategies from the precontemplation and contemplation stages.
- Assist the individual in setting goals to gradually increase physical activity levels.
- Encourage the individual to track progress with a physical activity log that details activity type, amount, duration, and frequency.
- Suggest the individual join an exercise class or club.

Action

The goal at the action stage is for individuals to begin making physical activity a regular part of their life.

- Praise all efforts of the individual.
- Work with the individual to develop a specific plan for tracking progress and setting short-term physical activity goals.
- Suggest the individual try new activities or train for an upcoming exercise event (such as walking or a bicycle race).
- Limit suggestions for additional changes to 1 or 2.
- Encourage the individual to begin to anticipate barriers.

Maintenance

The goal at the maintenance stage is for individuals to prepare for possible setbacks and find ways to continue to increase enjoyment with the personalized physical activity program.

- Praise all efforts of the individual.
- Use strategies from the action stage.
- Help the individual find ways to avoid boredom, such as varying exercise routines.
- Promote relapse-prevention strategies—distinguish between a lapse (slight slip) and a relapse (return to former behavior patterns) by having the individual identify potential high-risk situations and develop a plan to deal with them.
- Encourage the individual to reflect on the benefits achieved with regular physical activity.

Keep in mind that most people are not successful with their first attempt at increasing and maintaining new levels of physical activity. Some individuals may need 3 or 4 attempts before physical activity becomes a long-term habit. Individuals will progress through the stages as they learn from past attempts and successes and try different methods for increasing activity. The more an individual takes action to become more physically active, the better his or her chances of progressing forward. The role of the diabetes educator is to support the individual in all stages and apply appropriate intervention strategies as needed.

Using Motivational Interviewing

Motivational interviewing is an individual-centered directive method of communication for enhancing intrinsic motivation to change by exploring and resolving ambivalence.[95,96] This technique can be used with individuals to help increase motivational readiness to make positive behavior changes in physical activity.[16] (See also chapter 3.) Individuals with type 2 diabetes may be more receptive to motivational interviewing, given that its approach is more patient-centered and empowering than traditional care.[97] Key strategies that diabetes educators can use with individuals experiencing ambivalence with physical activity participation include the following[16,95,96]:

- ◆ Emphasize the individual's autonomy and freedom to choose not to be physically active.
- ◆ Encourage the individual's acceptance of responsibility for change and consequences of not changing activity habits.
- ◆ Use strategic feedback, reflections, and questions to help the individual develop internal discrepancies for remaining inactive.
- ◆ Use decisional balance scales to help the individual weigh being more active against remaining inactive or being less active.
- ◆ Obtain permission from the individual before providing information or offering advice.

A key tool of motivational interviewing is the use of rulers to explore importance and raise the individual's confidence regarding his or her exercise behaviors.[16,95,96] Start by asking the individual to rate on a 10-point scale how important the exercise behavior is and how confident he or she is about the behavior, such as walking 3 times a week for 15 minutes. After the individual chooses a number, ask why that specific number was chosen, versus a higher number. See the sidebar for an example of how this technique is implemented.

Summary

This chapter reviewed current physical activity and exercise guidelines for individuals with diabetes and discussed a variety of strategies to assist individuals, both those with diabetes and those at risk for diabetes, in becoming more active. The basic elements of the exercise prescription serve as a guide to creating safe and effective physical activity programs, even when complicated by the presence of diabetes-related health issues. However, the true art of program planning lies in the effective use of behavior-change strategies to tailor the program to each individual's health status, personal preferences, abilities, goals, and stage of readiness.

Readers are also referred to chapter 17, on exercise prescription. Whereas this chapter focused on strategies for promoting self-care behaviors relevant to being active, chapter 17 provides a good deal of fundamental information about physical activity and exercise prescriptions for those with diabetes or prediabetes. Readers learn about current fitness terminology, the physiological responses to physical activity related to blood glucose levels, and the effects of the various modes of physical activity on diabetes management and chronic complications, including prevention. Medical considerations regarding chronic complications are reviewed, hypoglycemia and hyperglycemia as they relate to physical activity are discussed, and more information on the exercise prescription and considerations for children and older adults is available there.

Using Behavior-Change Rules

Importance Rulers

1. On a scale of 0 to 10, how *important* is it for you to begin walking 3 times a week for 15 minutes?

The answer given helps determine the individual's readiness to change physical activity patterns.

2. And why are you a 2 and not a 6?

The individual's answer elicits conversation regarding behavior change.

Confidence Rulers

1. On a scale of 0 to 10, how *confident* are you that you could walk 3 times a week for 15 minutes?

The answer given helps determine the individual's confidence regarding increasing physical activity.

2. And why are you a 4 and not a 7?

The answer given elicits conversation regarding the individual's ability to be more active.

Case Wrap-up

A thorough interview with MT to discuss her personal beliefs, past experiences, preferences, and concerns about being more active helped the diabetes educator gain a better understanding of MT's view of physical activity.

Education Goals

Education focused on the importance of monitoring blood glucose before and after exercise and carrying a form of carbohydrate during activity. The educator also advised MT to start with low-intensity exercise and progress slowly with structured activities to avoid developing activity-related injuries, exercise nonadherence, or lack of motivation, with a goal of increasing her amount of physical activity gradually over a period of weeks to months as she is able and willing to do so.

Exercise Program Goals

- *Activity:* The initial focus was on lifestyle physical activity using low- to moderate-intensity forms of physical activity, particularly focusing on those activities she enjoys doing.

- *Frequency and duration:* Since MT is inactive, the educator encouraged short bouts of activity that could be incorporated into MT's daily routine. She was advised to start with a walking program consisting of 5 to 10 minutes of slow walking several times each day, 5 to 6 days a week. The exercise duration could then be gradually increased to 10 minutes per session, 3 times a day, and the walking speed could be increased slowly as she was able to do more.[24] In addition, MT should be encouraged to engage in more daily movement and break up her sedentary time whenever possible.

- *Progression:* Long-term exercise goals focused on progressively increasing amounts and frequency of activity to minimum recommended levels (150 minutes of moderate or vigorous exercise spread throughout the week).

Tools and Strategies

- *Activity Pyramid:* MT identified activities from the base of the pyramid that she might try incorporating into her daily lifestyle.

- *Pedometer:* A pedometer was suggested as a way for MT to obtain feedback about her activity levels, with a goal of increasing her number of baseline steps over a period of weeks or months.

- *Stages of change:* Behavior-change strategies appropriate for the contemplation and preparation stages were used, including offering information on the benefits of physical activity, discussing the pros and cons of increasing physical activity, helping identify and build a support system, and identifying barriers to physical activity and brainstorming possible solutions.

- *Self-efficacy through SMART goals:* The educator helped MT build self-efficacy by helping her set SMART goals she was likely to achieve, such as making a list of 5 ways to be more active throughout the day and trying 1 of them the next week.

- *Motivational interviewing:* MT was encouraged to ask questions and come up with ideas and suggestions for becoming more active, to promote autonomy and build confidence.

Focus on Education

Teaching Strategies

⊘ **Perform a pre-exercise evaluation.** Individuals who have or are at risk for vascular or cardiac complications need a pre-exercise evaluation. Once the evaluation is completed, a tailored program can be developed. Aerobic activities are recommended over other forms of exercise to start, but individuals must be evaluated for enrollment, and goals should include the incorporation of resistance training at some point.

⊘ **Set goals using the SMART approach.** Goals are set to achieve positive outcomes. Using the SMART approach (goals that are specific, measurable, attainable, realistic, and time-specific) encourages positive outcomes and helps establish lifelong habits. Encourage a plan for activity that is enjoyable, safe, and effective. Role-model your own activity plan, and wear and encourage use of a pedometer. Plan a group program such as a walking club or an exercise class; track activity and outcomes.

↻ **Use theory to guide interventions.**   Be familiar with theories to tailor and individualize interventions (eg, stage-matched strategies, goal setting, and motivational interviewing techniques).

↻ **Identify protocols and professional exercise resources.**   Contact exercise physiologists or clinical specialists for advice, consultation, and/or participation in your program. Shadow them during a work session for an exercise prescription and testing. With permission, videotape your session with the exercise physiologist and have this professional review and offer recommendations.

↻ **Monitor progress and impact of exercise on metabolic control.**   Patients can record and quantify daily physical activities and their impact on glycemic control. Exercise can be a therapeutic strategy for daily glucose control.

Messages for Patients

↻ **Establish a routine for physical activity.**   Physical activity is a vital part of improved or continued diabetes control, and it has a positive effect on blood pressure and blood cholesterol. It also aids in prevention of type 2 diabetes. Choose an activity you enjoy! Involve family or friends in a swim class, biking or hiking trip, or neighborhood street dance.

↻ **Identify health issues.**   Contact your healthcare provider for approval of an exercise plan if you have high blood pressure or any other complications (such as neuropathy or arthritis).

↻ **Practice safety first.**   Wear identification. Test blood glucose before and after activity. Wear clothing that fits well to prevent injury. Dress in layers so that you can easily adjust what you are wearing. Stop the activity if you are lightheaded or short of breath. If you are on medications for diabetes, be sure to carry a rapid-acting carbohydrate product. Consider carrying fluids to stay hydrated during physical activity.

↻ **Establish an exercise support network.**   Create a network of friends and family who will support you, keep you accountable, partner with you, and motivate you to get going. Make sure to talk to your healthcare professional team about your physical activity routine, any pain associated with it, any challenges, and the impact on your health.

↻ **Assess exercise relapse.**   Your usual physical activity routine can be interrupted for several days and consequently discontinued. Provide strategies for relapse prevention and its management. Also, reassess your physical activity routine and its impact annually.

Health Literacy

↻ **Low health literacy affects your patients' ability to locate proper health services, share personal information with providers, perform self-care behaviors, adopt healthy behaviors, make judgments, obtain tests, and follow up.**   Consider all of those elements in developing realistic physical activity education. Your education approach needs to be so much more than just providing information on what to do and how to do it.

↻ **Use low-literacy educational materials.**   It is recommended that health education material be written toward a sixth-grade level. However, the majority of diabetes education materials are written at a ninth-grade level or above. Even college-level readers prefer materials written in easy-to-read formats. Use handouts with pictures that demonstrate each stage of the desired physical activity, its duration, and when to progress to the next stage. You can use a calendar with prompts to adjust the routine or to keep people motivated. The illustrations and text should focus on desired behavioral strategies rather than medical facts.

→ **Use effective communication strategies with your patients.** Assume all of your patients have a low literacy level. Everyone, regardless of literacy level, deserves to be engaged in meaningful and strategic communication.

→ **Focus on high-priority behaviors first, but make sure that they are as important to your patient as they are to you.**

→ **Use concrete examples of activities, places, and times.**

→ **Limit the number of topics covered in one session.**

→ **Use the teach-back method to demonstrate adequate comprehension.**

→ **Address health numeracy by having patients identify methods of monitoring their physical activity with time, intensity, and duration.** Also, health numeracy can affect the patient's understanding of the impact of exercise on glucose readings and how to quantify its health benefits. One of the strategies used to understand the benefits is to have your patients check their blood glucose before and after physical activity. They can also use the "how do I feel" scale of 1 to 10 for days with exercise versus no exercise versus less exercise. Some patients might not understand the difference between "set" and "repetition" in weight lifting.

→ **Let your patient know that you will follow up by e-mail or with a phone call within the next few days to provide support and troubleshoot.**

→ **Use analogies or stories to increase comprehension.** You can relate that exercise works like medicine by showing a medication bottle with the name of the exercise, its benefits, and side effects. Share other patients' stories on overcoming a challenge or demonstrating success. Normalize obstacles by sharing your own strategies and your daily routine.

Focus on Practice

→ **Pre-exercise needs.** In the absence of known cardiovascular complications, requiring a pre-exercise evaluation may be a deterrent to physical activity and unnecessary prior to starting exercise programs involving only mild or moderate walking (ie, brisk walking or lower intensity exercise). Make sure you have access to proper footwear for weight-bearing activities like walking.

→ **Socioeconomic barriers.** A lower socioeconomic status may affect exercise opportunities because of cost (eg, joining an exercise facility), limited availability (neighborhood unsafe for walking), or time involvement (such as when economic pressures may necessitate working more than one job). Certain cultural traditions also downplay physical activity.

→ **Community assets.** Develop and maintain a referral list of appropriate exercise programs and other fitness resources available in your community that can be shared with patients to facilitate their involvement. Online information about exercise recommendations and precautions is available at http://www.health.gov/paguidelines and other sources.

→ **Physical inactivity is associated with an increased risk of chronic diseases.** Various physical activity interventions should be part of any healthcare system. Physical activity interventions reduce disease incidence, are cost-effective, and offer good value for the money. Provide choices and variety in exercise programs and interventions.

References

1. Kirk AF, Mutrie N, Macintyre PD, Fisher MB. Promoting and maintaining physical activity in people with type 2 diabetes. Am J Prev Med. 2004;27(4):289-96.

2. Morrato EH, Hill JO, Wyatt HR, Ghushchyan V, Sullivan PW. Physical activity in U.S. adults with diabetes and at risk for developing diabetes, 2003. Diabetes Care. 2007;30(2):203-9.

3. Kriska A. Can a physically active lifestyle prevent type 2 diabetes? Exerc Sports Sci Rev. 2003;31(3):132-7.

4. Diabetes Prevention Program (DPP) Research Group. Reduction in the incidence of type 2 diabetes with lifestyle intervention or metformin. N Engl J Med. 2002;346(6): 393-403.

5. Diabetes Prevention Program (DPP) Research Group. The Diabetes Prevention Program (DPP): description of lifestyle intervention. Diabetes Care. 2002;25(12):2165-71.

6. Diabetes Prevention Program (DPP) Research Group. Achieving weight and physical activity goals among diabetes prevention program lifestyle participants. Obes Res. 2004;12(9):1426-34.

7. Ryan DH; Diabetes Prevention Program (DPP) Research Group. Diet and exercise in the prevention of diabetes. Int J Clin Pract Suppl. 2003;134:28-35.

8. Castaneda C. Diabetes control with physical activity and exercise. Nutr Clin Care. 2003;6(2):89-96.

9. Hamman RF, Wing RR, Edelstein SL, et al. Effect of weight loss with lifestyle intervention on risk of diabetes. Diabetes Care. 2006;29(9):2102-7.

10. Dube JJ, Allison KF, Rousson V, Goodpaster BH, Amati F. Exercise dose and insulin sensitivity: relevance for diabetes prevention. Med Sci Sports Exerc. 2012;44:793-9.

11. George ES, Rosenkranz RR, Kolt GS. Chronic disease and sitting time in middle-aged Australian males: findings from the 45 and Up Study. Int J Behav Nutr Phys Act. 2013;10:20.

12. Bankoski A, Harris TB, McClain JJ, et al. Sedentary activity associated with metabolic syndrome independent of physical activity. Diabetes Care. 2011;34:497-503.

13. Wilmot EG, Edwardson CL, Achana FA, et al. Sedentary time in adults and the association with diabetes, cardiovascular disease and death: systematic review and meta-analysis. Diabetologia. 2012;55:2895-905.

14. Dunstan DW, Kingwell BA, Larsen R, et al. Breaking up prolonged sitting reduces postprandial glucose and insulin responses. Diabetes Care. 2012;35:976-83.

15. Kilpatrick ES, Rigby AS, Atkin SL. Insulin resistance, the metabolic syndrome, and complication risk in type 1 diabetes: "double diabetes" in the Diabetes Control and Complications Trial. Diabetes Care. 2007;30:707-12.

16. American College of Sports Medicine. Resource Manual for Exercise Testing and Prescription. 7th ed. Baltimore: Williams & Wilkins; 2013.

17. Sigal RJ, Kenny GP, Wasserman DH, Castaneda-Sceppa C. Physical activity/exercise and type 2 diabetes. Diabetes Care. 2004;27(10):2518-39.

18. American Diabetes Association. Physical activity/exercise and diabetes. Diabetes Care. 2004;27:S58-62.

19. Sigal RJ, Kenny GP, Wasserman DH, et al. Physical activity/exercise and type 2 diabetes: a consensus statement from the American Diabetes Association. Diabetes Care. 2006;29(6):1433-8.

20. Colberg SR, Albright A, Blissmer B, et al; for the American College of Sports Medicine and American Diabetes Association. Exercise and type 2 diabetes: position stand. Med Sci Sports Exerc. 2010;42(12):2282-303.

21. Haskell WL, Lee IM, Pate RR, et al. Physical activity and public health: updated recommendation for adults from the American College of Sports Medicine and the American Heart Association. Med Sci Sports Exerc. 2007;39(8): 1423-34.

22. Nelson ME, Rejeski WJ, Blair SN, et al. Physical activity and public health in older adults: recommendation from the American College of Sports Medicine and the American Heart Association. Med Sci Sports Exerc. 2007;39(8): 1435-45.

23. Garber CE, Blissmer B, Deschenes MR, et al; American College of Sports Medicine. American College of Sports Medicine position stand. Quantity and quality of exercise for developing and maintaining cardiorespiratory, musculoskeletal, and neuromotor fitness in apparently healthy adults: guidance for prescribing exercise. Med Sci Sports Exerc. 2011;43:1334-59.

24. Physical Activity Guidelines Advisory Committee. Physical activity guidelines advisory committee report, 2008. Washington, DC; 2008. 683 p.

25. Hawley JA, Lessard SJ. Exercise training-induced improvements in insulin action. Acta Physiol (Oxf). 2008;192(1): 127-35.

26. Winnick JJ, Sherman WM, Habash DL, et al. Short-term aerobic exercise training in obese humans with type 2 diabetes mellitus improves whole-body insulin sensitivity through gains in peripheral, not hepatic insulin sensitivity. J Clin Endocrinol Metab. 2008;93(3):771-8.

27. Hansen D, Dendale P, Jonkers RA, et al. Continuous low- to moderate-intensity exercise training is as effective

as moderate- to high-intensity exercise training at lowering blood HbA(1c) in obese type 2 diabetes patients. Diabetologia. 2009;52:1789-97.

28. Manders RJ, Van Dijk JW, van Loon LJ. Low-intensity exercise reduces the prevalence of hyperglycemia in type 2 diabetes. Med Sci Sports Exerc. 2010;42:219-25.

29. Little JP, Gillen JB, Percival ME, et al. Low-volume high-intensity interval training reduces hyperglycemia and increases muscle mitochondrial capacity in patients with type 2 diabetes. J Appl Physiol. 2011;111:1554-60.

30. Colberg SR, Swain DP, Vinik AI. Use of heart rate reserve and rating of perceived exertion to prescribe exercise intensity in diabetic autonomic neuropathy. Diabetes Care. 2003;26(4):986-90.

31. Boulé NG, Kenny GP, Haddad E, Wells GA, Sigal RJ. Meta-analysis of the effect of structured exercise training on cardiorespiratory fitness in type 2 diabetes mellitus. Diabetologia. 2003;46(8):1071-81.

32. Eriksen L, Dahl-Petersen I, Haugaard SB, Dela F. Comparison of the effect of multiple short-duration with single long-duration exercise sessions on glucose homeostasis in type 2 diabetes mellitus. Diabetologia. 2007;50:2245-53.

33. Umpierre D, Ribeiro PA, Kramer CK, et al. Physical activity advice only or structured exercise training and association with HbA1c levels in type 2 diabetes: a systematic review and meta-analysis. JAMA. 2011;305:1790-9.

34. Ross R, Dagnone D, Jones PJ, et al. Reduction in obesity and related comorbid conditions after diet-induced weight loss or exercise-induced weight loss in men. A randomized, controlled trial. Ann Intern Med. 2000;133(2):92-103.

35. Ross R, Janssen I, Dawson J, et al. Exercise-induced reduction in obesity and insulin resistance in women: a randomized controlled trial. Obes Res. 2004;12(5):789-98.

36. Boulé NG, Haddad E, Kenny GP, Wells GA, Sigal RJ. Effects of exercise on glycemic control and body mass in type 2 diabetes mellitus: a meta-analysis of controlled clinical trials. JAMA. 2001;286(10):1218-27.

37. O'Gorman DJ, Karlsson HK, McQuaid S, et al. Exercise training increases insulin-stimulated glucose disposal and GLUT4 (SLC2A4) protein content in patients with type 2 diabetes. Diabetologia. 2006;49(12):2983-92.

38. Castaneda C, Layne JE, Munoz-Orians L, et al. A randomized controlled trial of resistance exercise training to improve glycemic control in older adults with type 2 diabetes. Diabetes Care. 2002;25:2335-41.

39. Dunstan DW, Daly RM, Owen N, et al. High-intensity resistance training improves glycemic control in older patients with type 2 diabetes. Diabetes Care. 2002;25(10):1729-36.

40. Snowling NJ, Hopkins WG. Effects of different modes of exercise training on glucose control and risk factors for complications in type 2 diabetic patients: a meta-analysis. Diabetes Care. 2006;29(11):2518-27.

41. Gordon BA, Benson AC, Bird SR, Fraser SF. Resistance training improves metabolic health in type 2 diabetes: a systematic review. Diabetes Res Clin Pract. 2009;83(2):157-75.

42. Dunstan DW, Daly RM, Owen N, et al. Home-based resistance training is not sufficient to maintain improved glycemic control following supervised training in older individuals with type 2 diabetes. Diabetes Care. 2005;28(1):3-9.

43. Willey KA, Singh MA. Battling insulin resistance in elderly obese people with type 2 diabetes: bring on the heavy weights. Diabetes Care. 2003;26(5):1580-8.

44. Smith SC Jr, Allen J, Blair SN, et al. AHA/ACC guidelines for secondary prevention for patients with coronary and other atherosclerotic vascular disease: 2006 update: endorsed by the National Heart, Lung, and Blood Institute. Circulation. 2006;113(19):2363-72.

45. Herriott MT, Colberg SR, Parson HK, Nunnold T, Vinik AI. Effects of 8 weeks of flexibility and resistance training in older adults with type 2 diabetes. Diabetes Care. 2004;27(12):2988-9.

46. Morrison S, Colberg SR, Mariano M, Parson HK, Vinik AI. Balance training reduces falls risk in older individuals with type 2 diabetes. Diabetes Care. 2010;33:748-50.

47. Sigal RJ, Kenny GP, Boulé NG, et al. Effects of aerobic training, resistance training, or both on glycemic control in type 2 diabetes: a randomized trial. Ann Intern Med. 2007;147(6):357-69.

48. Marcus RL, Smith S, Morrell G, et al. Comparison of combined aerobic and high-force eccentric resistance exercise with aerobic exercise only for people with type 2 diabetes mellitus. Phys Ther. 2008;88(11):1345-54.

49. Church TS, Blair SN, Cocreham S, et al. Effects of aerobic and resistance training on hemoglobin A1c levels in patients with type 2 diabetes: a randomized controlled trial. JAMA. 2010;304:2253-62.

50. Yardley JE, Kenny GP, Perkins BA, et al. Effects of performing resistance exercise before versus after aerobic exercise on glycemia in type 1 diabetes. Diabetes Care. 2012;35:669-75.

51. Yardley JE, Kenny GP, Perkins BA, et al. Resistance versus aerobic exercise: acute effects on glycemia in type 1 diabetes. Diabetes Care. 2013;36:537-42.

52. Wang JH. Effects of Tai Chi exercise on patients with type 2 diabetes. Med Sport Sci. 2008;52:230-8.

53. Lee MS, Choi TY, Lim HJ, Ernst E. Tai chi for management of type 2 diabetes mellitus: a systematic review. Chin J Integr Med. 2011;17:789-93.

54. Tseng CL, Brimacombe M, Xie M, et al. Seasonal patterns in monthly hemoglobin A1c values. Am J Epidemiol. 2005;161(6):565-74.

55. Pena KE, Stopka CB, Barak S, et al. Effects of low-intensity exercise on patients with peripheral artery disease. Phys Sportsmed. 2009;37(1):106-10.

56. Zwierska I, Walker RD, Choksy SA, et al. Upper- vs lower-limb aerobic exercise rehabilitation in patients with symptomatic peripheral arterial disease: a randomized controlled trial. J Vasc Surg. 2005;42(6):1122-30.

57. Johansen KL. Exercise and chronic kidney disease: current recommendations. Sports Med. 2005;35(6):485-99.

58. Painter P, Carlson L, Carey S, Paul SM, Myll J. Physical functioning and health-related quality-of-life changes with exercise training in hemodialysis patients. Am J Kidney Dis. 2000;35(3):482-92.

59. Lemaster JW, Reiber GE, Smith DG, Heagerty PJ, Wallace C. Daily weight-bearing activity does not increase the risk of diabetic foot ulcers. Med Sci Sports Exerc. 2003;35(7):1093-9.

60. Lemaster JW, Mueller MJ, Reiber GE, Mehr DR, Madsen RW, Conn VS. Effect of weight-bearing activity on foot ulcer incidence in people with diabetic peripheral neuropathy: feet first randomized controlled trial. Phys Ther. 2008;88(11):1385-98.

61. Balducci S, Iacobellis G, Parisi L, et al. Exercise training can modify the natural history of diabetic peripheral neuropathy. J Diabetes Complications. 2006;20(4):216-23.

62. Vinik AI, Ziegler D. Diabetic cardiovascular autonomic neuropathy. Circulation. 2007;115(3):387-97.

63. Loimaala A, Huikuri HV, Koobi T, Rinne M, Nenonen A, Vuori I. Exercise training improves baroreflex sensitivity in type 2 diabetes. Diabetes. 2003;52(7):1837-42.

64. Chomentowski P, Dubé JJ, Amati F, et al. Moderate exercise attenuates the loss of skeletal muscle mass that occurs with intentional caloric restriction-induced weight loss in older, overweight to obese adults. J Gerontol A Biol Sci Med Sci. 2009;64(5):575-80.

65. Donnelly JE, Blair SN, Jakicic JM, Manore MM, Rankin JW, Smith BK. American College of Sports Medicine position stand. Appropriate physical activity intervention strategies for weight loss and prevention of weight regain for adults. Med Sci Sports Exerc. 2009;41(2):459-71.

66. Jakicic JM, Marcus BH, Gallagher KI, Napolitano M, Lang W. Effect of exercise duration and intensity on weight loss in overweight, sedentary women: a randomized trial. JAMA. 2003;290(10):1323-30.

67. Practice ACO. ACOG Committee opinion. Number 267, January 2002: exercise during pregnancy and the postpartum period. Obstet Gynecol. 2002;99(1):171-3.

68. Zavorsky GS, Longo LD. Exercise guidelines in pregnancy: new perspectives. Sports Med. 2011;41:345-60.

69. Ceysens G, Rouiller D, Boulvain M. Exercise for diabetic pregnant women. Cochrane Database Syst Rev. 2006;3(CD004225).

70. Corsino L, Rocha-Goldberg MP, Batch BC, Ortiz-Melo DI, Bosworth HB, Svetkey LP. The Latino Health Project: pilot testing a culturally adapted behavioral weight loss intervention in obese and overweight Latino adults. Ethn Dis. 2012;22:51-57.

71. Cogbill SA, Thompson VL, Deshpande AD. Selected sociocultural correlates of physical activity among African-American adults. Ethn Health. 2011;16:625-41.

72. Harley AE, Odoms-Young A, Beard B, Katz ML, Heaney CA. African American social and cultural contexts and physical activity: strategies for navigating challenges to participation. Women Health. 2009;49:84-100.

73. Dutton GR, Tan F, Provost BC, Sorenson JL, Allen B, Smith D. Relationship between self-efficacy and physical activity among patients with type 2 diabetes. J Behav Med. 2009;32(3):270-7.

74. Delahanty LM, Conroy MB, Nathan DM. Psychological predictors of physical activity in the diabetes prevention program. J Am Diet Assoc. 2006;106(5):698-705.

75. McAuley E, Blissmer B. Self-efficacy determinants and consequences of physical activity. Exerc Sport Sci Rev. 2000;28(2):85-8.

76. King DK, Glasgow RE, Toobert DJ, et al. Self-efficacy, problem solving, and social-environmental support are associated with diabetes self-management behaviors. Diabetes Care. 2010 Feb 11. [Epub ahead of print]

77. Allen NA. Social cognitive theory in diabetes exercise research: an integrative literature review. Diabetes Educ. 2004;30(5):805-19.

78. Di Loreto C, Fanelli C, Lucidi P, et al. Validation of a counseling strategy to promote the adoption and the maintenance of physical activity by type 2 diabetic subjects. Diabetes Care. 2003;26(2):404-8.

79. Koenigsberg MR, Bartlett D, Cramer JS. Facilitating treatment adherence with lifestyle changes in diabetes. Am Fam Physician. 2004;69(2):309-16.

80. Gleeson-Kreig J. Social support and physical activity in type 2 diabetes: a social-ecologic approach. Diabetes Educ. 2008;34(6):1037-44.

81. Armit CM, Brown WJ, Marshall AL, et al. Randomized trial of three strategies to promote physical activity in general practice. Prev Med. 2009;48(2):156-63.

82. Balducci S, Zanuso S, Fernando F, et al. The Italian diabetes and exercise study. Diabetes. 2008;57 Suppl 1:A306-7.

83. Rhodes RE, Warburton DE, Murray H. Characteristics of physical activity guidelines and their effect on adherence: a review of randomized trials. Sports Med. 2009;39(5):355-75.

84. Williams DM. Exercise, affect, and adherence: an integrated model and a case for self-paced exercise. J Sport Exerc Psychol. 2008;30(5):471-96.

85. Bravata DM, Smith-Spangler C, Sundaram V, et al. Using pedometers to increase physical activity and improve health: a systematic review. JAMA. 2007;298(19):2296-304.

86. Tudor-Locke C, Bell RC, Myers AM, et al. Controlled outcome evaluation of the First Step Program: a daily physical activity intervention for individuals with type II diabetes. Int J Obes Relat Metab Disord. 2004;28(1):113-9.

87. Ainsworth BE, Haskell WL, Herrmann SD, et al. 2011 Compendium of Physical Activities: a second update of codes and MET values. Med Sci Sports Exerc. 2011;43:1575-81.

88. Catenacci VA, Grunwald GK, Ingebrigtsen JP, et al. Physical activity patterns using accelerometry in the National Weight Control Registry. Obesity (Silver Spring). 2011;19:1163-70.

89. Marcus BH, Simkin LR. The transtheoretical model: applications to exercise behavior. Med Sci Sports Exerc. 1994;26:1400-4.

90. Marcus BH, Selby VC, Niaura RS, Rossi JS. Self-efficacy and the stages of exercise behavior change. Res Q Exerc Sport. 1992;63:60-6.

91. Kim CJ, Hwang AR, Yoo JS. The impact of a stage-matched intervention to promote exercise behavior in participants with type 2 diabetes. Int J Nurs Stud. 2004;41(8):833-41.

92. Clark M, Hampson SE, Avery L, Simpson R. Effects of a tailored lifestyle self-management intervention in patients with type 2 diabetes. Br J Health Psychol. 2004;9:365-79.

93. Kirk AF, Higgins LA, Hughes AR, et al. A randomized, controlled trial to study the effect of exercise consultation on the promotion of physical activity in people with type 2 diabetes: a pilot study. Diabet Med. 2001;18(11):877-82.

94. Koch J. The role of exercise in the African-American woman with type 2 diabetes mellitus: application of the health belief model. J Am Acad Nurse Pract. 2002;14(3):126-9.

95. Rollnick S, Mason P, Butler C. Health Behavior Change: A Guide for Practitioners. New York: Churchill Livingstone; 1999.

96. Miller WR, Rollnick S. Motivational Interviewing: Preparing People for Change. 2nd ed. New York: Guilford Press; 2002.

97. Dellasega C, Anel-Tiangco RM, Gabbay RA. How patients with type 2 diabetes mellitus respond to motivational interviewing. Diabetes Res Clin Pract. 2012;95:37-41.

CHAPTER 6

Taking Medication

Devra K. Dang, PharmD, BCPS, CDE, FNAP

Key Concepts

◆ Self-care behaviors related to taking medication are important to develop, evaluate, and enhance adherence. The diabetes educator plays an important role in this.

◆ The diabetes educator must have the ability to recognize potential barriers that could interfere with an individual's adherence to his or her medication regimen. An important part of the educator's job is to assist the person with diabetes in identifying and addressing these barriers.

◆ The diabetes educator must be well versed in medication-taking considerations (eg, administration technique, dosing, frequency, potential adverse reactions, possible drug interactions) for each type of prescription diabetes medication and be able to convey this information clearly to the person living with diabetes.

◆ The diabetes educator should also be familiar with basic concepts for common categories of nonprescription medications and dietary supplements that persons with diabetes may use.

Introduction

Medication taking is a crucial self-care behavior that contributes to optimal diabetes control. In this chapter, considerations related to medication use in persons living with diabetes are discussed. Special focus is on the diabetes educator's role and opportunities to reinforce self-care behaviors related to taking diabetes medications. The chapter begins by examining what enhances the individual's ability to follow the regimen and what enhances the actual administration of the medication. Risk factors and warning signs for the diabetes educator to recognize are summarized. This section describes the following:

◆ Promoting the use of medication administration aids that enhance the individual's ability to follow the medication plan
◆ Choosing medication delivery methods and treatment regimens appropriate to the individual
◆ Addressing cost (affordability)

Strategies to improve individuals' ability to follow their medication regimens and derive the intended benefit of the medications are also discussed.

Next, the chapter describes clinical considerations relevant to specific medications used in diabetes control, with an emphasis on patient education strategies. In regard to this, each of the following is discussed separately:

◆ Sulfonylureas and meglitinides
◆ Biguanides
◆ Thiazolidinediones
◆ Dipeptidyl peptidase-4 inhibitors
◆ Sodium-glucose co-transporter 2 inhibitors
◆ Alpha-glucosidase inhibitors
◆ Dopamine receptor agonists
◆ Bile acid sequestrants
◆ Insulin
◆ Glucagon-like peptide-1 agonists
◆ Amylin analogs

The discussion of insulin includes consideration of delivery method options and regimen choices. An outline of basic and advanced education topics is presented, along with a summary of teaching topics regarding insulin use. Strategies to overcome barriers of injection and fears related to taking insulin are presented to promote better medication-taking behaviors.

Other drugs that the individual with diabetes may be taking are considered next. Drug interactions and use of the following nonprescription medications and products are addressed:

- Alcohol- and sugar-free products
- Cough and cold products
- Pain and fever products
- Products for gastrointestinal ailments
- Dietary supplements
- Topical and dermatologic products
- Products for oral hygiene and dental care
- Ophthalmologic products

The chapter also provides an overview of the unique needs of children, adolescents, and the elderly with regard to medication taking.

Case—Part 1

You are a diabetes educator working at a primary care clinic. AB is a 53-year-old African-American woman diagnosed with type 2 diabetes 15 years ago. She has also been diagnosed with hypertension and hyperlipidemia. She is currently prescribed glyburide twice daily, metformin three times daily with meals, pioglitazone once daily, lisinopril once daily, hydrochlorothiazide once daily, and atorvastatin once daily. AB's A1C readings in the past year have ranged from 8.5% to 9.5%, and AB's primary care provider is interested in initiating her on insulin. However, he is concerned that she may not be adhering to the current medication regimen. You meet AB, and she immediately states that she is very reluctant to start insulin because within 2 years after her father went on insulin, he went blind and was also started on dialysis. AB wants to know if there is another "pill" she can take to control her diabetes instead.

Medication Adherence in Diabetes

Following a prescribed medication program is integral to the success of most medical treatment plans, and in the management of a chronic condition such as diabetes, following the medication regimen is crucial self-care behavior. Following the medication plan includes not only taking prescribed medications but also taking them on time, at the right time to get the best effects, and at the correct frequency and utilizing appropriate medication administration techniques. Although medication nonadherence is typically viewed as not taking medication, or not taking enough doses, it is important to remember that medication nonadherence also encompasses taking too much medication. Long-term adherence to oral glucose-lowering agents has been reported as ranging from 36% to 93%, with insulin adherence in persons with type 2 diabetes ranging from 62% to 80%.[1,2] The Diabetes Attitudes, Wishes, and Needs study found that a third of those with diabetes reported feeling tired of following their medication regimen.[1] Poor medication adherence has been shown to correlate with worse glycemic and lipid control.[2,3]

Risk Factors for, and Warning Signs of, Poor Medication-Taking Behavior

Awareness of the risk factors for, and warning signs of, poor medication adherence is the first step in resolving this problem. Warning signs of an individual's poor adherence with the medication and treatment plans include the following[3]:

- Uncontrolled diabetes
- Erratic fluctuations in blood glucose
- Lack of adherence with office visits and/or recommended clinical testing
- Lack of adherence with self-monitoring of blood glucose or with reporting these results

A review of the prescription refill history from the community pharmacy can provide clues to medication adherence. For example, if an individual is refilling medications too early, he or she may be taking more medication than prescribed due to elevations in blood glucose. Although the medication refill history pattern can be quite helpful in assessing medication adherence, it should be remembered that this record does not always accurately reflect medication-taking behavior. Many community pharmacies offer an automatic refill service whereby prescriptions are automatically refilled on the day they are due based on the day supply of the original prescription, thereby making it appear that the person is perfectly adherent. A multifaceted approach to assessing medication-taking behavior should be utilized. Risk factors for poor medication-taking behavior include the following[2,4-6]:

- Age—the elderly and adolescents are at the highest risk
- Medication dosing frequency and complexity of the regimen
- Number of medications the patient is taking
- Presence of other concurrent medical conditions
- Presence of depression or other psychiatric disorders
- The individual's understanding of the treatment regimen and its potential side effects
- Perception of the severity of the disease
- Socioeconomic status
- Health insurance status
- Cost of medications
- Poor family dynamics or lack of social support
- Poor patient-provider relationship
- Duration of diabetes

There are also medication-related and provider- or system-related barriers to medication adherence. Table 6.1 summarizes the patient-, medication-, and provider- or system-related barriers to medication adherence in the management of diabetes. Health literacy is another significant barrier to medication taking and is discussed in the Focus on Education section at the end of this chapter.

Strategies to Improve Medication-Taking Behavior

An interprofessional approach is crucial in the management of diabetes. The entire team of physicians, nurses, pharmacists, dietitians, physician assistants, social workers, and others can share information to increase the likelihood of positive clinical outcomes. Collaboration with the pharmacist can optimize both identification and resolution of medication-related problems, including but not limited to adherence barriers. Consultation with the pharmacist regarding medication formulations, frequency, pharmacology, pharmacogenomic factors, and cost can optimize efficacy and minimize adverse drug reactions and drug interactions, leading to improved medication adherence and clinical outcomes.

Relationship and Communication

Establishing a trusting, nonjudgmental relationship between the healthcare professional and the person with diabetes is a crucial component in enhancing the individual's adherence with medications and the treatment plan. The person with diabetes should feel that he or she has a level of control over treatment

TABLE 6.1 Adherence Barriers to Diabetes Mellitus Medication Use		
Patient Factor	*Medication Factor*	*Provider or System Factor*
Fears: disease worsening, hypoglycemia, needles, social stigma, weight gain	Complexity of regimen (eg, more than 1 diabetes medication or other drugs, splitting tablets, drawing up insulin)	Fear that patient will not be able to use therapy
Knowledge, understanding, and skill: education	Frequency of dosing (2 or more times daily results in poorer adherence)	Knowledge: medications, use of insulin, monitoring, diabetes treatment
Self-efficacy	Cost	Skill: able to demonstrate proper use of devices
Health beliefs	Adverse effects	Inadequate educational support
Depression		Inadequate follow-up resources
Lack of confidence in immediate or future benefits of the medication		Clinical inertia
Remembering doses and refills		

Source: Adapted from PS Odegard, K Capoccia, "Medication taking and diabetes: a systematic review of the literature," *Diabetes Educ* 33 (2007): 1014-29; discussion 1030-1.

decisions, including medication therapy, and that his or her wishes are viewed as important. He or she should feel comfortable expressing any concerns about medication therapy. It can be easy for healthcare professionals to forget that persons living with diabetes don't always share the same view and understanding of the efficacy and necessity of medications that they do.

The diabetes educator should explain to the person with diabetes the expected benefits and rationale of the medication and treatment plans. The educator should help the person understand the natural course of diabetes, how the prescribed medication(s) works to prevent complications of uncontrolled diabetes, and why frequent monitoring and intensification of therapy are needed to prevent these complications. The diabetes educator should also acknowledge the potential for adverse drug reactions and discuss the expected likelihood that these may occur, ways that the individual can minimize or avoid these reactions, what the healthcare team is doing to monitor for these reactions, and how the individual can actively participate in this via self-monitoring. When applicable, the educator should also explain why more than 1 drug is often needed in order to address the multiple pathophysiologic processes of diabetes and associated complications. Cultural and religious beliefs and socioeconomic factors should also be taken into consideration when communicating about the treatment plan.

Regimen Changes and Adjustments

Some simple strategies specific to medication formulation that can enhance an individual's ability to follow the medication plan include the following:

- ◆ Decreasing the frequency of medication administration—by using once-daily medications whenever possible
- ◆ Decreasing pill burden—by using combination tablets
- ◆ Utilizing diabetes therapies that target multiple pathophysiologic processes and have a synergistic effect
- ◆ Utilizing therapies that have proven micro- and macrovascular benefits

Combination tablets are available for glucose-lowering drugs (see Table 6.2) and many antihy-

TABLE 6.2 Combination Oral Glucose-Lowering Medications	
Generic Name	*Trade Name*
Alogliptin-metformin	Kazano®
Alogliptin-pioglitazone	Oseni®
Glipizide-metformin	Available as generic only
Glyburide-metformin	Glucovance®
Linagliptin-metformin	Jentadueto®
Pioglitazone-metformin	ACTOplus met® and ACTOplus met® XR
Pioglitazone + glimepiride	Duetact®
Repaglinide-metformin	PrandiMet®
Rosiglitazone-glimepiride	Avandaryl®
Rosiglitazone-metformin	Avandamet®
Sitagliptin-metformin	Janumet® and Janumet XR®
Saxagliptin-metformin XR	Kombiglyze™ XR

pertensive drugs, including various combinations of an angiotensin-converting enzyme (ACE) inhibitor or angiotensin II receptor blocker (ARB) plus the diuretic hydrochlorothiazide. Combinations of some calcium channel blockers and ACE inhibitors, such as amlodipine plus benazepril (Lotrel®, Novartis), or a calcium channel blocker and a 3-hydroxy-3-methylglutaryl-coenzyme A reductase inhibitor, such as amlodipine plus atorvastatin (Caduet®, Pfizer), are also available. It is important to recognize that cost may be a barrier, as some of these combination tablets are available as brand only or have a higher co-pay tier on insurance formularies. (Lotrel® and Caduet® are both generically available now.)

Product Aids

A variety of medication administration aids are available from pharmacies, via online Web sites, and directly through manufacturers. Administration aids may help the individual follow the medication plan and include the following:

- ◆ Pill organizers
- ◆ Medication reminders, including alarms and mobile apps
- ◆ Medication calendars
- ◆ Blister packaging
- ◆ Insulin injection aids

One study found that 80% of adults with diabetes use at least 1 form of an adherence aid, including use of a pill organizer in 50% of patients.[7] The diabetes educator should be aware of the different types of administration aids available in order to help persons with diabetes select the most appropriate product.

Addressing Medication Cost

No matter how effective a medication's clinical effects may be, those who cannot afford to have the prescription filled cannot benefit from it. In a study in adults with diabetes, 19% of those surveyed reported decreasing medication use due to cost, and 28% reported going without food or other essentials in order to afford medications.[8]

Strategies to Reduce Cost

Occasionally, the use of more expensive medications is necessary due to factors such as intolerable adverse drug reactions or to obtain clinical benefit, and less expensive medications may be less desirable. However, this rarely occurs today with the choices of medications available and the different strategies available to decrease medication cost. For those who have health insurance, selecting a medication that is not only on the insurance plan's formulary but also at the lowest co-pay tier (eg, generics) is one option. For those without medication insurance, various national and local pharmacy chains run medication discount programs whereby generic medications can be purchased for approximately $4 to $16 for 30 to 100 tablets/capsules. At least one of the national community pharmacy chains also offers selected nonprescription medications through the same discount plan. Some community pharmacy chains also advertise that they provide metformin, second-generation sulfonylureas, lancets, and insulin syringes at no cost. Prescription savings cards that enable the holder to receive a discount at participating pharmacies are also available to those who belong to various organizations (eg, the American Automobile Association's Prescription Savings program). If a person with diabetes chooses to utilize more than one pharmacy to obtain medications due to cost considerations, the diabetes educator should educate the person that the complete list of medications should be provided to both the healthcare team and the community pharmacists to ensure that there are no duplicate or interacting medications.

Individuals who are uninsured and meet income qualifications can overcome the cost barrier by using manufacturer-sponsored medication assistance programs. A listing of such programs is available from the Partnership for Prescription Assistance (http://www.pparx.org), a national program sponsored by pharmaceutical research companies, and the nonprofit NeedyMeds (http://www.needymeds.com). Other resources include some local and state health departments, which carry a limited formulary of medications for lower income individuals, and free clinics, where medical care and medications are provided free or at a minimal cost (usually based on a sliding scale based on income). Seniors and others who qualify for Medicare are able to purchase prescription drug coverage insurance through Medicare Part D; these individuals should be encouraged to sign up as soon as they are eligible. They should review their Part D plan once a year to determine whether the particular plan selected the previous year still provides adequate coverage and at an acceptable co-pay level for their current medication regimen, especially if they were initiated on new medications during the year. The Medicare Prescription Drug Plan Web site contains a section where the individual can compare prescription medication plans available in his or her zip code (https://www.medicare.gov/find-a-plan/questions/home.aspx).

Patient Education and Clinical Considerations for Diabetes Medications

The diabetes educator should be well versed in the potential efficacy, adverse drug reactions, and patient education points for all medications prescribed for hyperglycemia management. A review of patient education points specific to optimizing medication-taking behavior is provided below. More detailed information on the pharmacology, adverse reactions, and other factors for each drug and drug class is provided in chapter 18, on pharmacotherapy for glucose management.

Sulfonylureas and Meglitinides

Only second-generation sulfonylureas should be used, due to the lower potency and higher risk for hypoglycemia with first-generation sulfonylureas. The second-generation sulfonylureas are glipizide (Glucotrol® and Glucotrol XL®, Pfizer), glyburide (Diabeta®, Sanofi Aventis; Glynase® PresTab®, Pharmacia and Upjohn), and glimepiride (Amaryl®, Sanofi Aventis). All of the second-generation sulfonylureas are dosed once or twice daily. The XL version of glipizide should not be cut in half, because doing so may cause the medication to be released faster than intended and increase the risk of hypoglycemia. Sulfonylureas achieve their maximum glucose-lowering effect at half the maximum daily dose.[9] Nonsulfonylurea secretagogues—repaglinide (Prandin®, Novo Nordisk) and nateglinide (Starlix®, Novartis)—are given immediately prior to meals to specifically lower postmeal glucose elevations. Unlike sulfonylureas, which can be given once or twice daily, meglitinides must be given up to 3 times a day due to their short half-life, which may adversely affect medication adherence. However, this property is an advantage in persons who have an erratic meal schedule, as they can skip the dose if the meal is not eaten or delay the dose if the meal is delayed. Discussion of the risks of hypoglycemia and weight gain should be provided to persons taking either drug class. See also the more detailed discussions on these medications in chapter 18, on pharmacotherapy for glucose management.

Biguanides

The only medication currently available in this drug class is metformin. Metformin (Glucophage® and Glucophage® XR, Bristol-Myers Squibb; Fortamet®, Sciele Pharma; Glumetza®, Depomed, Inc; Riomet®, Ranbaxy Laboratories) is the first-line agent for the treatment of type 2 diabetes in most patients, and it has several advantages over the other oral medications for hyperglycemia (does not cause weight gain, has no risk of hypoglycemia in most persons when used as monotherapy, allows for lower doses of insulin, etc). Thus, every therapeutically appropriate effort should be made to maintain metformin as a viable treatment option in treating persons with type 2 diabetes.

In clinical practice, an oft-cited reason for discontinuation of metformin is intolerance to the gastrointestinal side effects. In many cases, these side effects are due to titrating the dose too quickly. Metformin should be initiated at the lowest dose (500 mg once or twice daily) and titrated slowly (eg, 500 mg per week) to decrease the risk of gastrointestinal side effects such as diarrhea, nausea, vomiting, and abdominal discomfort. Taking metformin with meals also minimizes the risk of these side effects. In most persons, gastrointestinal side effects, if they occur, are mild and typically abate with time. However, if a person is taking the full daily dose of metformin and stops taking it for more than several days, the medication should be re-titrated when it is restarted. Another reason for "intolerance" and/or nonadherence to metformin therapy is the very large tablet size, especially for the 1000-mg strength. Also, some formulations of metformin tablets emit a very strong odor that has been likened to "old locker-room sweat socks" or "fishy," and that in itself may lead to nausea and self-discontinuation of the drug.[10] Both of these barriers can be overcome by using liquid metformin (Riomet®, Ranbaxy Laboratories), which is available as a 500-mg/5-ml oral solution with a nonoffensive cherry flavor and odor. One drawback to the liquid form is that a person cannot rely on a pill organizer as an adherence aid. Using the film-coated, extended-release formulation can decrease the offensive odor while still allowing the person to place the tablets in a pill organizer, but it does not overcome nonadherence due to tablet size. Some manufacturers of metformin advertise that their formulation of metformin does not have the offensive odor. The diabetes educator can consult a pharmacist for recommendations on the formulation and manufacturer. Persons taking any formulation of metformin should be advised to report the use of this medication to all of their healthcare providers, as its use is contraindicated in most hospitalizations and during surgery, acute illness, administration of intravenous contrast media, and other conditions that predispose the individual to the risk of renal failure or lactic acidosis. See also the more detailed discussion of metformin in chapter 18, on pharmacotherapy for glucose management.

Thiazolidinediones

Persons taking a thiazolidinedione (TZD) should understand that the maximum glucose-lowering effect of this medication may not be apparent until after 8 to 12 weeks of use. Products available are pioglitazone (Actos®, Takeda) and rosiglitazone (Avandia®, GlaxoSmithKline). Those starting one of these medications need to be encouraged to keep taking it until a full effect can be determined. Persons taking TZDs should be educated about the risks of fluid retention and weight gain and how to self-monitor for these adverse events. The diabetes educator should ask about any concerns regarding side effects that persons taking a TZD may be displaying, as the potential adverse events associated with TZDs are receiving ongoing regulatory and media attention. See also the more detailed discussion of TZDs in chapter 18, on pharmacotherapy for glucose management.

Dipeptidyl Peptidase-4 Inhibitors

Medications in the dipeptidyl peptidase-4 (DPP-4) inhibitors class currently available in the United States are alogliptin (Nesina®, Takeda Pharmaceuticals America, Inc), linagliptin (Tradjenta®, Boehringer Ingelheim), saxagliptin (Onglyza™, Bristol-Myers Squibb), and sitagliptin (Januvia®, Merck), with various others currently in development. Persons taking one of these medications should be advised to monitor for symptoms of pancreatitis and seek medical attention immediately should these occur. See also the more detailed discussion of DPP-4 inhibitors in chapter 18, on pharmacotherapy for glucose management.

Alpha-Glucosidase Inhibitors

Alpha-glucosidase inhibitors work by delaying the absorption of carbohydrates from the intestinal tract, which reduces the rise of postprandial blood glucose. Products available are acarbose (Precose®, Bayer) and miglitol (Glyset®, Bayer). Normally, hypoglycemia is not a risk with monotherapy of these medications. However, when hypoglycemia does occur due to concomitant administration with other glucose-lowering drugs, the person needs to understand that only glucose tablets can be used for treatment, due to the mechanism of action of these drugs. See also the more detailed discussion on alpha-glucosidase inhibitors in chapter 18, on pharmacotherapy for glucose management.

Sodium-Glucose Co-transporter 2 Inhibitors

Sodium-glucose co-transporter 2 (SGLT2) inhibitors are the newest class of oral glucose-lowering medications available for the management of type 2 diabetes. Canagliflozin (Invokana™, Janssen Pharmaceuticals, Inc) and dapagliflozin (Farxiga™, AstraZeneca) are available in the United States in this drug class at the time of writing. A number of potential adverse drug reactions have been described with these agents and should be discussed with the person with diabetes. In particular, genital mycotic infections in both sexes, urinary tract infection, increased urination, and hypotension are potential adverse drug reactions that may be quite distressing to the individual prescribed this medication and lead to nonadherence. A potential benefit is weight loss. See also the more detailed discussion of SGLT2 inhibitors in chapter 18, on pharmacotherapy for glucose management.

Dopamine Receptor Agonists

Bromocriptine (Cycloset®, VeroScience) is the only medication in this drug class that has been approved by the US Food and Drug Administration (FDA) at the time of writing. Bromocriptine should be taken with food within 2 hours of waking in the morning. A potential adverse reaction is orthostatic hypotension and syncope and may be especially problematic in those who take concomitant antihypertensives. This medication can also cause somnolence and very rare episodes of sudden sleep onset during daily activities without awareness or warning signs. The medication's labeling advises caution while driving or operating heavy machinery.[11] See also the discussion of bromocriptine in chapter 18, on pharmacotherapy for glucose management.

Bile Acid Sequestrants

The main use of bile acid sequestrants is in the management of hyperlipidemia, but colesevelam (Welchol®, Daiichi Sankyo) has an additional FDA-approved indication for the management of type 2 diabetes as an adjunct to lifestyle changes. Bloating, nausea, and constipation are the main adverse reactions with this class of medication, and they can interfere with absorption of other medications the person with diabetes is taking and the fat-soluble vitamins (A, D, E, and K). Therefore, these affected medications should be taken at least 4 hours prior to colesevelam administration, which can adversely affect adherence in those juggling multiple medications. Another factor that may affect adherence with administration is that colesevelam tablets are large, and a dose is 6 tablets once daily or 3 tablets twice daily. The large tablets may cause dysphagia or esophageal obstruction, and the medication should be taken with food and liquid. An oral powder for suspension formulation (to be mixed with water, juice, or diet beverages) is available.[12] See also the more detailed discussion of colesevelam in chapter 19, Pharmacotherapy: Dyslipidemia and Hypertension.

Insulin

Insulin is essential for treatment of type 1 diabetes and is also used in persons with type 2 diabetes, especially in those with glucose toxicity or ineffective beta cell function. Insulin can be used at any time during the lifespan of type 2 diabetes and is no longer considered a "last resort." Insulin is available in formulations that differ in their onset, peak and length of action, and source. In addition to therapeutic considerations, the choice of which insulin regimen to use should be individualized based on the person's daily schedule, willingness to check blood glucose levels, and the number of daily insulin injections the individual is willing to receive or administer.

The most physiologic insulin regimen is the so-called basal-bolus regimen, which uses a long-acting insulin as the basal dose and a rapid-acting insulin as the bolus dose given at meals. Advantages of this regimen include a lower risk of hypoglycemia and the ability to adjust the dose of the rapid-acting insulin according to meal content and timing.

Premixed insulins may be chosen over a basal-bolus regimen due to the person's preference for no more than twice-daily insulin injections, the individual's inability to calculate mixed doses and/or changing doses of insulin, or financial constraints.

Whether insulin is administered with a syringe, pen device, pump, or needle-free jet injector is determined by the individual's personal choice, physical

limitations, insurance coverage, educational level, and/or financial resources.

Fears of Insulin

Taking insulin can be a particularly challenging self-care behavior for people with diabetes. Resistance to insulin (to initiation of insulin therapy, adherence with current insulin therapy, or both) due to fears and other beliefs has been described extensively in the literature. This "psychological insulin resistance" is a significant barrier to treatment and may be due to many factors—fear of needles and injections, fear of adverse reaction (hypoglycemia, weight gain), concern about alterations in lifestyle/schedule, concerns about ability to self-manage the demands of an insulin regimen, misconceptions about insulin including lack of efficacy, and perceived failure of self-management of diabetes are but a few examples.[1,13] Fear of insulin and misconceptions about insulin are fairly common in clinical practice, but these beliefs are not always shared with the healthcare team. The diabetes educator needs to be able to elicit concerns about insulin from the person with diabetes and assist the healthcare team in addressing these beliefs. One way to do this is through the establishment of a trusting relationship and open communication, as discussed earlier, as well as the use of motivational interviewing techniques. A thorough discussion of motivational interviewing is beyond the scope of this chapter. Welch et al provide a good review of motivational interviewing in diabetes.[14] In brief, motivational interviewing "instructs us to appreciate the limits of a direct-persuasion, advice-giving model of clinician influence, guides toward a strong appreciation of the role of ambivalence in behavior change and the value of eliciting patient change talk, and models the use of effective listening skills to build rapport, engage, understand, and facilitate behavior change" (p. 10).[14]

Explanations of the benefits of insulin and its crucial role for glycemic control, and hence potential prevention of long-term complications of diabetes, need to be carefully communicated. Some prescribers inadvertently communicate the need for insulin therapy to persons with diabetes as a "have to" medication (eg, "If you are not able to get your diabetes under control with diet, exercise, and the oral pills, I will have to put you on insulin"). The diabetes educator should strive to avoid any type of tone and wording that impart a negative connotation to the use of insulin.

Fear of hypoglycemia can be a particularly strong barrier to initiation of, and adherence to, insulin therapy. The fear of hypoglycemia because of past experiences with insulin (by the person or by a close friend or relative) may be ingrained in a person's mind. The educator should make such persons aware of the availability of insulin analogs that, compared with the older insulins, more closely mimic the body's natural release of insulin and have been shown to decrease the incidence and severity of hypoglycemia. Detailed education regarding steps to avoid hypoglycemia, recognition of symptoms of hypoglycemia, and corrective actions to take should it occur should always be provided to those prescribed insulin. Some people also associate insulin initiation with the development of long-term complications of diabetes, such as nephropathy and dialysis. The diabetes educator should explain that the complication was most likely present before the insulin was initiated and may have been avoided if insulin initiation to improve glucose control had not been delayed.

Showing the person the different options for administration (which may, as appropriate, include short needles or an insulin pen device or needle-free jet injector) may help alleviate some of the fears about injections and allow the person to make some choices in how to improve individual outcomes. Some people associate injections, especially with syringes, with drug abuse and do not want to be associated with this. The use of insulin pens may be more acceptable to those with this belief. Again, the diabetes educator should thoroughly discuss insulin administration and its crucial role in diabetes management with the individual.

Education Topics for Persons Taking Insulin

Minimal skills to be taught to those on insulin therapy are the following:

◆ Proper storage of insulin
◆ Preparation of dose
◆ Correct administration, including site selection, injection site rotation, and gently rolling the vials or inverting the pens for suspended insulin formulations prior to administration
◆ Priming insulin pens before each injection

◆ Removing the pen needle from the pen cartridge after each administration
◆ Strategies to avoid inadvertent needlesticks
◆ Safe disposal of syringes or needles
◆ Recognition of hypoglycemia symptoms and corrective actions to take
◆ Hypoglycemia prevention
◆ Timing of prandial insulin in relation to meals

To minimize potential adverse events, the individual's understanding of and ability to perform these skills should be assessed before the medication is prescribed.

The following are more advanced skills that are also important to teach. However, not all persons with diabetes will be able to learn and manage all of these skills:

◆ Mixing 2 insulins in the same syringe
◆ Pattern management
◆ Insulin adjustments for physical activity, sick days, and differing amounts of carbohydrate intake

The diabetes educator must individualize the educational strategies and message to each person's educational and coping levels. A number of chapters in this book address these topics individually (see index). See also the sections on hypoglycemia and insulin in chapter 18, on pharmacotherapy for glucose management.

Overcoming Insulin Administration Problems

As with other aspects of diabetes management, matching the insulin delivery device to the unique needs of the individual with diabetes is important. Any mismatch will increase the likelihood that the device or equipment will not be used as prescribed and the individual may be at increased risk for hypoglycemia or hyperglycemia. Chapter 18 describes insulin delivery devices: syringes, insulin pumps, jet injectors, pen devices, and potential new modalities including inhaled insulin and implantable pumps.

Individuals with dexterity problems or visual impairment may have difficulty drawing up a dose of insulin. The use of different injection aids (eg, syringe magnifying guide) or devices that are easier to use, such as an insulin pen, may be helpful for some. A list of insulin injection aids for those using the syringe and vial is published every January in the American Diabetes Association's *Diabetes Forecast Consumer Guide* magazine.

Persons with diabetes may be pleasantly surprised to learn that needle length and diameter are much smaller than they may have anticipated. The length of needles for insulin injection typically ranges from 4 mm (for pen needles) or 6 mm (for syringes) to 12.7 mm (for both pen needles and syringes). Shorter needles are often more acceptable to most individuals with diabetes, but healthcare providers may not be aware of the existence of these shorter pen and syringe needle lengths. In particular, providers have traditionally prescribed the longer needle lengths (8 mm and 12.7 mm) for obese individuals to ensure that the insulin delivered reaches the subcutaneous fat. However, while the thickness of the subcutaneous tissue varies significantly by body mass index, body site, and sex, it has been demonstrated among adults with diabetes that the average skin thickness at the 4 common insulin injection sites (abdomen, thigh, buttock, and arm) varies by only 0.5 mm between the thinnest (thigh) and the thickest (buttock) site.[15] Furthermore, the difference in skin thickness is not clinically different among those with different body mass index, race, or age.[15] The average thickness of the skin at the thickest site (buttock) in the study was 2.4 mm; therefore, a needle as short as 4 mm is adequate to reach past the epidermis and dermis into the subcutaneous fat layer, while at the same time minimizing risk of intramuscular administration. Recent studies have demonstrated equivalent glycemic control and

less pain with the shorter needles compared with the longer needles.[16–19]

The international Third Injection Technique Workshop in Athens (TITAN)—a conference consisting of 127 physicians, nurses, diabetes educators, and psychologists from 27 countries who provide evidence-based consensus recommendations on injection techniques for insulin and glucagon-like peptide-1 agonists—recommended that children, adolescents, and adults with diabetes use a 4-, 5-, or 6-mm needle and concluded that "there is no medical reason" for recommending needles longer than 8 mm.[20] Table 6.3 provides recommendations for insulin injection with different needle lengths.

The gauge of the needle is also important for comfort. Most insulin syringes are available in the smaller 30 or 31 gauge, which may make the injection less painful. The unit markings on the side of the syringe differ, depending on whether the syringe holds 30 units (3/10 cc), 50 units (1/2 cc), or 100 units (1 cc). Individual markings may be in 1/2-unit, 1-unit, or 2-unit increments. If a person is injecting less than 30 units for a dose, using a syringe that closely matches the dose, in this case a 3/10 cc syringe, will allow the person to see the units easier than using a 1-cc syringe. However, the risk for error in administration may be increased if the insulin dose is increased and the person is prescribed a different syringe size with a different unit increment but not given education regarding this. Insulin pens are typically easier to use and more discreet, and the unit markings may be easier to read than the markings on a vial and syringe; thus, they can provide greater accuracy and are usually preferred by persons on insulin

TABLE 6.3   Tips for Angle of Injection and for Pinching a Skinfold Prior to Injection
1. Most needles should be inserted at a 90° angle; however, a 45° angle is advised for frail elderly or cachexic adults or children.
2. Patients using 6-, 8-, or 12.7-mm needles do need to pinch a skinfold for the medication to reach its intended absorption site.
3. Four- or five-millimeter needles may be used by any patient, including lean or obese children and adults. Patients do not need to pinch a skinfold when using 4- or 5-mm needles. *Exception:* Children and adults with lesser amounts of subcutaneous fat who use their arms or thighs for injection sites are advised to pinch a skinfold when using 4- or 5-mm needles.

Source: Reprinted with permission from R Saltiel-Berzin, M Cypress, M Gibney, "Translating the research in insulin injection technique: implications for practice," *Diabetes Educ* 38 (2012): 635-43.

therapy.[21] The thinnest pen needle currently available is 32 gauge.

Key Points on Insulin Use: What to Review With Patients

- Determine what barriers to, and misconceptions of, insulin therapy exist. These may include fears of injection, complications, and hypoglycemia; fear that insulin initiation signals that the diabetes is end-stage; social concerns; cost; and weight gain.

- Show the person when and how the insulin is working to lower blood glucose levels and discuss with him or her the proven clinical benefits of insulin therapy. Printed educational materials and information from the insulin manufacturer's Web site, the American Diabetes Association, and the AADE may be beneficial.

- Explain how to properly administer the insulin, including proper mixing and resuspension (if appropriate), appropriate injection sites, site rotation, and storage.

- Educate the person about the potential for hypoglycemia, recognition of hypoglycemic symptoms, and specific corrective actions that can be taken if it occurs. Discuss risk factors for hypoglycemia, including missed or irregular meals, and hypoglycemia after exercise or physical activity. Discuss how to minimize or prevent the occurrence of hypoglycemic episodes. Educate the individual and family members and any caregivers about hypoglycemia unawareness and the use of a glucagon emergency kit for treating severe hypoglycemia. Educate family members and caregivers about how to recognize signs and symptoms of hypoglycemia.

- Properly match the amount and timing of food to the type and dose of insulin to minimize hypoglycemic events. If the person is able to perform carbohydrate counting, carbohydrate-to-insulin ratios should be developed with persons using basal-bolus regimens.

- Educate the person about what to do when engaging in exercise or sports.

- Educate the person about what to do when eating out or traveling.

- Discuss the disposal of syringes, pen needles, and testing supplies. This varies by city, county, and state.

- Discuss methods to avoid accidental needlesticks. One practice that is universal is to teach people not to recap syringes and pen needles after use.

- Discuss reusing syringes and pen needles and whether this is recommended. This should normally be avoided in most persons. Discuss that refrigerating the syringes for reuse later and wiping the needle off with alcohol are not recommended. Reusing needles dulls the needle tip and removes the lubricated coating, making the injection more painful. Discuss sick-day management and development of a sick-day plan (see chapter 22).

- Avoid potential medication prescribing and dispensing errors by educating all persons taking insulin products on both the brand and generic names for their insulins; those taking insulin mixes should know the generic names of both insulin components.

Glucagon-Like Peptide-1 Agonists and Amylin Analog

When the glucagon-like peptide-1 (GLP-1) agonists exenatide (Byetta®, Bydureon®, Amylin) and liraglutide (Victoza®, Novo Nordisk), and the amylin analog pramlintide (Symlin®, Amylin) are prescribed, the diabetes educator should explain the difference between these medications and insulin. Persons using these medications should understand that they are not a substitute for insulin in those who require insulin for glycemic control, as they may mistakenly think they are trading one type of injectable medication for another. The fact that exenatide, liraglutide, and pramlintide are associated with weight loss may be especially appealing for those individuals with diabetes who are overweight/obese and insulin resistant.

Those who are prescribed these injectable therapies should be carefully taught how to administer them, including differences in dosing units compared with insulin. Pramlintide is taken before meals and snacks that contain at least 250 calories or at least 30 g of carbohydrates and should be skipped if a meal is skipped or if the person is experiencing hypoglycemia. Persons taking pramlintide should also know that the mealtime insulin doses will need to be decreased by 50% initially. Education about the potential for hypoglycemia, recognition of hypoglycemic symptoms, and specific corrective actions that can be taken if it occurs should be provided. In addition, the potential for drug-induced nausea and vomiting should also be acknowledged. Persons taking exenatide and liraglutide should be advised to monitor for symptoms of pancreatitis and seek medical attention immediately should these occur. Those prescribed the once-weekly formulation of exenatide should clearly understand the very specific instructions for what to do if a dose is missed, as they can be confusing to some. See also the discussions on these medications in chapter 18, on pharmacotherapy for glucose management.

Drug Interactions

Persons living with diabetes often take a number of medications concurrently for comorbid conditions such as hypertension, hyperlipidemia, coronary artery disease, and heart failure. They may also take medications to treat long-term complications of diabetes such as peripheral neuropathy. Thus, the diabetes educator should be aware of the potential for drug interactions and increased adverse drug reactions and help the person with diabetes and the healthcare team monitor for these. A complete discussion of the many potential drug interactions and medication-related problems that may occur is beyond the scope of this chapter. A brief discussion of medications that can adversely affect glycemic control is included in the paragraphs that follow. Chapter 18 also briefly discusses drug-drug, drug-disease, and drug-food interactions of concern when using medications for diabetes control. Consultation with a pharmacist and/or inclusion of a pharmacist into the healthcare team helps reduce the potential for medication misadventures.

Many medications have the potential to induce hyperglycemia and worsen glycemic control. Commonly prescribed medications in this category include glucocorticoids, protease inhibitors, atypical antipsy-chotics, thiazide diuretics, beta-adrenergic blocking agents (beta-blockers), and niacin. Worsening of pre-existing diabetes, new-onset diabetes, impaired fasting glucose, and impaired glucose tolerance have all been reported with these medications. Proposed mechanisms for hyperglycemia vary by drug class but include decreased peripheral insulin sensitivity and insulin secretion and increased gluconeogenesis and insulin resistance. Atypical antipsychotics can also cause weight gain and dyslipidemia. Protease inhibitors can cause dyslipidemia and lipodystrophy. The risk of hyperglycemia may vary among drugs within a class. For example, clozapine (Clozaril®, Novartis) and olanzapine (Zyprexa®, Eli Lilly) appear to have the highest association with hyperglycemia, although any of the atypical antipsychotics may adversely affect blood glucose levels. The risk of hyperglycemia is also dependent on other factors such as the dose administered (as with glucocorticoids and niacin) and the route of administration (eg, lower risk with inhaled and topical formulations of glucocorticoids compared with oral and intravenous formulations).[22]

Use of Nonprescription Medications

In the United States, nonprescription medications, also known as over-the-counter (OTC) drugs, are reviewed by the US Food and Drug Administration (FDA).[23] There are more than 300,000 marketed OTC drug products on the market; the FDA reviews the active ingredients and the labeling of the 80+ therapeutic categories of drugs only, not each individual OTC product.[23] Some of the more frequent ailments that are treated with nonprescription products include cough, cold and flu, pain and fever, allergy and sinus complaints, dermatologic conditions, gastrointestinal distress, and musculoskeletal pain. People with diabetes may want to treat a common ailment but may take something that adversely affects their blood glucose or blood pressure. The labeling of the product should always be checked prior to administration, as nonprescription products are frequently reformulated and ingredients may change. Diabetes educators need to be knowledgeable about the ingredients in these products in order to assist in selecting appropriate self-care therapies. Due to the complexity involved (eg, multitude of drug ingredients and formulations, adverse drug reactions, contraindications to self-care,

You acknowledge AB's fears about insulin initiation and help her realize that it was most likely the delay in controlling her father's blood glucose by insulin initiation that led to the retinopathy and nephropathy he experienced. You also help AB understand the risks of both short-term and long-term hyperglycemia and inform her that insulin is the most effective medication currently available to treat hyperglycemia. You educate AB, in lay language, that insulin is not a strange or foreign substance but a natural hormone made by all living persons to maintain glucose homeostasis, and that the pancreas of persons with diabetes either does not make any insulin or does not make enough to control the hyperglycemia. You also help AB recognize that insulin can resolve the symptoms of hyperglycemia (excessive thirst, polyuria, blurry vision) that she is experiencing. These explanations seem to help AB feel more comfortable with initiating insulin, and she states that she is willing to try it. However, she is concerned about remembering to take "so many" different medications and admits to not remembering to take all of her medications each day. You consult with the pharmacist team member and AB's primary care provider and recommend several ways to decrease pill burden:

1. A combination tablet of pioglitazone and a different sulfonylurea, glimepiride (Duetact®, Takeda Pharmaceuticals), is available.

2. Switching AB to extended-release metformin will allow her to take the full dose just once daily.

3. A combination tablet for lisinopril and hydrochlorothiazide is also available; although if AB is currently taking the usual doses of 40 mg of lisinopril and 25 mg of hydrocholorthiazide, she will still need to take 2 tablets, as the combination only comes as lisinopril-hydrocholorthiazide 20 mg-12.5 mg or 20-25 mg.

4. A combination tablet of amlodipine and atorvastatin is available (Caduet®, Pfizer).

5. Alternatively, a combination tablet of amlodipine and an angiotensin II receptor blocker (ARB) (either valsartan, telmistartan, or olmesartan) is also available.

6. Another alternative is to switch the ACE inhibitor to valsartan and combine it with the amlodipine and hydrochlorothiazide into the triple combination tablet (Exforge HCT®, Novartis).

7. The sulfonylurea can be discontinued once the optimal dose(s) of insulin is reached. You also advise AB to purchase a pill organizer to help her remember which doses have already been taken for the day and to associate the medication taking with a regular daily activity such as eating breakfast.

AB is especially interested in taking "natural herbal products" to control hyperglycemia. What should you tell her?

---

and the potential for drug-drug, drug-disease, and drug-food interactions), consultation with a pharmacist prior to commencing use is especially important.

Alcohol-Free and Sugar-Free Products

Whether a person with diabetes needs to exclusively use alcohol-free and sugar-free products depends on the person's glycemic control, medications, and comorbid medical conditions. Individuals taking insulin or insulin secretagogues should be advised against using products with alcohol. If a product contains carbohydrates, the carbohydrate count needs to be added into the number of grams of carbohydrates the person consumes. The dosage of these products varies by product; therefore, just as with foods, labels have to be read carefully to prevent hyperglycemia or hypoglycemia. The amount of carbohydrate in some products may be so small that the potential increase in blood glucose is minimal. The illness being treated with the OTC product itself may also increase blood glucose levels, so this needs to be considered. Information on the carbohydrate content of products may be found on each product's Web site or by calling the consumer toll-free phone number listed on the package. The alcohol content of many nonprescription products can also be found this way and is also given in the ingredients list on the product's label (listed as an inactive ingredient).

Cough and Cold Products

One common mistake people make when self-treating with OTC products is taking a multi-symptom remedy when only a single symptom needs to be treated. For example, a person attempting to self-treat nasal congestion may purchase a product that has both a decongestant and a cough suppressant. Most OTC products marketed to treat cough and cold symptoms contain more than 1 active ingredient. They also may contain ingredients that adversely affect blood glucose and blood pressure. This effect varies by product and formulation. Selecting a product that treats only the symptom(s) present, and being cognizant of the carbohydrates and alcohol content (especially with liquid formulations), allows individuals with diabetes to better select products for self-care. In most cases, tablet and gelcap formulations to treat cough and cold symptoms do not contain any, or contain only a limited amount of, carbohydrate and alcohol. Nasal sprays used to treat nasal congestion and allergies should have limited systemic effects if used according to the directions on the label and with proper administration techniques. Oral decongestants such as pseudoephedrine or phenylephrine should be used with caution and under medical supervision, mainly due to their effects on increasing blood pressure and heart rate. They may be given to persons with well-controlled hypertension only if directed by a prescriber, and at the lowest dose possible for the shortest duration. Two major contraindications for the use of these medications are in those with coronary artery disease and those with arrhythmia. The labeling for oral and nasal decongestant products includes a warning against use in persons with diabetes, unless with medical supervision, since these sympathomimetic agents may increase blood glucose.

Pain and Fever Products

Pain and fever are commonly treated with nonprescription medications. Examples include acetaminophen and nonsteroidal anti-inflammatory drugs (NSAIDs) such as ibuprofen and naproxen. The person with diabetes should be aware that, unless directed otherwise by a healthcare professional, NSAID use should be avoided in those with renal impairment, hypertension, or heart failure. Some OTC pain reliever products contain large quantities of sodium and should be avoided in persons with hypertension and heart failure. For example, at the time of writing, Alka-Seltzer® Antacid and Pain Relief Effervescent Tablets (Bayer) contain 567 mg of sodium per tablet, along with 325 mg of aspirin, and the directions instruct adults to take 2 tablets per dose.[24] Aspirin may increase the risk of hypoglycemia when taken with sulfonylureas due to displacement of the sulfonylurea from plasma protein-binding sites. Aspirin also appears to possess hypoglycemic actions (proposed mechanisms include increasing pancreatic insulin secretion and insulin sensitivity and decreasing gluconeogenesis). However, these effects are usually only clinically relevant at higher (anti-inflammatory) doses.[22]

Products for Gastrointestinal Ailments

The diabetes educator should inquire about use of nonprescription products for gastrointestinal ailments, as this may be a sign that the person with diabetes is experiencing gastrointestinal autonomic neuropathy. Many nonprescription products for the treatment of gas, heartburn, constipation, and diarrhea do not contain noticeable amounts of carbohydrate or alcohol and do not possess any mechanisms of action that would adversely affect blood glucose levels. Most antacids contain magnesium, aluminum, a combination of the 2, or calcium carbonate.

Products containing aluminum should be avoided in persons with impaired renal function or those at risk for constipation. Calcium antacids (and supplements), as well as products containing iron, may also cause constipation. Nonprescription agents for treating constipation include bulk-forming laxatives (eg, psyllium), osmotic agents (eg, magnesium citrate or hydroxide, glycerin, polyethylene glycol 3350), stimulant laxatives (eg, bisacodyl, senna, aloe), and stool softeners (docusate). Differences in these products include the onset of action and potential adverse drug reactions. These products do not affect blood glucose, but the stimulant laxatives and osmotic agents may lead to electrolyte imbalances, especially with overuse. Senna, aloe, and mineral oil are not recommended due to the potential for many adverse drug reactions.

The nonprescription agents approved by the FDA for the treatment of diarrhea include loperamide (eg, Imodium® A-D, McNeil) and bismuth subsalicylate (eg, Pepto-Bismol®, Procter and Gamble). These do not adversely affect blood glucose levels. Products containing bismuth subsalicylate may interact with other medications that persons with diabetes take, such as aspirin and other antiplatelet drugs, NSAIDs, and anticoagulants, but generally do not adversely affect blood glucose levels in recommended nonprescription doses. As with all nonprescription products, a careful review of the ingredients list should be made each time an OTC product is purchased, even if the person believes he or she is buying the same product because the name of the product is the same. Due to frequent reformulations of OTC products, the risk of adverse events or lack of efficacy is increased if the person takes an OTC product with an ingredient or ingredients that are inappropriate for his or her current medication regimen or medical condition(s). For example, in the first decade of the 21st century, the Kaopectate product that used to contain attapulgite, an ingredient to treat diarrhea, was reformulated so that Kaopectate® Anti-Diarrheal (Pfizer Consumer Healthcare) contained bismuth subsalicylate. However, Kaopectate® Stool Softener (Pfizer Consumer Healthcare) actually contained docusate. Adverse effects are likely to occur if the person buying the product to self-treat an episode of diarrhea inadvertently selects this product (due to paying attention only to the brand name of the product and not reading the actual ingredients list) instead of the Kaopectate® Anti-Diarrheal. At the time of writing, the formulation containing docusate is called Kaopectate® Surfak® Stool Softener, with the wording for Surfak® in larger font than the Kaopectate® to minimize confusion.

In the past decade, 2 prescription proton pump inhibitors (omeprazole [Prilosec® OTC, AstraZeneca] and lansoprazole [Prevacid® 24 Hour, Novartis]), along with all of the prescription histamine-2 receptor blockers, became available as OTC medications. The medications are indicated for the self-treatment of heartburn. The OTC proton pump inhibitors are indicated for self-treatment for no more than a 14-day course, and each course may be repeated no more frequently than every 4 months, unless directed differently by a healthcare provider. There is not a maximum time limit on the labeling for the OTC histamine-2 receptor blockers, although there is a warning to ask a physician before use if heartburn symptoms have been present for over 3 months. The diabetes educator should help the person with diabetes who is using these products understand how to monitor his or her symptoms and when to seek medical attention, as gastrointestinal symptoms may be a sign of underlying gastrointestinal autonomic neuropathy. All of these medications are substrates and/or inhibitors of the cytochrome P450 (CYP450) enzyme system that metabolizes many prescription medications;

consultation with a pharmacist is advised if the person is also taking other medications. Especially problematic among the OTC histamine-2 receptor blockers is cimetidine, which inhibits most of the CYP450 isoenzymes, increasing the risk for drug interactions and adverse drug reactions.

Dietary Supplements

It is important that diabetes educators be aware of alternative remedies people may be using and how those therapies interact with recommended or prescribed treatments.

Dietary supplements may include herbs, vitamins, minerals, and nutritional supplements. Unlike prescription products, dietary supplements are not regulated by the FDA, and product quality may vary among manufacturers or even among lots of the same product. Some product manufacturers have voluntarily submitted to testing and verification by the US Pharmacopeia (USP; http://www.usp.org/USP Verified/dietarySupplements/supplements.html), the organization responsible for setting standards and quality control for all FDA-approved prescription and nonprescription medications. Evidence-based information about dietary supplements can be found via the Natural Medicine Comprehensive Database (http://www.naturaldatabase.com), the Natural Standard database (http://www.naturalstandard.com), and the National Center for Complementary and Alternative Medicine (http://nccam.nih.gov).

Persons with diabetes who wish to use an herbal product to help with glycemic control should be educated that the scientific evidence for effectiveness of these agents is equivocal and that these products cannot substitute for FDA-approved glucose-lowering medications. If a person still wishes to use these products, a careful check for potential drug interactions and adverse drug reactions should be completed. The diabetes educator should advise the person to use only USP-verified products, as noted above. Chapter 20, on biological complementary therapies, provides more information to assist educators and those with diabetes in evaluating complementary products.

Topical and Dermatologic Products

Persons with uncontrolled diabetes are at risk for fungal infections, dry skin, and possible skin ulcerations.

Trauma to the skin from wearing ill-fitting shoes can lead to blisters. Education regarding proper foot care, discussed in chapters 10, 23, and 28 (on reducing risks, chronic complications, and diabetic neuropathies), should be provided.

Tinea pedis, or "athlete's foot," is common in many persons with diabetes. Nonprescription antifungal products may take up to 4 weeks of continuous treatment to resolve the problem. Many people do not use these products long enough, which leads to recurrent or unresolved tinea infections. Therefore, education regarding adherence with the duration of therapy is key. If there is not significant improvement, systemic antifungal prescription medications may be needed. Fungal infections of the nails (onychomycosis), especially toenails, are also a frequent condition in those with diabetes. A number of nonprescription products are advertised for this condition, but persons affected by this condition should be educated that onychomycosis can be effectively treated only with systemic prescription medications.

Yeast infections may occur in the folds of the skin and vaginally. Antifungal products for treating vaginal yeast infections are available as creams, ointments, and suppositories and vary by the number of days (1-7) required for treatment. Self-treatment for vaginal yeast infections can be recommended only if the person has symptoms consistent with those of an episode previously diagnosed by a healthcare professional and if the person has had fewer than 4 infections per year.[25]

Autonomic neuropathy and polyuria caused by hyperglycemia may lead to dry skin. Various moisturizers containing glycerin, mineral oil, and lanolin are available to prevent and treat dry skin. Those containing alcohol should be avoided, as the alcohol promotes drying of the skin.

Nonprescription products marketed for the removal of corns and calluses should not be used, because excessive damage to the skin may occur due to the high salicylic acid content (12%-40%).[26]

Products for Oral Hygiene and Dental Care

Gum disease and dental caries may occur more frequently in people with inadequately controlled blood glucose. Proper brushing, flossing, and regular dental appointments as well as achieving and maintaining good glycemic control will minimize the risk of gum disease and dental caries in most people. Many mouth rinses contain large amounts of alcohol and should be avoided, even if the rinse is not swallowed, since they can lead to dry mouth, which can promote dental caries. Many people have problems with ill-fitting dentures if they have gingivitis. Candidiasis may occur in persons with poorly controlled blood glucose and may be prevented with adequate blood glucose control and removal of dentures at bedtime. Dentures should be cleaned as directed and rinsed thoroughly to prevent contact irritation. See also the discussion on oral care in chapter 23, on chronic complications.

Ophthalmologic Products

The use of nonprescription moisturizing eyedrops containing only lubricants is usually safe. As with all nonprescription medications, labels should be read carefully, as some products may contain more than 1 drug. Ophthalmic decongestants such as phenylephrine, naphazoline, oxymetazoline, or tetrahydrozoline are vasoconstrictors and are contraindicated in persons with angle-closure glaucoma. Medical supervision is advised when using these products, as incorrect administration or overuse may lead to appreciable systemic absorption and subsequent increases in blood pressure, heart rate, or blood glucose. Some ophthalmic decongestants are coformulated with ophthalmic antihistamines (eg, pheniramine) for the treatment of allergic conjunctivitis. Ophthalmic antihistamines are also contraindicated in angle-closure glaucoma.[27] The labeling for ophthalmic products containing an

---

Case—Part 3

Utilizing motivational interviewing techniques, you discuss with AB how she thinks herbal supplements would be helpful to her. You share with AB that the herbal products marketed for diabetes have not been adequately studied for both efficacy and safety. In addition, these products are not regulated by the FDA, and the contents of the products are not guaranteed to be manufactured under the stringent conditions that prescription medications are subject to. You also advise AB that some of these herbal products may interact with the medications she is currently prescribed, which could put her at risk for hypoglycemia. You discuss with AB that if she still feels strongly about taking an herbal product, or any OTC products, she should check with a pharmacist or other healthcare professional before purchasing the product.

antihistamine also recommends consultation with a prescriber before taking if the person has difficulty urinating due to an enlarged prostate.

Considerations in Children, Adolescents, and Older Adults

Children and Adolescents

Medication administration for children can be challenging, with different challenges at different ages—when children are young, when they are of school age, and when they become adolescents. Medication administration away from home can affect young children in day care as well as school-aged children and can sometimes still be a factor in the teen years. Psychosocial challenges related to medication taking must also be considered.

Appropriate Insulin Type

The availability of rapid-acting insulin analogs has allowed parents of young children who are fussy eaters to be able to both give insulin after the child decides to eat and adjust the dose based on the amount of carbohydrates the child actually ate. Prior to the availability of these insulins, a dose of short-acting insulin was prepared based on the child's blood glucose and the amount of carbohydrate for the meal. Since this type of insulin had to be administered 30 minutes before the meal, the risk of hypoglycemia was present if the child decided not to eat or did not consume the entire meal.

Medication Administration by Others

Some medications, including some regimens of insulin, may require administration at school and in care settings away from home. Education of school, day care, and camp staff is key to successful management. Another potential challenge is that different insulin schedules may be used on different days, depending on the level of physical activity typical for that day. Children who usually take a mixed dose of neutral protamine Hagedorn (NPH) and a rapid-acting analog insulin may, on occasion, be advised to use a premixed insulin, such as Humalog® Mix 75/25™ (lispro protamine suspension/lispro, Eli Lilly), to allow for simpler administration (not requiring mixing) away from home. Some children may be prescribed pre-mixed insulin to allow for administration to occur only at home. This may not provide the child with optimal blood glucose control, but it may be a way to ensure that the insulin is given and given correctly. In all children taking glucose-lowering medication(s), both the child and personnel at school, day care, and camps need to be able to recognize the signs and symptoms of hypoglycemia and perform the necessary corrective actions. Parents and personnel at school, day care, and camps also need to be educated on when to use glucagon to treat hypoglycemia. Teachers may try to administer this to conscious children, causing unnecessary fear and anxiety. Chapter 14, on type 1 diabetes, discusses information relevant to challenges that children with diabetes face when they are at school, when they are away from home at other care settings, and when they are physically active, such as when participating in sports.

Adolescent Considerations

The combination of having diabetes and managing it well during adolescence can be challenging for a child with diabetes, the family, and others involved in the individual's care and well-being. This period of growth, with its hormonal changes, poses a challenge to even those teens and parents who are firmly committed to managing diabetes well. Unfortunately, adolescents with chronic medical conditions, including diabetes, have been reported to exhibit poor adherence of treatment plans.[2,28] Teenagers need to be educated about the dangers of omitting their insulin doses. Some teenagers may feel that their parents are too protective and may become rebellious and seek attention through hospitalization. Teenagers trying to lose weight may purposely omit their insulin to improve their self-image. Teenagers also need to be educated on the detrimental effects of alcohol or illicit drug use on their medical condition and medications. Severe hypoglycemia may occur if they binge drink and pass out from intoxication. Referral to a psychologist or family counselor may be necessary for some families. Healthcare providers should be aware that insulin requirements will increase during puberty. See chapters 12 and 14 for more information on topics in adolescence relevant to taking medication. See chapter 9 for psychological and mental health issues, such as eating disorders and depression, which may also have a bearing on medication-taking behavior.

Insulin Administration

Insulin syringes have been improved to provide for "painless injections." The advent of 4-mm and 5-mm needles allows some children to inject their insulin at a 90° angle; these shorter needles are also less intimidating (see Table 6.3). Insulin pens may be a better option for children who have a fear of syringes as well as trouble operating the syringe and vial. Insulin injection aids (a list is published every January in the American Diabetes Association's *Diabetes Forecast Consumer Guide* magazine) can help those who need to inject via a syringe and vial. Various products for hiding the needle of the syringe and decreasing the injection sensation are available. Advances in insulin pens allow for more discreet insulin delivery. For children using an insulin pump, a variety of insertion sets with variable lengths of needles and cannulas are available to match individual preference for comfort and to promote best insulin absorption. The child with diabetes, the parents of the child, caregivers, and school/day care/camp personnel need to be educated on how to address problems that may occur with pump use. No matter which delivery devices and injection aids are used, careful education and monitoring of insulin administration must always be provided.

Type 2 Diabetes

For many years, the assumption was that the only type of diabetes that children could develop was type 1 diabetes, and terminology such as "juvenile-onset diabetes" was used. It is now known that children may develop both type 1 diabetes and type 2 diabetes. At the time of writing, the only oral glucose-lowering agent approved by the FDA is immediate-release metformin (in children 10 years of age and older with type 2 diabetes).[29] These children may not need to have medication administered at school, since this medication can be given twice daily. In teenagers with type 2 diabetes treated with metformin, the risk of lactic acidosis and binge drinking needs to be discussed. Insulin is required for some children with type 2 diabetes, and potential challenges with medication taking and administration discussed earlier should be taken into consideration.

Coping Skills

Social support and education about coping skills should be provided to the child and his or her family members. The diabetes educator should also recognize psychosocial risk factors for poor diabetes control, which include the presence of other medical conditions, poor school attendance, learning disabilities, and emotional and behavioral disorders in the child. Family-related risk factors include a single-parent home, chronic physical or mental health problems in close relatives, a recent major life change for the parent, lack of adequate health insurance, complex child-care arrangements, health/cultural/religious beliefs affecting adherence with treatment plans, and having a parent with diabetes.[30]

Healthcare professionals should understand the effect of these factors on self-management of diabetes and help children with diabetes and their families overcome these barriers. Resources such as support groups and summer camps are available in some communities, but finding one that is age-appropriate, meets the needs of the family, and is within an acceptable geographic location may be a barrier. See chapter 9 for more on healthy coping.

Older Adults

Older individuals with diabetes who are living at home are at increased risk for medication-related adverse events due to multiple factors, including polymedication, multiple comorbidities, cost, and psychosocial barriers. Adherence aids (such as medication planners and schedulers and pill organizers) and administration aids (such as insulin pens and injection guides) can help older people remember to take their medications and to administer them correctly. However, medication administration may still prove to be difficult due to decreased manual dexterity, decreased vision and mobility, or cognitive impairment. In addition, if inadequately or improperly trained, family members and other caregivers may give medication at the wrong time or in the wrong dosage. Involving them in the education session or discussing by phone can be critical in preventing errors from occurring. The use of combination tablets, of both oral glucose-lowering medications and cardiovascular medications, can decrease the pill burden in those taking multiple medications.

The risk of falls should always be assessed in all older persons, and those living with diabetes may be at an even higher risk. Many factors, such as visual impairment, gait instability from arthritis, or peripheral neuropathy, play a role. Another important contributing factor to the risk of falling in older persons with diabetes is medication side effects. Older persons with diabetes may have to contend with hypoglycemic symptoms from glucose-lowering agents, dizziness from antihypertensive medications and medications acting on the central nervous system (CNS), sedation and confusion from CNS-acting agents and psychotropics, and blurred vision from a variety of medications. The diabetes educator can remind the prescriber to assess for fall risk and assist in the discussion for fall prevention with both the person living with diabetes and any family member or caregiver. The diabetes educator should have an open discussion with these same parties about any concerns regarding the risk of falling due to side effects of prescribed medications that may lead to nonadherence.

Community-dwelling older persons with diabetes are more likely to be admitted to a long-term care facility than their counterparts without diabetes. Although this may present a difficult situation for the person with diabetes to accept, it provides an opportunity for members of the healthcare team to collaborate and work closely with the resident, family, and long-term care staff, so problems with medication taking can be avoided.

The elderly and people residing in assisted-living facilities may also have impaired liver and kidney function. They may be taking multiple medications that increase the risk of drug-drug interactions. Defects in the metabolism and excretion of medications can lead to episodes of hypoglycemia and hyperglycemia. Sulfonylureas and meglitinides are metabolized in the liver and excreted in the urine. People with hepatic or renal impairment have an increased risk of hypoglycemia, especially if the individual has irregular eating habits. If a sulfonylurea is chosen, glimepiride or glipizide is the drug of choice due to minimally active or inactive metabolites, respectively. On the other hand, given that the mechanism of action of both sulfonylureas and meglitinides is to stimulate insulin release from functioning pancreatic beta cells, older persons with long-standing diabetes may find that they no longer receive any benefit from these medications. Metformin is excreted by the kidneys, and renal function should be monitored before therapy is started and periodically, especially in the elderly and in those with known mild renal impairment. In persons with renal insufficiency using insulin, the

insulin dose will usually need to be adjusted downward as renal function worsens. The dose of sitagliptin, saxagliptin, and alogliptin should be adjusted based on the degree of renal insufficiency. Caution is advised with the use of exenatide and liraglutide in those with renal impairment. Thiazolidinediones can precipitate new-onset heart failure or worsen existing heart failure and may also precipitate or worsen diabetic macular edema. Sudden weight gain, edema, and difficulty in breathing should be brought to the healthcare provider's attention. Body weight should be closely monitored in those receiving these medications. Use of the TZDs may also lead to increased bone fracture risk. See chapter 18 for more details on renal and hepatic considerations with diabetes medications. Finally, decreased thirst and hunger mechanisms in the elderly increase the risk for dehydration, malnutrition, and swings in blood glucose levels, including the risk for a hyperglycemic hyperosmolar state. (Chapter 22, on hyperglycemia, describes a case study with an elderly adult in a hyperglycemic hyperosmolar state of care and provides more information.) For a detailed review of overall diabetes management considerations in older adults, see the consensus report by the American Diabetes Association and the American Geriatric Society available at http://www.americangeriatrics.org/files/documents/ADA_Consensus_Report.pdf.

Summary

There are many ways to ensure that optimal clinical outcomes are achieved with minimization of significant adverse effects when people who have diabetes and other conditions take prescription and nonprescription products. The person with diabetes, family members, caregivers, and healthcare professionals all need to contribute to the process. The diabetes educator should assess medication-taking and adherence behaviors for each agent, prescribed and OTC, in all persons living with diabetes and assist them in developing strategies to overcome identified barriers in order to take their medications safely. Using an interprofessional approach to identify and correct barriers to therapy can also increase the likelihood of optimal clinical success. Most importantly, persons living with diabetes should be active participants in their own care and be included in all healthcare decisions.

Focus on Education

Teaching Strategies

→ **Show and tell/demonstrate and discuss.** Construct the information/presentation by function/category of drug, relating the information to how the drug affects the body and blood glucose (sensitizers, secretagogues, and so on). Pictures of how the medications are used in the body and what the medicine looks like are useful. A poster board display of actual pills helps identify actual dosing and aids in recognition. Involve family and others to assist with learning drug names (brand and generic), dosing, frequency of administration, potential side effects (including how to monitor for them and what to do if they occur), and other important information.

→ **Assess medicines prescribed and barriers to taking them.** Have the person bring all medications to the appointment to determine the date of each prescription, dose, prescriber, pharmacy used, and other pertinent details. Ask the person to also bring nonprescription medications and alternative medicines. Have the person describe how he or she takes each medication and if there are any concerns and/or adherence challenges with taking prescribed medications. Work with the pharmacist to check for trade and generic duplication, outdated medicines, contraindicated medications, and other medication-related problems. Pharmacists can create a medication care plan to address both medication-related problems (eg, drug interactions or adverse effects) and medication adherence.

Messages for Patients

→ **Safety.** Establish one local pharmacy or mail-order pharmacy for consistency in medication refills. Ask if there is any lab work to be done once you have started taking a medication (to monitor for both therapeutic effects and potential side effects). Keep an up-to-date listing of medications including OTC vitamins, minerals, dietary supplements, and other products, and bring this list to all healthcare appointments, including specialist appointments, hospital visits, or procedures for review by the healthcare provider at each visit. Nonprescription products and dietary supplements may interact with your prescription medications or your conditions. Before taking any of these products, check with the prescriber or pharmacist.

→ **Side effects.** All medications have the potential for a side effect. Follow the prescription. Do not add medications on your own, including taking medications prescribed to others. Remind the prescriber of current medications you are taking, including any OTC medications, vitamins, and herbal supplements. When a new medication is prescribed, ask how the medicine will work with any current medicines you are taking, exactly how the medicine should be taken (such as before or after meals, with milk, at bedtime), and how to monitor for any potential side effects. Ask also what happens if illness occurs or if a procedure is scheduled that requires fasting overnight; if under those circumstances, ask whether you should take the medication or skip the dose and when to restart the drug. When in doubt, contact your healthcare team for instructions.

→ **Family and caregiver involvement and education.** Have a key member of your family, significant other, roommate, or close friend attend healthcare visits or classes with you to learn about the medications you take. Give this person a list of medications, side effects, treatment, and healthcare phone numbers in case of an emergency. Have the person demonstrate use of blood glucose testing equipment, discuss use of glucagon, and describe the number of glucose tablets used in case of low blood glucose.

Health Literacy

→ **Assessment.** Be vigilant for signs that the person may have low literacy and low health literacy. Some signs that the person may not be able to read, and therefore not able to correctly follow the directions on the label of the medication bottle, include the following: If the person does not know the names of the medications and what the directions say when asked but instead opens the bottle and relies on recognizing the shape and color of the medication in order to provide this information, or if the person is not able to read patient education handouts or fill out forms because he or she "forgot to bring my glasses" to healthcare appointments. Inspection of the medication bottles may show that the labels have symbols and other markings that indicate how to take the medications. When the dose is changed but a new prescription does not need to be provided at the appointment (such as when the dose is decreased from 2 tablets to 1 tablet), the person unable to read or write may ask the healthcare professional to make a mark on the medication bottle instead of writing the actual directions on the label. The problem of low literacy also extends to those who are able to read and write but at a level inadequate for optimal adherence to the medication and treatment plan. The diabetes educator should assess how well the person understands the messages being delivered by all members of the diabetes care team, including those delivered by both oral and written communications.

⊙ **Strategies to overcome health literacy problems relevant to medication taking.**   In persons unable to read, use of symbols, colors, and pictures can assist with correct administration of medications. United States Pharmacopeia has a library of pictograms related to medication taking that can be downloaded from http://www.usp.org/usp-healthcare-professionals/related-topics-resources/usp-pictograms. Be certain to explain the meaning of the pictogram to avoid any misinterpretation. In persons with low health literacy, avoiding the use of technical jargon is crucial in effectively conveying the educational message. Using the "teach-back" method is key in the education of all persons living with diabetes and doubly so both in those who are unable to read/write and in those with low health literacy. Involvement of caregivers and family members, including accompanying the person to healthcare appointments, should also be encouraged.

References

1. Skovlund SE, Peyrot M; DAWN International Advisory Panel. The Diabetes Attitudes, Wishes, and Needs (DAWN) program: a new approach to improving outcomes of diabetes care. Diabetes Spectr. 2005;18:136-42.

2. Cramer JA. A systematic review of adherence with medications for diabetes. Diabetes Care. 2004;27:1218-24.

3. Pladevall M, Williams LK, Potts LA, Divine G, Xi H, Lafata JE. Clinical outcomes and adherence to medications measured by claims data in patients with diabetes. Diabetes Care. 2004;27:2800-5.

4. Leichter SB. Making outpatient care of diabetes more efficient: analyzing noncompliance. Clin Diabetes. 2005;23:187-90.

5. Lin EH, Katon W, Von Korff M, et al. Relationship of depression and diabetes self care, medication adherence, and preventive care. Diabetes Care. 2004;27:2154-60.

6. Rubin RR. Adherence to pharmacologic therapy in patients with type 2 diabetes mellitus. Am J Med. 2005;118 Suppl 5A:27S-34S.

7. Littenberg B, MacLean CD, Hurowitz L. The use of adherence aids by adults with diabetes: a cross-sectional survey. BMC Fam Pract. 2006;7:1-5.

8. Piette JD, Heisler M, Wagner TH. Problems paying out-of-pocket medication costs among older adults with diabetes. Diabetes Care. 2004;27:384-91.

9. Inzucchi SE. Oral antihyperglycemic therapy for type 2 diabetes: scientific review. JAMA. 2002;287:360-72.

10. Pelletier AL, Butler AM, Gillies RA, May JR. Metformin stinks, literally. Ann Intern Med. 2010;152:267-8.

11. Cycloset [package insert]. Tiverton, RI: VeroScience; 2010.

12. Welchol [package insert]. Parsippany, NJ: Daiichi Sankyo, Inc; 2013.

13. Polonsky W. Psychological insulin resistance: the patient perspective. Diabetes Educ. 2007;33 Suppl 7:241S-4.

14. Welch G, Rose G, Ernst D. Motivational interviewing and diabetes: what is it, how is it used, and does it work? Diabetes Spectr. 2006;19:5-11.

15. Gibney MA, Arce CH, Byron KJ, Hirsch LJ. Skin and subcutaneous adipose layer thickness in adults with diabetes at sites used for insulin injections: implications for needle length recommendations. Curr Med Res Opin. 2010;26:1519-30.

16. Schwartz S, Hassman D, Shelmet J, et al. A multicenter, open-label, randomized, two-period crossover trial comparing glycemic control, satisfaction, and preference achieved with a 31 gauge × 6 mm needle versus a 29 gauge × 12.7 mm needle in obese patients with diabetes mellitus. Clin Ther. 2004;26:1663-78.

17. Hirsch LJ, Gibney MA, Albanese J, et al. Comparative glycemic control, safety and patient ratings for a new 4 mm × 32G insulin pen needle in adults with diabetes. Curr Med Res Opin. 2010;26(6):1531-41.

18. Kreugel G, Keers JC, Kerstens MN, Wolffenbuttel BHR. Randomized trial on the influence of the length of two insulin pen needles on glycemic control and patient preference in obese patients with diabetes. Diabetes Technol Ther. 2011;13(7):737-41.

19. Hirsch LJ, Gibney MA, Li L, Bérubé J. Glycemic control, reported pain and leakage with a 4 mm 32 G pen needle in obese and non-obese adults with diabetes: a post hoc analysis. Curr Med Res Opin. 2012;28:1305-11.

20. Frid A, Hirsch L, Gaspar R, et al. New injection recommendations for patients with diabetes. Diabetes Metab. 2010; 36:S3-18.

21. Pearson TL. Practical aspects of insulin pen devices. J Diabetes Sci Technol. 2010;4:522-31.

22. Dang DK, Pucino F, Ponte CD, Calis KA. Drug-induced glucose and insulin dysregulation. In: Tisdale JE, Miller DA, eds. Drug-Induced Diseases: Prevention, Detection, and Management. Bethesda, Md: American Society of Health Systems Pharmacists; 2010:365-78.

23. US Food and Drug Administration, US Department of Health and Human Services. Drug applications for over-the-counter (OTC) drugs. Last updated 2012 Oct 18 (cited 2014 Apr 10). On the Internet at: http://www.fda.gov/Drugs/DevelopmentApprovalProcess/HowDrugsareDevelopedandApproved/ApprovalApplications/Over-the-CounterDrugs/default.htm.

24. Bayer HealthCare. Alka-Seltzer® Original. 2012. On the Internet at: http://www.alkaseltzer.com/as/as_original.html.

25. Shimp LA, Lodise NM. Vaginal and vulvovaginal disorders. In: Berardi RR, DeSimone EM, Newton GD, et al, eds. Handbook of Nonprescription Drugs. Washington, DC: American Pharmacists Association; 2009:159-80.

26. Coffey CW, Foster KT. Minor foot disorders. In: Berardi RR, DeSimone EM, Newton GD, et al, eds. Handbook of Nonprescription Drugs. Washington, DC: American Pharmacists Association; 2009:1037-60.

27. Fiscella RG, Jensen MK. Ophthalmic disorders. In: Berardi RR, DeSimone EM, Newton GD, et al, eds. Handbook of Nonprescription Drugs. Washington, DC: American Pharmacists Association; 2009:659-89.

28. Kyngas H. Compliance of adolescents with chronic disease. J Clin Nurs. 2002;9:249-56.

29. George MM, Copeland KC. Current treatment options for type 2 diabetes mellitus in youth: today's realities and lessons from the TODAY study. Curr Diab Rep. 2013;13:72-80.

30. Silverstein J, Klingensmith G, Copeland K, et al. Care of children and adolescents with type 1 diabetes: a statement by the American Diabetes Association. Diabetes Care. 2005;28:186-212.

Monitoring

Mary M. Austin, MA, RD, CDE, FAADE
Nancy D'Hondt, RPh, CDE

Key Concepts

- Identify the role self-monitoring plays in supporting self-care behaviors and decision making.

- Review the important role of routine, accurate testing in achieving target blood glucose levels for prevention of complications.

- Examine testing schedules for glucose monitoring that are necessary to interpret the relationships and effects that food, physical activity, and medication have on glycemic control.

- Review the importance of blood glucose monitoring in providing data for glucose pattern management, with continuous glucose monitoring becoming a useful tool for filling in glucose data gaps.

- Review the benefits of monitoring for the complications and chronic conditions that often accompany diabetes.

- Recognize the value of monitoring as a tool for prevention and early diagnosis and to delay progression of the related complications and comorbidities that result in disabilities that may compromise effective self-management and reduce quality of life.

- Know the key teaching components and skill set requirements of blood glucose and ketone monitoring, blood pressure testing, weight measurement, routine lab visits, and the operational and interpretive aspects of each.

Introduction

Monitoring is one of the AADE7 Self-Care Behaviors™ and thereby is recognized as an important component of the treatment plan for persons with diabetes. Although diabetes is mostly a self-managed disease, the patient still needs to rely on healthcare professionals for assistance as the disease progresses and relates with other chronic and acute conditions. Healthcare professionals need to understand the parameters that require monitoring, as well as recognize those that must be monitored by them and those that are or can be self-monitored by the patient.[1] American Diabetes Association (ADA) clinical practice recommendations and standards of medical care in diabetes are helpful for guidance and direction regarding how to best manage people with diabetes.

When monitoring people with diabetes, it is important to start with a baseline evaluation. This should include a comprehensive medical and medication history, physical exam, and standard lab tests. A comprehensive medical and medication history is needed to make an appropriate assessment and implement a safe and effective care plan.

Key information includes the age of the person and characteristics of the onset of diabetes (eg, diabetic ketoacidosis [DKA], asymptomatic laboratory finding), the type of diabetes the person has (eg, type 1 diabetes, latent autoimmune diabetes of adults, or type 2 diabetes), and the person's understanding of his or her diabetes. Lifestyle habits must also be assessed, including eating patterns, physical activity habits, nutritional status, and weight history (such as weight gain or weight loss). In addition, the growth and development of children and adolescents with diabetes should be reviewed.

A thorough review of the person's diabetes education history should include a review of previous treatment regimens and the person's response to that therapy (A1C records). The healthcare professional needs to obtain the person's current treatment plan, including medications and medication adherence, meal plan, physical activity patterns, and self-monitoring of blood glucose (SMBG) patterns and readings (including how the person uses the data).

Next, a review of the person's history of diabetes-related complications should be obtained. The healthcare professional needs to review the person's history of acute and chronic complications for how often the person experiences DKA (including the severity and cause) and for microvascular complications such as retinopathy, nephropathy, and neuropathy (sensory [including history of foot lesions] and autonomic [including sexual dysfunction and gastroparesis]). The healthcare professional also needs to assess the person's history of macrovascular complications, such as chronic heart disease, cerebrovascular disease, and peripheral artery disease. Finally, any additional chronic complications should be discussed, such as psychosocial problems and dental disease.

A complete lab evaluation should be done to establish baseline of the person's lab parameters. This includes an A1C; fasting lipid profile with LDL, HDL, and triglycerides; liver function tests; serum creatinine and calculated glomerular filtration rate (GFR); and thyroid-stimulating hormone in persons with type 1 diabetes or dyslipidemia, or in women over 50.

Children with type 1 diabetes should be screened for celiac disease, since there is a genetic link between type 1 diabetes and celiac disease. Additional parameters that need to be monitored or assessed periodically are often referred to medical specialists. These include an annual dilated eye exam, family planning for women of reproductive age, medical nutrition therapy (MNT) from a registered dietitian, diabetes self-management education and support (DSMES) from a recognized or accredited education program, a dental examination, and, if needed, referral to a mental health professional.

Monitoring checklists can be helpful to the healthcare professional and the patient. See Tables 7.1 and 7.2.

As previously mentioned, diabetes is largely a self-managed disease, so diabetes self-management education (DSME) is critical for people with diabetes. Diabetes self-management education can educate a patient on how and what to check, as well as how often to check.

TABLE 7.1 Monitoring Checklist for Healthcare Professionals	
Clinical	• A1C
	• Lipids
	• Blood pressure
Microvascular	• Neuropathy
	• Nephropathy
	• Retinopathy
Macrovascular	• Smoking
	• Antiplatelet
DSMES	• Nutrition
	• Activity
	• Support
	• SMBG
	• Medication adherence
Acute complications	• Hypoglycemia
	• DKA
	• Hyperosmolar hyperglycemic state
Psychosocial	• Depression
	• Preconception planning
	• Transitional care

TABLE 7.2 Self-Monitoring Checklist for Patients
• SMBG
• Blood pressure
• Daily foot exam
• Daily dental care
• Acute complications
• Ketones, if appropriate
• Chronic complications

Monitoring of all these parameters is valuable. The first part of this chapter primarily focuses on blood glucose monitoring performed by the person with diabetes. The other aspects of diabetes management that require monitoring are outlined in the latter half of this chapter and are also discussed in appropriate chapters throughout this book. Assisting persons with diabetes in behaviors and issues related to appropriate and useful monitoring is an area of diabetes care that clearly combines the diabetes educator's skills of management and education.

Self-Monitoring of Blood Glucose

Self-monitoring of blood glucose provides people with diabetes the information they need to assess how food, physical activity, and medications affect their blood glucose levels. Persons performing SMBG and utilizing SMBG results need to understand how to properly operate the meter, interpret the results, and take appropriate action. Self-monitoring of blood glucose in itself is not a therapeutic intervention. The action taken as a result of utilizing the SMBG data becomes the therapeutic intervention.

Diabetes educators are pivotal in guiding individuals to select the meter most appropriate for them. The 2006 American Association of Diabetes Educators (AADE) position statement on SMBG states, "Health care professionals providing diabetes care and education should encourage and support the use of SMBG in all individuals with diabetes. Safe and appropriate blood glucose monitoring methods need to be taught, including self-management skills that incorporate and use the data obtained from blood glucose monitoring for an individualized program of self-care" (p. 836).[2]

Additionally, in 2010 the AADE maintained the following positions related to SMBG:

- "The diabetes educator incorporates education in the regular performance of SMBG as a means of facilitating diabetes self-management for optimal results.
- SMBG provides the person with diabetes with immediate feedback on the consequences of recent activity, including medication taking,

meals, and physical activity and should be included in the DSME/T. Diabetes educators help people with diabetes take advantage of this feedback to control their diabetes, and address barriers that may affect their ability and willingness to implement SMBG.
- Accurate SMBG readings are important to clinical decision-making and healthcare outcomes. Diabetes educators help people with diabetes to obtain, report, and use accurate data safely and effectively.
- Diabetes educators understand and address the barriers that may affect ability and willingness to implement SMBG. Community resources can help overcome barriers such as cost and limited access to diabetes education.
- The diabetes educator teaches people with diabetes how to recognize when blood glucose levels are out of range, how to adjust their therapy and behaviors based on the SMBG result, and how to then verify the effects of these adjustments by performing subsequent SMBG tests" (p. 4)[3]

Self-monitoring of blood glucose provides immediate feedback and data. Obtaining and using these data help one with the following[4]:

- Achieving and maintaining target goals for blood glucose
- Preventing and detecting hypoglycemia, including hypoglycemia unawareness
- Preventing and detecting hyperglycemia and avoiding DKA or hyperosmolar hyperglycemic state (HHS)
- Evaluating the glycemic response to types and amounts of food and physical activity
- Determining appropriate insulin-to-carbohydrate ratios, correction factors, and basal insulin rates for intensive management (multiple daily injections and insulin pumps)
- Adjusting treatment in response to changes in lifestyle and the need to add, subtract, increase, or decrease dosages or types of pharmacologic therapies
- Determining the need for adjustment in insulin dosages during illness
- Determining the need for insulin therapy in gestational diabetes

Two skill sets are required in order to successfully perform SMBG with the goal of improving diabetes outcomes. The person performing SMBG must be competent and confident in (1) operating the meter and (2) interpreting the SMBG data to make behavior changes. The latter is considered a "problem-solving" self-care behavior. Depending on how, when, and where the person initially receives a blood glucose meter, the diabetes educator may or may not be directly involved in teaching both of these skill sets. However, it is important for the diabetes educator to assess both of these skill sets at the time of diabetes education and to be aware of potential barriers to implementing SMBG.

Using the Meter—Operational Skills

As with other self-care behaviors, if individuals with diabetes are to integrate and embrace SMBG as part of their diabetes management, they must first learn the operational (technical) skills, understand their value, and be able to replicate the skill sets, as applicable.[5] The checklist for SMBG education outlines the operational skills required for successful SMBG (see Table 7.3).

Select a Meter

Choice of meter will depend on factors such as insurance coverage, an assessment of manual dexterity and visual acuity, and the individual's unique needs or desires. The diabetes educator can assist individuals with meter selection by reviewing the following factors that affect choice:

- *Availability and cost:* specific meter(s) covered by insurance or governmental plans, coverage for cost of strips and meter, and out-of-pocket expense
- *Overall size and shape of the meter and strips*
- *Ease of use:* physical dexterity, number of steps to check blood glucose, size of the readout, and required blood sample size
- *Optional features:* readout size and backlighting, memory capacity, required blood sample size, calibration (no coding), computer download features, average glucose data display, and flagging of events
- *General patient preference*

More often than not, for those who have healthcare insurance, either private or governmental, meter

TABLE 7.3 Checklist for SMBG Education	
Using the Meter— Operational Skills	*Using the Data— Interpretation Skills*
• Select a meter • Ensure meter accuracy • Obtain adequate blood sample • Document the SMBG data • Address individual needs	• Know blood glucose targets or goals • Understand frequency and timing of tests • Use pattern management

selection is limited to certain meters covered by the health insurance plan. Checking which meters are covered prior to the diabetes education visit saves time and prevents frustration. Some insurance plans provide coverage for a variety of meters and supplies. If this is the case, several meters can be demonstrated and the person with diabetes can be given the opportunity to "practice" using them.

It is important for the diabetes educator to evaluate whether the choice of meter itself is potentially a barrier to the patient using the meter. This may be the case when healthcare plans switch persons to different meters and strips. Without additional training and education, the patient might feel less comfortable and confident in using the replacement meter, which may compromise his or her ability to continue performing SMBG.

Medicare Coverage   If individuals have Medicare Part B coverage, the following supplies are covered for all people with diabetes: blood glucose meters, blood glucose strips, lancet devices and lancets, and glucose control solutions for checking the accuracy of testing equipment and test strips. Medicare will cover blood glucose self-testing equipment and supplies only if individuals have a prescription from their doctor that includes the following information: the individual's diagnosis of diabetes, the kind of meter needed and why (eg, a special meter because of vision problems), whether the individual uses insulin, and how often the individual should test his or her blood glucose.

It is important for diabetes educators to be aware of continual changes to Medicare regulations regarding coverage of meters, strips, and supplies. Starting July 1, 2013, the Centers for Medicare and Medicaid

Services (CMS) implemented a national mail order program for diabetes testing supplies. This is part of a larger effort to change the way Medicare pays for items considered as durable medical equipment (DME; ie, wheelchairs, oxygen, hospital beds, etc).[6] The intent of the program is to lower the out-of-pocket expense for the user. Educators should always ask the individual at each visit if there has been a change in the blood glucose meter he or she is using. This is an opportunity for training or retraining on the meter. The practice advisory Mail Order Program for Diabetes Testing Supplies—Information for Diabetes Educators was issued by the AADE on July 1, 2013, and can be found on the AADE Web site, http://www.diabeteseducator.org/export/sites/aade/_resources/pdf/general/PracticeAdvisoryDTS.pdf.

Private Insurance   Most private insurance plans follow Medicare guidelines for diabetic supply coverage. Some insurance plans consider the meter and testing supplies as part of an individual's pharmacy benefit while others consider them a DME benefit. Individuals may be directed by their insurance carrier to obtain their meter and supplies from a local pharmacy or place an order with a DME supplier that will ship the supplies directly to the individual. Refills for subsequent mailed supplies need to be requested by the individual; auto shipment of supplies is not allowed.

Individuals should be encouraged to learn about the specifics of their insurance plan coverage for blood glucose meters and supplies. Obtaining the meter and supplies from the insurance plan's specified supplier will ensure that the testing supplies are covered. This should be a cost savings for the individual, which will help reduce the financial barrier to blood glucose monitoring.

Ensure Meter Accuracy

Meaningful utilization of SMBG is dependent on the accuracy of the measurement, which depends on multiple factors.[7,8] The International Organization for Standardization (ISO) sets minimum accuracy requirements for blood glucose meters. ISO 15197:2003 requires 95% of meter results >75 mg/dL to be within ±20% of the true value, as measured by a standardized laboratory blood glucose test system. Below 75 mg/dL, 95% of meter results must be within ±15 mg/dL of the true value.[9] The

US Food and Drug Administration (FDA) requires that glucose meters meet the performance requirements of the ISO standard. Recently the ISO released ISO/FDIS 15197:2013: In Vitro Diagnostic Test System—Requirements for Blood-Glucose Monitoring Systems for Self-Testing in Managing Diabetes Mellitus. The updated standard requires that 95% of readings be (1) within +15% of reference for glucose levels >100 mg/dL and (2) within +15 mg/dL of the reference for glucose levels <100 mg/dL. Additionally, 99% of readings must be within Zones A and B of the survey-derived consensus grid for type 1 diabetes.[9,10] The ISO has suggested a 36-month transition period be instituted before requiring compliance with the revised 2013 standard. Meter accuracy is an important factor as new blood glucose monitoring technologies are developed. For example, calibration of currently available continuous glucose monitoring (CGM) systems is dependent on SMBG. Currently CGM is viewed as an adjunct to care, but as it evolves to become a standard of care, SMBG accuracy will be even more critical.[11,12]

Human errors can contribute to inaccurate data. To ensure meter accuracy, individuals should be encouraged to do the following:

- Use a properly stored meter and strips (avoid temperature extremes, high humidity, or open vial).
- Use in-date, compatible, and defective-free test strips.
- Code the meter (aligning strip lot and meter), if required.
- Perform control solution checks on a regular basis and when starting a new box of strips.
- Use a clean meter free of dried blood or debris.
- Apply an adequate size blood droplet.
- Use clean, dry fingers.

Other factors that may influence blood glucose results are listed in Table 7.4.

The safety of patients is always foremost when evaluating glucose test results. If physical symptoms are not consistent with blood glucose results (eg, hypoglycemic symptoms with in-target SMBG values), a repeat SMBG check should be performed. However, if hypoglycemic symptoms persist regardless of SMBG values obtained, the individual should treat the hypoglycemia promptly.

TABLE 7.4   Common Factors Affecting Accuracy of Blood Glucose Results

Problem	Result	Recommendation
Sensor strip not fully inserted into meter	False low	Always be sure strip is fully inserted into meter
Sample site (eg, the fingertip) is contaminated with a glucose source (eg, juice)	False high	Always clean test site before sampling
Not enough blood applied to strip	False low	Repeat test with a new sample
Batteries low on power	Error codes	Change batteries and repeat sample collection
Test strips/control solution stored at temperature extremes	False high/low	Store kit according to directions
Person is dehydrated	False high	Stat venous sample on main lab analyzer
Person is in shock	False low	Stat venous sample on main lab analyzer
Squeezing fingertip too hard because blood is not flowing	False low	Repeat test with a new sample from a new stick
Sites other than fingertips	High/low	Results from alternative sites may not match finger-stick results
Test strip/control solution vial cracked	False high/low	Always inspect package for cracks, leaks, etc
Anemia/decreased hematocrit	False high	Venous sample on main lab analyzer
Polycythemia/increased hematocrit	False low	Venous sample on main lab analyzer

Source: US Food and Drug Administration (FDA), "Common problems with the use of glucose meters at the point of care" (updated 2013 Mar 21; cited 2014 Apr 1). On the Internet at: http://www.fda.gov/MedicalDevices/Safety/AlertsandNotices/TipsandArticles onDeviceSafety/ucm109449.htm.

TABLE 7.5   Guidelines for Teaching Individuals How to Operate a Blood Glucose Meter

- Use universal precautions: change lancets, end-caps, and gloves for each person seen. Additionally, follow your institution's policies regarding use of a multiuse/patient device with regard to device quality checks.
- Encourage the individual to lance the finger or alternative site at the beginning of the session to minimize anxiety about the discomfort involved.
- Demonstrate how to check blood glucose using control solution first and then using the individual's blood.
- After demonstrating this technique, ask the individual to provide a return demonstration before you begin teaching about control solution, calibration, cleaning, and using the logbook.
- Explain how to dispose of lancets in an appropriate sharps container.
- Demonstrate how to document blood glucose in a logbook or download software to retrieve blood glucose data.
- Evaluate the individual's technique at every opportunity.
- Consider using a "demo only" meter using control solution only.

Source: American Association of Diabetes Educators, "Position statement: educating providers and persons with diabetes to prevent the transmission of bloodborne infections and avoid injuries from sharps," *Diabetes Educ* 23 (1997): 401-3.

Details on the use of test strips, control solution, and meters as well as the correct technique for obtaining the blood sample are given in the paragraphs that follow.

Guidelines for teaching individuals how to operate their blood glucose meters are summarized in Table 7.5.

Identifying Barriers to SMBG

Potential patient barriers to implementation of SMBG are important to identify up front so discussion of how to resolve these barriers may ensue. Table 7.6 provides examples of potential barriers and possible solutions.

TABLE 7.6 Identifying Barriers to SMBG		
Type of Potential Barrier	*Description*	*Possible Solution (depends on the real cause of the barrier)**
Physical	Lack of manual dexterity or visual deficits	• Select meter and strips that are easy to handle and maneuver • Select meter with large numbers and backlighting or specialty meter for visually impaired
Financial	Inadequate or lack of insurance coverage for testing supplies	• Focus testing times to maximize use of strips • Ensure testing technique does not waste strips • Explore programs offered by meter companies and social service agencies to provide supplies • Find a pharmacy or medical equipment supplier that is enrolled in Medicare (as applicable) and accepts assignment
Cognitive	Cognitive deficits that make it impossible to carry out the testing procedure without assistance	• Engage significant others or assistants in education and provide written directions at the level of the user and assistants • Adjust testing time and frequency to fit schedule of the assistants • Suggest reminder aids
Time constraints	Real or perceived lack of time to perform blood glucose checks	• Review operational skills to increase confidence in technique • Reinforce that the SMBG results are not a "test" but rather feedback to be used along with other information • Engage others to help perform the blood glucose check
Health literacy/ numeracy[1]	Difficulty understanding steps, recording SMBG data, and interpreting results	• Ask patient how to do SMBG and record the description using the patient's own words and/or pictures • Practice completing a logbook that the patient designs with you • Assess patient's numeracy skills[2]
Inconvenience	Choosing not to stop current activity to check blood glucose, limited access to hand-washing facilities, working in climate extremes that make access to blood glucose meter challenging	• Problem-solve what would help the individual to do the blood glucose check • Provide suggestions to keep the meter and strips within recommended temperature guidelines
Emotional	Fear of performing SMBG checks due to anticipated pain, fear of being noticed as being different, denial of diabetes, lack of support from family or caregivers	• Listen to patient fears and concerns and acknowledge that others have felt the same way • Suggest the patient access support by joining a diabetes support group or by receiving counseling to address concerns

*Be sure to determine the root cause of the barrier to ensure the solution addresses the appropriate need. Additionally, ask the individual how he or she feels about doing the blood glucose check and whether he or she is confident in performing the test and using the results. Determine whether the individual has the basic operational and interpretive skills necessary for successful SMBG.

Sources:

1. Osborn CY, Cavanaugh K, Wallston KA, White RO, Rothman RL. Diabetes numeracy: an overlooked factor in understanding racial disparities in glycemic control. Diabetes Care. 2009 Sept;32(9):1614-9. Epub 2009 Apr 28.
2. Cavanaugh K, Huizinga MM, Wallston KA, et al. Association of numeracy and diabetes control. Ann Intern Med. 2008;148:737-46.

American Association of Diabetes Educators[©]

Use of Strips

To yield accurate results, the strips must be compatible with the meter being used, stored according to the manufacturer's guidelines, and not be out of date.

All meters have companion strips made by the same manufacturer. Generic or "third-party" strips are made by a different manufacturer and are typically less expensive. It is important that the generic strips work with the meter for which they are used. The generic strip may *look* like the meter manufacturer's strip, but that does not mean it is compatible with the meter. If inconsistent results occur when using generic strips, it may be better to use the manufacturer's strips so it can be determined whether the strips are the problem or whether the inconsistent results are due to some other reason.

The expiration date of the strips should be checked prior to use, as expired strips may be inaccurate and the manufacturer will not guarantee or warrantee the accuracy of the results. Strips should be stored appropriately. Users should be instructed to store the strips in a dry place and to always make sure the strip bottle is properly sealed so strips are not exposed to light, moisture, and temperature variations. Additionally, to avoid introducing moisture into the strip vial, fingers should be completely dry when dispensing strips. Each meter and set of strips has its own storage requirements, and these should be reviewed with the individual.

Code the Meter

Coding is performed to align strip lot and meter. Coding the meter is also necessary to ensure the most accurate results. Some meters do this automatically, whereas other meters require setting a code or inserting a chip or strip. If this is required, coding should be performed with each new box of strips per manufacturer instructions.

Control Solution

Control solution is a product provided by manufacturers to verify the integrity of the test strips. The control solution has a known level of glucose, and a control check should be performed every time a new box of strips is opened. This is an underused method of verifying strip accuracy. A drop of control solution is placed on a test strip, or enters the test strip, in the same manner as when a drop of blood is used. Every manufacturer provides at least 1 control solution vial, and some have low-, normal-, and high-level control solutions to test the meter at extremes.

Follow-up discussions or initial visits with a person newly referred for education may reveal that the person has not been using control solution for a variety of reasons: its use or importance was not explained, the person did not want to "waste" a strip (because strips are costly) that could have been used to test his or her own blood, or the person's insurance plan does not cover the cost of the control solution. It is important that the individual's prescription for monitoring include not only the meter, strips, and lancets but also an order for control solution. An insurance plan that covers control solution will do so only with a prescription for it. The diabetes educator can discuss these needs with the person and problem solve regarding this aspect of ensuring meter accuracy.

Care of Meter

With some meters, the blood sample intended for the strip may come into contact with the meter and obstruct the optic window. This will yield inaccurate results. Manufacturers provide instructions for cleaning the meter.

When traveling, the individual should take extra care to keep the meter and all other monitoring supplies safe. The cargo compartments of buses, airplanes, and trains, as well as automobile trunks, may be too hot or too cold to store a meter and supplies. Extreme temperatures may damage the meter or cause a delay in its readiness to function (requiring several hours for the meter to warm up in very cold weather). Current Transportation Security Administration (TSA) regulations allow meters, test strips, lancets, alcohol swabs, control solution, and sharps disposal containers past the security checkpoint after screening.[13]

Obtain an Adequate Blood Sample

It is important that the individual provide an adequate blood sample. Some meters reject an inadequate sample, whereas other meters have a feature (usually an error message) that signals the user when the blood sample is not large enough to provide an accurate reading. Unfortunately, this feature creates a false sense of security because users assume that if they do not get an error message, they have given an adequate sample. The meter will only signal the user about a blood sample it cannot process; any other sample, even an inadequate one, registers a reading, but the reading can be inaccurate. At every opportunity, the educator should ask the individual to demonstrate his or her meter techniques. This demonstration gives the educator an opportunity to verify technique, provide advice, or clean a soiled unit.

Some individuals have difficulty securing a drop of blood and may require guidance in obtaining an adequate blood droplet, in choosing a lancing device, and/or in selecting a puncture depth. Most lancing devices are spring-loaded and release a lancet at the push of a button. The smaller the lancet needle's gauge and the shallower its penetration, the less pain occurs. Lancets are intended for onetime use and will dull with repeated use, resulting in more pain and possible inadequate blood sample. Careful and safe disposal of used lancets is critical. Used lancets should be disposed of in an appropriate sharps container (regulations vary from state to state). When monitoring blood glucose away from home, people can place their used lancets in an empty pill bottle for appropriate disposal later. Providing individualized guidance for each person's needs minimizes waste of test strips due to inadequate blood sample size and promotes a positive approach to blood glucose monitoring.

Securing an Adequate Blood Sample

Each person should be taught to follow specific directions for securing an adequate blood sample.[14] For example, when using the fingertips as a puncture site, the person should be aware of the following procedures to help increase sample size:

- Vigorously wash hands with warm water to increase circulation to fingertips.
- Hang the hand at your side for 30 seconds so blood pools in that hand.
- Shake the hand to be pricked as though you were shaking down a thermometer.
- Use either a larger gauge lancet or a lancing device or end-cap that will allow a deeper puncture.
- Puncture the sides of the fingertips rather than the pads in the center of the fingers, as this produces less pain.

- After your finger is punctured, gently milk the blood from the bottom to the tip of the finger until the blood sample is the correct size. Milking the finger with a press/release, press/release repetition assists blood flow, whereas just squeezing the fingertip may obstruct blood flow.

Use Alternative Sites Appropriately

Some meters and strips are designed to use alternative sites such as the forearm, palm of the hand, upper arm, or thigh for puncture. However, a few precautions are important for users to understand.

There is wide discordance between fingertip and alternative-site samples when blood glucose levels are changing rapidly due to circulatory physiology. Blood circulation in the skin of the fingers and palm of the hand is distinctly different from that in the arms and legs. The blood flow through the arteriovenous shunts in the fingertips proceeds at a higher velocity than the flow through other capillaries of the skin. Therefore, the transient difference between the alternative site and the fingertip during rapid blood glucose changes is a result of this decreased velocity of blood flow to sites such as the forearm. When blood glucose concentration is falling rapidly, this lag between the alternative site and the fingertip could cause a delay in detection of hypoglycemia if an alternative site is being used for measuring glucose levels. In preprandial monitoring, glucose levels are in a relatively steady state, so the difference between alternative-site and fingertip samples is small and often not clinically significant; but for up to 2 hours postprandial, the blood glucose is in flux.[15] The following are key points about when to use alternative sites:

- Alternative sites should not be used when the person is hypoglycemic, if the person is prone to hypoglycemia (during peak activity of a short- or intermediate-acting injected insulin or up to 2 hours after injecting rapid-acting insulin), after exercise, during illness, during a time when blood glucose levels are rapidly increasing or decreasing (such as any time less than 2 hours after a meal), before driving, or during pregnancy.
- Persons with a history of hypoglycemic unawareness should not use alternative sites.

Because between-site differences of up to 100 mg/dL (5.6 mmol/L) have been reported, the person performing the blood glucose check must document not only the result, time, medication, and relevant comments, but also the sampling site used.[16] Some pediatric endocrinologists prefer that children and adolescents use only the fingertips as puncture sites because of the rapid changes in blood glucose levels often seen in these age groups due to spontaneous activity and glucose uptake into the muscle.

Document Results

Some meter manufacturers provide complimentary logbooks or forms to record blood glucose results. Individuals should be encouraged to use a documenting system they are comfortable with, which enables assessment of relationships of food, activity, and medications, if taken. This will be critical when the individual begins to interpret the blood glucose results, as the results need to be readily available and in a format that is easily reviewed. During meter training, the diabetes educator should observe the individual document blood glucose results to ensure that the data (ie, date, time, and actual result) are correctly entered. Many meters have a memory feature that the educator can use to verify the accuracy of the individual's documentation. The memory feature is not intended to replace the logbook, but rather to provide the option of recording readings at a later date. Some meters have data download and analysis capabilities as well.

Although a written record and graph of blood glucose readings yield important information, recording comments or explanations can be more helpful for teaching the impact of certain decisions related to food, activity, and medication, if taken. Additionally, the individual, healthcare provider, and diabetes educator may find that documenting food intake and physical activity provides greater insight as to how these variables affect blood glucose. This is especially important for people who are new to monitoring. The person who finds value in performing SMBG will be more likely to continue to monitor.

It is important to remind individuals to bring their meter and logbook to every medical visit and present their logbook to their healthcare provider for review. The meter can be cleaned, the strips and control solution can be tested, codes can be verified, and an actual blood glucose measurement can be performed. Ask if more than 1 blood glucose meter is being used. Some individuals prefer the convenience of having an additional meter at their workplace. Results of SMBG will be most consistent if the same meter model is used each time. If an individual chooses to use more than 1 type of meter, the readings obtained from each should be identified as such in their logbook. Correctly and consistently performing SMBG and documenting blood glucose results lay the foundation for pattern management (described later in this chapter).

Meet Individual Needs for Operational or Interpretation Skills

Certain populations of people with diabetes have unique needs relating to meter selection and use. Issues specific to the elderly, children, the visually impaired, and those with special needs are discussed in the paragraphs that follow.

Elderly   Elderly adults with diabetes remain an underserved population despite the prevalence of diabetes in this population. Age should not be the sole criterion for decisions concerning SMBG. Indeed, research has shown that many older individuals perform equally as well as, and in some cases better than, younger individuals in their follow-through with SMBG. The elderly are a heterogeneous population requiring personalized therapy and monitoring schedules. Educators need to consider the unique needs of some of the elderly that may influence the choice of products, such as potential limitations in manual dexterity, slowed reaction time, or fluctuating vision.[17] For example, individually wrapped strips may be more difficult for some people to handle than strips dispensed from a vial. How an elderly person receives meter supplies may also influence adherence to the SMBG regimen. Many elderly individuals find that receiving meter supplies through mail order is both convenient and cost-effective. Reordering of meter supplies must be requested and/or authorized by the individual, as auto shipment of meter supplies no longer complies with current Medicare regulations. A relative or caregiver may need to help obtain the needed supplies.

Children   Children also have unique needs that influence product choice. Children especially benefit from strips that require a small sample of blood and lancing devices that hide the lancet and minimize discomfort. Parents often prefer meters that yield results quickly, have a backlight (for testing in the middle of the night), and store multiple values in memory. At a very young age, many children begin to take responsibility for doing their blood glucose "pokes" or "checks." When speaking with children, these terms are preferred over "tests," which often has a pass/fail or good/bad negative connotation. Emphasize the value of the information the numbers provide, "like clues of a puzzle." It is important that children be verbally praised for participating in this critical part of their diabetes management. However, even after children have mastered the technique, it is important for parents and other caregivers to supervise the testing procedure so that data are recorded for use in treatment and pattern management.

Visually Impaired Persons with diabetes who are visually impaired, including those with fluctuating vision and nonfunctional vision, need products that are fully accessible for them. Beneficial equipment features include tactile markings on the strip; clear speech output on a small, portable meter; and a method of consistent placement of the blood sample.[18] A limited number of products are currently available that meet these recommendations. The National Federation for the Blind continually evaluates and provides updates on products and services for people with diabetes who are blind. For the most current list of available products, contact the National Federation for the Blind.

Special Needs It is also important to recognize that due to age limitations, physical or cognitive disabilities, and other factors, some individuals may need to rely on family members or caregivers to help them with or to perform these tasks. Prior to the initial teaching session, the diabetes educator should ask who may be involved with facilitating diabetes management so that the appropriate individuals may be invited to attend the initial and subsequent sessions. These individuals must be part of the teaching and skills process. Also, as life's circumstances change, so does the level of involvement by others. For example, as the young child with type 1 diabetes grows and matures, the parents and other caregivers release increasingly greater amounts of the diabetes

management skills to the child; conversely, as older adults age, physical limitations such as a decline in visual acuity or manual dexterity may result in the need for more assistance by others.

Using the Blood Glucose Data— Interpretation Skills

Many persons with diabetes are trained in the mechanics of operating a meter and in how to record the blood glucose results, but not on how to use the data or why they are of value. Harris and associates found that the frequency of monitoring was related to having attended a diabetes patient education class.[19] Diabetes patient education was associated with an almost threefold increase in the probability that subjects would monitor their blood glucose at least once per day.

Once individuals are competent and confident in their ability to operate a blood glucose meter, diabetes education on utilizing or interpreting the blood glucose data to improve glycemic control can begin. Performing blood glucose checks without either the individual or the healthcare provider using the data obtained is of no value and a waste of resources.

Diabetes education on SMBG should provide the individual with guidance on blood glucose targets, monitoring frequency, and interpretation of the results in order to see a link between blood glucose values and factors known to contribute to glucose variability (eg, food, physical activity, stress, and medication), as well as reinforce positive outcomes. Criteria for more frequent monitoring are shown in Table 7.7.

Blood Glucose Targets

Individuals need to be clear regarding their blood glucose goal targets. It is not uncommon to find individuals dutifully performing SMBG but not be aware of their target blood glucose goals. Target goals for fasting, premeal, and postmeal times should be determined based on recommended guidelines. Table 7.8 lists 2 organizations' therapeutic goals for glycemia for nonpregnant adults. (See chapter 24 for specifics on blood glucose targets for pregnancy.) However, more or less stringent glycemic goals may be appropriate; goals should be individualized based on multiple factors such as duration of diabetes,

TABLE 7.7	Criteria for More Frequent Monitoring

SMBG may need to be performed more frequently in the following situations:

- Identifying and treating hypoglycemia
- Making decisions concerning food intake or medication adjustment when exercising
- Determining the effect of food choices or portions on blood glucose levels
- Managing intercurrent illness
- Managing hypoglycemia unawareness
- Prior to performing critical tasks, eg, driving
- Monitoring recommended glucose control during preconception and pregnancy

TABLE 7.8 ADA and AACE Target Blood Glucose Goals for Nonpregnant Adults

	American Diabetes Association (ADA)	*American Association of Clinical Endocrinologists (AACE)*
A1C	<7.0%. Individualized based on duration of disease, age/life expectancy, comorbid conditions, known CVD or advanced microvascular complications, hypoglycemia unawareness, individual patient considerations. • More (<6.5%) or less (8.0%) stringent glycemic goals may be appropriate for individual patients.	≤6.5% for most. Individualized based on age, comorbidities, duration of disease. • Closer to normal for healthy • Less stringent for "less healthy"
Fasting and preprandial blood glucose*	70–130 mg/dL (3.9–7.2 mmol/L)	<110 mg/dL (<6.1 mmol/L)
Postprandial blood glucose*	<180 mg/dL (<10.0 mmol/L) at "peak" levels, 1–2 hours after start of meal • Postprandial glucose may be targeted if A1C goal not met despite reaching preprandial glucose goals.	<140 mg/dL (<7.8 mmol/L) 2 hours after start of meal

*Capillary plasma glucose values

Sources: Adapted from American Diabetes Association, "Standards of medical care in diabetes 2013," *Diabetes Care* 36 Suppl. 1 (2013): S19-21; American Association of Clinical Endocrinologists, "AACE diabetes care plan guidelines," *Endocr Pract* 17 Suppl. 1 (2011): S12.

age/life expectancy, comorbid conditions, hypoglycemia unawareness, known cardiovascular disease (CVD) or microvascular complications, and individual patient considerations.

Target blood glucose differs between the ADA and the American Association of Clinical Endocrinologists (AACE). The glycemic guidelines of the ADA can be applied to all persons given that more stringent individualized targets are possible within its recommendations. The ADA postprandial "peak" level can best be explained to individuals as aiming for a blood

glucose value no higher than 180 mg/dL, 1 to 2 hours after the start of a meal. For individuals who find it difficult to check their blood glucose exactly 2 hours after the start of a meal, the "peak" provides a target limit within the 1- to 2-hour postmeal window.

All meters use a drop of whole blood on the test strip, and results are expressed as plasma glucose levels; this allows for easy comparison with a laboratory's plasma results.

Encourage individuals to write their target goals in their logbook or on their form; this helps remind them of their target goals while at the same time reinforcing them. Some glucose meters allow for setting individual target ranges which are then used in personalized graphic printouts.

Frequency of Monitoring The timing (the "when") and frequency (how often) of glucose checks depend on multiple factors. There are no universally accepted standard guidelines; professional organizations such as the ADA and the AACE have made their own recommendations, which are regularly revised and updated.

In general, SMBG is viewed from 2 perspectives: (1) SMBG results utilized by the individual to make behavior and lifestyle changes related to diet and exercise and (2) results utilized by the individual and the healthcare provider to adjust medications, usually insulin. These perspectives affect timing and frequency recommendations. The current consensus is that SMBG should be utilized by persons who use multiple daily insulin injections (MDI) or insulin pump therapy. However, within this therapy group, the frequency recommendation for SMBG differs. The ADA recommends that blood glucose testing be done prior to meals and snacks, occasionally postprandial, at bedtime, prior to exercise, when low blood glucose is suspected, after treating a hypoglycemic event until normalized, and prior to performing critical tasks such as driving. This recommendation may require testing 6 to 8 times per day or more. Additionally, the ADA recommends that persons who are prescribed SMBG receive instruction in and routine follow-up evaluation of SMBG technique and their ability to use the data to adjust therapy. The AACE recommends a minimum of twice-daily testing and ideally at least before any insulin injection. It also recommends more testing if the person has frequent hypoglycemia, is not at A1C target, or has symptoms.

For persons with type 2 diabetes using less intensive insulin regimens such as basal insulin, the ADA does not give a specific frequency regimen but does state that a number of studies have indicated that fasting SMBG provides guidance for the titration of basal insulin. Additionally, the ADA states that when SMBG is prescribed as part of a broader educational context, SMBG results may be helpful to guide treatment decisions and/or patient self-management. The AACE recommendation is less specific to basal insulin but states that all persons using insulin should perform SMBG at least twice per day and ideally before any insulin injection.

For persons with type 2 diabetes who are not on oral medications or non-insulin injections, there is less clarity regarding the timing and frequency of SMBG. Neither the ADA nor the AACE gives any specific SMBG frequency or timing recommendations. The ADA states that SMBG *may be helpful* to guide treatment decisions and/or patient self-management. The AACE states that these persons *may benefit* from SMBG, especially if the results are utilized to provide feedback about the effects of lifestyle and medications.[20,21] Numerous studies on the use of SMBG in persons with non-insulin type 2 diabetes and the positive effect on clinical outcomes, particularly A1C, have been published.[22–26] Recent studies found that SMBG in non-insulin-using individuals correlated positively with weight loss and ultimately better diabetes control (A1C) when SMBG results were utilized to promote adherence to dietary recommendations.[27,28]

Monitoring schedules are based on the person's needs, desires, and use of the data. It is important that the diabetes educator assess how SMBG results are going to be used by the person with diabetes. Is the intent of SMBG to use the results to guide behavior and lifestyle change, to guide medication efficacy, or both?

From a practical point of view, the number of blood glucose checks performed per day is often based on the number of strips covered by health insurance plans. The following factors should be considered when helping individuals determine their testing frequency and time:

- Type of diabetes
- Individual's willingness to perform SMBG
- Level of diabetes control
- Medication regimen
- Lifestyle and daily schedule with regard to activity, food, and work
- Physical ability to check blood glucose
- Ability to problem solve and take action
- Financial limitations
- Comorbid conditions

In type 1 diabetes, or in individuals on an MDI regimen, checking blood glucose levels 3 or more times per day is an accepted standard. Typically, these individuals are encouraged to check their fasting and premeal blood glucoses prior to mealtime insulin dosing. Additionally, postprandial glucose checks may be performed to monitor the glucose-rising effects of meals. Any hypoglycemic symptom also warrants performing a blood glucose check. Some individuals check their glucose level prior to bedtime and before driving to ensure their safety. More frequent monitoring is beneficial during insulin dose adjustment, illness, pregnancy, and heavy periods of exercise or physical activity and when an oral medication and/or injectable medications or insulin is prescribed. There is little doubt of the value of SMBG for individuals who take multiple insulin injections per day, as the SMBG results are used to dose insulin or detect hypoglycemia.

In type 2 diabetes, most diabetes educators find SMBG a valuable tool, even for those not treated with insulin. There is evidence that SMBG data can be used in this population to reinforce therapy decisions and therapeutic lifestyle changes. A study by Schwedes et al showed that meal-related blood glucose monitoring within a structured counseling program significantly improved glycemic control in the majority of non-insulin-using individuals with type 2 diabetes.[26] Utilizing SMBG also resulted in improvement in A1C in persons with type 2 diabetes on oral glucose-lowering medications in a study by Barnett et al.[29]

The 2009 IDF Guideline for Self-Monitoring of Blood Glucose in Non-Insulin Treated Type 2 Diabetes suggests that "SMBG should be used only when individuals with diabetes (and/or their caregivers) have the knowledge, skills, and willingness to incorporate SMBG monitoring and therapy adjustments into their diabetes care plan in order to attain agreed treatment goals."[30] In terms of frequency and timing of SMBG, the IDF guideline suggests numerous "focused" SMBG regimens based on what blood glucose information is desired. For example, a 5- or 7-point blood glucose profile (ie, preprandial and postprandial plus bedtime blood glucose performed in 1 day) repeated for 1 to 3 days can provide insight as to when out-of-target blood glucoses are occurring on a given day. If an individual is not willing to perform 5 to 7 blood glucose checks per day for 1 to 3 days, a "staggered" SMBG regimen where

1 mealtime is selected and premeal and postmeal blood glucose checks are performed can be useful. A different mealtime is selected on subsequent days. Over the course of a week, the individual has 2 premeal and postmeal blood glucose values for each meal to evaluate in light of blood glucose goals. Both the 5- or 7-point regimen and the staggered frequency regimen are considered meal-based regimens. Individuals can use the results from these regimens to gain insight into the effects of their meals on blood glucose excursions. A 3-point SMBG regimen—whereby fasting, pre-largest-meal, and post-largest-meal blood glucoses are taken—can be very helpful to an individual newly diagnosed with type 2 diabetes. This regimen provides information regarding glycemic control at fasting and the glycemic response to the largest meal of the day.[31]

Ideally, individuals who find their postmeal blood glucose values out of target range will have the opportunity to work with a registered dietitian, who can evaluate the meal composition and corresponding blood glucose results to individualize a meal plan. A more detailed discussion on the significance of checking postprandial blood glucose can be found in the glucose pattern management section of this chapter. See the examples in Figure 7.1. This approach is in stark contrast to what is often seen in non-insulin-using individuals with type 2 diabetes who are directed to check their blood glucose once a day, fasting, first thing in the morning. For individuals with type 2 diabetes whose fasting values are typically in target range, checking only fasting blood glucose offers little insight into overall blood glucose control.

A term that is becoming more commonly used when discussing SMBG testing schedules is "structured" testing. This refers to a testing schedule that is specifically prescribed to discover the effects of food, medication, or physical activity. The SMBG profiles provided in Figure 7.1 are examples of structured testing regimens. A number of studies have used structured testing in their research protocol to determine the effects of SMBG on clinical outcomes.[23–25,32,33] In a recent consensus report regarding the use of SMBG in non-insulin-using type 2 diabetes, the panel recommended that SMBG be performed in a structured format and used to guide treatment. Additionally, the panel noted that both patients and healthcare

3-point SMBG profile to check fasting and effect of largest meal

	Pre-breakfast	Post-breakfast	Pre-lunch	Post-lunch	Pre-supper	Post-supper	Bedtim
Monday	X				X	X	
Tuesday	X				X	X	
Wednesday	X				X	X	
Thursday	X				X	X	
Friday	X				X	X	
Saturday	X				X	X	
Sunday	X				X	X	

5-point SMBG profile

	Pre-breakfast	Post-breakfast	Pre-lunch	Post-lunch	Pre-supper	Post-supper	Bedtime
Monday	X	X		X	X	X	
Tuesday	X	X		X	X	X	
Wednesday							
Thursday							
Friday							
Saturday							
Sunday	X	X		X	X	X	

7-point SMBG profile

	Pre-breakfast	Post-breakfast	Pre-lunch	Post-lunch	Pre-supper	Post-supper	Bedtime
Monday							
Tuesday							
Wednesday							
Thursday	X	X	X	X	X	X	X
Friday	X	X	X	X	X	X	X
Saturday	X	X	X	X	X	X	X
Sunday							

"Staggered" SMBG profile

	Pre-breakfast	Post-breakfast	Pre-lunch	Post-lunch	Pre-supper	Post-supper	Bedtime
Monday	X	X					
Tuesday			X	X			
Wednesday					X	X	
Thursday	X	X					
Friday			X	X			
Saturday					X	X	
Sunday	X	X					

FIGURE 7.1   **Examples of SMBG Regimens**   *(continued)*

Meal-based SMBG profile (less intensive)							
	Pre-breakfast	Post-breakfast	Pre-lunch	Post-lunch	Pre-supper	Post-supper	Bedtime
Monday	X	X					
Tuesday							
Wednesday			X	X			
Thursday							
Friday							
Saturday					X	X	
Sunday							

SMBG profile to assess or detect fasting hyperglycemia							
	Pre-breakfast	Post-breakfast	Pre-lunch	Post-lunch	Pre-supper	Post-supper	Bedtime
Monday							X
Tuesday	X						
Wednesday							X
Thursday	X						
Friday							X
Saturday	X						
Sunday							

Note: Ensure that the patient's food and activity tracking are consistent in order to appropriately interpret the glucose data.

FIGURE 7.1   Examples of SMBG Regimens *(continued)*

Source: Type 2 Diabetes BASICS Curriculum Guide, 3rd ed (Minneapolis, Minn: International Diabetes Center, 2009).

providers require education on how to respond to SMBG data in order for SMBG to be an effective tool.[34]

Regardless of the ideal structured testing recommendation, it is key to keep in mind that the person with non-insulin-using type 2 diabetes will most likely have only 100 strips over 3 months available as a covered benefit, unless the physician prescribes and justifies the need for a greater quantity. The diabetes educator should work with the individual to determine how the strips will be used to gain the most actionable information; there will be days where blood glucose testing is not performed.

Interpreting SMBG Results—Utilizing Glucose Pattern Management

Blood glucose monitoring data provide the individual and the healthcare team with information to make lifestyle or therapeutic decisions. While some decisions (eg, treating hypoglycemia or determining the need for a snack) require instant feedback for taking action, most decisions require reviewing 3 to 4 readings to identify a glucose pattern (eg, adjusting medication dosages, changing the meal plan, or recognizing the impact of exercise). Glucose pattern management (GPM) is the process of recognizing, analyzing, and acting on out-of-target readings to move them into target range. This is also referred to as "pattern control" or "glucose pattern control."[35] The process requires the application of a systematic review and analysis of data by both persons with diabetes and their healthcare team in the daily, weekly, and long-term management of blood glucose levels. Integrating SMBG and GPM into a DSME program requires 3 essential components: (1) a guiding belief that SMBG and GPM are necessary for the understanding of the effects of food, physical activity, and medications on daily glucose levels (and ultimately on A1C); (2) a staff with expertise on how to teach patients to interpret and use glucose data to problem solve behaviors related to food, physical activity, and medication taking; and (3) tools that guide data collection and interpretation. A checklist for integrating SMBG and GPM into a DSME program has been developed by Powers et al.[36]

Steps in GPM As one begins to interpret the recorded SMBG data, a series of questions need to be asked: What medications are currently being taken, and what are their intended effects on blood glucose? (see Table 7.9). Have enough blood glucose checks been recorded? Are they accurate? Are contributors to the glucose result consistent (ie, food intake, physical activity, dosing of medication)? Are at least 3 blood glucose checks taken at the same time of day to spot a trend? Are activities, food, feelings, or unusual events recorded?

Table 7.10 provides additional questions to consider when analyzing blood glucose data. The timing of the blood glucose check provides insight as to where to direct efforts or make changes (see Table 7.11).

The process of reviewing the data can be made easier by encouraging persons to record blood glucose data in the logbook, with the testing time and results recorded in linear and vertical fashion, or to download the data utilizing available [...] example is shown in the sample blood glu[...] in Figure 7.2. The 3 fasting blood glucose [...] within target range, but the post-breakfast bl[...] coses are all out of range; no food records wer[...] able. Prior to making medication recommendat[...] the carbohydrate composition of the breakfast m[...] needs to be determined, and additional pre- and post-breakfast blood glucose checks need to be taken. The individual may find that small changes in the breakfast meal will result in in-target post-breakfast blood glucoses. Only 1 pre-dinner blood glucose is taken, and it is out of range; no conclusions can be drawn from 1 blood glucose number. Additional pre-dinner checks should be suggested to see if there is a trend. Also, only 1 in-target pre-lunch blood glucose number is recorded. One cannot assume from just 1 blood glucose number that pre-lunch blood glucoses are within target range, either. Regarding the Friday post-dinner blood glucose of 65, the individual revealed that he felt "shaky." He checked his blood glucose and treated himself for hypoglycemia. Hypoglycemia needs to be treated when it occurs. However, if blood glucose data reveal a trend for hypoglycemia, preventive action needs to be taken to reduce further episodes.

TABLE 7.9 Medication Effects on Blood Glucose		
Medication	*Fasting*	*Postprandial*
Biguanides (metformin)	X	X (mild)
Insulin secretagogues:		
• Sulfonylureas (glyburide, glimepiride, glipizide)	X	X
• Meglitinides (nateglinide, repaglinide)		X
Alpha-glucosidase inhibitors (acarbose, miglitol)		X
Thiazolidinediones (pioglitazone)	X	X
Sodium-glucose co-transporter 2 (SGLT2) inhibitors (canagliflozin, dapaglifozin)	X	X
Incretin mimetics:		
• GLP-1 receptor agonists (exenatide, liraglutide)	X (mild)	X
• Amylin analogs (pramlintide)		X
• DPP-4 inhibitors (sitagliptin, vildagliptin, linagliptin, saxagliptin, alogliptin)		X
Insulin:		
• Premeal insulins (lispro, aspart, glulisine, regular)		X
• Basal insulins (glargine, detemir, NPH, Ultralente)	X	X (mild)
• Premixed insulins (NPH/regular—70/30; NPH/lispro—75/25 or 50/50; NPH/aspart —70/30)	X	X

American Association of Diabetes Educators©

TABLE 7.10	Framework for Interpreting Blood Glucose Records			
	Sample Questions to Consider			
Step	*Food Plan*	*Physical Activity*	*Medications*	*Other*
1. Obtain sufficient data.	• Is a food plan being followed? • Are carbohydrates counted correctly? • If no food data, determine why	• Is a physical activity plan being followed? • If no physical activity data, determine why	• Are medications taken as prescribed? • If medication dose not available, determine why	• Are reasons for out-of-target glucoses noted? • If low glucoses are noted, how are they treated? How often do they occur and when? • Are more blood glucose checks needed? If so, when are they needed? • Can the patient offer insight into schedule or lifestyle variations? Are there trends or fluctuations?
2. Identify all possible interpretations.	• Does the patient understand and follow the food plan? • Could meals be spaced more appropriately? • Are meals consistent in size and composition? • Are regular snacks eaten?	• Has there been a change in physical activity? • Is physical activity irregular?	• If medication is taken, is the person taking the correct dose and at the correct time? • Are the medications expired? • Does the diabetes medication provide adequate or inadequate coverage at meal times?	• Are testing supplies in date? • Has the patient verified accuracy of the meter by using control solution that is not expired? • Has the patient's operation of the meter been observed for any concerns?
3. Collaborate with patient to integrate data and make individualized recommendations.	• Could changes be made to the food plan? Timing of intake to make it easier to follow? • Are carbohydrate amounts noted? • Could changes be made to carbohydrate amounts or timing to make the plan easier to follow?	• Could physical activity be more regular, increased, or decreased?	• Could the medication regimen be adjusted or simplified? • Could a different type or amount be taken at a different time?	• What changes would the patient be willing to make? • Should the target glucose goals be changed?

Source: Adapted from MA Powers, *Handbook of Diabetes Medical Nutrition Therapy* (Rockville, Md: Aspen Publishers, 1996).

TABLE 7.11 Information Provided by Timing of Blood Glucose Check	
Timing of Blood Glucose Checks	*Information Provided*
Fasting	Assesses overnight effect of meds: • If fasting is higher than bedtime—possible nocturnal hypoglycemia or dawn effect
Premeal	Assesses basal insulin therapy needs
Postmeal	Assesses adequacy of premeal medications (rapid- or short-acting insulin, orals) in light of meal eaten • If not taking medications—assesses effect of meal
Bedtime	Assesses the effect of evening meal and basal therapy needs
Random	Can help determine if presenting symptoms are due to blood glucose fluctuations (hypoglycemic event)

Target range 70–130 mg/dL fasting and premeal, <180 at 2 hours postmeal

	Pre-breakfast	Post-breakfast	Pre-lunch	Post-lunch	Pre-dinner	Post-dinner	Bedtime
Monday	128	256			188		
Tuesday	114	248					
Wednesday	118	212	122				
Thursday							
Friday						65	
Saturday							

FIGURE 7.2   **Sample SMBG Record**

Being aware of the factors that raise or lower blood glucose is key when interpreting blood glucose results, taking action, and/or modifying lifestyle behaviors (see Table 7.12).

Postprandial Glucose Postprandial monitoring is an essential part of diabetes self-management and has gained more attention in recent years. In general, a measurement of plasma glucose 2 hours after the start of the meal provides a reasonable assessment of postprandial hyperglycemia. Dietitians implementing MNT find assessing postprandial blood glucose results particularly valuable in assessing food intake and guiding nutrition recommendations. Postprandial monitoring is effective for teaching the impact of food portions and meal composition on blood glucose levels. For example, an individual may choose a meal high in carbohydrate content and have an elevated blood glucose reading 2 hours later, whereas after eating the same foods in smaller portions, the person may find the postprandial reading to be within goal range.

TABLE 7.12 Factors Which May Raise or Lower Blood Glucose	
Factors Which May Raise Blood Glucose	*Factors Which May Lower Blood Glucose*
• Insulin/oral agent—not enough	• Insulin/oral agent—too much
• Other medications	• Other medications
• Physical activity	• Physical activity
• Stress (dehydration, etc)	• Stress
• Carbohydrate—more than usual	• Carbohydrate—less than usual

Postprandial plasma glucose targets have been defined (see Table 7.8). Specific clinical conditions such as gestational diabetes or pregnancy complicated by diabetes may benefit from the measurement of blood glucose 1 hour after a meal.[37]

There has been interest in determining the contribution of fasting and postprandial glucose increments to overall hyperglycemia. Monnier and colleagues tested the effect of postprandial glucose on overall glycemic control itself. They analyzed the diurnal glycemic profiles of persons with type 2 diabetes and investigated different levels of A1C. They concluded that as A1C levels approach 7%, postprandial glucose levels contribute more to the A1C level (~70%), while fasting glucose levels (30%) contribute less. The study showed that in persons with fair control of their diabetes, the relative contribution of postprandial glucose excursions is predominant.[38]

The take-away message for the diabetes educator is that if individuals are aiming for an A1C of less than 7%, blood glucose monitoring efforts should focus on reaching postprandial glucose targets.

One of the most common barriers to postprandial monitoring is not remembering to check after a meal because there is no trigger to remind the person. With so many types of technology available today, the diabetes educator may suggest that people set the alarm feature on their insulin pump or glucose meter to sound or vibrate, program an alert message into their smartphone or tablet, or simply write a reminder in their appointment book and highlight it. Postprandial testing provides the person with diabetes information on the effect of the meal, the efficacy of the medication, and the impact of physical activity.

Diabetes Educators and SMBG

Successful behavior change results from the education interchange between the diabetes educator and the person with diabetes and the self-management efforts he or she implements. Educators and clinicians rely on SMBG to teach problem-solving skills, which are the essence of diabetes self-management, and complex management skills such as blood glucose pattern awareness and insulin dose adjustment. Diabetes educators use SMBG as a tool to link abstract principles of management with daily decision making. Educators can use blood glucose results to teach the concept of post-exercise, late-onset hypoglycemia and the behaviors necessary to prevent this condition. Behavior change concerning food choices or portions is facilitated by relating the food or portion to the postprandial blood glucose result.[39,40]

For persons with type 2 diabetes who may be asymptomatic for hyperglycemia, the need for behavior change becomes personally relevant when they monitor and record blood glucose levels.

Educators use SMBG to identify and influence psychosocial adaptations. Self-monitoring of blood glucose can influence self-efficacy.[41] For example, persons with diabetes report increased confidence in their problem-solving abilities as a result of using SMBG. The act of monitoring can also have emotional consequences when an individual is confronted with an unacceptable number. This phenomenon, called "monitor talk," can help identify psychosocial needs and direct future learning.[42] Educators can discourage value judgment and replace the notion of good and bad readings with the terms "in range" or "out of range." Reference to blood glucose tests can be replaced with the terms "checks" or "measurements."

Self-monitoring of blood glucose can be used to allay anxiety about hypoglycemia, especially parental anxiety, and is a critical tool for treating fear of hypoglycemia.[43] Although the influence of stress and stress management techniques on glycemic control varies among individuals, it may be beneficial for individuals to assess their blood glucose levels during such times to determine how they respond to psychological stress.

Tables 7.13 and 7.14 summarize how blood glucose monitoring can be utilized in problem solving, which can impact all 7 of the AADE7 Self-Care Behaviors™.

Educator's Role in SMBG Adherence

Even when the diabetes educator has presented the case for SMBG to the person with diabetes, this is not sufficient, nor is it any assurance that a person will consistently monitor blood glucose. Indeed, it is the job of the diabetes educator to not only explain "why" and "how" to perform SMBG but also help individuals identify barriers that may prevent them from continuing this activity and making it a habit.[44]

If the person has stopped monitoring, investigate. Common causes are emotional reactions to elevated or fluctuating readings, consistent readings within range, discomfort related to lancing the skin, emotional response to the sight of blood or skin piercing, cost, inconvenience, and the healthcare team not reviewing and using the data. As part of the assessment, simply ask, "Is it helpful?"[45]

A person may understand the value of SMBG but perceive multiple challenges to actually performing

TABLE 7.13 Blood Glucose Monitoring Problem Solving Tool for the Person With Diabetes

Blood Glucose Monitoring Problem Solving Tool—*For the Person with Diabetes . . .*

Why is my blood sugar out of the target range? These things can make your blood sugar go up or down. Do you se anything that might explain your blood sugar? Are blood sugars out of range for several days at the same time?

Eating	Physical Activity	Monitoring Blood Sugar	Taking Medication	Coping Skills	Problem Solving	Complications or Risks
Blood Sugar Too High—Questions to Ask						
Ate more food? Ate out or special occasion? Snacking or nibbling on food? Drank alcohol? Type of food?	Got less exercise? Changed schedule? BG was >300 mg before starting exercise?	Missed checking? Got off schedule? Not enough blood? Hands were not clean?	Took after eating? Missed meds/insulin? Problems drawing up insulin? Took too little? Need more oral medication? Insulin too hot/cold?	Stressed out? Family problems? Financial problems? Depressed? Work problems?	Been sick? Got a sore? Over treated low blood sugar?	Stomach problems? Chest pain? Hard to draw up insulin with poor vision? Pregnant?
Blood Sugar Too Low						
Ate less food? Drank alcohol? Missed snack? Delayed or missed meal?	Changed schedule? Got more exercise? Exercise was more intense? BG low before exercise?	Missed checking? Got off schedule? Not enough blood? Meter/strips too hot or cold?	Problems drawing up insulin? Took too much? Need less medication? Took wrong insulin at wrong time?	Stressed out? Took extra insulin to cover high BG from stress?	Over treated high blood sugar?	Stomach problems? Kidneys are failing? Hard to draw up insulin with poor vision?

Source: Developed by Donna Tomky, MSN, RN, CNP, CDE, FAADE and Sue Perry, PhD, CDE for the New Mexico Department of Health, Diabetes Prevention & Control Program. Version 2006. Reprinted with permission.

the monitoring. Barriers to SMBG were mentioned previously in this chapter. Use of the AADE7 Self-Care Behaviors™ Goal Sheet (part of the AADE7 System™ product) combines data in a format that the person with diabetes and the diabetes educator can use for problem solving and decision making.

There are times when diabetes educators need to acknowledge the challenge and frustrations related to the daily management and care of diabetes. However, these individuals have the ability to influence and address these issues in a positive way without negating the difficulties. A model for doing so comes from the Appreciative Inquiry literature.[46] This model of addressing change focuses on asking positive questions

that elicit a sense of power and empowerment. Many educators will understand the examples provided in Table 7.15, yet it is common to revert to a negative focus when in a counseling session unless a concerted effort is made to focus positively. Practice and observing patient responses will help highlight the advantages of positive questioning.

Data Management Systems

A variety of data management systems are available to help manage data from glucose monitoring meters and CGM devices. Data can be downloaded from monitoring meters/devices via computer connections

TABLE 7.14 Blood Glucose Monitoring Assessment Tool for the Diabetes Educator

Blood Glucose Monitoring Assessment Tool—*For the Diabetes Educator . . .*

More reasons to consider why the patient's blood glucoses are out of target ranges. Review several days of BG levels and look for patterns.

Eating	Physical Activity	Monitoring Blood Sugar	Taking Medication	Coping Skills	Problem Solving	Complications or Risks
Blood Glucose Too High—Questions to Ask						
Gastroparesis? Inaccurate carb counting? Snacking? Large or high-fat meal with slow digestion?	Insufficient insulin with counter-regulatory hormones release? Intense workout with elevated BG?	Integrity of strips? Meter/technique? Data accuracy? Insufficient data? Somogyi or dawn phenomenon?	Lipohypertrophy? Timing of meds/insulin? Absorption of meds or insulin? Insulin/pill integrity?	Stress hormones? Memory loss/forgetfulness? Untreated psych disorder?	Recent infection? Silent infection? Oral or injection of steroids? Pubertal or growth hormones? Hyperthyroidism?	2nd or 3rd trimester of pregnancy? Recent myocardial infarction? Visual acuity? Dexterity problems? Gastroparesis?
Blood Glucose Too Low						
Inconsistent carb intake? Inaccurate carb counting? Alcohol consumption? High-fat meal with rapid insulin absorption, and slow digestion?	Injection site near active extremity? Timing of med or insulin in relationship to activity? Weight loss?	Data accuracy? Integrity of strips? Meter/technique? Insufficient data?	Timing of insulin? Wrong med? Inconsistent taking of meds/insulin? No access to medication?	Depression? Anxious? Memory loss/forgetfulness? Untreated psych disorder?	Hypoglycemia unawareness? Missed other meds, ie steroids? Hypothyroidism?	1st trimester of pregnancy? Gastroparesis? Visual acuity? Dexterity problems? Renal insufficiency?

Source: Developed by Donna Tomky, MSN, RN, CNP, CDE, FAADE and Sue Perry, PhD, CDE for the New Mexico Department of Health, Diabetes Prevention & Control Program. Version 2006. Reprinted with permission.

using cables, or wirelessly using Bluetooth technology or wireless transfer via satellites and mobile phones. Data can be reported in a variety of ways, from lists of numbers similar to a typical written logbook to plotted graphs and pie charts. This visual review and summarization can advance the interpretation of blood glucose data so that therapies can be best matched to each individual. Glucose data may be used to not only provide guidance on medication therapy but also make recommendations regarding food intake and physical activity. Some meter systems have the capability to input information about food and activity. The goal of such systems is to support pattern review and decision making about therapeutic interventions related to food, activity, and medication.

Manufacturers of glucose monitoring devices provide information about compatible computer software on their Web sites. Several data management systems are being developed to accommodate data from a variety of devices. These universal systems aim to increase their usability by eliminating the need for a variety of software and cables, offering the same data reports for all devices, and including more features that promote improved data interpretation. Having one universal glucose data reporting system would be similar to the universal report obtained

TABLE 7.15 **Positive Glucose Questioning**	
Instead of	*Consider*
What is the most difficult part of blood glucose monitoring?	What is the easiest part of blood glucose monitoring for you?
	What would make blood glucose monitoring easier for you?
	How would you know when you were successful with blood glucose monitoring?
Why did you forget to test in the morning?	What helps you remember to test?
Your numbers are running high in the morning; what do you think you are doing wrong?	Look how great your numbers are on these days (or times). Let's talk about what you do then.
Why aren't you checking your blood glucoses?	How important is blood glucose monitoring to you?
Why are your post-dinner blood glucoses always high?	Tell me about your dinner meal.
	Tell me about what happens the hour or two before dinner.
Why are you checking only fasting blood glucose?	Tell me what your fasting blood glucoses are telling you.
Why aren't you checking your blood glucose at least twice per day?	What part of your day would you most like to know something about your blood glucose results?
	How often do you think you would want to look at (check) your blood glucose results in a week?
Do you think checking your blood sugar 3 times a day is realistic?	On a scale of 1–10, how confident are you that you can check your blood glucose 3 times a day every day of the week? (If not confident, ask the patient if she or he would like to change the goal to one in which she or he felt confident.)

from all 12 EKG machines, resulting in increased ease of use and interpretation.

Systems that transfer real-time glucose data to healthcare providers are available, and additional systems are under development. Such systems need to comply with the Health Insurance Portability and Accountability Act (HIPAA) and legal regulations governing patient information. It is expected that the use of technology to improve the care of persons with diabetes will rapidly expand and be more widely available in the upcoming years. That said, it is important to note that patient data should be used by patients; thus, the data need to be easily available for patient use. Educators contribute greatly to a patient's ability to interpret data for his or her own care and can be at the forefront of utilizing new technologies to improve diabetes care and outcomes.

Continuous Glucose Monitoring

Continuous glucose monitoring devices are, for the most part, simple to use and well tolerated by people with diabetes. Data from these devices have proved useful in projecting trends in glucose profiles and guiding therapy adjustments to enable people to better manage their diabetes. The new generation of CGM technology not only offers the data in a variety of formats but also offers alarms for high and low blood glucose levels and has the potential to fulfill the promise of improved glycemic control.

Continuous glucose monitoring systems monitor glucose from interstitial fluid. A short, thin sensor that lasts for 3 to 7 days is inserted into the skin with an insertion device. The sensor measures the glucose levels, which are converted to an electronic signal. These glucose data are then transmitted to a hand-held receiver that continuously acquires the data. Each CGM system has its own methodology and timing for reporting glucose data, resulting in hundreds of glucose data points in a day. Data are viewed on the receiver and can be downloaded for reports that are similar to an SMBG download. Reports that provide data and visuals related to glucose exposure, stability, and variability are valuable in therapy decision making.[47,48]

The continuous data provide a robust description of the glycemic response to food, activity, and medication as well as other diabetes-related situations.

Such a description can include the postprandial area under the curve, time to peak glucose, time to return to preprandial glucose, maximum peak glucose, and maximum peak glucose for a given time period.[49] This postprandial timeframe could be 2 or more hours, as the data are continuously available through these devices and do not rely on individuals to constantly perform capillary blood glucose tests. The postprandial information obtained from a CGM system can assist users and healthcare professionals in making more informed decisions about adjustments to diabetes management.[50]

Data can be viewed retrospectively or in real time for therapy decisions. Trend arrows on the receiver settings tell patients whether their glucose level is rising or falling, slowly or rapidly, which assists in immediate management decisions. Data also can help identify previously unrecognized hypoglycemia and improve insulin-to-carbohydrate ratios, the effects of specific foods or meals, absorption in gastroparesis, and the effects of dialysis on glucose levels. By evaluating glucose patterns, adjustments can be made that will decrease fear of nighttime hypoglycemia and increase comfort with intensive plans.[51]

The FDA has approved a few CGM systems, and more are under development with advancements in smaller size and extended data collection periods. Current devices are only approved for use in persons using insulin and are not to be used for treatment decisions. They need to be periodically calibrated with a conventional blood glucose meter. To date, CGM has been primarily used by people with type 1 diabetes, but some healthcare professionals are starting to explore its value for persons with type 2 diabetes. Although the future appears positive, wider adoption depends on improved reliability, ease of use, comfort, integration with other products, and affordability.[52] Those aspects are being addressed with each new version of the devices.

Other Glucose Monitoring Methods and Measurements

Noninvasive Monitoring
Noninvasive monitoring involves measuring the concentration of glucose in the blood without puncturing the skin to obtain a drop of blood.[53] No noninvasive monitoring devices are commercially available today. The only FDA-approved noninvasive monitoring device, the GlucoWatch G2 Biographer, was available for a short period of time and is no longer manufactured.

1,5-Anhydroglucitrol Blood Test (GlycoMark™)
The 1,5-Anhydroglucitrol (1,5-AG) blood test, more commonly known as the GlycoMark™ test, provides insight about short-term glycemic control and glycemic excursions, particularly for individuals with an A1C below 8%.[54,55] Neither an A1C test nor occasional blood glucose monitoring captures the frequency of blood glucose excursions (ie, glucose variability). Glucose variability has been identified as a determinant of microvascular complications.[56] The test assesses the amount of time over a 2-week period that glucose exceeds the renal threshold (>180 mg/dL), which correlates with the ADA "peak" postprandial blood glucose target. The test measures a glucose-like sugar called 1,5-AG found in most foods. During times when blood glucose is well controlled, most of the 1,5-AG is reabsorbed in the renal proximal tubules and the 1,5-AG levels stay high. In people without diabetes, the median 1,5-AG is above 20 ug/mL. During times of hyperglycemia, the excess glucose blocks the reabsorption of 1,5-AG and is excreted in the urine. Whenever the blood glucose is over 180 mg/dL, the body loses 1,5-AG. The more often the glucose spikes, the lower the 1,5-AG results will be. This test could distinguish whether extreme frequent glucose peaks occur or whether a high baseline glucose overall exists. In the first instance, the 1,5-AG value would be low, and in the latter instance, it would be high. Knowing whether you are trying to address postmeal glucose peaks or an overall elevated glucose would help guide more appropriate therapy. The validity of the test is limited by stage 4 or 5 kidney disease, advanced liver disease, and during pregnancy. Additionally, acarbose and sodium-glucose co-transporter 2 inhibitors may cause a low 1,5-AG value. Additional information can be found at http://www.glycomark.com.

Fructosamine Measurement
Fructosamine: glycosylated serum (fructosamine), a glycated serum protein test, measures glycemic control over 2 to 3 weeks. Normal ranges vary among

the different methods of measurement. Fructosamine values are used in short-term follow-up of interventions that have been recently implemented to lower blood glucose or when there is a discrepancy between A1C level and the individual's reported blood glucose readings.[4]

Urine Ketone Testing

Urine ketone testing was the original method of monitoring glycemic control and continues to be used in some underdeveloped countries where blood glucose meters are not available. However, since the advent of blood glucose monitoring, urine testing is no longer recommended in the United States. This is because urine ketone testing provides retrospective information and does not reflect current blood glucose. Some individuals may, however, still use urine ketone testing due to very limited financial resources or because they are adamant in their refusal to do an invasive testing procedure.

Urine testing for glucose has several distinct disadvantages:

- It will not detect hypoglycemia.
- It is limited to testing for elevated glucose levels.
- Elevated renal thresholds—that is, blood glucose >180 mg/dL (>10 mmol/L)—that occur with age will give false negative results.
- Renal thresholds may be low in pregnancy.
- It gives a delayed picture of what is happening in the blood, so is not indicated in flexible insulin therapy.
- False results (negative or positive) may occur with ingestion of certain medications (cephalosporins, large amounts of ascorbic acid).

Ketone Tests

Ketones are produced in the body when someone is severely depleted of carbohydrate or has inadequate insulin levels. The level of ketones can be measured in the blood or urine. The most accurate measurement of metabolic status is to measure 3-B-hydroxybutyrate in the blood. Currently, the only home blood ketone testing meter, a combination glucose/ketone meter, is the Precision Xtra®. Urine ketone tests measure acetoacetate and are done with a test strip. The level of acetoacetate in the urine is influenced by one's hydration level and may lag a couple hours behind the blood ketone levels. Thus, urine ketone tests are not reliable for diagnosing or monitoring treatment of ketoacidosis.[57]

Situations where it is important to monitor whether ketones are present include illness, consistently elevated blood glucose levels ≥250 mg/dL with type 1 diabetes,[58] infection, and pregnancy. Ketones should be routinely tested during illness by all individuals with diabetes. Individuals with type 2 diabetes can become ketotic during severe stress precipitated by infections or trauma.[59] For those using an insulin pump, ketonuria or ketonemia in the presence of hyperglycemia may indicate failure of the insulin delivery system.

Patient education regarding ketone testing should include the reason why ketone spillage would occur, due to lack of adequate insulin and the body burning its own fat, of which ketones are a by-product. Teaching must also make clear that during ketone spillage, fluid replacement—as well as carbohydrate replacement—is very important. Insulin users must be taught that they should continue taking their insulin and that additional insulin is often required to treat the accompanying hyperglycemia.

See also the section on ketone testing in chapter 14, on type 1 diabetes.

Long-Term Monitoring of Metabolic Control

A1C Measurement

A1C, which is expressed as a percentage of hemoglobin that is glycated, is the most widely accepted assay of glycemic control. The term "A1C" is the current preferred term in the United States, evolving from hemoglobin A1C and HbA1c. A1C, the most abundant minor hemoglobin component in the red blood cell, increases in proportion to the blood glucose level over the preceding 3 to 4 months. Glycosylation occurs as glucose in the plasma attaches itself to the hemoglobin component of the red blood cell; this process is irreversible. Because the red blood cell has a life span of 90 to 120 days, the measurement of A1C reflects the blood glucose concentration over that period of time. The more glycosylation that occurs, the higher the value. It is important to note that the

National Glycohemoglobin Standardization Program (NGSP) sought to standardize worldwide the assays which were used in the Diabetes Control and Complications Trial (DCCT), which established the relationship between A1C level and risk for developing long-term complications of diabetes. A1C measures long-term glycemic control, is the standard for guiding therapy, and is considered the surrogate for the risk of complications.[60,61] Until recently, the A1C did not reflect the average blood glucose but the weighted mean over a period of time.

Because A1C is expressed as a percentage (%) of hemoglobin that is glycated, and day-to-day glucose monitoring is expressed as milligrams per deciliter (mg/dL) or millimoles per liter (mmol/L), this can be a source of confusion for both the individual and the healthcare professional. The International Federation of Clinical Chemistry (IFCC) sought to develop a global standardization that expressed long-term glycemic control (A1C) and average glucose in the same units (ie, in the same units of glucose measurements reported in self-monitoring and laboratory reports). The results of the A1C–Derived Average Glucose (ADAG) study provided the IFCC with the data to determine the relationship between A1C and average glucose, and a simple linear relationship between average glucose and A1C levels was developed. The correlation between A1C and average glucose was 0.92.[62,63] The estimated average glucose (eAG) as it relates to A1C value can be obtained by the following formula:

$$eAG(mg/dL) = (28.7 \times A1C) - 46.7$$

For example, an A1C of 8% = (28.7 × 8) = 229.6; 229.6 − 46.7 = 182.9 (183) mg/dL. Table 7.16 lists the correlation between A1C levels and eAG levels based on data from the ADAG study. This new way of reporting A1C uses the same units that are seen on a glucose meter or laboratory report; thus, it will require educating, or reeducating, the person on the meaning of A1C as an average blood glucose value.

It is important to discuss with patients that both finger-stick checks and A1C testing are important to give day-to-day and longer term pictures of glycemic control. The A1C indicates mean plasma glucose over the last 2 to 3 months, providing a long-term view of blood glucose control. However, one is

TABLE 7.16 A1C to eAG Conversion Chart		
	Estimated Average Glucose (eAG)	
A1C (%)	*mg/dL*	*mmol/L*
5.0	97	5.4
5.5	111	6.2
6.0	126	7.0
6.5	140	7.8
7.0	154	8.6
7.5	169	9.4
8.0	183	10.2
8.5	197	11.0
9.0	212	11.8
9.5	226	12.6
10.0	240	13.4
10.5	255	14.2
11.0	269	14.9
11.5	283	15.7
12.0	298	16.5

Source: Adapted with permission from the American Diabetes Association, "Standards of medical care in diabetes, 2013," *Diabetes Care* 36 Suppl 1 (2013): S19.

not able to determine individual glucose excursions from an A1C value. Additionally, A1C doesn't provide day-to-day or immediate feedback on the following variables: food eaten, exercise regimen, and medications taken. Self-monitoring of blood glucose results provide real-time feedback on glucose control and, when performed premeal and postmeal, can detect glucose excursions. Self-monitoring of blood glucose provides tangible information which can be used to change behavior in order to improve glycemic control. Self-monitoring of blood glucose requires training and education in order to be utilized successfully.[64]

Frequency of A1C Testing

Regular measurements of A1C permit timely detection of departures from the target range. In the absence of well-controlled studies that suggest a definite testing protocol, both the ADA[5] and the AACE suggest A1C testing at least once or twice a year for persons with a history of stable glycemic control, and at least quarterly for those whose therapy has changed or who are in poor control.[65] Many facilities use point-of-care A1C testing, which allows for timely decisions on therapy changes. Additionally, this provides the opportunity to directly address therapy changes during the visit with the individual and allows for discussion on glycemic goals. At-home A1C testing is also available. Most products are certified by the NGSP. Insurance reimbursement varies with the insurance plan and the type of product.

A1C Targets

It is recommended that glycemic targets be individualized for each person with diabetes. The DCCT conclusively demonstrated, however, that the risk of retinopathy, nephropathy, and neuropathy in individuals with type 1 diabetes is reduced by intensive treatment regimens, as compared with conventional treatment regimens.[66] These benefits were observed with an average A1C of 7.2% (normal range being 4.0% to 6.0%) in the intensively treated group. The reduction in risk of these complications correlated continuously with the reduction in A1C produced by intensive therapy.[4] In the epidemiologic analysis of the UK Prospective Diabetes Study (UKPDS) data, the risk for occurrence of microvascular and macrovascular complications was shown to increase at A1C values of 6.5% or more.[67]

Table 7.8, appearing earlier in the chapter, lists the glycemic goals established by the ADA and the AACE. For the person with diabetes, an A1C result within the nondiabetic reference range may reflect frequent hypoglycemia and requires further evaluation.

The A1C is a strong indicator of blood glucose control when compared with SMBG results. In 2010, the ADA added to its diagnostic criteria that an A1C of >6.5% can also be used as a diagnostic criterion for diabetes. The test should be performed in a laboratory that is NGSP certified and standardized to the DCCT assay. In the absence of unequivocal hyperglycemia, the A1C test should be repeated, or another diagnostic test for diabetes should be performed.[68] The AACE supports the ADA's recommendation for a confirmed A1C as an available option for the diagnosis of diabetes with a number of additional recommendations, including using A1C as an additional option criterion, not as a primary criterion.[69]

A1C can be used as a teaching tool as well as a marker of metabolic control. If an individual monitors only fasting blood glucose levels and finds values in the normal range but has an A1C result of 9.8% (normal range being 4.0% to 6.0%), the educator can encourage this individual to monitor at other times of the day (especially postprandial readings) to uncover periods of elevated blood glucose and identify factors that may be associated with the elevated results.

Monitoring: A Comprehensive Approach to Patient Care Beyond Glycemic Management

Daily SMBG provides people with diabetes the information they need to assess how food, physical activity, and medications affect their glucose levels. The needs of people with diabetes, however, are not limited solely to adequate glycemic control; they also include learning to identify and prevent the related complications that result in disability and reduced quality of life. In keeping with these expanding patient needs, the role of the diabetes educator has evolved to address the global aspects of chronic disease management. Diabetes education should include both monitoring for the comorbidities and complications that frequently accompany diabetes and supporting patient-centered self-management education and training in those areas.

Diabetes education should include helping patients understand the risks for and the benefit of the identification and treatment of the complications of diabetes. Monitoring parameters of the various accompanying disease states should include common signs and symptoms, timing and frequency of testing, target values and goals, instruction on self-monitoring and devices, and interpretation and use of information and results. Today's educator is charged with knowing what information is needed, how often it should be evaluated, and how best to help support positive self-management behaviors in all areas of monitoring. This aspect of management is as crucial as glycemic control in improving outcomes in the chronically ill individual with diabetes.

Complications and Comorbidities

The importance of protecting the body from the effects of hyperglycemia cannot be overstated. The direct and indirect effects on the vasculature are the major sources of morbidity and mortality in both type 1 diabetes and type 2 diabetes. Typically, the injurious effects of diabetes are identified as either microvascular or macrovascular complications and include diabetes nephropathy, retinopathy, neuropathy, coronary artery disease, peripheral arterial disease, and stroke. There are, however, several other complications and disease states that have been associated with diabetes and should be included in risk assessment and routine monitoring to include: periodontal disease, thyroid disorders, mental health and depression, osteoporosis, sleep apnea, and immunizations. Monitoring parameters for common complications and comorbidities will be discussed as they relate to the role of the diabetes educator in assessment, follow-up, and patient self-management skills.

Initial Assessment

When monitoring people with diabetes, it is important to start with a baseline evaluation. This should include a comprehensive medical and medication history, physical exam, and standard lab tests.

The physical exam should include height, weight, and body mass index (BMI) as well as blood pressure (including orthostatic measurements when indicated), fundoscopic examination, thyroid palpation, skin examination, and comprehensive foot exam.

A complete lab panel should also be performed that includes A1C, fasting lipid profile, liver function tests, serum creatinine, and calculated GFR. Measurement of thyroid-stimulating hormone (TSH) should be included in persons with type 1 diabetes or dyslipidemia, or in women over 50 years of age. Children with type 1 diabetes should be screened for celiac disease, since there is a genetic link between type 1 diabetes and celiac disease.

The initial assessment and lab profile will be important points of reference for the healthcare provider when evaluating disease progression, assessing lifestyle and therapeutic interventions, and making future recommendations.

Macrovascular

People with diabetes should be regularly assessed for cardiovascular risk factors and the presence of macrovascular disease. The assessment should include an inquiry about symptoms of macrovascular disease, follow-up on recommended testing and monitoring

parameters, an evaluation of goals, and patient education and support.

Blood Pressure

Hypertension is a common comorbidity among persons with type 2 diabetes which magnifies the risk of diabetes-related complications. The aggressive treatment of high blood pressure decreases the incidence of CVD as well as microvascular complications.[21]

According to the ADA, blood pressure should be measured routinely to a goal of <140/80 mm Hg for most people with diabetes. A lower systolic target of <130 mm Hg may be appropriate for certain individuals, such as younger people with diabetes, if this can be achieved without undue treatment burden.[20]

Because hypertension often presents without symptoms, the accurate measurement of blood pressure is fundamental to both the diagnosis and effective management of the disease.[21] In light of this, specific procedures have been developed that describe the proper method for obtaining the most accurate blood pressure reading possible. These procedures, as outlined in Table 7.17, should be followed for both in-office and home blood pressure measurement.

The most common error in blood pressure measurement is the use of an inappropriately sized cuff. Considerable overestimation of readings can occur if the cuff is too small. To determine the correct cuff size, use a cloth measuring tape to measure the circumference of the arm that will most often be used

---

TABLE 7.17   Home Blood Pressure Monitoring Tips and Procedures

- The patient sits quietly for at least 5 minutes before the blood pressure is taken.
- Caffeine, smoking, and exercise are avoided for at least 30 minutes before the reading.
- Patient sits with back supported and both feet on the floor, legs uncrossed.
- The arm is supported at heart level.
- Outer garments are removed; avoid rolling sleeves if this will cause constriction.
- Talking is avoided during the reading.
- Place the lower edge of the cuff about 1 inch above the bend of the elbow.
- Record the reading.
- Take another reading, and record the second reading.

TABLE 7.18 Sizing Blood Pressure Cuffs	
Distance Around the Arm	*Blood Pressure Cuff Size*
7–9 inches	Small adult cuff
9–13 inches	Standard adult cuff
13–17 inches	Large adult cuff

for blood pressure measurements. Place the tape around the upper arm, midway between the elbow and the shoulder. Refer to the chart in Table 7.18 for appropriate sizing.

In-office blood pressure measurements are subject to a high degree of variability[70]; therefore, readings should be performed by trained individuals, using validated equipment to ensure consistency in measurements. With rare exceptions, blood pressure machines found in supermarkets and pharmacies are usually not properly maintained and should not be used. For home blood pressure monitoring, the American Heart Association recommends using an automatic cuff-style upper-arm monitor. Wrist and finger monitors are not recommended, because they yield less reliable readings. Electronic home monitors are easy to use, are cost-effective, and may improve therapeutic compliance. Additionally, home blood pressure monitoring may help identify patients with nocturnal hypertension, white-coat hypertension, or masked hypertension. Patients should be encouraged to purchase devices that have been tested, validated, and approved by the Association for the Advancement of Medical Instrumentation, the British Hypertension Society, and the International Protocol for the Validation of Automated BP Measuring Devices.[3] A list of validated monitors is available on the Dabl Educational Trust Web site (http://www.dableducational.org/).

Blood pressure is typically measured twice daily—once in the morning before taking any medications, and once in the evening. Two or three readings taken 1 minute apart should be taken at the same time each day and all of the results recorded. Blood pressure may vary throughout the day and is typically higher in the morning. *Orthostatic hypotension* may be identified by lightheadedness when standing, and if the blood pressure falls by >20 mm Hg systolic or >10 mm Hg diastolic from baseline upon standing.

Review of in-office and home blood pressure readings will provide information to help assess treatment goals, therapies, and patient options. The diagnosis of hypertension, as well as changes in therapy, will usually require confirmation of elevated blood pressure readings on a separate day or visit. Patients should understand their blood pressure numbers and the importance of blood pressure control to reduce complications and maximize quality of life. Diabetes self-management education and training (DSME/T) should include discussions around medications and adherence, critical blood pressure values, and development of a plan for identifying and managing hypertensive crisis.

Cholesterol: Lipids

Diabetes is correlated with a high risk for CVD. Management of the dyslipidemia of diabetes is a key element in the multifactorial approach to preventing CVD in persons with type 2 diabetes. The most typical lipoprotein pattern in type 2 diabetes consists of a moderate elevation in triglyceride levels, low HDL cholesterol values, and increased small dense LDL particles. This pattern has been associated with insulin resistance and may present even before the onset of type 2 diabetes.

An annual fasting lipid profile is recommended for most adults with diabetes.[20,71] However, patients with low-risk lipid values (LDL-C <100 mg/dL, HDL-C >50 mg/dL, and TGs <150 mg/dL) may be eligible for screenings every 2 years.[20] More frequent monitoring may be indicated after initiation or intensification of lipid-lowering therapies.[72,73]

In the absence of severe hypertriglyceridemia, lowering LDL-C to target is the first priority for most people with diabetes. The recommended treatment goal is LDL-C <100 mg/dL for patients without overt CVD and <70 mg/dL for patients with overt CVD. For patients on high-dose statin therapy who are unable to achieve the LDL-C goal, a 30% to 40% reduction in LDL-C from baseline is an acceptable alternate target.[20]

A lipid panel consisting of total cholesterol (TC), HDL-C, LDL-C, and triglycerides is most accurate if performed after a 9- to 12-hour fast, and if alcohol is avoided for 24 hours before the test. Concurrent conditions such as nephrotic syndrome[70] and hypothyroidism may cause elevated

TC and/or LDL-C, while the presence of infection or inflammation results in lower HDL-C values and/or increased triglycerides.[74] Additionally, lipid levels may be altered after an acute myocardial infarction, making a lipid panel vital within the first 24 hours after the infarct.[75]

Healthcare providers should be monitoring to ensure the required lipid panels and follow-up are completed. Assessment should include a review of goals, therapeutic adherence, patient barriers, and the importance of risk reduction. For patients not at goal, consider lifestyle modifications and initiation or intensification of medications. When intensification of statin therapy is warranted to reach the LDL-C goal, a doubling of the current dose generally achieves a modest, incremental reduction in the LDL-C of 5% to 6%,[76] a pattern that should be considered when escalating statin therapy to get to goal. Those patients on statins or fibrates should be monitored for possible medication side effects and counseled on the signs and symptoms of myositis and rhabdomyolysis.

Antiplatelet Therapy
The ADA recommends the use of low-dose aspirin, 75 to 162 mg per day, as a primary prevention strategy in persons with type 1 diabetes or type 2 diabetes at increased risk for CVD.

At each visit, the educator should monitor for all of the following: adherence to the antiplatelet therapy, signs and symptoms of gastrointestinal (GI) bleed, and concomitant therapies that may increase the risk of bleed. Symptoms of upper GI bleeding can include bright red blood, dark clots, and/or coffee-ground-like emesis, and/or black, tar-like stools. Symptoms of lower GI bleeding may include passing bright red or maroon blood alone or mixed in the stool. The use of enteric-coated aspirin may help alleviate stomach irritation but does not decrease the risk of GI bleed.

Smoking Cessation
Smoking cessation is associated with substantial health benefits.[77] Screening all patients at every visit for tobacco use and providing those who do smoke with behavioral counseling and advice on pharmacologic interventions are valuable preventive strategies. While the benefits of smoking cessation far outweigh the risks, the healthcare provider should be prepared to discuss the possible symptoms of nicotine withdrawal in order to maximize the likelihood that the patient will succeed. These include insomnia, anxiety, weight gain, depression, restlessness, and poor concentration. The most effective way to promote smoking cessation is to combine pharmacologic and behavioral interventions with ongoing support from the trained staff available through quit lines.

Microvascular

Hyperglycemia is an important risk factor for the development of microvascular disease in people with diabetes and has been supported in several observational studies.[78,79] Intensive glycemic control can reduce the risk of microvascular complications including progression of nephropathy, manifestation and progression of retinopathy, and retinal photocoagulation.

Retinopathy
Diabetic retinopathy is the most common ophthalmic complication of poorly controlled glucose and blood pressure and can eventually lead to blindness.[79] It occurs when blood vessels in the retina swell and leak fluid or become completely blocked. In some cases, abnormal new blood vessels grow on the surface of the retina. These ocular manifestations of diabetes affect up to 80% of all people who have had diabetes for 10 years or more.[80] Despite these intimidating statistics, research indicates that at least 90% of these new cases could be reduced through proper and vigilant treatment and monitoring of the eyes.[81] Early detection and treatment is critical because the risk of developing eye problems increases with the amount of time an individual has diabetes.[82]

An initial dilated and comprehensive eye examination by an optometrist or ophthalmologist is recommended in persons with type 1 diabetes within 5 years of diagnosis. In people with type 2 diabetes, the eye exam should be performed shortly after diagnosis because this population is more likely to have retinopathy at diagnosis.[20,83] Annual comprehensive follow-up exams are recommended after the initial evaluation; however, more frequent follow-up may be required if retinopathy is progressing. Less frequent exams (every 2-3 years) may be considered following 1 or more normal eye exams.[20] Retinal fundus photography may serve as a screening tool

TABLE 7.19   Risk Factors for Development of Diabetic Retinopathy
• Duration of diabetes
• High blood pressure
• Hyperlipidemia
• Pregnancy
• Use of tobacco products

for retinopathy, but it is not a substitute for a comprehensive eye exam.

Women with preexisting diabetes who are pregnant or are planning pregnancy should have a comprehensive eye examination and should be counseled on the risk of development and/or progression of diabetic retinopathy. The eye examination should occur in the first trimester with close follow-up throughout pregnancy and for 1-year postpartum.[20] Risk factors for the development of diabetic retinopathy are included in Table 7.19.

There are 4 stages of retinopathy progression: mild non-proliferative, moderate non-proliferative, severe non-proliferative, and the advanced stage, proliferative retinopathy. The early stages of the disease are often symptom-free; however, monitoring for blurred vision, blocked vision, floaters, or bleeding in the eyes should be done at each visit. Patients with or at high risk for retinopathy should be counseled to avoid heavy lifting and jarring exercise that could lead to microvascular retinal bleeding and possible retinal detachment. Educational and behavioral interventions should focus on reducing risks and adherence to regular eye examinations.

Nephropathy

In healthy individuals, protein (albumin) is typically not found in the urine, because the spaces in the glomerular membrane of the kidney are too small to allow protein molecules to escape. If the membrane is damaged, however, these molecules can leak through into the urine. People with diabetes are at significant risk of kidney damage leading to increased albumin in the urine and possible progression to diabetic nephropathy (DN). Reduced renal blood flow and the presence of albumin in the urine make the body retain excess amounts of water and salt, which may manifest in symptoms such as weight gain, ankle swelling, fatigue, and loss of appetite.

Diabetic nephropathy affects 20% to 40% of people with diabetes. It is the leading cause of end-stage renal disease (ESRD) in the United States,[84] and people at all stages of DN have a significantly increased risk of heart disease.[85,86] There are usually no symptoms in the early stages of DN, so the only sign of kidney damage may be small amounts of protein in the urine, referred to as microalbuminuria or moderately increased albuminuria.

Screening for DN is done by measuring the albumin-to-creatinine ratio on a spot urine specimen or total urinary albumin in a 24-hour collection. The spot urine test is the most practical method to assess the albumin-to-creatinine ratio because it is easy to perform and collection errors occur less frequently. The 24-hour urine collection can be burdensome and adds little predictive value or accuracy to the results.[87,88] Measurement of a spot urine for albumin only, without measuring urine creatinine, is somewhat less expensive but is more susceptible to yielding false-negative and false-positive results. Falsely elevated urine protein levels may be produced by conditions such as urinary tract infections, exercise, and hematuria. Abnormalities of albumin excretion are defined in Table 7.20.

Because of variability in urinary albumin excretion (UAE), 2 of 3 specimens collected within a 3- to 6-month period should be abnormal before considering a patient to have crossed one of these diagnostic thresholds. Exercise within 24 hours, infection, fever, congestive heart failure, marked hyperglycemia, and marked hypertension may elevate UAE over baseline values. False positives can also result from an improperly collected or stored specimen.

TABLE 7.20 Abnormalities of Albumin Excretion	
Category	*Spot Collection (μg/mg creatinine)*
Normal	<30
Microalbuminuria or moderately increased albuminuria (early diabetic nephropathy)	30–299
Macroalbuminuria or severely increased albuminuria	≥300

Microalbuminuria rarely develops in persons with type 1 diabetes during the first few years of the disease. For this reason the ADA recommends an annual test to assess UAE begin 5 years after diagnosis.[20,89] Persons with type 2 diabetes are more likely to have albuminuria at diagnosis because of the long duration of abnormal glucose metabolism that often precedes diagnosis. Thus, persons with type 2 diabetes should begin an annual UAE at the time of diagnosis.[20,89] Serum creatinine should be measured at least annually in all adults with diabetes regardless of the degree of UAE. The serum creatinine should be used to estimate GFR and stage the level of chronic kidney disease (CKD) if present.[20,89]

Treatment is rigorous glycemic control combined with blood pressure control. An angiotensin-converting enzyme (ACE) inhibitor, an angiotensin II receptor blocker (ARB), or both should be used to treat hypertension at the earliest sign of microalbuminuria or even before, because these drugs lower intra-glomerular blood pressure and thus have renal protective effects. Diabetes self-management education and support should focus on routine assessment to include monitoring for symptoms, regular testing, follow-up, and referral to a specialist as needed as well as ongoing education and support in line with patient needs and goals.

Neuropathy

Neuropathies are the most common complication of diabetes, characterized by a progressive loss of nerve fiber function. People with diabetes can, over time, develop nerve damage throughout the body, to which the clinical manifestations will depend on what nerves are affected, sensory or autonomic. Diabetic neuropathy can result in significant disability that may impair daily self-management activities, lower quality of life, and increase the risk of death.[90]

The prevalence of neuropathy increases with the duration of diabetes and severity of hyperglycemia, and while it is considered a progressive disease, patients may present without symptoms. For this reason, comprehensive screening for both distal symmetric polyneuropathy and diabetic autonomic neuropathy should take place annually beginning 5 years after diagnosis for people with type 1 diabetes, and at diagnosis for people with type 2 diabetes.[20]

Management of diabetic neuropathy has 2 approaches: therapies that help relieve symptoms and therapies that may slow progression of the disease. Of all the available treatments, optimal glycemic control is probably the most important for slowing the progression of neuropathy.

Peripheral Neuropathy It is estimated that approximately half of the people with diabetes will develop neuropathy during their lifetime.[91] Diabetic peripheral neuropathy (DPN) is the most common form of neuropathy in this population, with the most common presentation being distal symmetrical polyneuropathy, a stocking-and-glove pattern of numbness, pain, tingling, or weakness.

All people with diabetes should receive routine visual inspection of their feet at each diabetes-related visit with their healthcare provider and an annual comprehensive foot exam.[20] The routine visual foot inspection is used to detect the presence of acute problems as well as reinforce the importance of preventive strategies and self-care behaviors for foot health. The exam should include all areas indicated in Table 7.21.

Beyond the routine visual inspection, an annual comprehensive foot exam should be performed[20] to assess risk status and disease progression, and to determine the need for referral and prescription footwear. The annual exam should include both visual inspection of the feet and the use of some simple, in-office tests that assist in revealing decreased sensation to vibration, pressure, and superficial pain.[92]

A simple vibratory sensation exam consists of a 128-Hz tuning fork placed on the bony prominence at the dorsum of the great toe using the following steps:

1. Strike the tuning fork to initiate vibration.
2. Touch the tuning fork to the medial aspect of the great toe (avoid callused areas).
3. Ask the patient to state when he or she first feels the vibration and when it stops. If the patient indicates the vibration has stopped before the vibration has stopped in the examiner's hand, the test is abnormal (–).
4. Document the results as (+) for normal or (–) for abnormal.

Pressure sensation can be assessed using a simple clinical test such as the Semmes-Weinstein monofilament exam. The Semmes-Weinstein 5.07 monofilament nylon wire exerts 10 g of force when bowed

TABLE 7.21   **Routine Visual Foot Inspection**
• Inspect feet, heels, and between the toes.
• Check for signs of compromised blood flow such as thin and shiny skin, bluish-colored skin, or lack of hair.
• Check for wounds, calluses, blisters, ulcers, or deformities.
• Inspect nails for thickening, appropriate length, and signs of fungal or bacterial infection, and look for any ingrown nails.
• Check socks for discharge or blood.
• Check shoes for wear and for foreign objects.
• Check footwear for appropriate materials and support.
• Educate patients about daily foot inspections and self-care of the feet.
• Refer patients to healthcare provider or specialist as needed.

into a C shape against the skin for 1 second. Patients are asked if they detect the sensation. Patients who can't reliably detect application of the monofilament to designated sites on the plantar surface of their feet are considered to have lost protective pressure sensation. When performing this exam, the healthcare provider should follow these guidelines:

1. Place the patient in either a supine or sitting position with shoes and socks removed.
2. Touch the monofilament wire to the patient's skin on the arm or hand to demonstrate what the touch feels like.
3. Have the patient close his or her eyes and keep toes pointed straight upward during the exam.
4. Have the patient say "yes" or "now" each time he or she feels the pressure of the monofilament on the foot during the exam.
5. Hold the monofilament perpendicular to the patient's foot and press it against the foot, increasing the pressure until the monofilament bends into a C shape. (The patient should sense the monofilament by the time it bows.)
6. Hold the monofilament in place for about 1 second.
7. Repeat 2 to 3 times and then move to the next spot.
8. Test both feet on the locations according to the diagram. Avoid callused areas.
9. Record responses on a foot screening form with "+" for yes and "−" for no.

Neuropathy usually starts in the first and third toes and progresses to the first and third metatarsal heads.

These areas will likely be the first to have negative results with the Semmes-Weinstein monofilament exam.

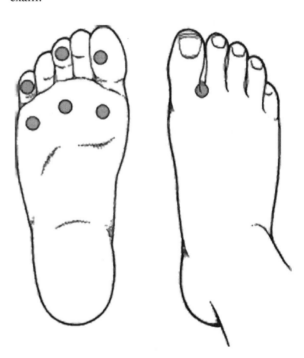

Superficial pain sensation is tested with a pinprick. The test is performed with a pin or needle gently applied to an area of skin that the subject cannot observe. The application of the pin is alternated with the pressing of a dull object against the skin, and the patient is asked to report pain.

Monofilament examination, vibration testing with a tuning fork, and superficial pain sensation testing have similar efficacy in detecting neuropathy.[91] Patients' mobility, gait, and balance should also be assessed because patients with DPN and balance problems have a two- to threefold increased risk of fall.[93]

Foot examinations can assist the healthcare provider with identification of risk factors and early detection and treatment, as well as provide an opportunity to reinforce healthy self-management behaviors. Self-management education should include encouraging patients to perform daily foot inspections and to contact their healthcare provider with any concerns. Use of a mirror or a support person can help in visual self-examination. The routine, in-office inspection offers the educator the opportunity to discuss appropriate footwear and foot care, and to reinforce the importance of glycemic control. People who receive foot self-management education and have a foot examination performed by a healthcare provider are significantly more likely to regularly check their feet than people who do not receive such services.[94]

Autonomic Neuropathy   Diabetic autonomic neuropathy (DAN) is a form of polyneuropathy affecting the nonvoluntary, non-sensory nerves, leading to damage mostly to the internal organs such as the bladder, cardiovascular system, digestive tract, and genital organs. Risk factors include duration of diabetes, increasing age, female sex, and higher BMI.[95]

The diagnosis of DAN is difficult given the number of organs that can be affected and the similarity of symptoms with other medical conditions. Clinical symptoms generally do not develop for many years after the onset of diabetes, so clinicians must rely on quantitative functional testing to help identify DAN. Healthcare providers should include assessment of risk as well as routine screening for symptoms associated with these complications. Some common clinical manifestations and symptoms of DAN may include those listed in Table 7.22.

Hypoglycemic unawareness can pose a serious threat to the person with diabetes. Persons with autonomic neuropathy may not experience the typical symptoms of low blood glucose, such as shakiness, making detection of hypoglycemia more difficult.

Persons showing symptoms of DAN should be referred to the primary care provider or specialist for a complete physical assessment and follow-up. Diagnostic tests that evaluate autonomic function include tests that measure heart rate variability, response of heart rate and blood pressure to breathing exercises such as the Valsalva maneuver, and the tilt-table test.

Additional assessment tools include gastric-emptying evaluation, thermoregulatory sweat test, urinalysis, ultrasound, and bladder function testing.

When DAN is undiagnosed or left untreated, the impact can be serious, resulting in complications ranging from discomfort and pain to heart attack and death. Identification of persons at risk for neuropathy in conjunction with routine monitoring for possible signs and symptoms is critical to preventing the onset of the disease and slowing disease progression. Strict glycemic control can slow the onset of DAN and sometimes reverse it.

Peripheral Arterial Disease

Peripheral arterial disease (PAD) is a narrowing of the arteries resulting in reduced blood flow to the extremities. People with diabetes are at an increased risk of developing this disease. Hyperglycemia, hypertension, dyslipidemia, and tobacco use are known risk factors for PAD. Screening for PAD should be done at diagnosis and then annually, and should include patient history of claudication as well as assessment of pedal pulses.

Early signs of PAD in persons with diabetes are the onset of lower extremity pain associated with walking and cold feet. A physical exam may reveal the presence of muscle atrophy, bruits, cool skin, thickened toenails, and possibly ulcers and gangrene. The ankle-brachial index (ABI) provides a simple, reliable, and noninvasive means for screening and diagnosing PAD. It is recommended that the ABI be performed on any person with diabetes over the age of 50 or who has positive risk factors that include the following:

- Duration of diabetes >10 years
- Tobacco use
- High blood pressure
- Hyperlipidemia

The ABI is the ratio of systolic blood pressure in the ankle to systolic blood pressure in the arm using a hand-held Doppler and a blood pressure cuff. A normal ABI value is from 0.9 to 1.2. Any value less than 0.9 is indicative of PAD.

Additional Areas to Monitor

Depression/Cognitive Assessment

Depression is an often unrecognized comorbid condition in persons with diabetes.[96] It is important for

TABLE 7.22   Common Symptoms of DAN by Affected Organ

Site	Monitoring/Assessment	Symptoms
Cardiovascular	Blood pressure	• Persistent or resting tachycardia (>100 beats per minute) • Orthostatic hypotension (a drop in systolic blood pressure of >20 mm Hg upon standing) • Syncope/light-headedness
	Heart rate	• Exercise intolerance where heart rate remains unchanged in response to changing activity levels
Gastrointestinal	Gastrointestinal function	• Constipation (may lead to bloating and esophageal reflux) • Diarrhea • Abdominal pain • Nausea or vomiting • Loss of appetite
	Swallow evaluation	• Difficulty in swallowing
	Gastric emptying	• Gastroparesis (delayed gastric emptying)
Genitourinary	Bladder function	• Urinary incontinence • Difficulty starting urination • Frequent urinary tract infections
	Sexual dysfunction	• Female sexual dysfunction • Vaginal dryness • Erectile dysfunction
Sudomotor	Perspiration	• Heat intolerance • Heavy sweating • Absence of perspiration • Gustatory sweating
	Skin hydration	• Dry or cracked skin • Skin infections
Pupillary	Vision problems	• Pupil response to light (difficult to adjust to changes in light/brightness) • Problems driving at night

Sources: D Ziegler, "Cardiovascular autonomic neuropathy: clinical manifestations and measurement," *Diabetes Reviews* 7 (1999): 342-57; DA Johnson, AI Vinik, "Gastrointestinal Disturbances," in *Therapy for Diabetes Mellitus* (Alexandria, Va: American Diabetes Association, 1998).

healthcare providers to monitor for signs of depression in their patients with diabetes. Signs of depression may include poor glycemic control despite ongoing adjustments, insomnia or hypersomnia, changes in weight by more than 5% within the last month, and crying spells.

According to the ADA, it is reasonable to include psychological and social assessments of the patient as part of diabetes management. Screening and follow-up may include attitudes about diabetes, management expectations, mood, quality of life, and financial, social, and emotional resources, as well as psychiatric history. In the presence of poor self-management, monitoring for depression, anxiety, eating disorders, and cognitive impairment is recommended.[20]

Many validated tools for screening for depression are available; however, obstacles, including length, cost, and degree of expertise required for use and interpretation, preclude inclusion in routine assessments. The Patient Health Questionnaire-2, or PHQ-2, is one tool that has been reported to be effective in determining the individuals who might benefit from a more complete evaluation for depression.[97] This quick assessment tool can easily be incorporated into the diabetes educator's routine follow-up as it consists of only 2 questions:

> Over the past 2 weeks, have you often been bothered by:
> 1. Little interest or pleasure in doing things?
> 2. Feeling down, depressed, or hopeless?

An affirmative answer to *either* question is a provisional positive screen and does not establish a final diagnosis or determine depression severity.

For an individual with a positive screening, the healthcare provider

- ◈ May ask the patient to complete a more robust screening tool
- ◈ Should report the findings to the referring primary care provider
- ◈ Should provide a list of resources available for referral to a mental health professional

Depression and cognitive impairment screening and treatment should become routine components of diabetes care. Integrating simple screening tools for depression into DSMES is likely to be the most effective means for ensuring their routine use. Diabetes educators are in a key position to monitor for depression in adults with diabetes, and can help ensure appropriate referral, coordinate follow-up care, and develop goals aimed at optimizing individuals' self-care of both their depression and diabetes.

Monitoring Weight

In persons with diabetes, controlled weight loss using nutritional interventions and increased physical activity is associated with many beneficial effects. For persons with type 2 diabetes mellitus, weight loss has been linked to reductions in insulin resistance and subsequent insulin levels. Conversely, high insulin resistance and obesity have been associated with higher insulin levels. Since insulin is anabolic and promotes fat storage, reductions in insulin levels may augment weight loss.

While intentional weight loss in persons with diabetes is usually safe, unintentional weight loss may be associated with uncontrolled glucose levels or other underlying conditions. The educator should monitor weight at every visit and assess whether there has been a substantial change. Factors that could be attributed to weight loss include hyperglycemia, dehydration, thyroid disease, and cancer. Causes of weight gain should also be explored to include medication use or nonadherence, thyroid disease, and nutritional sources.

The educator should be alerted if a patient suddenly develops significant involuntary weight loss, especially if it is accompanied by pronounced thirst or an increased need to urinate. Patients should be encouraged to weigh themselves once or twice a week and record these values in a log for comparison. Diabetes self-management education and training should include identification of patient weight goals and education around the safe and appropriate loss of body mass as well as weight loss programs, support, and surgical options.

Thyroid

People with diabetes have a higher prevalence of thyroid disorders than the general population. Up to 30% of women with type 1 diabetes have some form of autoimmune thyroid disease, and postpartum thyroiditis is 3 times more common in women with type 1 diabetes.[98–100] A number of reports have indicated a higher occurrence of thyroid diseases, particularly hypothyroidism, among people with type 2 diabetes.

Abnormal thyroid function may have profound effects on blood glucose control. Hyperthyroidism is typically associated with worsening glucose control and increased insulin requirements. The rapid heart rate resulting from excessive thyroid stimulation can worsen heart problems, and prolonged, untreated hyperthyroidism can exacerbate osteoporosis and risk of bone fractures. Hypothyroidism, however, rarely causes changes in blood glucose levels but can reduce clearance of insulin, warranting reductions in insulin doses. Low thyroid function may result in lipid abnormalities, including elevated triglyceride and LDL-C levels—changes that can further increase the risk of CVD.

The diagnosis of abnormal thyroid function in people with diabetes based solely on clinical manifestations is difficult. Routine screening for thyroid function abnormalities in all patients allows for early detection and treatment. Measurement of anti-thyroid peroxidase (anti-TPO) antibodies may detect subclinical hypothyroidism because those who are antibody positive have a higher risk of developing overt thyroid disease.[101] For persons with type 1 diabetes, it is recommended to test for anti-TPO antibodies at diagnosis. If anti-TPO antibodies are present, it is recommended that clinicians perform annual TSH screenings. In persons with type 2 diabetes, it is recommended that clinicians measure TSH at diagnosis of diabetes and every 5 years thereafter.[98] The AACE recommends TSH screening in women of childbearing age before pregnancy or during the first trimester.[21]

The educator plays an important role in ensuring routine testing and follow-up of thyroid function as well as monitoring for symptoms of thyroid dysfunction. The signs and symptoms of hypothyroidism tend to be more subtle than those of hyperthyroidism and include dry skin, cold sensitivity, fatigue, muscle cramps, weight gain, and constipation. Symptoms commonly associated with hyperthyroidism include rapid heart rate, sweating, weight loss, shortness of breath, skin thickening on knees and elbows, and in women, changes in menstruation.

Treatment goals include initiating levothyroxine therapy when applicable, ongoing diabetes education and support, and improving glycemic control.

Given the low therapeutic index for thyroid medications and the diversity of available products, it is recommended that patients be maintained on the same brand of levothyroxine throughout the course of their therapy. In the event they are switched to another brand or generic product, measurement of serum TSH in 6 weeks to make adjustments is indicated.

Vitamin D

Vitamin D and its active metabolite, calcitriol, are important regulators of serum calcium and bone health. Vitamin D deficiency is present in a large portion of the population, and there have been several suggested links between vitamin D status and diabetes.[102] For persons with type 1 diabetes, this relationship is mediated by the effects of vitamin D on the immune system; in type 2 diabetes, vitamin D has

been associated with improved beta cell activity as well as insulin sensitivity.[103] Dialysis patients, many of whom have diabetes, are especially at risk for vitamin D abnormalities.

The most accurate way to determine vitamin D status is to measure a 25-hydroxy vitamin D level, with the optimal range typically between 25 and 80 ng/ml. Although vitamin D deficiency is prevalent, routine measurement of serum 25(OH)D levels is expensive. Therefore, it has been suggested that healthcare providers routinely monitor for vitamin D deficiency only in those patients at risk for severe deficiency. This would include patients with musculoskeletal symptoms such as bone pain or myalgia, those who have low bone mineral density (BMD) or prior fracture, those at risk for falls, and patients with CKD.[104,105]

The diabetes educator should assess patients who may be at high risk for vitamin D deficiency and recommend follow-up monitoring with the primary care provider or specialist for diagnostic testing if applicable. The diabetes educator can play an important role in helping patients select an appropriate vitamin D supplement, encouraging mealtime dosing of supplements, and recommending dietary sources of vitamin D.

Osteoporosis

Osteoporosis is a condition in which bone loses density and becomes fragile and more likely to fracture. There is growing evidence that people with diabetes are at increased risk of nontraumatic fracture and that poor glycemic control may contribute to deterioration of bone health.[106] People with type 1 diabetes typically have lower BMD, resulting in an increased risk of fractures, while vision problems, nerve damage, and hypoglycemic events heighten the propensity for falls. People with type 2 diabetes and complications were once thought to be protected from osteoporosis because of their higher BMD, but they may actually be at higher risk of fracture.[107,108] This may be attributable to the high rate of obesity and sedentary lifestyles in this population.

The routine care of people with diabetes should include an assessment of bone health. Specialized tests known as BMD tests measure bone density in various body parts. These tests not only detect existing osteoporosis but also predict risk for a future

TABLE 7.23	T-Score Risk Assessment
+1 to −1	Indicates normal bone density
−1 to −2.5	Indicates low bone mineral density (osteopenia)
−2.5	Indicates osteoporosis

TABLE 7.24   Risk Factors for Falls and Osteoporotic Fracture

Non-modifiable risk factors for osteoporotic fracture

Age

Female gender

Race: Caucasian and Asian at greater risk than African American

Weight: less than 127 pounds

Bone structure: small framed

Early menopause (natural or surgical) and amenorrhea

Family and personal history of fracture as an adult

Medications (glucocorticoids, excessive thyroid hormone, anticonvulsants, gonadotropin-releasing hormones, methotrexate, cyclosporine A, heparin, and cholestyramine)

Diseases: type 1 diabetes, gastrointestinal and malabsorption

Modifiable risk factors for osteoporotic fracture

Cigarette smoking

Excessive caffeine intake

Excessive alcohol use

Inadequate intake for weight maintenance and bone health

Inadequate calcium or vitamin D

Disordered eating and low body weight

Insufficient weight-bearing exercise

Risk factors for falls more common with diabetes

Hypoglycemia

Hyperglycemia causing polyuria (nocturnal frequency when balance is impaired)

fracture. The most widely recognized BMD test is the dual-energy X-ray absorptiometry (DEXA or DXA) test, which measures bone density at the hip or spine. It is a noninvasive test that typically takes less than 15 minutes and is repeated every 1 to 2 years. The results are reported as a T-score, and risk assessment is based on this value. The lower the T-score, the lower the bone density, as indicated in Table 7.23.

Although there is no cure for osteoporosis, treatment options are available. Treatment includes a balanced diet rich in calcium and vitamin D, an exercise plan and healthy lifestyle, and prescription therapies. Osteoporotic medications are divided into 2 categories: anti-resorptive medications and bone-forming medications. The anti-resorptive class includes the bisphosphonates, calcitonin, and the selective estrogen receptor modulators (SERMs). There is presently only 1 bone-forming medication marketed as a synthetic version of parathyroid hormone.

The diabetes educator is afforded opportunities within the traditional assessment to evaluate patient risk for osteoporosis and fracture and provide appropriate intervention and referral. A comprehensive assessment should include key indicators that can help identify those at greatest risk (see Table 7.24).[109] The diabetes educator should work with the patient to achieve optimal glycemic control, improve nutritional status, make lifestyle changes, and create an exercise program to help improve bone health and decrease the chance of falls and fracture. Referral to specialists may include endocrinologists, bone specialists, podiatrists, ophthalmologists, occupational and physical therapists, and home care providers.

Immunizations

People with diabetes may have abnormalities in immune functions, putting them at risk for increased morbidity and mortality from infection. Therefore, immunization against influenza and pneumococcal disease is an important part of preventive services. An annual influenza vaccine should be recommended beginning on September 2 of each year for persons with diabetes 6 months of age or older.[110] Given that the influenza virus can be transmitted from person to person, vaccination of healthcare workers and family members of persons with diabetes may be justified. The flu vaccine does not contain a live virus, so the most frequent side effect is mild soreness at the injection site. Caution should be used for patients with a chicken egg allergy.

People with diabetes are also susceptible to pneumococcal infections and are at increased risk for bacteremia from this organism.[110] Additional risk is associated with patients 65 years of age or older who have chronic cardiovascular, pulmonary, and renal disease. Pneumococcal vaccination is recommended for persons with diabetes aged ≥2 years. A onetime revaccination is encouraged in patients over 64 years of age if they were previously immunized at an age of <65 years, and if it has been more than 5 years since their last pneumococcal dose. Repeat vaccination is also encouraged in patients with nephrotic syndrome, chronic renal disease, or other immune-compromised states. Common side effects include mild flu-like symptoms lasting less than 48 hours.

Hepatitis B vaccination should be administered to unvaccinated adults with diabetes aged 19 to 59 years and considered in unvaccinated adults ≥60 years old. Tetanus boosters should be repeated every 10 years.

Effective immunization strategies should include targeting the patient and family members. The diabetes educator visit should include monitoring and updating patient vaccination records, as well as education on the importance of immunizations. Finding community resources that provide immunizations and that are both accessible and affordable remains an important intervention.

Sleep Apnea

Sleep apnea is a common, yet potentially serious sleep disorder in which breathing repeatedly stops and starts. Obstructive sleep apnea (OSA), the most common form, occurs from relaxation of the throat muscles. Breathing pauses can last from a few seconds to minutes and may occur in excess of 30 times per hour. Typically, normal breathing restarts with a loud snort or choking sound. This chronic condition disrupts normal sleep patterns, resulting in poor quality of sleep and subsequent excessive daytime sleepiness. Risk factors for OSA are listed in Table 7.25. Type 2 diabetes and OSA share several clinical findings—obesity, hypertension, and impaired glucose tolerance—and OSA may be an under-recognized comorbidity of diabetes mellitus.[111]

The possibility of OSA should be considered in the assessment of all persons with type 2 diabetes and the metabolic syndrome. Monitoring for symptoms associated with sleep apnea can easily be incorporated into routine assessments and follow-up visits. Symptoms may include the following:

◆ Excessive daytime sleepiness (hypersomnia)
◆ Loud snoring, which is usually more prominent in OSA
◆ Episodes of breathing cessation during sleep witnessed by another person

TABLE 7.25   Risk Factors for OSA
• Excess weight
• Large neck circumference
• Being male—males have twice the risk of OSA than females
• Age >60 years
• Family history
• Ethnicity—in persons <35 years, African Americans are at increased risk
• Use of alcohol or sedatives
• Smoking—smokers are 3 times more likely to have OSA than nonsmokers
• Nasal congestion or allergies

Source: K Diaz, P Faverio, A Hospenthal, MI Restrepo, ME Amuan, MV Pugh, "Obstructive sleep apnea is associated with higher healthcare utilization in elderly patients," *Ann Thorac Med* 9 (2014): 92-8.

◆ Awakening with a dry mouth or sore throat
◆ Abrupt awakenings accompanied by shortness of breath, which more likely indicates central sleep apnea
◆ Difficulty staying asleep (insomnia)
◆ Morning headache
◆ Attention problems

One available screening tool that could easily be applied in the primary care setting as a means of identifying persons with type 2 diabetes mellitus who are likely to have sleep apnea is the Berlin Questionnaire.[111] This questionnaire asks about risk factors for sleep apnea, namely, snoring behavior, wake-time sleepiness or fatigue, and the presence of obesity or hypertension. It can serve as a valuable screening instrument to help recognize patients at increased risk of OSA who may benefit from further diagnostic studies and treatment. Considering the serious adverse health and quality-of-life consequences of OSA, efforts to expedite diagnosis and treatment are needed. The diabetes educator can play a critical role in improving screening for, and early diagnosis and treatment of, this potentially disabling condition.

Periodontal Disease

People with diabetes are at increased risk for periodontal (gum) disease, an infection of the gum and dental bone that hold the teeth in place. Periodontal disease can often lead to mouth pain, difficulty chewing, and possible loss of teeth. People with diabetes may also experience decreased flow of saliva and increased glucose in the saliva and the fluid between the teeth and gums, which can lead to increased plaque formation and contribute to a higher risk for caries. Xerostomia or dry mouth can contribute to the development of candidiasis, which may necessitate the use of antifungal agents for management. The management of oral burning symptoms can include maintaining adequate oral hydration and restricting intake of caffeine and alcohol.

Preventive measures for infection and delayed wound healing need to be monitored and reinforced by the diabetes educator. Preventive measures include daily brushing and flossing, regular dental visits, good glucose control, and the avoidance of compounding risk factors such as smoking. People with poor blood glucose control get gum disease more often and more severely than people whose diabetes is well controlled.[112] Just as the diabetes educator will closely monitor persons with diabetes for glucose control, compliance, and overall systemic health, he or she will do the same for oral health, because periodontal disease can be monitored and controlled with careful attention to home care and regular visits to the dentist.

Summary

The management of diabetes is multifaceted. Successful diabetes management requires monitoring multiple aspects of the disease, in addition to glucose control, in order to reduce complications of the disease and improve quality of life.

The success of SMBG is dependent on its utilization by individuals and their healthcare providers in taking action to improve glucose control. This requires that the educator teach not only the operational skills of SMBG but also the interpretive skills, and that the SMBG schedule be personalized and embedded in a diabetes management plan.

Diabetes self-management education should include self-monitoring beyond the single focus of glycemic management. Diabetes educators can teach individuals to approach all monitoring data as information which they can use to reinforce their active role in the self-management of their disease. Monitoring provides a comprehensive approach to the prevention, recognition, and management of the comorbidities and complications that frequently accompany this disease. Table 7.26 provides a comprehensive monitoring checklist.

TABLE 7.26 Monitoring Checklist				
Monitoring Parameter	*Goals*	*How Often*	*Patient Monitoring Behaviors*	*Professional Monitoring Parameters*
Macrovascular				
Blood pressure (BP)	• <140/80 mm Hg • <130/80 mm Hg may be appropriate in some patients	Each visit	• Home BP check • Once to twice daily • Validated home blood pressure monitoring • Upper arm measurement • Goals	• Office BP every visit • Check for orthostatic hypertension • Check home BP machine • Medication adherence • Self-management education
Lipids	Low risk • LDL <100 mg/dL • HDL >50 mg/dL • TG <150 mg/dL Overt CVD • LDL <70 mg/dL	Annually	• Lifestyle changes and healthy eating habits • Monitor for muscle pain, soreness, or weakness if on statin	Annual lipid panel • Repeat more frequently if not at goal or to assess treatment regimen • Low-risk patients may repeat every 2 years For statin/fibrates, monitor: • Lipid function tests baseline and as needed • CK (myositis)

TABLE 7.26	**Monitoring Checklist** *(continued)*				
Monitoring Parameter	*Goals*	*How Often*	*Patient Monitoring Behaviors*	*Professional Monitoring Parameters*
Antiplatelet	Reduce CV risk: • 75–162 mg per day low-dose aspirin primary prevention in at-risk type 1 diabetes mellitus (T1DM) and type 2 diabetes mellitus (T2DM)	Each visit	• Recognize and report symptoms of GI bleed	• Patient criteria for use • Therapy adherence • Bleeding
Smoking cessation	• Avoid smoking and all tobacco products	Every visit	• Smoking cessation counseling, treatment, and support	• Advise not to smoke • Assess readiness to quit • Discuss therapeutic options • Encourage use of quit lines
Microvascular				
Retinopathy	• Early detection/slow progression • Avoid permanent vision loss	Each visit Annually	• Glycemic control: avoid glycemic excursions	• Monitor at each visit for vision changes/disturbances • Support risk reduction strategies • Pregnancy and postpartum exams • Referral to specialist • Comprehensive eye exam • Referral as needed
Nephropathy	• Albumin: creatinine level <30	Each visit Annually	• Control BP • Good glycemic control	• Monitor weight gain, peripheral edema, fatigue, loss of appetite • Treatment adherence: ACE-I or ARB • Annual UAE ratio, serum creatinine, and calculated GFR
Neuropathy: Peripheral	• Avoid infection, complications, and loss of sensation • Slow progression	Each visit Annually	• Daily visual foot inspection • Appropriate footwear selection • Sensory changes • Glycemic control	• Visual foot inspection • Check footwear • Sensation testing • Assess gait, balance, and motor skills • Self-management support • Referral if needed • Comprehensive foot exam • Referral if needed
Neuropathy: Autonomic	• Prevention, early identification, and treatment	Each visit	• Monitor for various symptoms	• Risk assessment • Identification of symptoms • Support glycemic control: DSMES • Referral for quantitative testing and treatment

(continued)

American Association of Diabetes Educators©

	TABLE 7.26 Monitoring Checklist *(continued)*			
Monitoring Parameter	*Goals*	*How Often*	*Patient Monitoring Behaviors*	*Professional Monitoring Parameters*
Peripheral arterial disease	• ABI 0.9–1.2	Each visit Annually	• Therapeutic lifestyle changes • Avoid tobacco • Control glucose, BP, lipids • Pain associated with walking and cold feet	• Reinforce annual testing • Monitor for symptoms • Inspect lower extremities • Reinforce glycemic, BP, and lipid management • Encourage smoking cessation • Referral as needed • Perform ABI • Referral as needed
		Other		
Depression/ cognitive assessment	• Early recognition and treatment • Support self-management	Each visit	• Recognize and report symptoms	• Monitor for signs and symptoms of depression or compromised cognitive skills • PHQ-2 • Possible PHQ-9 • Help identify "support" systems • Referral to specialist
Weight	• Attain/maintain "healthy" weight • Planned weight loss only	Each visit	• Weight taken 2–3 times weekly • Goal for planned weight loss 2–3 lb week	• Monitor for sudden weight change • Nutrition counseling for healthy weight loss • Referral
Thyroid	• Early diagnosis and treatment • TSH within normal limits (check with local lab)	Variable for T1DM Every 5 years for T2DM	• Medications • Heart rate • Blood glucose • Recognize symptoms	• Anti-TPO antibodies in at-risk T1DM • Annual TSH level for T1DM if anti-TPO positive • Pregnancy and postpartum monitoring • T2DM every 5 years • Monitor heart rate, weight, glucose control, medication adherence • Patient education • Referral
Vitamin D	• 25-hydroxy vitamin D level 25–80 ng/ml (check with local lab)	As appropriate based on risk factors		• Monitor for risks: bone pain, low BMD, prior fracture, high risk for fall, CKD • 25-hydroxy vitamin D level if high risk

TABLE 7.26   Monitoring Checklist (continued)

Monitoring Parameter	Goals	How Often	Patient Monitoring Behaviors	Professional Monitoring Parameters
Osteoporosis	• T-score +1 to −1	DEXA every 1 to 2 years	• Balanced diet with calcium and vitamin D • Avoid activities that increase risk for fall • Optimal glycemic management • Medications if prescribed	• Assess risk factors for falls and/or fracture • Nutrition assessment and support • BMD testing • Referral • Medication adherence if applicable
Immunizations		Annual	• Keep records • Plan for yearly influenza vaccine	• Annual flu vaccine • Pneumococcal ≥2 years old • Repeat if ≥65 or CVD, chronic obstructive pulmonary disease, chronic renal failure • Hepatitis B 19–59 years old • Tetanus every 10 years • Education and support
Obstructive sleep apnea	• Early recognition and treatment	Each visit	• Report snoring/snorting, daytime sleepiness • Use of continuous positive airway pressure machine if ordered	Risk assessment: • Obesity, large neck, alcohol use, smoking, allergies • Symptoms: snoring, sleep disturbances • Berlin Questionnaire for at-risk patients • Refer to specialist for follow-up/sleep studies/treatment
Periodontal disease	• Early recognition and treatment	Each visit	• Brush and floss twice a day • Regular dental visits • Report oral bleeding or pain	• Monitor for dry mouth, pain, difficulty chewing • Education and support of overall dental hygiene • Encourage regular visits to dentist • Referral as needed

---

Focus on Education: Pearls for Practice

Teaching Strategies

⊘ **Appreciate a global definition of "monitoring."** Monitoring activities in diabetes care include not only blood glucose but also those activities related to metabolic control and the chronic complications associated with diabetes.

⊘ **Demonstrate empathy for the additional work of patients embracing this tool.** Monitoring the many aspects of diabetes management can be an overwhelming task, even for the most dedicated and goal-directed individuals with diabetes. At clinic appointments and outpatient visits, recognize and acknowledge the work that those you are serving have done in checking and recording blood glucose levels.

⊙ **Teach not just "how" but "why."** The diabetes educator's job is to teach those with diabetes not only the "how" of using a blood glucose meter but also the "why" so individuals with the disease are empowered to use the knowledge gained to make healthy, informed choices in their food intake, exercise, medication adjustments, and sick-day and stress management.

⊙ **Be aware of the words used to describe monitoring.** "Testing" may be interpreted as passing or failing. Terms such as "monitor," "check," or "measure" are value neutral and may be more acceptable to individuals. "Good" or "bad" blood glucose values may subconsciously be viewed as personal value judgments; instead, consider using "above or below target" or "above or below range."

⊙ **Use appreciative inquiry techniques when questioning individuals about their monitoring habits.**

⊙ **Facilitate goal setting.** Consider what data will best serve the individual in making informed decisions about diabetes management and obtaining a specific yet big-picture view of his or her glycemic control.

Messages for Patients

⊙ **Make the data work for you.** Blood glucose monitoring is a tool that puts diabetes management in your hands, with some assistance by others. Take advantage of the technology available to make informed decisions and improve your blood glucose control.

⊙ **Try something different.** Use SMBG to determine what happens when you are more or less active or try a new restaurant.

⊙ **Know your numbers.** Diabetes care involves more than just glucose numbers. Discuss with your healthcare team other numbers that need to be monitored besides glucose numbers.

⊙ **Monitor progress.** Keep track of your laboratory values, exam results, and other elements of diabetes care. Observing progress or trends will give you more control of your condition and self-management efforts.

Health Literacy

⊙ **Self-monitoring of blood glucose frequency is not independently associated with health literacy.**[113] The patient can monitor his or her blood glucose no matter what his or her health literacy is. The important issue is to make sure that the results are used to improve glycemic control: Patients need to use the numbers to adjust lifestyle or medications. Other research indicates that patients with limited health literacy show similar or better improvement in self-management behaviors compared with those with adequate health literacy after DSME.[114]

⊙ **Self-monitoring is not just about numbers.** Numeracy is defined as the ability to understand and use numbers and math skills in daily life. Your patients might not understand the meaning of the numbers if they are not familiar with quantitative description terms such as the following: small, decrease, weight, reduce, and chance.[115]

⊙ **Everyone can benefit from low health literacy education methods.** Everyone appreciates when information is simple, practical, and usable. When providing education, consider the following strategies for low literacy:
  • Introduce one concept at a time. Use one strategy per sentence. Make sure the concept is comprehended and then add additional applications. Instead of "If you have hypoglycemia, which is classified when your glucose is 70 mg/dL or below, have 2 to 5 glucose tablets, ½ cup (4 oz) of fruit juice, or ½ cup of a regular soft drink to raise your blood glucose," say, "Your blood glucose is considered too low when it is lower than 70 mg/dL." Then pause and ask, "What would you do if

your blood glucose got that low?" Add additional concepts, one step at a time. Evaluate comprehension and actual applications of the information.

- Demonstrate/illustrate the information. You can draw a picture, use analogies, show physical representations of quantity, encourage patients to create their own images, use vivid language, and teach with stories. Even drawing images on the white board when you explain the concepts can provide more time to think through the process and its applications (this is much more effective than briefly showing them complex pictures of complex processes).

Focus on Practice

⟳ **Self-monitoring of blood glucose is considered a therapeutic intervention only when the results are interpreted and appropriate interventions adjusted.** Create opportunities to work with patients to review the SMBG results and provide specific feedback and recommendations. Evaluate the effectiveness of the corresponding recommendations/adjustments.

⟳ **System integration of SMBG.** All healthcare team members involved in diabetes care need to agree on the SMBG methods, targets, and patient support methods. Patients feel more supported when the SMBG support is consistent among all providers. Trend management systems can allow for data tracking and guide decision making.

⟳ **Clinical information systems need to work together.** The systems that help integrate data from a wide range of systems will allow for healthcare professionals to offer efficient services. Healthcare professionals need to be able to access and share information quickly in order to work more efficiently and make better decisions.

References

1. Peeples M, Mulcahy K, Tomky D, Weaver T; National Diabetes Education Outcomes System (NDEOS). The conceptual framework of the National Diabetes Education Outcomes System (NDEOS). Diabetes Educ. 2001;27:547-62.

2. Austin MM, Haas L, Johnson T, et al; American Association of Diabetes Educators. Self-monitoring of blood glucose: benefits and utilization (position statement). Diabetes Educ. 2006;32(6):835-47.

3. American Association of Diabetes Educators. The American Association of Diabetes Educators position statement: self-monitoring of blood glucose. 2010 May (cited 2014 Apr 1). On the Internet at: http://www.diabeteseducator. org/export/sites/aade/_resources/pdf/research/Self Monitoring2010.pdf.

4. American Diabetes Association. Self monitoring of blood glucose (consensus statement). Diabetes Care. 1994;17:81-6.

5. Mulcahy K, Maryniuk M, Peeples M, et al. Diabetes self-management education core outcomes measures. Diabetes Educ. 2003;29:768-88.

6. Centers for Medicare & Medicaid Services. Fact sheet: expansion of competitive bidding program will increase competition, maintain quality, and save Medicare billions. 2013 Jan 30 (cited 2013 Jun 8). On the Internet at: http://www.cms.gov/Newsroom/MediaReleaseDatabase/ Fact-Sheets/2013-Fact-Sheets-Items/2013-01-302.html.

7. Heinemann L. (Analytical) accuracy of blood glucose meters and patients: how do they come together? J Diabetes Sci Technol. 2013;7:1-3.

8. Lajara R, Magwire ML. Accuracy considerations for self-monitoring of blood glucose: practical tools for primary care physicians. Prac Diabet. 2013;32(2):6-24.

9. International Organization for Standardization. ISO 15197: 2003: in vitro diagnostic test systems—requirements for blood-glucose monitoring systems for self-testing in managing diabetes mellitus. Geneva, Switzerland: International Organization for Standardization; 2003.

10. International Organization for Standardization. ISO/FDIS 15197:2013: in vitro diagnostic test systems— requirements for blood-glucose monitoring systems for self-testing in managing diabetes mellitus. Geneva,

Switzerland: International Organization for Standardization; 2013.

11. Garg SK, Reed K, Grey J, Westerman A. Possible impact of new accuracy standards of self-monitoring of blood glucose. US Endocrinol. 2013;9(1):28-31.

12. Hirsch IB. Clinical review: Realistic expectations and practical use of continuous glucose monitoring for the endocrinologist. J Clin Endocrinol Metab. 2009;94: 2232-8.

13. Transportation Security Administration. Travelers with disabilities and medical conditions. Last revised 2014 Jan 14 (cited 2014 Mar 24). On the Internet at: http://www.tsa.gov/traveler-information/travelers-disabilities-and-medical-conditions.

14. Peragallo-Dittko V. The lowdown on lancets and lancing devices. Diabetes Self Manag. 1999;16(3):64-71.

15. Peragallo-Dittko V. How accurate is your meter? Diabetes Self Manag. 2000;17(5):78-85.

16. Jungheim K, Koschinsky T. Risky delay of hypoglycemia detection by glucose monitoring at the arm (letter). Diabetes Care. 2001;24:1303-6.

17. Peragallo-Dittko V. Clinical and educational usefulness of SMBG with the elderly. Diabetes Spectr. 1995;8:17-9.

18. Bartos BJ, Cleary MJ, Kleinbeck C, Petzinger RA, Whittington A, Williams AS. Diabetes and disabilities: assistive tools, services and information. Diabetes Educ. 2008; 34(4):600-5.

19. Harris MI, Crowe CC, Howie LJ. Self-monitoring of blood glucose by adults with diabetes in the United States population. Diabetes Care. 1993;16:1116-23.

20. American Diabetes Association. Clinical Practice Recommendations 2013: Standards of Medical Care in Diabetes—2013. Diabetes Care. 2013;36 Suppl 1:S11-66.

21. American Association of Clinical Endocrinologists. Diabetes Care Plan Guidelines. Endocr Pract. 2011;17 Suppl 2.

22. Shiraiwa T, Takahara M, Kaneto H, et al. Efficacy of occasional self-monitoring of postprandial blood glucose levels in type 2 diabetic patients without insulin therapy. Diabetes Res Clin Pract. 2010;90(3):e91-2.

23. Polonsky WH, Fisher L, Schikman CH, et al. Structured self-monitoring of blood glucose significantly reduces A1C levels in poorly controlled, noninsulin-treated type 2 diabetes: results from the Structured Testing Program study. Diabetes Care. 2011;34(2):262-7.

24. Kempf K, Kruse J, Martin S. ROSSO-in-praxi: a self-monitoring of blood glucose-structured 12 week lifestyle intervention significantly improves glucometabolic control of patients with type 2 diabetes mellitus. Diabetes Technol Ther. 2010;12(7):547-53.

25. Franciosi M, Lucisano G, Pellegrini F, et al; ROSES Study Group. ROSES: role of self-monitoring of blood glucose and intensive education in patients with type 2 diabetes not receiving insulin. A pilot randomized clinical trial. Diabet Med. 2011;28(7):789-96.

26. Schwedes U, Siebolds M, Mertes G. Meal-related structured self-monitoring of blood glucose: effect on diabetes control in non-insulin treated type 2 diabetic patients. Diabetes Care. 2002;25:1928-32.

27. Zhang D, Katznelson L, Ming L. Postprandial glucose monitoring further improved glycemia, lipids, and weight in persons with type 2 diabetes mellitus who had already reached hemoglobin A1c goal. J Diabetes Sci Technol. 2012;6(2):289-93.

28. McAndrew LM, Napolitano MA, Pogach LM, et al. The impact of self-monitoring of blood glucose on a behavioral weight loss intervention of patients with type 2 diabetes. Diabetes Educ. 2013;39(3):397-405.

29. Barnett AH, Krentz AJ, Strojek K, et al. The efficacy of self-monitoring of blood glucose in the management of patients with type 2 diabetes treated with a gliclazide modified release-based regimen. A multi-centre, randomized, parallel-group, 6-month evaluation (DINAMIC 1 study). Diabetes Obes Metab. 2008;10(12):1239-47.

30. International Diabetes Federation. Guideline: Self-monitoring of blood glucose in non-insulin treated type 2 diabetes. Brussels, Belgium; 2009. On the Internet at: http://www.idf.org/webdata/docs/SMBG_EN2.pdf.

31. Type 2 Diabetes BASICS Curriculum Guide. 3rd ed. Minneapolis, Minn: International Diabetes Center; 2009. On the Internet at: http://www.internationaldiabetes center.com.

32. Bosi E, Scavini M, Ceriello A, et al. Intensive structured self-monitoring of blood glucose and glycemic control in noninsulin-treated type 2 diabetes: the PRISMA randomized trial. Diabetes Care. 2013;36(10)2887-94. Epub 2013 June 4.

33. Duran A. Benefits of self-monitoring blood glucose in the management of new-onset type 2 diabetes mellitus: the St Carlos study, a prospective randomized clinic-based interventional study with parallel groups. J Diabetes. 2010;2(3):203-11.

34. Klonoff D, Blonde L, Cembrowki G, et al. Consensus report: the current role of self-monitoring of blood in non-insulin-treated type 2 diabetes. J Diabetes Sci Technol. 2011;5(6):1529-48.

35. Blood Glucose Pattern Control: A Guide for People Who Use Insulin. 3rd ed. Minneapolis, Minn: International Diabetes Center at Park Nicollet; 2008. On the Internet at: http://www.idcpublishing.com/Blood-Glucose-Pattern-Control/productinfo/2058-816A/.

36. Powers M, Davidson J, Bergenstal R. Glucose pattern management teaches glycemia-related problem-solving skills in a diabetes self-management education program. Diabetes Spectr. 2013;26(2):91-7.

37. American Diabetes Association. Postprandial blood glucose (consensus statement). Diabetes Care. 2001;24: 775-8.

38. Monnier L, Lapinski H, Colette C. Contributions of fasting and postprandial plasma glucose increments to the overall diurnal hyperglycemia of type 2 diabetic patients. Diabetes Care. 2003;26(3):881-5.

39. Babione L. SMBG: the underused nutrition counseling tool in diabetes management. Diabetes Spectr. 1994;7: 196-7.

40. Ahern JA, Gatcomb PM, Held NA, Petit WA Jr, Tamborlane WV. Exaggerated hyperglycemia after a pizza meal in well-controlled diabetes. Diabetes Care. 1993;16:578-80.

41. Rubin RR, Peyrot M, Saudek CD. The effect of a diabetes education program incorporating coping skills training on emotional well-being and diabetes self-efficacy. Diabetes Educ. 1993;19:210-4.

42. Price MJ. Qualitative analysis of the patient-provider interactions: the patient's perspective. Diabetes Educ. 1989;15:144-8.

43. Cox DJ, Irvine A, Gonder-Frederick L, Nowacek G, Butterfield J. Fear of hypoglycemia: quantification, validation and utilization. Diabetes Care. 1987;10:617-21.

44. Austin MM. A call for standardized SMBG education. Endocrine Today. 2009 Apr;7(6):24.

45. American Association of Diabetes Educators. Diabetes Education Curriculum: Guiding Patients to Successful Self-Management [CD-ROM]. Zamudio Lange V, ed. Chicago: American Association of Diabetes Educators; 2009.

46. Hammond SA. The Thin Book of Appreciative Inquiry. 2nd ed. Bend, Ore: Thin Book Publishing Co.

47. Mazze RS, Strock E, Wesley D, et al. Characterizing glucose exposure for individuals with normal glucose tolerance using continuous glucose monitoring and ambulatory glucose profile analysis. Diabetes Technol Ther. 2008;10:149-60.

48. Mazze R, Strock E, Morgan B, Wesley D, Cuddihy R, Bergenstal R. Diurnal glucose patterns of Exenatide Once Weekly: a 1 year study using continuous glucose monitoring and Ambulatory Glucose Profile analysis. Endocr Pract. 2009;15(4):326-34.

49. Powers MA, Cuddihy RM, Wesley D, Morgan B. Continuous glucose monitoring reveals different glycemic responses of moderate- vs. high-carbohydrate lunch meals in people with type 2 diabetes. J Am Diet Assoc. 2010; 110(12):1912-5.

50. Block JM. Continuous glucose sensing technology: the latest in the evolution of glucose trend detection. On The Cutting Edge, DCE. 2005;26(4).

51. Halford J, Harris C. Determining clinical and psychological benefits and barriers with continuous glucose monitoring therapy. Diab Technol Ther. 2010;12:201-2.

52. Brauker J. Continuous glucose sensing: future technology developments. Diab Technol Ther. 2009;11:S25-36.

53. Klonoff DC. Noninvasive blood glucose monitoring. Diabetes Care. 1997;20:433-7.

54. Hirsch I, Brownlee M. Beyond hemoglobin A1C—need for additional markers of risk for diabetic microvascular complications (commentary). JAMA. 2010;303(2):2291-3.

55. Rubinow K, Hirsch I. Reexamining metrics for glucose control (commentary). JAMA. 2011;305(11):1132-3.

56. Brownlee M, Hirsch I. Glycemic variability: a hemoglobin A1C–independent risk factor for diabetic complications. JAMA. 2006;295(14):1707-8.

57. American Diabetes Association. Hyperglycemic crises in diabetes. Diabetes Care. 2004;27 Suppl 1:S94-102.

58. American Diabetes Association. Tests of glycemia in diabetes: clinical practice recommendations. Diabetes Care. 2004;27 Suppl 1:S91-3.

59. Fajans SS. Classification and diagnosis of diabetes. In: Porte D Jr, Sherwin RS, eds. Ellenberg and Rifkin's Diabetes Mellitus: Theory and Practice. 5th ed. Stamford, Conn: Appleton and Lang; 1997:357-72.

60. Diabetes Control and Complications Trial Research Group. The effect of intensive diabetes treatment on the development and progression of long-term complications in insulin-dependent diabetes mellitus: Diabetes Control and Complications Trial. N Engl J Med. 1993;329:978-86.

61. DCCT Research Group. The association between glycaemic exposure and long-term diabetic complications in the Diabetes Control and Complications Trial. Diabetes. 1995;44:968-83.

62. Consensus Committee. Consensus statement on the worldwide standardization of the hemoglobin A1C measurement: the American Diabetes Association for the Study of Diabetes, International Federation of Clinical Chemistry and Laboratory Medicine, and the International Diabetes Federation. Diabetes Care. 2007;30: 2394-9.

63. Nathan DM, Kuenen J, Borg R, Zheng H, Schoenfeld D, Heine R; A1C-derived Average Glucose (ADAG) Study Group. Translating the A1C assay into estimated average glucose values. Diabetes Care. 2008;31(8):1-6.

64. Saudek CD, Derr RI, Kalvani RR. Assessing glycaemia in diabetes using self-monitoring blood glucose and hemoglobin A1c. JAMA. 2006;295:188-97.

65. American Association of Clinical Endocrinologists. Medical guidelines for clinical practice for the management of diabetes mellitus. Endocr Pract. 2007;13 Suppl 1:16-34.

66. Boland E, Monsod T, Delucia M, et al. Limitations of conventional methods of self monitoring of blood glucose. Diabetes Care. 2001;24(11):858-62.

67. Stratton IM, Adler AI, Neil HA, et al. Association of glycaemia with macrovascular and microvascular complications of type 2 diabetes (UKPDS 35): prospective observational study. BMJ. 2000;321:405-12.

68. American Diabetes Association. Clinical practice recommendations, 2010. Diabetes Care. 2010;33 Suppl 1:S13.

69. AACE/ACE statement on the use of A1C for the diagnosis of diabetes. 2010 Feb (cited 2013 Aug 25). On the Internet at: https://www.aace.com/files/position-statements/a1cpositionstatement.pdf.

70. Wang J, Zgibor J, Matthews J, Charron-Prochownik D, Sereika S, Siminerio L. Self-monitoring of blood glucose is associated with problem-solving skills in hyperglycemia and hypoglycemia. Diabetes Educ. 2012;38(2):207-14.

71. Jellinger PS, Smith DA, Mehta AE, et al. American Association of Clinical Endocrinologists' guidelines for management of dyslipidemia and prevention of atherosclerosis. Endocr Pract. 2012;18 Suppl 1:1-78.

72. National Kidney Foundation. KDOQI clinical practice guideline for diabetes and CKD: 2012 update. Am J Kidney Dis. 2012 Nov;60(5):850-86.

73. Joven J, Villabona C, Vilella E. Abnormalities of lipoprotein metabolism in patients with nephrotic syndrome. N Engl J Med. 1990;323:579–84. doi: 10.1056/NEJM199008303230905.

74. Alvarez C, Ramos A. Lipids, lipoproteins and apolipoproteins in serum during infection. Clin Chem. 1986;32:142–5.

75. Ryder RE, Hayes TM, Mulligan JP, Kingswood JC, Williams S, Owens DR. How soon after myocardial infarction should plasma lipid values be assessed? BMJ. 1984;289:1651-3. doi: 10.1136/bmj.289.6459.1651.

76. Illingworth DR. Management of hypercholesterolemia. Med Clin North Am. 2000 Jan;84(1):23-42.

77. Rigotti NA. Clinical Practice. Treatment of tobacco use and dependence. N Engl J Med. 2002;346:506.

78. Mayo Clinic Staff. Diabetic retinopathy. Last updated 2012 Mar 27 (cited 2013 Jul 30). On the Internet at: http://www.mayoclinic.org/diseases-conditions/diabetic-retinopathy/basics/definition/con-20023311.

79. Diabetic retinopathy. Diabetes.co.uk (cited 2013 Aug 2). On the Internet at: http://www.diabetes.co.uk/diabetes-complications/diabetic-retinopathy.html.

80. Kertes PJ, Johnson TM, eds. Evidence Based Eye Care. Philadelphia: Lippincott Williams & Wilkins; 2007.

81. Tapp RJ, Shaw JE, Harper CA, et al. The prevalence of and factors associated with diabetic retinopathy in the Australian population. Diabetes Care. 2003;26(6):1731-7.

82. MacEwen C. Diabetic retinopathy. Last updated 2011 Mar 2 (cited 2013 Aug 2). On the Internet at: http://www.netdoctor.co.uk/diseases/facts/diabeticretinopathy.htm.

83. Fong D, Aiello L, Gardner TW, et al. Retinopathy in diabetes. Diabetes Care. 2004;27 Suppl 1: S84-7.

84. Excerpts from the United States Renal Data Systems 2002 annual report: atlas of end-stage renal disease in the United States. Am J Kidney Dis. 2003;41(4 Suppl 2):v-ix, S7-254.

85. Valmadrid CT, Klein R, Moss SE, Klein BE. The risk of cardiovascular disease mortality associated with microalbuminuria and gross proteinuria in persons with older-onset diabetes mellitus. Arch Intern Med. 2000;150:1093-100.

86. Gall MA, Hougaard P, Borch-Johnsen K, Parving HH. Risk factors for development of incipient and overt diabetic nephropathy in patients with non-insulin dependent diabetes mellitus: prospective, observational study. BMJ. 1997;314:783–8.

87. Eknoyan G, Hostetter T, Bakris GL, et al. Proteinuria and other markers of chronic kidney disease: a position statement of the National Kidney Foundation (NKF) and the National Institute of Diabetes and Digestive and Kidney Diseases (NIDDK). Am J Kidney Dis. 2003; 42:617–62.

88. Levey AS, Coresh J, Balk E, et al; National Kidney Foundation. National Kidney Foundation practice guidelines for chronic kidney disease: evaluation, classification, and stratification. Ann Intern Med. 2003;139:137–47.

89. Molitch ME, DeFronzo RA, Franz MJ, et al. Nephropathy in diabetes. Diabetes Care. 2004;27 Suppl 1: S79-83.

90. Vinik AI, Mitchell BD, Leicher SB, Wagner AL, O'Brian JT, Georges LP. Epidemiology of the complications of diabetes. In: Leslie RDG, Robbins DC, eds. Diabetes: Clinical Science in Practice. Cambridge: Cambridge University Press; 1995:221-87.

91. Maser RE, Steenkiste AR, Dorman JS, et al. Epidemiological correlates of diabetic neuropathy: report from Pittsburgh Epidemiology of Diabetes Complications Study. Diabetes. 1989;38:1456-61.

92. Perkins BA, Olaleye D, Zinman B, Bril V. Simple screening tests for peripheral neuropathy in the diabetes clinic. Diabetes Care. 2001;24:250-6.

93. Agrawal Y, Carey JP, Della Santina CC, Schubert MC, Minor LB. Diabetes, vestibular dysfunction, and falls: analyses from the National Health and Nutrition Examination Survey. Otol Neurotol. 2010;31:1445-50.

94. De Berardis G, Pellegrini F, Franciosi M, et al; QuED Study Group—Quality of Care and Outcomes in Type 2 Diabetes. Are type 2 diabetic patients offered adequate foot care? The role of physician and patient characteristics. J Diabetes Complications. 2005 Nov-Dec;19(6):319-27.

95. Ko SH, Park SA, Cho JH, et al. Progression of cardiovascular autonomic dysfunction in patients with type 2 diabetes: a 7-year follow-up study. Diabetes Care. 2008;31:1832.

96. Kessler RC, Berglund P, Demler O, et al. The epidemiology of major depressive disorder: results from the National Comorbidity Survey Replication (NCS-R). JAMA. 2003;289:3095-105.

97. Osborn CY, Kozak C, Wagner J. Theory in practice: helping providers address depression in diabetes care. J Contin Educ Health Prof. 2010;30(3):172-9. Epub 2010 Sept 28.

98. Wu P. Thyroid disease and diabetes. Clin Diabetes. 2000;18:38-9.

99. Stagnaro-Green A. Postpartum thyroiditis: prevalence, etiology, and clinical implications. Thyroid Today. 1993;16:1-11.

100. Alvarez-Marfany M, Roman SH, Drexler AJ, Robertson C, Stagnaro-Green A. Long term prospective study of postpartum thyroid dysfunction in women with insulin dependent diabetes mellitus. J Clin Endocrinol Metab. 1994;79:10-6.

101. Hossein GR, Tuttle M, Baskin HJ, Fish LH, Singer PA, McDermot MT. Subclinical thyroid dysfunction: a joint statement on management from the American Association of Clinical Endocrinologists, the American Thyroid Association, and the Endocrine Society. J Clin Endocrinol Metab. 2005;90(1):581-5.

102. Takiish T, Gysemans C, Bouillon R, Mathieu C. Vitamin D and diabetes. Endocrinol Metab Clin North Am. 2010;39:419.

103. Mathieu C, Gysemans C, Guilietti A, Bouillon R. Vitamin D and diabetes. Diabetologia. 2005;48:1247.

104. Chapuy MC, Arlot ME, Duboeuf F, et al. Vitamin D_3 and calcium to prevent hip fractures in elderly women. N Engl J Med. 1992;327:1637-42.

105. Bischoff-Ferrari HA, Willett WC, Wong JB, Giovannucci E, Dietrich T, Dawson-Hughes B. Fracture prevention with vitamin D supplementation: a meta-analysis of randomized controlled trials. JAMA. 2005;293:2257-64.

106. Nicodemus KK, Folsom AR; Iowa Women's Health Study. Type 1 and type 2 diabetes and incident hip fractures in postmenopausal women. Diabetes Care. 2001;24:1192-7.

107. Tuominen JT, Impivaara O, Puukka P, Ronnemaa T. Bone mineral density in patients with type 1 and type 2 diabetes. Diabetes Care. 1999;22:1196-200.

108. Weinstock RS, Goland RS, Shane E, Clemens TL, Lindsay R, Bilezikian JP. Bone mineral density in women with type II diabetes mellitus. J Bone Miner Res. 1989;4:97-101.

109. Kemmis K, Stuber D. Diabetes and osteoporotic fractures: the role of the diabetes educator. Diabetes Educ. 2005;31:187-96.

110. Advisory Committee on Immunization Practices (ACIP). Prevention and control of influenza; recommendations of the Advisory Committee on Immunization Practices (ACIP). MMWR. 1997;46:1-25.

111. Cass AR, Alonso WJ, Islam J, Weller SC. Risk of obstructive sleep apnea in patients with type 2 diabetes mellitus. Fam Med. 2013;45(7):492-500.

112. Pucher J, Stewart J. Periodontal disease and diabetes mellitus. Curr Diab Rep. 2001;4(1):46-50.

113. Mbaezue N, Mayberry R, Gazmararian J, Quarshie A, Ivonye C, Heisler M. The impact of health literacy on self-monitoring of blood glucose in patients with diabetes receiving care in an inner-city hospital. J Natl Med Assoc. 2010 Jan;102(1):5-9.

114. Kim S, Love F, Quistberg DA, Shea JA. Association of health literacy with self-management behavior in patients with diabetes. Diabetes Care. 2004 Dec;27:2980-2.

115. Cavanaugh K, Huizinga MM, Wallston KA, et al. Association of numeracy and diabetes control. Ann Intern Med. 2008;148:737-46.

CHAPTER 8

Problem Solving

Ginger Kanzer-Lewis, RN, BC, Ed M, CDE, FAADE

Key Concepts

◆ Problem solving is a core outcome of diabetes self-management education (DSME). Problem-solving skills are not only difficult skills to teach but also difficult skills to learn.

◆ Diabetes educators use both direct instruction and problem-solving skills when identifying and assessing problems and barriers that impact diabetes self-management.

◆ The problems that affect diabetes self-management occur on 3 levels: (1) clinical issues and emergencies, (2) problematic self-management behaviors, and (3) problems affecting self-management.

◆ The assessment can identify the problems and barriers affecting the patient's behaviors leading to resistance to change.

◆ The diabetes educator can choose the right approach to problem solving, plan for problem solving, and identify effective methods to use for each person.

◆ When working in a group setting, the diabetes educator can select the appropriate problem-solving strategy based on an assessment of the individuals or the specific characteristics of the group.

Introduction

Problem solving is an essential tool for diabetes self-management and for facilitating behavior change. As 1 of the AADE7 Self-Care Behaviors™, problem solving can be applied to the other 6 behaviors: healthy eating, being active, taking medication, monitoring, healthy coping, and reducing risks. Problem solving is a skill that can be learned and applied to all diabetes self-care behaviors. However, problem-solving skills can be the most challenging for the educator to teach[1] and for the patient to learn.[2]

Problem solving is not a onetime event. It is a complex, fluid process that involves active engagement from both the patient and the diabetes educator. What makes problem solving a unique behavior is that it cuts across all AADE7 Self-Care Behaviors™, which is why it is such an important skill for patients to master in order to better manage their diabetes.

This chapter discusses the application of problem-solving education by diabetes educators so that individuals with diabetes can effectively learn problem-solving skills for their own diabetes self-management.

What Is Problem Solving?

Problem solving is a core outcome of diabetes self-management education and support (DSMES) and is defined as follows:

A learned behavior that includes generating a set of potential strategies for problem resolution, selecting the most appropriate strategy, and evaluating the effectiveness of the strategy (pp. 790-1).[3]

Theoretical Model

Theories and models provide the building blocks for teaching and practicing problem-solving techniques with individuals and groups. Problem solving is often conceptualized as a process involving these steps:

1. Identify the problem.
2. Develop alternative solutions.
3. Select, implement, and evaluate the solution.

However, the ability of the person with diabetes to effectively execute these steps is affected by a number of components, as described in Table 8.1.

The problem-solving components described in Table 8.1 exist within a specific setting and context within which the problem occurs. This includes the individual's social and physical environment and the characteristics of the problem itself.

As part of the assessment process, the educator can use the components as a guide for determining how best to work with the individual to improve his or her problem-solving abilities.

Using Problem Solving in Diabetes Self-Management

While knowledge is necessary, it is insufficient for effective and maintained self-management. Problem solving requires more than just knowledge or skill acquisition.[3] The educator must determine whether an individual's issue requires direct knowledge/instruction or problem solving.

Direct Instruction Versus Problem Solving

Direct instruction refers to specific directions for patients to follow. This can be used when there is a specific course of action to follow and it would be too great a risk for the patient to consider alternatives. For example, if there is only one way to use a specific blood glucose meter, then there is no need to generate alternative solutions. The patient must follow the instructions to learn the proper usage of the meter.

Direct instruction—rather than problem solving—is recommended for problems meeting these criteria:

- Problem is well defined and straightforward[4]
- Problem has a single best strategy for resolution[4]
- Problem has a known, specific course of action that the individual with diabetes should take for problem resolution
- Use of trial and error could be detrimental or life threatening

Treating acute complications of hypoglycemia or hyperglycemia, and illness/sick days meet these criteria.

TABLE 8.1	Components of Problem Solving		
	Component	*Effective for Problem Solving*	*Ineffective for Problem Solving*
Environment The setting and context within which the problem occurs.	Approach to problem solving	Rational, logical	Impulsive, careless, avoidant
	Motivation toward managing problems	Positive attitude	Negative attitude
	Ability to learn from prior experience and apply that learning to new situations	Able to learn from experiences and transfers this learning to new situations in an appropriate manner	Unable to learn from experiences and transfers this learning to new situations in an inappropriate manner
	Knowledge base	Sufficient, accurate, and applicable	Insufficient, inaccurate, and not applicable

Source: F Hill-Briggs, "Problem solving in diabetes self-management: a model of chronic illness self-management behavior," *Ann Behav Med* 25, no. 3 (2003): 182-93.

Detecting Hypoglycemia and Hyperglycemia

When the situation involves detecting hypoglycemia or hyperglycemia, or sick-day management, a combination of direct instruction and problem solving may be warranted.

- *Direct instruction.* This includes education about the symptoms of hypoglycemia and hyperglycemia, how to monitor one's blood glucose and/or ketone levels, and the blood glucose levels that indicate hypoglycemia or hyperglycemia for that patient.
- *Problem solving.* This includes identifying specific and reliable symptoms the individual experiences during hypoglycemia or hyperglycemia, identifying any barriers to detection such as blood glucose unawareness, determining barriers to monitoring with appropriate frequency, and problem solving how these data can be used to act appropriately and adjust one's regimen with regard to medication, eating, and/or activity.

Preventing Hypoglycemia and Hyperglycemia

In the case of preventing hypoglycemia and hyperglycemia, problem solving is a particularly important strategy to employ. Selecting the most appropriate and effective strategies for a given individual to integrate and maintain in his or her lifestyle will result from effective problem solving. Problem solving can focus on identifying the unique situations that tend to lead to these acute complications in the individual's life, devising tailored strategies for prevention, developing strategies to address both daily and long-term resolution of barriers to effective self-management, and planning for ongoing adjustment or maintenance of self-management behaviors.

Identifying and Assessing Problems and Barriers

The initial step in problem solving is identifying the problems and barriers preventing the person with diabetes from solving or managing the problem.

Types of Problems

Problem identification occurs on 3 levels:

Level 1: Clinical markers and emergencies
Examples: Suboptimal blood glucose control, acute complications, ER visits

Level 2: Problematic self-management behaviors
Examples: Unhealthy diet, sedentary lifestyle, medication noncompliance

Level 3: Problems impacting self-management
Examples: Lack of self-management knowledge and skills, personal issues, and interpersonal issues

When a person is referred for consultation due to difficulties with disease control (a level 1 problem), assessment is needed to determine the individual's use of self-management behaviors (level 2). (See chapter 2 for more on assessment.) To provide education and counseling to improve these behaviors, level 3 factors must be determined. Once the level 3 problems are identified, they become the target for problem-solving education or counseling.

Whether a problem exists on level 1, 2, or 3, it becomes essential to both identify and manage the barriers to addressing the problem.

Types of Barriers

In working to better understand the variety of barriers the patient may be facing when trying to resolve his or her self-management problems, it can be helpful to think of barriers in 3 broad categories:

1. Personal: Emotional well-being and depression,[5,6] physical disabilities, poor coping styles, inaccurate health beliefs, and poor health literacy and numeracy skills
2. Interpersonal: Family conflict, lack of rapport with diabetes educator or others on the healthcare team
3. Environmental: Financial barriers for middle-aged and older adults[7,8]; social pressures for children and adolescents[9]; socioeconomic, language, and knowledge barriers for minorities[8,10,11]

For the healthcare educator, assessing and understanding these barriers is essential for ensuring that the problem-solving intervention is appropriate for the unique barrier the individual is experiencing.

Barriers to problem solving must be identified in order to provide culturally sensitive care and to make sustainable change.

Each state, Washington, DC, and the US territories have a diabetes prevention and control program available to help educators identify community resources. The educator should be aware of local resources including referral to the appropriate agencies and professionals. Conduct an Internet search on "Diabetes Prevention and Control Program & Your State/DC/territory" to find your locale's Web site.

Common Problem Areas and Associated Barriers

People   Self-management decisions can be influenced in both positive and negative ways by people in the patient's life. A patient's family, friends, employer, healthcare team, and others can have an impact on the patient's behavior. For example, an educator might discover that what appears to be a patient's unwillingness to adjust his or her eating habits stems from the patient's perception that such a change would be an inconvenience to others in the family. Sometimes the problem may be family members who are not supportive or healthcare professionals who give patients incorrect information. Educators need to work with the patient to identify the real issue and anyone else in the patient's life who may be involved.

Resources   What kind of resources does the patient need to manage his or her diabetes? Does the patient have access to these resources? Is the educator knowledgeable about the resources available within the patient's community or on the patient's healthcare team? (See Table 8.2.)

Financial   Diabetes equipment and supplies can be expensive. Can the patient afford them? Does the patient have insurance? Does the patient's insurance cover the equipment and supplies? Is the educator aware of agencies or resources that can provide assistance?

Scheduling   Are classes available at appropriate times when patients can attend them? Are weekend and evening classes available? Are the classes located near public transportation? How does the diabetes educator resolve scheduling problems?

TABLE 8.2   Who Is on the Healthcare Team?
The following are some of the people who can be on the healthcare team of the person with diabetes. All should be considered as resources when problem solving with your patient.
Person with diabetes and his or her family
Primary care provider (eg, physician, nurse-practitioner, advanced nurse practitioner)
Certified diabetes educator®
Nurse educator
Registered dietitian
Pharmacist
Eye doctor
Foot doctor
Dentist
Social worker
Psychologist
Psychiatrist
Marriage/family therapist
Exercise physiologist

Source: Adapted with permission from G Kanzer-Lewis, *10 Steps to Better Living With Diabetes* (Alexandria, Va: American Diabetes Association, 2007), 17.

Choice of Action   Problems can arise when the patient does not want to follow a specific course of action that may be of help to him or her. For example, is the patient unwilling to change from oral meds to injections? Will the patient agree to try an insulin pump? An educator can help the patient assess his or her options by creating a decision tree. Decision trees are discussed later in this chapter.

Strategy Based on Patient Assessment   Does this person need individual teaching or group classes? Will the patient be able to adjust to changes in his or her life? How can the educator help and support the patient to make that happen?

Communication/Comprehension   Each person is an individual with his or her own history and beliefs. How does the diabetes educator explain issues in a way in which each person will understand *and* learn methods to solve his or her problems?

Constraints   Are there other issues that prevent the problem from being solved? Does the patient have literacy or numeracy issues that affect his or her ability to manage the medication regimen? Perhaps the patient has physical conditions that will not allow him or her to inject his or her own insulin. See the following example.

> AM is a married woman with a number of adult children who were very supportive of their mother's need to manage her diabetes. The whole family attended every class and physician visit. AM was injecting her own insulin and doing well, but she had a stroke and is unable to use her right hand to inject her insulin. The diabetes educator decided she could teach AM to use an insulin pen with her left hand. However, her family was adamant that her culture and religion did not allow her to use the "dirty hand" for administering medication. In her culture the right hand is for eating and for "clean tasks" such as brushing teeth and taking medication, and the left hand is the "dirty" hand for toileting. Initially, the educator was concerned that the family was setting rules that AM did not understand, but she spoke to AM and asked what she wanted to do. AM agreed with her family.
>
> When working with a patient, educators need to keep in mind that what may not appear to be a barrier or constraint to self-care to the educator may be so to the patient. The goal is to find a suitable solution, not to try to convince the patient that there is no barrier or constraint.

Identifying and Assessing Problems and Barriers: Gather the Facts

- What is the *real* problem? Sometimes the actual issue is hidden within many smaller problems.
- Who is affected? Aside from the person with diabetes, are others affected by the problem? Are they a barrier or can they be part of the solution?
- Who should be involved in the decisions? Does the educator need to include family members in the discussion?

Table 8.3 provides examples of level 3 problems and associated barriers to effective self-management.

Create an Environment That Encourages Problem Solving

The diabetes educator can support a patient's problem-solving skills by creating an environment in which the patient is comfortable honestly discussing the barriers he or she faces in trying to self-manage his or her diabetes.

- *Give patients permission to ask questions.* Patients may avoid asking questions unless they are encouraged to ask them. Educators can encourage patients to keep a list of things they want to know about their diabetes and to bring the list with them to appointments. Remember to provide adequate detail, encourage additional questions, and request feedback to ensure they understand the meaning.
- *Collaboration, not confrontation.* Patients may withhold information or lie to healthcare providers either because they fear they will be criticized or lectured by the educator or because they are concerned that they will disappoint their educator.[12] By establishing an environment that recognizes that the patient will have setbacks and challenges, the educator and the patient can be honest with each other and focus on collaborative problem solving rather than confrontation.
- *Confirm understanding.* The diabetes educator should be aware that patients may not understand the language of diabetes and health care in the same way that the educator does. What does fasting mean? Does it mean no meat on Friday or no water or food for 24 hours? Does it mean don't take your pills before the test or take only your blood pressure pills and not your blood glucose pills? For example, telling patients that their blood test is good is meaningless if they are asked what their A1C is in an emergency room. Patients need to know and understand the significance of the values.
- *Ask, don't tell.* If the diabetes educator tells a patient what to do without asking the patient what he or she is willing to do, the educator may inadvertently create additional problems.

TABLE 8.3   Barriers to Diabetes Self-Management Behaviors

AADE7 Self-Care Behaviors™	Barriers	Strategies for Addressing Barriers
Taking Medication	Personal: "My grandmother died after taking insulin, so insulin will hurt me, not help me"	Cognitive Behavior Therapy to assist in new cognitions
	Interpersonal: "My family will think I'm weak if I take medication"	Discuss and examine beliefs about family perceptions in a family meeting
	Environmental: "I don't own a car, so I can't drive to the pharmacy to pick up my medications"	Identify alternatives and assist in choosing solutions to obtain medication
Monitoring	Personal: "I can just feel what my glucose is. I don't need to poke myself again"	Seek understanding of why patient does this, and challenge with an actual blood glucose test to compare the actual number with the patient's guess
	Interpersonal: "My wife gets woozy at the sight of blood, so I don't check my blood glucose for her sake"	Acknowledge concern for spouse, challenge the excuse, and help find alternative locations to check blood glucose
	Environmental: "I'm not allowed breaks at work to check my blood glucose"	Identify and role-play discussion points to be had with supervisor
Healthy Eating	Personal: "Health food tastes bad"	Explore what health food means to them
	Interpersonal: "My mother cooks true to our culture and she won't change her cooking style for me"	Listen, seek clarification about what the patient eats, discuss family's willingness to change, and suggest a family meeting
	Environmental: "My school doesn't offer healthy options in the cafeteria"	Appreciate the challenge, create list of alternatives
Being Active	Personal: "I'm not athletic"	Promote discussion of the patient's perception of being active versus being an athlete
	Interpersonal: "I am committed to taking care of my family and don't have time to exercise"	Explore the patient's ambivalence about caring for self and others and discuss solutions
	Environmental: "I don't live in a safe neighborhood so I can't exercise outside"	Explore the perception of being active and help the patient create alternatives

This may place the patient in conflict with the educator and result in the patient not learning what is needed to self-manage his or her diabetes.

◆ *Prioritize.* Once problems and barriers have been identified, consider prioritizing the problems that need to be addressed first based on importance for both the patient and the educator. Willingness to change is increased when both are able to agree and to collaborate on the goals. It is important to consider patient readiness for change and to be clear about the process and the goal. Some problems and barriers require action by the patients, others require action by the educator, and others require collaboration. See the following section for more information

on determining when a problem should be solved by the diabetes educator, the patient and the educator, or the patient.

Applying Problem Solving in Diabetes Education

There are different ways that problem solving might be used within an education or counseling session:

1. Clinical problem solving by the diabetes educator
2. Patient as observer or partial partner to problem solving by the diabetes educator
3. Patient and educator as collaborators
4. Patient as problem solver facilitated by the diabetes educator

Clinical Problem Solving by the Diabetes Educator

In this scenario, the diabetes educator is the problem solver.[13,14] The educator diagnoses the problem, plans a course of action or treatment, and evaluates the effectiveness.

Patient as Observer or Partial Contributor to Problem Solving

In this scenario, the patient may provide some input, but the educator takes the active role as the problem solver.[15] This approach should be used carefully and only under special circumstances, such as when time or other constraints of the education session necessitate a more directive role by the diabetes educator,[3,4,15] or when the person with diabetes is not able or prefers not to assume an autonomous role in decision making (see the section on special considerations later in this chapter). For example, some elderly patients may need and prefer clear directions on how to manage a situation due to declining cognitive abilities such as memory.

Patient and Professional Collaboration

Once a patient receives his or her initial diabetes education, the patient and educator collaborative approach is preferred in helping a patient feel engaged in the treatment. This team approach, where the health professional has the ideal diabetes information and the patient has the self-knowledge of whether it can be implemented, facilitates clarity and a feeling of equalizing power. They are joining each other in a common direction, as shown in the following example:

> **Diabetes Educator (DE):** I see your A1C has been a bit high lately.
> **Patient (Pt):** Yes, after I went to college I vowed I wouldn't have any more lows. So I've been running it high; it's safer.
> **DE:** So, how are you feeling?
> **Pt:** A bit crabby, not too sharp, but I'm not having lows.
> **DE:** You know there might be some other ways to not run so high and still stay safe. Do you know what I'm talking about?

> **Pt:** You mean like test more?
> **DE:** That is one way, or take a little more insulin, wear a pump, watch your carbs a bit closer. Are you open to any of these?
> **Pt:** I'm not doing the pump!
> **DE:** I'm not saying that is the only choice; I'm saying you have a number of choices, based on what you're OK with. I know lows are unpleasant, and being in college you need to stay safe, but a high A1C isn't safe either. Let's work together to come up with a plan.

Problem Solving by Patient Facilitated by Diabetes Educator

In this scenario, the person with diabetes is the problem solver.[3,4,15] The diabetes educator, through skillful patient-centered questions and responses, guides the person in using a problem-solving process to come up with his or her own solution(s)[16] or uses instructional methods to train the person in problem solving to resolve problems independently.[17] This approach is illustrated in the following example:

> **Pt:** I've been having a hard time remembering to take my long-acting insulin at bedtime, and I end up high in the morning and feel terrible.
> **DE:** What do you think gets in your way of remembering?
> **Pt:** I don't know, it gets late and I want to go to bed and just forget. My mom used to remind me, but now that I'm on my own I don't have that reminder.
> **DE:** How do you remember to get up in the morning, or go to class, and work?
> **Pt:** I just set the alarm on my cell. I suppose I could give that a try for reminding myself to take my insulin.

Therapeutic Relationship

Maintaining a therapeutic rapport is essential throughout all stages of self-management education and counseling. The way in which problem solving is used can be a source of conflict between the individual and the diabetes educator. One study of such conflict described the perspectives of diabetes educators and individuals regarding different approaches to problem solving.[15] In this study, when the diabetes educator rather than the individual was in the role of problem solver, individuals viewed professionals as not understanding their difficulties and as unable to help them resolve problems. In contrast, when both the professional and the individual agreed that the individual ought to take the problem-solver role, mutuality and the potential for supportive change by the individual were fostered. A model of the problem-solving conflict is shown in Table 8.4.

Use of communication methods from empowerment[18,19] and solution-focused therapy approaches[16] also facilitates maintenance of a therapeutic relationship in which persons with diabetes feel valued, supported, and autonomous. To learn more about empowerment and solution-focused approaches, see chapter 3, on motivational interviewing and patient empowerment.

Empowering the Person With Diabetes as Problem Solver

Planning for Problem-Solving Training and Intervention

The planning process for designing any training or intervention begins with assessing a patient's needs and assets, which should include an assessment of his or her knowledge, skills, and beliefs. Understanding an individual's problem-solving skills is integral to designing problem-solving training and selecting intervention techniques.

Problem-Solving Assessment Strategies and Measures

Assessing problem solving in the context of self-management education provides useful information regarding the problem-solving skills or styles of the individual. This information helps guide the problem-solving training or education. In practice, interviewing (discussed in chapter 2, on assessment) is often used by the diabetes educator to determine an individual's intervention needs; however, formal measures are also valuable. Formal measures have the advantage of standardizing the problem-solving assessment, while quantifying the patient's problem-solving ability. Problem-solving assessment also allows for outcomes measurement to determine the impact of the intervention on an individual's problem-solving ability.[20]

Healthcare educators who have the resources to conduct a large-scale self-management intervention may consider using diabetes-specific or generic measures in evaluating their educational program. However, the majority of healthcare educators intervene on an individual or small group basis and rely solely on regular clinical measures (HbA1c, body mass index [BMI],

TABLE 8.4 Conflict Between Patient and Diabetes Educator: Influence of Problem-Solving Approaches		
Problem-Solving Approach	*Professional's Perception of the Patient*	*Patient's Perception of the Professional*
Failure-expecting approach Conflict deadlocked	"Patient is a problem"	"My diabetes educator has tried to help but has not been able to do so"
Compliance-expecting approach Conflict unchanged	"Patient has a problem that we can solve"	"My diabetes educator has decided how I should manage my diabetes but she has no idea how hard it is for me"
Mutuality-expecting approach Conflict resolved; situational reflection takes advantage of a potential for change in different points of view	"Patient is a problem solver"	"My diabetes educator understands how difficult it is for me to manage diabetes and has helped me problem solve how I can control my blood glucose levels"

Source: Adapted with permission from Sage Publications Inc. V Zoffman, M Kirkevold, "Life versus disease in difficult diabetes care," *Qual Health Res* 15, no. 6 (2005): 758.

blood pressure, blood lipids, etc) and self-administered questionnaires to assess impact and outcomes.

Diabetes-Specific Measures

A majority of studies examining associations between problem solving and diabetes self-management behaviors or blood glucose control have used diabetes-specific measures.[10,20-24] These measures can be administered in different formats (interviews, questionnaires), include various response formats (multiple choice, open-ended, Likert scales), and address different content (diabetes-specific knowledge-based problem solving, specific problem-solving style or ability).

Diabetes-Specific Problem-Solving Training

Research studies have used a variety of methods to train individuals in diabetes-specific problem-solving techniques. Some of these techniques include the use of visual media,[25-27] computer-based education,[28,29] and discussion group formats.[30,31] Interventions have also been conducted in a variety of different settings that include routine DSME classes,[32] diabetes summer camps,[25,33] and primary care offices.[28,34] Some studies have incorporated problem solving as part of a more comprehensive intervention approach,[35,36] while others have focused on problem-solving skills training or problem resolution as the core intervention.

Problem Solving in Group Settings

In many ways the characteristics of working with a group are similar to the characteristics of working with individuals: The educator builds rapport, answers questions, and helps the patient develop and implement goals. But in a group setting, the patient, the educator, and the group help evaluate the goals.

In some cases, the group setting may be the first time the educator meets the patient; however, an individual assessment should still be completed. This can be done before the class starts or in a telephone conversation before or after the group class; the patient could also complete an assessment form and bring it to class. The educator should know about each patient in order to individualize the group class and meet the needs of all participants.

Using an exercise, such as in the example below, at the beginning of the group program can be an effective tool for determining diabetes knowledge gaps among the group members.

Example: Game to Identify Knowledge Deficit

At the beginning of the class, the diabetes educator can play a game similar to Jeopardy!® with the group members. The members answer questions about diabetes and obtain a score. At the end of the class or course the game is repeated and the scores are compared as an outcome measurement tool. The educator can then identify, on the assessment tool, the lack or gain in cognitive knowledge.

The group quiz game allows the entire group to identify problems and then help solve them. The educator can develop exercises or activities that allow him or her to learn things about the patients and that help him or her revise the teaching plans for that individual or group.

Remember—a test or quiz only measures knowledge, not skills or attitudes.

Another problem-solving tool that can be effective in one-on-one settings as well as group settings is a decision tree. A decision tree is a graphical representation of all possible outcomes of a decision. The purpose of the decision tree is to show how the user's initial decision will impact later outcomes.

In the example in Figure 8.1, the person with diabetes doesn't want to take his medications. Rather than telling him why he needs to take the medications, the educator creates a decision tree with him so he can see, step-by-step, the consequences of a decision not to take his medications. The decision tree in Figure 8.1 starts with the question "Should I take meds?"

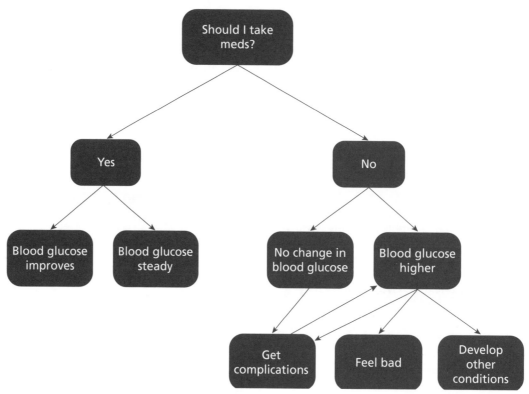

FIGURE 8.1   **Decision Tree: Should I Take Meds?**

In Figure 8.2, the educator is using the decision tree tool to work with a patient who does not want to monitor her blood glucose.

Special Considerations for Problem Solving

One reason problem solving is considered to be among the most difficult skills to teach and learn is that it is influenced by a number of factors. These factors should be considered when planning or implementing problem-solving-based education.

Factors That Influence Problem Solving

1. Cognitive impairment: Because problem solving is a cognitive skill involving knowledge, some individuals may not understand enough to solve problems independently. These patients may require the diabetes educator or their support structure to develop solutions to their problems.

2. Age: Children and adolescents solve problems differently, and problem-solving efforts should be aligned with the maturity level and cognitive development of each individual. There is no one right answer for each age group. The educator should work with the child, family, and support structure and healthcare team to decide what will work best for each child.

3. Age: Older adults may have multiple physical conditions and psychosocial conditions to manage, in addition to diabetes, which may further complicate their lives. This may make problem solving more difficult and sometimes frightening. End-stage-of-life issues may result in family conflicts and confusion. Patients should always be made aware and have input into decisions involving their care, even if they cannot participate fully.

4. Education: Higher levels of educational attainment or literacy and numeracy do not necessarily mean the person has good problem-solving skills. It is important to evaluate each individual

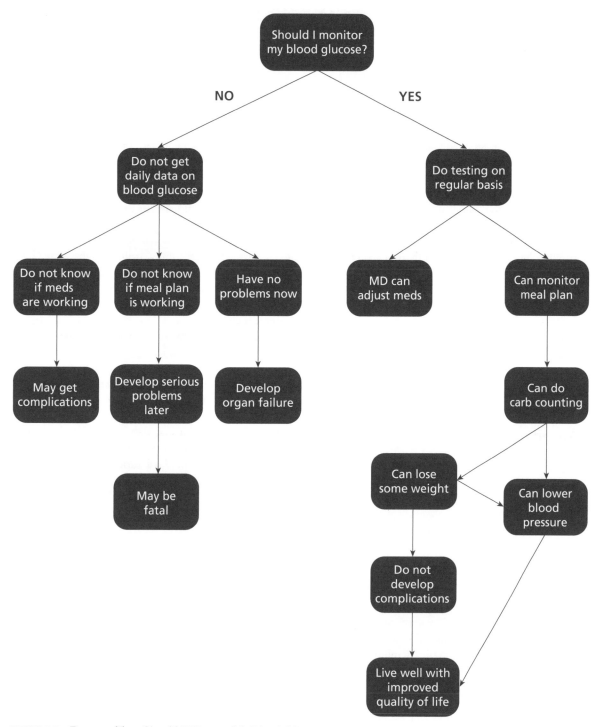

FIGURE 8.2   **Decision Tree: Should I Monitor My Blood Glucose?**

patient's ability to comprehend knowledge about their diabetes as well as their willingness and ability to address the problems and issues involved.

5. Cultural issues: To date, neither the diabetes scale nor intervention studies have examined whether diabetes-related problem-solving differences are related to ethnicity or culture. The educator should remember that factors including cultural appropriateness, education, and literacy should guide selection of strategies and materials for best outcomes.

American Association of Diabetes Educators©

Case: Pharmacotherapy Nonadherence Due to Beliefs

RC is a 68-year-old African-American man who was diagnosed with type 2 diabetes 3 years earlier. He was prescribed medications for diabetes and for hypertension at that time. RC stopped taking all the medications over 2 years ago because, as he said, "they make me sick." He also has not returned to see the internist who was treating his diabetes since he stopped taking the medications. A cardiologist referred RC for counseling and education due to poorly controlled diabetes and hypertension and refusal to take his diabetes and antihypertensive medications. RC was treated surgically by the cardiologist 6 years earlier for congestive heart failure stemming from a congenital heart defect. RC felt he had done a good job of controlling his health independently by making wise food choices.

Physical Assessment Results:

- Height: 68 in
- Weight: 182 lb
- BMI: 27.7
- Blood pressure: 161/81 mm Hg

Lab Results:

- A1C: 9.7%
- Fasting blood glucose: 199 mg/dL
- LDL-C: 102 mg/dL
- HDL-C: 44 mg/dL

RC reports that when he was diagnosed with diabetes, his internist prescribed oral medications for him. He was not sure what the medications were, but "the names were long" and he had difficulty finding out information about them. He reported that the medications made him feel sick, so he stopped taking them. When he told his internist of this concern, the internist reminded him of the importance of continuing to take the medications. RC then decided that he would not return for follow-up visits, since he was planning not to take the medications anyway.

He reports a family history of diabetes. Both parents had diabetes. RC's father suffered a stroke and his mother suffered a heart attack. Both are deceased. He said his father always told him to be careful about medications because they "do more harm than good." RC believes strongly, as his father taught him, that medications are designed to help pharmaceutical companies make a profit and that the properties of medication and the side effects are harmful and should be avoided. RC does not believe that medications are good for the human body.

RC states that he controls his diabetes and blood pressure through healthy foods and natural supplements. He reports that he does not add salt to foods. He shops for low-salt versions of foods like crackers and snacks. For breads, he relies on wheat and whole grains. RC does the cooking in his household. He often cooks large meals for his son and for neighbors, but he does not eat them "because I'm not supposed to have all that fried food." He often makes himself his favorite meal, spaghetti and meat sauce. He cooks with olive oil, prepares spaghetti sauce from a jar, and usually uses ground turkey instead of ground beef. He doesn't eat fresh fruits and vegetables, but buys canned vegetables that he cooks with seasoning salt for flavor. He eats canned fruits in light syrup. His weakness is candy bars, which he craves in the evenings. He states that he generally is able to resist his craving, but he keeps a few bars in his nightstand drawer in case he needs extra energy.

RC quit smoking 6 years earlier when diagnosed with congestive heart failure. He has arthritis that limits his ability to do rigorous exercise, but he does get physical activity through routine walking. He doesn't own a car, so getting from one point to another always involves some walking—either to and from the bus or to and from the destination itself. He feels confident that with his healthy eating and his walking he can control his health without medication. He says, "What I can't do, I will turn over to God."

RC is divorced and lives with his adult son. He is retired from his job in a steel factory. He completed education through the tenth grade and reads at a sixth-grade level, assessed using the Wide Range Achievement Test (WRAT-3). RC has some vision problems and needs to read materials in a very large-print format.

RC feels very confident that he is on the right track. He is hopeful about his ability to take control of his health. He states that he plans to live to see his 100th birthday. The cardiologist wants to see RC learn more about behavioral methods for controlling his blood glucose and blood pressure. He also hopes RC will return to see an internist, who will resume medications if RC's metabolic control has not shown any improvement in 3 to 6 months' time.

Questions for Consideration

1. RC is disengaged from a problem-solving process because he feels he is already on the right track and doing a good job. Moreover, although his diabetes educator considered his refusal to take medication a problem, RC does not. Using components of the problem-solving model, how might you select ways to reengage him?

Assess Diabetes-Specific Knowledge

RC's level of control does not match his stated understanding of diabetes and health behaviors—or his goal of seeing his 100th birthday. The discrepancy is an opportunity to establish that there is a problem to be worked on. What can be done? To help him evaluate whether he is fully on the right track and identify goals to work on, review target numbers for A1C, blood pressure, and BMI. Have him compare his current results with those targets. Ask if he knows why it is important for his numbers to be close to target. Share the connection between being in the target range and diabetes outcomes/complications; emphasize the importance of diabetes and blood pressure control for his heart. Provide information on how—and what—medications can help. Keep in mind that factors such as reduced literacy and difficulty seeing may have impeded his understanding of health information he received previously. Make sure wording and materials are at or below a sixth-grade reading level and in large-print format.

Assess Problem-Solving Skills

Problem solving can be introduced as a self-management tool that will help RC figure out what's going on and what he can change. What can be done? Help RC look at his current approach to dealing with his diabetes self-management (rational/logical, impulsive, careless, or avoidant). Reinforce that taking a logical, step-by-step approach will help him make the best decisions regarding his health and self-management behaviors.

Assess Problem-Solving Motivation

What can be done? Connect controlling his diabetes and blood pressure to his goal of living to see his 100th birthday. Reinforce that problem solving is an opportunity for him to work on new tools for managing his diabetes—ones that could give him a better shot at reaching his goal.

Discuss Transfer of Past Experience/Learning

RC has learned quite a bit about diabetes and managing diabetes from his parents and from his experiences. Unfortunately, what he has learned is likely to maintain suboptimal self-management. This is an opportunity for RC to look at what he learned from his parents' situations and what happened to them. What can be done? Encourage him to learn from both his parents' experiences and his own experiences so that his outcome will be different from theirs. Encourage him to think about modifying those things that have not been working as well as he thought.

2. Identifying the problem and where to begin to make changes can be clarified by breaking his situation down into level 1, level 2, and level 3 problems. What would be the most immediate problems at each level?

Level 1

- Suboptimal blood glucose control, elevated blood pressure control

Level 2

- Desire not to take medication
- Suboptimal medical follow-up
- Some unhealthy eating patterns

Level 3

- Identify differences regarding the issue of medication taking.
- Although RC has stopped adding table salt to foods, he continues to have a high sodium intake through canned and jarred foods and seasonings.
- He is consuming more carbohydrate from canned fruit than he was aware of and keeps candy bars readily available for when he has cravings.

Barriers

- Personal: Beliefs about taking medications and about canned sodium in foods; likes candy bars
- Interpersonal: Cooks for others and they like fried foods; lack of communication or follow-up with internist
- Environmental: Support people don't focus on his needs. The educator needs to include family in DSME classes.

3. Considering the 3 levels of problems can help clarify goals to be set. Level 1 goals were stated in the referral (improvement in control of blood glucose and blood pressure in 3 to 6 months). Level 2 has 3 areas for goals (medication taking, appointment keeping, and healthy eating). How might you help RC set level 2 goals?

- Have him choose which level 2 problem he is willing to work on first.
- Help him set a goal for the problem that is specific, easily measured, and realistic. (See chapter 2 for more on goal setting.) Give information about label reading and discuss the sodium content of canned food as opposed to frozen or fresh food.

(continued)

Case: Pharmacotherapy Nonadherence Due to Beliefs (continued)

4. Discuss with RC what he might want to change to meet his goal of living a long life.

   - Help him identify what would give him the biggest payoff and motivate him to keep going
   - Help him consider what he is most confident about being able to do
   - Discuss his choices to help meet his overall goal, and let him identify what he can do given new facts about food and medications

5. How might you help RC generate alternative solutions?

   - Have him brainstorm as many ideas as possible, without worrying about whether they will work, and then add additional ideas he might not have thought of. Then ask him what worked/did not work before.

6. How might you help RC select an alternative to try?

   - Have him consider what is most likely to work (stress desired outcomes while minimizing undesired outcomes) and to have the biggest payoff for his efforts
   - Have him consider what is most doable and what he feels most confident about trying

7. How would you help RC evaluate the outcome of his goals?

   - Ask him what would be a sign that he was achieving some success with his goals and what would be a sign that he was not achieving his goals?
   - Have him keep a record of what he is trying and the outcomes; use worksheets to help RC commit to his chosen action plan and then evaluate whether it worked and why.

8. How would you plan a follow-up for RC?

   - See him for follow-up appointment(s) preferably through completion of all identified goals, but at least through completion of the first identified goal. Ideally, follow-up visits would extend over the 3- to 6-month time frame stated in the referral.
   - Use the time between follow-up visits to make check-in phone calls for him to report on progress or reevaluation.
   - If possible, between visits have him fax worksheets that document what he is working on and the outcomes of those efforts.

Summary

In this chapter, you learned that problem solving is defined as "a learned behavior that includes generating a set of potential strategies for problem resolution, selecting the most appropriate strategy, applying the strategy, and evaluating the effectiveness of the strategy."[3]

Problem-solving techniques can be used to overcome problems and barriers encountered in day-to-day self-management, especially those that may have several possible solutions. However, direct instruction should be used for problems where the patient must follow a specific course of action.

Prior to problem solving with a patient, the educator should have a conversation with the patient in order to assess what he or she is doing well and what problems and barriers are affecting the patient's self-management. Problems fall into 1 of 3 levels: clinical markers and emergencies, problematic self-care behaviors, and problems impacting self-management. It is essential to identify and understand the barriers in order to better comprehend the nature of the patient's self-care problems. Barriers fall into 3 broad categories: personal, interpersonal, and environmental.

Another approach to problem solving is the decision tree. This may be useful and can be more engaging and fun to do with patients. It is also a skill that may help the diabetes educator make decisions about their diabetes education program, job, and indeed their own life.

Once problems and barriers are identified, patients and providers should collaborate to prioritize them based on importance and readiness to change. Identified problems require action by the patient, action by the provider, or collaborative action by both.

Information gathered from the patient (eg, personal, interpersonal, and environmental barriers) can be used to design a tailored, solution-focused approach to problem solving. It may be helpful to use a motivational interviewing style in counseling patients in problem solving.

Many diabetes educators work with patients in group settings. It can be challenging to work with several patients at once; however, by establishing rapport with the group and effectively facilitating discussion, groups can feel empowered by having the opportunity to be the experts. As an individual presents a problem, other group participants can weigh in and learn to find their own answers/solutions.

In order to provide effective care for either individuals or groups, it is important to take into account several factors that affect the cognitive process of problem solving, such as cognitive impairment, age, education, cultural issues, and urgent situations. Being aware of these factors will help the healthcare educator plan the most effective problem-solving counseling interventions.

Problem solving is not a onetime event. It is a complex, fluid process that involves active engagement from both the patient and the diabetes educator. What makes problem solving a unique behavior is that it cuts across all AADE7 Self-Care Behaviors™, which is why it is such an important skill for patients to master in order to better manage their diabetes.

Focus on Education

Teaching Strategies

↷ **When to use problem solving?** Problem solving is best used when there are a variety of options or courses of action from which to choose. Patients will appreciate a collaborative approach that fits with their preferences, lifestyle, and goals. Remember, it is their life.

↷ **Interviewing techniques.** Use a variety of interviewing techniques and skills to identify problems and barriers that will be the focus of problem solving. Identify the problem-solving ability of the individual—for example, by role playing or discussing alternatives to real-life situations. Trying new techniques like games and exercises to assess patients instead of formal interviewing sessions can be more interesting for you as well as the patient. It can be useful in assessing your own classes and teaching techniques as well as patient knowledge.

↷ **Techniques for empowering the patient.** Work with the patient's goals, not just the diabetes educator's goals. Assist patients with identifying what is most important to them and setting realistic goals that fit with their priorities. Make sure you know how to create and set goals that are measurable, realistic, sustainable, and clear. Goals should be attainable and meaningful; avoid setting goals that are impossible to reach. Empower the patient by building on successes.

↷ **Tailored approaches to problem solving.** Approaches need to fit the capability and preference of the individual. Using motivational interviewing styles and skills can help the patient feel more empowered and competent. A patient who believes that the educator is supportive and truly understands him or her is more apt to work to solve problems.

↷ **Patient-focused.** The patient knows the diabetes educator cares about him or her and sometimes, in an effort to please, will not always tell the truth. If the patient does not achieve the goals that were set or continue the activities he or she was taught, the goals can be reevaluated. Patients should be told that they are in control of their lives and that the educator's job is to provide them all the information they need to make decisions that work for them to succeed in their diabetes self-management.

Messages for Patients

↷ **Problem solving is a learned skill.** Through practice, discussing alternatives, and brainstorming solutions, you can develop effective problem-solving skills.

↷ **Identifying potential problems and the variety of possible solutions takes time.** To broaden possible solutions, discuss, role-play, and consider the experiences of others (caregivers, for example) and the different approaches they may offer. This collaboration will strengthen problem-solving skills when unusual situations are present, such as traveling, rotating work schedules, snowstorms, illness, and other situations that alter the daily routine.

Health Literacy

↷ **Patient-focused education versus content-driven teaching.** People with diabetes need to learn new information and skills by a method that allows them to retain the content and apply it in practice. Patient-focused methodology allows patients to interpret the content/information in their own way. Patients need to internalize the information and come up with their own strategies to implement it. In order to internalize the information, patients need to have the opportunity to hear it, think about it, and verbalize their understanding of the information.

↷ **What can patients teach educators?** A traditional "noncompliant" patient knows why he or she was not able to implement or do what he or she should be doing. It is counterproductive for the educator to keep on teaching the same information in the same way while knowing that it does not work for that patient. The educator should ask patients the following questions: What do you think you can do to . . . ? What might you have done differently to . . . ? What are you going to do about this challenge . . . ? How will you know if you have succeeded with this task . . . ?

↷ **Educator versus facilitator.** Diabetes educators need to teach patients information that they need to know in order to manage their diabetes. As facilitators, educators assist in making the learning process easier. They need to navigate the teaching process, focus on the patient's agenda, and give the patient an opportunity to process the content. It is not about educators and what they know, but about patients and what they know and are willing to learn.

↷ **Education is all about retention and application of information.** When working with patients, information needs to be explored by answering the questions what, why, and how. People learn best when they practice, perform, and work with new knowledge, skills, and attitudes. Self-reflection is also an important part of learning. A follow-up visit should allow patients to verbalize what they have done, how they feel about it, and what their strategy is to keep the momentum.

Focus on Practice

↷ **The diabetes education delivery systems need to align with the assumption of andragogy, or the art and science of helping adults learn[37]:**

- *Changes in self-concept:* As people develop with age, so does their perception on life and self-care. People with diabetes need to be given continuous opportunities to self-reflect on existing circumstances and how diabetes fits within them.
- *The role of experience:* As people mature they define who they are by their environment at that time. They may be influenced by their coworkers, church, children, or financial status, as well as factors such as well-being, health, and pain management.
- *Readiness to learn:* As people mature, their perspective on learning progresses from "ought to" because of their biological and academic development to "need to" because of the development phases they are approaching in their roles as workers, spouses, parents, leaders, leisure time users, and so forth.
- *Orientation to learning:* Most of the learning among children is subject-centered, whereas among adults it is problem-centered.

References

1. Bonnet C, Gagnayre R, d'Ivernois JF. Learning difficulties of diabetic patients: a survey of educators. Patient Educ Couns. 1998;35(2):139-47.

2. Bonnet C, Gagnayre R, d'Ivernois JF. Difficulties of diabetic patients learning about their illness. Patient Educ Couns. 2001;42(2):159-64.

3. Mulcahy K, Maryniuk M, Peeples M, et al. Diabetes self-management education core outcomes measures. Diabetes Educ. 2003;29(5):790-1.

4. King EB, Schlundt DG, Pichert JW, Kinzer CK, Backer BA. Improving the skills of health professionals in engaging patients in diabetes-related problem solving. J Contin Educ Health Prof. 2002;22(2):94-102.

5. Hill-Briggs F, Cooper DC, Loman K, Brancati FL, Cooper LA. A qualitative study of problem solving and diabetes control in type 2 diabetes self-management. Diabetes Educ. 2003;29(6):1018-28.

6. Ciechanowski PS, Katon WJ, Russo JE. Depression and diabetes: impact of depressive symptoms on adherence, function, and costs. Arch Intern Med. 2000;160(21):3278-85.

7. Hill-Briggs F, Gary TL, Hill MN, Bone LR, Brancati FL. Health-related quality of life in urban African Americans with type 2 diabetes. J Gen Intern Med. 2002;17(6):412-9.

8. Schoenberg NE, Drungle SC. Barriers to non-insulin dependent diabetes mellitus (NIDDM) self-care practices among older women. J Aging Health. 2001;13(4):443-66.

9. Thomas AM, Peterson L, Goldstein D. Problem solving and diabetes regimen adherence by children and adolescents with IDDM in social pressure situations: a reflection of normal development. J Pediatr Psychol. 1997;22(4):541-61.

10. Lawton J, Ahmad N, Hanna L, Douglas M, Hallowell N. 'I can't do any serious exercise': barriers to physical activity amongst people of Pakistani and Indian origin with type 2 diabetes. Health Educ Res. 2006;21(1):43-54.

11. Samuel-Hodge CD, Headen SW, Skelly AH, et al. Influences on day-to-day self-management of type 2 diabetes among African-American women: spirituality, the multi-caregiver role, and other social context factors. Diabetes Care. 2000;23(7):928-33.

12. Kanzer-Lewis G. Ten Steps to Better Living With Diabetes. Alexandria, Va: American Diabetes Association; 2008:18.

13. Taylor C. Problem solving in clinical nursing practice. J Adv Nurs. 1997;26(2):329-36.

14. Taylor C. Clinical problem-solving in nursing: insights from the literature. J Adv Nurs. 2000;31(4):842-9.

15. Zoffmann V, Kirkevold M. Life versus disease in difficult diabetes care: conflicting perspectives disempower patients and professionals in problem solving. Qual Health Res. 2005;15(6):750-65.

16. Davis ED, Vander Meer JM, Yarborough PC, Roth SB. Using solution-focused therapy strategies in empowerment-based education. Diabetes Educ. 1999;25(2):249-7.

17. D'Zurilla TJ, Nezu AM. Problem-Solving Therapy: A Social Competence Approach to Clinical Intervention. 2nd ed. New York: Springer Publishing Co; 1999.

18. Anderson RM, Funnell MM, Barr PA, Dedrick RF, Davis WK. Learning to empower patients: results of professional education program for diabetes educators. Diabetes Care. 1991;14(7):584-90.

19. Anderson B, Funnell MM. The Art of Empowerment: Stories and Strategies for Diabetes Educators. Alexandria, Va: American Diabetes Association; 2000.

20. Glasgow RE, Toobert DJ, Barrera M Jr, Strycker LA. Assessment of problem-solving: a key to successful diabetes self-management. J Behav Med. 2004;27(5):477-90.

21. Johnson SB, Pollak RT, Silverstein JH, et al. Cognitive and behavioral knowledge about insulin-dependent diabetes among children and parents. Pediatrics. 1982;69(6):708-13.

22. Cook S, Aikens JE, Berry CA, McNabb WL. Development of the diabetes problem-solving measure for adolescents. Diabetes Educ. 2001;27(6):865-74.

23. Hill-Briggs F, Yeh HC, Brancati FL. Development of the diabetes problem-solving scale. Ann Behav Med. 2005;30 Suppl:S-091.

24. Hill-Briggs F, Gary TL, Yeh HC, Batts-Turner M, Brancati FL. Validity of a novel diabetes problem-solving scale. Diabetes. 2005;54 Suppl 1:A471.

25. Schlundt DG, Flannery ME, Davis DL, Kinzer CK, Pichert JW. Evaluation of a multicomponent, behaviorally oriented, problem-based "summer school" program for adolescents with diabetes. Behav Modif. 1999;23(1):79-105.

26. Lucey D, Wing E. A clinic based educational programme for children with diabetes. Diabet Med. 1985;2(4):292-5.

27. Pichert JW, Snyder GM, Kinzer CK, Boswell EJ. Sydney meets the ketone challenge—a videodisc for teaching diabetes sick-day management through problem solving. Diabetes Educ. 1992;18(6):476-7, 479.

28. Glasgow RE, Toobert DJ, Hampson SE, Noell JW. A brief office-based intervention to facilitate diabetes dietary self-management. Health Educ Res. 1995;10(4):467-78.

29. Glasgow RE, La Chance PA, Toobert DJ, Brown J, Hampson SE, Riddle MC. Long-term effects and costs of brief behavioural dietary intervention for patients with diabetes delivered from the medical office. Patient Educ Couns. 1997;32(3):175-84.

30. Cook S, Herold K, Edidin DV, Briars R. Increasing problem solving in adolescents with type 1 diabetes: the choices diabetes program. Diabetes Educ. 2002;28(1): 115-24.

31. Halford WK, Goodall TA, Nicholson JM. Diet and diabetes (II): a controlled trial of problem solving to improve dietary self-management in patients with insulin-dependent diabetes. Psychol Health. 1997;12:231-8.

32. Rubin RR, Peyrot M, Saudek CD. Effect of diabetes education on self-care, metabolic control, and emotional well-being. Diabetes Care. 1989;12(10):673-9.

33. Kaplan RM, Chadwick MW, Schimmel LE. Social learning intervention to promote metabolic control in type I diabetes mellitus: pilot experiment results. Diabetes Care. 1985;8(2):152-5.

34. Anderson BJ, Wolf FM, Burkhart MT, Cornell RG, Bacon GE. Effects of peer-group intervention on metabolic control of adolescents with IDDM: randomized outpatient study. Diabetes Care. 1989;12(3):179-83.

35. Wysocki T, Harris MA, Greco P, et al. Randomized, controlled trial of behavior therapy for families of adolescents with insulin-dependent diabetes mellitus. J Pediatr Psychol. 2000;25(1):23-33.

36. Grey M, Boland EA, Davidson M, Li J, Tamborlane WV. Coping skills training for youth with diabetes mellitus has long-lasting effects on metabolic control and quality of life. J Pediatr. 2000;137(1):107-13.

37. Knowles M, Holton EF, Swanson RA. The Adult Learner: The Definitive Class in Adult Education and Human Development. 7th ed. Oxford, UK: Butterworth-Heinemann; 2011:138, 140.

CHAPTER 9

Healthy Coping

Joseph B. Nelson, MA, LP, CST
Katherine I. Nelson Ward, MPH, CHES

Key Concepts

- Understanding healthy coping within the context of diabetes helps healthcare professionals on the diabetes care team work collaboratively with individuals with diabetes, their families, and caregivers toward successful diabetes self-management.

- Mental health, stress, illness adjustment, and coping, as well as related concepts of self-efficacy, perceived control, and coping styles, are important for diabetes educators to understand.

- Successful self-management of diabetes depends on mastery of the medical regimen as well as coping with the emotional and social demands of living with diabetes.

Introduction

The diagnosis of a chronic disease, such as diabetes mellitus, is often an unanticipated life event for an individual and his or her family. Even when known risk factors exist, such as family history of type 2 diabetes or gestational diabetes, most individuals are caught off guard when they are diagnosed with diabetes. The initial response is often one of disbelief or doubt regarding the accuracy of the diagnosis.

Individual responses to chronic disease are varied and depend on multiple personal, interpersonal, and environmental factors. Personal, familial, and societal views, beliefs, and attitudes about the meaning of a chronic disease all factor into an individual's response to a diagnosis. These factors may create conflict and emotional distress that distract or discourage one from diabetes self-management. This begins the process of coping, which is continuous and defined by appraisal of and response to emotions and situations generated by living with a chronic disease.

The chronic phase of a disease or illness has been defined as the time span between initial diagnosis and a readjustment period involving various coping responses. In Rolland's Toward a Psychosocial Typology of Chronic and Life-Threatening Illness, this time span is characterized by periods of constancy, progression, or episodic change that require the individual and family to cope with the psychological and organizational changes brought about by the nature of the condition.[1] Because diabetes requires daily self-management behaviors and decision making, individuals and families may need to be guided through the coping process at each stage in order to make necessary lifestyle adjustments. The core learning outcomes defined by the American Association of Diabetes Educators (AADE) for diabetes self-management education (DSME) include the development of problem-solving and coping skills.[2] Implementing these skills helps the person with diabetes improve overall health status by overcoming barriers and practicing self-management behaviors.[2] The goal of developing coping and problem-solving skills involves regularly assessing these skills in the patient and determining whether there is a need for intervention.

Depression, Diabetes Distress, and Other Mental Health Concerns

Clinical care and research have helped us understand that people with diabetes are at greater risk for mental health issues such as depression, diabetes distress, anxiety, and eating disorders.[3-5] These issues are often mistaken for behavioral problems in diabetes; consequently, if these issues are not identified and treated, they may affect one's coping, behavior change, and diabetes outcomes. It is important that people with diabetes be screened regularly to identify whether these concerns need to be addressed.

Depression

Depression is characterized by depressed mood, loss of interest in activities usually found pleasurable, poor energy, difficulty concentrating and sleeping, appetite problems, and, often with diabetes, difficulty in following through with self-management behaviors. The assessment of depression is complicated by the fact that the neurovegetative signs of depression are very similar to symptoms of poorly controlled diabetes, and, thus, depression is often confused with diabetes distress. For example, an individual with diabetes who is depressed will probably not be able to engage in healthy diabetes behaviors. Assessment of diabetes-specific distress can be clarified by having a clinical conversation or by using the Diabetes Distress Scale.[6-9] Due to recent research that indicates a bidirectional relationship between diabetes and depression, the need to assess and offer treatment for depression is essential.[10]

Different types of depression include dysthymia, a low-grade depression that affects care but is usually not disabling, and major depressive disorder (MDD), which is often disabling and highly likely to make life with diabetes very difficult. Seasonal affective disorder (SAD) is cyclic, and individuals may be more depressed during certain times of the year, which can affect diabetes care during those times.

Often in conversation the diabetes educator may sense that the patient is experiencing "the blues" or that the patient is not feeling well. At times "the blues" can be normal, but unless the educator asks, it can be difficult to discern whether the patient is experiencing a temporary down period or if it is a more serious, longer

term problem. If this down period is related to diabetes distress, the educator might be able to help the patient use the time to problem solve the issues. If it appears more complicated and possibly related to depression, the Patient Health Questionnaire-2 (PHQ2) could be used to conduct a preliminary screening for depression. The PHQ2 asks the following 2 questions:

1. "Over the last two weeks have you been feeling down, depressed or hopeless?"
2. "Over the last two weeks have you lost interest in doing the things that usually bring you pleasure?"

Each question is scored on a 0 to 3 scale: 0 for no days, 1 for several days, 2 for more than half the days, and 3 for nearly every day. If the total for both questions is 3 or more, further assessment should take place with referral to a qualified mental health professional. Helping the patient with the referral process is critical. This might include contacting a professional or assisting in making the appointment. Keep in mind that someone who is depressed may lack the energy or focus to follow up on seeking this help, even if he or she wants to get better. Mental health professionals may suggest counseling, medication, exercise, or meditation. By helping those who suffer from depression access this treatment, the educator is helping them move closer to better diabetes management.

Anxiety

Anxiety is characterized by irrational fears that may lead to feeling overwhelmed and potentially cause avoidant behavior.[11] Some diabetes-specific issues do have a rational basis for fear or concern, such as low glucose, high glucose, or long-term complications. These types of issues are likely to lead individuals to be vigilant about how they eat, exercise, and monitor their glucose. Those with anxiety are more likely to have greater fear of these issues and exhibit more extreme behavior. Examples include someone who intentionally runs high glucose to prevent lows, or someone who ignores diabetes completely in order to not feel the anxiety related to developing long-term complications. On the other end of the anxiety continuum are those who check their glucose excessively out of fear of having hypoglycemia. Those with anxiety might also run intentionally low glucoses to the point of experiencing numerous episodes of severe hypoglycemia in order to achieve optimal glycemic control to prevent long-term complications. Brief anxiety measures can be used to detect generalized anxiety, but for diabetes-specific distress, the Diabetes Distress Scale[7] or the Problem Areas in Diabetes (PAID)[12] can be used to measure these concerns and to stimulate discussion about how one is dealing with diabetes overall.

Stress

Stress is the body's response to any demand made on it. Stress can be perceived as positive or negative. Stressors are expected and unexpected events that upset our balance. The crises of the diagnosis of diabetes and the resulting demands of disease self-management place numerous stressors on the individual and his or her family.

Stress not only affects individuals psychosocially but also includes a biochemical response in the body. The biochemical (hormonal) stress response can significantly impact metabolic control in persons with diabetes, which is why learning to manage and cope with stress is so important.

Common diabetes-related stressors occur on 3 levels:

1. Personal
2. Interpersonal
3. Environmental

Stress, whether temporary or chronic, results in physiological and behavioral reactions that can affect diabetes self-management. Behavioral responses can have a positive or negative influence on eating, testing, and exercise self-care activities. The consequence will have an impact on physiological measures like glucose control as well as psychosocial well-being.

Table 9.1 offers helpful questions in screening for depression and diabetes distress. Referring patients to appropriate and qualified mental health professionals may be necessary after you have covered these questions.

Diabetes, Drugs, and Alcohol

It would seem obvious that a metabolic disease like diabetes mixed with mind- and body-altering substances would be counteractive to self-care. The temptation for people who have diabetes is no less than

TABLE 9.1   Diabetes-Related Stress, Depression, and Anxiety Disorders: Informal Screening Questions
Depression
In the past 2 weeks, did you consistently feel depressed or down?
Have you had difficulty with feeling sad or blue?
Has your mood interfered with taking care of your diabetes?
Anxiety Disorders
Anxiety
What concerns do you have about your diabetes?
Tell me about the aspects of diabetes you worry about.
Avoidance
What parts of your diabetes self-care are the hardest for you to do?
Are there situations or activities you avoid because of your diabetes?
Fear
What is scary about diabetes for you?
Are there things about diabetes that frighten you?
Worry
What do you worry about regarding your diabetes?
Tell me some of the thoughts that run through your head about diabetes.
Diabetes-Related Stress
Identification of Specific Stressors
What drives you crazy about your diabetes?
Describe your typical day for me, starting when you wake up and ending when you go to sleep. What stressors do you face on a typical day?
Assessment of Stress Levels
How high has your stress level been since our last appointment?
On a scale from 0 to 10, with 0 being no stress and 10 being the worst stress imaginable, what number would you give your stress level today?
Assessment of Diabetes Burnout
Do you ever feel frustrated, fed up, overwhelmed, or burned out by diabetes?
I've noticed that lately you've had a hard time managing your diabetes. Do you think stress may play a role?

it is for anyone else who desires an altered state of consciousness. In fact, some who have not adjusted well to having diabetes may be more likely to have a desire for something different. The consequences for such behavior, however, are likely to be more dangerous. Alcohol abuse can cause difficulties with tracking blood glucose, unpredictable fluctuation in glucose, and potentially serious lows that could be mistaken for passing out. These side effects could result in hospitalization or potential death if the individual does not receive proper care. Regular and chronic abuse of alcohol can lead to overall poor self-care, lack of follow-up to diabetes treatment, and a self-destructive attitude. Significant others and families can also be dramatically affected. Alcoholism has a serious effect that is much broader than just the individual and needs to be addressed with proper treatment and follow-up.

Drug use can be harmful as well. Hard drugs like methamphetamine, cocaine, and heroin take a toll on the individual's way of thinking, significantly impacting self-care. Marijuana can also have a negative effect with unpredictable eating binges as well as forgetful behavior leading to poor self-care.

Moderate alcohol use in adults is considered to be reasonable. However, it needs to be accompanied by planful behavior that includes eating, testing, and self-monitoring of amounts. The legalization of marijuana use in some states is likely to introduce a similar recommendation for its use as well. A mindful approach to moderating alcohol and marijuana use may in fact be appropriate to avoid creating an "all or nothing" type of thinking.

For people with diabetes it's appropriate to have occasional discussions about use of these substances, particularly if their diabetes control seems questionable. Additionally, it's important to simply check in as part of the education process.

Eating Disorders

The diabetes educator needs to be aware of symptoms of eating disorders and the potential need for assessment and referral for treatment. What are the major eating disorders?

The American Psychiatric Association has 3 diagnostic categories for eating disorders[13]:

- Anorexia nervosa
- Bulimia nervosa
- Binge eating disorder

Anorexia Nervosa
The primary clinical features of anorexia nervosa are the following[13]:

- Restriction of energy intake relative to requirements

- Intense fear of becoming fat even though underweight
- Body image issues

In addition, people with anorexia may display unusual eating habits, such as cutting their food into very small pieces or not eating in front of others, and they often obsess about food.[13]

Bulimia Nervosa
The primary clinical signs of bulimia nervosa include the following[13]:

- Repeated episodes of binge eating involving a sense of loss of control and an amount of food consumed in a 2-hour period that is larger than what would be typical for most people in a similar amount of time
- Compensatory behaviors to prevent weight gain, such as self-induced vomiting, fasting, and excessive exercise and/or misuse of diuretics, laxatives, enemas, or other medications for weight-loss purposes
- The binge eating and compensatory behaviors occur on average once a week for 3 months
- Body image issues
- The behavior does not occur during episodes of anorexia nervosa

Binge Eating Disorder
While purging is not associated with binge eating disorder (BED), many of the challenges that someone with BED faces are similar to those of bulimia nervosa. Unwanted weight gain is often a symptom of the disorder. Many people live in a combination cycle of bingeing and starving, so they do not quite meet the criteria for anorexia nervosa but are still doing serious damage to their physical and mental health.

Table 9.2 lists diagnostic criteria for anorexia nervosa, bulimia nervosa, and BED.

Eating Disorders and Diabetes
Several aspects of diabetes and its treatment may make people with diabetes more vulnerable to eating disorders.[9] For example, the initial weight loss associated with the onset of type 1 diabetes followed by weight gain with the initiation of insulin may increase the risk of an eating disorder. This is

TABLE 9.2 Anorexia Nervosa, Bulimia Nervosa, and Binge Eating Disorder: Diagnostic Criteria		
Anorexia Nervosa	*Bulimia Nervosa*	*Binge Eating Disorder*
A Restriction of energy intake relative to requirements leading to a significant low body weight in the context of age, sex, developmental trajectory, and physical health. Significantly low weight is defined as a weight that is less than minimally normal, or, for children and adolescents, less than that minimally expected. B Intense fear of gaining weight or becoming fat, or persistent behavior that interferes with weight gain even though at a significantly low weight. C Disturbance in the way in which one's body weight or shape is experienced, undue influence of body weight or shape on self-evaluation, or denial of the seriousness of the current low body weight. D *Specify Type:* *Restricting Type:* During the last 3 months, the person has not regularly engaged in recurrent episodes of binge-eating or purging behavior (ie, self-induced vomiting or the misuse of laxatives, diuretics, or enemas). *Binge-Eating/Purging Type:* During the last 3 months, the person has regularly engaged in recurrent episodes of binge-eating or purging behavior (ie, self-induced vomiting or misuse of laxatives, diuretics, or enemas).	A Recurrent episodes of binge eating. An episode of binge eating is characterized by both of the following: 1. Eating, in a discrete period of time (eg, within any 2-hour period), an amount of food that is definitely larger than most people would eat during a similar period of time and under similar circumstances. 2. A sense of lack of control over eating during the episode (eg, a feeling that one cannot stop eating or control what or how much one is eating). B Recurrent inappropriate compensatory behavior in order to prevent weight gain, such as self-induced vomiting; misuse of laxatives, diuretics, enemas, or other medications; fasting; or excessive exercise. C The binge eating and inappropriate compensatory behaviors both occur, on average, at least once a week for 3 months. D Self-evaluation is unduly influenced by body shape and weight. E The disturbance does not occur exclusively during episodes of anorexia nervosa.	A Recurrent episodes of binge eating. An episode of binge eating is characterized by both of the following: 1. Eating, in a discrete period of time (eg, within any 2-hour period), an amount of food that is definitely larger than most people would eat during a similar period of time and under similar circumstances. 2. A sense of lack of control over eating during the episode (eg, a feeling that one cannot stop eating or control what or how much one is eating). B The binge-eating episodes are associated with at least 3 of the following: 1. Eating much more rapidly than normal 2. Eating until feeling uncomfortably full 3. Eating large amounts of food when not feeling physically hungry 4. Eating alone because of being embarrassed by how much one is eating 5. Feeling disgusted with oneself, depressed, or very guilty after overeating C Marked distress regarding binge eating. D The binge eating occurs, on average, at least 2 days a week for 6 months. E The binge eating is not associated with the regular use of inappropriate compensatory behaviors (eg, purging, fasting, excessive exercise) and does not occur exclusively during the course of anorexia nervosa or bulimia nervosa.

Source: Reprinted with permission from the American Psychiatric Association, *Diagnostic and Statistical Manual of Mental Disorders,* 5th ed., text revision (Washington, DC: American Psychiatric Association, 2013). Copyright 2013. American Psychiatric Association.

American Association of Diabetes Educators©

especially true in those who have body image issues or weight concerns. In addition, routine dietary recommendations may challenge the vulnerabilities of those prone to eating disorders. Such individuals may interpret recommendations in an extreme manner. For example, a recommendation to monitor intake of simple carbohydrates may be interpreted as "never eat sweets," and a recommendation to get regular physical activity may be interpreted as "exercise every day for 2 hours." Restrained eating in response to weight concerns or perceived dietary restrictions might make people with diabetes more vulnerable to binge eating. One study found, notably, that about 90% of people with type 2 diabetes reportedly developed their eating disorders prior to the diagnosis of diabetes[10]; this suggests that these factors are associated with related binge eating disorders even in the absence of diabetes.

Over time some individuals with type 1 diabetes learn they can alter their weight through omitting insulin injections or reducing the amount they take, and thereby discover a unique way to purge. This is often referred to as "diabulimia." While not accepted in the fifth edition of the Diagnostic and Statistical Manual of Mental Disorders as a specific eating disorder, it clearly meets the criteria. This is especially true when used in combination with bingeing behavior. The consequences can be quite dramatic, with an increased risk of hospitalization from diabetic ketoacidosis (DKA) and the risk of chronic complications. The elevated glucose levels also contribute to difficulty in performing daily tasks and an increased risk of depression. Diabulimia is also more difficult to treat because persons with this disorder experience the sensations of hypoglycemia when they begin taking the required insulin, in spite of having more normalized glucoses. They are then tempted to reduce insulin again to rid themselves of the physical discomfort of hypoglycemia and bloating from water weight gain.

Table 9.3 provides questions that can be used to screen for eating disorders in people with diabetes. Educators can facilitate referrals to qualified mental health professionals if an eating disorder is suspected.

Coping

Successful self-management of diabetes depends on mastery of the medical regimen as well as coping

TABLE 9.3   Eating Disorders: Informal Screening Questions

Weight Concerns
  How do you feel about your weight?
  Do you think you are overweight or worry about becoming overweight?
  Do you avoid getting on the scale?
  Would you weigh yourself in front of others?

Body Image Issues
  How do you feel about your appearance? Weight? Shape? Body size?
  What is your ideal body weight?

Binge Eating
  Are there certain foods you try to totally avoid eating? (Ask for details.)
  How often do you binge eat? (May need to define.)
  Describe your last binge episode.
  Do you ever feel as though you cannot control your eating?

Compensatory Behaviors
  Have you ever induced vomiting or taken laxatives, diuretics, or enemas to lose weight?
  Have you ever reduced or skipped an insulin dose for weight purposes?
  Do you exercise regularly? (Ask for details.)

Weight History
  What was your lowest and highest adult weight? (Ask about weight during adolescence when appropriate.)
  At what weight are you happiest?
  Have you experienced any rapid weight changes? (Ask for details.)

Unusual Eating Behaviors
  Are you uncomfortable eating in front of others?
  Do you have any eating habits your friends or family have told you were unusual?

with the emotional demands of living with a chronic disease.

Illness Adjustment

The process of healthy coping involves actions that are needed to restore order and a sense of well-being. In order for self-management to occur, integration of the chronic illness has to be incorporated into the individual's self-awareness. For the patient, the question is, "How do I take this new information and apply it to what I know about my life in order to live the way I want?"

Frequently, however, such adjustment is difficult due to societal or self-imposed stigmas that are often associated with having a chronic condition. This gets at the core of an individual's personal identity.

Personal Identity

Personal identity comprises the following: the material self, the psychological self, the cognitive-affective self, the social self, and the ideal self.[14] Each of these components focuses on specific aspects of the self and is affected by coping with a chronic illness and is potentially redefined by the individual's responses. The components of personal identity are defined as follows:

- *Material self:* The physical body
- *Psychological self:* Attitudes, beliefs, judgments
- *Cognitive-affective self:* Thinking, imagining, experiencing
- *Social self:* Roles and labels
- *Ideal self:* Aspirations

Table 9.4 shows the types of questions and concerns a person with diabetes might have and to which

TABLE 9.4 Personal Identity and Concerns About Diabetes		
Component of Personal Identity	*Aspects of Component*	*Questions/Concerns*
Material self	Physical body	Individuals may have concerns or questions about their body. For those diagnosed with type 1 diabetes, the question may be: Why is my body not functioning as it should? For children and adolescents with type 1 diabetes, the question may be: How can I be "normal" with my insulin pump? For individuals diagnosed with type 2 diabetes, the question may be: Why is my body not working as it used to?
Psychological self	Attitudes	Individuals may have concerns, and questions can range from the healthcare system to the reactions of their family and friends to the diagnosis. Kids and adolescents may have attitudes about receiving help from parents, teachers, and friends. Adults may have attitudes toward accessing medical care. Ask: What do they feel toward doctors? People who have diabetes? Has anyone in their family had diabetes and what are their attitudes toward this person?
	Beliefs	Individuals may question their beliefs. Are they going to suffer the same fate as the person in their family who had diabetes? Do they believe they are different and will have a different fate? What are their beliefs about the need for them to control their food?
	Judgments	Individuals may blame themselves for having the disease. "I deserve this because I'm fat." "I can't tell anyone about this because they will treat me differently." "I can't be honest with the educator or she will know how bad I've been."
Cognitive-affective self	Thinking	Individuals may have concerns about how their diabetes will affect their plans for the future. "I have to be perfect or diabetes will kill me." "I can't be perfect so why even try?"
	Imagining	Individuals may have concerns about how their diabetes will affect their plans for the future. "I planned on serving in the military, and I guess I can't now. I might go blind." "What does this mean if I want to have children? Can I have children? Will my children have diabetes?"
	Experiencing	Individuals may have concerns about how their diabetes will affect their current activities and interests. "I have to be more responsible than everyone else." "Why can't I go to the sleepover?" "Do I have to quit scuba diving because I use insulin?"
Social self	Roles and labels	Individuals may have concerns about how their diabetes will affect their relationships with their family, friends, colleagues, or classmates. "My family is always watching what I eat." "I feel so out of control when I have a low reading." "I don't want the people at work to know that I have diabetes because they'll treat me differently." "I hate it when my children have to help me out of a low."
Ideal self	Aspirations	Individuals may have concerns about how their diabetes will affect their view of themselves. "This really changes how I see myself as a healthy person." "I hate having to depend on anything, even insulin." "This really changes how we see our son. We know he's not different, but somehow how we see him has changed."

component of personal identity these questions and concerns are related.

Further, one's cultural identity and affiliation often provide the foundation for personal identity and subsequent behaviors. Cultural identity is composed of the learned and shared beliefs, values, and lifestyle norms of a given group that have been passed down from one generation to another, which influences the thinking and behaviors of its members.[15] For instance, spiritual and/or religious traditions often foster distinct healthcare practices and beliefs across and within ethnic groups affected by diabetes. Such beliefs may cause individuals to ask why they have been burdened with the diagnosis of diabetes or diabetes-related complications despite their adherence to spiritual and religious beliefs and practices.[16] Many religions are based on a belief in a higher power, and some members believe and accept that this higher power has ultimate control over their lives.[17] Such beliefs can sometimes result in a less proactive coping style, so perceived control over diabetes self-management outcomes can be low. Educators can acknowledge the beliefs and devise strategies to facilitate a higher level of self-management.

Some cultural and ethnic groups among Asian, Hispanic, and Native American populations view illness as caused by an imbalance between the individual and the environment that may involve not only spiritual but also emotional, social, and/or physical factors.[17,18] The diabetes healthcare professional should acknowledge such views and beliefs and incorporate them into motivational strategies for DSME that will assist with restoring balance between the individual and the environment.

The Diabetes Educator's Role in Coping

The diabetes educator can play a major role in guiding a patient through coping and stress management. This role begins with assessing and identifying mental health issues early in the treatment process. Once these issues are managed, the educator can begin working with a patient to generate a diabetes self-management plan that includes various coping strategies.

Assessment

Perceptions of how to fit daily diabetes self-management into an already busy or demanding life may cause emotional distress, anxiety, or depressive symptoms. Perceptions of "fit" affect all aspects of personal identity and in particular the *social self*. Because stress responses and coping strategies are based on a complex set of personal health beliefs, perceptions, motivations,[19,20] and support relationships, it is important to assess these issues to determine how they impact the individual.

Developmental Age and Stage

It is critical to understand and appreciate how developmental stages play a role in the way an individual adapts to the demands of diabetes. For example, a school-aged child may take pride in being able to do his or her own injections even though the child's healthcare team is encouraging the parents to give the injections. A teenager may seem willing to do all of his or her own injections, but not do so when peers are present. All are normal behaviors, but without understanding this, parents can become quite distressed.

The most obvious aspect of life stage interacting with diabetes care occurs in the ages between infancy and early adulthood. This is a time of growth and change that is most dramatic for human growth physically, mentally, socially, and emotionally.

When considering the developmental challenges of the infant and toddler—trust and mistrust coupled with autonomy and dependence—having parents be the source of physical pain can challenge a positive resolution. The need exists to not only understand how the stage of development might interact with the necessary aspects of diabetes care, but also give careful thought to how the educator or parent might approach the child with awareness of these issues. This can be complicated by the fact that parents have their own feelings about their child having diabetes, which also need to be in balance so they can communicate this acceptance to the child. While some of these developmental stages can be challenges, some can be used as resources. The opportunity for a family to join together in support of the infant or toddler by changing familial behaviors can provide support for the child and the parents, ultimately strengthening the family bonds.

School-aged children's developmental focus is to be industrious, and they are interested in performing to please parents and teachers. This energy might be guided toward focusing on their diabetes and their own courage to deal with it as something positive and potentially teach others.

The teen years can be a bit more complicated, as the development task has to do with identity and intimacy. Given the very nature of diabetes, which requires a focus on the body and how it doesn't work quite perfectly, this is not exactly something of which the teen wants to be more aware. Teenagers prefer to go through life automatically, and diabetes requires far more thought than they want to give. The teen's need for growing independence and the parent's need to maintain a "safe container" for this growth to occur should be negotiated. While negotiation is not an automatic strength for the teen, it can be an opportunity for both parent and teen to get what they want—for example, "If I, as the parent, get an assurance that you, as the teen, will provide a minimum of the data I need to be comfortable, then you will get the freedom (keys, curfew, contact with friends) you are seeking." While this isn't fail-safe, it is an opportunity to work with the emerging adult. This stage can be difficult given the risky behavior common to teens. However, it is critical to keep the developmental stage in mind as a normal aspect of growing up.

Often young adulthood is an opportunity for the person with diabetes to accept responsibility for the disease and sort out how to live with it. This is also an opportunity for the educator to open a dialogue that is appropriate for someone who can take full responsibility and may be willing to look honestly at how diabetes can fit into his or her life.

Adults between the ages of 25 and 55 will be different depending on the type of diabetes as well as where they are with their overall developmental process. Each individual will be influenced somewhat differently by his or her developmental stage, and also by the physical, emotional, and social impact of diabetes.

The personal and developmental aspects of the elderly will be moderated by who they are and how they have lived their lives; overall health, complications from the disease, and degree of needed support will all have an effect. Ultimately, questions for this group are how are they feeling about their involvement in life, and does diabetes limit in any way their social world or ability to be involved in life as they would like. Their responses can influence their diabetes self-care if it is viewed as interfering or as not affecting them at all. In either case, it is important to address how they perceive diabetes and whether this perception needs to be altered.

The bottom line is that the developmental life stage will interact with diabetes. It might be negative or positive, and educators can influence this by being aware of it and encouraging those involved to use this awareness to facilitate a positive approach.

Psychosocial Factors of Social Support

Social support may be one of the most influential aspects of dealing with diabetes. Support systems may include friends, classmates, family members, significant others, and support group members. A support system that understands the demands of diabetes and is willing to provide the support that the person with diabetes requests serves a helpful purpose. A person who takes on a social support role should ask himself or herself the key question, "What does the person with diabetes want in the way of support?" Is the person with diabetes able to verbalize his or her needs clearly? If so, is the support system willing to give the person with diabetes the requested support? This type of honest communication is necessary for both the person with diabetes and the people who support him or her. Diabetes educators can facilitate this discussion.

The Family System and Related Roles and Responsibilities

Family systems vary dramatically. The system can range from being too close (enmeshed) to being too distant (disengaged). Family systems also involve levels of structure that are provided by the parents, which can range from rigid (inflexible) to overly flexible. The points of balance here have to do with levels of structure that use rules and guidelines in a clear fashion that the family understands. With diabetes it is important to have family systems that have useful structure and caring that is clear and present. Without the proper structure for a child or adult, diabetes can be lonely and very confusing.

Financial Resources and Insurance Coverage

Diabetes can be a costly disease, so it is important for diabetes educators to ask about and understand each person's or family's financial situation. Families that are struggling financially may need help accessing resources.

Process of Coping With a Chronic Disease

The stages of denial, anger, bargaining, depression, and acceptance that Kübler-Ross[21] described for the process of grief in dying are similar to what an individual facing a new diagnosis of diabetes may feel. Table 9.5 describes how these stages may appear in an individual with a chronic disease. Basic to both of these demanding life situations—living with a chronic illness or living with dying—is the process of coping. It is important to keep in mind that the

TABLE 9.5 Adaptation to the Emotional Stages of a Chronic Disease: Therapeutic Approaches		
Stage	*Presentation*	*Approach*
Denial	May question diagnosis and treatment, especially if asymptomatic. Attempts to seek alternative diagnosis or may "doctor shop."	Work with patient to help him or her see the connection between the medical data and his or her beliefs. If possible, let the patient come to his or her own conclusion. Limit teaching to survival skills and reinforcement of basic principles. Denial is a normal coping defense, usually needed until the person is emotionally ready to deal with the crisis.
Anger	Anger, anxiety, and guilt are common. Cognitive confusion results in the need for repeated instructions. Family conflict may arise. "Why me?" "I can't do that." Anger is often suppressed, and it may be important to give the person opportunities to identify it.	Indicates that awareness is taking place. Learning begins at this stage. Provide clear, concise instructions. Patients may need to talk about the existential question of "Why" and have opportunities to talk about feelings about this new issue. Reading children stories about other kids with diabetes may be helpful.
Bargaining	May involve magical attempts to cure diabetes. Compulsive behavior to "make up" for prior non-adherence is common. "If I lose 20 pounds, can I go off insulin?"	Identifies with others; group classes and support groups may be helpful. Education needs to focus on what the patient wants to know. Patient may need to have small, safe experiments to test the reality of diabetes mellitus (eg, have a treat and then test 1 and 2 hours afterward).
Depression and frustration	Can occur at any time. Difficulty establishing or maintaining self-management. Feelings of anxiety, hopelessness, and loss of control. "I can't handle this. No matter how hard I try, my blood sugar stays high." Some of this is normal; however, if it becomes protracted a referral may be required.	Patient reaches a point of resignation to diabetes diagnosis and treatment; there are no vacations or breaks. Make mental health referrals as needed. Emphasize positive changes and accomplishments but appreciate the sadness that comes with this resignation.
Acceptance and adaptation	Becomes actively involved in management plan. Asks questions and seeks more information. "I never realized this." "What do you mean by that?" "What should I do?"	Indicates acknowledgement of condition and a sense of responsibility for care/self-management. This is not a permanent state, as new challenges always come along. Grief is a cycle; expect its return.

Adapted from readings and lectures by E Kübler-Ross, M Peyrot, WH Polansky, and RR Rubin.

process of coping has no set order as to when and how each task of coping is accomplished. It is also important to note that not everyone goes through these stages.

Coping Styles

Coping styles, based on individual traits or dispositions, have been said to determine coping strategies and outcomes.[22] Individuals who adapt well despite serious stress or stressors usually possess the following[23–26]:

- Strong internal resources
- Sense of meaning and purpose
- Strong sense of confidence
- Overall hardiness
- An optimistic rather than pessimistic view

Of these coping styles, optimism has been studied most extensively and has been shown to affect behavior-change outcomes.[26] In addition to optimism, information-seeking and avoidance coping styles have also determined coping outcomes. Depending on their coping style, some individuals will need to avoid or minimize the extent of information seeking in order to cope with the stress confronting them. Initially, this can be a healthy coping response that eases an individual forward in the process. This type of coping also happens to fit with what was identified earlier as denial, a defense that helps prevent one from becoming overwhelmed emotionally. However, if continued for an extended period, such avoidance or minimizing can be maladaptive and affect diabetes self-management and related outcomes.

Problem-Focused Coping

Problem-focused coping can be characterized as a style that involves identifying various problem areas that need solutions. This often involves what has been identified as a problem-solving approach. This is a useful approach when there are specific issues that need to be addressed and a resolution that will solve the concern. This style tends to be consistent with the acute care medicine view that diagnoses the problem, identifies the best solution, applies the solution, and resolves the problem.

How to Work With This Style

The problem-focused coping style is conducive to working with a problem-solving approach. This style is particularly useful when there is a "best response" to a problem area, and it is easily taught since educators can usually help the patient identify life experiences in which he or she successfully resolved a problem. With this style, the educator may be able to do more guiding and coaching rather than directing, and this often feels very collaborative and cooperative to both the educator and the patient. Consult chapter 8 for more on the problem-solving approach.

Emotion-Focused Coping

The emotion-focused coping style can be characterized as using emotion-based decision making (ie, choosing what feels right). The patient may be doing what feels best rather than using a more thought-out, logical process. This can be frustrating for educators, who are trained to think through the problem and come to a rational decision that can be planned and measured. Emotion-focused copers may not be able to provide a clear explanation as to why they act the way they do. They will need to process their feelings about diabetes and the issues associated with it.

How to Work With This Style

Emotion-focused copers will likely need to process their feelings about diabetes before they can conduct the problem solving needed to achieve better self-management. This style requires that the educator be willing to listen to the patient and validate his or her emotions. By doing so, the educator is not confirming that this is how to make decisions regarding treatment. Rather, the educator is simply confirming that these emotional experiences are normal and that it is acceptable to have these emotions. This may open the door to a collaborative approach and invite a discussion of how the patient can use his or her emotions to work with the problem to be addressed. For example, the diabetes educator might say, "That anger is very strong. I wonder how you might use that energy to work with diabetes struggles?" The main challenge for the diabetes educator is to acknowledge the patient's emotions but not acquiesce to this style as the only way to cope with the challenges of self-management.

Information-Seeking Coping

Some educators and patients prefer the information-seeking style of coping since it is primarily a question-and-answer process, which supports the traditional roles of the diabetes educator as the expert and the patient as the student. Patients with this style may look at diabetes as primarily a disease for which there are always right answers. They often seek information online, so this may challenge the educator, particularly when the patients get poor or contradictory information from the Internet. While patients with this coping style often treat the diabetes educator as the expert, this can be a setup for the educator to simply give information and the patient to passively receive it.

How to Work With This Style

The information-seeking style is likely to be the most used coping style early in the diagnosis since most of the information will be new and the patient is more likely to be passive. As time passes, this style can become difficult if the patient does not assume responsibility and do some of his or her own thinking and problem solving. It becomes important for the educator to be prepared to not only give information but also elicit interaction and responses from the patient's perspective. By using the approaches described in motivational interviewing, the patient's involvement becomes part of the educational goal and this coping style can be used appropriately. (See chapter 3 for more on motivational interviewing.)

Avoidance Coping

The avoidance coping style is characterized as doing only the bare minimum and ignoring or blocking additional information that is beyond the scope of survival skills alone. Avoidance is often attached to the emotion-focused coping style. The avoidance of diabetes tasks and information is primarily associated with the emotional discomfort that comes with fear, anxiety, the inability to be perfect, anger, shame, or any number of uncomfortable feelings the patient may have. If the patient learns to manage the discomfort associated with these feelings, he or she will be more likely to be open to expanding the scope of his or her information base.

How to Work With This Style

Avoidance coping can be a difficult style with which to work because the mere fact that the diabetes educator may broach the topic of diabetes creates discomfort in the patient. The approach here is one of combining honesty about the issue with some work on self-soothing skills needed to help calm the patient's anxiety or fears. An open discussion of what the person is feeling is a first step in working with an avoidance coping style. It is important to keep in mind that the strong feelings the patient has are not the diabetes educator's problems to solve. These feelings are information that is acting as a barrier to the patient getting the care required. It is ultimately the patient's responsibility to deal with these emotions. The educator can listen, validate, and help show the person how to manage the anxiety associated with these feelings. Part of anxiety management can be helpful for diabetes care (eg, using breathing techniques to relax). Educators also may make a referral to a mental health professional. It is important to remember that the patient will act only when he or she is ready. If educators push too hard too soon, they may lose any follow-up with that patient.

The coping style a person uses is likely due to what has worked in the past. If being optimistic and using a problem-focused style of coping worked before, the person will likely move in that direction first. If it was helpful to use denial and avoidance to get past the early stage of fear at another time in life, the person may do this again until emotionally ready to address the issues related to his or her self-management. Whatever style of coping people use initially is not necessarily what they will continue to use as they learn to manage their diabetes. Educators need to be careful not to judge any particular style as bad or inappropriate. It is likely that most patients do not use just one style of coping. The style may change given different situations. People likely have patterns in their life of when and how they have used these different coping processes. Uncovering these patterns will be useful for the diabetes educator in planning how to work with the patient.

Stress Management

The association between stress and diabetes self-management is multilayered. The first layer has to do with the direct impact of stress on the person's glucose. It is typical for the glucose to rise during or after a stressful event. Long-term stress may also have a longer-term effect of causing problems with glycemic control. The second layer is that stress can act as a distraction, which may take away from the focus or energy necessary to deal with diabetes management tasks. The third layer is that the behaviors used to manage stress may work against optimal glycemic control. Overeating, drinking alcohol, watching too much TV, or playing video games may be used to combat the effects of stress but will not help with diabetes management. It is clear that stress has a negative impact on diabetes self-care. It will be helpful early in the relationship for the diabetes educator to discuss what stress is, how the patient usually experiences stress (symptoms the patient has), the impact of stress on diabetes, and whether the patient knows how stress affects his or her own diabetes and self-care. It is helpful to ask about the usual stressors in a patient's life and to revisit this question at least once every 6 months. It is important that the educator be able to assess for stress, help the patient identify the impact that stress has on him or her, and identify helpful methods to manage stress that lower the impact on diabetes management.

Assessing for Stress

Stress shows up in most people as the following symptoms:

1. Physical symptoms, such as headaches, gastrointestinal concerns, muscle tension, teeth grinding, fatigue, elevated glucose, lower glucose, and loss of appetite or increased appetite
2. Emotional symptoms, such as increased anger or hostility, sadness, increase in fears or anxiety, frustration with diabetes, and a feeling of just being burned out with managing the disease
3. Interpersonal symptoms, such as lack of patience, more arguments, distancing from usual contacts, lack of interest in sex, avoidance of follow-up with healthcare providers, and missing meetings

In assessing for diabetes distress, the Diabetes Distress Scale[7] and PAID[12] are useful in identifying specific areas where the patient is having difficulty.

Use of these questionnaires can also help initiate a conversation with the patient about the nature of stress and how it impacts diabetes care. These questionnaires can be given annually to keep this type of communication open and to note any changes.

Diabetes educators who don't want to use these questionnaires may assess diabetes distress by asking simple, open-ended questions such as the following:

- "What emotions have you been experiencing lately?"
- "How would you describe your energy level over the past week/month?"
- "What noticeable physical problems have you experienced lately that might be connected to stress (eg, stomachaches, headaches, or pain in the neck or lower back)?"
- "What changes in your glucose have you noted when you are under stress?"
- "Describe recent feelings of tenseness or irritability—what was the trigger for these feelings?"

All of these questions are specific to symptoms, but if the person is attuned to his or her own stress-related symptoms, a simple question like, "How has your stress been?" might suffice as an assessment. If an educator sees that stress is having an impact and the patient agrees and would like some help dealing with it, the next question is, "What are your stress triggers?" This may seem like an easy question, but as with problem solving, educators need to continue to drill down to find the origin of the stress. Since the stress associated with diabetes cannot be eliminated, it needs to be balanced. Once the educator knows what the stressor is and the current impact of the stress on the patient, the educator will have a better idea of what type of intervention will be most useful.

Physiologic Reaction to Stress

Often the physiology of stress can prevent people from dealing with the circumstance rationally. If a person is angry, heart rate and blood pressure rise and brain chemistry hormones are elevated in a way that inhibits clear thinking. The rule of thumb is if your heart rate is above 80, step away from the battle and settle down first, get your heart rate back to normal, consider the circumstance and methods to manage it, and then go back to the discussion. Because stress affects the mind/body process, learning to first lower the physical reactivity and then identify what to do about the stressor is a helpful skill for patients.

Methods to deal with physical reactivity include deep breathing, self-hypnosis, meditation, deep muscle relaxation, and biofeedback. All of these techniques have one thing in common: using the breath to establish calmness. These simple techniques have the ability to calm the brain and the body's reactivity when a person becomes stressed. They are generally simple to do, but do require practice in order to be useful. If not practiced regularly, these techniques may not be useful when someone is experiencing a stressful event.[22,23]

Another method of dealing with physiological reactivity is to do something physical, such as the following:

◆ Walking or running
◆ Swimming, riding a bike, lifting weights
◆ Yoga, tai chi, Qigong, Pilates

These activities to manage stress can have the added benefit of helping the patient manage his or her weight and the prolonged impact of diabetes on the body.

Identifying and Managing Stress

The next series of questions is designed to get at the nature of the stressor and identify methods to deal with it and what the educator can do to help.

Can something be done to deal with or eliminate the stressor? This question has implications with problem solving, and we might use a problem-solving approach here. (See chapter 8 for more on problem solving.)

It also may be as simple as identifying how to make a stressor go away by changing the situation. For example, "I'm worried about what my blood glucose is. I'm feeling a little funny." Stress solution: test blood glucose. In essence, if something can be done to change the situation that is causing stress and the person can take charge of it, then direct action is fitting here.

If something cannot be done to directly affect the stressor, can the patient change his or her mind about the stressful situation? If so, this would be a good place for an intervention called cognitive behavioral treatment (CBT) or cognitive reframing (CR).

Cognitive behavioral treatment is a counseling technique that helps the patient recognize that his or her thinking or beliefs are at the center of the stress experience. For example, someone thinks, "My friends are going to think I'm weird and won't want to hang out with me if I tell them I have diabetes." This person experiences anxiety because the belief is that this is what his or her friends think, regardless of whether there is any evidence or facts to support the belief. The diabetes educator may want to use this as an opportunity to help the individual explore alternative possible outcomes. The educator may ask, "What other reactions do you think your friends might have if you tell them you have diabetes?" The educator can ask this several times to show the person how beliefs and reaction to beliefs can change. Cognitive behavioral treatment can help the person see that internal beliefs have an impact on behavior, actions, and outcomes in different situations. As a stress management technique, CBT can be quite useful when the stressor is internal.

The following are examples of internal stressors that can be responsive to CBT:

◆ Perfectionism
◆ Anxiety over complications
◆ Fear of knowledge about blood glucose results
◆ "I can't" beliefs related to eating, exercise, blood glucose monitoring, injections, lab blood testing, or doing anything that is clearly within the capabilities of the person
◆ Internal messages of "I can't change"

Stress management process:

◆ Assess for diabetes-specific distress every 6 months
◆ Assess for general stress issues every 6 months
◆ Increase patient's awareness of stress symptoms
◆ Educate as to stress awareness
◆ Identify stressors

If a stressor cannot be changed or if a person cannot change his or her view of the stressor, the next option is to explore "letting it go." This requires the ability to accept that the stressor cannot be altered or is something that is simply out of one's control. The educator can help the patient focus on what he or she *can* do instead of what he or she can't do or change.

This is an appropriate time to seek support from a group of peers. Those who live with diabetes will from time to time feel exhausted by the effort it takes to keep doing what needs to be done. To sit in a group with others who are experiencing the same issues can be reassuring. It also may be a place to share ideas for coping with the challenges of managing diabetes. People can benefit from being in a support group where they can express themselves and not feel judged when they are struggling with self-care issues.

Relapse Prevention Strategies

Patients who have changed their behavior and intend to continue with the change need to understand that old behaviors don't go away; they simply "lie in wait" for an opportunity to return. This requires knowledge of relapse prevention and preparation to deal with temptation.

One component of prevention is self-awareness. For behavior change to occur, one must be aware of and acknowledge his or her risky behavior, such as knowing a personal tendency to overeat or smoke when stressed. Next, the patient should have a plan to deal with stressful situations—for example, having a plan to combat negative thinking with positive thoughts, or calling a friend or family member when feeling tempted to engage in risky behavior. Substituting positive thoughts or behaviors can be a useful prevention strategy.

Using these strategies, individuals who are stressed or anxious can find new ways of responding to stressors. It is important to keep in mind that these new responses may require extraordinary commitment and planning in order for patients to change their behavior, because they may be used to automatically responding in another way.

The stress management techniques described earlier are particularly helpful because the physiological arousal when stressed leads to a desire for immediate relief. Negative behaviors such as overeating, drinking alcohol, and smoking may have given the patient immediate relief from stressors in the past. Practicing and using the stress management strategies can help in reducing the physiological reaction and may also allow the person to make better choices.

The following are ways to deal with risky behavior:

- Acknowledge the risky behavior and when it is most likely to happen
- Identify what is likely to happen (ie, what is the patient's scenario)
- Identify the factors that contribute to this risky behavior (eg, stress, conflict, fatigue, hunger, being alone)
- Find ways to combat these behaviors at higher risk times (eg, alternative solutions like finding support)
- Develop a plan to follow

Considerations for Special Populations
Age: Children and Adolescents

Anxiety is the most common mental health disorder among children and adolescents in the general US population.[27] It is unclear whether youth with diabetes are at greater risk for anxiety disorders, but it is known that anxiety is associated with poor metabolic control. In addition, youth with type 1 diabetes have significantly higher rates of depression compared with the general US population.[28] Both anxiety and depression play a significant role in the ability of children and adolescents to cope with diabetes stressors. Eating disorders, such as anorexia nervosa, bulimia nervosa, BED, and diabulimia, often co-occur with anxiety and/or depression. Diabetes educators should be able to recognize the signs and symptoms of eating disorders and make appropriate referrals, as eating disorders can negatively impact one's ability to manage diabetes. (See assessment of eating disorders earlier in chapter.) Anxiety, depression, and eating disorders are serious mental health conditions that require professional psychiatric treatment.

Children and adolescents are exposed daily to stressors in school and at home, and youth with diabetes have the added stress of managing their disease. For the diabetes educator, helping youth cope with these stressors may begin with understanding the importance of peer relationships. Peer conflict has been shown to increase the likelihood of poor metabolic control among girls with type 1 diabetes, whereas positive peer interactions are associated with fewer depressive symptoms and better self-care behaviors.[29]

There are 2 mental health conditions that may affect a person's lifelong ability to effectively cope with the daily stressors associated with diabetes: attention deficit disorder/attention-deficit hyperactivity disorder (ADD/ADHD) and autism. These conditions are among the most common mental disorders in children and adolescents in the general population,[27] but there is no evidence showing a link between ADD/ADHD and diabetes. It should be noted, however, that certain ADD/ADHD medications can cause a lack of appetite, which can have significant implications for blood glucose levels in youth with diabetes. Attention deficit disorder/attention-deficit hyperactivity disorder primarily affects an individual's ability to focus, which can be quite challenging for a diabetes educator. Autism is a spectrum disorder, meaning it is a group of disorders with common features (ADD/ADHD is on this spectrum), and no 2 people have the same symptoms.[27] Autism typically affects an individual's ability to communicate and connect emotionally with others. With all of the conditions listed above, youth with diabetes and their families face several challenges of coping with both diabetes and another serious, lifelong condition.

Age: Adults

About 7% of all adults in the United States have been diagnosed with MDD.[27] Depression, which often co-occurs with anxiety disorders, affects adults with diabetes significantly more often than the general population.

Age: Elderly Adults

In working with elderly patients, diabetes educators should be cognizant of the impact of dementia and Alzheimer's disease. Both dementia and Alzheimer's disease affect an individual's memory, problem-solving ability, and control over his or her moods. Therefore, patients with dementia or Alzheimer's disease may struggle significantly with self-care behaviors. Diabetes educators may need to work with these patients in coping with their frustrations and their emotional distress. Recent research has shown that cognitive training may improve self-management behaviors in older adults with diabetes.[30]

Increasing age is the greatest risk factor of both dementia and Alzheimer's disease, with onset most commonly occurring after the age of 65. People with type 2 diabetes are at an elevated risk for developing Alzheimer's disease,[31] so it is important for diabetes educators to be able to identify early signs and symptoms of the disease among their aging patients.

Veterans

A mental disorder commonly occurring in adulthood, although it can manifest earlier, is posttraumatic stress disorder (PTSD). Posttraumatic stress disorder is more common among combat veterans than among the general population[32] and affects veterans of all ages and sexes. Studies have found a link between PTSD and diabetes, but it is unclear which one precedes the other. The comorbidity of diabetes and PTSD is especially prevalent among veterans.[33] Posttraumatic stress disorder in veterans is commonly accompanied by depression, substance abuse, or other anxiety disorders, all of which can contribute to poor glycemic control.[33]

Gender

Both anxiety disorders and MDD affect women twice as much as men, in addition to PTSD and eating disorders affecting women disproportionately.[27]

Eating disorders commonly co-occur with anxiety or depression. About half of those with BED are depressed. Women with diabetes are 2.4 times more likely than women without diabetes to develop an eating disorder.[3]

Diabetes during pregnancy puts both the mother and the baby at risk of negative health outcomes. In addition, self-management is complex and behaviorally demanding. For those with preexisting diabetes, the management of diabetes may be intensified with additional glucose self-tests and insulin shots.[34] For those who are newly diagnosed, there is the need to learn all about diabetes and its management as well as adhere to the complex daily self-care regimen. The regimen, either intensified or new, may be accompanied by emotional and behavioral challenges. To date, however, few controlled studies have focused on psychosocial aspects of diabetes during pregnancy.

The few controlled studies that have been conducted have indicated that pregnant women with diabetes, especially those newly diagnosed with gestational diabetes, may experience an initial increase in negative emotions, such as anxiety and hostility.[35] In one study, mothers with gestational diabetes had nearly double the odds of experiencing depression during pregnancy compared with those without diabetes and with women with preexisting diabetes.[36]

These symptoms often do not reach clinical levels and usually improve and return to baseline levels over time during the pregnancy and the early postpartum period.[35,37–40] A few studies have examined stress in pregnant women with diabetes. Findings suggest that women with higher levels of stress have associated elevations in glucose levels.[41]

More information on pregnancy complicated by diabetes can be found in chapter 24.

Ethnicity

Ethnic minorities commonly experience economic inequality, racism, and discrimination, all of which increase the risk for anxiety and depression. People in the lowest strata of income, education, and occupation are 2 to 3 times more likely to have a mental disorder compared with those in the highest strata.[42] Many ethnic minority groups in the United States are less likely than white Americans to seek care for mental health disorders due to financial and/or cultural and linguistic barriers, causing mental health

disorders to be underreported in many minority communities. In many cultures, mental health problems are seen as shameful, have different symptom manifestations, and are attributed to the spiritual world.

African Americans

Rates of mental health disorders are higher among the homeless, the incarcerated, children in foster care and child welfare systems, and people exposed to violence. African Americans constitute a disproportionate amount of each of those groups. While the prevalence of diabetes is higher among African Americans than among whites, the same cannot be said for common co-occurring mental disorders: There is no significant difference between African Americans and whites regarding rates of depression and anxiety.[27,42]

American Indians and Alaska Natives

American Indians and Alaska Natives have the highest prevalence of diabetes of any minority group. While currently there is little evidence linking diabetes and mental health disorders in this particular minority group, it should be noted that American Indians and Alaska Natives have a suicide rate that is 50% higher than the national rate.[27,42] Diabetes educators working with this population should become familiar with the warning signs of suicide.

Asian Americans and Pacific Islanders

Asian Americans and Pacific Islanders have a relatively low incidence of mental health disorders. However, elderly Asian-American women have the highest suicide rate among all women over the age of 65. Diabetes educators working with refugees from Southeast Asian countries such as Cambodia, Vietnam, or Laos should be mindful that PTSD is very common among immigrants from these war-torn countries.[27,42]

Hispanic Americans

Hispanic Americans are the fastest-growing minority group in the United States. On average, Hispanic-American adults are known to have very few reported mental health disorders due to resilience and good coping skills. Hispanic-American youth, however, experience higher rates of depressive and anxiety disorders, suicide ideation, and suicide attempts compared with white youth.[27,40,42]

Case: A Maladaptive Coping Strategy

LP is a 56-year-old woman who has had diabetes for 10 years. She came in to the diabetes center because her blood glucose control had worsened over the past 6 months. Her daughter, a nurse, accompanied her. LP lives alone, but her daughter lives nearby in the same city. LP admitted to poor dietary intake, skipping meals, and eating whatever was available when she did eat. While LP was reporting her dietary intake, her daughter encouraged her to give more details about what she was eating and drinking. With some hesitation, LP reported that she drinks alcohol and asked if that was a problem.

Assessment

The diabetes educator could have responded to the question by providing knowledge about how alcohol can increase blood glucose and predispose one to hypoglycemia. However, an approach that will help the educator know best what knowledge to impart and to facilitate coping will be the most helpful in understanding the drinking behavior.

- Is this something new, or did LP drink in the past?

- How much and what is LP drinking?

- When does the drinking occur, daily or episodically?

- Does LP drink with others or alone?

- Can LP recall a time when the drinking began to increase? If so, was there any reason that triggered the increased drinking?

Understanding the Behavior

One or more of these assessment questions might lead to an understanding of the issues LP was attempting to address.

LP responded to the questions, saying that in the past she only drank socially, but now she drinks when she is alone. She stated that she begins drinking in the afternoon and continues into the night, usually skipping lunch but having some supper. She stated that her drinking increased in the past year, since her husband, sister, and mother had died.

LP is clearly trying to cope, but using a maladaptive strategy of alcohol abuse. It will be important to either discuss whether LP thinks she is depressed or ask the 2-question assessment. The drinking has resulted in increased isolation and disengagement from others as well as lack of motivation for diabetes self-management. Before LP can achieve better diabetes control, she needs to deal with her grief. The diabetes educator needs to ascertain whether LP is depressed and whether she wants to change her drinking behavior. If so, LP can be referred for further assessment of her depression or alcohol consumption to identify whether she needs treatment. Discussion of her grief process may help determine whether a support group or therapy might be helpful in getting through her losses. LP should meet with the diabetes educator more frequently until optimal glucose control can be achieved and LP demonstrates she is using positive strategies for coping with her losses and diabetes self-management.

Outcomes

As psychosocial behavioral interventions within DSME, coping strategies and processes of CBT and coping skills training may help individuals achieve and, more importantly, maintain disease self-management goals. These interventions may be particularly valuable given the multiple, and often stressful, competing demands of life.

Coping skills training for diabetes self-management has been tested in adolescents with type 1 diabetes[38-40] and in adults with type 2 diabetes.[43-46] In these studies, both adolescents and adults benefited from coping skills development using the strategies of problem identification, problem exploration, and problem solving. Significant improvements in glycemic control, quality of life, and self-efficacy

and decreased diabetes-related emotional distress were demonstrated.

The report of the Psychosocial Therapies Working Group provides further rationale and evidence for the importance of assessing psychosocial factors and providing interventions that will ensure optimal psychosocial functioning for optimal health and quality of life.[47] Positive outcomes of stress moderation or elimination and modified stress response can result in restoration and maintenance of physiological and psychosocial well-being. The coping appraisal and strategies used in psychosocial interventions such as coping skills training and CBT in the context of DSME are consistent with the AADE7 Self-Care Behaviors™ and core outcomes and serve as a guide for the assessment, intervention, and evaluation of stress and coping in individuals with diabetes and their families.

Focus on Education

Teaching Strategies

⊘ **Meet basic needs first.**   Understand that basic survival needs must be met before the process of identifying stressors and barriers can take place. This is key to problem solving and will affect motivation for higher order needs. For example, the basic needs for physical comfort and safety must be met, as well as the goal of stabilizing blood glucose, before introducing higher level problems to solve. This includes appreciating the family system, acknowledging the stage of development, and determining whether the person is experiencing depression.

⊘ **Special circumstances related to the individual.** Individual, cultural, spiritual/religious, and family traditions have an impact on beliefs and practices that shape future decision making. Before introducing problem-solving and coping skills, assist individuals with identifying stressors and treatment plans for optimal coping and illness adjustment based on individual, cultural, and religious influences.

⊘ **Be aware of different focuses.**   It is critical for diabetes educators to understand the process that is typical for an individual patient or family and to do their best to work within the framework of that orientation. Whether they have a problem-focused orientation or are more emotionally focused, it is important for educators to be nonjudgmental in their approach. The overall goal is to achieve a working relationship that fosters a collaborative approach.

⊘ **Support the individual's mental health.**   At each contact, promote good nutrition, regular physical activity, and proper sleep habits and offer problem solving to assist with adherence to medication regimens.

⊘ **Seek team collaboration.**   Maintaining ongoing communication with all members of the diabetes care team and mental health professionals is crucial for the appropriate care of individuals with mental health problems.

⊘ **Regularly incorporate screening.**   Be familiar with screening tools and comfortable in initiating screening for symptoms of mental health problems during the education and care process. Be comfortable with the referral process and establish communication lines with mental health professionals.

Messages for Patients

⊘ **Start a medical regimen.**   Begin testing the basic treatment plan and ask for assistance and clarification from the healthcare team. Frequent calls, e-mails, and clinic visits are expected in the first several weeks of a new plan while comfort with the plan is mastered.

⊘ **Develop coping skills.**   Skills are developed through experience and information, trial and error. Learning coping skills is a process and can be encouraged by family, friends, and health professionals. An example of the process is problem solving: Define a problem or concern and discuss possible individualized solutions; consider the solutions and implement one plan; evaluate the plan and decide whether to modify, change, or adopt it; practice the plan. If it is working, develop a relapse prevention plan.

⊘ **Discuss disorders openly.**   Individuals with diabetes may experience diabetes distress, depression, anxiety, or eating disorders. Talking about the possibility of this and creating awareness may offer quicker recognition and allow treatment opportunities to be scheduled sooner.

⊘ **Consider mental health part of good diabetes control.**   Assessing diabetes distress and understanding how it can interfere with diabetes self-management and diabetes control may help improve the provider-patient relationship and facilitate better care. Periodically monitoring mental health and feelings is an important part of routine diabetes care.

American Association of Diabetes Educators©

→ **Seek available help.**   Persons dealing with both diabetes and matters of mental health need to know they are not alone. Help and support are available. Ask your diabetes educator for handouts or Web site addresses with information on where to find additional support. Make an appointment with a mental health professional as the need arises.

Health Literacy

→ **Health literacy and mental health.**   Health literacy includes the ability to recognize specific issues/disorders and seek mental health information; knowledge of risk factors and causes, and self-management and professional help available; and attitudes that promote recognition and appropriate help-seeking.[48]

→ **Picture stories.**   Consider using a visual approach when screening for depression or other conditions. Picture storyboards can be used with patients with low literacy skills or when language barriers are present. Picture stories are designed to be safe, impersonal prompts that allow patients to discuss difficult topics, ask questions, and obtain information. For an example, see Picture Stories for Adult ESL Health Literacy (http://www.cal.org/caela/esl_resources/Health/healthindex.html#Depress).

References

1. Rolland JS. Toward a psychosocial typology of chronic and life-threatening illness. Fam Syst Med. 1984;2(3):245-62.

2. Mulcahy K, Maryniuk M, Peeples M, et al. Diabetes self-management education core outcomes. Diabetes Educ. 2003;29(5):1-25.

3. Goebel-Fabbri AE. Detecting and treating eating disorders in young women with type 1 diabetes. In: Anderson BJ, Rubin RR, eds. Practical Psychology for Diabetes Clinicians. 2nd ed. Washington, DC: American Diabetes Association; 2002.

4. Lustman PJ, Clouse RE. Depression in diabetic patients: the relationship between mood and glycemic control. J Diabetes Complications. 2005;19(2):113-22.

5. Grigsby AB, Anderson RJ, Freedland KE, Clouse RE, Lustman PJ. Prevalence of anxiety in adults with diabetes: a systematic review. J Psychosom Res. 2002;53(6):1053-60.

6. Golden SH, Lazo M, Carnethon M, et al. Examining a bidirectional association between depression symptoms and diabetes. JAMA. 2008;299(23):2751-9.

7. Polonsky WF. Assessing psychological stress in diabetes: development of the Diabetes Distress Scale. Diabetes Care. 2005;28:626-31.

8. Pan A, Lucas M, Sun Q, et al. Bidirectional association between depression and type 2 diabetes mellitus in women. Arch Intern Med. 2010;170(21):1884-91.

9. Chen PC, Chan YT, Chen HF, Ko MC, Li CY. Population-based cohort analyses of the bidirectional relationship between type 2 diabetes and depression. Diabetes Care. 2013;36(2):376-82.

10. Petrak F. Diabetes and depression. Curr Opin Psychiatry. 2009;22(2):211-7.

11. Howe CJ, Ratcliffe SJ, Tuttle A, Dougherty S, Lipman TH. Needle anxiety in children with type 1 diabetes and their mothers. MCN Am J Matern Child Nurs. 2011;36(1):25-31.

12. Polonsky WH, Anderson BJ, Lohrer PA. Assessment of diabetes-related distress. Diabetes Care.1995;18(6):754-60.

13. American Psychiatric Association. Diagnostic and Statistical Manual of Mental Disorders. 5th ed., text revision. Washington, DC: American Psychiatric Association; 2013.

14. Dimond M, Jones S. Chronic Illness Across the Lifespan. Norwalk, Conn: Appleton-Century-Crofts; 1983:165-76.

15. Leininger M. What is transcultural nursing and culturally competent care? J Transcult Nurs. 1999;10(1):9.

16. Melkus GD, Newlin K. Cultural considerations in diabetes care. In: Childs B, Cypress M, Spollett G, eds. Nursing Care of Persons With Diabetes. Alexandria, Va: American Diabetes Association; 2005:207-19.

17. Minarik PA. Diversity among spiritual and religious beliefs. In: Lipson JG, Dibble SL, Minarik PA, eds. Culture & Nursing Care: A Pocket Guide. San Francisco: UCSF Nursing Press; 1996:11-22.

18. Still O, Hodgkins D. Navajo Indians. In: Purnell LD, Paulanka, BJ, eds. Transcultural Health Care. 2nd ed. Philadelphia: FA Davis; 2003:40-53.

19. Miller R, Rollnick S. Meeting in the middle: motivational interviewing and self-determination theory. Int J Behav Nutr Phys Act. 2012;9(25):1.

20. Deci EL, Ryan RM. Self-determination theory in healthcare and its relation to motivational interviewing: a few comments. Int J Behav Nutr Phys Act. 2012;9:24.

21. Kübler-Ross E. On Death and Dying. New York: Touchstone; 1969.

22. Lazarus RS. Coping theory and research: past, present, and future. Psychosom Med. 1993;55:234-47.

23. Antonovsky A. Health, Stress and Coping. San Francisco: Jossey-Bass; 1979.

24. Kobasa SC. Stressful life events, personality and health: an inquiry into hardiness. J Pers Soc Psychol. 1979;42:168-77.

25. Pollack SE. The hardiness characteristic: a motivating factor in adaptation. ANS Adv Nurs Sci. 1989;11(2):53-62.

26. Maciejewski PK, Prigerson HG, Mazure CM. Self-efficacy as a mediator between stressful life events and depressive symptoms: differences based on history of prior depression. Br J Psychiatry. 2000;176:373-8.

27. National Institute of Mental Health. The numbers count: mental disorders in America. Washington, DC: National Institutes of Health; 2009 (cited 2010 Nov 18). On the Internet at: http://www.nimh.nih.gov/health/publications/the-numbers-count-mental-disorders-in-america/index.shtml.

28. Kanner S, Hamrin V, Grey M. Depression in adolescents with diabetes. J Child Adolesc Psychiatr Nurs. 2003;16(1):15-24.

29. Dantzer C, Swendsen J, Maurice-Tison S, et al. Anxiety and depression in juvenile diabetes: a critical review. Clin Psychol Rev. 2003 Nov;23(6):787-800.

30. Vianna Paulo DL, Sanches Yassuda M. Elderly individuals with diabetes: adding cognitive training to psychoeducational intervention. Educ Gerontol. 2012;38(4):257-70.

31. Arvanitakis Z, Wilson RS, Bienias JL, et al. Diabetes mellitus and risk of Alzheimer disease and decline in cognitive function. Arch Neurol. 2004 May; 61(5):661-6.

32. Taneilian T, ed. Invisible Wounds of War: Psychological and Cognitive Injuries, Their Consequences, and Services to Assist Recovery. Santa Monica, Calif: RAND Corporation; 2008.

33. Trief PM, Ouimette P, Wade M, Shanahan P, Weinstock RS. Post-traumatic stress disorder and diabetes: co-morbidity and outcomes in a male veterans sample. J Behav Med. 2006 Oct;29(5):411-8.

34. Tuffnell DJ, West J, Walkinshaw SA. Treatments for gestational diabetes and impaired glucose tolerance in pregnancy (review). Cochrane Database Syst Rev. 2003;(3):CD003395.

35. Langer N, Langer O. Emotional adjustment to diagnosis and intensified treatment of gestational diabetes. Obstet Gynecol. 1994;84:329-34.

36. Kozhimannil KB, Pereira MA, Harlow BL. Association between diabetes and perinatal depression among low-income mothers. JAMA. 2009;301(8):842-7.

37. Daniells S, Grenyer BF, Davis WS, et al. Gestational diabetes mellitus: is a diagnosis associated with an increase in maternal anxiety and stress in the short and intermediate term? Diabetes Care. 2003;26:385-9.

38. Langer N, Langer O. Pre-existing diabetics: relationship between glycemic control and emotional status in pregnancy. J Matern Fetal Med. 1998;7:257-63.

39. Spirito A, Williams C, Ruggiero L, et al. Psychological impact of the diagnosis of gestational diabetes. Obstet Gynecol. 1989;73:562-6.

40. York R, Brown LP, Persily CA, et al. Affect in diabetic women during pregnancy and postpartum. Nurs Res. 1996;45:54-6.

41. Barglow P, Hatch R, Berndt D, et al. Psychosocial childbearing stress and metabolic control in pregnant diabetes. J Nerv Ment Dis. 1985;173:615-20.

42. Public Health Service. Mental health: culture, race, and ethnicity, a supplement to mental health: a report of the Surgeon General. Washington, DC: Department of Health and Human Services; 2001.

43. Grey M, Boland EA, Davidson M, et al. Coping skills training for youths with diabetes on intensive therapy. Appl Nurs Res. 1999;12:3-12.

44. Rubin R, Peyrot M, Saudek C. The effect of a comprehensive diabetes education program incorporating coping skills training on emotional well-being and diabetes self-efficacy. Diabetes Educ. 1993;19(3):210-4.

45. Peyrot M, McMurry J. Stress-buffering and glycemic control: the role of coping styles. Diabetes Care. 1992;15(7):842-6.

46. Surwit RS, van Tilburg MAL, McCaskill CC, et al. Stress management improves long-term glycemic control in type 2 diabetes. Diabetes Care. 2002;25(1):30-4.

47. Delamater AM, Jacobson AM, Anderson B, et al. Psychosocial therapies in diabetes: report of the Psychosocial Therapies Working Group. Diabetes Care. 2001;24(7):1286-92.

48. Provincial Health Services Authority. Towards Reducing Health Inequities: A Health System Approach to Chronic Disease Prevention. A Discussion Paper. Vancouver, BC: Population & Public Health, Provincial Health Services Authority; 2011.

CHAPTER 10

Reducing Risks

Ann Constance, MA, RD, CDE, FAADE

Key Concepts

◆ All people with diabetes should be knowledgeable about the tests, exams, and interventions contained within the Standards of Care, including the frequency with which they are to be performed. Inclusion and monitoring of these can help reduce risks for diabetes complications.

◆ Targeted, therapeutic goals are recommended for people with diabetes to reduce risks of complications. To best meet an individual's needs and to optimize health, these goals need to be personalized.

◆ People with diabetes should receive preventive healthcare services to maximize their health.

◆ To reduce their risks for diabetes complications, people with diabetes must be supported in learning and implementing skills that help them develop and maintain healthy behaviors.

◆ Reviewing the approaches to dealing with barriers to risk reduction is valuable to a diabetes educator's practice.

◆ Identifying and linking to other health system, community-based, or technology-driven programs or resources, especially for ongoing behavior-change support, may also assist with risk reduction.

Introduction

Reducing risks, as contained in the AADE7 Self-Care Behaviors™, means that people with diabetes implement effective risk-reduction behaviors to prevent or slow progression of diabetes complications and maximize health and quality of life.[1] One of the roles of the diabetes or health educator is to assist the person with diabetes in understanding what risk reduction truly means. To this end, those involved in diabetes education are charged with helping those with diabetes acquire the appropriate skills, identify and overcome barriers to implementation, and adopt preventive behaviors. In addition, linking people with diabetes to other sources of support and services may help reduce the risks of developing complications.[2]

The threat of complications is one of the greatest burdens that people with diabetes carry each day.

People respond to this burden in many ways. Some responses facilitate the learning process and behavior change, while others may have negative effects. The person with diabetes must be actively involved in preventing complications; therefore, the educator should revisit the person's coping strategies (see chapter 9—Healthy Coping) periodically to determine whether other types of care or support may be helpful. Ongoing assessment of a person's family and community support is also important.

This chapter discusses the knowledge content areas, skills, and barriers that should be addressed when guiding people with diabetes through behavior changes that reduce their risk for complications and maximize their health. The focus is on risk factors that people have the ability to modify. Due to the broad scope of this topic, references are often made to other chapters of the book where specific risks and approaches to reducing them are discussed in more detail.

Knowledge Content Areas

To practice behaviors that minimize the risk of developing complications, knowledge of the Standards of Medical Care, preventive care services, and ways to gain ongoing support and education is important for people with diabetes. In addition, it is recommended that people with diabetes work with their healthcare teams to develop personal therapeutic goals. To enhance effectiveness, this information should be presented in ways that engage the person with diabetes, and it should be sensitive to learning preferences, culture, language, and health literacy levels.

Standards of Care: Diabetes

The Standards of Medical Care in Diabetes provide a comprehensive list of preventive-care practices (eg, assessments, physical examinations, laboratory tests, interventions) and describe how frequently each should be recommended to all people with diabetes. The American Diabetes Association (ADA) is the primary organization responsible for developing the Standards of Medical Care in Diabetes and publishes them annually as part of the Clinical Practice Recommendations.[3] These are formulated from a thorough review of the literature and rating of the scientific evidence currently available.

The Standards of Care include information on several topics, such as the following: diabetes detection, diagnosis and classification of diabetes, prevention or delay of type 2 diabetes, diabetes care, prevention or management of complications, diabetes care in special populations, diabetes care in specific settings, and strategies for improving diabetes care.[3] While all of the information in the Standards of Care is valuable, the information that specifically pertains to reducing risks for diabetes complications is the focus of this chapter. Table 10.1 summarizes the Standards of Care relevant to risk reduction. Refer to the chapters in this text on self-care behaviors related to monitoring (chapter 7), healthy eating (chapter 4), being active (chapter 5),

problem solving (chapter 8), and healthy coping (chapter 9) for additional information.

Glycemic Control

The results of the Diabetes Control and Complications Trial (DCCT)[4] and the UK Prospective Diabetes Study (UKPDS)[5,6] have demonstrated that intensive glycemic control is associated with decreased rates of retinopathy, nephropathy, and neuropathy. This effect (known as the "legacy effect") has been shown to persist in previously intensively treated subjects even though their glycemic control returns to that of the standard treated group.[7,8] Randomized controlled trials of intensive versus standard glycemic control have not shown a significant reduction in cardiovascular disease (CVD) during the initial trial, but long-term follow-up from the DCCT and UKPDS suggests that A1C targets around 7% or below in years soon after diagnosis are associated with a long-term reduction in risk of macrovascular disease.[9,10] The results of 3 recent large trials in those with type 2 diabetes and either a history of a CVD event or a significant CVD risk suggested no significant reduction in CVD events with intensive glycemic control.[11]

Glycemic control is best gauged by the combination of results from self-monitoring of blood glucose (SMBG) and the results from A1C testing (see chapter 7 for more information on monitoring). Self-monitoring of blood glucose is most useful when individuals with diabetes learn how to use the monitoring information to assist with diabetes management. This can be reinforced by including individuals in a review of the results and showing them how the results can be used in making treatment decisions.

The frequency and timing of SMBG are based on the needs and goals of each person living with diabetes. While there are data that demonstrate the importance of SMBG in diabetes self-management, the available studies used multifactorial interventions, which makes it difficult to provide evidence to support a specific frequency or timing of SMBG.[4-6,12] It is important that patients receive initial instruction and routine follow-up evaluation of the SMBG technique and use data to adjust treatment. The Standards of Care recommend the following[3]:

◆ Blood glucose monitoring should occur before each meal and snack for people using multiple insulin injections or insulin pump therapy.

TABLE 10.1 Summary of Standards of Care*	
Test/Exam/Service	*Frequency*
Psychosocial assessment	Routine screening as part of ongoing care.
Comorbid conditions	Assess need to screen for depression, fatty liver disease, obstructive sleep apnea, cancer, fracture, cognitive changes, hearing impairments, and in men, low testosterone levels. Specifically, people with type 1 diabetes may need to be screened for celiac disease and thyroid dysfunction.
Self-monitoring of blood glucose (SMBG)	Those using multiple insulin injections or insulin pump therapy: For many, that will mean at least 6–8 times per day. Those using less frequent insulin injections or noninsulin therapies: As needed to meet treatment goals
A1C	At least twice per year if at goal. Quarterly if treatment changes or not meeting goals. Note: More timely changes in treatment can occur when point-of-care testing is employed
Renal status	Annual test to quantitate urine albumin excretion. At least once a year measure serum creatinine and use to calculate glomerular filtration rate (GFR)
Weight	Each regular diabetes visit
Blood pressure	Every routine visit
Lipids	Fasting profile at least yearly (every 2 years with low-risk lipid values)
Dilated eye exam	Yearly (every 2–3 years may be considered following 1 or more normal eye exams; more frequent exams needed if retinopathy is progressing)
Comprehensive foot exam	At least yearly
Medical nutrition therapy (MNT)	Individualized as needed to meet treatment goals
Diabetes self-management education (DSME) and support	At diagnosis and as needed following initial DSME. Note: DSME should be delivered according to National Standards for DSME and support
Physical activity plan	Assess at least annually
Immunizations	Influenza vaccination annually for those at least 6 months of age. Pneumococcal vaccination at least once for those at least 2 years of age (revaccination may be needed). Hepatitis B vaccination in adults aged 19–59 (consider administering to those aged 60 and older)
Dental care	Comprehensive periodontal examination by dentist at least once a year
Tobacco use status	As part of routine care

*Standards listed are for adults with diabetes; some standards are different for children living with diabetes.

Source: Adapted from American Diabetes Association, "Standards of medical care in diabetes, 2014," *Diabetes Care* 37, Suppl 1 (2014): S14-80.

Other times to use SMBG include prior to driving (or participating in potentially dangerous activities), when blood glucose may be low, following treatment of low blood glucose, before physical activity, when not feeling well or when ill, and at bedtime. It may also be helpful to periodically check postprandial levels.

◆ For those using less frequent insulin injections, noninsulin therapies, or medical nutrition therapy (MNT) alone, monitoring should be done frequently enough to help patients meet their treatment goals. At this time there are insufficient data to make recommendations about how often these patients should be using SMBG.

A1C testing should be conducted at least twice a year in people who are meeting treatment goals and quarterly in those whose therapy has changed or who are not meeting glycemic goals.[3]

Continuous glucose monitoring (CGM) in conjunction with intensive insulin therapy can be a useful tool to lower A1C in selected adults (age 25 years or over) with type 1 diabetes.[4] Continuous glucose monitoring may be helpful in children, teens, and younger adults, although there are less data, and success correlates with ongoing use of the device.[3]

Preventing Complications

The Standards of Care are important, but therapeutic goals must be determined specifically for and in collaboration with each individual.

Medical Nutrition Therapy

Medical nutrition therapy is a key component of diabetes management and one that can require significant time and attention (see chapters 16 and 4, respectively, for more information on nutrition therapy and self-care behaviors related to healthy eating). Food is not only a means of nourishing the body and providing fuel, but also an integral part of one's personal being and culture. Food is often closely tied to celebrations, stress, and coping.

The Standards of Care recommend that people with diabetes receive MNT as needed to achieve treatment goals, preferably provided by a registered dietitian familiar with the components of diabetes MNT.[3,13] There is also no one diet plan that is suitable for all with diabetes, so individualization is critical.[13] For children and adolescents with type 1 diabetes, the Standards of Care recommend that MNT be provided at diagnosis, and regularly thereafter, by a healthcare professional experienced with the nutritional needs of growing children and adolescents and the behavioral issues that often impact their diets.[3] The Diabetes Nutrition Practice Guidelines (NPGs), developed through the Academy of Nutrition and

Dietetics, provide information for healthcare professionals regarding the recommended process to follow when conducting MNT for adults living with type 1 diabetes or type 2 diabetes.[14] The NPGs were tested and validated by registered dietitians and are discussed further in chapter 16.

The goals of MNT that apply to adults with diabetes include the following[13]:

- Attain and maintain blood glucose, lipid, and blood pressure goals, which are individualized for each person.
- Modify diet and lifestyle to prevent or delay the development of diabetes-related complications and to achieve and maintain body weight goals.
- Address individual nutritional needs, taking into consideration personal and cultural preferences and lifestyle, while respecting the individual's wishes and willingness to change. Numeracy and health literacy levels as well as foods an individual has access to should also be taken into consideration.
- Use only scientific evidence to limit food choices and work to make eating enjoyable.
- Provide person with tools that will help him or her develop a personalized eating plan.

Weight Management

Overweight and obesity are strongly linked to type 2 diabetes. In addition, obesity is an independent risk factor for hypertension, dyslipidemia, and CVD. Moderate weight loss improves glycemic control, improves some of the risk factors linked to CVD, and helps decrease insulin resistance. However, the Look AHEAD trial, which explored the role of long-term weight control in controlling glucose and preventing strokes and heart attacks for adults living with type 2 diabetes, was ended early, after 11 years, as no significant difference in cardiovascular events was noted between the control group and the intervention group. The Look AHEAD weight loss group showed cardiovascular risk factor reduction, used fewer medications, and reported an improved quality of life.[15] For these reasons and other documented positive changes, weight loss continues to be a recommended treatment for those with diabetes or prediabetes who are overweight.

The Standards of Care recommend that body weight be measured at each diabetes visit.[3] Weight (in kilograms) and height (in meters) are measured to calculate body mass index (BMI). Weight loss is recommended for all overweight (BMI 25.0-29.9 kg/m²) or obese (BMI ≥30.0 kg/m²) adults with diabetes.[3]

The primary approach for achieving weight loss is a lifestyle change that includes a reduction in energy intake, an increase in physical activity, and behavioral strategies.[3] Reduction in caloric balance (500-1000 calories per day) results in a slow but progressive weight loss of about 1 to 2 lb per week. Low-carbohydrate, low-fat, and Mediterranean-style diets have all been shown to be effective in assisting with short-term weight loss (less than 2 years); additional monitoring of lipids, protein intake, and renal function and possible medication adjustment are recommended for those choosing low-carbohydrate plans. Physical activity should be increased gradually, working to achieve 30 to 45 minutes of aerobic activity most days (150 minutes per week). Activity levels of 1 hour per day of moderate activity or 30 minutes of vigorous activity may be needed for long-term maintenance of weight loss. Because weight loss can be difficult to achieve and maintain, the educator must work with overweight individuals in a sensitive and supportive manner. Emphasizing modest weight loss (5% of body weight) as the goal is especially important.

Bariatric surgery may be an option for adults with type 2 diabetes and a BMI >35 kg/m², especially if the diabetes or related comorbidities are difficult to control with lifestyle and medications.[3] However, the surgery does come with both short- and long-term risks. A study from the Veterans Affairs Medical Center, over almost seven years of follow-up, did not find reduced mortality in those patients who received bariatric surgery.[16] Another study found that laparoscopic adjustable gastric banding surgery seems to have poor long-term outcomes.[17]

Physical Activity

Regular physical activity provides numerous benefits to people with diabetes. It has been shown to improve glucose control in those with type 2 diabetes, reduce cardiovascular risk factors, contribute to weight management, and improve well-being.[18,19] A regular physical activity program, adapted if complications are present, is recommended in the Standards of Care for all people with diabetes who are capable of participating.[3] See chapters 5 and 17 for additional information on physical activity. The Standards of Care recommend the following:

- Adults with diabetes should strive to get 150 minutes of moderate-level activity per week on 3 or more days. In addition, they should go no more than 2 days in a row without activity.
- If not contraindicated, at least 2 days of resistance training is recommended for adults with type 2 diabetes.
- Youth should strive for at least 60 minutes of physical activity each day. Those with type 1 diabetes will need more frequent blood glucose monitoring, especially with the addition of new activity, with carbohydrate and insulin adjustments.[20]

Psychosocial Assessment and Care

People with diabetes are likely to be psychologically vulnerable at diagnosis and when their medical status changes (eg, intensification of treatment or when complications are diagnosed).[21,22] The DAWN (Diabetes Attitudes, Wishes, and Needs) study indicated that more than 4 out of 5 people living with diabetes are not adhering to prescribed treatments. In addition, at diagnosis and 15 years after diagnosis, the majority of people with diabetes were still experiencing distress linked to living with diabetes. Even if individuals are equipped with accurate knowledge and sufficient skills to reduce their risks, the ability to carry out healthy behaviors can be significantly impacted by their psychological and social state.[23]

Regarding psychosocial assessment and care, the Standards of Care recommend the following[3]:

- Assessment of psychological and social situation should be included as an ongoing part of diabetes management.
- Psychosocial screening should include attitudes about illness, medical management expectations, affect or mood, general and diabetes-related quality of life, resources (financial, social, and emotional), and psychiatric history.
- Screening for psychosocial problems such as depression, eating disorders, and cognitive impairment is needed when adherence to the medical regimen is poor.
- Incorporating psychological treatment into routine care is preferred over waiting for

identification of a specific problem or deterioration in psychological status.

Refer to chapter 8 for information on problem solving and chapter 9 for information on healthy coping. Chapters 4 and 9 cover eating disorders and depression.

Standards of Care: Complications

This section discusses risk reduction and prevention and management of the following chronic complications:

◈ Cardiovascular disease
◈ Retinopathy
◈ Nephropathy
◈ Foot problems

Preventive services of importance in diabetes care, specifically for the following, are also discussed:

◈ Immunizations for influenza, pneumonia, and hepatitis B
◈ Dental care
◈ Prepregnancy counseling

The importance of personalizing therapeutic goals is emphasized. Blood pressure and lipid levels for adults with diabetes, as well as for children and adolescents with diabetes, are summarized.

Cardiovascular Disease

Cardiovascular disease is the leading cause of mortality for people with diabetes.[24] Research studies support reducing cardiovascular risk factors to prevent or slow CVD. The following modifiable CVD risk factors are topics for diabetes education:

◈ Hypertension[25]
◈ Dyslipidemia[26]
◈ Smoking[27]
◈ Increased platelet adherence[28]

Blood Pressure   Hypertension is a major risk factor for cardiovascular and cerebral vascular disease as well as for microvascular complications including diabetic nephropathy and retinopathy.[3,29] Consequently, emphasis must be placed on ensuring that people with diabetes know their blood pressure values and how to use MNT, physical activity, and, when necessary, medication to keep blood pressure values at their therapeutic goals (see Therapeutic Goals section). The Standards of Care recommend that blood pressure be measured at every routine diabetes visit; elevated levels should be confirmed on a separate day. Goals of therapy for people with diabetes and hypertension, according to the ADA, are the following[3]:

◈ *Adults.* Treat systolic blood pressure to less than 140 mm Hg and diastolic pressure to less than 80 mm Hg. A lower systolic blood pressure (less than 130) may be appropriate for some.
◈ *Children and adolescents.* Hypertension in childhood is defined as an average systolic or diastolic blood pressure greater than or equal to the 95th percentile for age, sex, and height percentile or over 130/80 mg/dL on a regular basis and should be immediately treated pharmacologically.[3] "High-normal" blood pressure is defined as average systolic or diastolic blood pressure greater than or equal to the 90th percentile but less than the 95th percentile for age, sex, and height percentile. Treat with lifestyle measures for 3 to 6 months, followed by medication if goals are not met.[3]

Lipids   Lipid abnormalities are more common in people with type 2 diabetes than in those with type 1 diabetes or those without diabetes. Although there is less data on lipid-lowering therapy in type 1 diabetes, this intervention should be considered in those with cardiovascular risk factors in addition to their diabetes.[30] Lipid management should target lowering LDL-C, raising HDL-C, and lowering triglycerides. In addition, the 2014 ADA Standards of Care recommend that statin therapy be initiated in all people with diabetes who have overt heart disease and in those who are over age 40, do not have overt heart disease, but have one or more cardiovascular risk factors such as smoking, hypertension, history of CVD, albuminuria, or dyslipidemia.[31] The various lipid tests and their corresponding values should be explained to people with diabetes in terms that are easy to understand and that emphasize the importance of this matter. Instructions should be provided on MNT, physical activity, weight loss (if overweight), smoking cessation, and medication (if necessary) to keep lipids at their therapeutic goals (see Therapeutic Goals section). The Standards of Care recommend the following[3]:

◆ *Adults.* Adults with diabetes should be tested for lipid disorders at least annually. In adults with low-risk lipid values (LDL-C less than 100 mg/dL [5.55 mmol/L], HDL-C greater than 50 mg/dL [2.77 mmol/L], and triglycerides less than 150 mg/dL [8.33 mmol/L]), lipid assessment may be done every 2 years.[3]

◆ *Children and adolescents.* A fasting lipid profile should be drawn for all children over 2 years of age at the time of diagnosis (after glucose control has been established) if there is a family history of hypercholesterolemia or a history of a cardiovascular event before age 55, or if family history is unknown. Otherwise, the first lipid screening should be performed at puberty (≥10 years of age). If diabetes is diagnosed in puberty, the first lipid screening should be done at diagnosis. If values are within the accepted range (LDL-C less than 100 mg/dL [5.55 mmol/L]) for children and adolescents, a lipid profile may be repeated every 5 years. If lipids are abnormal, annual monitoring is recommended.[3,32]

Smoking Cessation Cigarette smoking is the most important modifiable cause of premature death for those with and without diabetes. Studies of people with diabetes have repeatedly found an increased risk of morbidity and premature death associated with the development of macrovascular complications among smokers.[33] Smoking is also related to earlier development of microvascular complications.[3]

Large, randomized clinical trials that were not focused specifically on people with diabetes have shown that smoking cessation counseling is efficacious and cost-effective in reducing tobacco use.[34] There is no reason to believe these results do not also apply to those with diabetes. Routine assessment of tobacco use is an important part of preventing smoking or encouraging cessation. However, there is currently not enough evidence to support tobacco status assessment or treatment in the primary care setting for youth.[34] The Standards of Care recommend the following[3]:

◆ Advise all people with diabetes not to smoke or use other tobacco products.

◆ Include smoking cessation counseling and other forms of treatment as a routine component of diabetes care.

The educator should address the issue of smoking cessation in a nonjudgmental and supportive way. There are many programs (eg, telephone help lines for counseling) and tools (eg, gum and patches) available to assist with cessation efforts. Special consideration should be given to assessing the level of nicotine dependence, which is associated with the difficulty of quitting and relapse. Often several attempts are required for success with smoking cessation.[35]

Aspirin Therapy Aspirin therapy has been shown to be effective in reducing cardiovascular morbidity and mortality in high-risk people with previous myocardial infarction (MI) or stroke (secondary prevention).[36,37] The benefit of aspirin in primary prevention among people with no previous cardiovascular events is controversial, both for those with diabetes and those without diabetes.[38]

Recommendations in the Standards of Care for the use of aspirin include the following[3]:

◆ *Secondary prevention:* Use aspirin therapy (75-162 mg per day) as a secondary prevention strategy in those with diabetes who have a history of CVD.

◆ *Primary prevention:* Consider aspirin therapy (75-162 mg per day) as a primary prevention strategy in those with type 1 diabetes or type 2 diabetes at increased cardiovascular risk. This includes most men >50 years of age or women >60 years of age who have at least 1 additional major risk factor (family history of CVD, hypertension, smoking, dyslipidemia, or albuminuria).

◆ *Contraindications:* People with contraindications should not take aspirin, but other antiplatelet agents should be considered.

◆ *Younger adults and children:* Aspirin therapy is not recommended for those under 21 years of age, as it is linked to an increased risk of Reye's Syndrome.[20]

When reviewing medications with the person with diabetes, the educator must also ask about aspirin use.

Retinopathy

Diabetic retinopathy is considered the leading cause of new cases of blindness among adults aged 20 to 74 years.[24] The prevalence of retinopathy increases with the duration of diabetes. In addition to targets for optimal glycemic and blood pressure control, the Standards of Care include the following recommendations[3]:

- *Type 1 diabetes.* Adults and children aged 10 years or older with type 1 diabetes should have an initial dilated and comprehensive eye exam by an ophthalmologist or optometrist within 5 years of the onset of diabetes.
- *Type 2 diabetes.* People with type 2 diabetes should have an initial dilated and comprehensive eye exam by an ophthalmologist or optometrist shortly after diagnosis of diabetes.
- *Follow-up.* Subsequent examinations for those with type 1 diabetes or type 2 diabetes should be repeated annually by an ophthalmologist or optometrist. Less frequent exams (every 2-3 years) may be considered following 1 or more normal eye exams. Eye exams will be required more frequently if retinopathy is progressing.

Women Planning a Pregnancy   When planning a pregnancy, women with preexisting diabetes should have a comprehensive eye exam and be counseled on the risk of development and/or progression of diabetic retinopathy. Women with diabetes who become pregnant should have a comprehensive eye exam in the first trimester and close follow-up throughout pregnancy and for 1 year postpartum.

The educator must ensure that the woman with diabetes receives the necessary referral or assistance for scheduling an eye exam. The educator can help prepare the woman for the eye care visit. Explaining what to expect when the eyes are dilated is important. These exams can be uncomfortable, and some individuals are reluctant to follow through with an exam for this reason. Also, the woman needs to be prepared to arrange a ride home after the exam. People can be tempted to ignore eye care, believing there are no problems because they have not noted any changes in vision. The importance of these exams in saving vision cannot be emphasized enough. Ask the woman about barriers to having an exam and work with her to overcome them (barriers are discussed more completely toward the end of the chapter).

Nephropathy

Diabetic nephropathy is the leading cause of end-stage renal disease (ESRD).[24] Consistent albuminuria of 30 to 299 mg per 24 hours (also known as microalbuminuria) is the earliest stage of diabetic nephropathy in type 1 diabetes and serves as a marker for the development of nephropathy in type 2 diabetes.[3] Persistent albuminuria of 30 to 299 mg per 24 hours is also a marker of increased risk for CVD.[39,40] Those who develop high levels of albuminuria (300 mg or greater per 24 hours) are at high risk for progressing to ESRD.[41,42]

In addition to optimal glycemic and blood pressure control for the prevention or treatment of chronic kidney disease (CKD), MNT, with protein restriction for some, and medication may be used in the treatment of CKD. The Standards of Care include the following[3,20]:

- Assess urine albumin excretion annually in individuals who have had type 1 diabetes for 5 years or more and in all individuals with type 2 diabetes, beginning at diagnosis. Continued monitoring of urine albumin excretion is recommended to track the response to therapy and progression of the disease.
- Measure serum creatinine at least annually in all adults with diabetes. Use serum creatinine level to calculate estimated glomerular filtration rate (GFR) and stage level of CKD, if present.
- In younger children with type 1 diabetes, annual screening for microalbuminuria, with random spot urine sample for microalbumin-to-creatinine ratio, should be initiated once the child is 10 years of age and has had diabetes for 5 years.

Since people are asymptomatic throughout the early stages of diabetic nephropathy, the educator plays a key role in helping them understand the importance of routine tests to assess kidney function. Since various tests can be done to assess kidney function, the educator should be sure that individuals understand the particular test that has been prescribed. In addition, a variety of other factors, such as infections, congestive heart failure, elevated glucose levels, high blood pressure, or exercise within the previous 24 hours, can influence urinary albumin screening. Hence, repeat testing is needed to confirm elevated albumin excretion levels.

Foot Care

Diabetes is the leading cause of nontraumatic lower limb amputations.[24] Amputation and foot ulcerations are the most common consequences of diabetic peripheral neuropathy.[3] The Standards of Care for a foot examination include the following[3]:

◈ Perform a visual inspection, assess foot pulses, and test for loss of protective sensation (10-g monofilament plus testing of the following: vibration using 128-Hz tuning fork, pinprick sensation, ankle reflexes, or vibration perception threshold).

◈ Educate all individuals, especially those whose risk factors include smoking or prior lower extremity complications, about the risk and prevention of foot problems and reinforce self-care behaviors. In addition, those at high risk for foot problems should be referred to foot care specialists (see Skills section).

◈ Perform a comprehensive foot exam annually to identify risk factors predictive of foot ulcers and amputations. Perform visual inspection of an individual's feet at each routine visit.

◈ Screen for peripheral arterial disease (PAD), which includes history of claudication and measurement of pedal pulses and may include ankle-brachial index (ABI). Those with positive ABI or significant claudication would benefit from vascular assessment; in addition, medication, exercise, and surgery may be necessary.

Many educators are responsible for performing diabetic foot exams. The educator must be appropriately trained to perform foot exams and refer individuals to foot care specialists when appropriate.

Resources to Aid in Implementing Standards of Care

Because of the significant amount of information contained in the Standards of Care, various public health programs (ie, state- and territorial-based diabetes prevention and control programs funded by the Centers for Disease Control and Prevention [CDC]) facilitate implementation by organizing the information in user-friendly formats. The following link takes you to state diabetes control Web sites where additional tools may be available: http://www.cdc.gov/diabetes/states/. The National Diabetes Education Program is another source of educational resources and tools that the busy educator may find helpful; the Web site address is http://ndep.nih.gov/.

Therapeutic Goals

People with diabetes not only must understand the necessary tests and exams and other components in the Standards of Care, but also must relate these to their own personalized therapeutic goals. For example, the person with diabetes not only needs to know to get an A1C test 2 to 4 times per year but also needs to know his or her A1C target value. Both the ADA[3] and the American Association of Clinical Endocrinologists[43] have developed recommended therapeutic goals for A1C, preprandial and postprandial plasma blood glucose, blood pressure, and lipids (see Table 10.2). The variation in the goals suggested by each is the result of different interpretations of the literature and variation in expert opinion. Too many people with diabetes are currently not at the targets recommended by either organization. Consequently, either set of therapeutic goals can serve as the targets for most people with diabetes.

Although the ADA-recommended therapeutic goals are the key guide, goals must be individualized based on the person's unique needs and capabilities. The educator must conduct a thorough assessment of needs (see chapter 2) and work with the individual and other members of the healthcare team to determine appropriate and achievable goals. Circumstances where the goals may need to be less stringent include the following[3]:

◈ Limited life expectancy
◈ History of severe hypoglycemia or hypoglycemia unawareness
◈ Advanced microvascular or macrovascular complications
◈ Presence of comorbid conditions that make the recommended targets unsafe

TABLE 10.2   Therapeutic Goals for Nonpregnant Adults

	American Diabetes Association	*American Association of Clinical Endocrinologists*
A1C	<7.0%*	≤6.5% or lower for most
Preprandial capillary plasma glucose	70–130 mg/dL (3.88-7.22 mmol/L)	<110 mg/dL (6.11 mmol/L) (fasting)
Peak postprandial capillary plasma glucose	<180 mg/dL (10 mmol/L) (1–2 hours after the beginning of a meal)	<140 mg/dL (7.77 mmol/L) (2 hours postprandial)
Blood pressure		
Systolic	<140 mm Hg[†]	<130 mm Hg
Diastolic	<80 mm Hg	<80 mm Hg
Lipids		
LDL-C	<100 mg/dL (6.11 mmol/L) (without CVD)	<100 mg/dL (6.11 mmol/L) (high risk)
	<70 mg/dL (3.88 mmol/L) (with overt CVD)	<70 mg/dL (3.88 mmol/L) (highest risk)
HDL-C	*Men:* >40 mg/dL (2.22 mmol/L)	*Men:* >40 mg/dL (2.22 mmol/L)
	Women: >50 mg/dL (2.77 mmol/L)	*Women:* >50 mg/dL (2.77 mmol/L)
Triglycerides	<150 mg/dL (8.33 mmol/L)	<150 mg/dL (8.33 mmol/L)

*Goal adjusted based on individual factors.

[†]Lower systolic blood pressure appropriate for some.

Sources: American Diabetes Association, "Standards of medical care in diabetes, 2014," *Diabetes Care* 37, Suppl 1 (2014): S14-80. American Association of Clinical Endocrinologists, "Medical guidelines for clinical practice for the management of diabetes mellitus," *Endocr Pract* 17, Suppl 2 (2007): 1-53.

The decision to modify the therapeutic goals needs to be mutually determined by the person with diabetes and the healthcare professional.

Children and Adolescents

Blood Glucose   Glycemic control in children and adolescents with type 1 diabetes must consider the unique risks of hypoglycemia in young children. Most children younger than 6 or 7 years of age have immature counterregulatory mechanisms, which result in a form of hypoglycemia unawareness. In addition, young children do not have the cognitive capacity to recognize and respond to hypoglycemia.[3] The A1C level attained in the "intensive" adolescent cohort in the DCCT was 1% above that achieved by adult participants.[4] The therapeutic goals for plasma blood glucose premeal and bedtime/overnight as well as A1C are listed by age in Table 10.3.[3] As in adults, postprandial SMBG is recommended when A1C values are not reaching target despite achievement of premeal SMBG goals.

Blood Pressure   The definitions of hypertension and "high-normal" blood pressure for children were given earlier in this chapter. Information on normal blood pressure levels for age, gender, and height and methods for determinations are available online at http://www.nhlbi.nih.gov/health/prof/heart/hbp/hbp_ped.pdf. The therapeutic target for LDL-C in children is less than 100 mg/dL (5.55 mmol/L).

Preventive Care Services

In addition to the tests, exams, and interventions that are important for reducing risks for microvascular and macrovascular complications, there are other preventive care services that people with diabetes should receive to improve their health:

- Influenza, pneumococcal, and hepatitis B immunizations
- Dental care
- Prepregnancy counseling

Immunizations

Influenza and pneumonia are associated with high mortality and morbidity in the elderly and in those with chronic diseases. These common infectious

TABLE 10.3 Plasma Blood Glucose and A1C Goals for Type 1 Diabetes by Age Group			
Plasma blood glucose goal range (mg/dL [mmol/L])			
Values by age (years)	*Before meals*	*Bedtime/overnight*	*A1C*
Toddlers and preschoolers (0–6)	100–180 (5.55-10)	110–200 (6.11-11.11)	<8.5%*
School age (6–12)	90–180 (5-10)	100–180 (5.55-10)	<8%†
Adolescents and young adults (13–19)	90–130 (5.55-7.22)	90–150 (5.55-8.33)	<7.5%‡
Key concepts in setting glycemic goals: Goals should be individualized, and lower goals may be reasonable based on benefit-risk assessment. Blood glucose goals should be higher than those listed above in children with frequent hypoglycemia or hypoglycemia unawareness. Postprandial blood glucose values should be measured when there is a disparity between preprandial blood glucose values and A1C levels.			

*A lower goal (<8.0%) is reasonable if it can be achieved without excessive hypoglycemia.

†A lower goal (<7.5%) may be appropriate if it can be safely achieved.

‡A goal of <7% may be appropriate for some if it can be safely achieved.

Source: Reproduced with permission from the American Diabetes Association; American Diabetes Association, "Standards of medical care in diabetes, 2014," *Diabetes Care* 37, Suppl 1 (2014): S14-80.

diseases are preventable. Safe and effective vaccines are available and can reduce the complications from influenza (seasonal and other) and pneumococcal disease. Influenza vaccine has been shown to reduce diabetes-related hospital admissions by as much as 79% during flu epidemics.[44]

In addition, hepatitis B virus (HBV) vaccinations are now recommended as part of preventive care for many previously unvaccinated adults with diabetes. Among the general population over age 23, HBV is 2 times more common in those living with diabetes, and multiple HBV outbreaks have occurred in long-term care facilities and hospitals among people with diabetes. Hepatitis B virus is stable for long periods of time on lancing devices and glucose meters; receiving assistance with testing glucose in a location where others are also being tested increases the likelihood of spreading HBV.[45]

The ADA provides the following recommendations[3]:

◈ Provide an influenza vaccine annually to all people with diabetes 6 months of age or older.
◈ Provide at least 1 lifetime pneumococcal vaccine for people with diabetes who are at least 2 years of age. A one-time revaccination is recommended for individuals over 64 years of age previously immunized when they were less than 65 years of age if the vaccine was administered more than 5 years ago. Other indications for repeat vaccination include nephrotic syndrome, chronic renal disease, and other immunocompromised states such as after organ transplantation.
◈ Individuals between the ages of 19 and 59 should receive HBV vaccination shortly after diagnosis of diabetes if they have not been previously vaccinated for HBV. Consider vaccination for those over the age of 59.

Individuals may express a belief that the flu shot gave them the flu in the past and that it is something they do not really need. The educator must address these concerns and explain the benefits of getting immunizations as recommended (a helpful resource from the CDC is at http://www.cdc.gov/flu/diabetes/). Also, the influenza nasal spray vaccinations are not recommended for people with diabetes.[46]

Confirming that the person does not have any contraindications for receiving the vaccine is also important. Precautions and contraindications to vaccinations are listed at http://www.cdc.gov/vaccines/recs/vac-admin/contraindications-vacc.htm. The following general guidelines are given for the HBV, influenza, and pneumococcal vaccinations:

1. Use caution when giving the vaccination to someone who has a moderate or acute illness, with or without a fever.
2. Don't give the vaccination to anyone who has had a previous severe allergic reaction to the vaccination or any component in the vaccination in the past.

Dental Care

While periodontal disease does not seem to occur more often in people with diabetes, it tends to be more serious.[47] Oral hygiene, regular dental care, and improved metabolic control may reduce the risk of periodontal disease.

People with diabetes should see a dentist every 6 months and more frequently if periodontal disease exists. Periodontal disease is often asymptomatic, so it is important that the educator raise this issue. During routine medical visits, people with diabetes should be assessed for signs of periodontal disease, including redness of gums, swelling or bleeding of gums, foul odor, loose teeth, and pain.[48] The importance of effective brushing and flossing should be reinforced. If patients are apprehensive about dental procedures, the educator should help them express this anxiety and reduce their fears by explaining what to expect and reinforcing the positive outcomes of dental care.

Prepregnancy Counseling

Preconception care has been shown to reduce the risk of congenital malformations. Several nonrandomized studies have compared rates of malformations in infants between women who participated in preconception diabetes care and women who initiated intensive diabetes management after they were already pregnant.[49-53] The preconception care programs were multidisciplinary and trained participants in diabetes self-management with MNT, intensified insulin therapy, and SMBG. In all studies, the incidence of major congenital malformations in infants was much lower in those who participated in preconception care than in those who did not participate.

Standard care for all women with diabetes in their reproductive years with childbearing potential should include the following[3]:

◈ Starting in puberty, preconception counseling should be incorporated into the routine diabetes care visit.
◈ Medications should be evaluated in those who are or may become pregnant, as some medications used to treat women with diabetes are not recommended during pregnancy (ie, statins, angiotensin II receptor blockers [ARBs], angiotensin converting enzyme [ACE] inhibitors, and most noninsulin glucose-lowering medications).

Women contemplating pregnancy should be seen frequently by a multidisciplinary team experienced in managing diabetes before and during pregnancy. The goals of preconception care are as follows[54,55]:

◈ To integrate the patient into the management of her diabetes
◈ To achieve the lowest A1C test results (<7%) possible without excessive hypoglycemia
◈ To ensure effective contraception until stable and acceptable glycemia is achieved
◈ To identify, evaluate, and treat long-term complications of diabetes (retinopathy, neuropathy, nephropathy, and CVD)

Skills

To practice behaviors that minimize the risk of developing complications, people with diabetes must master skills that include SMBG (see chapter 7 for additional information), self-monitoring of blood pressure, self-examination of the feet, and maintaining a personal care record.

Self-Monitoring of Blood Glucose

Self-monitoring of blood glucose is considered an important component of effective therapy[56] and one of the Standards of Care described earlier in this chapter. Educators must refrain from limiting their teaching about SMBG to the achievement of correctly performed finger-stick checks. People with diabetes must be taught how to use this information to make treatment decisions by monitoring their responses to food, medication, physical activity, and stressors of various types. Chapter 7 reviews this topic.

Self-Monitoring of Blood Pressure

In addition to blood pressure monitoring by a healthcare professional during each diabetes visit, some individuals may benefit by self-monitoring their blood pressure. While this issue has not been specifically studied in people with diabetes, a meta-analysis found that home monitoring, or self-monitoring, of blood pressure improved blood pressure in those with essential hypertension.[57] If the healthcare professional and the person with diabetes determine that this level of monitoring is important, the individual may choose to use a home blood-pressure monitor.

The educator should have the person with diabetes bring the home blood-pressure monitor to a diabetes care appointment to be sure that he or she understands how to use it. It is also valuable to note the differences in readings between the home monitor and the office equipment. Having the person demonstrate use of the monitor is a good way to assess the individual's skills and provide feedback and support.

Self-Examination of Feet and Foot Care

Lower extremity complications of diabetes result from a combination of factors including neuropathy, ischemia, trauma, ulceration, faulty wound healing, infection, and gangrene.[58–60] Careful foot care and proper patient education have been shown to reduce the amputation rate associated with diabetes by 50%.[61]

During the foot exam, the importance of the individual's foot care and self-examination can be stressed. Additionally, this is a time when the educator can assess an individual's vision and mobility to determine whether they will pose difficulties in performing self-exams. If the person with diabetes has poor vision, a manual palpation may be substituted for the visual inspection. If mobility is impaired, making it difficult to reach the feet, a regular or magnifying mirror can be used to help visualize the plantar surface and other areas of the feet. When both vision and mobility are severely impaired, another individual may need to assist with foot inspections.[58]

Before teaching foot exam and foot care skills, the educator needs to assess the person's present knowledge, behaviors, beliefs, and abilities by finding out what the individual is currently doing for foot care and examination. The following foot exam and foot care skills should be taught to all persons with diabetes[58]:

◆ Look at both feet (top, bottom, and sides) and between the toes daily. This can be done when putting on or taking off socks and shoes. Look for cuts, calluses, blisters, thick or ingrown toenails, and signs of infection such as redness, swelling, or pus. Seek prompt medical attention for any problems.

◆ Wash and dry feet thoroughly, especially between the toes. Avoid routine foot soaks. To avoid hot water burns, test the temperature of bath and shower water with an elbow before stepping in.

◆ Moisturize dry skin (except between the toes) with an emollient such as lanolin or a hand or body lotion. Avoid using lotions that contain alcohol, as this can dry the skin.

◆ Cut toenails straight across and file the sharp corners to match the contour of the toe.

◆ Inspect shoes daily by feeling the insides for torn linings, cracks, pebbles, nails, or other irregularities that may irritate the skin. Get in the habit of shaking out shoes before putting them on. Changing shoes during the day can limit repetitive local pressure.

◆ Avoid going barefoot or sock-footed. Wear footwear at the pool or beach and apply sunscreen to avoid burns.

Having the person with diabetes perform a self-examination of the feet is important. This will allow the educator to provide positive reinforcement for those aspects that have been successfully done and to point out areas that need additional attention.

Personal Care Record

A personal care record is a valuable tool for people with diabetes to keep track of their therapeutic goals and the tests and exams that are recommended in the Standards of Care. These records come in various formats and sizes, and individuals should select a type according to their personal preferences. Some may prefer a pocket-sized, paper tool while others may use a smartphone app or a Web-based record to monitor and record care. Self-monitoring of blood glucose may be done several times per day, and thus a separate log for SMBG is usually more practical. In addition, many blood glucose meters come with software that allows results to be downloaded to personal computers or personal digital assistants.

The personal care record is a great way to teach people with diabetes about the Standards of Care. It provides a concise listing of the necessary tests, exams, and interventions and should include places for the person to record his or her measured values. Educators can assist people with diabetes in keeping their personal care record up to date and using it to help them determine whether they are getting all of the necessary Standards of Care and meeting treatment goals. Reviewing the personal care record is a useful way to guide this discussion in a logical and complete manner.

Barriers

To successfully attain and, of equal importance, maintain risk-reduction behaviors, the educator must work with the person with diabetes to address barriers and ways to overcome them. Barriers can be organized into 3 broad categories[23]:

- ◆ *Personal:* Includes depression, physical disabilities, poor coping styles, and inaccurate health beliefs
- ◆ *Interpersonal:* Includes family conflict and lack of rapport with healthcare professionals
- ◆ *Environmental:* Includes financial constraints and other competing priorities

Many of the barriers that people with diabetes face do not have simple answers and can be disheartening for both the individual and the healthcare professional. The first step toward helping people deal with barriers is to listen to their concerns in a nonjudgmental way. It is also important to provide culturally competent care. Sometimes a difficulty may seem overwhelming or be poorly defined if the individual has not had the chance to discuss the issue in a safe environment. The educator can assist a person in clearly defining barriers and developing an action plan to deal with the problems.[23] For more discussion regarding barriers, problem solving, and coping skills, see chapters 8 and 9.

The educator should be knowledgeable about community resources that may help people deal with such barriers as financial issues and physical disabilities. The diabetes prevention and control programs located in each state, the District of Columbia, and the 8 US territories may be able to assist educators in identifying these community resources (http://www.cdc.gov/diabetes/states/index.htm). Although there are gaps in services and limitations in program resources, there may be programs and services that individuals qualify for but need assistance accessing. Some areas have 211 numbers to provide assistance in locating social and medical resources.

Summary

Reducing risks, the seventh of the AADE7 Self-Care Behaviors™, is multifaceted and influenced by family, friends, cultural background, community, and societal pressures. As the final self-care behavior, it incorporates aspects of the preceding 6 self-care behaviors. Reducing risks involves helping people with diabetes gain knowledge and understanding about the necessary tests, exams, interventions, and achievement of therapeutic goals that can help them reduce their likelihood of developing complications of diabetes. In addition, those living with diabetes must acquire self-care skills and develop strategies that will maximize their level of health and quality of life.

Reducing risks can be a challenging aspect of self-care behavior to address; the individual must be encouraged by the healthcare professionals on the diabetes care team to take steps to address potential problems. Yet practicing preventive behaviors may not always be a priority in the face of current life demands. The delicate balance the educator must strike falls between helping people with diabetes gain an understanding of and appreciation for the future benefits linked to preventive behaviors and employing methods that do not undermine self-efficacy. The evidence is strong that following the Standards of Care and achieving therapeutic goals greatly reduce the likelihood of diabetes complications. The educator plays a vital role in partnering with the person with diabetes, family members, and the other members of the healthcare team to translate the evidence supporting risk-reduction behaviors into practice.

Case: Risk Reduction in a Man With Type 2 Diabetes

AJ is a 49-year-old Hispanic man who was diagnosed with type 2 diabetes 5 years earlier during a visit to the clinic for back pain. At the time of diagnosis, his weight was 179 lb and he complained of blurry vision. In a follow-up appointment after his diabetes diagnosis, AJ and his physician discussed his therapeutic goals for A1C (<7.0%), fasting blood glucose (70-130 mg/dL [3.88-7.22 mmol/L]), blood pressure (<140/80 mm Hg), and lipids (LDL-C <100 mg/dL [5.55 mmol/L], HDL-C >40 mg/dL [2.22 mmol/L], and triglycerides <150 mg/dL [8.33 mmol/L]). AJ indicated he was okay with these, but he was overwhelmed by his diagnosis. Although AJ's first language is Spanish, he is fluent in English.

Current Physical Assessment

- Height: 66 in
- Weight: 182 lb
- BMI: 29.4
- Blood pressure: 132/84 mm Hg

Current Lab Values

- A1C: 8.2%
- Fasting blood glucose: 139 mg/dL (7.72 mmol/L)
- Triglycerides: 147 mg/dL (8.16 mmol/L)
- LDL-C: 103 mg/dL (5.72 mmol/L)
- HDL-C: 48 mg/dL (2.66 mmol/L)

AJ is married and has 4 adult children. He is a manager in a manufacturing plant and often feels very stressed due to the demands of his job and the financial responsibilities he and his wife have taken on to ensure their children graduate from college. AJ copes with his stress by smoking a pack of cigarettes a day and snacking on a bag of potato chips and a half carton of dip in the evening while catching up on paperwork he brings home from the office.

His doctor started him on 500 mg of metformin twice daily. This was increased to a current dosage of 1000 mg twice daily, taken before the breakfast and evening meals. At his diagnosis, he received general nutrition and physical activity guidelines and was encouraged to lose some weight and get a dilated eye exam. AJ's physician discussed with him whether he needed to do SMBG, and they decided he would since he has a hectic schedule and would feel more confident if he could check his blood glucose levels. No specific SMBG monitoring schedule was determined at that time.

AJ has been irregular in his medical visits due to his busy schedule. However, he attended a community education program where he learned more about the possible risks he might be facing for diabetes complications. This prompted him to consider changing some of his lifestyle habits. His mother and paternal grandfather had type 2 diabetes, and he worries he will suffer a future like that of his family members, which includes kidney failure and a premature heart attack. While AJ is interested in changing some of his current habits, he is feeling overwhelmed and is not sure where to start.

Case—Part 2: Questions for Consideration

1. What are AJ's modifiable risk factors for diabetes complications?

   - Hyperglycemia as reflected in both A1C and fasting blood glucose measures
   - Overweight
   - Prehypertension
   - LDL-C (2014 ADA Standards of Care recommend statin therapy for those with diabetes who have not been diagnosed with CVD, are over age 40, and have at least one CVD risk factor, which includes smoking and hypertension)[3]
   - Smoking
   - Stress

2. Which Standards of Care are being met for AJ, and which ones need improvement?

   While current laboratory values are available for A1C, blood pressure, lipids, and weight, it is possible AJ has not been getting these tests/exams on the others as recommended in the Standards of Care since he has been irregular in his medical visits. A paper or electronic flow sheet in his medical record would allow easy monitoring to determine the frequency and values of his tests and exams in the Standards of Care. If his A1C, blood pressure, lipids, and weight are being measured as recommended, then attention should be given to microalbumin, serum creatinine with calculated GFR, a dilated eye exam, a comprehensive foot exam, immunizations, and dental care. It is also very important for AJ to meet with the registered dietitian to develop a food plan and physical activity program to help him meet realistic weight-loss goals.

3. Which therapeutic goals have been met, and which ones deserve attention?

   AJ's current lab values indicate he is on target for triglycerides and HDL-C and very close to his LDL-C goal (but 2013 AHA/ACC guidelines indicate statin therapy). It would be helpful to review his goals for A1C, fasting blood glucose, blood pressure, and weight. His efforts to lose 5% of his body weight (10 lb) through modifications in his food intake and an increase in his physical activity are critical first steps in helping him meet his therapeutic goals. Smoking is also a significant health concern that should be addressed.

4. Which skills does AJ need to learn or review?

   AJ would benefit from reviewing his SMBG skills and working with a diabetes educator to determine a reasonable frequency of testing. A review of his skills and a discussion about the best times to test would help him better use this information and not just randomly test. He would also benefit from learning how to inspect his feet and what signs to report to his healthcare team. AJ is under a lot of stress, which impairs his ability to carry out any of the self-care behaviors necessary to reduce the risk of diabetes complications. He would benefit from learning some coping skills and stress reduction techniques (in addition to physical activity).

5. What community and educational resources would you suggest for AJ?

   AJ is fluent in English, but it is important to assess whether he prefers to receive information in Spanish or English. His language preference could impact the community and educational materials selected. Since AJ is a pack-a-day smoker, it is very important that this habit be addressed and carefully monitored. Local smoking cessation programs might be an option, along with the national Smoker's Helpline (1-800-QUIT-NOW), which refers callers to phone-based counseling cessation programs in their state. The American Lung Association offers a low-cost online smoking cessation program (http://www.ffsonline.org). AJ may be given a health record card or assisted with using an electronic method to track his tests and exams. He should also be encouraged to continue attending community education programs since he found the one he attended helpful. He might benefit from going to the ADA Web site (http://www.diabetes.org) and using the Diabetes Personal Health Decisions (PHD) to insert his information and see how lifestyle changes would help him reduce his risk for complications. Other online tools might also be of assistance since he has limited time for events or meetings.

6. What barriers does AJ face as he works to reduce his risk for diabetes complications, and what are some suggested strategies?

   The barriers that AJ faces primarily fall in the categories of personal and environmental. Personal barriers include his use of tobacco products and consumption of high-fat snacks late in the evening to cope with stress. These coping strategies are a detriment to his health and increase his risk for diabetes complications. He would benefit from learning problem-solving and coping skills that offer a healthier alternative to his current coping strategies. Financial concerns and long work hours are environmental barriers. While these are not easy to solve, AJ might see if there are any community lectures or online resources for time management to help him better organize his workload. He might also benefit from talking to a financial planner about strategies to help fund his children's education.

Focus on Education

Teaching Strategies

⟳ **Establish the importance.** Help people with diabetes gain an appreciation for the importance of risk-reduction behaviors by partnering with them to make these behaviors personal and meaningful. Tailor information, appealing to the individual's learning preferences, culture, language, and educational level.

⟳ **Deliver risk information.** Use as much interactive teaching as possible, such as asking the person with diabetes to suggest specific actions he or she will take to reduce personal risk for complications and poor health. Ask individuals to demonstrate skills related to diabetes management to be sure they are performed correctly. Directly and specifically address feelings and concerns in addition to knowledge and skills acquisition. Use phrases like, "What might stop you (hold you back) from trying this?"

⟳ **Achieve targets.** While there may be some differences in the glycemic therapeutic goals recommended by various associations and groups, too many people with diabetes are living far above any of the targets. Evidence from further studies may help elucidate this issue, but the focus should be on helping people achieve the goals (with any adjustments needed for their individual circumstances).

⟳ **Keep records.** Personal care records are a valuable tool for engaging people with diabetes in risk-reducing self-care behaviors. They provide a list of the recommended tests, exams, and interventions based on the Standards of Care and help people with diabetes track their results. Encourage individuals to use a record-keeping tool that includes reminders for visits, follow-up lab testing, and immunizations and to consider keeping it in their purse or billfold for quick reference or use a smartphone or Web-based tool.

Messages for Patients

⟳ **Learn the skills.** Learn all that is needed to be a master in diabetes self-management. Knowledge alone is not enough for behavior change, but it is an important first step. Identify any barriers that can interfere with risk-reduction behaviors. Ask the healthcare team to assist in identifying gaps in information and skills. Try not to be worried about or afraid of admitting the need for help.

⟳ **Realize that it's a lot of work!** Diabetes management is a lot of work, but you and your health are worth it! Take advantage of the knowledge and recent advances in diabetes research to keep yourself healthy and reduce your risk for complications in the years to come.

⟳ **Envision a healthier future.** Focus on making your future a healthier one. There is no better time than the present to begin reducing your risk for diabetes complications and living a long and healthy life. Every day, month, and decade that your blood glucose, blood pressure, and blood cholesterol levels are closer to target range, you are building a healthier future.

⟳ **Keep records.** Work closely with your diabetes team to track blood glucose levels, blood pressure, and blood lipids. Make time for the recommended visits to associated healthcare providers and for suggested exams and immunizations. Keep a record of the results of your diabetes tests and exams and your medications (and changes). Bring this information to each clinic visit, educational class, or urgent care visit.

Health Literacy

⟳ **Health literacy can negatively impact the interactions and the relationship between patients and healthcare providers.** Communicating meaningfully with patients with low health literacy levels will maximize concordance. Often low-literacy patients are considered noncompliant. Learning more about ways to effectively communicate with those who may have low health literacy can improve the ability of persons with diabetes to make lifestyle changes and adhere to medical treatment. All persons with diabetes should be assessed for literacy issues, including the use of numbers.

↻ **Choose words that people understand.** The main purpose of patient education is to help patients own the information so that they can improve their health. Choose words that patients can relate to and translate into action. For example, instead of asking, "What are your goals?" ask, "What will you do differently till the next time I see you?"

↻ **Low health literacy affects what happens during healthcare appointments, after the visit, and in potential future concordance.** Existing miscommunications and, consequently, inaccurate perceptions about self-care among patients can prevent adequate future risk-reduction behaviors. Some patients may be intimidated by the overwhelming amount of information it takes to

manage the new diagnosis of diabetes and may be resistant to preventive care. Craft your messages with empowered but realistic expectations of what it really takes to manage diabetes effectively at each stage. Use supplemental tools like videos, pictures, and models to assist with teaching. In addition, be certain to use demonstration and the teach-back method to ensure patient understanding of information.

↻ **Teach patients what questions to ask their healthcare providers:** What is my main problem? What do I need to do about it? And why is it important for me to do it?

↻ **There are online courses to help individual clinicians or health systems improve their dealings with those living with low literacy levels.** Examples include the following:
- A free online continuing education course on health literacy through the Health Resources and Services Administration is at http://www.hrsa.gov/publichealth/healthliteracy/.
- An overview of initiatives going on across the country to address low health literacy is at http://www.cdc.gov/healthliteracy/.

Focus on Practice

↻ **Integrate the clinical preventive services and chronic disease management through the delivery of usual care among doctors, physician assistants, nurse practitioners, nurses, and administrators at their practice sites.** Every clinical encounter creates an opportunity to inspire, support, and encourage patients in preventive care and management. Use of brief, targeted messages through verbal communication, visuals, or media can bring up important issues at the right time and the right place for those who are ready to receive them.

↻ **Utilize health status trend management systems.** There are many risk assessment programs that allow people to learn which habits will reduce their healthcare costs and increase their life span.

People can weigh in on the cost and benefits of behavior change and risk-reduction activities.

↻ **Create access to wellness and the environment to support it.** Risk reduction among people with diabetes is part of a general community well-being that includes healthy social interactions, parks, bike trails, sidewalks, morning tai chi, people-watching at the local café, Sunday choir, family dinners, book clubs, and healthy, affordable food at local stores. It is all about opportunities for people to interact with healthy people. Healthy behaviors need to become a norm and part of society in order to be considered desirable and not part of medical treatment.

References

1. Boren SA, Gunlock TL, Schaefer J, Albright A. Reducing risks in diabetes self-management: a systematic review of the literature. Diabetes Educ. 2007;33:1053-77.

2. Stange KC, Nutting PA, Miller WL, et al. Defining and measuring the patient-centered medical home. J Gen Intern Med. 2010 (cited 2013 May 16);25(6):601-12. On the Internet at: http://www.ncbi.nlm.nih.gov/pmc/articles/PMC2869425/.

3. American Diabetes Association. Standards of medical care in diabetes—2014. Diabetes Care. 2014;37:S14-80.

4. The Diabetes Control and Complications Trial Research Group. The effect of intensive treatment of diabetes on the development and progression of long-term complications in insulin-dependent diabetes mellitus. N Engl J Med. 1993;329:977-86.

5. UK Prospective Diabetes Study (UKPDS) Group. Intensive blood-glucose control with sulphonylureas or insulin compared with conventional treatment and risk of complications in patients with type 2 diabetes (UKPDS 33). Lancet. 1998;352:837-53.

6. UK Prospective Diabetes Study (UKPDS) Group. Effect of intensive blood-glucose control with metformin on complications in overweight patients with type 2 diabetes (UKPDS 34). Lancet. 1998;352:854-65.

7. Martin CL, Albers J, Herman WH, et al, DCCT/EDIC Research Group. Neuropathy among the diabetes control and complications trial cohort 8 years after trial completion. Diabetes Care. 2006;29:340-4.

8. Holman RR, Paul SK, Bethel MA, Mathews DR, Neil HA. 10-year follow-up of intensive glucose control in type 2 diabetes. N Engl J Med. 2008;359:1577-89.

9. Duckworth W, Abraira C, Moritz T, et al, VADT Investigators. Glucose control and vascular complications in veterans with type 2 diabetes. N Engl J Med. 2009;360:129-39.

10. Nathan DM, Cleary PA, Backlund JY, et al, Diabetes Control and Complications Trial/Epidemiology of Diabetes Interventions and Complications (DCCT/EDIC) Study Research Group. Intensive diabetes treatment and cardiovascular disease in patients with type 1 diabetes. N Engl J Med. 2005;353:2643-53.

11. Skyler JS, Bergenstal R, Bonow RO, et al, American Diabetes Association, American College of Cardiology Foundation, American Heart Association. Intensive glycemic control and the prevention of cardiovascular events: implications of the ACCORD, ADVANCE and VA diabetes trials: a position statement of the American Diabetes Association, American College of Cardiology Foundation and the American Heart Association. Diabetes Care. 2009;32:187-92.

12. Farmer A, Wade A, Goyder E, et al. Impact of self monitoring of blood glucose in the management of patients with non-insulin treated diabetes: open parallel group randomised trial. BMJ. 2007;335:132.

13. Evert AB, Boucher JL, Cypress M, et al. Nutrition therapy recommendations for the management of adults with diabetes. A position statement of the American Diabetes Association (cited 2013 Nov 16). On the Internet at: http://care.diabetesjournals.org/content/early/2013/10/07/dc13-2042.full.pdf.

14. Leontos CJ, Franz MJ, Holzmeister LA, Kulkarni K, Monk AM, Powers MA, American Dietetic Association. American Dietetic Association Diabetes Type 1 and 2 Evidence-Based Nutrition Practice Guideline for Adults. Chicago: American Dietetic Association; 2008.

15. NIH News. Weight loss does not lower heart disease risk from type 2 diabetes. 2012 Oct 19 (cited 2013 May 28). On the Internet at: http://www.nih.gov/news/health/oct2012/niddk-19.htm.

16. Maciejewski ML, Livingston EH, Smith VA, et al. Survival among high-risk patients after bariatric surgery. JAMA. 2011;305:2419-26.

17. Himpens J, Cadière GB, Bazi M, Vouche M, Cadière B, Dapri G. Long-term outcomes of laparoscopic adjustable gastric banding. Arch Surg. 2011;146:802-7.

18. Colberg SR, Sigal RJ, Fernhall B, et al. Exercise and type 2 diabetes; The American College of Sports Medicine and the American Diabetes Association: joint position statement. Diabetes Care. 2010;33:12. e147-67.

19. Mullooly CA, Kemmis KL. Diabetes educators and exercise prescription. Diabetes Spectr. 2005;18(2):108-13.

20. Silverstein J, Klingensmith G, Copeland K, et al. Care of children and adolescents with type 1 diabetes: a statement of the American Diabetes Association. Diabetes Care. 2005;28(1):186-212.

21. Anderson RJ, Freedland KE, Clouse RE, Lustman PJ. The prevalence of comorbid depression in adults with diabetes: a meta-analysis. Diabetes Care. 2003;24(6):1069-78.

22. Young-Hyman D. Psychosocial factors affecting adherence, quality of life, and well-being: helping patients cope. In: Bode BW, ed. Medical Management of Type 1 Diabetes. 4th ed. Alexandria, Va: American Diabetes Association; 2004:162-82.

23. Skovlund SE, Peyrot M. The Diabetes Attitudes, Wishes and Needs (DAWN) program: a new approach to improving outcomes of diabetes care. Diabetes Spectr. 2005;18(3):136-42.

24. Centers for Disease Control and Prevention. National diabetes fact sheet: general information and national estimates on diabetes in the United States, 2007. Atlanta: US Department of Health and Human Services; 2008.

25. Arauz-Pacheco C, Parrott MA, Raskin P. The treatment of hypertension in adult patients with diabetes. Diabetes Care. 2002;25:134-47.

26. National Institutes of Health. Detection, evaluation and treatment of high blood cholesterol in adults: third report of the National Cholesterol Education Program. 2002.

27. Fagard RH, Nilsson PM. Smoking and diabetes—the double health hazard! Prim Care Diabetes. 2009;3(4):205-9.

28. Ong G, Davis TME, Davis WA. Aspirin is associated with reduced cardiovascular and all-cause mortality in type 2 diabetes in a primary prevention setting: the Fremantle Diabetes Study. Diabetes Care. 2010;33(2):317-21.

29. UK Prospective Diabetes Study (UKPDS) Group. Tight blood pressure control and risk of macrovascular and microvascular complications in type 2 diabetes (UKPDS 38). BMJ. 1998;317:703-13.

30. Collins R, Armitage J, Parish S, Sleigh P, Peo R, Heart Protection Study Collaborative Group. MRC/BHF Heart Protection Study of cholesterol-lowering with simvastatin in 5963 people with diabetes: a randomized placebo-controlled trial. Lancet. 2003;361(9374): 2005-16.

31. Stone NJ, Robinson J, Lichtenstein AH, et al. 2013 ACC/AHA guideline on the treatment of blood cholesterol to reduce atherosclerotic cardiovascular risk in adults: a report of the American College of Cardiology/American Heart Association task force on practice guidelines. Circulation. 2013 (cited 2013 Nov 21). On the Internet at: http://circ.ahajournals.org/content/early/2013/11/11/01.cir.0000437738.63853.7a.citation.

32. The Expert Panel of Blood Cholesterol Levels in Children and Adolescents. Treatment recommendations of the National Cholesterol Education Program Report of the Expert Panel on Blood Cholesterol Levels in Children and Adolescents. Pediatrics. 1992;89:525-84.

33. American Diabetes Association. Smoking and diabetes (position statement). Diabetes Care. 2004;27 Suppl 1:S74-5.

34. US Preventive Services Task Force. Primary care interventions to prevent tobacco use in children and adolescents (cited 2013 May 29). On the Internet at: http://www.uspreventiveservicestaskforce.org/uspstf12/tobacco/tbacfinalrs.htm.

35. Larzelere MM, Williams DE. Promoting smoking cessation. Am Fam Physician. 2012 Mar 15;85(6):591-8.

36. Hayden M, Pignone M, Phillips C, Mulrow C. Aspirin for the primary prevention of cardiovascular events: a summary of the evidence for the U.S. Preventive Services Task Force. Ann Intern Med. 2002;136:161-72.

37. US Preventive Services Task Force. Aspirin for prevention of cardiovascular disease: US Preventive Services Task Force recommendation statement. Ann Intern Med. 2009;150:396-404.

38. Buse JB, Ginsberg HN, Bakris GL, et al, American Heart Association, American Diabetes Association. Primary prevention of cardiovascular disease in people with diabetes mellitus: a scientific statement from the American Heart Association and the American Diabetes Association. Diabetes Care. 2007;30:162-72.

39. Garg JP, Bakris GL. Microalbuminuria: marker of vascular dysfunction, risk factor for cardiovascular disease. Vasc Med. 2002;7:35-43.

40. Klausen K, Borch-Johnson K, Feldt-Rasmussen B, et al. Very low levels of microalbuminuria are associated with increased risk of coronary heart disease and death independently of renal function, hypertension, and diabetes. Circulation. 2004;110:32-5.

41. Gall MA, Hougaard P, Borch-Johnson K, Parving HH. Risk factors for development of incipient and overt diabetic nephropathy in patients with non-insulin-dependent diabetes mellitus: prospective, observational study. BMJ. 1997;314:783-8.

42. Ravid M, Lang R, Rachmani R, Lishner M. Long-term renoprotective effect of angiotensin-converting enzyme inhibition in non-insulin-dependent diabetes mellitus: a 7-year follow-up study. Arch Intern Med. 1996;156:286-9.

43. Handelsman Y, Mechanick JI, Blonde L, et al. American Association of Clinical Endocrinologists medical guidelines for clinical practice for the management of diabetes mellitus. Endocr Pract. 2011;17 Suppl 2:1-53.

44. Smith SA, Poland GA. Use of influenza and pneumococcal vaccines in people with diabetes. Diabetes Care. 2000;23:95-108.

45. Centers for Disease Control and Prevention. Use of hepatitis B vaccination for adults with diabetes mellitus: recommendations of the Advisory Committee on Immunization Practices (ACIP). MMWR Morb Mortal Wkly Rep. 2012;60:1709-11.

46. Centers for Disease Control and Prevention. Seasonal influenza (cited 2013 May 22). On the Internet at: http://www.cdc.gov/flu/about/qa/nasalspray.htm#not-vaccinated.

47. Khader YS, Dauod AS, El-Qaderi SS, Alkafajei A, Batayha WQ. Periodontal status of diabetics compared with nondiabetics: a meta-analysis. J Diabetes Complications. 2006;20(1):59-68.

48. Hunt C. Skin and dental care. In: Franz MJ, ed. A Core Curriculum for Diabetes Education: Diabetes and Complications. 5th ed. Chicago: American Association of Diabetes Educators; 2003:89-96.

49. Kitzmiller JL, Gavin LA, Gin GD, Jovanovic-Peterson L, Main EK, Zigrang WD. Preconception care of diabetes: glycemic control prevents congenital anomalies. JAMA. 1991;265:731-6.

50. Goldman JA, Dicker D, Feldberg D, Yeshaya A, Samuel N, Karp M. Pregnancy outcome in patients with

insulin-dependent diabetes mellitus with preconceptional diabetic control: a comparative study. Am J Obstet Gynecol. 1986;155:293-7.

51. Rosenn B, Miodovnik M, Combs CA, Khoury J, Siddiqi TA. Pre-conception management of insulin-dependent diabetes: improvement of pregnancy outcome. Obstet Gynecol. 1991;77:846-9.

52. Tchobroutsky C, Vray MM, Altman JJ. Risk/benefit ratio of changing late obstetrical strategies in the management of insulin-dependent diabetic pregnancies: a comparison between 1971-1977 and 1978-1985 periods in 389 pregnancies. Diabetes Metab. 1991;17:287-94.

53. Willhoite MB, Bennert HW Jr, Palomaki GE, et al. The impact of pre-conception counseling on pregnancy outcomes: the experience of the Maine Diabetes in Pregnancy Program. Diabetes Care. 1993;16:450-5.

54. Kitzmiller JL, Buchanan TA, Kjos S, Combs CA, Ratner RE. Preconception care of diabetes, congenital malformations, and spontaneous abortions. Diabetes Care. 1996;19:514-41.

55. American Diabetes Association. Preconception care of women with diabetes (position statement). Diabetes Care. 2004;27 Suppl 1:S76-8.

56. Polonsky WH, Fisher L, Schikman CH, et al. Structured self-monitoring of blood glucose significantly reduces A1C levels in poorly controlled noninsulin-treated type 2 diabetes. Diabetes Care. 2011;34(2):262-7.

57. Cappuccio FP, Kerry SM, Forbes L. Blood pressure control by home monitoring: meta-analysis of randomized trials. BMJ. 2004;329:145-51.

58. Ahroni JH. Diabetic foot care and education. In: Franz MJ, ed. A Core Curriculum for Diabetes Education: Diabetes and Complications. 5th ed. Chicago: American Association of Diabetes Educators; 2003:67-86.

59. Pecoraro RE, Reiber GE, Burgess EM. Pathways to diabetic limb amputation: basis for prevention. Diabetes Care. 1990;13:513-21.

60. Edmonds ME, Blundell MP, Morris ME, Thomas EM, Cotton LT, Watkins PJ. Improved survival of the diabetic foot: the role of the specialized foot clinic. Q J Med. 1986;60:763-71.

61. Boulton AJ, Armstrong DG, Albert SF, et al, American Diabetes Association, American Association of Clinical Endocrinologists. Comprehensive foot examination and risk assessment: a report of the task force of the foot care interest group of the American Diabetes Association, with endorsement by the American Association of Clinical Endocrinologists. Diabetes Care. 2008;31:1679-85.

Diabetes Education Program Management

Melinda Maryniuk, MEd, RD, CDE, FADA

Key Concepts

◆ Diabetes educators have opportunities to establish and manage diabetes self-management education (DSME) programs, but they may need to augment their skill set to manage the operational and business aspects of the program.

◆ The process of establishing and managing a DSME program is similar to the 5-step process of DSME: (1) assessment, (2) goal setting, (3) planning, (4) implementation, and (5) evaluation/monitoring.

◆ Whether starting a new DSME program or managing an existing program, the business skills required include program financial management, strategic planning, human resource management, integration of technology, marketing, quality improvement, and outcomes management.

◆ Because managing an education program usually involves completing an application for accreditation from the American Association of Diabetes Educators (AADE) or recognition from the American Diabetes Association (ADA), awareness of critical components in this process is helpful for program managers for appropriate resource allocation.

Introduction

Access to quality, formal diabetes education should be a right of all Americans with diabetes. The government-sponsored initiative Healthy People 2020 continues to have as one of its key objectives, "to increase the proportion of persons with diagnosed diabetes who receive formal diabetes education." Currently, only 57% of adults with diabetes reported ever receiving some sort of formal diabetes education.[1]

Thus, there is an opportunity for diabetes educators to establish, operate, and manage effective and efficient quality DSME programs. While diabetes educators are experts in the subject of diabetes, they may be less comfortable with their skills as a program manager when it comes to the overall management and business operations of a program. The purpose of this chapter is to highlight the essentials of program operations. It is intended to be relevant for the diabetes educators who find themselves starting a new program or who are being asked to manage an existing program. In this chapter, the term "program" is used broadly to include DSME in all delivery models, ranging from a small service provided by one educator in a physician office, to a large multidisciplinary comprehensive program delivered in an academic medical center, and everything in between, including diabetes education delivered in retail pharmacies, local health clinics, and independent practices. The term "program manager" is used to describe the educator with program management responsibilities. This term applies to both educators for whom program management is a full-time job and educators who are solo practitioners filling all roles, including counseling patients on all relevant topic areas as well as overseeing the operations of the program.

The process of starting and running a diabetes education program is very similar to the 5-step process of DSME as described in the *AADE Guidelines for the Practice of Diabetes Self-Management Education and Training*.[2] The steps for providing DSME are as follows:

1. Assessment
2. Goal setting
3. Planning
4. Implementation
5. Evaluation/monitoring

Keeping these steps in mind will help organize the process for the program manager. This chapter is organized into 3 sections. It first addresses the steps involved in starting a DSME program (assessment, goal setting, and planning). Then it moves into operating and maintaining a program (implementation) and concludes with program evaluation and monitoring.

As access to education services increases and more people with diabetes are able to take advantage of diabetes education programs, the nation will come closer to not only meeting but exceeding the Healthy People 2020 goals.

Starting a Diabetes Self-Management Education Program

Assessment

As part of good patient care, the diabetes educator understands the importance of a thorough assessment to design the best education intervention for the patient. Similarly, to design a successful diabetes education program, the diabetes educator in the role of program manager must also do a thorough assessment. Questions such as the following will need to be answered as part of the assessment:

What are the expectations for the program?
What resources exist?
Who is the target population and what are their needs?
Are there similar programs in the region, and how might this program be similar or different?

Assess Expectations and Guidelines

If the program is part of a larger organization or business (such as a hospital, pharmacy, or medical office), it is important to make sure that the expectations of the administrators are understood. Does the senior leadership expect a program that will reach a certain target population? Break even in terms of expenses? Contribute revenue to other departments? It is critical for the program manager to understand as fully as possible what expectations are held by the executive team. If expectations are not realistic, the program manager needs to discuss with the leaders what may actually be possible, instead of focusing on what is *not* likely to happen.

A thorough understanding of the National Standards of Diabetes Self-Management Education and Support (NSDSMES) is essential to starting and running a quality diabetes education program.[3] The National Standards are guidelines designed to define quality DSME and to assist diabetes educators who work in a variety of settings to provide evidence-based diabetes education. The most recent review and revisions acknowledge the importance of ongoing support for sustaining behavior change, and thus the name of the standards was revised to emphasize this. Table 11.1 provides a summary of the 10 standards. To receive Medicare reimbursement for services, the program manager must demonstrate that every standard has been met.

Assess Available Resources

As part of the assessment process, the program manager must determine what is available in terms of existing resources and what needs to be acquired (purchased) or developed. As a first step, the program manager may assess his or her own competencies, skills, and experience and compare them with those outlined in the AADE *Competencies for Diabetes Educators*. Within that resource, 5 competency domains are described, including a domain of knowledge called Program and Business Management.[4] A series of objectives for both program and business management provides the newly appointed program manager with specific guidance for skills and knowledge he or she may need to acquire in order to be successful in the role. See Table 11.2 for examples.

TABLE 11.1	National Standards of Diabetes Self-Management Education and Support (NSDSMES)
Standard 1: Internal structure	The provider(s) of DSME will document an organizational structure, mission statement, and goals. For those providers working within a larger organization, that organization will recognize and support quality diabetes DSME as an integral component of diabetes care.
Standard 2: External input	The provider(s) of DSME will seek ongoing input from external stakeholders and experts in order to promote program quality.
Standard 3: Access	The provider(s) of DSME will determine who to serve, how best to deliver diabetes education to that population, and what resources can provide ongoing support for that population.
Standard 4: Program coordination	A coordinator will be designated to oversee the DSME program. The coordinator will have oversight responsibility for the planning, implementation, and evaluation of education services.
Standard 5: Instructional staff	One or more instructors will provide DSME and, when applicable, diabetes self-management support (DSMS). At least one of the instructors responsible for designing and planning DSMS will be either a registered nurse, registered dietitian, or pharmacist with training and experience pertinent to DSME, or another professional with certification in diabetes care and education, such as a certified diabetes educator (CDE) or board certified–advanced diabetes manager (BC-ADM). Other health workers can contribute to DSME and provide DSMS with appropriate training in diabetes and with supervision and support.
Standard 6: Curriculum	A written curriculum reflecting current evidence and practice guidelines, with criteria for evaluating outcomes, will serve as the framework for the provision of DSME. The needs of the individual participant will determine which parts of the curriculum will be provided to that individual.
Standard 7: Individualization	The diabetes self-management, education, and support needs of each participant will be assessed by one or more instructors. The participant and instructors will then together develop an individualized education and support plan focused on behavior change.
Standard 8: Ongoing support	The participant and instructor(s) will together develop a personalized follow-up plan for ongoing self-management support. The participant's outcomes and goals and the plan for ongoing self-management support will be communicated to the other members of the healthcare team.
Standard 9: Patient progress	The provider(s) of DSME and DSMS will monitor whether participants are achieving their personal diabetes self-management goals and other outcome(s) as a way to evaluate the effectiveness of the educational intervention(s), using appropriate measurement techniques.
Standard 10: Quality improvement	The provider(s) of DSME will measure the effectiveness of the education and support and look for ways to improve any identified gaps in services or service quality using a systematic review of process and outcome data.

Source: L Haas, M Maryniuk, J Beck, et al, "National standards for diabetes self-management education and support," *Diabetes Care* 35, no. 11 (2012): 2393-401.

Look for ways to develop and launch a program that makes the most efficient use of resources as possible. Ask questions that assess the program's finances: Has a budget been allocated for the program? Will the program manager be able to control the budget and plan for allocation of resources for staff, materials, continuing education training, marketing, materials development, etc? The most expensive resource is staff. It may sound ideal to have a full-time nurse educator, a full-time dietitian, and a full-time secretary, but can the volume of patients you are projecting justify the staff desired? It is better to start small with part-time staff and ramp up as needed. Likewise, it may be ideal to have your own classroom or your own equipment (such as a projector), but this can also be costly. Can space and equipment be shared with other departments or programs? Ensure the resources necessary to meet the program expectations of senior leadership are available. For example, if the leaders requesting a DSME program are expecting to review clinical outcomes on the entire population of patients getting

TABLE 11.2	Example Objectives for Program and Business Management

Domain V: Program and Business Management

Competency: Applies principles of program and/or business management to create a climate that supports successful self-management of diabetes

Level 2 Practitioner	*Program Management*
	1. Directs and/or manages all aspects of a diabetes education program
	2. Incorporates program strategies that lead an interdisciplinary care team toward achievement of optimal patient and family outcomes
	3. Develops and integrates a variety of problem-solving strategies aimed at improving diabetes self-management for individuals and families
	4. Anticipates, plans for, and manages patient transitions within the healthcare system to ensure care continuity
	5. Displays creativity to find and use healthcare resources to meet expected and unanticipated patient needs
	6. Develops, selects, and evaluates resources for use within the agency
	7. Serves as a role model of leadership, effective communication, and collaboration to the interdisciplinary/multi-professional care team
	8. Provides coaching and/or mentorship to other members of the diabetes care team
	9. Identifies areas of research need and assists with diabetes-related research
	Business Management
	1. Applies business management processes to create and manage a diabetes education program
	2. Identifies system failures and inefficiencies
	3. Uses principles of continuous quality improvement (CQI) to seek opportunities to improve quality and efficiency of program services
	4. Balances competing demands on time and financial resources
	Note: It is assumed that competency requirements are cumulative throughout the 3 levels.

Source: Adapted from American Association of Diabetes Educators, *The AADE Guidelines for the Practice of Diabetes Self-Management Education and Training (DSME/T)* (Chicago: American Association of Diabetes Educators; 2009).

DSME, an electronic health or education record of some sort will be a necessary investment.

It may be helpful to keep your scope of services narrow at first, so the program does not have to acquire too many resources or stretch the staff too thinly. For example, the logical place to start may be to serve a population of adults with diabetes, with a focus on the major minority group in your community that has a high incidence of diabetes. Adding services for pediatrics or gestational diabetes, or adding other languages may have to wait until the program is well established. It may be to the program's advantage financially to have a registered dietitian on the team who can also bill for medical nutrition therapy

(MNT), as that allows for another set of services to be offered.

Assess Community Needs

When an educator conducts an assessment of patient needs in order to understand the patient's diabetes skills and knowledge of diabetes education, the educator does the best he or she can given the limited timeframe. The educator does not go live in the patient's home and follow him or her around. Likewise, understanding the needs of the community where the program will be based is essential, but it can be done in a practical manner. Many program managers make the mistake of overinterpreting the NSDSMES and turn what was intended to be a quality guideline into something far too complex and unnecessary. For example, Standard 3 of the NSDSMES states that "the providers of DSME will determine who to serve, how best to deliver diabetes education to that population , and what resources can provide ongoing support for that population." It does not say that a 10-item survey needs to be designed, validated, and mailed to all residents with diabetes in a 20-mile radius for a scientific analysis. Getting input from several potential referring providers in the community about the kinds of patients they see and the barriers in skills/knowledge/behaviors they hope a diabetes program will address will fill this requirement quite adequately.

In addition to assessing the needs of the patients in a community, it is equally valuable to assess the needs of the providers (physicians and nurse practitioners) who will be referring patients to the program. Ask if they currently refer patients for diabetes education services and if not, why not. What would make them more likely to refer? How do they want to receive communication from the diabetes education program? How much involvement would they like you to have in terms of adjusting medications? The success of a diabetes education program is largely based on the satisfaction of referring providers (and the subsequent volume of patients they refer), so aim to keep them happy.

Finally, a program manager will be well served by taking time to assess the competition. What other programs are in the area? Whom do they serve? What features do they have? Don't be deterred from building a diabetes education program just because there may already be one in the community. When you consider the size of the population that may have diabetes, there are usually plenty of potential clients, even in small communities. Chances are, by learning about the competition, you can find ways to collaborate with and complement each other rather than compete with each other.

Assess Resources for Ongoing Support

While DSME alone is effective, it is even more effective when coupled with some sort of ongoing diabetes self-management support (DSMS) to help reinforce behavior change. Diabetes self-management support is part of the minimum quality standards (see

Table 11.1, Standard 8) and can be behavioral, educational, psychosocial, or clinical.[3] While the DSME program does not need to provide formal support, it does need to be familiar with resources that could serve this function. Diabetes self-management support can be provided through one-on-one interaction such as with a trained peer counselor or community health worker, or via a telephone call with a nurse case manager or lifestyle coach that is part of the patient's insurance plan. A growing number of online healthy living programs and apps include some kind of ongoing support and encouragement to stick with new behaviors and assist with goal setting. Patients can also receive ongoing support through their own primary care team, something that has become possible with the organization of patient-centered medical homes in many practices. Diabetes self-management support can involve joining a community-based program such as a mall walking group or weight management program. It might even involve strengthening an existing relationship with a community pharmacist who can chat with the patient about his or her goals and progress. But no matter the method of ongoing support, the DSME instructor and patient must agree on a plan together, which is communicated back to the referring provider in writing at the end of the formal education program.

Goal Setting

Goal setting for DSME requires knowing the plans of the referring provider and balancing them with the patient's own goals. It is important that goal setting be collaborative among the provider, the patient, and the diabetes educator. The same applies to the goal-setting process for program management. Begin with defining the program mission (and ensure there is agreement on the mission from all stakeholders) and then define more specific, measurable program goals. Just as with patient education, make sure the goals that are set are realistic and are clearly agreed upon by all parties (eg, institutional administrators, advisory board, and program staff). The business plan for a program is like the education plan for a patient in that it must describe what is expected to be done for the upcoming year of operations. All goal-setting activities should be assessed annually and revised as needed.

Define the Program Mission

The development and adoption of a mission statement is something a program manager can draft and present to the advisory group for discussion. A good mission statement may be short and state the obvious, but it helps focus the direction and clarifies the purpose of your program. Mission statements should be reviewed annually and edited as needed to ensure they remain relevant. Two sample mission statements that could serve as a starter for your advisory group to review and refine are as follows:

- The mission of ABC Diabetes Program is to provide comprehensive diabetes medical care and self-management education to individuals with diabetes and prediabetes.
- The mission of ABC Pediatric Diabetes Program is to provide the highest-quality diabetes education services to children with diabetes seen at XYZ Health Clinic and their families and thus help them better manage their disease and reduce their risks of complications.

Define the Program Goals

Establishing program goals is a good way for the program manager to stay accountable to the mission and help measure success. Written program goals are part of an annual program plan and should be reviewed annually both to assess progress on the previous year's goals and to modify the upcoming year's goals accordingly. Ensure goals have input from all stakeholders (such as institutional administrators) and are well understood by the instructional staff. The following are examples of first-year goals:

- To provide diabetes education services to patients from at least _____ different referring providers (or to increase the number of referring providers by _____ percent)
- To deliver services that meet patient needs by having at least _____ percent of patients complete the program
- To demonstrate success in moving patients toward achieving behavioral goals by at least _____ percent of patients showing progress toward the goal
- To operate a financially responsible program by showing a break-even budget at the end of the first operating year

Write a Business Plan

A written business plan and pro forma statements including budgets help establish clear expectations for the diabetes program. The business plan should be aligned with the program mission and goals. The term "pro forma" means "as a matter of form" and is applied to the process of presenting financial projections for a specific period in a standardized format. Pro forma statements are used for decision making, program management, and plans for expected expenses and revenues by which the program can be managed and evaluated. Essential to the development of a useful business plan is having a set of realistic assumptions in terms of expenses (salary, educational materials, and other operating supplies) and revenues (number of patients expected to be seen, expected revenues based on reimbursement rates, etc).

In addition to financial projections, the business plan may include the marketing plan as well as a plan for annual educational activities—or these may all be separate documents. Table 11.3 outlines key elements to think about in a business plan, including the following:

1. Defining the program overview
2. Describing program activities and timeline
3. Preparing the budget
4. Identifying marketing plans
5. Planning for program evaluation

Planning

Develop a Budget Based on Expected Income and Expenses

An important way to measure the financial success of the diabetes education program is to track the direct expenses of the program that are related to patient care and the revenue associated with those activities. In the case of diabetes education programs, salaries are the largest expense. Revenue is defined as cash you are entitled to receive once any contract discounts you have agreed on are taken into consideration. Dividing revenue by expenses gives you an indicator that is referred to as your return on investment (ROI), which helps determine whether expenses are being covered and, ideally, returning something to the hospital or larger organization or yourself. This overage can be used to cover expenses such as rent, or it can be reinvested in improving the operations. For

TABLE 11.3 **Sample Business Plan for a Diabetes Education Program**	
A business plan is a written document that helps you chart your course and follow it. Use this template as a guide to help you think about the steps involved in launching a successful diabetes education program.	
Program Overview	Organizational structure: • Reporting relationships • Sponsoring organization Mission/Goals: What is the purpose of the program?
	Target Audience (both patients/referring providers): • Who is the program aimed at reaching? Will you be providing gestational diabetes education, prediabetes education, insulin pump training, and continuous glucose monitoring system training in addition to general education for individuals with type 1 diabetes or type 2 diabetes? • What are the needs as expressed by potential referring providers? • Will you have resources to address the culturally and socioeconomically diverse needs of your target population, including resources needed by individuals with varying literacy levels and language needs?
	Staff/Team: • Who is on your planning/support team? • Who will deliver services? • Who is on the advisory board? • Who else do you need to connect with to build support? • Can you afford the staff size that you think is ideal? If not, what compromises might need to be made? What staff-to-patient ratios are reasonable and justify staff time?
	Resource Needs and Accessing Local Specialists/Community Resources: What resources are needed? (instructional, AV aids, etc) Program evaluation and continuous quality improvement: • Proposed dates for key activities (eg, advisory group meetings, large community events, continuing education programs) If you need to refer to others, do you know where to find a: • Podiatrist • Registered dietitian who offers MNT • Mall walking group • Reduced-cost exercise program • Weight management program • Mental health provider with expertise in chronic disease or diabetes
	Location/Space: • Where will the program be held? • What preprogram preparations are needed? • Is the classroom large enough to handle the numbers of registrants needed to meet your budget, as well as provide space for guests or interactive activities? • How often will you offer group classes, and how long will they be? Will you offer any support groups?

(continued)

American Association of Diabetes Educators©

TABLE 11.3 Sample Business Plan for a Diabetes Education Program (continued)	

Program Activities and Timeline	• What program activities and materials need to be developed? Examples include:
	  – Curriculum
	  – Documentation and referral forms
	  – Patient handouts and resources
	  – Plan for continuous quality improvement
	• When do the program activities need to be completed?
	• How soon can you submit to an accreditation/recognition program for review?

Program Budget	**Overview:** • Do you plan to have the program make a profit, break even, or operate at a loss? • How will patients be charged? • How will you get paid? • What are the expectations of the senior administrators for the program budget (are your expectations aligned? realistic?) • What is the landscape of the insurance companies in the region regarding covering diabetes education services? Is there a state mandate to cover diabetes education? Income: (see Table 11.4) Expenses: (see Table 11.4)
Marketing	**Building an Audience:** How do you plan to market the program? What are free/low-cost sources of spreading the word?
Evaluation	How will you know if the program is successful?

your program to be financially viable, covering direct expenses, it should produce an ROI of at least 1.

As part of the process of developing the budget, explore the following questions:

- What are the expectations of administrators for the program?
- Does there need to be a break-even budget or one that yields a profit, or will the program be partially subsidized by the hospital or physician's office as a service to patients?
- In addition to billing for patient visits (group and one-on-one), are there additional opportunities to generate revenue through conducting professional education programs, charging fees for educators' speaking engagements, selling books or educational resources, or billing for lab tests such as point-of-care A1C in the education office?

- If your center offers both medical and educational services, would a program of shared medical visits provide both a patient support benefit and clinical and financial benefits?

Use the budget planning worksheet in Table 11.4 to help think about sources of income and expenses. Plan for the practice to build over time. While breaking even in the first year may be difficult, a budget can be designed to show increasing revenues over the first several years, until a break-even point or profit is realized in the second or third year.

How the money will be collected needs to be determined. You can capture more revenue if you consistently collect co-pays up front. In addition, you can maximize revenue if you operate a cash-only program and have patients submit a bill to their insurance company on their own.

TABLE 11.4   Diabetes Education Budget Planning Worksheet

Use this worksheet as a guide to help you think about expenses you might have. Look for ways to decrease expenses or increase income by sharing expenses and seeking donations in the form of goods (AV equipment and patient education material from pharmaceutical companies) or services (volunteer time to help organize patient packets).

Projected expenses: _____

Item	Considerations	Dollar Amount
Staff	This is your largest expense: • Do you need to include only salary, or benefits as well? • Can any of the staff be part-time?	
Space/Overhead	• Do you need to pay for the space, or will it be donated by the sponsoring organization (hospital or physician's office)? Keep in mind that space cannot be "free" or donated to the program if Medicare is being billed for the education services, or it will violate kickback laws. • How will services such as electricity, heat, telephone, and postal services be covered? • You may need to pay for coding/billing support in your overhead expenses.	
Program materials	• This includes curricula, handouts, and teaching materials as well as AV aids (such as an LCD projector or flipcharts). See if you can share resources or seek donations from pharmaceutical companies for some items.	
Marketing	• This not only includes activities to promote your program, such as placing ads and mailing flyers, but also includes costs of printing things like stationery and brochures. • Plan time to make referral development visits to provider offices to describe your services and leave behind referral pads and/or other helpful information.	
Professional fees	• Do you need to generate enough revenue to cover expenses like continuing education unit credit hours and meeting attendance, professional association membership, and journal subscription? • Budget for application fees for AADE accreditation or ADA recognition.	

Projected income: _____

Source	Considerations	Dollar Amount
Patient revenue	• Will you bill the patient directly and have him or her submit to insurance? • If you will accept insurance, which plans cover DSME and MNT and at what reimbursement rate? • What patient volume will you need to see to meet your expenses? • What percentage is billable time? • What percentage is scheduled time? • How will you account for no-shows and what no-show rate do you anticipate?	
Sales of books/educational materials	• Will you sell any books and educational materials at a break-even cost or at a profit?	
Special events	• Fees can be charged for special events such as a continuing education program for healthcare providers or diabetes prevention and awareness classes and/or classes for grandparents or caregivers (as they are not billable to insurance).	

American Association of Diabetes Educators©

Establish an Advisory Group

The NSDSMES require that the advisory group include, at a minimum, a health professional, a person affected by diabetes, an individual representing the community, and other stakeholders. It is important to give careful thought to members and include not only obvious program supporters (such as a local endocrinologist) but also people who might be somewhat resistant to the program and would be advantageous to win over (such as a doctor from a group practice where a medical assistant who has diabetes herself is doing all the teaching). Advisory group members found to be helpful include people who have an "in" with marketing opportunities (staff member of a local newspaper), people who may be potential sources of referrals (local podiatrists, a retail pharmacist from the corner drugstore, or a representative from the community health clinic), and individuals who might have knowledge of competitive programs in the area (pharmaceutical industry representatives). Community leaders who can influence patients and providers to use your service are additional stakeholders to consider.

The standards are intentionally vague on how often an advisory group should meet, and the review criteria require, at a minimum, only annual input from the group. There is no requirement that the meeting be conducted face-to-face. However, it has been the experience of many program managers that well-planned meetings that tap into the ideas and expertise of advisors can really help shape the program and identify possible problems and barriers to growth before they arise. In fact, an excellent education program the author recently visited had 4 advisory board meetings each year, and each meeting focused on the review of certain standards. In addition to other routine business, the first meeting reviewed Standards 1 through 5, the second was devoted just to the curriculum (Standard 6), the third reviewed individualization and ongoing support (Standards 7 and 8), and the fourth meeting focused on patient progress and quality improvement (Standards 9 and 10).

Adopt, Adapt, or Create a Curriculum

The NSDSMES require that a program have a defined curriculum that is reviewed and updated annually and covers all required content areas (see Table 11.5). A curriculum includes learning objectives, methods

TABLE 11.5 DSME Curriculum Content Areas Required by the NSDSMES
1. Diabetes disease process and treatment options
2. Nutrition
3. Physical activity
4. Medications
5. Monitoring blood glucose and other parameters
6. Acute complications
7. Chronic complications
8. Psychosocial issues and concerns
9. Strategies to promote health and behavior change

Source: L Haas, M Maryniuk, J Beck, et al, "National standards for diabetes self-management education and support," *Diabetes Care* 35, no. 11 (2012): 2393-401.

of delivery, and criteria for evaluating learning for the populations served. It is not a set of slides and handouts sorted by topic area. The curriculum must define teaching approaches that are interactive and tailored to individual needs. Ideally, activities will involve problem solving so learners can practice application in real-world situations.

Evaluate whether it is more cost-effective for the program to build or buy. In other words, is it better to create everything, including learning objectives, teaching materials, and patient handouts, or purchase a complete program and tailor it to fit your needs? While commercial comprehensive curricula such as Healthy Interactions Conversation Maps can be useful, time must be allowed to annually review and update the objectives, content outlines, and support materials as needed and make any needed adaptations to fit the target population. Take care to identify resources that can meet a variety of literacy needs.

Determine Realistic Space Needs

In addition to traditional space options in hospital outpatient clinics and physician offices, explore other locations including community centers, public library meeting rooms, and shopping mall conference rooms. Think about accessibility issues, parking, and safety factors. If you have access to a classroom in a medical clinic, share it with other groups to minimize costs. Keep in mind that if you plan to bill for services and you use another health facility or physician office not owned by your institution, you will need to pay fair market value for use of the space to avoid violating kickback laws.

Identify Instructional and Support Staff

A common problem is overstaffing and not maximizing the use of group education. Having both a nurse and a dietitian work in a center may be ideal but not financially realistic. If only one education discipline is represented, consider identifying educators from other disciplines who might contribute to your advisory board, accept referrals, and deliver programs such as a special topics lecture. Hiring support staff may be desired, but it may not always be feasible. Tap into the hospital volunteer network or consider using former patients as volunteers who can help with mailings or preparing class materials. Maintain a written list of specialists and resources available within the community for referrals as needed, such as for experienced mental health providers, exercise physiologists, and specialty medical providers (eg, endocrinologists, podiatrists, and psychiatrists). Identify community pharmacists who have a special interest in diabetes and might be able to help with medication therapy management. In addition, maintain a list of support services that may be suggested to program participants, such as weight management programs, fitness or mall walking groups, diabetes support groups, and healthy cooking classes.

To best ensure program sustainability, program managers should ensure all staff are working at the top of their license. With training and mentoring from experienced educators, primary care offices can involve other office staff in education programs, including medical assistants and licensed practical nurses.[5] Many programs have found that involving community health workers or trained peer support counselors can be very valuable, especially with patient populations that represent diverse ethnic and cultural backgrounds.[6] When well trained and managed, these individuals can effectively work closely with the diabetes educators to deliver elements of the diabetes education classes, provide real-world examples to facilitate behavior change within unique community settings, and take leadership roles in programs offering ongoing support.

While having educators with additional certifications such as CDE (certified diabetes educator) or BC-ADM (board certified–advanced diabetes manager) may be ideal, it is not required for billing or reimbursement purposes. Obtaining such certifications has other benefits, however; individuals who hold either of these credentials do not need to provide detailed documentation of continuing education hours. Two significant changes have been made to broaden eligibility to apply for the CDE credential: (1) a new group of professionals, masters certified health education specialists (MCHES), may now sit for a CDE exam, and (2) volunteer hours working in DSME may now count toward the total 1000 practice hours needed before applying for the credential.[7]

Determine Information Technology Needs

Technology is a powerful tool, and program managers need to be aware of how it can be used within their programs. Evaluating information technology (IT) needs, available resources, and the kinds of data that program leaders are expected to analyze will help the program manager decide what kinds of IT resources need to be built and/or purchased.

Program managers are responsible for reporting patient and program outcomes and identifying methods for collecting individual and population-based data. Useful IT systems include the following:

- Electronic medical records (EMRs)
- Personal health records
- Diabetes data management systems and external large-scale Web programs through diabetes organizations, the government, and/or insurers

Information technology capabilities to aggregate, analyze, and report robust data need to be taken into consideration along with patient information security.

Implementation: Operating and Maintaining a DSME Program

Once all the assessment, goal-setting, and planning activities have been completed, the next step is program implementation. Like the fourth step in the DSME process for patient education, the implementation process for a diabetes program involves many components. The program manager oversees all operations related to the diabetes program, but turns to the advisory group whenever possible as a sounding board or for advice and recommendations. As part of day-to-day program operations, a review of key roles and responsibilities in the following 6 areas will help both new and experienced program managers improve the implementation process for their programs:

1. Managing staff
2. Communications
3. Front-end operations
4. Metrics and data
5. Marketing
6. Meeting the NSDSMES

These roles and responsibilities need to be reviewed regardless of program size, as they apply to both one-person operations and large multidisciplinary specialty centers. Program management of a diabetes center can sometimes feel like a lonely job (you don't have others in your institution who do that same job), but know that there are others across the country who are often happy to network and share ideas.

Managing Staff: The Most Important Resource for Overall Program Success

Staff development is a critical role for successful program coordinators. Whether the staff is just a team of 2 or a large team including educators and support staff, part of the coordinator's job is to keep the team members motivated, aligned in their goals, and competent in their overall roles and responsibilities. Program staff is the most important resource from the standpoint of the budget as well as from program delivery. Care must be taken to select the right person for the job and to make sure that tasks are clearly assigned (see Clear Communication section below) and that all employees are used to their maximum capacity (see Metrics and Data section below). Clear and frequent feedback to employees (including lots of praise when things are going well) helps shape appropriate behaviors. The program coordinator will be aware of where staff need further development, both for job satisfaction and job performance, and will identify ways to help each employee obtain those additional skills for growth and continuous quality improvement (CQI). Finally, the program coordinator will likely be the individual to maintain necessary

records of updated clinical licenses, registration, CDE credential status (if appropriate), and records of continuing education for all clinical employees.

Clear Communication: Enhances Overall Program Operations

The importance of documentation and clear communication as a basis for a well-functioning program is emphasized within the NSDSMES. Policies and procedures that are understood by the team and reviewed with the advisory board are an integral part of a quality process. Referrals to the education program from the medical care provider need to be documented in the medical record, as does communication back to the referring provider reporting on achievement toward goals and plans for ongoing support. The diabetes educator will need to document that the needs for self-management education have been assessed in all content areas, and that those areas found lacking are addressed in the education plan. Responsibilities and expectations for care must be clarified between the educator and the referring provider. For example, educators should assume only those roles within their scope of practice related to medication adjustment if operating under clear orders or guidelines from the referring provider. The referring provider should not expect the educator to handle routine phone follow-up unless it has been built into the budget. Discussing roles and clarifying expectations are an important part of accepting referrals and developing a collaborative care model with the patient.

In addition to clear communications within the team regarding clinical care, the program manager needs to ensure that all team members understand their productivity goals. Keep in mind that if the job can't be done in a cost-effective manner, it may not be done at all. Thus, to help ensure employment security (and to reach the maximum number of patients in a timely fashion), each healthcare provider should know what is expected of him or her in terms of numbers of patients needed to be seen in order to generate revenue to meet the program budget.

Although the NSDSMES require that an advisory group convene only once a year, most experienced program managers will agree that regular communication with members of this group can greatly enhance program operations. Advisory group members should be selected based on their connections with the wider community and ability to represent different points of view. Advisory group members bring the most value when they are kept in the loop regarding program activities and periodically asked for input or advice. Maximize the use of the advisory group members and the program will benefit.

Programs that are larger than a one-person operation will benefit by creating written policies or guidelines on a variety of topics to ensure clear communications. The program manager will want to guide the implementation and annual review of policies and procedures on clinical care topics such as the handling of medical emergencies (such as hypoglycemia) and medication adjustment guidelines. Operational policies are also needed, such as when and how to refer to other educators (especially if the program is only offered by a single educator representing one discipline, such as nutrition) and how to handle patients who miss appointments, along with policies related to billing and collection.

Finally, remember to keep the widest audience in mind when evaluating ways to enhance communication and keep everyone informed. In larger multidisciplinary programs, all too often formal communication is only between the healthcare providers, and the front/back office team is left out of the loop. Look for ways to obtain feedback from patients as well as from other customer groups (such as referring providers) to assess satisfaction with program services and operations. Ensuring clear and effective communications will help ensure effective program operations. Take the time to assess whether all systems are working as well as they can be or if there is room for improvement.

In addition to communicating with the team and referral sources, the program manager is responsible for communicating with the regional Centers for Medicare and Medicaid Services (CMS) and other government insurers, such as Tricare, to provide copies of accreditation/recognition certificates as soon as the program is approved. In addition, the program manager is responsible for ensuring that these agencies have NPI (national provider identifier) numbers for any dietitian instructors, especially if they plan on

billing for MNT. It would be prudent for the program manager to find out who his or her contact is at these agencies and keep communication lines open.

Front-End Operations: An Integral Part of the Overall Program

Even though many diabetes educators prefer to steer clear of anything related to the business operations of a diabetes program, it has to be recognized that good business is good medicine. The program manager must stay abreast of all operational aspects of the program, including the following:

- ◆ Scheduling
  - —Are schedules filled tightly and efficiently?
  - —Is a waiting list maintained in the event of a cancellation?
- ◆ Registration and patient data collection
  - —Are new patients asked how they were referred to the center?
  - —Are names of referring providers analyzed to assess impact of marketing efforts?
- ◆ Billing and collection information
  - —Are co-pays consistently collected at the time of visit?
  - —Are reports summarizing collection rates being run?

Regardless of whether the front-end operations are handled within the diabetes education program or by employees who are off-site (or within another department as part of hospital operations), the program manager should do his or her best to communicate and collaborate with these essential team members so they fully understand their role in the overall diabetes education program.

Individuals who are the "voice" of the program on the phone should have a very thorough understanding of the diabetes education program. Ideally, invite them to go through one or more of the classes. Help them understand the high value of diabetes education services. Offer a written script for training so receptionists can accurately articulate the services, benefits, and expectations for a new patient appointment.

The program manager is responsible for understanding all aspects of accurate billing and coding for the services provided, including DSME and MNT.

Even if these services are handled by another department within the institution, it is important that the program manager oversee what is happening to help maximize revenue opportunities.

Metrics and Data: Assess Program Operations and Impact

Ensuring clinical quality in a diabetes education program should be obvious. The NSDSMES require CQI, so educators will review performance metrics to demonstrate improvement in clinical and/or behavioral outcomes. However, while not required for a quality DSME program, operational metrics such as monthly patient visits (new and follow-up) and analysis of number of referrals by providers are essential to track in order to continuously improve program operations, thus ensuring its survival. In addition, the program coordinator often is responsible for budget planning and a monthly review of revenue and expense reports. If careful projections are not done for developing budgets, managing expenses, and increasing revenue streams, there will be no program.

To keep a diabetes program operating, there has to be clear expectations and accountability for revenue and expenses. Schedules for patient visits need to be built to maximize productivity and meet revenue goals. At Joslin Diabetes Center (and all of its affiliated programs), the standard has been set for 2 metrics. Joslin productivity data evaluate "outpatient hours billed as a percent of paid time" as well as "percent of time spent treating billable outpatients" (also known as face-to-face time). The goal for educators is to achieve 100% each month for the first metric and 60% for the second. For example, consider Chris, a CDE who in 1 week saw 20 hours of one-to-one appointments and conducted two 2-hour classes, each with 6 patients (resulting in 24 billable hours). Chris kept that same schedule for the whole month (4 weeks), resulting in 80 billable one-to-one hours plus 96 group hours for a total of 176 billable patient care hours during the 4-week period. If that number is divided by the standard number of working hours in a month (173), Chris is considered to be very productive by this standard, as she is billing for 102% of her time.

Using the same figures, how much time is Chris actually face-to-face with patients? This calculation provides an estimate of educator efficiency and productivity. The goal is to aim for 60% of an educator's time to be face-to-face with patients either one-to-one or in a group. Using the figures above, in a typical week, Chris sees patients for 24 hours (or 96 hours in a month). This calculates to 55% face-to-face time, which nearly meets the goal of 60%. It is clear that by seeing patients in groups, educators can be more productive.

One way to assess and improve productivity is to have educators complete a time study.[8] Ask educators to document for at least 2 weeks exactly how much time is spent in the following activities: billable patient care (group versus one-to-one), charting, phone calls, meetings, and other (be specific). By tracking exactly how time is spent, the program manager can assess whether the highest and best use is made of the resources. Are diabetes educators doing tasks that could be handled by the medical assistant or receptionist? How much time is spent on nonbillable patient care activities—and can that be reduced? The results are often surprising, as most educators are always very "busy" but not necessarily doing valuable billable activities. An analysis of diabetes educator productivity in 22 sites demonstrated that, on average, educators were billing 0.55 hours of education (one-to-one or group) for each hour of salary they were paid (range 0.19-1.21) but spent only 25% of their time on billable activities (range 11%-46%).[9] Findings such as this do not justify the types of salaries that educators are paid. Thus, educators not only need to be clear on what their productivity goals are for patient visits, but also need to participate in systems improvements to make sure they can meet or exceed those expectations.

Marketing: Ensuring Ongoing Program Growth

A large part of what most program managers do is related to ensuring a consistent flow of new patients into the education program and helping retain them for ongoing care and follow-up. Marketing activities do not necessarily mean that high-priced ads need to be placed in regional newspapers or magazines or heard over the radio, although that does help. Many things should be done on an ongoing basis to keep the patient schedules filled. A few tips are discussed below.

Focus Attention on Referring Provider

Referring providers are the most reliable source of patients and well worth the time it takes to make personal visits to primary care providers or endocrine groups to ensure they know about the diabetes education services offered. In addition to explaining the services of the diabetes education program and asking for referrals, it may be appreciated if you offer some services to the office staff, such as providing handouts on treating hypoglycemia or foot care guidelines, or conducting a lunchtime diabetes education program. Educating the office staff about diabetes will usually result in more referrals as they begin to understand that the disease is more complex than they first realized.

Don't Overlook the Obvious Often diabetes education programs are part of a larger institution such as a hospital or multispecialty outpatient medical practice. These days, everyone knows someone with diabetes, so make sure all employees know about the diabetes program. Offer an annual open house for staff, conduct diabetes awareness activities in March and November in the employee cafeteria, and see where posters or brochures promoting program activities can be distributed. Consider having patients who complete the education program mail a preprinted "thank you for referring me" postcard to their healthcare provider and share a flyer with a friend. A happy customer is a great source of referrals.

Keep Existing Patients in the System All too often, patients come for a comprehensive class series or a set of one-to-one counseling visits but return only in the event of a crisis. As part of the initial education program, help patients understand that because diabetes is a chronic disease, education also should be ongoing. The assistance a diabetes educator offers over time becomes even more valuable as it moves from providing vital survival-skills information that is part of the initial diagnosis to more complex problem-solving skills and ongoing DSMS. Take advantage of the Medicare reimbursement benefit that allows for up to 2 hours of education annually for DSME (after the initial 10 hours in the first year) and 2 hours of MNT (after the initial 3 hours in the first year). This can also be incorporated into a system of providing DSMS and thus keeping the patient engaged and supported over time.

No matter what strategies are used to market the program, keep all team members informed of the different initiatives so that they can help track the results and evaluate the effectiveness of the activity. For example, if spending a day at a health fair resulted in only 1 new patient, it may not be worth repeating that activity next year. On the other hand, if the front desk receptionists handling new callers are aware that the program manager has been working to build a relationship with the new internal medicine practice in town, they can provide reports on the numbers of patients coming from the practice and the program manager can respond with timely "thank you" acknowledgements for the referrals. Once again, communication is key.

Meets the Standards (NSDSMES)

There are 2 organizations that accredit or recognize diabetes education programs that meet quality standards as outlined by the NSDSMES.[10] The AADE and the ADA offer accreditation or recognition status to programs meeting established criteria. The Joint Commission provides accreditation for inpatient diabetes management. Ensuring that a diabetes education program meets minimum standards as outlined by the NSDSMES is important for 3 reasons:

1. It helps ensure a high level of quality.
2. It protects consumers with diabetes by helping them identify programs that meet the standards.
3. It is required in order for a program to be eligible for Medicare reimbursement.

Despite the detailed instructions prepared by each organization regarding the program guidelines and application process, there are many misunderstandings. Table 11.6 outlines some of the common myths and reports the facts for each topic.

AADE: Diabetes Education Accreditation Program (DEAP): http://www.diabeteseducator.org/

ADA: Education Recognition Program (ERP): http://professional.diabetes.org/

Evaluation and Monitoring

Evaluation is defined in the broad sense as a method of determining the significance or value of something by careful appraisal and study. An essential

TABLE 11.6 Myths versus Facts about Program Accreditation and Recognition	
Myth	*Fact*
All 9 content areas must be documented as taught in order for a patient to have completed the program.	It is true that there must be documentation to assess the patient's skills, knowledge, and behavior in all 9 content areas, but the patient only needs to be taught in areas that the assessment deems necessary.
At least 1 CDE needs to be on staff for a program to be accredited or recognized.	Having a CDE on staff is not required. However, an advantage to having a CDE or BC-ADM on staff is that he or she does not have to maintain documentation of all continuing education hours.
Accreditation or recognition will automatically guarantee reimbursement.	Accreditation or recognition is required for Medicare reimbursement of the G codes for diabetes self-management training (DSMT). Accreditation or recognition does not, however, guarantee reimbursement. Although most payers require that a DSME/T program have accreditation or recognition, reimbursement criteria vary.
A comprehensive education program should take about 10 hours.	Do not confuse what Medicare has agreed to cover in terms of diabetes education (up to 10 hours in the first year) with how long a program "should" be.

and ongoing step in the process of providing quality DSME is for the educator to evaluate his or her programs on an individual (patient) level, a program level, and a system level. The terms frequently referred to in DSME programs are "outcome measurement," "evaluation," and "continuous quality improvement." To ensure that all of the evidence-based standards and program requirements have a mechanism for evaluation, it would be wise to use and refer to each standard in the NSDSMES. The standards direct baseline and repeated measurements to assess the impact of DSME for individual patients as well as programs or populations. The design of DSME programs varies widely, and reliance on the standards and respective measures provides a framework for evaluating practice consistently. In this chapter, evaluation will be addressed from the program level.

Program-Level Evaluation

Evaluation helps determine which interventions are most appropriate and will produce the best outcomes for the population served by the DSME program. Just as patient education is not considered complete until outcomes are reviewed and evaluated, a program cannot be considered comprehensive if the overall clinical effectiveness and operational metrics are not routinely assessed. Regardless of whether the DSME service is provided by a single educator or a multidisciplinary team, the need for program

evaluation remains. The standards that address program structure and processes also require attention to evaluation.

Organizational Structure

Standard 1 requires that the DSME entity have documentation of its organizational structure, mission statement, and goals.[3] The mission statement sets the stage for the program and should be articulated, understood, and supported by the larger organization's stakeholders, administrators, staff, patients, volunteers, and community members. The DSME staff should review the mission statement annually with the advisory group or board to ensure its relevance and make modifications as necessary.

In accomplishing the mission, program goals and objectives first need to be identified and then monitored. The objectives can include statements regarding the target audience as well as metrics related to the reach and volume of patients to be seen. A review of the program goals and objectives should be conducted annually with the program's advisory board. It is essential to obtain an understanding of the program goals of the various program stakeholders. For example, don't assume that hospital administrators are only interested in program goals that demonstrate clinical excellence. They may be looking at goals that establish financial return or increased outreach to community providers. Take the time to understand the kinds of goals that are important to each of your stakeholders. Three sample program goals are as follows:

- To increase the percentage of patients discharged from the hospital who receive follow-up care in the diabetes program from 20% to 40%
- To increase the number of women with gestational diabetes seen at the center by 10%
- To increase the number of referring providers by 50%

Careful measurement and documentation of these goals is critical in meeting the program's mission.

Standard 2 mandates that the DSME entity appoint an advisory board to include broad participation of organization(s) and community stakeholders, including health professionals, people with diabetes, consumers, and other community groups.[3] The advisory board members are responsible for the development, ongoing planning, and outcomes evaluation process for the program.

It is the educator's responsibility to reassess the makeup of the board and participation of the members. Measures can include attendance records, member satisfaction surveys, and a review of meeting minutes to ensure active involvement. Focus groups led by a trained investigator also provide a unique opportunity to collect qualitative information about the community needs and program services. Advisory board members should be routinely polled to determine their preferences for meetings and communications (e-mail, face-to-face meetings, timing of meetings, etc).

Standard 3 refers to the identification of the diabetes education needs of the target population(s).[3] Thus, it is the responsibility of the educator to carefully assess the target population and determine its self-management education needs. The assessment process should identify the educational needs of all individuals with diabetes, not just those who routinely attend clinical appointments. Demographic variables, such as ethnic background, age, formal education level, and reading ability, and barriers to participation in education must be considered to maximize the effectiveness of DSME for the target population. Educators can assess this information using a variety of methods, including interviewing other providers in the target area, talking with the patients, and evaluating their own patient data, as well as reviewing epidemiological data available on federal and state Web sites. Surveys such as the Behavioral Risk Factor Surveillance System (http://www.cdc.gov/brfss/) and the National Health and Nutrition Examination Survey (NHANES) (http://www.cdc.gov/nchs/nhanes.htm) provide useful, reliable large-scale data.

Identification of access issues is an essential part of the assessment process. Although DSME is considered to be a critical component of diabetes care, the majority of individuals with diabetes do not receive DSME. It is the educator's responsibility to understand the barriers within the community. A thorough program evaluation process will help ensure that the education program reaches a wide audience. How are the services being marketed? How are programs being deployed? What is the effectiveness of the different marketing interventions? Tracking and evaluating the results of each type of marketing intervention can help assess its overall effectiveness in reaching the target audience and ideally result in increased visits.

Measuring patient satisfaction provides important insights from the population served. When evaluating patient satisfaction, it is helpful to have a core group of basic assessment questions as well as several questions that may be specific to a particular time period or need. For example, the standard patient evaluation assessment tool might always ask patients to respond on a scale from 1 to 5 how satisfied they were with the following:

- Diabetes care overall
- Ease of reaching someone in an emergency
- Lab tests reviewed and explained
- Concern, courtesy, respect, and sensitivity of the provider you saw
- Would you recommend your diabetes care provider if a family member or friend needed diabetes care?

Questions asked on a consistent basis are valuable for benchmarking progress across time. Many commercial patient satisfaction survey businesses benchmark results against similar institutions or programs that are also their customers. Optional questions that could be varied based on need might address issues related to parking, time of day for classes, interest in different kinds of support groups, or satisfaction with new educational materials being offered. It is valuable to regularly review your satisfaction survey and ensure you are obtaining information that can truly help effect program improvement and change as needed.

Remember that patients are not the only group that needs to be satisfied. Think about other consumers who influence the business of the diabetes program. Consider surveying referring providers to determine whether the education services are meeting their needs. It can also serve as a good marketing tool and reminder to the referring providers of the diabetes education program services. Other customer groups might include inpatient unit managers (Do they know of the diabetes consultation service? Are there improvements that could be made?) or hospital staff nurses and medical office assistants (Are there ways to improve their diabetes knowledge, skills, or awareness of services?).

Standards 4 and 5 attend to program staff.[3] A coordinator is designated to oversee the planning, implementation, and evaluation, while instructors are responsible for providing DSME. Careful evaluation of the credentials and skills of these individuals is critically important, and a mechanism must be in place to ensure that the participants' needs are met if those needs are outside the instructors' scope of practice and expertise. In addition to registered nurses, dietitians, and pharmacists, other health professionals (eg, physicians, behaviorists, exercise physiologists, ophthalmologists, optometrists, and podiatrists) and, more recently, lay health and community workers and peers provide information, behavioral support, and links with the healthcare system as part of DSME.

By assessing various operational metrics regularly, the educator can determine whether personnel and other resources are used efficiently. Without adequate operational data, it is difficult to justify the addition of new staff members or the expense of equipment such as practice management software and computers. An in-depth study of how educator time is used can guide the program administrator to ensure that the educators' time is put toward patient-centered, billable activities and that nonbillable or nonclinical tasks are delegated to others. Ultimately, the goal is to use the right person for the right task. Table 11.7 offers a tool that program managers and educators may use for setting goals, measuring baseline productivity, and tracking improvement.[10]

TABLE 11.7 Diabetes Educator Productivity Metrics						
Category	*Definition*	*Your Program Goals*	*Month 1 Actual Results*	*Month 2 Actual Results*	*Month 3 Actual Results*	*Quarterly Actual Results*
Educator paid hours	Total hours paid including hours worked and paid time off					
Billed 1:1 hours	DSMT and MNT provided ONLY if billed and ONLY for time billed					
Billed group hours	Total number of group hours times the number of patients in the group					
Total billed hours	Total billed 1:1 hours and total billed hours					
% paid hours billed	Divide the number of total billed hours by educator paid hours					
Group face time	Number of hours spent teaching billable group classes					
Total face time hours	Number of hours spent in billable interventions in front of patients. Total billed 1:1 hours and group face time					
% face time	Total face time hours divided by educator paid hours					

Standards 6 and 7 require a written evidence-based curriculum and an assessment tool.[3]

The content and questions within a standardized curriculum and assessment tool provide the foundation for direct evaluation measures. For example, if the curriculum content addresses nutrition strategies for women with gestational diabetes, specific questions should be developed regarding nutrition habits in the patients educated about gestational diabetes. If the assessment tool includes questions regarding cultural themes, a companion evaluation tool should include questions regarding the program's attention to culture and ethnicity. The use of evidence-based tools and outcome measures has been adopted by organizations and initiatives such as CMS, the National Committee for Quality Assurance (NCQA), the Diabetes Quality Improvement Project (DQIP), the Healthcare Effectiveness Data and Information Set (HEDIS), the Veterans Health Administration, and the Joint Commission.

The standards emphasize the importance of employing clear communication principles, avoiding jargon, making information culturally relevant, and using language- and literacy-appropriate education materials.

Health literacy is defined as the degree to which an individual can obtain, process, and understand basic health information and services needed to make appropriate health decisions. This involves both reading words and using numbers (numeracy).[11] It is estimated that 14% of adults have below basic literacy and an additional 22% have only basic literacy.[12] Limitations in literacy are most common in older adults, those with lower education levels, immigrants, and racial/ethnic minorities. Two questions which have been validated as effective as a basic literacy screen are the following:[11]

How often do you have someone help you read hospital materials?
Answers: always, often, sometimes, rarely, never (answers other than "never" may indicate a literacy concern)

How confident are you filling out medical forms by yourself?
Answers: extremely, quite a bit, somewhat, a little bit, not at all (answers other than "extremely" or "quite a bit" may indicate a literacy concern)

It has been shown that patients need ongoing DSMS to sustain behavior. Standard 8 refers to the development of a personalized DSMS follow-up plan.[3] A variety of innovative strategies are being made available for providing DSMS both within and outside the DSME entity. For example, nurse case managers, disease-management programs, trained peers and health community workers, community-based programs, use of technology, ongoing education and support groups, and MNT are providing this key service. Although many of these programs are expected to be effective, evaluation is crucial to informing healthcare practices and ultimately policy change and reimbursement. Educators would be wise to document follow-up processes, their frequency, and methods for delivery. Currently, it is not known which methodology is most effective in supporting DSME and in which environment.

The need to measure attainment of patient-defined goals and outcomes at regular intervals is the basis of Standard 9.[3] Measuring behavior change is the unique domain for DSME.[13] The AADE7 Self-Care Behaviors™ determine the effectiveness of diabetes education at the individual and group levels. Evaluation measures should be made at baseline and at regular intervals after the education program. Although systems to measure behavior change should be built into the education documentation systems and forms, educators may also consider tracking software that can help identify trends and progress.

Finally, Standard 10 states that the DSME program will use a CQI process to evaluate the effectiveness of the education experience provided, and determine opportunities for improvement.[3] Continuous quality improvement is a methodology used to evaluate how businesses and organizations deliver quality to customers. The first step toward providing a quality DSME program is reflected in these questions:

◆ Are your customers (patients) receiving the information/services they want?
◆ Are the methods used to provide these services effective and efficient?

A quality DSME program will evaluate its effectiveness (quality) on several levels:

◆ Process evaluation, which examines the degree to which recommended steps of care are currently being delivered

American Association of Diabetes Educators©

◆ Outcomes evaluation, which follows the impact of care on clinical indicators (glycated hemoglobin A1C, lipids, blood pressure) and on the general health and well-being of patients served

◆ Utilization review, which determines whether persons with diabetes are receiving appropriate care and treatment

Not only is CQI a mechanism to ensure the delivery of quality clinical and education services, it also is a valuable way to evaluate and improve a program's operational success and thus leads to an improved financial bottom line. Table 11.8 offers 2 sample CQI projects that are written following the AADE suggested format,[8] although there are several different formal processes for writing a CQI plan that may be used.

TABLE 11.8 CQI Case Examples	
CQI Case #1	
Determining whether behaviors actually change as a result of DSME	
1. Identify the problem	When the CDE manager was asked, "How effective is your program in changing behaviors?" she realized she did not have concrete data on which to base her reply. She decided to see if the team could get a better understanding of how often people actually do meet their behavioral goals by doing a chart review and phone survey.
2. Collect and analyze data	Charts were pulled from 20 patients who had completed the DSME program 3–6 months earlier (so there would have been time for a change to be assessed or documented in a behavioral goal). Two behaviors were chosen to study: 1. Increasing activity 2. Using a meal plan Data were available on 6 patients, either through an education follow-up visit documented in the medical record or via a follow-up phone call. Results showed 2 patients maintained or increased their activity level and 3 patients reported using a meal plan >75% of the time. The analysis revealed the following additional problems: • The percentage of patients available for follow-up analysis was lower than expected • Education records were not well designed to capture behavioral outcomes, and it took a long time to search for them • Some patients' goals were unrealistic and needed better oversight before they were documented in the chart
3. Consider possible solutions	The educators were disappointed in the results and brainstormed the following solutions: 1. Familiarize the staff with motivational interviewing and/or empowerment techniques to promote patient-generated realistic goals 2. Hire more staff just to do follow-up 3. Redesign education documentation tools to be easier to assess outcomes 4. Ask patients to provide a phone number where they can be reached in 3 months for a follow-up phone call (instead of using home numbers in the chart) 5. Conduct an additional class on writing measurable goals 6. Ask patients to self-address 2 reminder postcards to themselves. One would be sent about 6 weeks post program with an upbeat message of support. The other would be sent a week before the follow-up call to remind them that the call is coming and that if they are not available, they should call in. 7. Use an outcomes charting tool 8. Use a follow-up assessment form to remeasure behaviors

TABLE 11.8 CQI Case Examples (continued)	
4. Make recommendations	The CQI team narrowed the list down to choose 3, 5, and 7, as they appeared to be lower cost options (time and money).
5. Implement	The CQI team (including all staff) designed and printed the postcards and discussed exactly how the follow-up assessment tool would be used. (Patients would complete at last class and then again at follow-up, even if it was over the phone.) The CDEs were much more vigilant in reviewing patients' behavioral goal choices and suggesting modifications if they were too ambitious.
6. Evaluate	After 2 comprehensive programs, the new methods had been implemented with 20 patients. Eighty-five percent of the patients were reached at follow-up by phone or by clinic appointment. Of those, 80% met or exceeded their meal plan and exercise goal. The program could now say that at baseline, patients walked an average of 30 minutes a week and at follow-up they walked an average of 60 minutes a week. In addition, 80% of patients say they follow their meal plan >75% of the time, an increase from 20% saying they use a meal plan at baseline.
7. Have a maintenance plan	Patients reported liking the postcard reminders. The clinic found that address labels could be easily printed, so the patients only needed to affix the label to their cards. Goal sheets are kept on file but may be moved to a computerized record.
CQI Case #2	
Improving appointment scheduling at diabetes class	
1. Identify the problem	Although patients were encouraged as part of a group class to schedule a 1:1 follow-up appointment, they were leaving class before scheduling an appointment.
2. Collect and analyze data	At the monthly comprehensive class attended by 10 patients, the team determined that only 1 person made a follow-up appointment after class, and 1 more called before the next scheduled class. At the next class, each person was asked individually the reason an appointment was not made. Five of the 8 said "forgot" or "didn't understand that I was supposed to do it."
3. Consider possible solutions	The team brainstormed the following solutions: 1. Ask the secretary to come to class to schedule appointments 2. CDEs will call patients to schedule appointments 3. CDEs will write possible class dates on the board and each patient will select a date and turn it in 4. Mount a large piece of paper in front of the class listing date options for the follow-up class and invite patients to write their name next to the class they will attend
4. Make recommendations	The fourth choice above was selected since it not only requires the least amount of time but also empowers the patient to take the action and potentially join a class that a classmate/friend has signed up for.
5. Implement	For the next 2 series of classes, a large piece of poster paper was mounted in the front of the class with options for 3 different follow-up classes. The CDEs and scheduling staff met to discuss implementation. CDEs introduced the follow-up class sign-up at the beginning of the class and again at the end.
6. Evaluate	After the first class series, 7 out of 10 class members signed up for class, and 6 actually attended. After the second series, 9 out of 11 signed up and 8 attended.
7. Have a maintenance plan	The solution demonstrated an excellent improvement, without the staff needing to commit extra time. When class members sign up for a follow-up class, they are given the choice of 2 different kinds of classes, at 2 different times. They can also complete and take home a reminder card.

Source: Adapted with permission from "Diabetes Education Programs and the CQI Process: Recommendations for Joslin Education Programs," in *Education Program Planning Manual* (Boston: Joslin Diabetes Center, 2010).

Summary

As the epidemic of diabetes continues to escalate, the need for diabetes education programs remains high. However, in order to survive, programs must operate at a high level of efficiency. This means that the program manager not only needs to understand diabetes and chronic disease, but also needs to be skilled in business operations.

This chapter offered specific resources and suggestions to help program managers build and strengthen skills in program management and operations. The process of successful program management that was outlined follows the same 5 steps defined for DSME: (1) assessment, (2) goal setting, (3) planning, (4) implementation, and (5) evaluation/monitoring. Keeping these steps in mind will help organize the process for the program manager.

Focus on Education

Teaching Strategies

⊙ **DSME programs that produce good results share common qualities.** These include culturally relevant clinical approaches; adequate contact time; and treatment goals that are based on collaboration between the patient and the provider, involve competent diabetes education professionals, are group based, and have a strong foundation of collaboration between diabetes educators and physicians.

⊙ **Developing a learner-centered curriculum should be an ongoing process.**
- Use program evaluations to determine whether the content and delivery of diabetes education meet the needs of each patient. Adjust accordingly.
- Make sure that the curriculum is evidence based, both with teaching content and education methods.
- Align the curriculum with your teaching philosophy.
- Know which theories underpin your curriculum (eg, Common Sense/Health Belief Model, Social Learning/Self Efficacy, Dual Processing Theory).
- Assess how your teaching style works with the curriculum.
- Audit patient feedback and adjust the curriculum as needed.

⊙ **Design your teaching facility to bring out the best of the learning experience.** Create comfortable counseling and classroom spaces that are roomy enough for family members to join, have space for small group practice activities, yet feel private enough for intimate, personal conversations. To make waiting rooms more comfortable, consider adjusting the lighting and adding chairs for people of different sizes. Flowers and relaxing art are also a nice addition.

Messages for Patients

⊙ **Diabetes self-management education programs are designed to assist you in managing your diabetes.** Diabetes educators are skilled in teaching you about diabetes and how to incorporate diabetes self-management skills into your daily routine.

⊙ **Education is ongoing.** Diabetes education is not just a one-time event. Take as much time as you need to understand your options and make choices. As your life changes, so will your diabetes self-management. Your body changes, your diabetes changes, and your perspectives and ability to take care of your diabetes change. Adjust your diabetes self-management therapies accordingly.

⊘ **You are in charge of your diabetes.** You have the right and responsibility to ask questions, seek clarification, and make changes in managing your diabetes and overall health. You have a right to know all of your options and alternatives and the potential outcomes of your choices. You have the right to a second opinion, to ask your family or others for advice, and to take as much time as needed. And you have the right to receive information in a way that best matches your learning style, literacy level, and needs.

⊘ **You can learn about and manage your diabetes well regardless of your health literacy level.** *Education is the kindling of a flame, not the filling of a vessel—Socrates.* Socrates never told people what the correct answer was, but rather he engaged them in a conversation, asking questions that were designed to make them aware of their own beliefs and judge for themselves whether they were based on mistaken information or contradictions. Explore your own diabetes and solutions to your diabetes care.

Focus on Practice

⊘ **The NSDSMES set a foundation for developing and implementing a quality diabetes education program.** To receive Medicare reimbursement for services, a program manager must be able to demonstrate that every standard is implemented.

⊘ **There are 10 standards in the NSDSMES:** (1) organizational structure, mission statement, and goals; (2) advisory group; (3) target population(s); (4) a coordinator; (5) instructors; (6) curriculum; (7) individual patient assessment; (8) personalized follow-up plan; (9) measurement of patient-defined goals and patient outcomes; (10) CQI.

⊘ **There are 9 content areas of DSME:** (1) diabetes disease process and treatment options, (2) nutrition, (3) physical activity, (4) medications, (5) monitoring, (6) acute complications, (7) chronic complications, (8) psychosocial issues and concerns, (9) strategies to promote health and behavior change.

⊘ **Before you establish your DSME program, carefully assess the needs of all parties.** This includes patients, the community, providers, and financial stakeholders. Examine all existing available resources to either complement the existing services or provide a competitive edge. Set program expectations by defining program goals, its mission, and a business plan. Outline a strategy with a budget, advisory group, curriculum, office space, staffing, and IT needs.

⊘ **Effective implementation of a DSME program involves several factors:** ongoing marketing, clear operational communication, metrics collection, and meeting desirable accreditation standards, as well as a good understanding of coding and reimbursement for the services offered.

⊘ **Put a system in place in which providers are given consistent feedback on performance.** Feedback should be both quantitative (eg, A1C) and qualitative (eg, observations with patients) by the healthcare system and/or respected colleagues.

⊘ **Ask what the DSME program will do and how it will do what it is meant to do.** How will it improve patient care outcomes? How will it improve the delivery of care? How will it help the patient? How will it help the clinician?

⊘ **Review the requirements for accreditation/recognition of programs early in your planning so that you know what you will need to report and put in place to get your program approved in order to bill CMS.**

References

1. Department of Health and Human Services. Healthy People 2020 topics and objectives. On the Internet at: http://healthypeople.gov/2020/topicsobjectives2020/objectiveslist.aspx?topicid=8.

2. American Association of Diabetes Educators. AADE Guidelines for the Practice of Diabetes Self-Management Education and Training (DSME/T). Chicago: American Association of Diabetes Educators; 2009 (cited 2013 Jul 22). On the Internet at: http://www.diabeteseducator.org/export/sites/aade/_resources/pdf/PracticeGuidelines2009.pdf.

3. Haas L, Maryniuk M, Beck J, et al. National standards for diabetes self-management education and support. Diabetes Care. 2012;35(11):2393-401.

4. American Association of Diabetes Educators. Competencies for Diabetes Educators. Chicago: American Association of Diabetes Educators; 2009 (cited 2010 Nov 23). On the Internet at: http://www.diabeteseducator.org/export/sites/aade/_resources/pdf/competencies.pdf.

5. Maryniuk MD, Mensing C, Imershein S, Gregory A, Jackson R. Enhancing the role of medical office staff in diabetes care and education. Clin Diabetes. 2013;31:116-22.

6. Tang TS, Funnell MM, Oh M. Lasting effects of a 2-year diabetes self-management support intervention: outcomes at 1-year follow-up. Prev Chronic Dis. 2012;9:E109. Epub 2012 Jun 7.

7. National Certification Board for Diabetes Educators (NCBDE) (cited 2013 Aug 6). On the Internet at: http://www.ncbde.org/ncbde-announces-changes-regarding-initial-certification-effective-2014/.

8. Sullivan E. Educator productivity. In: AADE in Practice. Chicago: American Association of Diabetes Educators; Fall 2010.

9. Maryniuk MD, Moore T, Weinger K, et al. Diabetes educator productivity: an outpatient time study of daily activities. Diabetes. 2001;50 Suppl 2:A75.

10. American Association of Diabetes Educators. CQI: A Step-by-Step Guide for Quality Improvement in Diabetes Education. 2nd ed. Chicago: American Association of Diabetes Educators; 2008.

11. Powers BJ, Trinh JV, Bosworth HB. Can this patient read and understand written health information? JAMA. 2010;304(1):76-84.

12. Chew LD, Bradley KA, Boyko EJ. Brief questions to identify patients with inadequate health literacy. Fam Med. 2004 Sept;36(8):588-94.

13. Mulcahy K, Maryniuk M, Peeples M, et al. AADE position statement: standards for outcomes measurement of diabetes self-management education. Diabetes Educ. 2003;29:804-16.

CHAPTER 12

Transitional Care

Amy Hess Fischl, MS, RD, LD, BC-ADM, CDE
Christie A. Schumacher, PharmD, BCPS, BC-ADM, CDE

Key Concepts

- Transitional care occurs throughout the life span and settings, is continuously evolving, and must be tailored to each individual.
- There are important differences between children/adolescents/young adults and adults in diabetes education and management. Focusing on the methods of communication, teaching tools, and goals is key to successful transition.
- Education in the hospital can play an important role in diabetes management and should begin upon admission.
- Self-care and adherence should be encouraged through disease state education, and barriers

to inpatient and outpatient care should be identified early in the education process.
- The patient's knowledge should be assessed and continually reassessed throughout the transition to maintain an appropriate knowledge base and confirm important concepts.
- An individualized plan that promotes self-care should be developed for each person with diabetes.
- Communication among the person with diabetes, his or her family, and the healthcare team is a vital component of diabetes care. Confirm that everyone involved in the patient's care understands the goals and care plan.

Introduction

Transitional care has become an essential component of patient care within the inpatient and outpatient settings and at all ages and stages of life. Transitions for persons with diabetes are multifaceted throughout the life span since responsibilities are closely tied to age and maturity. The transition from pediatric to adult care has also become an integral element within diabetes education due to the competing demands of relationships and careers, as well as the psychological and physical changes.[1] A successful path for good diabetes self-management is founded on a collaborative approach with the healthcare team with the individual actively involved in the process from the beginning.

"Transitional care" is a diverse term. It includes the care of diabetes across the life span and transitions between different institutions and settings—all of which are an important part of patient care. It has been shown that one half of hospitalized patients experience

at least 1 medical error in medication management, diagnostic workup, or follow-up testing as they change between healthcare settings.[2] The majority of errors and adverse drug events can be attributed to lack of communication between healthcare providers at the different settings.[3] This is an important area for diabetes educators as they are in a position to facilitate communication and encourage self-care and adherence.

Infancy Through Young Adulthood

While children at different ages will be able to accomplish different tasks and accept different responsibilities, diabetes is a family condition. During this time, it is important not to expect more from children than they are able to do. Age does not always equal maturity, and increasing diabetes responsibility must be individualized. Table 14.3 in chapter 14 lists the normal developmental tasks for the developmental stages from infancy through age 19.

Pediatric Care: Infant to Age 3

Tips for managing diabetes in an infant include the following:

◆ Adjust insulin program around eating patterns.
◆ Use small lancets and small needles for blood glucose testing and injections.
◆ Use an auto-injector and numbing cream to help minimize the fear and pain of injections.
◆ Have supplies ready before blood tests and injections to minimize stress.
◆ Avoid glucose testing or injections in the child's bed (keep the bed a "safe" place).
◆ Use play as a teaching tool.
◆ Use the toes or heels for blood glucose testing.
◆ Distract the child with a game or song so that he or she is not focused on the task at hand.
◆ Speak in soothing tones so the infant is not frightened.

During this time of rapid growth and development, key motor and brain maturity is taking place[4,5]:

◆ Sitting—age 6 to 8 months
◆ Crawling—age 6 to 12 months
◆ Walking—age 12 to 18 months
◆ Language development

Diabetes tasks are essential components of healthy growth and development, and parents and caregivers must attempt to remove emotion from the equation while completing these tasks. Infants and toddlers can identify emotional cues from their caregivers. Most outbursts regarding diabetes care are due to an interruption in the child's activity rather than true pain. Infants and toddlers develop trust during this time, so it is important to combine the diabetes care with love and affection and make it part of the routine instead of an addition. Then, the child will accept it more readily. Since the child cannot independently perform self-care activities at this age, diabetes care is the responsibility of the parent. As the toddler demonstrates increased interest in participation, this interest should be fostered.

Once mobility begins, this may affect blood glucose levels due to more energy expenditure. At this age, hypoglycemia unawareness is more common, so symptoms may not be evident. It will be important to test blood glucose levels more frequently as well as adjust insulin doses or add more carbohydrate snacks to reduce the risk of hypoglycemia.[4,5]

Tips for managing diabetes in the toddler include the following:

◆ Align foods in blocks of time.
◆ Limit choices for food, injection sites, and blood test times to minimize stress.
◆ Have the child help with blood tests and injections, perhaps by placing the test strip in the blood glucose meter or placing the lancet in the lancing device.
◆ Have supplies ready before blood tests and injections to minimize stress; for example, Buzzy® devices assist children with pain management (http://buzzy4shots.com/children/).
◆ Use stories, books, and games as teaching tools.

School—Early and Middle School

Table 12.1 lists the average age for mastery of specific diabetes-related skills.

TABLE 12.1 Average Ages for Diabetes-Related Skills	
Skill	*Average Age of Mastery (Years)*
Hypoglycemia	
• Recognizes and reports	8–10
• Able to treat	10–12
• Anticipates/prevents	14–16
Blood glucose testing	8–10
Insulin injection	
• Gives to self (at least sometimes)	8–11
• Able to adjust doses	14–16
Meal planning	
• Can identify appropriate pre-excercise snack	10–12
• States role of meal planning	14–16
• Able to alter food in relation to blood glucose level	14–16

Source: T Wysocki, P Meinhold, DJ Cox, WL Clarke, "Survey of diabetes professionals regarding developmental changes in diabetes self-care," *Diabetes Care* 13, no. 1 (1990): 65.

Tips for managing diabetes in the preschooler include the following[6,7]:

◈ Allow the child to do his or her own blood glucose tests and push the plunger on the syringe.
◈ Use reward systems, such as a sticker chart, to help with compliance.
◈ Avoid labeling blood glucose test results as good or bad.
◈ Help the child identify feelings of low blood glucose.
◈ Involve the child in meal plan decisions.
◈ Use stories, books, and games as teaching tools.

Tips for managing diabetes in the school-aged child include the following:

◈ Incorporate school lunches, parties, and special events into the meal plan.
◈ Plan meal, activity, and insulin schedules around usual activities.
◈ Make sure the school understands and provides for the child's needs.
◈ Monitor school attendance and performance.

Adolescence

There are several differences in behavior and development between early, middle, and late adolescence, the time between 11 and 21 years of age. Characteristics of each of these stages are highlighted in Table 14.4 in chapter 14. Adolescence is a period of rapid growth and increasing physical, cognitive, and emotional maturity. These changes may occur slowly or rapidly and are determined by genetic familial factors, the economy, nutrition, health, and the environment. Diabetes affects normal adolescent development, but identity and self-image concerns can revolve around diabetes concerns such as the appearance of the injection site or self-identification as "a diabetic." Normal independence issues may be impeded as a result of parental protectiveness or the teen's failure to assume responsibility for self-care. Adolescents with diabetes can become particularly concerned about their growth and sexual maturation. Metabolic control tends to deteriorate in adolescence due to a multitude of factors. Attitudes of experimentation and rebellion and risk-taking behaviors normally associated with adolescence can affect diabetes issues such as taking insulin regularly, monitoring, and the quality and quantity of food

consumption.[8] See Table 14.4 in chapter 14 for developmental characteristics at each stage of adolescence.

The following are tips for helping the early adolescent with diabetes management:

◈ Incorporate a hectic lifestyle into the diabetes plan.
◈ Begin to work on problem-solving skills and work up to independence.
◈ Discuss treatment options (multiple daily injections [MDIs], insulin pump therapy, and meal planning).
◈ Allow independent visits with the healthcare team.
◈ Include sex education as part of diabetes education.
◈ Monitor school attendance and performance.
◈ Allow independence in problem solving.
◈ Be nonjudgmental (eg, there is no such thing as a "bad" blood glucose reading).
◈ Keep social issues separate from diabetes.
◈ Help establish realistic goals.
◈ Watch for risk-taking behaviors, such as not taking insulin or substance use.

Transition Care (Adolescence to Young Adulthood)

According to Blum et al, "Transition is a purposeful, planned movement of adolescents and young adults with chronic physical and medical conditions from child-centered to adult-orientated health care systems."[9]

In 2002, the American Academy of Pediatrics, the American Academy of Family Physicians, and the American College of Physicians–American Society of Internal Medicine created a consensus statement on healthcare transitions for young adults with special healthcare needs. This was designed to illustrate the critical first steps for successful transition care. These steps are as follows:

◈ Identify an adult healthcare professional who can meet the individual's needs and provide uninterrupted, comprehensive, and accessible care.
◈ Identify the core knowledge and skills needed for successful transition and make them a required knowledge skill for primary care professionals in practice.

- Create a detailed medical summary of the individual.
- Create a written transition plan by age 14.
- Apply the same guidelines to all individuals and identify resources needed for those with special healthcare needs.
- Ensure affordable and continuous healthcare coverage.[10]

To encourage safe and successful diabetes management into adulthood, transition care from the pediatric setting to the adult setting is essential. Typically, most pediatric practices transition the young person to adult care after age 18. However, some pediatric practices allow the person to remain until postsecondary education is completed. At this point, there are no established long-term guidelines in place.[11,12] However, healthcare professionals throughout the world understand the need for transition care. Many position statements and recommendations have been created around the world in order to create continuity in the process.[13–17] A research thesis from Sweden published in 2008 illustrated the need to focus on gender-specific needs and timing of the transition, as it may be different for each gender.[18] One particular study conducted follow-up of individuals post-transition.[19] The average age of transition for this group was over 21. Since the ideal timing for transition is after psychosocial maturity is reached, waiting until this time or later may be advantageous in successful transition.[20]

Additional research has shown that young adults who have gone through transition mention the following issues with the process: (1) the mean age for adult referral was 17; (2) transition was too abrupt; (3) there was very little accessibility when transferring to adult care, as compared with communication received in pediatric care; (4) lack of coordination for the transfer; and (5) difficulty reaching the adult provider to ask questions.[21,22] Another discussion with patients identified that in the development of a smooth transition, a patient's ideal situation would be to feel as though nothing has changed and that any transition was a "natural" process.[23] Recent research has found that instead of focusing on blood glucose control, the focus should be redirected to psychosocial support much earlier and more often with

diabetes self-management. It was found that diabetes self-care confidence and perception of diabetes as a problem could be a positive indication of follow-up appointment attendance and better transition.[24]

A metasummary conducted by Lugasi et al[25] discussed patient perspectives of transition as well as factors or "conditions" that can successfully facilitate transition to adult care. The first condition refers to the *meaning* given to transition by the individual and his or her family. It is important that the discussion reiterate that transition is normal and is not a punishment or form of abandonment by the pediatric healthcare providers. Transition should have a positive connotation. The second condition is related to the individual's *expectations* regarding transition. The goal of preparing for transition is to reduce the stress involved. Assessing the individual's thoughts regarding the process can help move the individual in the right direction and make this a positive experience with realistic expectations. The third condition is the individual's level of *knowledge and skills* before the transfer. Empowerment is key to diabetes care, and the earlier this can be fostered, the more likely this process will not need to be a "cram session" prior to transition. The fourth condition encompasses the actual *planning* itself. While timing of the transfer may vary depending on maturation and individual goals, it is essential that planning begin early and be embedded in the conversation every time the individual has an office visit. The final condition includes the *environment* and the resources necessary for continued success.[25]

Effective transition is essential for continued quality care and successful long-term follow-up. The earlier the conversation begins, the more prepared the individual and family can become. Regardless of the individual's age at transfer, it is important to include the individual in the decision-making process.[26] Table 12.2 provides age-specific decision points for diabetes self-care and management.

Recommendations and guidelines from around the world are summarized in Table 12.3.

Within the United States, the National Diabetes Education Program created a transition tool to aid teens, young adults, and healthcare professionals through the process. The Web site includes a planning checklist, which begins 1 to 2 years prior to transition

TABLE 12.2   Examples of Teaching Points/Objectives for Transitions/Topic Checklists

Ages 8–10:

- Begin to answer questions in clinic
- Why you need to attend clinic every 3 months
- The importance of A1C values and target goals
- What it means to have diabetes
- Why some people have diabetes and others do not
- Importance of testing blood sugar and learning to test blood glucose (if not already)
- How to administer insulin (if not already)
- How the body uses food
- Identify carbohydrates

- How to make healthy food choices using MyPlate (USDA; http://www.choosemyplate.gov)
- The causes and symptoms of hypoglycemia and its treatment
- The role of insulin during sick-day management
- Identification of insulin types
- The effect of the school day and scheduling on blood sugar levels
- How sports, outside play, and other types of physical activity affect blood sugar levels and insulin doses

Ages 11–12:

- Assume responsibility to check blood sugars on your own at specific times of the day
- Define healthy eating and how it fits into your meal plan. Discuss ways to make healthy choices at school, when eating out with friends, and at other special occasions. Also discuss how to incorporate "occasional" foods.
- Begin to understand how an illness like a cold or the flu can affect your body and blood sugar
- Begin to name insulin types taken, their actions, reasons for taking them, and the proper doses

- How sports (especially practices versus games), play, and other exercise (including gym class) affect your blood sugar levels and insulin doses
- How diabetes affects your school day
- Introduction to drinking, smoking, peer pressure, and diabetes
- Effects of growth, puberty, and sexual development on diabetes

Ages 13–15:

- Answer questions independently in clinic and meet alone with the certified diabetes educator for part of the visit
- Inject insulin/change insulin pump with minimal reminders
- Parents review blood sugar logs and help you think through and double-check insulin doses
- Let parents know when you need medications or supplies
- The significance of A1C, how the choices you make affect it, and how you can change it

- What are urine or blood ketones, what do they signify, and how to test for them
- Discuss the blood tests that are completed each year and why
- Effects of growth, puberty and sexual development, sexual activity, and reproduction on diabetes
- The impact of diabetes on driving and the importance of checking blood sugar levels prior to driving

Ages 16–17:

- Independent with monitoring and recording blood sugars
- Independent with all insulin doses without parents reminding you
- Begin to call/e-mail the diabetes team and speak directly with staff if there are changes in your health
- The impact of diabetes on driving, the importance of checking blood sugar levels prior to driving, and steps to take if blood sugar is low prior to getting behind the wheel

- Know your health history including major illnesses, surgeries, allergies, and healthcare providers (dentist, eye doctor, psychologist)
- The impact of college, work, and career choices on diabetes management

(continued)

American Association of Diabetes Educators©

TABLE 12.2   Examples of Teaching Points/Objectives for Transitions/Topic Checklists (continued)

Ages 18–21:

- Routinely call the diabetes team and speak directly with staff if there are changes in your health
- Understand reproductive choices and the impact on your diabetes and overall health
- Discuss long-term complications of diabetes, the need for routine follow-up and tests, and the importance of glucose control into adulthood
- Establish care with a primary care health professional and with an adult diabetes team

- Review the American Diabetes Association guidelines versus the American Association of Clinical Endocrinologists guidelines (http://www.aace.com/files/dm-guidelines-ccp.pdf) and the International Diabetes Federation guidelines (http://www.idf.org/diabetesatlas) for managing and controlling diabetes

Source: Curriculum created by A Hess Fischl for the University of Chicago Kovler Diabetes Center, 2006.

TABLE 12.3   Key Global Transition Recommendations/Guidelines

International Society for Pediatric and Adolescent Diabetes (ISPAD)[1]

- Appropriate age of transfer varies according to maturity of adolescent and availability of appropriate services
- Provide a joint pediatric and adult clinic working together to facilitate the transition process
- Liaison between the pediatric services and the adult services
- Discussion of transition well in advance of transfer, allowing the adolescent and family to choose the appropriate time

American Diabetes Association Transitions Work Group[2]

- Preparation of at least 1 year prior to transfer
- Preparation should focus on self-management skills with a gradual transfer of care from the parent to the teen
- Information regarding the differences between pediatric and adult care should be included in the preparation for transition
- Written summary of transfer needed for adult provider and patient

National Institute for Health and Clinical Excellence (NICE)[3]

- Should be allowed sufficient time to become familiar with the practicalities of transition from pediatric care to adult care in order to improve clinic attendance
- Age of transfer should depend on the individual's physical and emotional development and maturity
- Transition should occur at a time of relative stability in the individual's health and should be coordinated with other life transitions
- Young people with type 1 diabetes who are preparing for transition to adult services should be informed that some aspects of diabetes care will change at transition

Queensland Government—Sweet—The Diabetes Transition Program[4]

- Flexible timing of transfer
- Flexibility in provision of health services
- A key worker for each individual
- Preparation period
- Choice of adult provider
- Coordinated transfer
- Accessible medical summary

Step 1: Ages 12–13—Introduction to program

Step 2: Ages 12–13—Assess diabetes knowledge and provide diabetes education

Step 3: Age 15—Key adolescent issues (see individual without parents)

Step 4: Ages 16–17—Assign transition manager

Step 5: Ages 16–17—Fully self-managing care

TABLE 12.3   Key Global Transition Recommendations/Guidelines (continued)

Diabetes Care Program of Nova Scotia[5]

- Ages 13–16: Initiate transition process, knowledge and skills assessment
- Ages 15–17: Continue completion of skills and education review and reinforcement, initiate complications education
- Ages 17–18: Assess readiness for transition, fill knowledge gaps, begin transition but pediatric to continue with follow up, pediatric and adult "designate" (case manager) collaborate for transition
- Ages 18–19: Appointment with adult team and adult designate; communication between pediatric and adult designate

Sources:

1. Court J, Cameron F, Berg-Kelly K, Swift P. ISPAD Clinical Consensus Guidelines 2009 Compendium. Diabetes in adolescence. Pediatr Diabetes. 2009;10 (suppl 12):185-94.

2. Peters A, Laffel L; the American Diabetes Association Transitions Work Group. Diabetes care for emerging adults: recommendations for transition from pediatric to adult diabetes care systems. Diabetes Care. 2011;34:2477-85.

3. National Institute for Health and Clinical Excellence. Diagnosis and Management of Type 1 Diabetes in Children, Young People, and Adults. London: NICE; 2004. On the Internet at: http://www.nice.org/Guidance/CG15.

4. Queensland Government/Queensland Health. Best practice guidelines for health professionals for the effective transition of young people with diabetes from paediatric to adult care. Diabetes Transition Program. 2006. Draft copy available at http://www.sweet.org.au/docs/PDFS/bestpracticeguidelines.pdf.

5. Diabetes Care Program of Nova Scotia. Moving on . . . with diabetes: adolescent transition resources. March 2012. On the Internet at: http://diabetescare.nshealth.ca/guidelines-resources/healthcare-professionals/adolescent-transition.

Case: Transition to Young Adulthood

CT is a female who was diagnosed with diabetes at age 3. What are the expectations for self-care?

At the time of diagnosis, her parents were responsible for all her diabetes care. At this age she was not able to identify hypoglycemia, so her parents needed to test her blood glucose levels more than usual since typical outbursts of a 3-year-old and the symptoms of hypoglycemia are similar.

There were times when CT was not cooperative with her diabetes care. Her parents and caregivers made sure to incorporate the care into her usual routine so there was no disruption in her daily life or increased episodes of acting out.

CT's parents allowed her to participate in her care by allowing her to choose which finger to poke for blood glucose testing as well as which arm for her medication injection.

As CT grew older, more diabetes tasks were transferred to her, depending on her maturity level. At age 7, she was very willing to test her blood glucose on her own as well as give her own injections. While her mother in particular was worried about having CT begin injecting on her own, it was important to foster this independence. However, setting guidelines was important to maintain safety. She did not inject her own insulin doses until she discussed the dosage with an adult.

At age 15, CT enrolled in drivers education. Discussing the importance of blood glucose monitoring prior to driving was cornerstone to her current care. She learned that in the event her blood glucose is under 80 mg/dL (4.4 mmol/L), she must wait 30 to 60 minutes before driving. While most teenagers would not comply with this recommendation due to time constraints, it was important to set realistic expectations and suggest that she test her blood glucose at least an hour before driving so that she could safely increase it if needed. At this time, to foster independence, all questions were directed to CT during her quarterly diabetes visits.

As CT prepared for college, during the years leading up to fall enrollment, conversations regarding drinking, smoking, drugs, and sex were usual discussions during each visit with the diabetes educator. While the conversations were not an invitation to engage in these behaviors, they were an essential component of diabetes care and education to help her understand what can occur in these situations and how to stay safe.

CT has been enjoying her time in college and has joined an intramural soccer team. Unfortunately, she tore her ACL during one of the games and spent the night in the hospital undergoing surgery to repair it. She will be discharged tomorrow afternoon to a rehabilitation facility. The nurse reviewing CT's chart notices that CT has diabetes. At a minimum, what should the nurse make sure CT is educated on before she leaves the hospital?

to an adult provider. It also includes downloadable documents for the current team to use, including a clinical summary document to complete for the new healthcare team. The transition tool and information about it can be found at http://www.Yourdiabetes info.org/Transitions.

Children in Foster Care/ Residential Settings

A recent case study reviewing foster care in the Bronx revealed poor glycemic control and suboptimal social outcomes for the children's cases reviewed.[27] For any children or young adults in foster care or residential settings, it is important to incorporate the following strategies:

◈ Work with a social worker and maintain communication in between health visits.
◈ Require the foster family to be involved in all health visits.
◈ Provide access to health data, especially if the individual is frequently moved to different foster homes.[28]

Transition continues throughout the individual's lifespan. While transition from one age to another

comes with its own set of rules and responsibilities, transitions to and from acute and long-term care also present their own unique sets of challenges and obstacles. Since each of these types of transition includes unique variables, collaboration with multiple healthcare professionals is the key to successful transition from admission to discharge and all components in between.

Transition Into the Hospital

Upon admission to the hospital, it is important to establish the individual's outpatient diabetes control and his or her home regimen (see Table 12.4). Reviewing the admission laboratory values, especially the glycosylated hemoglobin (HbA1c) and blood glucose, is useful to gain a better understanding of the efficacy of the individual's home regimen.

Communication is also an important component to determine the efficacy of the medication regimen and the individual's knowledge of and satisfaction with his or her diabetes care. Patients may or may not bring in their medication bottles upon admission. It is important to ask the patient about a typical day and have him or her clarify which medications are taken at which time of day.

Case Wrap Up

CT should be able to perform basic survival skills. CT's medication regimen should be confirmed to make sure that she is taking each medication correctly, and she should be notified of any changes in her home regimen during her hospital stay. It should be confirmed that CT is capable of checking her blood glucose and able to recognize the signs and symptoms of hypoglycemia and how to treat it. CT should receive information regarding a follow-up appointment for her diabetes management. It is important that she schedule a follow-up appointment since her activity level will change, along with her food and insulin requirements. It is also important to provide CT with contact information of a member of the healthcare team whom she can call with questions.

After the surgery, CT will stay at a rehabilitation facility for 7 days and will participate in physical therapy 3 times daily. What education should be provided to CT to

assist her in managing her diabetes during her stay at the rehabilitation facility?

CT should receive education on checking her blood glucose before and 15 minutes after exercise and should be educated to record and understand the relationship between her physical therapy exercises and her blood glucose. She should check her blood glucose before exercising and have a modified exercise plan or consume a 15-g carbohydrate snack for a value of less than 100 mg/dL (5.5 mmol/L). If CT experiences hypoglycemia during physical therapy, she should target a higher blood glucose before exercise. CT should be advised to keep carbohydrate snacks with her during exercise in case she develops hypoglycemia during physical therapy. It is important to educate patients on the importance of meal planning around exercise to prevent excess caloric intake and weight gain during rehabilitation.

TABLE 12.4 Assessment of A1C and Blood Glucose on Admission

A1C	Blood Glucose	Explanation
↑	↑	Uncontrolled diabetes mellitus or prolonged reversible cause of hyperglycemia
↑	↔	Improved control of diabetes mellitus Possible recent medication change
↔	↑	Controlled diabetes mellitus with recent lack of adherence or stress hyperglycemia

The process of obtaining a medication history involves integration of information from several sources, including patient and caregiver recollections, a patient-provided medication list, prescription bottles, outpatient medical records, and prescription refill information from community pharmacies. Prescriptions are often updated, and the patient may be taking the medication differently than instructed on the prescription; this is most commonly seen with insulin therapy. Always ask the patient to confirm the dose he or she is taking. Any discrepancies should be resolved with the patient and the caregiver upon admission, and all medications and dose instructions should be put on a list and saved for comparison at discharge (see Table 12.5). It is also important to identify any adherence issues upon admission so that barriers to care can be appropriately assessed and addressed

TABLE 12.5 Assessment at Admission[29]

Important Questions to Ask the Patient on Admission	Explanation
Do you have prescriptions from more than 1 physician?	Patient may be receiving duplicate therapy from multiple providers.
Do you take medications that are not tablets or capsules, such as patches or inhalers?	Important to include all medication delivery systems in medication reconciliation.
Do you take the medications differently than written on the prescription label?	To confirm that patient is taking the medication in an effective manner. Also an opportunity to assess compliance with recommended therapy.
How long have you been taking the medication and when was the last dose administered?	To determine when it would be appropriate to administer next dose in the hospital.
Do you use any over-the-counter products and/or herbal or vitamin supplements?	Over-the-counter supplements and products may contribute to drug-drug, drug-supplement, or drug-disease interactions.
Which vaccines have you received?	Hospital admissions are an important time to assess vaccination status and administer appropriate vaccinations.
Do you have any medication allergies or intolerances?	To determine whether patient can tolerate recommended therapy to prevent nonadherence.
Did you miss any of your recommended medication doses last week?	Important to assess adherence upon admission, so barriers to compliance and optimal care can be addressed before discharge.

Source: S Kripalani, A Jackson, J Schnipper, E Coleman, "Promoting effective transitions of care at hospital discharge: a review of key issues for hospitalists," *J Hosp Med* 2, no. 5 (2007): 314-23.

accordingly upon discharge. If the patient is admitted from a nursing home setting, the institution should be contacted for confirmation of medication and medical history.[29]

Medication Use in the Hospital

Upon hospitalization, patients may be transitioned to insulin therapy and home medication regimens placed on hold during the hospital stay. Hospitalized patients may be at an increased risk for changes in fluid, electrolyte, and renal status; therefore, medications, such as metformin, may be discontinued during the hospital stay to minimize the risk of lactic acidosis. Sulfonylureas are not commonly used, because patients are at risk for worsening renal function, which may decrease the clearance of the medication and increase the risk of hypoglycemia. Many hospitalized patients also have reduced oral intake, which can increase the risk of hypoglycemia with sulfonylureas. Thiazolidinediones (TZDs) have the potential to cause fluid retention and are typically held in the hospital setting. There are limited studies establishing the safety and efficacy of newer agents such as glucagon-like peptide-1 (GLP-1) receptor agonists and dipeptidyl peptidase-IV (DPP-IV) inhibitors in the hospital setting, therefore limiting their use as well.

Patients started on insulin in the hospital who were controlled on non-insulin medications at home will need an insulin dose calculated that is based on their weight, age, and kidney function. The first step is to determine the patient's total daily dose.[30,31] This is illustrated in Table 12.6.

If the patient is eating regular meals, the total daily dose of insulin should be divided into 50% basal and 50% bolus components to match the patient's carbohydrate intake, and additional correction doses of insulin should be utilized to cover elevations in the patient's blood glucose. The use of sliding scale regimens provides suboptimal blood glucose control and is no longer recommended. Patients who were well controlled on non-insulin agents at home can be transitioned back to these agents at discharge as long as they are clinically stable. The use of insulin in the hospital does not suggest that the patient be transitioned to a home insulin regimen. Patients who present on insulin pumps may continue to use their pump and should be monitored according to a uniform hospital policy to ensure safety.[31,32]

Example: Transitioning From Intravenous (IV) Insulin Drip to Subcutaneous (SC) Insulin Injections[33–35]

SC total daily dose (TDD) is 80% of 24-hour insulin requirement

Example case: Converting IV to SC insulin therapy

Calculate an SC dose for a patient who received 5 units/hour of rapid-acting insulin IV over the previous 24 hours

Step 1: 80% of (5 units/hour × 24) = 96 units

Step 2: Basal dose is 50% of SC TDD: 96 units × 50% = 48 units of long-acting insulin

Step 3: Bolus total dose is the other 50% divided among meals: 48 units/3 meals daily = ~16 units with each meal if eating 3 meals daily

SC insulin should be given before the drip is discontinued in order to allow an overlap that takes into consideration the onset of action. The first dose of basal insulin should be given 2 hours before the insulin infusion is discontinued.

TABLE 12.6 Determining Patient's Total Daily Dose of Insulin	
Patient Characteristics	*Starting Dose*
Older, has a lean body mass, and/or a history of chronic kidney disease or acute kidney injury in the hospital	0.3 units/kg/day
Normal body weight and no risk factors for hyper- or hypoglycemia	0.4 units/kg/day
Obese or on a high dose of steroids	0.5 units/kg/day
If patient was receiving insulin before admission, he or she should be started on the same dose as the outpatient dose	• Half of the total daily dose will be given as basal insulin and half as rapid-acting insulin • Basal insulin should be given once daily at the same time every day • Rapid-acting insulin should be given in 3 equally divided doses before each meal and should be held if patient is not able to eat, in order to prevent hypoglycemia

Sources: D Wesorick, C O'Malley, R Rushakoff, et al, "Management of diabetes and hyperglycemia in the hospital: a practical guide to subcutaneous insulin use in the non-critically ill, adult patient," *J Hosp Med* 3, Suppl 5 (2008): 17-28; C Lansang, G Umpierrez, "Management of inpatient hyperglycemia in noncritically ill patients," *Diabetes Spectr* 21, no. 4 (2008): 248-55.

Discharge Planning: Transition to Outpatient Care

Hospitalizations are an important time to initiate education with patients to prevent complications and future hospitalizations. An adverse event after discharge occurs in about 20% of adult patients and is most commonly caused by an adverse drug event.[36]

An increase in communication between the hospital team and the patient or the primary care physician can reduce the risk of an adverse event.[29,36,37] The patient should be assessed upon admission to determine his or her baseline disease state knowledge, and patient education should commence during admission and continue throughout the entire stay.

Early education and counseling provide an opportunity to identify barriers and determine the patient's feelings and knowledge of the plan. Patients are more likely to retain the information if it is divided over the entire stay. It is also important to include family members if they will be assisting in the patient's care. Inpatient diabetes education focuses on basic skills and knowledge and should serve as a bridge to ongoing outpatient education centered on the AADE7 Self-Care Behaviors™.[38] Disease state education and proper medication therapy management can improve long-term diabetes care. Table 12.7 lists things to consider when a person with diabetes is transitioning from inpatient to outpatient care.

Discharge Counseling

The main focus of discharge counseling should be survival skills. At a minimum, the patient should have knowledge of the following:

- The diabetes disease state and treatments available
- How to take each medication (eg, drawing up and administering insulin) and any changes in the medication regimen from admission
- How to check blood glucose and record in logbook
  —Patients should be educated to check relative to meals
- Signs and symptoms of hypoglycemia and how to treat
- Basic meal planning with an emphasis on eating consistently
- Sick-day management
- Contact information for follow-up appointments and education
- When to call a member of the healthcare team and who to call with questions

American Association of Diabetes Educators©

TABLE 12.7 Transitioning From Inpatient to Outpatient Care	
Consideration	*Comments*
Goal of this patient's diabetes care	Care should be individualized and based on cognitive and physical ability. Also, the educator should assess the patient's readiness to learn at the beginning of the educational sessions and should inquire about patient's preferred learning style.
Past history of diabetes mellitus	Does the patient have a past history of diabetes mellitus, and are the A1C and blood glucose readings at diagnosis within target range? The patient's previous medical history and disease state control should play a role in the patient's discharge education and home regimen. Newly diagnosed patients will require more discharge education, and previously diagnosed patients who are not well controlled will need to be assessed for barriers to adherence, and if needed, an intensification in medication therapy.
Hypoglycemia risk factors	If the patient has declining physical ability and/or cognitive impairment and is living at home, consider a simplified regimen with low risk for treatment errors and hypoglycemia.
Patient's medication history	The patient's home medication regimen should be evaluated upon admission, and the medication summary should include: • Medications the patient was taking before hospitalization • Medications started during hospitalization • New medications to be taken upon discharge It is important to highlight new changes in the regimen and make sure the patient understands why the changes were made. Most confusion occurs when the patient is unable to distinguish which medications were discontinued prior to discharge and which medications he or she should take when at home. Consider asking the patient what a typical day is like and when he or she takes his or her medications, to assess compliance and accuracy of medication administration.
Patient's knowledge of diabetes and treatment recommendations	Always assess patient thoroughly and tailor education appropriately to match learning style. The focus of newly diagnosed patients should be "survival skills" with referral for outpatient follow-up.
Financial stability	Is the patient able to pay for the recommended and prescribed blood glucose monitoring supplies, medications, and healthy food choices?
Access to healthcare services	Does the patient have established care with a primary care physician and health insurance to pay for medications and follow-up appointments? Consider transportation issues and make sure the patient has transportation for the first follow-up appointment.
Available support	Consider the patient's home support system. Does the patient have family and friends who can offer support?

Lifestyle	Ability to perform self-care activities:
	
	• What is the patient's current level of self-care?
	
	Physical/cognitive barriers:
	
	• Does the patient have any physical limitations, such as diminished vision or neuropathies, and what is his or her anticipated activity level?
	• Assess mobility, visual acuity, hearing loss, and dexterity.
	  – Will the patient be able to check his or her blood glucose, draw up insulin from a syringe, or use an insulin pen?
	• Will the patient be able to remember to take the medications as instructed?
	  – Will the patient need a pill box or a log to record information to assist with adherence?

TABLE 12.7 **Transitioning From Inpatient to Outpatient Care (continued)**	
Consideration	*Comments*

Lifestyle (cont.)	Psychological/social barriers:
	
	 • Does the patient have social support at home?
	 • Is the patient capable of adhering to the care plan, or does the plan need to be simplified?
	 • Does the patient feel comfortable injecting insulin or checking his or her blood glucose in front of others?
	  – Will he or she skip doses with variations in his or her work or social schedule?
	  – Identify and address barriers to using insulin or checking blood glucose when not at home.

Culture	Ask the patient about diet restrictions and, if needed, assist the patient in planning for days of fasting.
Health literacy	Will the patient be able to comprehend the educational materials? The education provided should not exceed a fourth- or fifth-grade reading level.

Sources: C O'Malley, M Emanuele, L Halasyamani, A Amin, "Bridge over troubled waters: safe and effective transitions of the inpatient with hyperglycemia," *J Hosp Med* 3, Suppl 5 (2008): 55-65; S Rogers, "Inpatient care coordination for patients with diabetes," *Diabetes Spectr* 21, no. 4 (2008): 272-5; A Nettles, "Patient education in the hospital," *Diabetes Spectr* 18, no. 1 (2005): 44-8; A Brown, C Mangione, D Saliba, et al, "Guidelines for improving the care of the older person with diabetes mellitus," *J Am Geriatr Soc* May, 51 Suppl 5 (2003): S265-80; A Migdal, SS Yarandi, D Smiley, GE Umpierrez, "Update on diabetes in the elderly and nursing home residents," *J Am Med Dir Assoc* 12 (2011): 627-32.

Educational sessions should be short and should be structured to optimize learning and utilize active learning techniques.[38,39] Education should be divided over the length of the hospital stay to be less overwhelming for patients, to reinforce previously taught concepts, and to spread the responsibility to more providers.[7,33]

Always ask the patient if he or she foresees any barriers or reasons why he or she would not be able to follow through with the recommended plan. An assessment of potential barriers should be conducted to rule out any potential nonadherence issues.

Common barriers that may prevent a patient from following the recommended regimen include the following[40]:

- Association of needles and injections with pain
- Weight gain
- Fear of complications of diabetes
- Inconvenience
- Complex, time-consuming regimen
- Cost

The diabetes educator should provide written information in addition to verbal instruction because patients are unlikely to remember all verbal instructions at discharge. Written instructions for patients and family members are a useful tool to reinforce important self-care instructions. These materials should contain information written at a fourth- to fifth-grade reading level and should be written in patient-friendly language. The "teach-back" method should be used to confirm understanding. Through this method, the educator asks patients to repeat back what they understood from the discharge instructions and education.[29] Patients should be asked to demonstrate any new self-care tasks that they will be required to carry out at home, such as administering a subcutaneous injection. Open-ended questions should be utilized to confirm understanding and to allow the patient and family members to voice questions and concerns; avoid questions with "yes" or "no" responses.

When creating a home medication list for the patient, avoid stating "continue home medications" or "resume all medications." Patients should be provided with a complete list of all their medications to be taken at home with indications, highlighting new medications and medications that they were taking upon admission that have been changed. Patients should be educated extensively on any changes from their home regimen before admission and on their discharge medication list. To improve adherence to the recommended regimen, patients should understand why medications have been added or discontinued. The medication list should also include specific instructions for administration, including the times of day. It is also important to make sure the patient has prescriptions for blood glucose testing supplies and insulin pen needles or syringes so that he or she has all the supplies necessary to carry out the discharge plan.[29]

Adherence With Follow-up Appointments

Patients are more likely to adhere to their post-hospital follow-up appointments if they are given a set appointment that is reviewed before or at discharge. Another method to improve adherence to the discharge regimen is to conduct a telephone follow-up 2 to 3 days after discharge. The additional telephone follow-up allows patients to inquire about any new medication issues and to ask any questions that they may not have thought to ask during hospitalization. The call also provides an opportunity for the educator to assess compliance with the home regimen and determine whether there are any barriers to compliance with the prescribed regimen. Evidence shows that follow-up telephone calls improve patient satisfaction, increase medication adherence, decrease

preventable adverse drug events, and decrease the number of emergency room visits and hospital readmissions.[29] Additional considerations for improving transitions in patients with physical limitations are listed in Table 12.8.

Diabetes Medications at Discharge

Newly diagnosed patients should receive appropriate treatment based on the current guidelines.[35,41] Patients with a previous diagnosis of diabetes mellitus who had good control prior to hospitalization can be discharged on their home regimen. Treatment should be intensified if the patient does not have good glycemic control; however, changes in lifestyle and stressors in the hospital which may have influenced glycemic control, such as illness, decreased food intake, or glucocorticoid use, should be taken into consideration. Before reinitiating medications, such as metformin or TZDs, check the patient's electrolytes, renal function, liver function, cardiac stability, and nutritional status to reduce the risk of complications such as lactic acidosis.[35,42]

For patients discharged on oral diabetic agents, discontinue basal insulin 12 to 24 hours before discharge and use bolus insulin when starting oral agents if extra coverage is needed.[33,35] Consider the onset and duration of each medication. Sulfonylureas, meglitinides, metformin, DPP-IV inhibitors,

TABLE 12.8 Improving Transitions for Patients With Physical Limitations	
Consideration	*Comments*
Age-related changes	• Decreases in the olfactory system and subsequent loss of taste may result in loss of appetite and malnutrition. • Malnutrition can also result from poor dentition. Patients may no longer be able to eat solid foods as easily and may start substituting with meal replacement drinks. • Increased risk of dehydration, which can lead to hyperglycemic hyperosmolar state (HHS) as the kidneys are no longer able to concentrate urine in response to fluid deficit. • Cognitive changes such as confusion, depression, and social isolation may also lead to an inability to provide adequate self-care.
Diabetic neuropathies	• Patients may not want to check their blood glucose because they fear additional pain in their hands or may have tremors that make them unable to check their blood glucose or draw up insulin.
Visual deficits and retinopathy	• Visual deficits and retinopathy can also present a barrier to patient self-care. Patients with visual deficits may miss taking certain medications or draw up an inaccurate dose of insulin.

Source: C O'Reilly, "Managing the care of patients with diabetes in the home care setting," *Diabetes Spectr* 12, no. 3 (2005): 162-6.

and GLP-1 agonists will begin to work shortly after administration; however, pioglitazone has a delayed onset of 4 weeks, and full effect may not be seen until 12 weeks. Other important considerations when choosing a medication regimen include the setting in which the patient is being treated (home, skilled nursing facility, etc), physical and cognitive ability, and family and social support. To prevent hypoglycemia and improve adherence, a basic medication therapy regimen may be required for an elderly patient with declining physical and/or cognitive ability who lives alone.[35]

Hospitalizations can also serve as an important time to reinforce that the patient is taking the recommended preventive measures to decrease cardiac complications. Vaccination status should also be confirmed in patients.

Case Wrap Up

HK should discontinue basal insulin 12 to 24 hours before discharge. She may start metformin 500 mg twice daily with breakfast and dinner if her kidney function and electrolytes are stable. Metformin will begin to work within 1 to 3 hours after the first dose and can be taken concomitantly with insulin to achieve euglycemia in the hospital. Metformin is cost-effective, so cost should not be a barrier for HK; however, she may need a pillbox to help with adherence.

The main focus of discharge counseling should be survival skills. At a minimum, HK should learn basic survival skills. Since HK is newly diagnosed, she should be educated on the diabetes disease state and treatments available. HK should also be educated on how to take her medication and what to do if she misses a dose. She should learn how to check her blood glucose, and the diabetes educator should confirm that HK has the proper prescriptions for a glucometer, strips, lancets, and alcohol swabs to check her blood glucose at home. HK should know the signs and symptoms of hypoglycemia and how to treat, and she should learn basic meal planning. She should receive contact information for follow-up appointments and educational sessions and should be given contact information for a member of the healthcare team whom she can call with questions. HK's physical and cognitive ability should be assessed as well as family and social support. It may be beneficial for HK to have a family member or friend present when reviewing survival skills, since the initial education process may be overwhelming for patients—especially HK because she is also recovering from a urinary tract infection.

Transitioning to a Skilled Nursing Facility or Other Acute Care Hospital

Management of nursing home patients includes education similar to that given to the patient and caretaker when the patient is going home. Only 15% of nursing home facilities have an established algorithm for treating patients with diabetes, and 30.8% of nursing home facilities have blood glucose monitoring policies[43]; therefore, it is important that patients going to another institution receive the same education as a patient going home. It is important for the diabetes educator to evaluate the formulary, processes, and staffing issues and determine whether the facility is similar to a hospital versus the patient's home. Hypoglycemic events are common and reported in up to 48% of nursing home residents; it should not be assumed that patients receive full diabetes care in the nursing home.[33,37,43,44] The diabetes educator should provide patients with hypoglycemia education, including signs and symptoms and how to treat to prevent complications of hypoglycemia.

Meal planning, including carbohydrate counseling and diet education, is an important educational component in the elderly population. For patients who have a poor nutritional status, the focus should be on medication management and lifestyle rather than diet restriction. The risk of hypoglycemic events with intensive glucose control may precipitate complications, such as falls and cardiovascular events that are more harmful to the elderly population than hyperglycemia.[43] All of these factors should be considered when assessing an elderly patient at discharge.

Transition to a Correctional Institution

Correctional institutions have policies and procedures in place for the management of persons with diabetes and trained staff available; however, the transition to prison can be a new challenge for a person with diabetes, as he or she will have to learn how to manage diabetes mellitus with access to fewer resources. The transition to a correctional institution will require additional considerations in meal planning and medication use as people with diabetes may not be able to test their blood glucose as frequently and will have to learn how to count carbohydrates effectively to prevent hypoglycemia or hyperglycemia during times when food is not available.

The patient's medical history should be conveyed to the correctional institution as early as possible to prevent hypoglycemia or hyperglycemia and complications of uncontrolled diabetes. Other information that is important for the correctional institution to receive includes the following[45,46]:

- Type and duration of diabetes
- List of current therapy and date and time of last medication administration
- Identified barriers to self-care
- Presence of complications and concurrent illnesses
- Family history
- History of alcohol and drug use
- Behavioral health issues, such as depression, distress, and suicidal ideation
- Information regarding follow-up if patient needs transportation to a provider outside the facility
- Name and contact information of provider at transfer institution who can provide additional information to correctional facility if needed

Each correctional institution has its own formulary, which will not include all insulin preparations and medications. The diabetes educator should call the institution to determine which medications on the formulary would best fit the patient's care plan. Rapid-acting insulin should be avoided in most circumstances due to the inability to coordinate administration with the timing of food. If needed, the benefit versus the risk of using rapid-acting insulin within the correctional environment should be assessed, and a plan should be established to prevent hypoglycemia. See Table 12.9.

Insulin pumps may not be allowed in the correctional institution, so the individual with diabetes may need to change insulin delivery methods. Glucometers should be provided and patients will be allowed to use them in accordance with regulatory guidance that addresses security, logistical, and infection control issues. Individuals with diabetes should be well educated about carbohydrate counting because they may not have access to resources for rapid correction of low or high blood glucose. They may encounter situations where they have to

TABLE 12.9 Considerations When Planning for Optimal Insulin/Food Coordination in Prison Facilities
• The size of the dining hall and the number of inmates:
– It may take 1–3 hours for the patient to receive his or her food.
– When will the patient be able to access his or her medication relative to the meal?
• Type of meal being served:
– Is there adequate nutritional information for the patient to be able to count carbohydrates?
• If the patient administers his or her insulin dose and a lockdown or emergency situation occurs before the patient can eat his or her meal, is there a contingency plan to prevent hypoglycemia?
• Is the correctional staff trained to identify and treat hypoglycemic episodes?
• Are emergency meals prepared for individuals with diabetes who received their medication but were prevented from eating their regular meal?

Source: C O'Reilly, "Managing the care of patients with diabetes in the home care setting," *Diabetes Spectr* 12, no. 3 (2005): 162-6.

self-detect hypoglycemia because frequent blood glucose monitoring is unavailable. Meal planning and signs and symptoms of hypoglycemia should be an important focus of disease state education when transitioning to correctional facilities. Encourage persons with diabetes to buy extra food from the canteen to have with them in the event of hypoglycemia.[41]

Transition to Rehabilitation Facilities

Individuals with diabetes who are transitioning to rehabilitation facilities should receive previously discussed discharge education with an added focus on checking blood glucose during planned or unplanned exercise. Rehabilitation facilities will have a formal exercise program, and a person with diabetes will have to learn how to check his or her blood glucose and eat according to the rehabilitation exercise schedule. The person with diabetes will have to document and learn his or her body's relationship between exercise and blood glucose. It is also important for the diabetes educator to provide goal ranges for blood glucose relative to exercise and advice for meal planning around rehabilitation activities. Individuals with diabetes should be educated to check their blood glucose before exercise and should have a modified plan for a value of 100 mg/dL (5.6 mmol/L) or less. They should also be educated to look for blood glucose patterns in response to different exercise regimens. If the individual has a higher rate of hypoglycemia unawareness during exercise, a higher pre-exercise blood glucose level may be targeted to prevent it.[47]

Individuals with diabetes should also be instructed to check their blood glucose 15 minutes after exercise. Hypoglycemia can occur up to 24 to 48 hours after an exercise session, so individuals should be educated to keep carbohydrate snacks available to prevent its occurrence. To prevent hypoglycemia, a snack of 15 to 30 g of carbohydrates should be consumed every 30 to 60 minutes during continuous physical activity. Meal planning, nutritional intake during exercise, and treatment of hypoglycemia are important components to avoid unnecessary caloric intake and weight gain during rehabilitation.[47]

Summary

Transitional care is an important component of the diabetes disease state management process. It starts at diagnosis and continues throughout the life span of the patient. It is crucial to take a proactive role in educating the patient and his or her family about the various transitions that may occur throughout his or her lifetime. Successful management of diabetes mellitus is dependent on collaboration between the patient and the healthcare team and their communication strategies to create an individualized plan. The diabetes educator's role should include a combination of care coordination and education focusing on the following[38]:

- Using an interdisciplinary team approach incorporating a patient- and family-centered model across the continuum of care
- Collaborating closely with other disciplines as needed, including social workers, care managers, and home care coordinators
- Establishing means of communicating the status of the diabetes self-management education plan of care and medication reconciliation to the next provider
- Empowering the patient and caregivers to actively participate in the patient's care regardless of the setting
- Promoting self-care

Focus on Education

Teaching Strategies

(→) **Create a timeline of teaching points for children, adolescents, and young adults in order to increase independence and improve diabetes self-management skills.** The earlier you begin the checklist of skills, the easier the transition to an adult provider.

(→) **When transitioning adults from an inpatient to an outpatient setting, the best chance for success is focusing on survival skills first.** Once in the outpatient setting, more detailed education can be initiated, based on individual need.

Focus on Practice

(→) **Utilize checklists for education topics that are needed for adolescents and young adults to successfully transition to adult care.**

(→) **For inpatient education, work with inpatient nursing staff to encourage teachable moments regarding the survival skills that are needed upon discharge.**

References

1. Wolpert HA, Anderson BJ, Weissberg-Benchell J. Transitions in Care: Meeting the Challenges of Type 1 Diabetes in Young Adults. Alexandria, Va: American Diabetes Association; 2009.

2. Moore C, Wisnivesky J, Williams S, McGinn T. Medical errors related to the discontinuity of care from an inpatient to an outpatient setting. J Gen Intern Med. 2003;18:646-51.

3. Forster A, Murff H, Peterson J, et al. The incidence and severity of adverse events affecting patients after discharge from the hospital. Ann Intern Med. 2003;138:161-7.

4. American Academy of Pediatrics. Caring for Your Baby and Young Child: Birth to Age 5. 5th ed. Elk Grove Village, Ill: American Academy of Pediatrics; 2011.

5. Borzekowski DLG. Considering children and health literacy: a theoretical approach. Pediatrics. 2009;124 Suppl 3:S283-8.

6. Silverstein J, Klingensmith G, Copeland K, et al. Care of children and adolescents with type 1 diabetes: a statement of the American Diabetes Association. Diabetes Care. 2005;28(1):186-212.

7. American Diabetes Association. Standards of medical care in diabetes—2013. Diabetes Care. 2013 Jan;36 Suppl 1:S11-66.

8. Siminerio LM, Laffel L, Peters A. Initial evaluation and follow-up. In: Peters A, Laffel L, eds. American Diabetes Association/JDRF Type 1 Diabetes Sourcebook. Alexandria, Va: American Diabetes Association; 2013:78-9.

9. Blum RW, Garrell D, Hodgman CH, et al. Transition from child-centered to adult health care systems for adolescents with chronic conditions: a position paper of the Society of Adolescent Medicine. J Adolesc Health. 1993;14:570.

10. American Academy of Pediatrics; American Academy of Family Physicians; American College of Physicians–American Society of Internal Medicine. A consensus statement on health care transitions for young adults with special health care needs. Pediatrics. 2002;110(6):1304-5.

11. Peters A, Laffel L; American Diabetes Association Transitions Working Group. Diabetes care for emerging adults: recommendations for transition from pediatric to adult diabetes care systems. Diabetes Care. 2011;34(11):2477-85.

12. Court JM, Ramerson FJ, Berg Kelly K, Swift GGF. ISPAD clinical practice consensus guidelines 2009 compendium. Diabetes in adolescence. Pediatr Diabetes. 2009;10 Suppl 12:185-94.

13. Nakhla M, Daneman D, To T, Paradis G, Guthman A. Transition to adult care for youths with diabetes mellitus: findings from a universal health care system. Pediatrics. 2009;124(6):e1134-41.

14. Kipps S, Bahu Ong TK, Ackland FM, et al. Current methods of transfer of young people with type 1 diabetes to adult services. Diabet Med. 2002;19:649-54.

15. Beskine D, Owen P. Review of transitional care for young people with diabetes. J Diabetes Nurs. 2008;12(1):34-8.

16. Wysocki T, Hough B, Ward K, Green L. Diabetes mellitus in the transition to adulthood: adjustment, self-care, and health status. J Dev Behav Pediatr. 1992;13:194-201.

17. Lotstein DS, Seid M, Klingensmith G, et al; SEARCH for Diabetes in Youth Study. Transition from pediatric to adult care for youth diagnosed with type 1 diabetes in adolescence. Pediatrics. 2013;131(4):e1062-70.

18. Sparud Lundin C. Living with diabetes during transition to adult life—relationships, support of self-management, diabetes control and diabetes care: thesis summary. Int J Integr Care. 2008 (cited 2014 Mar 10);8:1-2. On the Internet at: http://www.ncbi.nlm.nih.gov/pmc/articles/PMC2581663/pdf/ijic2008-200871.pdf.

19. Nev A, Losch-Binder M, Ehehalt S, Schweizer R, Hub R, Serra E. Follow-up of adolescents with diabetes after transition from paediatric to adult care: results of a 10-year prospective study. Exp Clin Endocrinol Diabetes. 2010;118(6):353-5.

20. Weissberg-Benchell J, Wolpert HA, Anderson BJ. Transitioning from pediatric to adult care. A new approach to the post-adolescent young person with type 1 diabetes. Diabetes Care. 2007;30:2441-6.

21. Pacaud D, Yale JF, Stephune D, Trussell R, Dele Davies H. Problems in transition from pediatric care to adult care for individuals with type 1 diabetes. Can J Diabetes. 2005;29(1):13-8.

22. Busse FP, Hiermann P, Galler A, et al. Evaluation of patients' opinion and metabolic control after transfer of young adults with type 1 diabetes from a pediatric diabetes clinic to adult care. Horm Res. 2007;67(3):132-8.

23. Allen D, Cohen D, Robling M, et al. The transition from paediatric to adult diabetes services: what works, for whom and in what circumstances? Final report. London: NIHR Service Delivery and Organisation programme; 2010.

24. Kaye J, Rapley P, Babel G, Brown S. Healthcare transition risk assessment for emerging adults with diabetes type 1. J Diabetes Mellitus. 2013;3(2):62-70.

25. Lugasi T, Achille M, Stevenson M. Patients' perspective on factors that facilitate transition from child-centered to adult-centered health care: a theory integrated metasummary of quantitative and qualitative studies. J Adolesc Health. 2011;48:429-40.

26. Lewis K, Hermayer K. All grown up: moving from pediatric to adult diabetes care. Am J Med Sci. 2013;345(4):278-83.

27. Gangat M, Klein GW, Heptulla RA. Foster care and type 1 diabetes in the Bronx: a case series. J Pediatr Endocrinol Metab. 2012;25(7-8):775-9.

28. DiGiuseppe DL, Christakis DA. Continuity of care for children in foster care. Pediatrics. 2003;111(3):e208-13.

29. Kripalani S, Jackson A, Schnipper J, Coleman E. Promoting effective transitions of care at hospital discharge: a review of key issues for hospitalists. J Hosp Med. 2007 Sep; 2(5):314-23.

30. Wesorick D, O'Malley C, Rushakoff R, et al. Management of diabetes and hyperglycemia in the hospital: A practical guide to subcutaneous insulin use in the non-critically ill, adult patient. J Hosp Med. 2008 Sep;3 Suppl 5:17-28.

31. Lansang C, Umpierrez G. Management of inpatient hyperglycemia in noncritically ill patients. Diabetes Spectr. 2008;21(4):248-55.

32. Moghissi E, Korytkowski M, DiNardo M, et al. American Association of Clinical Endocrinologists and American Diabetes Association consensus statement on inpatient glycemic control. Diabetes Care. 2009 Jun;32(6): 1119-31.

33. O'Malley C, Emanuele M, Halasyamani L, Amin A. Bridge over troubled waters: safe and effective transitions of the inpatient with hyperglycemia. J Hosp Med. 2008 Sep;3 Suppl 5:55-65.

34. Bode B, Braithwaite S, Steed R, Davidson P. Intravenous insulin therapy: indications, methods, and transition to subcutaneous insulin therapy. Endocr Pract. 2004; 10 Suppl 2:71-80.

35. Peterson G. Transitioning from inpatient to outpatient therapy in patients with in-hospital hyperglycemia. Hosp Pract. 2011 Oct;39(4):87-95.

36. Forster AJ, Murff HJ, Peterson JF, et al. The incidence and severity of adverse events affecting patients after discharge from the hospital. Ann Intern Med. 2003;138:161-7.

37. Rogers S. Inpatient care coordination for patients with diabetes. Diabetes Spectr. 2008;21(4):272-5.

38. AADE Position Statement. Diabetes inpatient management. Diabetes Educ. 2012;38:142-6.

39. Nettles A. Patient education in the hospital. Diabetes Spectr. 2005;18(1):44-8.

40. Laverna F. Treating hyperglycemia and diabetes with insulin therapy: transition from inpatient to outpatient care. Medscape J Med. 2008;10(9):216.

41. Inzucchi SE, Bergenstal RM, Buse JB, et al; American Diabetes Association; European Association for the Study of Diabetes. Management of hyperglycemia in type 2 diabetes: a patient-centered approach: position statement of the American Diabetes Association (ADA) and the European Association for the Study of Diabetes (EASD). Diabetes Care. 2012;35(6):1364-79.

42. Magaji V, Johnston J. Inpatient management of hyperglycemia and diabetes. Clin Diabetes. 2011;29(1):3-9.

43. Feldman SM, Rosen R, DeStasio J. Status of diabetes management in the nursing home setting in 2008: a retrospective chart review and epidemiology study of diabetic nursing home residents and nursing home initiatives in diabetes management. J Am Med Dir Assoc. 2009;10:354-60.

44. Migdal A, Yarandi SS, Smiley D, Umpierrez GE. Update on diabetes in the elderly and nursing home residents. J Am Med Dir Assoc. 2011;12:627-32.

45. American Diabetes Association. Diabetes management in correctional institutions. Diabetes Spectr. 2005;18(3):151-8.

46. Federal Bureau of Prisons. Clinical Practice Guidelines. Management of diabetes. Washington, DC: Federal Bureau of Prisons; June 2012 (cited 2014 Mar 10). On the Internet at: http://www.bop.gov/resources/pdfs/diabetes.pdf.

47. Lopez-Jimenez F, Kramer V, Masters B, et al. Recommendations for managing patients with diabetes mellitus in cardiopulmonary rehabilitation. J Cardiopulm Rehabil Prev. 2011;32:101-12.

SECTION 2

The Science of Diabetes Self-Management Education

Associate Editor
Cindy Halstenson, RD, LD, CDE

> Education is the most powerful weapon which you can use to change the world.
>
> Nelson Mandela

Diabetes educators are expected to have a foundation of medical knowledge that encompasses a current understanding of the science of diabetes, its treatment options, and diabetes-related complications. There is a notable difference in the way educators use this information, in comparison with others on the team: The educator not only must understand the science and apply it in decision making, but also must be able to translate such medical concepts and information into messages that can contribute to effective diabetes self-management.

Levels of Learning

As healthcare professionals, diabetes educators develop their expertise in stages, moving from concrete facts to abstract thinking. Competency requires both knowledge and experience, and takes time to acquire. Bloom[1] revised definitions of the levels of abstraction to include remembering, understanding, applying, analyzing, evaluating, and creating. Learning skills progress from remembering, based on simple recall; to understanding, when knowledge is interpreted and

translated into a new situation or context; to applying information, concepts, and theories. Analyzing involves the ability to organize and recognize patterns, and evaluating is demonstrated by the ability to assess, discriminate between ideas, and verify the value of theories and evidence. Finally, creating is the ability to relate a body of knowledge into predictions and conclusions.

The chapters in this section show how learning progresses, how information is organized and integrated into problem-solving strategies. While diabetes educators may recognize this progression in themselves, they need to appreciate their patients' need to apply new and sometimes intricate knowledge into new situations, and apply information to become competent in self-management. Bloom's taxonomy not only provides educators with direction in diabetes self-management education (DSME), but also reminds them how complex this new knowledge can be for them and their patients.

From Medicine to Messaging

For the diabetes educator, the focus in this information-rich section of the *Desk Reference* is on understanding and using medical information to promote behavior change and self-management. These chapters emphasize how this body of scientific and medical knowledge is integrated into the educator's practice setting. In dealing with the constant changes of a chronic progressive disease, the diabetes educator is further challenged to continually modify and adapt self-management education. Case studies are used in many of the chapters to help elucidate the experience of the individual living with the disease and draw out important points for diabetes education. The cases follow the patient through descriptions of the symptoms, explanations of physiology, and treatment options. The authors then discuss how the health-care team member can use his or her own experience and knowledge to help the individual affected by the disease.

As healthcare professionals, diabetes educators learn about disease by studying the basic science and medical concepts and reading the published literature. As knowledge advances, educators must stay current with the literature and evolution of the practice. Using evidence-based practice, they synthesize the scientific evidence to improve the quality and effectiveness of health care and DSME. The science of medicine is transformed into the art of diabetes education when the educator is able to appropriately incorporate and translate medical concepts into assessments, plans, interventions, and interactions. The educator needs to listen to his or her patients, understand their needs and capacity to understand difficult concepts, and then translate complicated science into actionable information to help them make behavior changes for diabetes self-care.

Diabetes care is a multidisciplinary and interdisciplinary challenge in which healthcare professionals of multiple disciplines collaborate with non–healthcare professionals who all contribute their expertise to provide comprehensive care. The interdisciplinary approach is clearly evident in this section of the book; chapter authors incorporate knowledge from the various health specialties, but frame it in the context of diabetes education. Material is organized into 3 content areas: the disease itself, its therapies and management, and chronic complications. Chapters within each topic area review and summarize current knowledge and relate to points relevant for diabetes education.

Chapter 13 reviews the pathophysiology of diabetes, and understanding the pathophysiology

enables the educator to not only interpret the signs and symptoms experienced but be proactive in the way he or she portrays the significance of effective self-management. True to the book's focus, the authors detail how the disease presents in individuals. Chapters 14, 15, and 22 provide an excellent overview of diabetes throughout the life span as well as hyperglycemia as it appears in youths, teenagers, young adults, pregnancy, young adulthood, and later adulthood. Patients often ask why certain things are happening to their bodies, and these chapters provide some answers. With the current interest and research into alternatives to Western medicine and efforts to blend it with other approaches, chapters 20 and 21 offer valuable insight for healthcare professionals working in DSME for both biologically based practices and nonbiologically based therapies. Whether health professionals use or recommend these therapies is not as relevant in diabetes education as being aware of the alternative remedies people may be using and how those therapies interact with recommended or prescribed treatments. Emerging evidence on the use of such interventions may well change the way DSME is delivered.

Several chapters in this section of the text focus on the core of DSME, integrating food, activity, frequent monitoring, and medication prescription and management. These chapters summarize important technical knowledge pertinent to these self-management issues, and in each chapter, the science is presented, the research is discussed, and implications for diabetes education are highlighted.

The final chapters in this section of the *Desk Reference* remind us of the impact of diabetes, controlled or not, on the health and quality of life of people affected by this disease. Since comorbid conditions often affect the individual with diabetes, other chronic illnesses, specifically hypertension and dyslipidemia, are included.

Each chapter begins with an overview of the various physical and psychological systems affecting the individual with diabetes. Issues of chronic complications, macrovascular disease, pregnancy with diabetes, eye disease, nephropathy, and neuropathy are then dealt with in individual chapters. Current information on primary, secondary, and tertiary prevention is highlighted. The case study approach helps show how specific conditions can affect an individual and how the individual progresses; the cases consider current treatments and recommended therapies.

The Challenge to Change

As the profession of diabetes education continues to move from a strictly content-driven method of teaching to an approach that is individualized and outcome-centered, practitioners are urged to recognize that their own methods of learning must change as well. Personal philosophies and experiences, moral and ethical positions, and understanding and knowledge about science and behavior change all color and enrich the patient-provider interaction. The unique work of diabetes education, and its ultimate goal of positively affecting the person with diabetes, requires taking evolving diabetes knowledge and applying it to individuals and populations.

Competence in the science, theory, and research is an underpinning of diabetes education. With this grounding, those responsible for DSME begin the art of their work: using their talents, personalities, and gifts in a therapeutic manner and integrating personal meaning and values into meaningful interactions with patients and clients.[2,3] Readers are challenged to recognize how they and their patients learn so that they can best apply complex medical information in their delivery of DSME and collaborate with their patients on making appropriate behavior changes to manage their diabetes. The diabetes educator's success in translating, explaining, and interpreting difficult information enables those with diabetes to become experts in their own care.

References

1. Anderson LW, Krathwohl DR, Airasian PW, et al. Revision of Bloom's Taxonomy of Educational Objectives. Upper Saddle Ridge, NJ: Pearson; 2000.

2. Carper BA. Fundamentals patterns of knowing in nursing. In: Polifroni EC, Welch M, eds. Perspectives on Philosophy of Science in Nursing: An Historical and Contemporary Anthology. Philadelphia: Lippincott; 1999:12-9.

3. Chinn PL, Kramer ML. Integrated Knowledge Development in Nursing. St Louis, Mo: Mosby; 2004.

Pathophysiology of the Metabolic Disorder

Joan K. Bardsley, RN, MBA, CDE, FAADE
Michelle F. Magee, MD, MBBCh, BAO, LRCPSI

Key Concepts

◆ Diabetes is a disease characterized by abnormal metabolism of carbohydrates, proteins, and fats. An understanding of normal fuel metabolism and its hormonal control is necessary if one is to fully grasp the abnormalities that occur in diabetes.

◆ A progressive increase in our understanding of the hormones and systems that regulate the normal physiology of energy balance is increasing our knowledge of the pathophysiology of diabetes. This is leading to improved pharmacologic treatment options for diabetes.

◆ An estimated 8.3% of the US population (25.8 million people of all ages: 18.8 million diagnosed and 7 million undiagnosed) has diabetes, and, based on fasting glucose or hemoglobin HbA1c levels, 35% of US adults aged 20 years or older are predisposed to diabetes or prediabetes. These disorders are increasingly prevalent in both children and adults and have increased prevalence in certain racial and ethnic groups (Hispanics, Native Americans, African Americans, and Pacific Islanders).

◆ Reflecting the underlying pathophysiologic processes that result in diabetes, glycemic criteria are used to diagnose diabetes and prediabetes. The fasting blood glucose threshold for a diabetes diagnosis of ≥126 mg/dL (7 mmol/L) correlates with the value at which appearance of retinopathy has been observed. Upon 2-hour 75-g oral glucose tolerance testing, glucose ≥200 mg/dL (11.1 mmol/L) remains the diagnostic threshold. An HbA1c of >6.5% may now be used for diagnosis. The

diagnostic test should be performed using a method certified by the National Glycohemoglobin Standardization Program (NGSP) and standardized to the Diabetes Complications and Control Trial (DCCT).

◆ Diabetes includes 4 clinical classes, which result from a variety of underlying pathophysiologic processes. These are type 1 diabetes, type 2 diabetes, gestational diabetes, and other specific types of diabetes (eg, caused by genetic defects in beta cell function or insulin action, diseases of the exocrine pancreas, or medications).

◆ Type 1 diabetes results from autoimmune beta cell destruction, leading to absolute insulin deficiency. Both genetic and environmental factors are implicated in type 1 diabetes. Type 1 diabetes is characterized by the abrupt onset of clinical signs and symptoms associated with marked hyperglycemia and a strong propensity for ketoacidosis.

◆ Type 2 diabetes results from multihormonal pathophysiologic abnormalities, the hallmark features of which are a progressive insulin secretory defect and insulin resistance. This disease progresses from an early asymptomatic state with insulin resistance, to mild postprandial hyperglycemia, to clinical diabetes requiring pharmacologic intervention, typically over many years. Obesity, weight gain in adulthood, and physical inactivity are environmental factors affecting this pathologic progression. The evidence for familial aggregation of both type 2 diabetes and obesity is substantial.

State of the Problem

Diabetes is a chronic, progressive metabolic disorder characterized by abnormalities in the ability to metabolize carbohydrate, fat, and protein, leading to a hyperglycemic state. This chronic metabolic dysregulation is associated with long-term damage to various organ systems, including the eyes, kidneys, nerves, heart, and blood vessels.

Diabetes is an epidemic in the United States, with 25.8 million people (8.3% of the population) affected by the disorder. Approximately 18.8 million people are diagnosed, while 7 million people are unaware they have the disease.[1]

Epidemiology: Race and Ethnic Differences in the Prevalence of Diagnosed Diabetes

After adjusting for population age differences, the national survey data from 2007 to 2009 for all Americans aged 20 years or older include the following prevalence of diagnosed diabetes by race/ethnicity[2]:

- 7.1% non-Hispanic white
- 8.4% Asian American
- 12.6% non-Hispanic black
- 11.8% Hispanic

Among Hispanics, rates are as follows:

- 7.6% for Cubans
- 13.3% for Mexican Americans
- 13.8% for Puerto Ricans

Table 13.1 provides a breakdown of diagnosed and undiagnosed diabetes among people aged 20 years or older in the United States in 2010.

An increase in body mass index (BMI) is generally associated with a significant increase in the prevalence of diabetes mellitus, hypertension, and dyslipidemia. The prevalence of diabetes mellitus and hypertension increases in an observable, linear fashion as BMI levels increase. Two national surveys, SHIELD and NHANES, showed the prevalence of diabetes mellitus was highest among morbidly obese individuals (BMI ≥ 40 kg/m^2), with rates of 25% (SHIELD) and 27% (NHANES).[3]

The maps in Figure 13.1 show the trend in the age-adjusted prevalence of obesity and diagnosed diabetes among US adults aged 18 years or older from 1994 through 2010. During this period, the prevalence of obesity and diagnosed diabetes rose in all states. In 1994, all but 2 states had a prevalence of obesity less than 18%, and no state exceeded 22%. In 2010, no state had a prevalence of obesity less than

TABLE 13.1 Diagnosed and Undiagnosed Diabetes Among People Ages 20 Years or Older, United States, 2010	
Group	*Number or Percentage Who Have Diabetes*
Ages 20 years or older	25.6 million, or 11.3% of all people in this age group
Ages 65 years or older	10.9 million, or 26.9% of all people in this age group
Men	13.0 million, or 11.8% of all men ages 20 years or older
Women	12.6 million, or 10.8% of all women ages 20 years or older
Non-Hispanic whites	15.7 million, or 10.2% of all non-Hispanic whites ages 20 years or older
Non-Hispanic blacks	4.9 million, or 18.7% of all non-Hispanic blacks ages 20 years or older

Note: Sufficient data are not available to estimate the total prevalence of diabetes—diagnosed and undiagnosed—for other US racial/ethnic minority populations.

Source: National Diabetes Information Clearinghouse (NDIC), National Institute of Diabetes and Digestive and Kidney Diseases (NIDDK), National Institute of Health (NIH), "Fast facts on diabetes," National Diabetes Health Statistics, 2011, NIH publication no. 11-3892 (Bethesda, MD, 2011; last updated 2013 Sep 9, cited 2014 Apr 9), on the Internet at: http://diabetes.niddk.nih.gov/dm/pubs/statistics/index.aspx#fast.

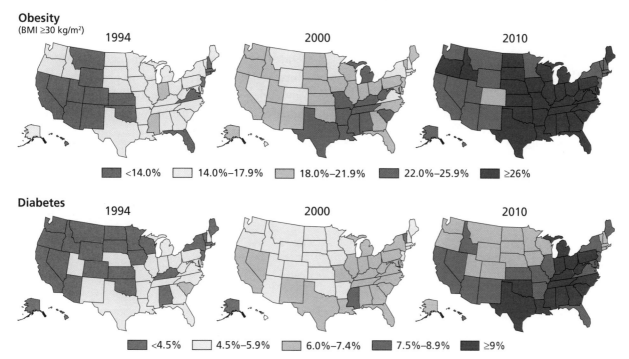

FIGURE 13.1   Maps of Trends in Diagnosed Diabetes and Obesity, 1994–2010 Trends

Source: Centers for Disease Control and Prevention, "Diabetes interactive atlas" (cited 2014 Apr 9), on the Internet at: http://www.cdc.gov/diabetes/atlas/.

18%, and all but 2 states exceeded 22%. Similarly for diagnosed diabetes, in 1994, almost all states had a prevalence less than 6.0%. In 2010, all states exceeded 6.0%; 15 of those exceeded 9.0%.

Overweight and especially obesity, particularly at younger ages, substantially increase lifetime risk of diagnosed diabetes, while their impact on diabetes risk, life expectancy, and diabetes duration diminishes with age.

The prevalence of type 2 diabetes is 3 to 7 times higher in obese adults than in normal-weight adults, and those with a BMI >35 kg/m² are 20 times more likely to develop diabetes than those with a BMI between 18.5 and 24.9 kg/m².[4]

Characteristics used to identify people at risk for type 2 diabetes and prediabetes include the following:

- Obesity
- Sedentary lifestyle
- Hypertension
- Dyslipidemia
- Family history of diabetes
- Gestational history
- Race/ethnicity
- Age

These risk factors may be assessed by various means, including community health screening, media campaigns, annual health maintenance exams, and risk assessment tools. Diabetes risk assessment tools have been validated for their ability to predict the likelihood of developing type 2 diabetes.[5,6] A variety of organizations, including the American Diabetes Association (http://www.diabetes.org), the National Diabetes Education Program (http://ndep.nih.gov), and the Harvard School of Public Health (http://www.hsph.harvard.edu), provide diabetes risk surveys on their Web sites.

Clinic-based reports and regional studies indicate that type 2 diabetes is becoming more common among American Indian, African-American, Hispanic, and Latino children and adolescents.[7] Data from the 2009 Indian Health Service indicate that 14.2% of American Indians and Alaska Natives aged 20 years or older who received care from the Indian Health Service had diagnosed diabetes.[7] Type 1 diabetes may account for 5% to 10% of all diagnosed cases of diabetes in adults.[1] Risk factors for type 1 diabetes include genetic, autoimmune, and environmental factors.

Fuel Homeostasis: 5 Phases

An understanding of the phases of fuel homeostasis (Figure 13.2) will enable the diabetes educator to more fully understand how hormonal physiology is relevant to and must be considered in glycemic control efforts undertaken with the patient. The following description is adapted from *Joslin Diabetes Mellitus.*[8]

Phase I is the anabolic/fed state (0-3.9 hours after eating), in which circulating glucose predominantly comes from an exogenous source. Plasma insulin levels are high, glucagon levels are low, and triglycerides are synthesized in liver and adipose tissue. Insulin inhibits breakdown of glycogen and triglyceride reservoirs. The brain and other organs use some of the glucose that has been absorbed from the gastrointestinal tract, with the remaining excess glucose stored in hepatic, muscle, adipose, and other tissue reservoirs.

Phase II is the postabsorptive state (4-15.9 hours after food consumption), in which blood glucose

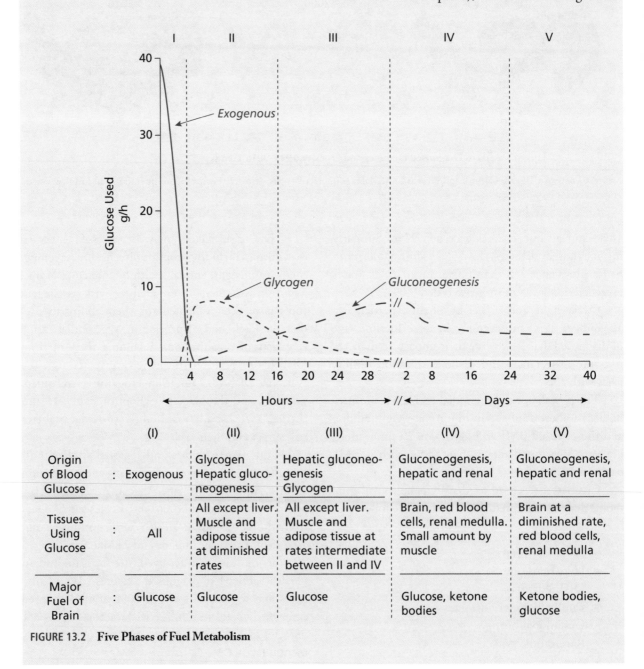

	(I)	(II)	(III)	(IV)	(V)
Origin of Blood Glucose	: Exogenous	Glycogen Hepatic gluco-neogenesis	Hepatic gluconeo-genesis Glycogen	Gluconeogenesis, hepatic and renal	Gluconeogenesis, hepatic and renal
Tissues Using Glucose	: All	All except liver. Muscle and adipose tissue at diminished rates	All except liver. Muscle and adipose tissue at rates intermediate between II and IV	Brain, red blood cells, renal medulla. Small amount by muscle	Brain at a diminished rate, red blood cells, renal medulla
Major Fuel of Brain	: Glucose	Glucose	Glucose	Glucose, ketone bodies	Ketone bodies, glucose

FIGURE 13.2   **Five Phases of Fuel Metabolism**

originates mainly from glycogen breakdown and hepatic gluconeogenesis. Plasma insulin levels decrease and glucagon levels begin to increase. Energy storage (anabolism) ends in this phase and energy production (catabolism) begins. Carbohydrate and lipid stores are mobilized. Hepatic glycogen breakdown provides maintenance of plasma glucose and ensures an adequate supply of glucose to the brain and other tissues. Adipocyte triglyceride begins to break down, and free fatty acids (FFAs) are released into the circulation and used by the liver and skeletal muscle as a primary energy source and as a substrate for gluconeogenesis. The brain continues to use glucose, provided mainly by gluconeogenesis (35%-60%), because of its inability to use FFA as fuel.

Phase III is the early starvation state (16-47.9 hours after food consumption), in which blood glucose originates from hepatic gluconeogenesis and glycogenolysis. Gluconeogenesis continues to produce most of the hepatic glucose. In this phase of starvation, lactate makes up half the gluconeogenic substrate. Amino acids, specifically alanine, and glycerol are other major substrates. Insulin secretion is markedly suppressed, and counterregulatory hormone (eg, glucagon, cortisol, growth hormone, and epinephrine) secretion is stimulated.

Phase IV is the preliminary prolonged starvation state (48 hours to 23.9 days after food consumption), in which blood glucose originates from hepatic and renal gluconeogenesis. By 60 hours of starvation, gluconeogenesis provides more than 97% of hepatic glucose output. Insulin secretion is markedly suppressed, and counterregulatory hormone (eg, glucagon, cortisol, growth hormone, and epinephrine) secretion is stimulated. In phases IV and V there is a progressive breakage of proteins as the effective fat stores are depleted. This results in a severe catabolic state represented by muscle wasting.

Phase V is the secondary prolonged starvation state (24-40 days after food consumption), in which blood glucose originates from hepatic and renal gluconeogenesis, the same source as in phase IV. In phase V, the rate of glucose being used by the brain diminishes, as does the rate of hepatic gluconeogenesis.

Normal Fuel Metabolism

To understand the abnormalities in fuel metabolism characterized by diabetes, a basic understanding of normal fuel metabolism is needed.[8] Humans have a constant requirement for energy but eat only intermittently. To offset this, food is ingested in excess of the immediate need of the vital organs and stored as extra calories in the form of hepatic and muscle glycogen, adipose tissue triglyceride, and to some extent tissue protein. In times of starvation and other stresses, these fuel stores are broken down to provide energy for organ metabolism and function.

The two main fuels in humans are glucose and FFAs. Glucose is stored as glycogen in the skeletal muscle and the liver. Free fatty acids are stored as triglycerides primarily in adipose tissue.

The energy stores are utilized and replenished in response to hormones, depending on whether one is in a fasting or fed state. In the fed or anabolic state, where fuels are stored in the tissues, insulin levels increase, promoting glycogen synthesis in the liver and muscle, lipid storage in adipocytes, and amino acid uptake and protein synthesis in most cells. The net result is movement of glucose from the circulation into storage depots. Insulin thus acts as an anabolic hormone. In the fasting state (8-12 hours without energy intake) or starvation (more than 12-24 hours), which occurs when the body no longer has any stored energy and begins breaking down fat and protein for an energy source, decreased insulin secretion enables glycogen breakdown, lipolysis, hepatic ketogenesis, and decreased synthesis and increased degradation of protein in order to meet the body's energy requirements.[9] Fasting and starvation represent a catabolic state where insulin secretion decreases, and glucagon, a catabolic hormone, enables glycogenolysis, lipolysis, and ketogenesis.

Counterregulatory hormones oppose insulin's actions. Glucagon and catecholamines stimulate glycogenolysis and gluconeogenesis in the liver, thereby raising blood glucose levels. Catecholamines are key regulators of lipolysis in adipose tissue and glycogenolysis in muscle and other tissues. Growth hormone and cortisol are also insulin counterregulatory hormones.

In normal glucose homeostasis, the balance between insulin and the counterregulatory hormones maintains normoglycemia. The serum glucose concentration depends on the rate at which the glucose enters and the rate at which it is utilized from the circulation. In adults without diabetes or impaired fasting glucose (IFG), the fasting plasma glucose (FPG) concentration remains within a narrow range of 70 to 100 mg/dL (3.88-5.55 mmol/L) despite varying rates of utilization. This maintenance occurs because glucose appearance and glucose disposal, which reflect the rate at which glucose is taken up by peripheral tissues, are well matched.

Insulin lowers plasma glucose levels both by stimulating glucose uptake in muscle and adipose tissue and by inhibiting hepatic glycogen breakdown and gluconeogenesis. The counterregulatory hormones balance these effects of insulin in order to maintain normogylcemia.[8]

The Role of Hormones

Multiple hormones play a key role in the regulation of fuel physiology. They may be broadly grouped as pancreatic (glucoregulatory), incretin (intestinal), and other hormones and factors affecting fuel metabolism. The knowledge and understanding of incretins and other hormones that diabetes educators need has grown. Therefore, the salient features relative to the role of each in the pathophysiology of diabetes will be reviewed below.

Pancreatic (Glucoregulatory) Hormones

Insulin   Insulin is produced by the beta cells in the pancreas. It is highly regulated by glucose and the incretinomimetic system, including glucagon-like peptide-1 (GLP-1) and glucose-dependent insulin-releasing polypeptide (GIP).

Insulin controls postprandial glucose via 2 mechanisms:

- Peripheral glucose utilization by insulin-sensitive tissues, mainly muscle and fat cells
- Direct inhibition of hepatic glucose production and glucagon secretion, thus further decreasing gluconeogenesis[10]

Amylin   The discovery of amylin has contributed to the understanding of postprandial glucose homeostasis. This 37–amino acid polypeptide hormone is co-secreted from the pancreatic beta cells with insulin in response to nutrient stimuli. It inhibits postprandial glucose exertions via 3 primary actions[11]:

- Regulation of food intake
- Slowing of gastric empting
- Inhibition of digestive secretions (gastric acid, pancreatic enzymes, and bile)

Glucagon   Glucagon is an alpha cell pancreatic hormone associated with maintaining glucose homeostasis. Glucagon increases glucose through gluconeogenesis during the fasting state and when blood glucose concentrations are low. Alpha cells are regulated by glucose, insulin, and the incretinomimetic system—mainly by glucagon-like polypeptide. Glucagon is secreted in response to low blood concentrations of glucose. Glucagon-like peptide-1 suppresses glucagon secretion.[11]

Incretin (Intestinal) Hormones

When meals are consumed, the gastrointestinal tract releases a number of hormones that aid in the absorption and disposition of nutrients. Among these hormones, GLP-1 and GIP are particularly important because of their regulation of hormone secretion. Glucagon-like peptide-1 and GIP augment glucose-stimulated insulin secretion, a process termed the *incretin effect*. The incretin effect accounts for approximately 50% of the insulin secreted after a meal and, therefore, has a prominent role in postprandial metabolism.[12] Figure 13.3 summarizes the effects of GLP-1 in humans.

In animal and in vitro studies, both GIP and GLP-1 also promoted beta cell proliferation and inhibited apoptosis, leading to expansion of beta cell mass. Glucagon-like peptide-1, but not GIP, controls glycemia via additional actions on glucose sensors, inhibition of gastric emptying, food intake, and glucagon secretion.

Glucose-Dependent Insulin-Releasing Polypeptide   Glucose-dependent insulin-releasing polypeptide is secreted by K cells from the upper small intestine. Along with GLP-1, GIP is released following a meal; together, these hormones act on the

GLP-1 Effects in Humans

Brain: Promotes satiety and reduces appetite

Intestines: GLP-1 is secreted upon the ingestion of food

Beta Cells: Enhance glucose-dependent insulin secretion

Alpha Cells: Lower postprandial glucagon secretion

Liver: Lowers glucagon and reduces hepatic glucose output

Stomach: Helps regulate gastric emptying

FIGURE 13.3   Antidiabetic Activities of GLP-1

Source: A Flint et al, *J Clin Invest* 101 (1998): 515-20; H Larsson et al, *Acta Physiol Scand* 160 (1997): 413-22; MA Nauck et al, *Diabetologia* 39 (1996): 1546-53; DJ Drucker, *Diabetes* 47 (1998): 159-69.

beta cells to increase their sensitivity to glucose. Glucose-dependent insulin-releasing polypeptide may help stimulate insulin secretion, but this is under study and not yet conclusive.[12]

Glucagon-Like Peptide-1   Glucagon-like peptide-1 is predominantly produced in the enteroendocrine L cells located in the distal intestine.[13] As noted above, it is released after a meal and works with GIP to increase beta cell sensitivity to glucose. Glucagon-like peptide-1 appears to be the major mediator of the incretin effect in humans, and it potentiates the glucose-stimulated insulin secretion following a carbohydrate meal.

In addition to its effects on insulin secretion, GLP-1 exerts other significant actions to modulate intermediary metabolism, including stimulation of insulin biosynthesis, inhibition of glucagon secretion and gastric emptying, reduced food intake, and trophic effects on the pancreatic islet cells.[14]

Dipeptidyl Peptidase-4   Both GIP and GLP-1 are rapidly metabolized in the circulation by the enzyme dipeptidyl peptidase-4 (DPP-4), which is produced by endothelial cells and circulates in the plasma. This protease cleaves the first 2 amino acids from GLP-1, leaving a metabolite that does not stimulate insulin secretion of glucose clearance. The half-life of the incretin in the circulation (1-2 minutes for GLP-1 and 7 minutes for GIP) is due to the presence of DPP-4.[15]

Other Hormones and Factors Affecting Fuel Metabolism

Peptide-YY   The hormone peptide-YY (PYY) is a 36–amino acid peptide secreted from the L cells of the gastrointestinal tract postprandially in proportion to the calorie content of the meal. This gut hormone reduces food intake via hypothalamic Y2 receptors in the brain. Preliminary data show that infusion of postprandial concentrations of PYY significantly decreases food intake at a buffet meal. Its site of action is the nucleus of the hypothalamus, an area known to be involved in regulating food intake.[16]

Leptin and Ghrelin—Leptin and ghrelin are 2 hormones that have been recognized as having a major influence on energy balance. Leptin is a mediator of long-term regulation of energy balance, suppressing food intake and thereby inducing weight loss. Ghrelin, on the other hand, is a fast-acting hormone, seemingly playing a role in meal initiation. As a growing number of people suffer from obesity, understanding the mechanisms by which various hormones and neurotransmitters have influence on energy balance has been a subject of intensive research. In obese subjects, the circulating level of the anorexigenic hormone leptin is increased, whereas, surprisingly, the level of the orexigenic hormone ghrelin is decreased. It is now established that obese patients are leptin resistant. However, the manner in which both the leptin and ghrelin systems contribute to the development or maintenance of obesity is not yet clear.[9]

Endocannabinoid System   The endocannabinoid system further contributes to the physiological regulation of energy balance, food intake, and lipid and glucose metabolism through both central and peripheral effects.[17]

Activation of the central endocannabinoid system increases food intake and promotes weight gain. The observation that endocannabinoid activation is not reversible with a 5% weight loss suggests that this activation may be a cause rather than a consequence of obesity. The endocannabinoid system is overactivated in response to exogenous stimuli, such as excessive food intake, leading experts to believe that overeating promotes more overeating.[18]

Exogenous cannabinoids and endocannabinoids increase food intake and promote weight gain by activating central endocannabinoid receptors. These normal endocrine processes provide the framework for research that may further our understanding of the pathophysiology leading to diabetes as well as insight into potential sites of pharmacologic intervention. Exploration of the potential for endocannabinoid blockers as diabetes and weight control agents is ongoing. To date, drugs investigated and/or under development have shown some promise; further investigation is under way.

Diabetes Diagnostic Criteria

International diabetes organizations have determined categorical cutoff points in glucose and A1C to define diabetes.[19] These cutoff points correlate with the epidemiologic risk of developing microvascular complications, particularly diabetic retinopathy. However, vascular problems may pose a threat to individuals even at glycemic levels that do not approach the diagnostic definition of diabetes. These glycemic levels represent a high predisposition to diabetes and have been termed "prediabetes." Prediabetes can be defined in terms of impaired glucose tolerance (IGT) or IFG, depending on which test is used. Progression of prediabetes to type 2 diabetes may be reduced by lifestyle intervention and by some pharmacotherapeutic strategies. One study showed that 8.1% of subjects whose initial abnormal fasting glucose was 100 to 109 mg/dL (5.55-6.06 mmol/L) and 24.3% of subjects whose initial abnormal fasting glucose was 110 to 125 mg/dL (6.11-6.94 mmol/L) (original IFG

subjects) developed diabetes. Added IFG subjects who progressed to diabetes did so within a mean of 41.4 months, a rate of 1.34% per year. Original IFG subjects converted at a rate of 5.56% per year after an average of 29.0 months. A steeper rate of increasing fasting glucose; higher BMI, blood pressure, and triglycerides; and lower HDL cholesterol predicted diabetes development.[20]

A diagnosis of diabetes is made when results of a screening test or presentation with a variety of clinical symptoms lead to confirmation of its presence by formal diagnostic glycemic criteria.

The glycemic thresholds used to diagnose diabetes have been modified over the years largely on the basis of the current understanding of the epidemiologic relationship between glucose levels and diabetes-specific microvascular complications (Table 13.2). As has been described earlier in this chapter, the processes by which diabetes occurs take place over a prolonged period of time, with a wide variety of compensating mechanisms. The disease is continuous, even though the glucose definitions are fixed.[19]

For decades, the diagnosis of diabetes has been based on glucose criteria, either an FPG or a 75-g oral glucose tolerance test (OGTT). In 1997, the first Expert Committee on the Diagnosis and Classification of Diabetes Mellitus revised the criteria using the association between FPG and the presence of retinopathy as the key factor with which to identify threshold glucose level. The additional analysis of FPG and

TABLE 13.2 Diagnosing Diabetes—4 Testing Options	
A1C	≥6.5%
Acute symptoms* plus casual plasma glucose†:	≥200 mg/dL (11.1 mmol/L)
Fasting plasma glucose‡:	≥126 mg/dL (7.0 mmol/L)
2-hour postprandial plasma glucose:	≥200 mg/dL (11.1 mmol/L) during OGTT (75-g glucose)

Note: Unless unequivocal symptoms of hyperglycemia are present, these criteria must be confirmed by repeat testing on a subsequent day.

*Classic symptoms of diabetes: polyuria, polydipsia, polyphagia, and unexplained weight loss.

†Casual implies any time of day without regard to time since last meal.

‡Fasting is defined as no caloric intake for at least 8 hours.

2-hour postprandial glucose set a new cutoff point of ≥126 mg/dL (7 mmol/L) for FPG and confirmed the long-standing 2-hour postprandial plasma glucose value of ≥200 mg/dL (11.11 mmol/L).[21]

In 2009 the International Expert Committee on the role of the A1C assay in the diagnosis of diabetes recommended the use of A1C ≥6.5% obtained using NGSP methodology for the diagnosis of diabetes.[22] The NGSP harmonized A1C test results to those of the DCCT and the UKPDS, which established the direct relationships between HbA1c levels and outcome risks in people with diabetes.[23] The decision to add A1C as a diagnostic criterion is now accepted by the major organizations involved in diabetes.[7] It is important to be aware that A1C levels are not reliable in a variety of clinical circumstances. In people who have hemoglobin variants such as HbS (sickle cell trait) or thalassemia, some A1C tests give falsely high or low readings that can lead to the over- or undertreatment of diabetes. Patients may be at risk for having a hemoglobin variant if they are of African, Mediterranean, or Southeast Asian heritage; members of their family have sickle cell trait or sickle cell anemia; the results of blood glucose tests or self-monitoring of blood glucose don't match the results of their A1C test; the A1C result is different from what was expected or is very high (above 15%); or the most recent A1C result is very different from the last A1C result.[24] A1C results may also be inaccurate in anemia due to other etiologies (eg, iron deficiency anemia) and in the setting of renal failure or liver disease. In addition, changes in A1C take place in pregnancy. A1C is significantly decreased early in pregnancy and further decreased in late pregnancy compared with age-matched nonpregnant women.[25]

The actual rate of diagnosis of type 2 diabetes remains poor, with almost 25% of those affected undiagnosed. Microvascular complications are found in approximately 20% of newly diagnosed individuals with type 2 diabetes. Type 2 diabetes may be present, on average, 6 to 12 years prior to identification and treatment. The prevalence of coronary artery disease in those with type 2 diabetes is twice that of the population without diabetes, and cardiovascular and total mortality are two- to threefold greater than that of individuals without diabetes.[26]

A diabetes diagnosis must be considered when encountering the classic acute symptoms associated with hyperglycemia, including blurred vision, excessive thirst and hunger, frequent urination, weight loss, fatigue, headache, and muscle cramps. A blood glucose ≥200 mg/dL (11.11 mmol/L) in the presence of these symptoms allows a formal diagnosis of diabetes. An acute presentation with diabetic ketoacidosis (DKA) or hyperglycemic hyperosmolar state (HHS) constitutes an endocrine emergency. The distinction between type 1 diabetes and type 2 diabetes generally can be made on the basis of laboratory testing at the time of such a presentation. However, increasing clinical evidence highlights significant overlap between type 1 diabetes and type 2 diabetes, and the classification into 2 main types has been challenged.

Diagnosis in Children

Distinguishing between type 1 diabetes and type 2 diabetes in children is important but can be difficult. Patient age at presentation is the main risk factor of delayed diagnosis, especially in children younger than age 2.[27] Ketosis may be present in those with otherwise straightforward type 2 diabetes (including obesity and acanthosis nigricans). Such a distinction at diagnosis is critical, because the natural history, treatment regimens, educational approaches, and dietary counsel markedly differ between the 2 diagnoses.

Children should be screened for diabetes if they are overweight; have a family history of type 2 diabetes; are of a minority population; and have 2 of the following risk factors, which are signs of insulin resistance or conditions associated with insulin resistance: acanthosis nigricans, hypertension, dyslipidemia, polycystic ovary syndrome, or small-for-gestational-age birth weight. Children also should be screened if their mother had gestational diabetes during their gestation. Testing should begin at age 10, or younger if puberty has already occurred. Testing should be repeated every 3 years.[19]

Confirmation of Diagnosis

With the addition of the A1C as a diagnostic tool (see Table 13.2), more information may be available than was previously routine for diagnosis. The test results that diagnose diabetes should be repeated unless there is strong clinical evidence, such as classic signs of diabetes or a hyperglycemic crisis. Ideally, the same test

---

Case: An African American Woman at Risk for Diabetes

CS, a 29-year-old African-American woman, was noted to have a random glucose of 125 mg/dL (6.94 mmol/L) on a blood test obtained as part of a visit to the local health clinic. She had no symptoms of diabetes and thought her blood glucose was okay during her last pregnancy. She had been told to "watch her sugars" and to exercise. She has been healthy but recently complained of frequent yeast infections. Her family history includes a mother and 2 older sisters with type 2 diabetes. Her grandmother died from diabetes after she was started on "the shot." CS smokes cigarettes, at a rate of a pack per day since age 18. She tried stopping because of the cost but has been unsuccessful. She works evenings, and her husband works days to cover child care. They have 2 children, ages 3 and 5 years old.

Physical Exam

- Height: 63 in
- Weight: 203 lb
- Blood pressure: 138/94 mm Hg
- Waist circumference: 40 in
- Skin: Acanthosis nigricans on neck, trace edema; otherwise normal
- A1C: 6.4%
- 1-hour postprandial glucose: 132 mg/dL (7.33 mmol/L)

---

should be used. However, if 2 tests are available for an individual and only 1 test's results are above the diagnosis point, the test that indicates results above the diagnostic point should be repeated. If the retest results are above the diagnostic point, then a diagnosis is made.

The emergency department may serve as a venue for the identification of previously unrecognized diabetes and/or prediabetes. Diagnostic criteria for use in people with diabetes and prediabetes presenting to the emergency department have not been well established. There are, however, some reports related to the potential for detection of these conditions in high-risk patients during emergency department visits.[28-30]

In the presence of signs and symptoms consistent with chronic hyperglycemia, including growth impairment; susceptibility to certain infections; and renal, retinal, macrovascular disease, connective tissue disorders, and neuropathic syndromes, it is contingent upon the provider to test for diabetes. Distinctions among the various conditions that encompass diabetes are described below.

Diabetes Classification

Prediabetes

The Expert Committee on Diagnosis and Classification of Diabetes Mellitus[21] recognized an intermediate group of individuals whose glucose levels do not meet criteria for diabetes yet are higher than those considered normal (Table 13.3). These individuals are referred to as being at high risk for developing diabetes. This condition has been described as prediabetes.

Impaired fasting glucose and IGT are not clinical entities but risk factors for diabetes as well as cardiovascular disease. They are associated with obesity (especially abdominal or visceral obesity), dyslipidemia with high triglycerides and/or low-density lipoprotein cholesterol (LDL-C), and hypertension.

Using an A1C test to screen for prediabetes was not formally defined when the recommendation was made to use A1C to diagnose diabetes. However, it was noted that those who have A1C levels above the laboratory normal (5.7%-6.4%) but below the diagnostic cutoff point are at high risk for developing diabetes.[22]

TABLE 13.3 Categories of Increased Risk for Diabetes (Prediabetes)	
IFG	100-125 mg/dL (5.55-6.94 mmol/L)
IGT	2-hour OGTT values of 140-199 mg/dL (7.77-11.06 mmol/L)
A1C	5.7%–6.4%

Type 1 Diabetes

People with type 1 diabetes generally present with acute symptoms associated with markedly elevated blood glucose. Because of the acute onset of symptoms, type 1 diabetes usually is detected soon after symptoms develop, although the autoimmune process causing the disease may precede the clinical presentation by many years.[31] Approximately three-quarters of all cases of type 1 diabetes are diagnosed in individuals younger than age 18.[1]

◆ Type 1 diabetes develops at any age, but in most cases is diagnosed before age 30.

◆ Type 1 diabetes is characterized by autoimmune destruction of the beta cells of the islets of Langerhans with resulting absolute insulin deficiency.

◆ Undiagnosed or untreated individuals experience significant weight loss, polyuria, and polydipsia characterized by the abrupt signs and symptoms associated with marked hyperglycemia and the strong propensity for the development of ketoacidosis.

◆ Subjects are dependent on exogenous insulin to prevent ketoacidosis and sustain life.

◆ Coma and death can result from delayed diagnosis and/or treatment.

Type 2 Diabetes

Type 2 diabetes frequently is not diagnosed until complications appear. This is because many of the symptoms are absent or attributed to other causes.[7]

◆ Approximately 90% of people in the United States with diabetes have type 2 diabetes, with disproportionate representation among the elderly and certain ethnic groups, including Native Americans, Alaskans and Hawaiian, South Asians, Hispanics, and African Americans.

◆ If present trends continue, as many as 1 in 3 adults in the United States will have diabetes in 2050.[4]

◆ Type 2 diabetes is usually diagnosed after age 30, but onset can occur at any age.

◆ Onset of type 2 diabetes in adolescence is becoming increasingly more common as obesity rates rise among youth. Type 2 diabetes now accounts for 30% to 50% of childhood-onset diabetes.[4]

◆ Type 2 diabetes is frequently asymptomatic at the time of diagnosis. As many as 20% of individuals may present with end-organ complications (eg, microvascular disease such as retinopathy, neuropathy, and nephropathy or macrovascular events such as stroke or myocardial infarction) due to delays in diagnosis of prediabetes and/or type 2 diabetes.

◆ Endogenous insulin levels may be normal, increased, or decreased, with a variable need for exogenous insulin.

◆ Insulin resistance occurs early and persists through prediabetes and subsequent clinical diabetes.

◆ Individuals with type 2 diabetes are not prone to ketosis except in rare cases of severe physiologic stress.

Test Selection

Which test to use is at the discretion of the healthcare professional. Factors to take into account include cost, practicality, and availability of the test.

Case—Part 2: Screening and Diagnostic Testing

With a random blood glucose of 125 mg/dL (6.94 mmol/L), CS did not meet the criteria for diabetes. However, she has several risk factors, physical evidence of insulin resistance, and an indication of hyperglycemia:

• High-risk racial group

• Family history of type 2 diabetes

• Obesity

• Acanthosis nigricans

• Recurrent yeast infections

Her family physician ordered a fasting blood glucose level:

• FPG: 112 mg/dL (6.22 mmol/L; when repeated, 108 mg/dL [6 mmol/L])

CS was identified as being at risk for diabetes and advised to lose weight and exercise.

Other Forms of Diabetes

Other forms of diabetes are diagnosed when diabetes occurs as a result of another disorder or treatment. Treatment of these underlying disorders or discontinuation of diabetogenic agents may result in amelioration of the diabetes. Frequently, however, reversing the underlying disorder or stopping the offending agent is not possible.[32] Therapy, then, is similar to diabetes therapy in general—using the modalities of medical nutrition therapy, physical activity, and medications. The following disorders are classified as other kinds of diabetes:

- ❖ Known genetic defects associated with maturity-onset diabetes of the young, glycogen synthase deficiency, and mitochondrial DNA markers
- ❖ Pancreatic disorders, such as hemochromatosis, chronic pancreatitis, and pancreatectomy
- ❖ Hormonal disorders, such as Cushing's syndrome (excess amounts of corticosteroids), pheochromocytoma (excess catecholamines), and acromegaly (excess growth hormone)
- ❖ Other disorders, such as cystic fibrosis, congenital rubella syndrome, and Down syndrome
- ❖ Concomitant diabetogenic medications (eg, atypical antipsychotics, glucocorticoids, protease inhibitors, and pentamidine)[1]

Gestational Diabetes

Gestational diabetes (GDM) was traditionally defined as a diagnosis that applied to women in whom glucose intolerance developed or was first discovered during pregnancy.[33] Although most cases resolved with delivery, the definition applied whether or not the condition continued after pregnancy, and did not address the possibility that the pregnant women had preexisting undiagnosed diabetes. This definition facilitated a uniform strategy for detection and classification of GDM, but its limitations were recognized for many years. As the ongoing epidemic of obesity and diabetes has led to more cases of type 2 diabetes in women of childbearing age, the number of pregnant women with preexisting type 2 diabetes diagnosed during pregnancy has increased.[33]

After deliberations in 2008 and 2009, the International Association of Diabetes and Pregnancy Study Groups (IADPSG), an international consensus group with representatives from multiple obstetrical and diabetes organizations, recommended that high-risk women found to have diabetes at their initial prenatal visit (using standard criteria) receive a diagnosis of overt, not gestational, diabetes.[34]

Gestational diabetes is associated with insulin resistance due to pregnancy and perhaps obesity and genetic predisposition.[35] Failure to augment beta cell insulin response to the insulin resistance is the hallmark of the disorder. The condition is usually asymptomatic but is dangerous for the developing fetus. Maternal risks include hypertension, polyhydramnios, and cesarean delivery. There is mounting evidence that treating even mild GDM reduces morbidity for both mother and baby.[36] See Chapter 24 for a complete discussion of GDM.

Pathophysiology
Type 1 Diabetes

Type 1 diabetes is an autoimmune disorder. It develops when the body's immune system generates antibodies that destroy the pancreatic beta cells, leading to the inability to produce the hormones insulin and amylin. Type 1 diabetes usually occurs in children and young adults, although disease onset can occur at any age. Type 1 diabetes is characterized by the abrupt onset of clinical signs and symptoms associated with hyperglycemia and a strong propensity for ketoacidosis. Decline in insulin secretion begins to develop long before the clinical signs become evident and may take place for as long as 9 years before the clinical presentation of type 1 diabetes. The 5 progressive stages of the natural history of the development of type 1 diabetes are shown in Table 13.4.

Genetic Propensity

There is a genetic propensity for type 1 diabetes. The risk of type 1 diabetes in the general population ranges from 1 in 400 to 1 in 1000.[1] That risk is substantially increased (from approximately 1 in 50 to 1 in 20) in the offspring of people with diabetes. Children with the HLA-risk genotypes HLA-DR3 and HLA-DR4 and DQ8 who have a family history of type 1 diabetes have more than a 1 in 5 risk for developing islet autoantibodies during childhood, and children with the

TABLE 13.4   Pathophysiologic Stages in the Development of Type 1 Diabetes

Stage	Physiology and Events	Comments
1	Genetic predisposition	Aggregates in families, but most do not have a relative with type 1 diabetes; strongly increased risk in monozygotic/identical twins
2	Precipitating event	Environmental trigger causes insulitis; congenital rubella, viruses implicated
3	Active autoimmunity	Antibodies to auto/self antigens lead to anti–islet cell antibodies which can be measured; insulin release remains normal
4	Progressive beta cell dysfunction	Progressive loss of beta cell function: loss of first phase of insulin release; glucose remains normal
5	Overt type 1 diabetes mellitus	C-peptide presents early, then lost; clinical onset of type 1 diabetes

Source: AK Steck, MJ Rewers, "Genetics of type 1 diabetes," *Clin Chem* 57 (2011): 176-85. doi: 10.1373/clinchem.2010.148

same HLA-risk genotype but no family history have approximately a 1 in 20 risk. Children born with the high-risk genotype HLA-DR3 and HLA-DR4 and DQ8 compose almost 50% of children who develop anti-islet autoimmunity by age 5 years.[37] Determining extreme genetic risk is a prerequisite for the implementation of primary prevention trials, which are now under way for relatives of individuals with type 1 diabetes.[38] The major susceptibility locus maps to the HLA class II genes at 6p21, although more than 40 non-HLA susceptibility genetic markers have been confirmed. The HLA class II alleles account for up to 30% to 50% of genetic type 1 diabetes risk. Multiple non–major histocompatibility complex loci contribute to disease risk with smaller effects; these include the insulin, PTPN22, CTLA4, IL2RA, IFIH1, and other recently discovered loci.[37]

Not all individuals at genetic risk for type 1 diabetes develop the disease. Although 40% of Caucasian individuals express the DR3 or DR4 haplotype, less than 1% develops diabetes. A 50% discordance rate of type 1 diabetes exists between identical twins, suggesting that specific genes are necessary but not sufficient conditions for disease development.[39]

A trigger is necessary for expression of the genetic propensity for type 1 diabetes; environmental triggers have long been suspected. The pathogenesis of type 1 diabetes is believed to involve T-cell mediated autoimmune processes directed against the pancreatic beta cell. Increasing evidence suggests that environmental factors, including toxins, food antigens, and particularly viral infections, are implicated in the induction of type 1 diabetes.[32]

Viral triggers, such as enteroviruses, rubella, mumps, rotavirus, parvovirus, and cytomegalovirus, have been investigated in both laboratory and clinical studies to attempt to define their roles in the pathogenesis of type 1 diabetes. Recent efforts have focused on enteroviruses, which are the most common cause of viral infection in humans worldwide. Enteroviruses have an affinity for islet cells and have been isolated from the islets of a person with type 1 diabetes and shown to be present in an individual concurrent with development of islet cell antibodies.[32] Recently, enteroviral antigen-positive islet cells were shown to be present in 44 of the 72 persons with recent-onset type 1 diabetes in an autopsy series.[40] All enterovirus serotypes (over 100) studied to date include strains with the ability to damage beta cells.[41] These findings reinforce the potential relevance of enteroviruses in the pathophysiology of this disease.

Bovine serum albumin (BSA), contained in cow's milk, has been reported as an environmental trigger. Antibodies specific to BSA have been found in the majority of children with newly diagnosed type 1 diabetes, leading to the hypothesis that early exposure to cow's milk may be a potential determinant of type 1 diabetes, with the potential to increase disease risk by as much as 1.5 times.[42] Structural similarities exist between BSA and an islet cell surface antigen referred to as ICA-69. The cross-reactivity of circulating anti-BSA antibodies with ICA-69 provides a link between the environmental trigger and subsequent development of autoimmunity. Longer duration of breastfeeding, exclusive breastfeeding in particular, and supplementation with vitamin D in infancy have been reported to confer partial protection against beta cell autoimmunity and type 1 diabetes.[43] Other researchers, however, have not been able to find data to support the hypothesis that infant diet is related to the occurrence of type 1 diabetes.[36]

Oxidative Stress

Some researchers suggest that type 1 diabetes may be resultant of oxidative stress, due to high local levels of nitric oxide (NO) and oxygen radicals (O_2) in the beta cells, which plays a role in their destruction.[44,45]

Furthermore, there is evidence suggesting that the incidence of type 1 diabetes is increased in both spring and fall and is coincidental with various viral disorders.[46]

One dilemma in identifying specific triggers for type 1 diabetes involves the apparent long latency period between the triggering of active autoimmunity and the subsequent clinical development of diabetes. Thus, identifying which specific insult over the past 7 to 10 years may have been the actual trigger of the disease process is challenging. It is also possible that a variety of viral or environmental agents play a role in triggering expression of the genetic predisposition to the disease.[32]

Autoimmunity

Regardless of the trigger, early type 1 diabetes is first identified by the appearance of active autoimmunity directed against pancreatic beta cells and their products. Fifty percent of relatives with high-titer islet cell antibodies (ICAs) have diabetes within 5 years of follow-up. Islet cell antibody negativity has a 99.9% probability of freedom from the development of type 1 diabetes. Additional ICAs that may play a permissive or pathologic role in the causation of type 1 diabetes include those related to insulin, glycolipids, ganglioside GT3, carboxypeptidase H, PM-1 polar antigen, additional islet cell proteins of varying sizes (37 kd or 40 kd, 38 kd, 52 kd, and 69 kd) and as yet undetermined function, peripherin, heat shock protein 65, insulin receptors, other endocrine cell antigens, cytoskeletal proteins (tubulin, actin, reticulin, nuclear antigens [single-stranded DNA and RNA]), and agonist islet tyrosine phosphatase (islet antigen A2 and A2 beta).[47]

Although the clinical onset of type 1 diabetes may be abrupt, the pathophysiologic insult occurs slowly and progressively. In the early stages of the disease, markers of immune destruction of the beta cells are found, including ICAs, insulin autoantibodies (IAAs), and autoantibodies to GAD. Beta cell destruction occurs at varying rates and is usually faster among younger patients, accounting for the classic abrupt clinical manifestation. Beta cell destruction is slower in adults, which sometimes leads to an incorrect diagnosis of type 2 diabetes.[48] Evidence suggests autoantibodies are predictive of type 1 diabetes and help distinguish autoimmune type 1 diabetes and latent autoimmune diabetes in adults (LADA) from non-autoimmune diabetes.[49] Positivity to increasing numbers of autoantibodies indicates that the individual's autoimmune response is spreading and that the disease is progressing. The predictive ability of autoantibody tests therefore increases with the number of autoantibodies detected in an individual and may be influenced by the autoantibody titer, as well. There also appears to be a hierarchy of diabetes relevance in the autoantibody response against different antigenic targets within and between islet autoantigens. Circulating islet autoantibodies are present in sera from approximately 5% of children with new-onset diabetes and provide evidence of an active and disease-specific B lymphocyte response. The best-validated and most widely used predictive markers are autoantibodies directed against the biochemically defined target antigens insulin (IAA), GAD65 (GADA), IA-2 (IA-2A), and the zinc transporter ZnT8 (ZnT8A). Hyperglycemia and symptoms consistent with diabetes develop only after more than 90% of the secretory capacity of the beta cells has been destroyed.[47]

At any time during the progressive decline in beta cell function, overt diabetes may be precipitated by either acute illness or stress, which increases insulin demand beyond the reserve of the damaged islet cells. Hyperglycemia will ensue until such time as the acute illness or stress is resolved; then, the individual may revert to a compensated state for a variable time period in which the beta cells are able to maintain normal glycemia. This honeymoon period is a variable period of noninsulin dependency following acute decompensation. Ongoing progression of beta cell destruction continues, leading to absolute insulin deficiency and the need for insulin treatment, typically over 3 to 12 months.[50]

Case—Part 3: Inattention to Modifiable Risk Factors

For 2 years CS felt fine. Despite being advised to exercise and lose weight, she had been unable to incorporate this into her busy life. That summer, however, she experienced progressive fatigue and found that she was often very thirsty. She assumed this was from the heat of summer. She noticed a shiny red patch of skin under her breasts and went to her local health clinic. A random blood glucose at that time was 203 mg/dL (11.27 mmol/L).

Type 2 Diabetes

The pathophysiology of type 2 diabetes is characterized as progressive and multifactorial. Both insulin resistance in the liver and muscle and impaired insulin secretion play a major role in its pathogenesis. Increased and inappropriate hepatic glucose production is a hallmark feature. Initially, in the basal state, the liver overproduces glucose despite high fasting insulin levels, which leads to fasting hyperglycemia. In addition, in the insulin-stimulated state after glucose ingestion, insulin resistance leads to reduction in muscle glucose uptake by more than 50%, which results in postprandial hyperglycemia.[51]

Pancreatic beta cell insulin secretory capacity while increased is impaired to compensate for the demands caused by insulin resistance. In the pancreas, in response to the hyperglycemia that results from increased hepatic glucose production and peripheral insulin resistance, beta cells increase their secretion of insulin. However, with persistent fasting hyperglycemia, the compensatory insulin response cannot be maintained, insulin secretion declines progressively, and diabetes emerges. About 70% of beta cell function has been lost when the 2-hour glucose value during the OGTT reaches 120 to 140 mg/dL (6.66-7.77 mmol/L). In addition, acquired defects in beta cell activity have been noted in response to hyperglycemia and are referred to as glucose toxicity. Beta cells chronically exposed to hyperglycemia and to increased FFAs become progressively less efficient in responding to subsequent glucose challenges. Thus, beta cell dysfunction may be either primary or acquired in the pathogenesis of type 2 diabetes. Further progression of the disease is marked in its later stages by an absolute insulin deficiency.[52]

The islet in type 2 diabetes is characterized by a deficit in beta cell mass, increased beta cell apoptosis, and impaired insulin secretion. Some but not all studies suggest that a decrease in beta cell mass contributes to the impaired insulin secretion of type 2 diabetes.[53] In sum, the beta cell mass is decreased in both obese and lean individuals with type 2 diabetes compared with their nondiabetic age- and weight-matched counterparts. The net change in beta cell mass leads to a decrease in beta cell function. People with prediabetes have decreased beta cell mass, suggesting that this is an early process and mechanistically important in the development of type 2 diabetes. Finally, the decrease in beta cell mass may be caused by an increase in the frequency of beta cell apoptosis with the rate of new islet formation being unaffected. Thus, in striving to prevent type 2 diabetes, strategies to avoid beta cell apoptosis may be useful. Also, in people with established type 2 diabetes, inhibition of this three- to tenfold increased rate of apoptosis may lead to restoration of beta cell mass, because islet neogenesis appears intact.[53]

Heredity plays a major role in the expression of type 2 diabetes. However, the function of genes may also be impacted through epigenetic changes that take place in the course of life. Epigenetic changes are described as external changes resulting from environmental influences that turn genes on or off. Epigenetic changes come about as a result of factors such as aging, chemicals, medication, diet, and exercise.[54]

Researchers have now demonstrated that half of the known genetic risk variants for type 2 diabetes can be influenced by epigenetic changes that in turn influence the function of the insulin-producing cells. Most cases of type 2 diabetes involve many genes contributing small amounts to the overall condition. As of 2011, more than 36 genes have been found to contribute to the risk of type 2 diabetes. All of these genes together account for only 10% of the total genetic component of the disease.[55]

Although there is no recognized human leukocyte antigen (HLA) linkage, offspring of individuals with type 2 diabetes have a 15% chance of developing the disease and a 30% risk of developing IGT.[6] A greater than 90% concordance rate exists between monozygotic twins if one has type 2 diabetes, suggesting the primacy of the genetic defect in this form of the disease.[56]

In addition, in type 2 diabetes, adipocytes (fat cells) are resistant to the antilipolytic effect of insulin and pour fat into the bloodstream, resulting in elevated plasma FFA levels. These processes are referred to as lipotoxicity. In this component of the pathophysiology of type 2 diabetes, the elevated FFA levels exacerbate liver and muscle insulin resistance, drive gluconeogenesis in the liver, and impair beta cell insulin secretion, further exacerbating the tendency toward hyperglycemia. The dysfunctional adipocytes produce multiple cytokines that contribute to inflammation and atherosclerosis as well as insulin resistance.[57]

Gastrointestinal incretin hormones have been implicated as a factor in the pathogenesis of type 2 diabetes. Glucagon-like peptide-1 is deficient in people with type 2 diabetes and prediabetes, contributing to excessive hepatic glucose production, failure to suppress postprandial glucagon, and unrestrained eating. Dipeptidyl peptidase-4 activity is increased in the fasting state in people with type 2 diabetes. This may be one reason type 2 diabetes may be associated with impaired postprandial GLP-1 secretion.[17]

Contributing to our understanding of the specific timing of changes in glucose metabolism before the occurrence of type 2 diabetes, a recent report characterizes the trajectories of fasting and postload glucose, insulin sensitivity, and insulin secretion in the Whitehall II cohort of British civil servants. This study compared those who developed type 2 diabetes and those who did not over a 13-year follow-up. The study shows changes in glucose concentrations, insulin sensitivity, and insulin secretion as much as 3 to 6 years before the diagnosis of diabetes. Such information may contribute to more accurate risk prediction models that use repeated measures taken at serial checkups.[58]

Obesity, aging, weight gain in adulthood, and physical inactivity are environmental factors affecting the progression of diabetes at all points along the continuum. Type 2 diabetes progresses from an early asymptomatic state with insulin resistance, to mild postprandial hyperglycemia, to clinical diabetes requiring pharmacologic intervention.

Prevention and Intervention

Identifying people at risk for diabetes is the first step in preventing the disease. The landmark Diabetes Prevention Program (DPP) screened over 14,000 high-risk individuals for the presence of prediabetes. Interventions with intensive lifestyle modifications (eating habits, exercise, and subsequent weight loss) versus a pharmacologic intervention using metformin to improve endogenous insulin action were aimed at ameliorating the specific defects prior to decompensation to diabetes. The DPP showed that lifestyle intervention reduced incidence by 58% and metformin by 31% (95% confidence interval, 17%, 43%), as compared with placebo; the lifestyle intervention was significantly more effective than metformin. To prevent 1 case of diabetes during a 3-year period, 6.9 persons would have to participate in the lifestyle intervention program, and 13.9 would have to receive metformin.[20] A 10-year follow-up to the DPP showed that diabetes incidence was reduced by 34% in the lifestyle group and by 18% in the metformin group.[59]

The DPP Research Group continues to publish on the persistence of the effects and benefits of the study's intervention. During the 10-year follow-up since randomization to the DPP, the original lifestyle group lost and then partially regained weight. The modest weight loss with metformin was maintained. During the DPP follow-up, incidence rates in the former placebo and metformin groups fell to equal those in the former lifestyle group, and the cumulative incidence of diabetes remained lowest in the lifestyle group. These data demonstrate that prevention or delay of diabetes with lifestyle intervention or metformin can persist for at least 10 years.[59]

The Look AHEAD (Action for Health in Diabetes) study was a multicenter randomized clinical trial to examine the effects of a lifestyle intervention designed to achieve and maintain weight loss in people with diagnosed diabetes through decreased caloric intake and increased exercise. The Look AHEAD study tested whether a lifestyle intervention resulting in weight loss would reduce rates of heart disease, stroke, and cardiovascular-related deaths in overweight and obese people with type 2 diabetes.[60] Researchers at 16 centers across the United States studied 5145 people, with half randomly assigned to an intensive lifestyle intervention and the other half to a general program of diabetes support and education. Both groups received routine medical care from their own healthcare providers. The intervention arm was stopped in 2012 because of the finding that the intervention did not reduce cardiovascular events. One positive finding was that both groups had a lower number of cardiovascular events compared with previous studies of people with diabetes. Data are currently being analyzed to help illuminate the reasons for the cardiovascular results.[60]

Look AHEAD did show other important health benefits of the lifestyle intervention, including decreasing sleep apnea, reducing the need for diabetes medications, helping to maintain physical mobility, and improving quality of life. Few, if any, studies of this size and duration have had comparable success in achieving and maintaining weight loss. Participants in the intervention group lost an average of more than 8% of their initial body weight after 1 year of intervention. They maintained an average weight loss of nearly 5% at 4 years, an amount that experts recommend to improve health. Participants in the diabetes support and education group lost about 1% of their initial weight after 1 and 4 years.[60]

Latent Autoimmune Diabetes in Adults

The clinical distinction between type 1 diabetes and type 2 diabetes is not always clear. There is increasing evidence that suggests significant overlap between type 1 diabetes and type 2 diabetes. It is important to note that both type 1 and type 2 diabetes are heterogeneous disorders and that LADA may account for as much as 10% of cases of insulin-requiring diabetes in older individuals and represents a slow, progressive form of type 1 diabetes that is frequently confused with type 2 diabetes. Persons with LADA may remain insulin-independent for many years even though they experience the autoimmune beta cell deterioration associated with classic type 1 diabetes.[61] Independent risk factors for progression of beta cell failure in LADA are sulfonylurea treatment, ICA positive periods, and initial body weight. Whether agents that preserve islet cell function, stimulate beta cell proliferation and survival, and/or improve insulin sensitivity can delay progression of LADA (ie, incretins and DPP-4 inhibitors) is being studied. Exenatide also may act as a regulator of the immune response in addition to its potential effects on beta cell proliferation.[62] When insulin therapy is required, the patient generally should be treated with a basal-bolus insulin regimen, as it is part of the treatment spectrum

for type 1 diabetes. The presence of autoantibodies suggests that LADA is, like type 1 diabetes, an autoimmune disease. There are, however, differences in autoantibody clustering, T-cell reactivity, and genetic susceptibility and protection between type 1 diabetes and LADA, suggesting important differences in the underlying disease processes. In LADA, diabetes occurs earlier in the process of beta cell destruction because a significant degree of insulin resistance is present.[63]

Persons with LADA are typically older than 35 years and nonobese. Their diabetes is controlled initially with diet. Within a relatively short period of time, months to years, a need for oral agents and progression to insulin treatment are required. The eventual clinical features include weight loss, propensity for ketosis, unstable blood glucose, and low C-peptide reserves. As immune system modulating therapies that slow or halt the progression of type 1 diabetes are developed, consideration of their potential role in the treatment of LADA will be necessary.[64]

Maturity-Onset Diabetes of the Young

Some rare forms of diabetes result from mutations in a single gene and are called monogenic. Monogenic forms of diabetes account for about 1% to 5% of all cases of diabetes in young people. Maturity-onset diabetes of the young (MODY) is a monogenic form of diabetes that usually first occurs during adolescence or early adulthood. People with MODY may have mild or no symptoms of diabetes and their hyperglycemia may be discovered only through routine blood tests. This form of diabetes may be confused with type 1 diabetes or type 2 diabetes. People with MODY generally are not overweight and do not have other risk factors for type 2 diabetes, such as high blood pressure or abnormal blood fat levels. While both type 2 diabetes and MODY can run in families, people with MODY typically have a family history of diabetes in multiple successive generations, meaning that MODY is present in a grandparent, a parent, and a child. Unlike people with type 1 diabetes, who always require insulin, people with MODY often can be treated with oral diabetes medications. Treatment varies depending on the genetic mutation that caused MODY.[65]

Identification of specific gene defects in certain groups with exceptionally high prevalence of type 2 diabetes has resulted in their designation as "other specific types of diabetes." These gene defects occur in a small percentage (<5%) of people with type 2 diabetes. Maturity-onset diabetes of the young is one monogenetic disorder that results from such defects. It is characterized by early onset and mild hyperglycemia. It is associated with distinct genetic defects of beta cell function and minimal or no defects in insulin action. Six genes on different chromosomes have been identified that cause MODY. Each abnormality leads to impaired insulin secretion. Numerous other specific mutations also have been identified in insulin, insulin receptor, and mitochondrial DNA that result in diabetes. Maturity-onset diabetes of the young can be suspected and recognized if a type 2 diabetes–like condition occurs in 2 or 3 or more generations and the pattern of inheritance is consistent with autosomal-dominant inheritance. The latter is the hallmark of MODY and distinguishes it from type 2 diabetes.[65]

Pathogenesis of Diabetes Complications

Although hyperglycemia plays a key modifiable role in the complications of diabetes (which are caused by abnormalities in the structure and function of blood vessels and nerves and the impact of hyperglycemia on various factors, including platelet aggregation, inflammatory processes, and coagulation factors), other major, and sometimes independent, factors contribute to its complications. In a comprehensive approach to preventing diabetes complications, the care team, including the person with diabetes, must proactively manage not only the hyperglycemia but also the complete spectrum of risk factors for complications. Other chapters in this book focus on management of nonglycemic risk factors.

Pathogenesis of Cardiovascular Disease in Diabetes

One cannot complete a discussion of the pathophysiology of the spectrum of diabetes as a metabolic disorder without mention of its links with cardiovascular disease (CVD). Diabetes clearly confers a strong increase in risk for CVD morbidity and mortality. While it is beyond the scope of this chapter to fully discuss this topic, further information may be found in chapter 25. Besides the coexistence of diabetes with other known risk factors for CVD, including family history, hypertension, dyslipidemia, and renal disease, hyperglycemia itself affects numerous processes that may be implicated in the pathogenesis of CVD. Hyperglycemia is pro-inflammatory and pro-thrombotic, causes platelet aggregation, impairs endothelial function and left ventricular function, and causes metabolic derangements, including an increase in FFAs. All these pathophysiologic mechanisms are closely interrelated and are responsible for premature CVD morbidity and mortality.[66]

The strength of the association between diabetes and CVD has led to a search for data demonstrating the definitive impact of lifestyle and therapeutic interventions on CVD outcomes in people with diabetes. Since the UKPDS first suggested a trend toward reduction in CVD events when targeted glycemic control was undertaken, definitive evidence that glycemic control can improve CVD outcomes has proven to be elusive. The ACCORD trial for type 1 diabetes[67] and the ADVANCE[68] and VADT[69] studies (see chapter 25) of type 2 diabetes each sought to demonstrate that intensive control of A1C would reduce cardiovascular events and death. In none of these studies was it clear that lowering A1C alone resulted in definitive improvement in cardiovascular endpoints.

These studies do, however, provide some insights that may prove useful in aiding our understanding of the relationship between glycemic control and CVD. The VADT showed that intensified diabetes control reduced the risk of CVD events provided that therapy was started early, suggesting that it is necessary to intervene early in the underlying pathophysiologic processes if one is to have an impact on the course of CVD. In ACCORD, while an increased risk of CVD death was observed in the intensively treated group, this increase was seen in those subjects with an A1C >7%, rather than in those reaching the intensive goal. It would appear that those who responded more readily, as measured by improved glycemic control, did better than those who were more refractory to therapy. This finding raises the possibility that the responsiveness of the individual to treatment, which would reflect the underlying pathophysiologic status of his or her diabetes, might be pivotal in determining CVD outcomes.[69]

Diabetes and Cancer Risk

Epidemiologic evidence suggests that people with diabetes are at significantly higher risk for many forms of cancer. Furthermore, evidence from observational studies suggests that some medications used to treat hyperglycemia in diabetes may have an impact on cancer risk.[70] This evidence is discussed in the chapters on each antihyperglycemic medication, including metformin, GLP-1 agonists, and insulins. In addition, type 2 diabetes and certain cancers share a variety of risk factors, including advancing age, male gender (cancers and diabetes occur more often in men overall), racial/ethnic propensity, being overweight or physically inactive, smoking, and drinking more than 1 alcoholic drink per day for women or 2

for men. Biologic links between diabetes and cancer, however, are not well understood.

The summary and recommendations from the 2010 joint consensus report of the American Diabetes Association and the American Cancer Society on diabetes and cancer are shown in Table 13.5.

Case Wrap-Up

There were numerous clues that, if dealt with earlier, may have prevented or delayed the onset of type 2 diabetes for CS. Diabetes education could have played a vital role in primary prevention in this case. Care should have included recognizing the clues and intervening early to counsel CS about her risk factors (and her children's risk), treating her high risk for diabetes, and emphasizing the need for follow-up. The fact that this did not occur caused continued and progressive metabolic abnormalities that may have resulted in decreased beta cell function. Early intervention prevents short- and long-term microvasculopathy, supporting the importance of early diagnosis and treatment.

TABLE 13.5 Summary and Recommendations of the Diabetes and Cancer Risk Consensus Report

Diabetes (primarily type 2) is associated with increased risk for some cancers (liver, pancreas, endometrium, colon and rectum, breast, bladder). Diabetes is associated with reduced risk of prostate cancer. For some other cancer sites, there appears to be no association or the evidence is inconclusive.
The association between diabetes and some cancers may be partly due to shared risk factors between the 2 diseases, such as aging, obesity, diet, and physical inactivity.
Possible mechanisms for a direct link between diabetes and cancer include hyperinsulinemia, hyperglycemia, and inflammation.
Healthful diets, physical activity, and weight management reduce risk and improve outcomes of type 2 diabetes and some forms of cancer and should be promoted for all.
People with diabetes should be strongly encouraged by their healthcare professionals to undergo appropriate cancer screenings as recommended for all people of their age and sex.
The evidence for specific drugs affecting cancer risk is limited, and observed associations may have been confounded by indications for specific drugs, effects on other cancer risk factors such as body weight and hyperinsulinemia, and the complex progressive nature of hyperglycemia and pharmacotherapy in type 2 diabetes.
Although limited, early evidence suggests that metformin is associated with a lower risk of cancer and that exogenous insulin is associated with an increased risk of cancer. Further research is needed to clarify these issues and evaluate whether insulin glargine is more strongly associated with cancer risk compared with other insulins.
Cancer risk should not be a major factor in choosing between available diabetes therapies for the average patient. For selected patients with very high risk for cancer occurrence (or for recurrence of specific cancer types), these issues may require more careful consideration.
Many questions remain regarding the association between diabetes and cancer risk.

Source: E Giovannucci, DM Harlan, MC Archer, "Diabetes and cancer: a consensus report," *Diabetes Care* 33, no. 7 (2010; cited 2014 Apr 9): 1674-85. doi: 10.2337/dc10-0666. On the Internet at: http://care.diabetesjournals.org/content/33/7/1674/T1.expansion.html.

Diabetes Complications Prevention and the Role of the Diabetes Educator

The diabetes educator must recognize that the pathophysiology of diabetes is a problem not only of carbohydrate metabolism but also of abnormalities in fat metabolism, feeding behavior, and vascular biology.

Although advances in medications, technology, and scientific knowledge are providing more tools to enable people with diabetes to attain an optimum physiologic state to enable prevention of complications, the diabetes educator needs to be aware that responsibility for the lifestyle and self-management practices needed to maintain optimum physiology lies primarily with the patient. The person with diabetes owns the daily decisions that play a large role in the course of the disease. Healthcare professionals are challenged to understand the impact self-management has on the outcome of disease management. The American Association of Diabetes Educators (AADE) has defined 7 self-care behaviors—the AADE7 Self-Care Behaviors™—as a framework for patient-centered diabetes education and care. Diabetes education focuses on these behaviors that are essential for health status and quality of life.[7] As understanding of the disease increases, health professionals must use this information to support clients in making their self-care behavior decisions.

In summary, knowledge of the pathophysiology of diabetes is increasing. Diabetes educators can use this new knowledge to guide their clients in managing their diabetes to ameliorate complications.

Focus on Education

Teaching Strategies

⟳ **As the diabetes epidemic broadens, the classic model of care has proven to be ineffective in controlling its spread.** Recognize how the Chronic Care Model needs to be implemented in order to effectively deal with all aspects of the continuum of care for those with or at risk for diabetes. Stay abreast of evolving concepts and new criteria.

⟳ **Know all specific signs, symptoms, and classifications of the different types of diabetes.** Recognize that the boundaries for traditional classifications are moving. More children are being diagnosed at a younger age. Teaching needs to be part of a widespread effort to focus on health in all parts of our community and society.

⟳ **Stay informed about pathophysiology and implications for treatment.** Attend local and national meetings and retain membership in organizations that provide frequent updates and the latest research. Bring this information back to the practice setting and inform peers and patients when teaching. Use the information for patient education.

⟳ **Heed diagnosing information.** The diagnosis of diabetes may have major life-altering implications. Thus, the following steps are essential: diagnostic criteria must be followed, testing must be completed, and test results with future implications (such as the need for follow-up or annual retesting) must be discussed.

Messages for Patients

⟳ **Early diagnosis and treatment are important.** Recognizing the risk of diabetes may be an opportunity to act. Lifestyle changes can prevent or delay diabetes. Healthy lifestyles should be integrated throughout the entire family. Recognize also that having diabetes or even having risk factors for diabetes increases the chances that relatives may also have the same problem. Healthy lifestyles can improve the future health of the entire family.

⟳ **You are part of the care team.** The more you know, the better prepared you are to be an active participant on the healthcare team. Being involved from the beginning is the first step toward implementing preventive medicine and is revolutionizing the concept of health management through lifestyle modification.

↗ **Staying up-to-date can help your health.**   Keep current with new ideas on diabetes management, treatment options, and other pertinent information. Attend educational sessions annually. Use Web sites, the educator on the team, and diabetes publications to learn the latest about diabetes management.

Health Literacy

↗ **"Simplicity is the ultimate sophistication"— Leonardo da Vinci.**   Information on the pathophysiology of the metabolic disorder is complex even for healthcare professionals. Patients need to understand what is happening in their bodies, how it relates to diabetes symptoms, and what can be done about it. It is hard for people with diabetes to follow recommendations and do all that needs to be done without understanding why and what will change as a result. Use analogies and a simple explanation of pathophysiology and how it affects glucose levels. For example, "Fueling your body with glucose . . . your car cannot drive without gasoline just as your body cannot operate without glucose." People need to visualize the connections between the functionality of the glucose regulations and their impact on the body and treatment.

↗ **"If you can't explain it simply, you don't understand it well enough"—Albert Einstein.**   Use simple language to communicate the relevant information about pathophysiology and how it affects diabetes management. Think about being on an elevator and having only 1 minute to convey important information about the pathophysiology of diabetes to a patient. What would you say? What would be the most important information to convey? How would you explain it?

↗ **It is better to have 3 important messages and repeat them 3 times than it is to have 9 messages but repeat them only once.**   Choose the most important concepts to understand and relate them to patients frequently to indicate the importance and increase recollection.

↗ **When communicating a lot of complex information, choose 3 or 4 messages that you think are most important for your listener to hear and remember.**   For each message, focus your audience by first stating the main point or "headline" (1 engaging statement), back up the message with facts or data, provide an anecdote to help your audience visualize what you are saying, use a personal example to humanize your story, and end by restating your main point or headline.

Focus on Practice

↗ **Utilize evidence-based interventions.**   Stay current on the pathophysiology of diabetes and how it relates to diagnosis and care. Create systems for addressing new advances in care and patients' expectations. Examine whether your healthcare system can efficiently support the advancements, their cost-effectiveness, and the expected outcomes.

↗ **Clinical leaders need to communicate with administrative departments and operational leaders to provide system integration of metabolic care.**   Monitoring and improving metabolic care

outcomes should be an ongoing and necessary process for every shift and corresponding department. Developing a continuous quality improvement plan with specific performance and markers of success indicators will provide a road map and destination points for all involved.

↗ **Existing healthcare systems are becoming competitive because of a focus on high quality, cost-effectiveness, and continuous improvement.**   Diabetes care clinicians must self-reflect on their practices and how they relate to the hospital, clinical, public health, and other applicable deliverables.

References

1. National Institute of Diabetes and Digestive and Kidney Diseases (NIDDK). NIH national diabetes statistics. 2013 Jun (cited 2014 Nov 13). On the Internet at: http://diabetes.niddk.nih.gov/dm/pubs/statistics/index.htm#pre-diabetes.

2. National Diabetes Information Clearinghouse (NDIC), National Institute of Diabetes and Digestive and Kidney Diseases (NIDDK), National Institute of Health (NIH). Fast facts on diabetes. NIH publication no 11-3892. Bethesda, Md, 2011 (last updated 2013 Sep 9; cited 2014 Apr 9). On the Internet at: http://diabetes.niddk.nih.gov/dm/pubs/statistics/index.aspx#fast.

3. Bays HE, Chapman RH, Grundy S, et al. The relationship of body mass index to diabetes mellitus, hypertension and dyslipidaemia: comparison of data from two national surveys. Int J Clin Pract. 2007 May 1;61(5):737-47. doi: 10.1111/j.1742-1241.2007.01336.x. PMCID: PMC1890993

4. Maps of trends in diagnosed diabetes and obesity. CDC's Division of Diabetes Translation. National Diabetes Surveillance System. 2011 Nov (cited 2014 Apr 9). On the Internet at: http://www.cdc.gov/diabetes/statistics/slides/maps_diabetesobesity_trends.pdf.

5. Heikes KE, Eddy DM, Arondekar B, Schlessinger L. Diabetes risk calculator: a simple tool for detecting undiagnosed diabetes and pre-diabetes. Diabetes Care. 2008; 31(5):1040-5.

6. Schulze MB, Hoffmann K, Boeing H, et al. An accurate risk score based on anthropometric, dietary, and lifestyle factors to predict the development of type 2 diabetes. Diabetes Care. 2007;30(3):510-5.

7. Centers for Disease Control and Prevention. National diabetes fact sheet (cited 2014 Apr 9). On the Internet at: http://www.cdc.gov/diabetes/pubs/estimates11.htm.

8. Ruderman NB, Myers M, Chipkin SR, et al. Hormone–fuel interrelationships: fed state, starvation, and diabetes mellitus. In: Joslin EP, Kahn CR, eds. Joslin Diabetes Mellitus. 14th ed. Baltimore: Lippincott Williams and Wilkins; 2005:128-44.

9. Klok MD, Jakobsdottir S, Drent ML. The role of leptin and ghrelin in the regulation of food intake and body weight in humans: a review. Obes Rev. 2007;8:21-34.

10. Ratner RE. Pathophysiology of the diabetes disease state. In: Franz MJ, ed. A Core Curriculum for Diabetes Education: Diabetes and Complications. 5th ed. Chicago: American Association of Diabetes Educators; 2003:3-18.

11. Heptulla RA, Rodriguez LM, Bomgaars L, et al. The role of amylin and glucagon in the dampening of glycemic excursions in children with type 1 diabetes. Diabetes. 2005;54:1100-7.

12. Jessen L, D'Alessio D. The incretins and beta-cell health: contrasting glucose-dependent insulinotropic polypeptide and glucagon-like peptide-1 as a path to understand islet function in diabetes. Gastroenterology. 2009;137:1891-4.

13. Baggio LL, Drucker DJ. Biology of incretins: GLP-1 and GIP. Gastroenterology. 2007;132:2131-57.

14. Gautier JF, Fetita S, Sobngwi E, et al. Biological actions of the incretins GIP and GLP-1 and therapeutic perspectives in patients with type 2 diabetes. Diabetes Metab. 2005; 31(3 pt 1):233-42.

15. Richter B, Bandeira-Echtler E, Bergerhoff K, et al. Dipeptidyl peptidase-4 (DPP-4) inhibitors for type 2 diabetes mellitus. Cochrane Database Syst Rev. 2008;2:CD006739.

16. Hung CC, Pirie F, Luan J, et al. Studies of the peptide YY and neuropeptide Y2 receptor genes in relation to human obesity and obesity-related traits. Diabetes. 2004;53:2461-6.

17. Di Marzo V, Bifulco M, De Petrocellis L. The endocannabinoid system and its therapeutic exploitation. Nat Rev Drug Discov. 2004;3:771-84.

18. Engeli S, Bohnke J, Feldpausch M, et al. Activation of the peripheral endocannabinoid system in human obesity. Diabetes. 2005;54:2838-43.

19. Standards of medical care in diabetes—2014. Diabetes Care. 2014;37 Suppl 1:S14-80. doi: 10.2337/dc14-S014

20. The Diabetes Prevention Program Research Group. The Diabetes Prevention Program: baseline characteristics of the randomized cohort. Diabetes Care. 2000;23:1619-29.

21. Expert Committee on the Diagnosis and Classification of Diabetes Mellitus. Report of the Expert Committee on the Diagnosis and Classification of Diabetes Mellitus. Diabetes Care. 1997;20:1183-97.

22. International Expert Committee. International Expert Committee report on the role of the A1C assay in the diagnosis of diabetes. Diabetes Care. 2009;32:1327-34.

23. NGSP. Harmonizing hemoglobin A1C testing. 2010 (cited 2014 Apr 9). On the Internet at: http://www.ngsp.org.

24. National Diabetes Clearinghouse, National Institute of Diabetes and Digestive and Kidney Disease, National Institutes of Health. For people of African, Mediterranean, or Southeast Asian Heritage: important information about diabetes blood tests (cited 2014 Apr 9). On the Internet at: http://diabetes.niddk.nih.gov/dm/pubs/traitA1C.

25. Nielsen LR, Ekbom P, Damm P, et al. HbA1c levels are significantly lower in early and late pregnancy. Diabetes Care. 2004 May;27:1200-1.

26. Baglia V, Sapsford R. Diabetes mellitus and heart failure: an overview of epidemiology and management. Diab Vasc Dis Res. 2009;6:164-71.

27. Pawłowicz M, Birkholz D, Niedźwiecki M, et al. Difficulties or mistakes in diagnosing type 1 diabetes in children?—demographic factors influencing delayed diagnosis. Pediatr Diabetes. 2009;10:542-9.

28. Charfen MA, Ipp E, Kaji AH, et al. Detection of undiagnosed diabetes and prediabetic states in high-risk emergency department patients. Acad Emerg Med. 2009;16:394-402.

29. Magee MF, Nassar C. Hemoglobin A1C testing in an emergency department. J Diabetes Sci Technol. 2011;5:1437-43.

30. Magee MF, Nassar CM, Copeland J, et al. Synergy to reduce emergency department visits for uncontrolled hyperglycemia. Diabetes Educ. 2013;39:354-64. doi: 10.1177/0145721713484593

31. Atkinson MA, Eisenbarth GS. Type 1 diabetes: new perspectives on disease pathogenesis and treatment. Lancet. 2010;358:221-9.

32. Vaarala O, Hyoty H, Akerblom HK. Environmental factors in the etiology of childhood diabetes. Diabetes Nutr Metab. 1999;12:75-85.

33. Feig DS, Hwee J, Shah BR, et al. Trends in incidence of diabetes in pregnancy and serious perinatal outcomes: a large, population-based study in Ontario, Canada, 1996–2010. Diabetes Care. Published online before print, April 4, 2014. doi: 10.2337/dc13-2717

34. International Association of Diabetes and Pregnancy Study Groups Recommendations on the Diagnosis and Classification of Hyperglycemia in Pregnancy. Diabetes Care. 2010; 33:676-82.

35. Lawrence JM, Contreras R, Chen W, et al. Trends in the prevalence of preexisting diabetes and gestational diabetes mellitus among a racially/ethnically diverse population of pregnant women, 1999-2005. Diabetes Care. 2008;31:899-904.

36. Sipetic S, Vlajinac H, Kocev N, Bjekic M, Sajic S. Early infant diet and risk of type 1 diabetes mellitus in Belgrade children. Nutrition. 2005;21:474-9.

37. Achenbach P, Warncke K, Reiter J, et al. Stratification of type 1 diabetes risk on the basis of islet autoantibody characteristics. Diabetes. 2004;53:384-92.

38. Protective effects of sitagliptin on beta cell function in patients with adult-onset latent autoimmune diabetes (LADA) (cited 2014 Apr 9). On the Internet at: http://clinicaltrialsfeeds.org/clinical-trials/show/NCT01159847.

39. Metcalf K, Hitman G. Concordance for type 1 diabetes in identical twins is affected by insulin genotype. Diabetes Care. 2001;21:838-42.

40. Dotta F, Censini S, van Halteren AG, et al. Coxsackie B4 virus infection of beta cells and natural killer cell insulitis in recent-set type I diabetic patients. Proc Natl Acad Sci USA. 2007;104:5115-20.

41. van der Werf N, Kroese FG, Rozing J, Hillebrands JL. Viral infections as potential triggers of type 1 diabetes. Diabetes Metab Res Rev. 2007;23:169-83.

42. Wasnuth HE, Kolb H. Cow's milk and immune-mediated diabetes. Proc Nutr Soc. 2000;59:573-9.

43. Knip M, Akerblom HK. Early nutrition and later diabetes risk. Adv Exp Med Biol. 2005;569:142-50.

44. Franco R, Panayiotidis MI. Environmental toxicity, oxidative stress, human disease and the "black box" of their synergism: how much have we revealed? Mutat Res. 2009;674:1-2. doi: 10.1016/j.mrgentox.2009.01.005

45. Lenzen S. Oxidative stress: the vulnerable beta-cell. Biochem Soc Trans. 2008;36(Pt 3):343-7. doi: 10.1042/BST0360343

46. Moltchanova EV, Schreier N, Lammi N, Karvonen M. Seasonal variation of diagnosis of type 1 diabetes mellitus in children worldwide. Diabet Med. 2009;26:673-8.

47. Knip M, Siljander H. Autoimmune mechanisms in type 1 diabetes. Autoimmun Rev. 2008;7:550-7.

48. Babaya N, Nakayama M, Eisenbarth GS. The stages of type 1A diabetes. Ann N Y Acad Sci. 2005;1051:194-204.

49. Palmer JP. Latent autoimmune diabetes in adults. J Clin Endocrinol Metab. 2009;94:4635-44.

50. Abdul-Rasoul M, Habib H, Al-Khouly M. 'The honeymoon phase' in children with type 1 diabetes mellitus: frequency, duration, and influential factors. Pediatr Diabetes. 2006;7:101-7.

51. Nichols GA, Hillier TA, Brown JB. Progression from newly acquired impaired fasting glucose to type 2. Diabetes Care. 2007;30:228-33.

52. Bays H, Mandarino L, DeFronzo RA. Role of the adipocyte, free fatty acids, and ectopic fat in pathogenesis of type 2 diabetes mellitus: per oxisomal proliferators-activated receptor agonists provide a rational therapeutic approach. J Clin Endocrinol Metab. 2004;28:463-78.

53. Triangle Butler AE, Janson J, Bonner-Weir S, et al. Beta-cell deficit and increased beta-cell apoptosis in humans with type 2 diabetes. Diabetes. 2003;52:102-10.

54. Lund University. New clues in hunt for heredity in type 2 diabetes. ScienceDaily. 2013 Mar 19 (cited 2013 Nov 10). On the Internet at: http://www.sciencedaily.com/releases/2013/03/130319091144.htm.

55. Drong AW, Lindgren CM, McCarthy MI. The genetic and epigenetic basis of type 2 diabetes and obesity. Clin Pharmacol Ther. 2012 Dec;92(6):707-15. doi: 10.1038/clpt.2012.149. Epub 2012 Oct 10.

56. Meigs J, Cupples LA, Wilson PW. Parental transmission of type 2 diabetes: the Framingham Offspring Study. Diabetes. 2000;49(12):2201-7.

57. Bauters C, Ennezat PV, Tricot O, et al. Stress hypergly-caemia is an independent predictor of left ventricular remodelling after first anterior myocardial infarction in non-diabetic patients. Eur Heart J. 2007;28:546-52.

58. Tabak AG, Jokela M, Akbaraly TN, et al. Trajectories of glycaemia, insulin sensitivity, and insulin secretion before diagnosis of type 2 diabetes: an analysis from the Whitehall II study. Lancet. 2009;373:2215-21.

59. Diabetes Prevention Rescue Group. 10 year follow up of diabetes incidence and weight loss in the DPP outcome. Lancet. 2009;374:1677-86.

60. The Look AHEAD Research Group. Cardiovascular effects of intensive lifestyle intervention. N Engl J Med. 2013;369:145-54.

61. Naik RG, Brooks-Worrell BM, Palmer JP. Latent autoim-mune diabetes in adults. Endocr Pract. 2009;94:4635-44.

62. Protective effects of sitagliptin on β cell function in patients with adult-onset latent autoimmune diabetes (LADA) (cited 2013 Nov 3). On the Internet at: http://www.bioportfolio.com/resources/trial/63001/Protective-Effects-Of-Sitagliptin-On-Cell-Function-In-Patients-With-Adult-onset.html.

63. Groop L, Tuomi T, Rowley M, et al. Latent autoimmune diabetes in adults (LADA)—more than a name. Diabetolo-gia. 2006;49:1996-8.

64. Pozzilli P, Di Mario U. Autoimmune diabetes not requir-ing insulin at diagnosis (latent autoimmune diabetes of the adult): definition, characterization, and potential preven-tion. Diabetes Care. 2001;24:1460-7.

65. Fajans SS, Bell GI. MODY: history, genetics, pathophysiol-ogy, and clinical decision making. Diabetes Care. 2011;34:1878-84.

66. Zarich SW. Mechanism by which hyperglycemia plays a role in the setting of acute cardiovascular illness. Rev Car-diovasc Med. 2006;7 Suppl 2:S35-43.

67. The Action to Control Cardiovascular Risk in Diabetes Study Group. Effects of intensive glucose lowering in type 2 diabetes. N Engl J Med. 2008;358:2545-59.

68. Patel A, MacMahon S, Chalmers J, et al; for the ADVANCE Collaborative Group. Intensive blood glucose control and vascular outcomes in patients with type 2 diabetes. N Engl J Med. 2008;358:2560-72.

69. Duckworth W, Abraira C, Moritz T, et al; for the VADT Investigators. Glucose control and vascular complications in veterans with type 2 diabetes. N Engl J Med. 2009;360:129-39.

70. Giovannucci E, Harlan DM, Archer MC, et al. Diabetes and cancer: a consensus report. Diabetes Care. 2010;33:1674-85.

Type 1 Diabetes Throughout the Life Span

Carolyn Banion, RN, MN, CPNP, CDE
Virginia Valentine, CNS, BC-ADM, CDE, FAADE

Key Concepts

- Clinical management of diabetes relies on patient and family self-management.

- Diabetes education is an essential and crucial component of the care and management of individuals with type 1 diabetes. Education must be ongoing throughout the course of the disease.

- There are important differences between children/adolescents and adults in diabetes education and management. Learning materials, content, demonstration of skills, and expectations must be appropriate for the age, abilities, and attention span of each child, adult, and family member.

- The primary goals of treatment are achievement of optimal glycemic goals, avoidance of acute and chronic complications, positive psychosocial adjustment to diabetes, and normal growth and development in children.

- To achieve the desired goals of diabetes management, the person with diabetes and the person's family must integrate a comprehensive and rigorous diabetes regimen into their daily lives. In caring for children and adolescents with diabetes, healthcare providers need to understand the importance of involving adults in diabetes management for these youths.

Introduction

Type 1 diabetes affects all ages, and management and education are ongoing processes throughout an individual's life span. There are a variety of issues, situations, and physical and emotional differences that present at distinct ages and life stages. The diabetes educator must appreciate that diabetes self-management education (DSME) in children, adolescents, and adults presents challenges. The goals for treatment are twofold: (1) to promote normal physical and psychological growth and development, and (2) to avoid both acute and chronic complications of diabetes. This chapter focuses on DSME in type 1 diabetes throughout the life span. Issues in providing care to children and teens are given primary attention. As appropriate, though, throughout the chapter, information pertinent to adults with type 1 diabetes is provided. Transition to adult care and development of type 1 diabetes in adults are addressed at the end of the chapter.

State of the Disease

Type 1 diabetes is an autoimmune disease in which hyperglycemia is secondary to insulin deficiency, which is caused by destruction of pancreatic beta cells. Type 1 diabetes accounts for 5% to 10% of all diagnosed cases of diabetes.[1] Age at diagnosis was the initial classification criterion used to describe what was clearly a distinct form of diabetes. Recent classification systems abandoned both age and treatment as criteria and now attempt to identify etiology of disease to classify different types of diabetes.[1]

Seventy percent of type 1 diabetes cases are diagnosed before the person reaches 30 years of age, but onset can occur at any age. Type 1 diabetes is one of the most common childhood illnesses, and in the United States approximately 1 in every 400 to 500 children and adolescents under 20 years of age has type 1 diabetes.[1] The worldwide prevalence and incidence of type 1 diabetes vary from one geographic location to another, with the highest incidence occurring in the Scandinavian countries of Sweden, Finland, and Norway, and the lowest incidence occurring in Japan. Evidence suggests that the incidence of type 1 diabetes is increasing globally at a rate of about 3% per year. In some regions, this increase is reported to be greater in children under the age of 5 years.[2] This trend has been speculated to be more likely related to environmental changes, such as exposure to viral infections, than to differences in genetic susceptibility.[3]

The current standards for diabetes management reflect the need to maintain glucose control as near to normal as safely possible in both children and adults. The Diabetes Control and Complications Trial (DCCT) and the follow-up Epidemiology of Diabetes Interventions and Complications (EDIC) study have shown that intensive treatment and maintenance of glucose concentrations close to the normal range clearly decrease the frequency and severity of the macrovascular and microvascular complications of diabetes.[4,5] These trials have involved adults and only a small cohort of adolescent patients. Evidence indicates that near normalization of blood glucose levels is not often attained in children and adolescents after

the honeymoon (remission) period.[6] Special consideration must be given to the unique risks of hypoglycemia in young children. Glycemic goals need to be modified because most children less than 6 to 7 years of age have a form of "hypoglycemic unawareness." Their counterregulatory mechanisms are immature, and they may lack the cognitive capacity to recognize and respond to hypoglycemic symptoms, placing them at greater risk for severe hypoglycemia and its sequelae. Children under the age of 5 years are at risk for permanent cognitive impairment following episodes of severe hypoglycemia.[7] The plasma blood glucose and A1C goals for type 1 diabetes in children are shown in Table 14.1. See also the section on type 1 diabetes in adults at the end of this chapter.

Diagnosis

The onset of type 1 diabetes is usually acute, with symptoms ranging from incidental glycosuria to life-threatening DKA. The diagnosis of diabetes in infants is rare, and children less than 4 years of age more often present in DKA than do older children or adults. About 25% of children with new-onset type 1 diabetes present in DKA, requiring intravenous rehydration and insulin.[8] Many require treatment in an intensive care unit. At the time of diagnosis, 80% to 90% of the beta cells have been destroyed. Most children present with complaints of nocturia and enuresis and a several-week history of polyuria, polydipsia, and weight loss. Adults with type 1 diabetes often present with polyphagia, but this is rarely seen in children. Other common symptoms include blurred vision, drowsiness, poor stamina, nausea and vomiting, frequent skin and bladder infections,

---

Case: Type 1 Diabetes—Infancy to Young Adulthood

JJ is a 22-year-old college student who was diagnosed with type 1 diabetes at 9 months of age.

- His diabetes was diagnosed when his parents took him to his primary care physician because he was waking frequently and soaking through many diapers during the night and would drink anything given to him.

- He was hospitalized at a children's hospital in moderate diabetic ketoacidosis (DKA) for metabolic stabilization, initiation of insulin therapy, and education of his family.

- Family history includes a maternal aunt with type 1 diabetes, who incidentally had been a subject in the DCCT before JJ's diagnosis.

The case study in this chapter follows a young male from diagnosis at infancy through young adulthood. Issues that the boy and his family faced at different stages are highlighted.

	Plasma Blood Glucose Goal Range (mg/dL)			
Values by Age	*Before Meals*	*Bedtime/ Overnight*	*A1C*	*Rationale*
Toddlers and preschoolers (<6 years)	100–180 (5.5–10.0 mmol/L)	110–200 (6.1–11.1 mmol/L)	<8.5% (but >7.5%)*	High risk and vulnerability to hypoglycemia
School age (6–12 years)	90–180 (5.0–10.0 mmol/L)	100–180 (5.5–10.0 mmol/L)	<8%*	Risk of hypoglycemia and relatively low risk of complications prior to puberty
Adolescents and young adults (13–19 years)	90–130 (5.0–7.2 mmol/L)	90–150 (5.0–8.3 mmol/L)	<7.5%*	Risk of hypoglycemia Developmental and psychological issues
Key Concepts in Setting Glycemic Goals: Adults: 70–130; 70–150; <7%				
Goals should be individualized, and lower goals may be reasonable based on benefit–risk assessment				
Blood glucose goals should be higher than those listed above in individuals with frequent hypoglycemia or hypoglycemia unawareness				
Postprandial blood glucose values should be measured when there is a disparity between preprandial blood glucose values and A1C levels				

TABLE 14.1 Plasma Blood Glucose and A1C Goals for Type 1 Diabetes in Children

*A lower goal (<7.0%) is reasonable if it can be achieved without excessive hypoglycemia.

Sources: American Diabetes Association, "Clinical practice recommendations 2013," *Diabetes Care* 36 Suppl 1 (2013): S40; "Hypoglycemia and diabetes: a report of a workgroup of the American Diabetes Association and the Endocrine Society," *Diabetes Care* 36 (2013): 1384-95.

and vaginitis in females. Laboratory values indicate hyperglycemia, glycosuria, and often but not always ketonemia and ketonuria.

Diagnosis of type 1 diabetes in children is usually clear-cut and requires little or no specialized testing. An elevated blood glucose concentration or A1C ≥6.5% must be documented to diagnose diabetes. The American Association of Clinical Endocrinologists (AACE) does not recommend the A1C as a diagnostic test for type 1 diabetes. The incidental discovery of hyperglycemia in the absence of classic symptoms does not necessarily indicate new-onset diabetes, especially in young children with acute illness.[6]

The criteria for the diagnosis of diabetes are presented in Table 14.2. In the absence of unequivocal hyperglycemia, these criteria should be confirmed by repeat testing on a different day. The oral glucose tolerance test (OGTT) is not recommended for routine clinical use, but may be required in the evaluation of patients when diabetes is still suspected despite a normal fasting plasma glucose.[7] Glucose tolerance testing is rarely required to diagnose type 1 diabetes, except in atypical cases or at the beginning of the disease. Because of the risk of rapid clinical deterioration, especially in untreated children with type 1 diabetes, unnecessary delays in the diagnosis must be avoided, and a definitive diagnosis should be made promptly.[6]

As the incidence of type 2 diabetes in children and adolescents increases, differentiating newly diagnosed type 1 diabetes from type 2 diabetes has become more important. In the slender prepubertal child, type 2 diabetes would be very unlikely. In the overweight adolescent, measurement of islet autoantibodies may be necessary to differentiate the diagnosis. Between 85% and 95% of individuals with type 1 diabetes have circulating antibodies directed against 1 or more islet cell components. Regardless of the type of diabetes, insulin will be required for the child who presents with significant fasting hyperglycemia, metabolic derangement, and ketonemia.[6]

TABLE 14.2 Diagnosing Type 1 Diabetes			
4 Options			
A1C*	**Fasting Plasma Glucose†**	**2-Hour Plasma Glucose**	**Acute Symptoms§ Plus Casual⁆ Plasma Glucose**
≥6.5%	≥126 mg/dL (7.0 mmol/L)	≥200 mg/dL (11.1 mmol/L) during OGTT (75 g glucose)‡	≥200 mg/dL (11.1 mmol/L)

Note: Unless unequivocal symptoms of hyperglycemia are present, these criteria must be confirmed by repeat testing on a subsequent day.

*Performed in a laboratory using a method that is NGSP (National Glycohemoglobin Standardization Program) certified and standardized to the DCCT assay. The AACE does not recommend the A1C as a diagnostic test for type 1 diabetes mellitus.

†Fasting is defined as no caloric intake for at least 8 hours.

‡See text for discussion of when the OGTT is appropriate.

§Classic symptoms of diabetes include polyuria, polydipsia, and unexplained weight loss.

⁆Casual is defined as any time of day without regard to time since last meal.

Source: American Diabetes Association, "Clinical practice recommendations 2013," *Diabetes Care* 36 Suppl 1 (2013): S11.

The diagnosis of diabetes, as in other chronic illnesses, often causes individuals to grieve the loss of their health, or parents to grieve the loss of their healthy child. Frequently, parents feel guilty about the diagnosis of diabetes in their child because of the genetic component of the disease. Parents may have numerous unexpressed questions, and they may fear they did something to cause the diabetes.

The diabetes educator can be instrumental in initiating discussion of and normalizing these feelings. Parents and family must be reassured that there is nothing they could have done to prevent the disease and that the combination of genes from both parents increases the risk for type 1 diabetes in their offspring. New technology, medications, and treatment strategies have changed diabetes management dramatically in recent years; explaining this to families is usually reassuring. The parents and family need to understand the difference in pathophysiology and treatment of type 1 diabetes and type 2 diabetes. Diabetes self-management education is essential for all individuals with newly diagnosed diabetes. Planning and provision of diabetes education should recognize the following:

Infants and preschoolers. Education is directed toward the parents and primary caregivers (babysitters, grandparents, older siblings). The tremendous responsibility of care and fear of hypoglycemia are extremely stressful for these families.[9]

School-aged children. Parents need to assume most of the responsibility, but the child will be able to learn some of the skills needed for self-management.

Adolescents. For most (depending on their cognitive and emotional development), education should be directed primarily toward the adolescent, with parents included.

Adults. Spouses or significant others should also receive self-management education.

Survival Skills: The Focus of the First Week

Because of the strong emotions (shock, anger, grief) felt at this time, most patients and their families do not comprehend much more than survival skills in the first week. Others may seem to adapt more quickly and move forward at a quicker pace; sometimes, however, these same families experience the grief and anger at a later time. The initial teaching focuses on the following survival skills:

- Testing blood glucose and urine or blood ketones
- Measuring and administering insulin
- Understanding insulin actions
- Performing insulin actions
- Meal planning
- Preventing, recognizing, and treating hypoglycemia

The education provided must be culturally appropriate, personalized to the needs of its recipients (child, individual, family), sensitive to family resources, paced to accommodate individual needs,

Case—Part 2: Provision of Family Education and Support

Once JJ's DKA was treated, the educational process with his family was initiated by a team of healthcare professionals, including a pediatric endocrinologist, diabetes nurse educator, dietitian, and medical social worker. JJ's parents experienced the usual shock, grief, anger, sadness, and denial that most parents do when their child is diagnosed. JJ's mother grew up with a sibling with type 1 diabetes, so she had some preconceived ideas about diabetes management. Due to the high prevalence of type 2 diabetes, other friends and family members who had experience with type 2 diabetes offered conflicting advice about the management of JJ's diabetes. This heightened JJ's parents' fears. Both parents had a real fear of hypoglycemia because of the increase in frequency of hypoglycemia the mother's sister had experienced with intensive insulin therapy during the DCCT. The diagnosis can be particularly devastating for families who have experienced the complications of diabetes. It is important for the healthcare team to know a family's past experience with diabetes.

Education needed to be individualized and communicated in a way that addressed the age and developmental stage of the child, family dynamics, past experiences with diabetes, and issues facing the entire family. In JJ's case, his family needed to understand that there are different types of diabetes and that everyone's experience with diabetes is different. The family needed to be reassured that they could not have prevented the diagnosis of diabetes. Diabetes education regarding survival skills was foremost, and this education included JJ's siblings and other caretakers, such as grandparents. The pace of teaching followed the progress the family was making in learning the necessary skills.

The art of diabetes education and care is in the delivery and effectiveness. Although the biomedical aspects of type 1 diabetes are similar across patients, the experience of having diabetes can be very different in different cultural and ethnic groups. The majority of people with type 1 diabetes are non-Hispanic whites, 10% are Hispanic, and 7% are other ethnic backgrounds.[10] Assessments should include cultural values and language skills including health literacy. Healthcare providers need to be familiar with the normative cultural values that may affect the health care of ethnic and cultural groups and be understanding about these values. For example, in some cultures, diabetes is seen as a death sentence, so why take care of it? Sometimes diabetes is thought to be the result of some traumatic event, and there is tremendous guilt. In some cultures, insulin is thought to be a drug that can cause blindness, kidney problems, amputations, or death.

To provide appropriate education for the family, the diabetes educator must carefully evaluate the meaning of the diagnosis, assess family members' comfort with using insulin, ensure that they understand that insulin is necessary, encourage the patient/family to share whether they are using any alternative therapies, and assess family routines and schedules. It is also important to have educational materials available to meet the language, cultural, and literacy needs of patients and families. Frequent contact in the weeks after the diagnosis and the initial education will be necessary.

and provided for all caregivers. Siblings should not be overlooked, as they sometimes feel left out because of the attention being given to the child with diabetes.

The educational process needs to be an open-ended, ongoing experience between the individual with diabetes and the individual's family, friends, and diabetes team.[11] Developing effective stress management/coping skills and problem-solving skills is considered as important to successful therapy as insulin administration, nutrition therapy, monitoring, and exercise.[12]

The content provided will be the same whether the individual with new-onset diabetes is in the inpatient or outpatient setting. About 75% of children with new-onset diabetes are not acutely ill and do not require hospitalization for medical management.[13] However, hospitalization may be an option for these children for initiation of insulin therapy and education. If there is an outpatient facility equipped to do outpatient education and management for individuals and their families, these children will not require hospitalization. To do this successfully, a multidisciplinary team must teach the patient and family how to safely use insulin at home, and be available to troubleshoot by phone if problems arise. Initial outpatient care and education costs are substantially lower than those associated with inpatient care.[13,14] Families may be directed to additional educational support through the American Association of Diabetes Educators (AADE) and the American Diabetes Association (ADA), which can refer them to a diabetes educator or diabetes education team.

American Association of Diabetes Educators©

To achieve the desired goals for glycemic control, patients and families must integrate a comprehensive and rigorous diabetes management plan into their daily lives.

Management of type 1 diabetes includes the following key components:

- *Monitoring:* Measurement of blood glucose 6 to 8 times per day
- *Taking medication:* Insulin infusion therapy or 3 to 4 injections of insulin per day
- *Healthy eating:* Attention to food intake
- *Being active:* Regular exercise

Monitoring
Blood Glucose Monitoring

Frequent monitoring of blood glucose levels is necessary for optimal glycemic control. In a number of studies, the frequency of blood glucose monitoring was strongly associated with glycemic control.[15,16] In a study of 7- to 16-year-olds, frequency of testing was the most important predictor of A1C levels.[17,18]

The ADA recommends blood glucose checks prior to meals and snacks, occasionally postprandially, at bedtime, prior to exercise, when the individual suspects low blood glucose, after treating low blood glucose until the individual is normoglycemic, and prior to critical tasks such as driving for patients using multiple daily injections (MDIs) or insulin pump therapy.[1]

Frequent monitoring (ie, 4 or more measurements) is essential in determining patterns of hypoglycemia and hyperglycemia and in enabling individuals to make adjustments in food, exercise, scheduling, and/or insulin.

- *Preprandial blood glucose*: To determine premeal insulin dose
- *Postprandial blood glucose:* Important in determining whether premeal insulin dose was correct
- *Overnight blood glucose:* Valuable in determining doses and detecting nocturnal hypoglycemia, especially after exercise that is greater than usual intensity, duration, or frequency; hypoglycemia; illness; or poor food intake
- *Frequent testing:* Essential in young children or anyone who has hypoglycemic unawareness

Meters

Many good blood glucose meters are available. Often, third-party payers dictate which meter the individual uses. The fingertips are the most frequently used site for blood samples. Some individuals may find alternate sites (forearm or palm of the hand) more acceptable. The results from fingertips and forearms are usually similar in the fasting state. Alternate-site testing may not reflect arterial glucose values as quickly as finger-stick capillary blood glucose measurements, so it is advised that fingertips be used when symptoms of hypoglycemia are present.[19,20]

Data Log

It is important for blood glucose test results to be documented in a logbook or downloaded from the meter. Almost all meters contain a memory chip that allows individuals and care providers to download blood glucose test results. Interpretation of results and use of this information for calculating insulin doses are essential in achieving good metabolic control. Individuals and families should be taught to review these data frequently to look for blood glucose patterns and make appropriate dose adjustments or call their healthcare provider for assistance.

Continuous Glucose Monitoring

Continuous glucose sensors track glucose levels every few minutes, 24 hours a day. These devices hold promise for improved metabolic control and the avoidance of hypoglycemia, which is often the most significant barrier to optimal control. As continuous glucose monitoring becomes more widely available, it is anticipated that lower blood glucose targets may be safely achieved, thus improving HbA1c levels without increasing hypoglycemia.[21] Continuous glucose monitoring devices may dramatically alter the management of type 1 diabetes in individuals who are motivated to use this technology and capable of incorporating it into their own daily diabetes management. Continuous glucose monitoring may be particularly useful in those with hypoglycemia unawareness, frequent episodes of hypoglycemia, nocturnal hypoglycemia, unexplained glucose excursions, or gastroparesis.[22]

Conventional blood glucose monitoring provides incomplete data, giving a snapshot of the blood glucose at that moment. Improvements in continuous blood glucose monitors will continue. The challenge for healthcare providers will be to learn how to interpret these data in an efficient way and teach patients how to respond to and use the data to achieve the best possible metabolic control. Chapter 7, on monitoring, discusses this new technology.

Ketone Testing

The general recommendation for ketone testing is to test when blood glucose levels exceed 250 mg/dL (13.9 mmol/L) and during illness.

Some centers advise routine ketone testing before breakfast as an indicator of overnight or antecedent insulin deficiency. Overnight (antecedent) insulin deficiency—referred to as the "dawn phenomenon"—is fasting hyperglycemia related to the normal rise in growth hormone, cortisol, and other hormones that can raise blood glucose levels in the absence of insulin.[23]

Ketones can be tested in either urine or blood. Blood ketone testing gives more current results, but the blood testing strips are more expensive than the urine testing strips. Testing the urine for ketones is a commonly taught skill; however, meters are now available that test both blood glucose and blood ketones.[1] Some families may find this meter more convenient for those times when obtaining a urine sample is difficult.

The presence of persistent moderate or large amounts of ketones in the urine or concentrations of greater than 0.6 mmol/L in the blood suggest the possibility of impending DKA and should prompt individuals to adjust their insulin or seek assistance from their healthcare provider. Additional fluids and/or insulin are often required to clear ketosis. See chapter 22 for more information on management of hyperglycemia.

Case—Part 3: Tools of Therapy

During baby JJ's hospitalization, his parents were taught survival skills for diabetes management.

Monitoring

- Blood glucose

- Blood or urine ketones

JJ's parents were instructed on the use of a blood glucose meter that uses a small sample of blood. They were also instructed on record keeping and the importance of using these data for pattern management.

Insulin Therapy

JJ was started on MDIs, using a long-acting insulin analog for basal insulin and a rapid-acting insulin analog with all food intake. JJ's parents were instructed on the measurement of insulin and the administration and rotation of insulin injections. When JJ's mother expressed reluctance because she did not want to hurt her baby, the educator had the parents practice giving each other saline injections.

Meal Planning

Ensuring adequate nutrition and calories was a primary consideration, as it is essential in the growing child. At the time JJ was diagnosed, JJ's parents met with a pediatric registered dietitian. Food was one of their biggest concerns, as is often the case for parents of infants and toddlers. The educator explained that because infants require a frequent feeding schedule, getting glucose values with even a 2-hour fast is often difficult, and "feeds" often do not match the peaks of insulin.

Physical Activity

The activity level of a 9-month-old, such as JJ at the time of his diagnosis, is unpredictable and in general cannot be planned for or controlled. That is one of the many challenges of managing diabetes in an infant. It was important for JJ's parents to understand how his activity level, sleep, and nap patterns affected his blood glucose levels so they could make appropriate adjustments in food and insulin.

Hypoglycemia

The fear of hypoglycemia is both one of the major barriers to achieving optimal glycemic control for all individuals with diabetes and one of the biggest fears of parents of children with diabetes. Severe hypoglycemia can affect the growing brain of the child, and recognizing the early warning signs of hypoglycemia in a very young child may be difficult. However, due to the seriousness of hypoglycemia, the importance of prevention and early adequate treatment must be stressed. JJ's parents were instructed on the signs, symptoms, and treatment of hypoglycemia, including the use of glucose gel and glucagon. They were encouraged to do frequent monitoring of blood glucose to validate hypoglycemic episodes.

When baby JJ was discharged from the hospital, his parents had learned an entire new set of skills and had the challenge of raising a child with diabetes.

Considerations for Insulin Injections in Children and Teens[24]

- Usual injection sites for young children are the legs, arms, and buttocks. Because children usually have less subcutaneous tissue than adults, appropriate sites must be used to ensure subcutaneous injection and avoid administration into underlying muscle. Abdominal injections may not be advisable in young children with little subcutaneous abdominal fat. Injections can be given in the abdomen of school-aged children and adolescents if they have adequate subcutaneous tissue.
- Rotating sites in a consistent manner (eg, legs in the morning, arms in the evening, buttocks at bedtime) may provide a more consistent rate of absorption. It may also prevent lipohypertrophy of sites.
- Avoid giving injections into hypertrophied areas, to achieve the best absorption possible.
- Use 31-gauge, short, or mini needles for more comfortable injections and to avoid intramuscular injection.
- Use the smallest barrel possible (eg, 30-unit syringe for doses less than 30 units, 50-unit syringe for doses between 30 and 50 units) for the most accurate dosing.
- Half-unit increments can now be measured on certain insulin syringes.
- Some insulin pens have the option of half-unit dosing. These are reusable pens that use only rapid-acting insulin.
- An automatic injector (Inject-Ease® or similar device) may be useful for some individuals.
- Needle phobias are common in children and adults (parents or patients). *Always* assess.
- By giving each other practice saline injections, parents can reassure themselves that giving insulin injections to their child is not the trauma they envision.
- For older children, seeing family members give themselves a practice saline injection may be supportive, making it less frightening for the child.

Taking Medication
Insulin Injection Therapy

Insulin is the mainstay of treatment of type 1 diabetes. Subcutaneous insulin injections are begun at the time of diagnosis, or once ketoacidosis is resolved in those in whom it was present. There are many different insulin preparations available. The various preparations are genetically engineered to have different onsets, peaks, and duration of activity (see chapter 18). These insulins are used in combination or individually and can be delivered by syringe, pen, or pump.

Regimen and Dose Determinations

For all patients with newly diagnosed diabetes, a basal/bolus regimen, consisting of a long-acting insulin plus rapid-acting insulin before meals, is recommended. Some patients are started on insulin pump therapy very soon after diagnosis.

Infants and Toddlers

Because of their need for frequent food intake, infants and toddlers may require frequent small injections. The small insulin needs of infants and toddlers may require diluted insulin to allow for more precise dosing and measurement of insulin in less than 1-unit increments. Diluents are available for specific types of insulin from the insulin manufacturers. Insulin can be diluted either at a pharmacy or at home, once parents are trained. Insulin pump therapy is another option since most pumps can infuse insulin in very small increments.

Children/Adolescents

In situations where a midday dose of insulin is impractical or impossible, an intermediate-acting insulin (NPH) can be used to cover food intake during the day.

Children's insulin requirements are based on body weight, age, and pubertal status. Children with newly diagnosed type 1 diabetes usually require an initial total daily dose of 0.5 to 1.0 units per kilogram. Younger and prepubertal children usually require lower doses, while the presence of ketoacidosis, use of steroids, and onset of puberty all dictate the need for higher doses.

Adults

Adults, on average, require 0.5 to 1 unit per kilogram per day.[1]

Decreased Insulin Needs During Honeymoon Period

Once blood glucose levels are normalized and endogenous insulin production increases during the first few weeks after diagnosis, most individuals with type 1 diabetes enter a honeymoon, or remission, period. During the honeymoon phase, insulin requirements will be less (0.2 to 0.6 units per kilogram of body weight per day) compared with the initial diagnosis of diabetes.[1] The duration of the honeymoon period varies, but it typically lasts between 3 and 12 months. Parents and patients need to be prepared for this period of decreasing insulin needs and minimal fluctuation in blood glucose values so they do not question the diagnosis of diabetes. Beta cell destruction continues during the honeymoon period. The end of this remission period is characterized by the following:

◆ Increased variability of blood glucose levels
◆ Increased insulin requirements
◆ Greater need to attend to diabetes management

Some patients who have had a prolonged and significant honeymoon period have described the end of this period as "getting diabetes all over again."

Increased Insulin Needs With Growth and Puberty

Insulin requirements increase with growth, and particularly during puberty. Insulin requirements during puberty may increase to as much as 1.5 units per kilogram per day due to the hormonal influences of increased growth hormone and sex hormone secretion. Insulin therapy regimens must be based on the individual needs of the child, adolescent, adult, and family, including meal, school, and work schedules, supervisory issues, and glycemic patterns.

Metabolic Control

The DCCT demonstrated that individuals on basal/bolus insulin therapy with MDI or a continuous subcutaneous insulin infusion (pump therapy) achieved better metabolic control compared with those on twice-daily insulin dosing.[4]

Regimen Flexibility

A basal/bolus insulin regimen uses a long-acting insulin analog (most often given at bedtime, although it can be given at other times) combined with a rapid-acting insulin analog given before meals and snacks. Using an insulin-to-carbohydrate ratio in determining the rapid-acting insulin dose before meals and snacks allows flexibility for the timing and amount of food consumed. Other factors involved in determining the dose are the current blood glucose level and the anticipated level of physical activity in the coming hours.

To prevent postprandial hyperglycemia, the premeal rapid-acting insulin analog should be given 10 to 20 minutes before the meal when the premeal blood glucose is at or above the target range. The higher the blood glucose, the further before the meal the insulin should be given so that it begins to lower the blood glucose before the meal is ingested. If the blood glucose is greater than 300 mg/dL (16.6 mmol/L), it may be necessary to give the insulin even more than 20 minutes before the meal. If premeal blood glucose is below target range, food may need to be consumed before insulin is administered.[25,26] This regimen must be individualized and may also need to be specific for meals. One of the most difficult times to control postprandial glucose is after the morning meal.

For children, whose intake is unpredictable, giving the insulin immediately after the meal,[27] so that actual food intake and insulin are matched more closely, may be efficacious in minimizing the potential for hypoglycemia. However, postprandial glucose control will not be as good when insulin is given after the meal.

The multiple snacks consumed by some children and adolescents may translate into multiple injections (5 or more) if the basal/bolus plan is strictly followed. The number of insulin injections may be a barrier to good control using an MDI regimen with carbohydrate counting, even though it allows flexibility of eating times and amounts. Omission of injections may increase when the regimen becomes too difficult. Some patients and families may consider insulin infusion therapy when injections are required too frequently.

Premixed Insulins

Commercially prepared, premixed insulins do not allow for the flexibility of daily dosage adjustment based on

---

Case—Part 4: Insulin Infusion Therapy to Improve Glycemic Control

When JJ was 14 years old, he was using MDIs, and his A1C was in the 8% to 9% range. He had 1 severe nocturnal hypoglycemic episode and was experiencing fairly frequent mild to moderate hypoglycemic episodes, often related to his competitive ski racing. JJ and his parents decided to pursue pump therapy (continuous subcutaneous insulin infusion).

Insulin pump therapy should be a joint decision by the patient, family, and diabetes management team. It requires more in-depth self-management education and performance of self-care behaviors. JJ and his family received extensive DSME, including adequate nutrition for his activity, the need for more frequent blood glucose monitoring, problem solving, calculating insulin dosages, and mechanics of the insulin pump. JJ had to demonstrate his ability to operate the pump and manage his diabetes safely and appropriately. With help from the diabetes management team, JJ learned to adjust his pump for his skiing and reduced the number of hypoglycemic episodes. JJ and his parents also discussed the use of pump therapy with JJ's ski coach.

---

blood glucose values and exercise levels, which are especially variable in children, and therefore may not be appropriate for people with type 1 diabetes. However, these insulins may be useful for those who are unable or unwilling to regularly adjust insulin doses.

Continuous Subcutaneous Insulin Infusion

Continuous subcutaneous insulin infusion (CSII) has been demonstrated to improve control, decrease fluctuations in blood glucose, decrease the risk of severe hypoglycemia, and allow more flexibility in food intake. These advantages make CSII a safe, effective, and appealing option for children and adults with type 1 diabetes. Results from several studies indicate that CSII is safe and effective in the pediatric population.[28-33] Some pump issues are unique to children, including use at school or camp and adjustments for sports.

Use at School, Day Care, or Camp

One issue with CSII is management of the pump in the school setting, at day care, or at camp. The child may need help counting carbohydrates, correctly bolusing, and troubleshooting the pump (eg, what to do for air bubbles, alarms, dislodgement of insulin infusion sets). Either the school nurse or other school or camp staff will require training to perform these tasks for or with the child. Camp counselors, camp nurses, and day care staff should be familiar with the mechanics of the insulin pump and know how to problem solve and who to contact if there is a problem with the pump.

Adjusting for Sports

Managing insulin infusion therapy during sports requires some special adjustments. For sports that require the pump to be disconnected (swimming, soccer, football, basketball, and hockey), the individual and his or her parents usually learn by trial and error how to adjust for the missed basal. If history proves that the blood glucose is above target after an activity, a starting place is to give one half of the missed basal prior to disconnecting. It is best if the pump is disconnected for no longer than 2 hours. If the pump must be disconnected for longer periods (eg, a day of water sports), it is possible to simultaneously use an insulin pump and a long-acting insulin analog by injection.[34] Frequent blood glucose monitoring is essential so that the individual can learn what adjustments work. For sports that do not require the pump to be disconnected, temporary basal rates and decreasing boluses usually work well.

Glycemic Control

Unfortunately, even with CSII, approximately 30% of subjects remain in suboptimal glycemic control.[32] In other words, nearly 1 in 3 pump users falls short of glycemic goals. The primary reasons for suboptimal glycemic control in children and adults using CSII are missed meal boluses and inadequate checking of blood glucose, resulting in blood glucose levels not being corrected.

Studies show that for every 4 to 5 missed meal boluses per week, the A1C increases by 1%.[4,35] The use of meal bolus alarms may be helpful, and in children an effective partnership between the child and the parent is essential. Adult supervision is often required while the child is away from parents. Children in preschool or day care need an adult to supervise pump programming; school-aged children, and in some instances adolescents, may require supervision as well.

Healthy Eating

Eating is usually one of the biggest concerns for all individuals with new-onset diabetes. Old wives' tales have instilled a fear in some people with diabetes that they will never again eat sweets or other foods they like. An important role of the educator is to help the patient and the patient's family understand how to incorporate foods the patient likes into a healthful food plan. The clinical goals of medical nutrition therapy (MNT) are the same for all individuals with type 1 diabetes, with the addition of maintenance of normal growth and development for children and adolescents.[36,37]

Medical Nutrition Therapy

All individuals with type 1 diabetes should receive individualized MNT as needed to achieve treatment goals. Nutrition recommendations are based on a nutritional assessment. This assessment involves evaluating parameters such as age, weight, height, growth percentiles on a growth chart for children and adolescents, body mass index (BMI), gender, recommended daily allowances (RDAs) for caloric range, schedules, treatment modalities, and blood glucose patterns for each individual.

Calorie Consumption and Normal Growth in Children

Children need sufficient calories for growth and pubertal development without excessive hypoglycemic episodes. The child's height and weight should be plotted on a growth chart at each visit to determine trends. If the child's growth patterns are appropriate for his or her age, then the child's meal plan includes calories adequate for growth and development. Children and teens who are of normal weight do not need to focus on weight-control issues, other than to follow prudent recommendations important for the general population. For children and adults who are above an ideal weight range, encouraging alterations in food selection and physical activity levels can help decrease possible insulin resistance and improve metabolic status.[36]

Meal Plans and Insulin Regimen

Meal plans must be individualized to match food preferences, cultural influences, family eating patterns and schedules, age, weight, activity level, and insulin action peaks. Insulin therapy can be integrated into usual eating and exercise habits. Therefore, it is important to determine the meal plan before determining an insulin regimen. The individual's appetite should be considered when determining the total caloric level provided in the meal plan.[24] Young children require smaller portions of food and need to eat more frequently than adults. Infants and toddlers have changing and unpredictable eating patterns.

Most children and adults newly diagnosed with type 1 diabetes have experienced some weight loss that will be restored with insulin initiation, hydration, and adequate energy intake. Once their weight is restored to normalcy, their appetite and caloric intake will decrease significantly.

When the patient recovers from the acute onset of diabetes and his or her appetite decreases, the insulin dose must be decreased to avoid hypoglycemia. The patient and/or family should be forewarned that this may occur and must be alerted to watch for this.

Adolescents, especially girls, are often pleased with the weight loss they incur as diabetes develops and do not want to regain the weight. As appropriate, these teens should be given guidance to help them minimize their weight gain.

Using an insulin-to-carbohydrate ratio for determining the premeal insulin dose allows for more flexibility in food intake, whereas food intake will need to be more consistent for individuals on fixed insulin regimens. In children, withholding food can feel punitive to the child and eventually promote reluctance to honestly report extra food or high glucose values. This can also result in inadequate caloric intake for growth. Forcing children to eat when they are not hungry or when they are no longer hungry should also be avoided.[24]

Carbohydrate-counting principles are the same for children and adults. Carbohydrate counting can allow greater flexibility and alternatives in meal planning in MDI and CSII (see chapter 16, on nutrition therapy, for more detail). Children under the age of 6 typically want 3 meals per day plus 3 snacks. Most children over the age of 6 want 3 meals per day plus midafternoon and bedtime snacks.[21] Additional carbohydrate intake is often needed before physical activity to decrease the risk of a hypoglycemic episode during or after exercise.

Chapters 4 and 16, on self-management behavior related to healthy eating and nutrition therapy, respectively, provide more information.

Being Active

Physical activity has many benefits, but in type 1 diabetes increased attention must be given to age, consistency, insulin dosing, and changes in blood glucose levels. Increased frequency in checking blood glucose is a requirement, as is education on how to respond before, during, and after the period of physical activity.

Adjusting for Activity Levels

The activity level of the very young child is unpredictable and in general cannot be planned for or controlled. That is one of the many challenges of managing diabetes in infants and children. Individuals of all ages with diabetes need to make adjustments in their diabetes regimen for changes in activity levels.

Benefits of Physical Activity

Intervention strategies that promote lifelong physical activity should be encouraged for all individuals with diabetes because of the health-promoting benefits of a regular exercise program. The benefits of exercise in type 1 diabetes are detailed in an ADA technical review[38] and include the following[38,39]:

- Lower plasma glucose levels
- Greater sense of well-being
- Weight management
- Improved physical fitness
- Improved cardiovascular fitness with lower pulse and blood pressure
- Improved lipid profile

These advantages apply to children as well as adults. All individuals with type 1 diabetes should adhere to the recommendation of the Centers for Disease Control and Prevention (CDC) and the American Academy of Sports Medicine[6]:

- *Recommendation:* At least 30 to 60 minutes of moderate physical activity daily

Hypoglycemia Prevention

More frequent blood glucose monitoring (before, during, and after exercise) may be necessary to avoid hypoglycemia during or after exercise. The decision of whether to adjust food or insulin is determined by the individual's diabetes management goals and is further affected by whether the exercise was planned. When exercise is planned sufficiently in advance, the preference is to adjust the insulin acting during the period of physical activity to minimize hypoglycemia risk.[40] If exercise is not planned far enough ahead to modify the relevant insulin dose, a carbohydrate snack should be consumed. Planning or predicting physical activity in very young children is especially difficult. For school-aged children and adolescents, the intensity and duration of a sports practice, physical education period, or sports game may vary greatly from day to day, so adjusting insulin may be difficult for them as well. With the increasing prevalence of obesity in all age groups, exercise is often important for weight management, and if additional food is consumed to cover increases in activity, the benefits of exercise for weight management are lost.

Depending on the glucose value at the start of exercise and the intensity and duration of the activity, carbohydrate intake may be necessary before, during, and/or after exercise.[40] Recommendations must be individualized, but a general guideline is to consume 10 to 20 g of carbohydrate for every 30 minutes of moderate activity.

In the pediatric population, 10% to 20% of hypoglycemic episodes are associated with exercise that is of greater-than-usual intensity, duration, or frequency. Increased hepatic glucose output in association with vigorous exercise secondary to both beta- and alpha-adrenergic stimulation may cause hyperglycemia during and immediately after exercise. Hypoglycemia may follow within 1 to 16 hours of completion of exercise due to glucose transport into skeletal muscle tissue and hepatic glycogen depletion.[41] School-aged children and adolescents are frequently involved in different sports at various times of the year, all requiring different adjustments in their diabetes regimen. Their activities are often during the late afternoon and evening, and the delayed hypoglycemia that can occur is likely to occur during the night if appropriate adjustments are not made in insulin or carbohydrate intake. Blood glucose monitoring at bedtime is crucial.

In a study examining the effect of exercise on overnight hypoglycemia in children with diabetes, 36% of the 50 study participants experienced nocturnal hypoglycemia even when their blood glucose was greater than 130 mg/dL (7.2 mmol/L) at bedtime.[42]

Consuming an electrolyte-containing sports drink or other source of a readily absorbable carbohydrate may be helpful in preventing hypoglycemia both during and after exercise. Chapter 17 offers more information on encouraging fluid intake.

See chapters 5 and 17 for more information on physical activity and self-management behaviors related to being active.

Healthy Coping

When a family has a child with type 1 diabetes, developing effective stress management/coping skills and problem-solving skills is as important as insulin administration, nutrition therapy, monitoring, and exercise. Many parents equate having a newly diagnosed child with diabetes with leaving the hospital with their firstborn child. The parents can be overwhelmed with fears and the stress of learning new skills and having new responsibilities associated with having a child with diabetes. The stressful, changed situation may create tension among family members. The mother and the father may argue, and siblings may feel frightened and can become resentful as all the attention is directed toward the family member with diabetes. The potential for family dysfunction is great. The diabetes educator can be instrumental in assisting families dealing with these issues by initiating discussion about these feelings and suggesting referral for family counseling. Many diabetes teams include a social worker or psychologist to help families deal with these issues. Including the entire family in the diabetes education process helps support all family members and provides everyone the opportunity to participate in the care of the person with diabetes.

Peer group activities such as diabetes camp, support groups, and group clinic visits may be helpful for both parents and children in improving acceptance of diabetes, management skills, quality of life, and glycemic control. Stress management, problem-solving, and coping skills training delivered in small groups of youths has been shown to reduce diabetes-related stress, improve social interaction, increase glucose monitoring, and improve glycemic control.[43]

Psychosocial issues for the patient and the entire family change throughout the child's lifetime. The diabetes educator needs to understand normal developmental tasks at different developmental stages in order to identify and circumvent potential problems. Major developmental issues and their effect on diabetes in children and adolescents are summarized in Table 14.3.

Psychosocial Issues: Infants and Toddlers

Normal characteristics in the development of young children must be taken into account when diabetes management regimens are determined. Normal growth and development for infants and toddlers (from birth to age 3) progress rapidly and predictably. An understanding of normal developmental tasks of children is essential when developing the diabetes management plan.

One of the developmental tasks of infancy is to build a trusting relationship with caregivers. Parents often worry that "hurting" their child (finger pokes and injections) will hamper this bonding process. Parents should be encouraged to develop a matter-of-fact attitude for the management tasks with the provision of incentives, like hugs, positive verbal reinforcement, or reading a book immediately after the poke or injection. Infants become much more mobile when they begin crawling at around 9 months of age and walking at about 10 to 15 months of age. Their energy expenditure increases greatly once they become mobile; insulin dose adjustments or extra snacks may thus be necessary to prevent hypoglycemia.[24]

In infancy, feedings not only provide nutrition to maintain life and physiologic well-being but also build a relationship. A positive feeding interaction

TABLE 14.3   Major Developmental Issues and Their Effect on Diabetes in Children and Adolescents

Developmental Stage (Approximate Ages)	Normal Developmental Tasks	Type 1 Diabetes Management Priorities	Family Issues in Type 1 Diabetes Management
Infancy 0–12 months	Developing a trusting relationship/"bonding" with primary caregiver(s)	Preventing and treating hypoglycemia Avoiding extreme fluctuations in blood glucose levels	Coping with stress Sharing the "burden of care" to avoid parent burnout
Toddler 13–36 months	Developing a sense of mastery and autonomy	Preventing and treating hypoglycemia Avoiding extreme fluctuations in blood glucose levels due to irregular food intake	Establishing a schedule Managing the "picky eater" Setting limits and coping with toddler's lack of cooperation with regimen Sharing the burden of care
Preschooler and Early Elementary School Age 3–7 years	Developing initiative in activities and confidence in self	Preventing and treating hypoglycemia Managing unpredictable appetite and activity Positive reinforcement for cooperation with regimen Trusting other caregivers with diabetes management	Reassuring child that diabetes is no one's fault Educating other caregivers about diabetes management
Older Elementary School Age 8–11 years	Developing skills in athletic, cognitive, artistic, social areas Consolidating self-esteem with respect to the peer group	Making diabetes regimen flexible to allow for participation in school/peer activities Child learning short- and long-term benefits of optimal control	Maintaining parental involvement in insulin and blood glucose monitoring tasks while allowing for independent self-care for "special occasions" Continuing to educate school and other caregivers
Early Adolescence 12–15 years	Managing body changes Developing a strong sense of self-identity	Managing increased insulin requirements during puberty Diabetes management and blood glucose control become more difficult Weight and body image concerns	Renegotiating parents' and teen's roles in diabetes management to be acceptable to both Learning coping skills to enhance ability to self-manage Preventing and intervening with diabetes-related family conflict Monitoring for signs of depression, eating disorders, risky behaviors
Later Adolescence 16–19 years	Establishing a sense of identity after high school (decisions about location, social issues, work, education)	Begin discussion of transition to a new diabetes team Integrating diabetes into new lifestyle	Supporting the transition to independence Learning coping skills to enhance ability to self-manage Preventing and intervening with diabetes-related family conflict Monitoring for signs of depression, eating disorders, risky behaviors

Source: Copyright © 2005 American Diabetes Association. Modified with permission from the American Diabetes Association. J Silverstein, G Klingensmith, K Copeland, et al, "Care of children and adolescents with type 1 diabetes: a statement of the American Diabetes Association," *Diabetes Care* 28 (2005): 186-212.

American Association of Diabetes Educators©

between the infant and the caregiver fosters the ingestion of an appropriate amount of food. Infants usually nurse or eat predictably, but for breastfed infants it is difficult to know how much breast milk they are getting. A feeding pattern that imitates family mealtimes should evolve by the end of the first year of life to incorporate the infant into the family's normal meal schedule.[24]

Toddlers develop a sense of mastery and autonomy, and they begin to separate and individuate, testing their separateness by saying "no" and behaving in an oppositional manner. Most parents know this as the "terrible twos." Providing choices can give the toddler with diabetes some control, but the choices need to be framed in such a way that the child is not allowed to make important decisions.[24] For example, asking, "Which finger shall we use?" works better than asking, "Do you want to do your blood test now?" Some families have "cute" names for finger pokes and injections. Naming the meter and decorating it with stickers can take some of the fear out of the testing procedure. Injections should not be called "shots," because children may confuse this with the shot of a gun.

Appetite may become erratic in toddlers when rapid growth begins to subside. Food can become problematic for parents and caretakers. If a toddler will not eat, favorite foods or alternatives can be offered, but parents should avoid becoming short-order cooks for a demanding toddler.[24] A basal/bolus regimen, adjusting insulin for food intake, and giving insulin immediately after consumption of food may work best. Insulin infusion therapy is also an option in this age group. Normal activity in toddlers is sporadic and spontaneous, interspersed with sudden bursts of whole body movement. To prevent hypoglycemia, activity needs to be balanced with extra food or beverages such as milk or juice.[41]

Hypoglycemia is a constant fear for parents of infants and toddlers with diabetes. Parents must rely on frequent blood glucose monitoring to distinguish normal infant and toddler behaviors from symptoms of hypoglycemia. Infants and toddlers are often defiant, demanding, sleepy, or cranky as part of their normal development.[24] Temper tantrums cannot be ignored until hypoglycemia has been ruled out with a blood test.

Psychosocial Issues: Preschool Years

The preschool years are from ages 3 to 5. Physical growth slows after the toddler stage but is still relatively rapid. Development of fine motor skills continues, and cognitive language is rapid. Children engage in magical thinking: they believe that if they think or wish something, they can cause it to happen.[44] Separation-individuation continues as children learn to distinguish themselves as separate from their parents. Body integrity and confidence in their ability to accomplish tasks are important. Fear of intrusive procedures is characteristic of this age, and children may act out their anxieties when insulin injections and blood testing are done. The use of adhesive bandages is helpful to the preschool child and helps address concerns about body integrity.[24] Even though they often lack the fine motor skills, cognitive development, and impulse control to do diabetes management tasks independently, allowing preschoolers to do "bits and pieces" of procedures is important; examples include placing the meter and lancing device on the table or getting the syringe out of the box.

Preschoolers have difficulty understanding the need for insulin injections and blood tests, particularly if they are feeling well. Describing the need in terms of "keeping you healthy" fosters a positive outlook. Allowing the child to have some control by providing limited choices can be helpful,[24] for example, asking, "Do you want mashed potatoes or macaroni for dinner?" Preschoolers need positive reinforcement for cooperating with the regimen; this may include verbal praise and/or sticker charts. Diabetes management tasks should not be used as rewards or punishment.

Children establish a balance between their inner life and reality by continually exploring and testing through their play. Guided play, or play therapy, provides a forum and vehicle for children to express their concerns. Play therapy provides a mechanism for emotional release by helping the child learn to deal with these issues through creative expression. Giving a child a "safe" syringe, family and health professional dolls, a meter, and other diabetes supplies provides an opportunity for the child to play out personal life issues and concerns about having diabetes. A stuffed bear with colored patches for injections and finger pokes is useful for this and is available from the Juvenile Diabetes Research Foundation (JDRF). Forms of artwork also help young children express themselves.[24]

A preschool child's appetite may be erratic and is often unpredictable. Variability in eating is not considered harmful but, rather, normal from a developmental point of view. Children may eat only a few foods or may want the same item meal after meal; for example, children may want to eat only bananas and peanut butter for days at a time, and then they will switch to grilled cheese sandwiches and apples. These eating patterns typically last a few days or weeks. When treated casually, the behaviors are forgotten after a brief period. Increased appetites tend to precede growth spurts, and food intake is usually balanced over a period of weeks. This erratic eating makes glucose control difficult for this age group, and parents worry about hypoglycemia when their child will not eat. Parents can allow the child some control over eating by providing reasonable choices without allowing the child to control eating situations. By giving young children limited choices, parents may avoid a battle of wills.[24]

Many preschool-aged children are able to identify symptoms of hypoglycemia and can at least alert adults that they do not feel well. This is especially important since many children are in preschool or day care settings at this age. Undetected hypoglycemia is still a risk in the preschool years and is especially worrisome to parents when their child is in the care of others.

The responsibility of caring for a young child with diabetes and the fear of hypoglycemia are extremely stressful for families.[9] In 2-parent families, both parents should be involved in the day-to-day management of the child's diabetes. In single-parent families, the parent needs to identify others who can provide support and respite care. Healthcare providers can often assist parents in identifying support systems that can be helpful in easing the burden of care and avoiding parental burnout. Professional organizations such as the ADA and the JDRF and local organizations may be a source of support for families, not only those with young children but those with children of all ages.

Psychosocial Issues: School-Aged Children

A school-aged child (6-11 years old) is physically well coordinated, has a vivid fantasy life, speaks fluently, has a conscience, and is able to share and cooperate. The child has concrete reasoning and likes repetition, which is played out in sports, games, and skills. Although the school-aged child has an increasing need for independence, the power and protection of the parent are very important to the child's well-being. One of the greatest drives of school-aged children is to avoid failure. They acquire strategies to keep from feeling different from peers.[24]

One study showed that mild depression and anxiety are common immediately following the diagnosis of diabetes in the school-aged child.[45] This usually resolves by 6 months after diagnosis.

Anxiety and depression are concerns for school-aged children with diabetes. After the first 1 to 2 years, symptoms of depression increase; anxiety decreases for boys but increases for girls over the first 6 years after diagnosis.[45] The increase in depression may be associated with the end of the honeymoon period, when children come to realize that the disease will not go away and that it is more difficult to manage.[44] Support groups, individual counseling, or diabetes camps can be useful in assisting the child in resolving these feelings. Determining the child's individual coping skills, supporting adaptive strategies, and providing interventions should be initiated early and should be part of follow-up care.[24] Chapter 9 provides more information on depression and anxiety in the child with diabetes.

Parent and Child Roles in Diabetes Management

The parent's role in diabetes management is to perform diabetes care tasks while moving the child toward independence through supervision, encouragement, and support. At times, the child may be willing and able to perform blood glucose monitoring, prepare his or her own snacks, and administer insulin (and may do so with supervision). At other times, a parent will need to perform the test or administer insulin. Parent-child sharing of these responsibilities is essential during the school-age years and beyond.[24] Several studies have shown that a child's early and independent participation in the diabetes regimen was significantly associated with poorer control.[46,47] Parents of the school-aged child with diabetes may be more protective than other parents. Although this is understandable, this attitude can make it difficult for the child with diabetes to attain the same level of independence as a child of the same age without diabetes. Diabetes management planning for special events and activities is important to promote independence and minimize differences. By planning ahead, most children with diabetes can safely participate in all childhood activities.[24]

Monitoring, eating special snacks, taking injections, and fearing that peers will witness symptoms of hypoglycemia can alter diabetes self-care routines and ultimately affect self-esteem. Helping the child fit diabetes management into normal routines both at home and at school can minimize feelings of being different. For example, a snack break can be implemented for all children in the classroom. Children who want to check their glucose in the classroom should be able to do so. However, school policies vary, and not all schools allow blood glucose testing in the classroom. Some are concerned about other children coming into contact with another student's blood and the school's liability if the blood test result is not reported correctly. Children should carry a source of fast-acting carbohydrate with them at all times and need to be able to treat hypoglycemia in the classroom. An adult or other student should accompany the student with diabetes to the clinic if the student is not feeling well.

Blood glucose values are often seen as "good" or "bad," and a child's level of control can also affect self-esteem. Because of their desire to please adults and their fear of failure, school-aged children sometimes falsify blood glucose results or report results when tests were omitted. When a child's A1C result is incompatible with the day-to-day glucose testing results, there is a high level of suspicion that this is occurring.

Care in School Settings

Because school-aged children spend a large portion of their day in school, expecting school personnel to become informed about diabetes care is reasonable. The school can either present significant challenges or be a source of support to the child with diabetes.[6] This topic is well covered in the ADA's position statement on diabetes care in the school and day care setting[48] and in another publication, Helping the Student With Diabetes Succeed: A Guide for School Personnel, by the National Diabetes Education Program, which is available on the Internet (http://ndep.nih.gov/diabetes/pubs/catalog.htm). School districts and personnel are obligated to provide an individualized plan to accommodate a child's special healthcare needs. Certain federal laws address these issues. The Education for All Handicapped Act of 1975, commonly referred to as Public Law No. 94-142, is a federal mandate that entitles all physically, developmentally, emotionally, and other health-impaired children to free, appropriate public education.[49] Any school that receives federal funding or a facility that is considered open to the public must reasonably accommodate the special needs of children with diabetes.[48] The other law, Section 504, is a more general civil rights law that makes it illegal for any agency or organization that receives federal funds to discriminate in any way against qualified people with disabilities.[50] See the sidebar summarizing key points on facilitating appropriate diabetes care in school settings.

The current standards for diabetes management reflect the need to maintain glucose control as near to normal as safely possible. To achieve this level of control, many children will be on intensified management. Intensified therapy requires the following: (1) 1 to 3 blood glucose checks during the school day, (2) insulin administration by injection or infusion pump, (3) attention to food intake and carbohydrate content of foods, and (4) knowledgeable school staff to observe for and treat hypoglycemia. This requires flexibility and close communication among the child, parents, school personnel, and the healthcare team.[48]

Each school year should begin with a conference involving the child with diabetes, his or her parents, and school personnel to establish a plan of care, communication, and a means of addressing important issues and concerns.

Key Points on Arranging Diabetes Care in School Settings

Information from parent. Parents need to provide the school with basic information about diabetes, the causes of hypoglycemia, the specific requirements of their child's daily management plan, and their child's usual signs and symptoms of hypoglycemia and hyperglycemia.

Plan of care. The information provided by the parents is used to develop a plan of care that satisfies the needs of the child, the child's parents, and school policies.[24] This written plan includes who will administer the care, the location of the supplies, and where the treatment will take place in the school setting.

Glucagon administration. The administration of glucagon must be provided if recommended by the student's healthcare provider.[48] When an order is issued by the healthcare provider, the school must designate a person to administer glucagon in the written plan of care.

Scheduling changes. When scheduling changes occur in the daily school routine (eg, field trips or parties), the school needs to notify parents prior to the event so appropriate care can be administered or arranged. However, parents cannot be required to attend all field trips.

Meal plan. A review of the food/meal plan basics provides school personnel with a general awareness of what the child eats. Providing a plan to enable the child to manage parties and snacks in school is also beneficial.[45] Some instruction on carbohydrate counting will be necessary if the student is using an insulin-to-carbohydrate ratio for calculating the insulin dose for lunch and snacks.

Psychosocial Issues: Adolescence

There are many differences in behavior and development between early, middle, and late adolescence, the time between 12 and 21 years of age. Characteristics of each of these 3 stages are outlined in Table 14.4.

Adolescence is a period of rapid biological change and increasing physical, cognitive, and emotional maturity. These changes may occur slowly or rapidly

TABLE 14.4   Developmental Characteristics at Each Stage of Adolescence
Early adolescence, 11–13 years old:
The child becomes acutely aware of body image
Dependent versus independent struggles begin between parent and child
There may be great vacillation between childlike and adult behaviors
There is less social involvement with family and more with peers
Parental criticism becomes difficult to accept
Turmoil and conflict within the parent-child relationship may begin
Middle adolescence, 14–18 years old:
Peer group allegiance develops
Greater experimentation and risk taking occurs
Physical and social activity increases
Opposite sex relationships emerge and are important
Formal operational thinking begins along with abstract reasoning
Late adolescence, 19–21 years old:
Teens and parents experience conflict in their relationship
Cognitive abilities and abstract morals develop
The peer group loses its primary importance
There is increasing separation from the family unit
Teens become future oriented
Conscience can stand without support or validity from others

Source: M Grey, ME Cameron, TH Lipman, et al, "Psychosocial status of children with diabetes in the first 2 years after diagnosis," *Diabetes Care* 18 (1995): 1330-6.

and are determined by genetic factors, the economy, nutrition, health, and habitat.

Identity and self-image concerns can revolve around diabetes concerns such as the appearance of the injection site or self-identification as "a diabetic." Normal independence issues may be thwarted as a result of parental protectiveness or the teen's failure to assume responsibility for self-care. Adolescents with diabetes can become particularly concerned about their physical growth and sexual maturation even though they usually display normal growth patterns and normal onset and progression of pubertal development.

Metabolic control tends to deteriorate in adolescence.[45] Attitudes of experimentation and rebellion and risk-taking behaviors normally associated with adolescence can affect diabetes issues such as taking insulin regularly, monitoring, and the quality and quantity of food consumption.

Risky Behaviors

Healthcare providers must be aware of and address issues of substance abuse (tobacco, alcohol, and drug use), use of steroids or other supplements to enhance muscle growth, and sexual practices and attitudes in their assessment of adolescent diabetes management. Risk taking and lack of health-promoting behaviors are widespread.[45] Alcohol use can result in severe hypoglycemia several hours after drinking if adequate food is not ingested. Some individuals may need to lower their basal insulin through the night. Alcohol can also affect judgment and impair an individual's ability to recognize and adequately treat the symptoms of hypoglycemia.

Eating Habits

Food intake becomes less consistent due to issues such as participation in athletics, busier schedules, preoccupation with body weight and/or appearance, and the search for self-identity. Proper eating habits are still important to ensure continued growth and development and to develop good practices over the lifetime. Adolescents give low priority to their nutritional needs regarding recommended amounts and types of food. Typical food-related behaviors include skipping meals, eating away from home, experimenting with fad diets, and attempting to change their weight.[45] Educating adolescents, especially boys, about the effect of poor metabolic control on growth can sometimes be a motivating factor for improving control.

Issues Involving Reproductive Health

Issues of sexuality, sexual functioning, and reproductive health should be addressed with teens and young adults, as well as adults, in a relaxed, comfortable manner. Reproductive health must be discussed in those of childbearing age. Comfort in discussing sexual topics comes with practice and a sense of control over the subject matter. The comfort level of the healthcare provider is communicated to the patient and sets the tone for discussions. Sex education should begin in the preteen years so that it becomes a routine part of diabetes assessment and education. Use of unbiased,

gender-neutral language is important when assessing sexual orientation, practice, frequency, use of contraceptives, and consistency of contraceptive practices.[45]

Females with diabetes must be taught the importance of planning pregnancy and meticulously using contraception to avoid an unwanted pregnancy. Their instruction should include a frank dialogue about the potential fetal/maternal health risks of an unplanned pregnancy in a woman with diabetes.[24] (See chapter 24, on pregnancy.)

Females may experience vaginal candidiasis, especially if metabolic control is less than optimal. Males may have concerns about sexual dysfunction, since this is a fairly common complication in adults with diabetes. Discussing this with them can sometimes be a motivating factor to strive for good control. Teens should be reminded that abstinence is the only 100% effective contraceptive method for preventing pregnancy, sexually transmitted diseases (STDs), and acquired immune deficiency syndrome (AIDS). They need to be taught that use of a condom during sexual activity will help prevent STDs and AIDS, but it is not the most effective method of preventing pregnancy.[24] Table 24.6, in chapter 24, summarizes the efficacy and safety of female contraceptive methods for those with diabetes.

Conditions Associated With Poor Glycemic Control and/or Health Outcomes[24]

- Biologically, the adolescent's heightened insulin resistance combined with earlier and greater epinephrine responses to drops in blood glucose concentrations may contribute to some of the lability in metabolic control.
- Adolescent rebellion/experimentation, a chaotic home environment, chronic family stress, parent-child conflicts, and parental over- or underinvolvement can contribute to poor metabolic control for children and adolescents. While adolescents can perform the tasks necessary for diabetes management, they may not always follow the treatment regimen and may still need help making decisions about insulin dose adjustments. Adolescents whose parents maintain some guidance and supervision in the management of diabetes have better metabolic control.[43,47]

- Developmental delays or learning disabilities in either the adolescent child or a parent may hamper understanding of diabetes care and thus self-management.
- Emotional disturbance can cause disequilibrium and precipitate frequent episodes of DKA. Insulin insufficiency may occur by insulin omission or in response to physical or emotional stress, resulting in overproduction of counterregulatory hormones.[43] Repeated episodes of DKA warrant investigation, as DKA can be deliberately induced to displace family tensions. Family patterns of interaction may reveal family enmeshment, rigidity, poor communication, and overprotectiveness.[49] Treatment may include family counseling and aggressive insulin therapy when illness, stress, or ketones appear. Adolescents sometimes develop DKA because they fail to take their insulin. Insulin doses can be missed when parents are not involved in an adolescent's diabetes management.[49,51]
- Adolescents and adults may decide to skip injections for the purpose of weight control, which is a variant of an eating disorder. This most often occurs in females but can also occur in males. Diabetes and the treatment regimen may provide the right conditions for those who are at risk of developing an eating disorder because of the focus on food and discipline required. Healthcare providers need to be aware of the possibility of pathologic eating behaviors, particularly among adolescent and young adult females.
- Needle anxiety occurs in almost everyone to some degree. If this anxiety is severe or persistent and left unresolved, diabetes control may suffer because of missed injections, inadequate testing, and avoidance of healthcare follow-up visits. When a parent has needle fears, the child will most likely have the same fears. Any patient who has a persistently high A1C should be evaluated for needle phobias. Desensitization therapy, biofeedback, assistance with relaxation, distraction, and use of an automatic injector (Inject-Ease® or similar device) have proven helpful.[52]

Case—Part 5: Acute Complications: Hypoglycemia and DKA

JJ was never hospitalized again in DKA. He did, however, experience 1 nocturnal hypoglycemic seizure, at the age of 13 years, after a very active day of skiing.

Driver Safety

Driving is a serious adult responsibility that can be given as a privilege to teens. The use of appropriate self-care skills and safety precautions must be taught and reinforced in teens and adults who drive themselves to school or work or otherwise operate a motorized vehicle. Healthcare professionals and parents of teens who are approaching legal driving age should begin discussions with the teen about the responsibility of safety when driving. Students heading off to college with a car should be frequently reminded to drive responsibly and take the self-care steps necessary to ensure safety of the driver, passengers, and those on the road. Guidelines for safety while driving are summarized in Table 14.5.

TABLE 14.5   Safe Driving for Persons With Diabetes
Issues to Discuss:
Practicing responsible diabetes self-care
Considering the safety of self and others
Monitoring blood glucose levels before driving
Stopping to check blood glucose at 2-hour intervals while driving
Carrying appropriate supplies, including fast-acting carbohydrates
Wearing a medical ID
Never driving with signs or symptoms of hypoglycemia

Source: JB Roemer, T McGee, "Type 1 diabetes in youth," in MJ Franz, ed, *A Core Curriculum for Diabetes Education: Diabetes Management Therapies,* 5th ed (Chicago: American Association of Diabetes Educators, 2003), 36-7.

Hypoglycemia

The fear of hypoglycemia is one of the major barriers to achieving optimal glycemic control for all individuals with diabetes, and it is one of the biggest fears for parents of children with diabetes. The definition of hypoglycemia is typically recognized as a blood glucose level less than 70 mg/dL (3.86 mmol/L) but studies have shown cognitive impairment at blood glucose concentrations of less than 60 mg/dL (3.3 mmol/L).[53] Mental function is reduced somewhat during the acute phase of hypoglycemia, and sometimes this persists beyond the acute phase. Hypoglycemia that interferes with normal thinking can make schoolwork difficult. It also makes riding a bicycle, driving a car, or operating machinery dangerous. While diabetes itself is not associated with cognitive deficits, some investigations have found an increase in cognitive dysfunction in individuals who have experienced repeated or prolonged episodes or severe hypoglycemia before the age of 5 years.[54-56] Glycemic goals are higher for children under 5 years of age because of the deleterious effects of hypoglycemia in this age group.

Hypoglycemia is more frequent in individuals with lower A1C levels, a prior history of severe hypoglycemia, or higher insulin doses and in younger children.[57] Frequent hypoglycemia, even if it is mild, can cause hunger and overeating, thus contributing to excessive weight gain and subsequent hyperglycemia. Repeated episodes of hypoglycemia or long diabetes duration may result in abnormality of the counterregulatory system and loss of adrenergic symptoms, leading to hypoglycemia unawareness. Frequent blood glucose monitoring is necessary to avoid recurrent episodes.

Hypoglycemia can be categorized according to severity. The precise blood glucose level at which patients develop symptoms or the level at which they experience a mild, moderate, or severe hypoglycemic episode is difficult to define. Symptoms generally occur when the blood glucose is less than 60 mg/dL (3.3 mmol/L).

Mild Hypoglycemia

Mild hypoglycemia is associated with mild adrenergic symptoms (sweating, pallor, palpitations, and tremors) and occasionally mild neuroglycopenic symptoms (headache and behavior change). Except in infants and toddlers, these can usually be self-treated with 10 to 15 g of easily absorbed carbohydrate, such as 3 to 4 glucose tablets or 4 oz of juice or regular soda. Additional intake of a more complex carbohydrate may be necessary, depending on timing for the next meal or snack. Treatment is individualized, and most individuals learn what and how much works best for them. Excessive intake should be avoided.

Moderate Hypoglycemia

Moderate hypoglycemia requires that someone else help with treatment, but the treatment can be administered orally. Typical symptoms are aggressiveness, drowsiness, and confusion. Usually, at least 15 to 30 g of an easily absorbed glucose in a gel form is required, with an additional snack to follow.

Severe Hypoglycemia

Severe hypoglycemia is associated with altered states of consciousness, including coma or seizure, and requires treatment with glucagon or intravenous glucose. Glucagon may be required when the patient cannot safely swallow, is combatant to efforts to intervene, or is unable to cooperate with treatment. Doses for infants and children are significantly different from those for adults. Table 14.6 lists recommended doses. Glucagon can be given intramuscularly or subcutaneously in the deltoid or anterior thigh region. Parents, roommates, spouses, and significant others should be taught how to mix, draw up, and administer glucagon.

Following a hypoglycemic episode, the plasma glucose threshold for autonomic activation is lowered, thus increasing the potential for further hypoglycemic events. Any severe episode of hypoglycemia should be reported to the healthcare provider so that changes in therapy can be made when indicated.

Also see the section on hypoglycemia in chapter 18, Pharmacotherapy for Glucose Management.

TABLE 14.6   **Recommended Doses for Glucagon**
Adults and children >20 kg:
1 mg subcutaneously (SQ) or intramuscularly (IM)*
Children <20 kg:
0.5 mg SQ or IM or 20–30 mcg per kilogram (9.1–13.6 mcg per pound) of body weight*

*If necessary, the dose may be repeated after 15 minutes.

Source: HP Chase, D Maahs, "Hypoglycemia," in *Understanding Diabetes,* 12th ed (Denver, Colo: Paros Press, 2011).

> **Case—Part 6: Associated Autoimmune Disorders**
>
> When he was 11 years old, JJ was diagnosed with hypothyroidism on a routine screening test. He denied symptoms (fatigue, dry skin, constipation), his physical exam did not reveal thyromegaly, and his linear growth was normal. He was started on thyroid replacement therapy. At age 13, he was diagnosed with celiac disease after 2 positive TG antibodies, which was confirmed by a gastroenterologist via a small-bowel biopsy. JJ also had no symptoms of celiac disease.
>
> The dietitian instructed JJ and his parents on a gluten-free diet. The diagnosis of another chronic illness can be difficult for patients and their families. The affected individual often feels that his or her entire body is failing. This may be especially difficult for adolescents, who are working to develop a strong sense of identity.

Diabetic Ketoacidosis

Diabetic ketoacidosis is a result of insulin deficiency leading to hyperglycemia, an accumulation of ketone bodies in the blood, dehydration, and subsequent metabolic acidosis. Diabetic ketoacidosis is potentially a life-threatening emergency and occurs in a variety of circumstances. Approximately 25% of children with new-onset diabetes present in ketoacidosis.[8] In the patient with known diabetes, the most common cause is omitted insulin injections or mismanagement of insulin infusion therapy. Diabetic ketoacidosis also results when inadequate dose adjustments are made for intercurrent illnesses, trauma, surgery, or other physiological stress. Recurrent episodes of DKA in the child or adolescent/adult are frequently due to insulin omission. These patients have a higher incidence of psychiatric illness, especially depression, and are more likely to omit insulin, come from single-parent homes, and be underinsured than their peers.[45]

Because of the significant morbidity and mortality associated with DKA, prevention is of paramount importance. Prevention can be achieved by the following:

- Public awareness of the signs and symptoms of untreated diabetes
- Education of friends, roommates, and other caregivers about the signs and symptoms of early DKA

- Increased recognition that insulin omission due to psychological problems and lack of financial resources is the most common cause of DKA in patients with established diabetes
- Improved detection of families at risk
- Education about ketone monitoring
- 24-hour telephone availability and encouragement to contact the healthcare team when blood glucose levels are high, when there is ketonuria or ketonemia, and especially during intercurrent illnesses[6]

Chapter 22 provides detailed information on hyperglycemia.

Associated Autoimmune Disorders

There are several autoimmune disorders associated with type 1 diabetes.

Thyroid Disorders

Thyroid disorders are the most common autoimmune disorder associated with type 1 diabetes, with an incidence of about 17%. Patients with thyroid autoimmunity may be euthyroid, hypothyroid (most common), or hyperthyroid.[58]

Individuals with type 1 diabetes should be screened for autoimmune thyroid disease shortly after diabetes diagnosis, when metabolic control has been established. Thyroid antibodies are measured to identify thyroid autoimmunity and patients at risk for developing thyroid disease. Measurement of thyroid-stimulating hormone (TSH) may be the most sensitive way to identify persons with thyroid dysfunction. Subclinical hypothyroidism has been associated with an increased risk of symptomatic hypoglycemia and with reduced linear growth. Patients with elevated TSH levels should be treated with thyroid replacement therapy. Patients with a normal TSH who have no thyromegaly or growth abnormality should be screened every 1 to 2 years.[6]

Celiac Disease

Celiac disease is an immune-mediated disorder that is also more common in individuals with type 1 diabetes, with a prevalence of 1% to 16%.[59] Individuals with type 1 diabetes should be screened for celiac disease by measuring tissue transglutaminase or antiendomysial antibodies, with documentation of normal serum IgA levels, soon after the diagnosis of diabetes. Testing should be repeated if growth failure, failure to gain weight, weight loss, or gastroenterolic symptoms occur. Consideration should be given to periodic rescreening of asymptomatic individuals.[7] In individuals with gluten intolerance, immune-mediated damage to the mucosa of the small intestine occurs after exposure to gluten, leading to destruction of the villi of the small intestine. Symptoms of celiac disease include diarrhea, constipation, weight loss or poor weight gain, growth failure, abdominal pain, chronic fatigue, irritability, an inability to concentrate, malnutrition due to malabsorption, and other gastrointestinal problems. In individuals with diabetes, the maldigestion and malabsorption of nutrients, vitamins, and minerals in the gastrointestinal tract may lead to unpredictable blood glucose levels, unexplained hypoglycemia, and deterioration in glycemic control. Although positive antibody test results can be supportive of a diagnosis, a small intestinal biopsy is the gold standard for the diagnosis of celiac disease.[60] Individuals with confirmed celiac disease should be provided guidance so they are able to follow a gluten-free diet to prevent unexpected hypoglycemia due to absorptive abnormalities and to prevent the other nutritional, metabolic, and oncologic consequences of celiac disease.[6]

There are no controlled trials to guide recommendations for asymptomatic individuals with elevated autoantibody levels and normal small-bowel biopsies.

Case—Part 7: Ongoing Care

JJ's most recent A1C was 6.9%. Over the years, he has had regular quarterly visits, and his parents have always been involved in his care. His most recent eye exam was normal, as were his urine microalbumin excretion tests. He is successfully using continuous insulin infusion therapy and has experienced infrequent hypoglycemia. He has been following a gluten-free diet. Since starting college, he has experienced some depression and has been taking an antidepressant.

Ongoing Care

Individuals with type 1 diabetes should see their diabetes healthcare provider every 3 months for evaluation of therapy and ongoing education. Studies suggest that delivery of intensive diabetes care management, telephone availability of the healthcare team, and regular in-person care improve A1C and decrease hospitalizations.[61-65] Knowledge and skills of the person with diabetes should be evaluated regularly by a diabetes educator. Frequency of hypoglycemia and the presence of hypoglycemia unawareness should be assessed at every visit. If hypoglycemia unawareness is present, blood glucose targets should be reassessed and continuous glucose monitoring may be an appropriate recommendation. For children, height and weight measurements are essential and should be plotted on growth charts at each visit. Poor diabetes control can lead to poor linear growth and poor weight gain, as well as a delay in pubertal and skeletal maturation. Poor growth with adequate metabolic control should raise suspicion of hypothyroidism or celiac disease.

Quarterly Follow-up With Healthcare Provider

Each quarterly follow-up visit with the healthcare provider should include the following:

- Height, weight, and BMI calculation (and comparison with age- and sex-specific norms)
- Blood pressure determination (and comparison with age-, sex-, and height-related norms)
- A1C determination
- Evaluation of results of blood glucose monitoring, ketone testing, and patient's use of data
- Physical examination with specific emphasis on injection or pump sites (lipoatrophy or lipohypertrophy) and finger or alternative sites for blood glucose testing; physical examination should also include funduscopic, oral, cardiac, abdominal (hepatosplenomegaly), hand/finger, foot, skin (acanthosis nigricans, necrobiosis lipoidica diabeticorum), and neurological examinations
- Interval history should include recent or current infections or illnesses; current or recent use of medications; frequency and treatment of hypoglycemia; presence of hypoglycemia

unawareness; physical activity and exercise habits; meal plan; psychosocial factors that may influence diabetes management; use of tobacco, alcohol, and/or recreational drugs; and contraception and sexual activity (if applicable)

- Review of symptoms should include gastrointestinal function (including symptoms of gluten intolerance) and symptoms of other endocrine disorders, especially thyroid and Addison disease
- Assessment of knowledge, skills, and coping level with referral to appropriate diabetes healthcare provider (diabetes nurse educator, dietitian, behavioral specialist) for intervention
- Assessment of emergency preparedness, including availability of glucagon to parents, roommates, and significant others knowledgeable about administering it; wearing of diabetes identification (wallet cards are not adequate); testing before driving, and the availability of a source of glucose in the car; for those living alone, identification of someone to check in if the individual fails to show for work or school

Yearly Assessments and Screenings

- Ophthalmologic evaluation: Starting at 10 years of age with diabetes duration of 3 to 5 years[6]
- Microalbuminuria: Starting at 10 years of age with diabetes duration of 5 years[6]
- Lipid profile: Starting at 2 years of age if positive or unknown family history for cardiovascular disease; starting at puberty if family history is negative
- Celiac and adrenal antibodies, TSH: Every 1 to 2 years (more frequently if symptomatic or poor growth)
- Depression screening: Starting at 10 years of age
- Diabetes nurse educator and dietitian: Yearly visit is the minimum; many individuals may benefit from this quarterly or even more frequently, especially during the first year of diagnosis
- Behavioral specialist: To enhance support and empowerment, to identify and discuss ways to overcome barriers in successful diabetes management, and, in pediatrics, to maintain family involvement in diabetes care tasks[6]

Vaccinations

Children and adults with type 1 diabetes should receive all immunizations in accordance with the recommendations of the CDC. This includes the annual influenza vaccine and a one-time pneumococcal polysaccharide vaccine to all individuals with diabetes over 2 years of age. A onetime revaccination is recommended for individuals over 64 years of age who were previously immunized when they were less than 65 years of age if the vaccine was administered more than 5 years ago.[7] Large studies have shown no causal relationship between childhood vaccination and type 1 diabetes.

Transition to Adult Care

The individual with diabetes, the family, the pediatric diabetes team, and the adult care providers should determine the appropriate time for the transition to adult care providers. Issues for adults with diabetes usually include college, marriage, family, employment and establishment of a career, and finances. Adult care providers may be more knowledgeable about dealing with these issues.

Primary Treatment Goals for All Individuals With Type 1 Diabetes

- To achieve optimal glycemic goals with a flexible, individualized diabetes management plan
- To avoid severe hypoglycemia, symptomatic hyperglycemia, and ketoacidosis
- To promote and maintain day-to-day clinical and psychological well-being[1]

Adults newly diagnosed with diabetes often employ a basal/bolus regimen, using a long-acting insulin plus a rapid-acting insulin before meals. Adults, on average, require between 0.4 and 1.0 units per kilogram per day.[1]

Type 1 Diabetes in Adults

Although type 1 diabetes is most frequently diagnosed in children, 30% to 50% of people are diagnosed over the age of 30, and the diagnosis can occur at any age. When diabetes is diagnosed in adults, differentiating type 1 diabetes from type 2 diabetes is sometimes more difficult. One way to identify the person with the autoimmune type of diabetes (type 1) versus the insulin-resistant form (type 2) is to look for the presence or absence of islet autoantibodies. Laboratory markers of immune destruction of the beta cell include islet cell autoantibodies, autoantibodies to insulin, and autoantibodies to glutamic acid decarboxylase (GAD$_{65}$). One and usually more of these autoantibodies are present in 85% to 90% of individuals when fasting hyperglycemia is initially detected.[66] See chapter 13, on pathophysiology, for a more in-depth discussion on latent autoimmune diabetes in adults (LADA).

The rate of beta cell destruction can be rapid in some adults (as it almost always is in infants and children) and slow in others. While some authors differentiate rapid-onset type 1 diabetes in adults from LADA,[67] most clinicians now recognize the term "LADA" to describe the adult form of type 1 diabetes. Adults with LADA have similar human leukocyte antigen (HLA) genetic susceptibility as well as autoantibodies to islet antigens. However, they may retain sufficient residual beta cell function so that treatment of their diabetes does not require insulin initially, and they appear to be clinically affected by type 2 diabetes. Adults with LADA usually require insulin for survival after about 6 years, and they are at risk for ketoacidosis at that time. At this latter stage of the disease, there is little or no insulin secretion, as manifested by low or undetectable levels of plasma C-peptide.[66]

Associated Autoimmune Disorders

Adults with type 1 diabetes are also prone to other autoimmune disorders, such as Graves disease, Hashimoto thyroiditis, Addison disease, vitiligo, celiac sprue, autoimmune hepatitis, myasthenia gravis, and pernicious anemia.[60] In one study, the proportion of patients testing negative for all autoantibodies was lower among the children than among the adults. The adults were characterized by a higher proportion of males, a longer duration of symptoms, and a lower frequency of infections during the preceding 3 months.[68]

Clinical Presentation

The clinical presentation of adults with rapid-onset type 1 diabetes and the initial management of their diabetes and treatment with insulin are similar to the presentation and management of children with new-onset diabetes, as discussed earlier in this chapter. The clinical presentation of the adult with LADA may include the following:

◆ Lean body mass
◆ Family history of type 1 diabetes or autoimmune disease
◆ Age 35 to 60 years

Diagnosis

In addition to the usual glucose diagnostic tests, the clinician may want to measure anti-GAD antibodies; if positive, this confirms the diagnosis of LADA. Subsequent measurement of C-peptide can delineate progression to insulin dependency. Attention should be paid to diagnose such individuals because therapy may influence the speed of progression toward insulin dependency, and in this respect, efforts should be made to protect residual C-peptide secretion.[69]

Treatment

No specific guidelines for management of LADA currently exist, but treatment to achieve normoglycemia to prevent complications is warranted. Most individuals with LADA become insulin dependent within 6 to 8 years, and many clinicians progress to insulin sooner rather than later, although in the initial stages, LADA can be managed with therapies used for type 2 diabetes.

Summary

Type 1 diabetes is not only a disease of the very young. It affects people throughout the life span and presents many challenges to both the person with diabetes and the family and friends of that person. The self-management behaviors and skill sets required to be successful and effective are very demanding, and this is in addition to the issues and stages that an individual goes through as he or she ages. It is important to not only make normal physical growth and development a goal for this population, but also address emotional growth and development. In addition, self-management depends on socioeconomic support as well as emotional and physical support. Wishing to participate in intensive management but not being able to afford the supplies needed may be one of many barriers the individual with type 1 diabetes and the family will face. More and more people with type 1 diabetes are reaching senior age and qualifying for Medicare and must learn to navigate the requirements for Medicare reimbursement. Seniors with type 1 diabetes face all the challenges of advancing age with the added complications of type 1 diabetes, such as labile glucose levels. Focusing only on blood glucose values and judging blood glucose numbers as "good" or "bad" will only lead to resentment and can affect self-esteem. The diabetes educator is a very important part of the diabetes care team and plays a crucial role in helping families cope with the many anticipated and unanticipated events and changes that occur.

Focus on Education

Teaching Strategies

- **Individualize self-management teaching plans and approaches.** There is no *one* right way to provide DSME in type 1 diabetes, whether working with children or adults. Focus on the "need to know" and "need to do" first. Build on practical and essential daily function needs to keep glucose levels within desirable ranges.

- **Focus on patient's needs and expectations.** Assess what is the most difficult daily diabetes management task. Explore reasonable solutions to the most challenging tasks so they come as routine. Evaluate the accomplishments in successful problem solving.

- **Provide age-appropriate clinical therapies and care.** Healthy growth, nutritional needs, and lifestyle trends need to be evaluated on an ongoing basis. Allow for a healthy relationship with food and diabetes self-care to develop.

- **Collaborate with family members to build needed assistance or support in care.** Whether it's a child, an adolescent, or an adult, each age group has a different support network. An infant, toddler, preschooler, older elementary child, early adolescent, or later adolescent is able to do different tasks at different stages. Parental involvement varies at different stages, and normal characteristics in the development of young children must be considered when determining needs and self-management strategies.

- **Respect that all persons have different desires, needs, and expectations.** Flexibility, creativity, and options for different learning styles and ages are needed—for example, use of games and puppets for small children; demonstrations and media-based materials (videos, handheld and electronic games) for teens and young adults; and models, problem-solving discussions, and demonstrations for adults.

- **Teach the person to become the "expert."** Coach children or adults to be the "expert" in their diabetes. Assist them in planning a topic-specific presentation in their school or support group (in a safe environment). Include family and friends. This teaching activity reinforces information and may help self-esteem.

Messages for Patients

- **Knowledge is power.** Learn as much as possible about taking care of diabetes. Attend classes offered through a local clinic or diabetes-affiliated organizations at every reasonable opportunity.

- **Change is inevitable.** Expect that at different stages of life and in different situations glucose control will change and require adjustments in how it is managed. The diabetes educator and care team will help with these unexpected or unanticipated events. Include your child with diabetes in care issues and teaching school personnel.

⊘ **Diabetes is often unpredictable.** Everything can be done "right," and still perfection is not achieved. Generally speaking, life is not perfect and often not predictable. The focus should not be on making life perfect and being in total control; rather, it needs to be more about how to cope with change and how to prioritize effectively. The same thing may be handled differently, under a different circumstance. Keep on strategizing and reevaluating the ability to handle things on an ongoing basis.

⊘ **Everyone needs support.** Use friends, family, and your medical team for support. Ask for help; ask for necessities to achieve short- and long-term goals. Use the diabetes educator and the health team as consultants. Diabetes care needs to be flexible, dynamic, and individualized. There are many different ways to achieve optimal control. If one method or plan does not work, try a different approach.

⊘ **Utilize peer-to-peer social support networks.** Sharing experiences with others can help both the patient and others. Other benefits may include learning effective and practical diabetes management strategies, validating assumptions, sharing successes, and getting others' perspectives on things. Everyone needs to be around peers and people who share similar interests.

⊘ **Embrace yourself and your diabetes.** Allow the challenges with diabetes to become opportunities. You can do what you desire in your life when managing diabetes. Remember that diabetes is manageable, and every day is a new day!

Health Literacy

⊘ **Health literacy in pediatrics, young adults, and adults with type 1 diabetes varies greatly as per multiple contributing factors.** It means that different age groups understand information about health, know how to perform daily self-care, and make good decisions differently based on their age.

⊘ **Everyone is at risk for low health literacy.** Be careful not to make assumptions about health literacy levels on the basis of an individual's age, race, ethnicity, education, or income.

⊘ **Regardless of health literacy level, there are 3 key things a person with diabetes should know.** Each individual should know where to get health information, understand the health information he or she finds, and apply the information to make good decisions about health.

⊘ **Assess your patient's attitude and belief system toward diabetes care.** The following questions will help patients explore their attitudes and focus on effective care:
- What is important to you about your diabetes?
- What would you like to be different about your diabetes?
- What is the most difficult thing for you about managing your diabetes on a daily basis?
- What can I do to help you accomplish your diabetes care goals?
- What are you going to do differently till I see you next time?
- How are you going to monitor your daily self-management?

⊘ **Effective communication with patients can minimize the challenge of health literacy:**
- Avoid miscommunication by finding the right words to say, as well as the right questions to ask
- Take the time to assess recall and comprehension in all patients
- Achieve true agreement with patients on goals and strategies to care for their diabetes
- Problem + Solution = Strategy
- Put a meaning to the numbers
- Use phrases to remember: simple, concrete, emotional
- Use real stories with real examples and demonstration/hands-on experience

Focus on Practice

⟳ **Type 1 diabetes affects all ages; consequently, management and education are ongoing processes throughout an individual's life span.** Healthcare professionals involved in care need to be specialized in clinical and age-appropriate behavioral therapies.

⟳ **Clinical management of type 1 diabetes relies on patient and family self-management.** Continuous reassessment of needs and the support network is part of ongoing DSME.

⟳ **The primary goals for type 1 diabetes management in children include glycemic control, avoidance of acute and chronic complications, positive psychosocial adjustment to diabetes, and normal growth and development.** The functionality of healthcare systems needs to provide access to the qualified healthcare team.

⟳ **Situational problem solving needs to be incorporated into all patient interactions.** Patients need to know how to handle daily glucose management emergencies and learn from each experience.

Proactive behaviors and attitudes need to be assessed on an ongoing basis.

⟳ **Type 1 diabetes self-management requires ongoing care with careful consideration of multiple factors such as the following: state of the disease, patient's age, survival skills, glucose management, insulin taking, healthy eating, carbohydrate counting, activity, sports, hypoglycemia, appetite changes, bedtime, school, parties, friends, peer pressure, glucagon, driving, anxiety, depression, DKA, short-term versus long-term metabolic control, thyroid disorders, celiac disease, ongoing care, screening, and vaccinations.** Diabetes educators are instrumental in helping patients maximize their potential in living a healthy and self-fulfilling life.

⟳ **Make a paradigm shift to the empowerment model of care by learning to ask questions instead of offering advice.** Time spent offering recommendations that are not relevant for patients or will never be implemented is time wasted.

References

1. American Diabetes Association. Clinical practice recommendations 2013. Diabetes Care. 2013;36 Suppl 1: S67.

2. DIAMOND Project Group. Incidence and trends in childhood type 1 diabetes worldwide 1990-1999. Diabet Med. 2006;34(8):857-66.

3. Libman IM, LaPorte RE. Changing trends in epidemiology of type 1 diabetes mellitus throughout the world: how far have we come and where do we go from here. Pediatr Diabetes. 2005;6:119-20.

4. Diabetes Control and Complications Trial Research Group. The effect of intensive treatment of diabetes on the development and progression of long-term complications in insulin-dependent diabetes mellitus: the Diabetes Control and Complications Trial Research Group. N Engl J Med. 1993;329:977-86.

5. The Epidemiology of Diabetes Interventions and Complications (EDIC) Study. Sustained effect of intensive treatment of type 1 diabetes mellitus on development and progression of diabetic nephropathy. JAMA. 2003;290: 2159-67.

6. Silverstein J, Klingensmith G, Copeland K, et al. Care of children and adolescents with type 1 diabetes. Diabetes Care. 2005;28:186-212.

7. American Diabetes Association. Clinical practice recommendations 2013. Diabetes Care. 2013;36 Suppl 1:S40-1.

8. Agus MS, Wolfsdorf JI. Diabetic ketoacidosis in children. Pediatr Clin North Am. 2005;52:1147-63.

9. Gonder-Frederick L, Nyer M, Shepard J, Vajda K, Clarke W. Assessing fear of hypoglycemia in children and their parents. Diabetes Manag (Lond). 2011;1(6):627-9.

10. Steck AK, Barrica KJ, Emery LM, Fiallo-Scharer RV, Gottlieb PA, Rewers MJ. Secondary attack rate of type 1 diabetes in Colorado families. Diabetes Care. 28;2: 296-300.

11. Boland E, Grey M. Coping strategies of school-age children with diabetes mellitus. Diabetes Educ. 1996;22: 592-7.

12. Drash A, Becker D. Behavioral issues in patients with diabetes mellitus with special emphasis on the child and adolescent. In: Rifkin H, Porte D Jr, eds. Ellenberg and Rifkin's Diabetes Mellitus Theory and Practice. 4th ed. New York: Elsevier Publishing; 1990:922-33.

13. Kostraba JN, Gay EC, Rewers M, et al. Increasing trend of outpatient management of children with newly diagnosed IDDM. Colorado IDDM Registry, 1978-1988. Diabetes Care. 1992;15:95-100.

14. Escobar O, Becker D, Drash A. Management of the child with diabetes. In: Lifshitz F, ed. Pediatric Endocrinology. 4th ed. New York: Marcel Dekker; 2004:653-67.

15. Mortensen HB, Hougaard P. Comparison of metabolic control in a cross-sectional study of 1,873 children and adolescents with IDDM from 18 countries. Diabetes Care. 1997;20:714-20.

16. Anderson B, Ho J, Brackett J, et al. Parental involvement in diabetes management tasks: relationships to blood glucose monitoring adherence and metabolic control in young adolescents with insulin-dependent diabetes mellitus. J Pediatr. 1997;130:257-65.

17. Helgeson V, Honcharuk E, Becker D, et al. A focus on blood glucose monitoring: relation to glycemic control. Pediatr Diabetes. 2011;12:25-30.

18. Miller KM, Beck RW, Bergenstal RM. Evidence of a strong association between frequency of self monitoring of blood glucose and hemoglobin A1C Levels in TID Exchange Clinic Registry Participants. Diabetes Care. 2013;36(7): 2009-24.

19. Greenhalgh S, Bradshaw S, Hall CM, et al. Forearm blood glucose testing in diabetes mellitus. Arch Dis Child. 2004; 89:516-8.

20. Fedele D, Corsi A, Noacco D, et al. Alternative site blood glucose testing: a multicenter study. Diabetes Technol Ther. 2003;5:983-9.

21. Rewers M, Pihoker C, Donaghue K, Hanas R, Swift P, Klingensmith GJ. Assessment and monitoring of glycemic control in children and adolescents with diabetes. Pediatr Diabetes. 2009;10 Suppl 12:71-81.

22. Valentine V. Continuous glucose monitoring has left the station: are you on board? Diabetes Educ. 2005;31:649-62.

23. Hanas R, Donaghue K, Klingensmith G, Swift PG. ISPAD clinical practice consensus guidelines 2009. Pediatr Diabetes. 2009;10 Suppl 12:1-2.

24. Roemer JB, McGee T. Type 1 diabetes in youth. In: Franz MJ, ed. A Core Curriculum for Diabetes Education: Diabetes Management Therapies. 5th ed. Chicago: American Association of Diabetes Educators; 2003:36-7.

25. Cobry BS, McFann K, Messer L, et al. Timing of meal insulin boluses to achieve optimal postprandial glycemic control in patients with type 1 diabetes. Diabetes Technol Ther. 2010;12:173-7.

26. Rassam A, Burge M, et al. Optimal administration of lispro insulin in hyperglycemic type 1 diabetes. Diabetes Care. 1999;22:133-6.

27. Rutledge KS, Chase HP, Klingensmith GJ, et al. Effectiveness of postprandial Humalog in toddlers with diabetes. Pediatrics. 1997;100:968-72.

28. Mack-Fogg JE, Orlowski CC, Jospe N. Continuous subcutaneous insulin infusion in toddlers and children with type 1 diabetes mellitus is safe and effective. Pediatr Diabetes. 2005;6:17-21.

29. Ahern JAH, Boland EA, Doane R, et al. Insulin pump therapy in pediatrics: a therapeutic alternative to safely lower HbA1c levels across all age groups. Pediatr Diabetes. 2002;3:10-5.

30. Fox LA, Buckloh LM, Smith SD, et al. A randomized controlled trial of insulin pump therapy in young children with type 1 diabetes. Diabetes Care. 2005;28:1277-81.

31. Wilson DM, Buckingham BA, Kunselman EL, et al. A two-center randomized controlled feasibility trial of insulin pump therapy in young children with diabetes. Diabetes Care. 2005;28:15-9.

32. Plotnick LP, Clark LM, Brancati FL, et al. Safety and effectiveness of insulin pump therapy in children and adolescents with type 1 diabetes. Diabetes Care. 2003;26:1142-6.

33. Maniatis AK, Klingensmith FJ, Slover RH, et al. Continuous subcutaneous insulin infusion therapy for children and adolescents: an option for routine diabetes care. Pediatrics. 2001;107:351-6.

34. Edelman S. The un-tethered regimen. Children With Diabetes. Last reviewed 2010 Jan 6 (cited 2012 May). On the Internet at: www.childrenwithdiabetes.com/clinic/untethered.htm.

35. Burdick JC, Chase HP, Slover RH, et al. Missed insulin meal boluses and elevated hemoglobin A1C levels in children receiving insulin pump therapy. Pediatrics. 2004;113: 221-4.

36. American Diabetes Association. Clinical practice recommendations 2013. Diabetes Care. 2013;36 Suppl 1.

37. Smart C, Aslander-van Vliet E, Waldron S. Nutritional management in children and adolescents with diabetes. Pediatr Diabetes. 2009;10 Suppl 12:100-117.

38. Wasserman DH, Zinman B. Exercise in individuals with IDDM. Diabetes Care. 1994;17(8):924-37.

39. Austin A, Warty V, Janosky J, et al. The relationship of physical fitness to lipid and lipoprotein levels in adolescents with IDDM. Diabetes Care. 1993;16:421-5.

40. American Diabetes Association. Intensive Diabetes Management. Alexandria, Va: American Diabetes Association; 2003.

41. Robertson K, Adolfsson P, Scheiner G. Exercise in children and adolescents with diabetes. Pediatr Diabetes. 2009;10 Suppl 12:154-68.

42. The Diabetes Research in Children Network (DirectNet) Study Group. Impact of exercise on overnight glycemic control in children with type 1 diabetes mellitus. J Pediatr. 2005;147:528-34.

43. Delamater AM. Psychological care of children and adolescents with diabetes. Pediatr Diabetes. 2009;10 Suppl 12:175-84.

44. Kovacs M, Iyengar S, Goldston D, et al. Psychological functioning of children with insulin-dependent diabetes: a longitudinal study. J Pediatr Psychol. 1990;15:619-32.

45. Grey M, Cameron ME, Lipman TH, et al. Psychosocial status of children with diabetes in the first 2 years after diagnosis. Diabetes Care. 1995;18:1330-6.

46. Fonagy P, Moran GS, Lindsay MK, et al. Psychological adjustment and diabetic control. Arch Dis Child. 1987;62:1009-13.

47. Follansbee DS. Assuming responsibility for diabetes management: what age? what price? Diabetes Educ. 1989;15:347-53.

48. American Diabetes Association. Clinical practice recommendations 2013. Diabetes Care. 2013;36 Suppl 1.

49. Mancuso E. Numbers That Add Up to Educational Rights for Children With Disabilities. Washington, DC: Children's Defense Fund; 1989.

50. Grey M, Boland EA, Yu C, et al. Personal and family factors associated with quality of life in adolescents with diabetes. Diabetes Care. 1998;21:909-14.

51. Rewers A, Chase HP, Mackenzie T, et al. Predictors of acute complications in children with type 1 diabetes. JAMA. 2002;287:2511-6.

52. Chase HP, Maahs D. Understanding Diabetes. 12th ed. Denver, Colo: Paros Press; 2011.

53. Ryan CM, Atchison J, Puczynski S, et al. Mild hypoglycemia associated with deterioration of mental efficiency in children with insulin-dependent diabetes mellitus. J Pediatr. 1990;117:32-8.

54. Northam EA, Anderson PJ, Werther FA, et al. Neuropsychological complications of IDDM in children 2 years after disease onset. Diabetes Care. 1998;21:379-84.

55. Rovet J, Alvarez M. Attentional functioning in children and adolescents with IDDM. Diabetes Care. 1997;20:803-10.

56. Bjorgaas M, Gimse R, Vik T, et al. Cognitive function in type 1 diabetic children with and without episodes of severe hypoglycemia. Acta Paediatr. 1997;86:148-53.

57. Davis EA, Keating B, Byrne GC, et al. Impact of improved glycaemic control on rates of hypoglycaemia in insulin dependent diabetes mellitus. Arch Dis Child. 1998;78:111-5.

58. Roldan MB, Alonso M, Barrio R. Thyroid autoimmunity in children and adolescents with type 1 diabetes mellitus. Diabetes Nutr Metab. 1999;12:27-31.

59. Holmes GK. Screening for celiac disease in type 1 diabetes. Arch Dis Child. 2002;87:495-8.

60. Green PH. Where are all those patients with celiac disease? Am J Gastroenterol. 2007;102:1461-3.

61. Beck JK, Logan KJ, Hamm RM, et al. Reimbursement for pediatric diabetes intensive case management: a model for chronic diseases? Pediatrics. 2004;113:e47-50.

62. Svoren BM, Butler D, Levine BS, et al. Reducing acute adverse outcomes in youths with type 1 diabetes: a randomized, controlled trial. Pediatrics. 2003;112:914-22.

63. Howells L, Wilson AC, Skinner TC, et al. A randomized control trial of the effect of negotiated telephone support on glycaemic control in young people with type 1 diabetes. Diabet Med. 2002;19:643-8.

64. Couper JJ, Taylor J, Fotheringham MJ, et al. Failure to maintain the benefits of home-based intervention in adolescents with poorly controlled type 1 diabetes. Diabetes Care. 1999;22:1933-7.

65. Mortensen HB, Tobertson KJ, Aanstoot HJ, et al. Insulin management and metabolic control of type 1 diabetes mellitus in childhood and adolescence in 18 countries. Hvidore Study Group on Childhood Diabetes. Diabet Med. 1987;15:752-9.

66. American Diabetes Association. Clinical practice recommendations 2010. Diabetes Care. 2010;33:S62-7.

67. Rosario PWS, Reis JS, Amim R, et al. Comparison of clinical and laboratory characteristics between adult-onset type 1 diabetes and latent autoimmune diabetes in adults. Diabetes Care. 2005;28:1803-4.

68. Sabbah E, Savola K, Ebeling T, et al. Genetic, autoimmune and clinical characteristics of childhood- and adult-onset type 1 diabetes. Diabetes Care. 2000;23:1326-32.

69. Pozzilli P, DiMario U. Autoimmune diabetes not requiring insulin at diagnosis (latent autoimmune diabetes of the adult). Diabetes Care. 2001;24:1460-7.

CHAPTER 15

Type 2 Diabetes Throughout the Life Span

Eva M. Vivian, PharmD, MS, CDE, BC-ADM, FAADE

Key Concepts

- Type 2 diabetes, while historically a disease affecting older individuals, is affecting children, teenagers, young adults, and older adults at alarming rates. Each age group has specific problems requiring specific strategies.

- Risk factors for developing type 2 diabetes include ethnic background, family history, obesity, and a sedentary lifestyle.

- Type 2 diabetes is also associated with hypertension, hyperlipidemia, and cardiovascular disease.

- Treatment primarily consists of physical activity, healthy eating, and multiple medications, which present challenges to the diabetes educator, the individual with diabetes, and family.

Introduction

The discussion of type 2 diabetes across the life span begins with the concept of diabetes as a progressive disease. A case study is used to provide a brief overview of the pathophysiologic deficits and diagnostic criteria for type 2 diabetes. Next, treatment is discussed, using the clinical practice recommendations of the American Diabetes Association (ADA). The basic principles of care are then outlined for 2 age groups with numerous special considerations: (1) elderly adults and (2) children and adolescents. Similarities and differences in approaches to care for each of these age-specific populations are explored.

State of the Problem

Clinical Presentation

Type 2 diabetes is a disease characterized by hyperglycemia. The dual defects of insulin resistance, primarily at the cell receptor sites of muscle tissue, and a progressive decrease in insulin secretory capacity result in hyperglycemia.[1]

The deficiency of pancreatic beta cell function, which progresses over time, limits insulin production. Without adequate amounts of insulin to compensate for insulin resistance, the transportation of glucose from the bloodstream into the cell cannot occur. Insulin resistance and a reduction in insulin production and secretion are present in varying degrees, depending on the duration of the disease.

- *Phase 1:* The natural progression of type 2 diabetes appears to start with insulin resistance and impaired insulin sensitivity, followed by compensatory insulin hypersecretion.
- *Phase 2:* Impairment of pancreatic beta cell secretion of insulin produces an abnormal rise in postmeal and fasting glucose levels (now referred to as prediabetes).
- *Phase 3:* Overt diabetes appears due to progressive impairment of beta cell insulin secretion and lack of insulin sensitivity accompanied by increased hepatic glucose production.[2]

In the third phase, fasting glucose levels are greater than or equal to 126 mg/dL (7.0 mmol/L); however, many people with type 2 diabetes are unaware they have the disease since the mild elevations in glucose levels do not produce physical signs and symptoms prompting medical evaluation. Because of the number of persons who have long-term complications at initial presentation, scientists have estimated that diabetes may have been present for 4 to 7 years prior to the clinical diagnosis.[3]

Unlike the abrupt onset of type 1 diabetes, which presents with the classic symptoms of polyuria, polydipsia, and polyphagia, type 2 diabetes is usually insidious and progresses gradually. The first symptoms may be fatigue, poor wound healing, dry mouth, blurred vision (patients are often diagnosed during or after a visit with their eye doctor and often have just gotten new glasses), or other poorly differentiated symptoms. Alternately, type 2 diabetes that has gone undetected for a period of time can present with many of the overt symptoms usually attributed to type 1 diabetes. This wide range of presenting symptoms reflects the level of insulin resistance and the degree of beta cell dysfunction at diagnosis.

Incidence and Prevalence

Diabetes is reaching epidemic proportions throughout the world. The Centers for Disease Control and Prevention (CDC) and the World Health Organization (WHO) estimate that by the year 2030, 366 million people will have diabetes, predominantly type 2. The greatest areas of growth are in Asia and Africa, where the shift to more industrialized economies, sedentary lifestyles, and Westernized diets has increased the incidence of type 2 diabetes dramatically.[4]

The 2011 National Diabetes Fact Sheet announced that 25.8 million people, or 8.3% of the US population, have diabetes. Approximately 7 million of these Americans are undiagnosed. Of those diagnosed, 85% to 90% have type 2 diabetes. The number of adults aged 20 years and older at risk for diabetes with prediabetes is 79 million. The assessment of the CDC, the National Institutes of Health (NIH), and the ADA put forth in the National Diabetes Fact Sheet predicts that 1.6 million new cases of diabetes are diagnosed in people aged 20 years and older each year.[5]

Generally Increases With Age

In looking at how type 2 diabetes affects the demographic groups, the fastest-growing segment of the population diagnosed with this disease is individuals aged 65 years and older. The prevalence of diabetes increases with age. In 2011 it was estimated that 10.9 million people aged 65 years and older (26.9% of all people in this age group) have diabetes.[4] The incidence may vary between the sexes from one population to another, but in general, men and women are afflicted equally.[5]

Children and Adolescents Now Also a Concern

The National Diabetes Fact Sheet 2011 indicates that type 2 diabetes in children is still rare but of growing concern.[5,6] Although type 2 diabetes typically presents in adults over 30 years old, diagnosis of children with type 2 diabetes, particularly among the high-risk ethnic groups (ie, Hispanic, African American, and Native American), continues to increase. The SEARCH study, which estimated diabetes mellitus (DM) incidence in youth under 20 years old according to race/ethnicity and DM type, found that while type 2 DM is still relatively infrequent among children under 10 years of age, the highest rates (17.0 to 49.4 per 100,000 person-years) were observed among adolescent minority populations.[7] Two million adolescents (or 1 in 6 overweight adolescents) aged 12 to 19 years have prediabetes.[4] As this explosion in the number of persons with diabetes reaches epidemic proportions, healthcare economics will be seriously affected. The healthcare system will be straining its capacity to effectively and efficiently diagnose, treat, and educate those affected. Prevention and early detection of diabetes play a significant role in controlling this epidemic.

Risk Factors for Type 2 Diabetes

The most important risk factors for type 2 diabetes are the following:

- Heredity, which is nonmodifiable
- Obesity, which is modifiable
- Physical inactivity, which is also modifiable

Family studies have revealed that first-degree relatives of individuals with type 2 diabetes are about 3 times more likely to develop the disease than individuals without a positive family history of the disease. It has also been shown that concordance rates for monozygotic twins, which have ranged from 60% to 90%, are significantly higher than those for dizygotic twins. Thus, it is clear that type 2 diabetes has a strong genetic component.[8,9]

Unlike type 1 diabetes, type 2 diabetes can generally be prevented by maintaining an age-appropriate body weight and engaging in physical activity.[8,9]

Obesity is also a heritable trait that arises from the interaction of multiple genes and lifestyle factors. Obesity is the most powerful predictor for the development of type 2 diabetes. In high-risk populations, such as the Pima Indians, members of the at-risk group who are not obese have a lower incidence of diabetes. The interplay of other risk factors, however, such as family history with obesity, can increase incidence.[9,10]

Habitual physical inactivity is a contributor to obesity and the rising rates of diabetes. Physical activity has been found to decrease insulin resistance, lower blood glucose levels, and decrease the risk of disease. Cohort studies have documented the lower risk of incident diabetes even for everyday activities such as walking.[11,12] Physical activity is now recognized as a major component of type 2 diabetes prevention.

The following list summarizes commonly accepted risk factors.[1] In addition, some public health experts and planners have noted that the economically disadvantaged have increased risk, and some groups are targeting public health programs to this group.

Testing should be considered in all adults who have the following factors:

- Overweight (body mass index [BMI] ≥25 kg/m[2*])
- Age of at least 45 years: The elderly especially have increased risk
- First-degree relative with diabetes
- Habitual physical inactivity
- Member of a high-risk ethnic population: African American, Hispanic, Native American, Asian American, Pacific Islander

---

*May not be correct for all ethnic groups. May need to adjust for Asian populations.

- Previously identified prediabetes: impaired glucose tolerance (IGT) or impaired fasting glucose (IFG)
- History of gestational diabetes mellitus or delivery of a baby weighing more than 4.1 kg (9 lb)
- Hypertension ≥140/90 mm Hg
- High-density lipoprotein level of up to 35 mg/dL or a triglyceride level of at least 250 mg/dL
- Polycystic ovarian syndrome
- A1C greater than or equal to 5.7%, IGT or IFG on previous testing
- Conditions associated with insulin resistance, such as acanthosis nigricans, a thickening of the stratum corneum that becomes pigmented (obesity)
- History of cardiovascular disease

Diagnosis of Type 2 Diabetes

The ADA has outlined 4 options for diagnosing type 2 diabetes. See Table 15.1 for a summary. Findings should be confirmed by repeat testing on a different day.

Treatment of Type 2 Diabetes

At diagnosis of type 2 diabetes, the person with diabetes and the healthcare professional work together to create an individually tailored management plan that focuses on the treatment of hyperglycemia present as well as the underlying physiologic deficits, self-management, and behavior change. The plan addresses the following:

- Healthy eating
- Being active
- Monitoring
- Taking medication
- Problem solving
- Healthy coping
- Reducing risks

This multifaceted approach requires that the patient and the provider consider a significant range of options. Much of the initial treatment aims to reduce troublesome symptoms such as polyuria and dry mouth and restore physiologic balance. Treatment should also include the psychosocial aspects of

TABLE 15.1 Diagnosing Type 2 Diabetes in Nonpregnant Adults			
4 Options			
A1C ≥6.5%*	**Acute Symptoms† Plus Casual‡ Plasma Glucose** ≥200 mg/dL (11.1 mmol/L)	**Fasting Plasma Glucose§** ≥126 mg/dL (7.0 mmol/L)	**2-Hour Postload Glucose** ≥200 mg/dL (11.1 mmol/L) during oral glucose tolerance test (75-g glucose)¶

Note: These results should be confirmed by repeat testing on a different day.

*Test is performed in a laboratory using a method that is NGSP (National Glycohemoglobin Standardization Program) certified and standardized to the DCCT (Diabetes Control and Complications Trial) assay.

†Classic symptoms of diabetes include polyuria, polydipsia, and unexplained weight loss.

‡Casual is defined as any time of day without regard to time since last meal.

§Fasting is defined as no caloric intake for at least 8 hours.

¶The oral glucose tolerance test is not recommended for routine clinical use.

Source: Data from the American Diabetes Association, "Diagnosis and classification of diabetes mellitus," *Diabetes Care* 36 Suppl 1 (2014): S81-90.

the diagnosis, which affect the patient as well as every member of the patient's family.

Lifestyle Interventions

For persons newly diagnosed with diabetes, medical nutrition therapy (MNT) is an essential first step in controlling glucose levels. Increasing physical activity is also important to reduce insulin resistance and manage weight. The case in this chapter exemplifies this; more information on these topics can be found in chapters 4 and 16 (on nutrition) and 5 and 17 (on physical activity).[1]

Reducing Complications

Cardiovascular disease (CVD) is the major cause of mortality and morbidity in persons with type 2 diabetes.[13] Adults with diabetes have heart disease death rates about 2 to 4 times higher than adults without diabetes. In 2004, heart disease was noted on 68% of diabetes-related death certificates among people aged 65 years and older.[5]

Both nutrition plans and exercise plans for individuals with type 2 diabetes must incorporate prevention of CVD. Reducing saturated fat, limiting sodium use, and encouraging physical fitness and weight reduction when appropriate are all components of a healthy-heart strategy. After the diagnosis of diabetes, screening for hypertension and hypercholesterolemia is appropriate; if these comorbidities are present, aggressive treatment is initiated.

The ADA recommendations for glycemic, blood pressure, and lipid control for adults with diabetes follow[1]:

- ◈ A1C: <7.0%*
- ◈ Blood pressure: <140/80 mm Hg
- ◈ Lipids: LDL cholesterol: <100 mg/dL†

Blood Glucose Control

The ADA established the following target goals to minimize the effects of the disease and its chronic complications[1]:

- ◈ *Preprandial capillary plasma glucose:* 70 to 130 mg/dL
- ◈ *Peak postprandial capillary plasma glucose:* <180 mg/dL‡
- ◈ *A1C:* below 7%

---

*Referenced to a nondiabetic range of 4.0% to 6.0% using a DCCT-based assay.

†In overt CVD, a lower LDL cholesterol goal of <70 mg/dL is an option.

‡These measures should be made 1 to 2 hours after the beginning of the meal.

The Diabetes Control and Complications Trial (DCCT)[14] and the UK Prospective Diabetes Study (UKPDS)[15] demonstrated that maintaining glycemic control with an A1C of <7% significantly reduced the microvascular complications associated with diabetes. Most of the microvascular complications of diabetes are related to the degree and length of exposure to hyperglycemia. New data from the follow-up study of the Diabetes Control and Complications Trial, the Epidemiology of Diabetes Intervention and Complications (DCCT/EDIC) study,[16] and the UKPDS stressed the importance of glycemic control early in the course of the disease and its value in prevention of later complications. The ongoing beneficial effects on diabetic complications after a period of improved glycemic control, even if followed by a return to usual (often poorer) metabolic control, have been described as representing "metabolic memory" by the DCCT/EDIC investigators and as a "legacy effect" by the UKPDS investigators.

Self-Monitoring   Self-monitoring of blood glucose (SMBG) is an essential component of self-care. It empowers those with diabetes to make needed adjustments in their daily care and gives them the necessary data to evaluate those changes.

See Table 7.8 in chapter 7 for a comparison of the ADA and the American Association of Clinical Endocrinologists (AACE) target blood glucose goals.

Case—Part 1: An Adult Develops Type 2 Diabetes

EB, a 46-year-old widowed Hispanic woman, noted that in the past year she gained 15 lb, had recurrent vaginitis, and tended to become fatigued after her main meal. She attributed these problems to her stressful life, which includes caring for both her ill mother and a new grandchild in her home. Her past medical history was significant for hypertension and dyslipidemia, notably an elevated triglyceride level and a decreased HDL level. Her social history revealed that she has never smoked and that she drinks red wine approximately 1 to 2 times per month. She has not been sexually active since the death of her husband 3 years prior. During the medical evaluation for urinary tract infection (UTI) and the subsequent follow-up laboratory testing, the following data were gathered:

- Urine analysis: glycosuria
- BMI: 35 kg/m^2
- Blood pressure: 130/85 mm Hg
- Skin: marked acanthosis nigricans in folds of neck and axillae
- Fasting glucose: 199 mg/dL and 233 mg/dL
- A1C: 8.2%

The lab data confirmed the diagnosis of diabetes. EB was upset but not surprised by the diagnosis. Her mother, 2 sisters, and a brother all have type 2 diabetes; in the past, she had wondered if she, too, had diabetes. During the course of the visit, EB stated she knew very little about managing diabetes and could not see herself incorporating changes in diet or exercise into her already busy life. She expressed fear at the possible development of blindness and kidney disease and is worried that her children will be burdened with her care.

Since coming to the United States from Puerto Rico 4 years ago, EB has been learning to speak English but still prefers to read in Spanish.

Discussion

The diagnosis of type 2 diabetes in EB signifies the increased incidence of the disease among certain ethnic groups, in this case among Hispanic Americans. With a significant family history, EB had a genetic predisposition: 4 first-degree relatives already diagnosed with diabetes. A history of obesity with further weight gain, diminished exercise, and significant life stressors may have been the environmental and behavioral triggers that led to the manifestation of type 2 diabetes. The presence of acanthosis nigricans, a thickening of the stratum corneum that becomes pigmented, was a marker for the presence of insulin resistance. This hyperinsulinemia promotes keratinocyte proliferation, resulting in acanthosis nigricans and/or skin tags.[1]

EB had a significant number of risk factors for diabetes. She was obese with a BMI of 35 kg/m^2 and, although active, rarely exercised. Her family history was strongly positive for diabetes, and her ethnicity further increased her risk. EB also had a past medical history of hypertension and elevated lipid values.

In those with underlying pathophysiologic changes indicative of prediabetes, the overt presentation of type 2 diabetes often occurs after an illness or other stressor. In EB's case, she had the physical stress and exhaustion of being a multigenerational caregiver. Determining whether

(continued)

the underlying and as-yet untreated diabetes exacerbated the urinary tract symptoms, which brought her to the clinic, or whether the UTI was an initial symptom of the diabetes is difficult. Often, UTI or vaginitis is the presenting symptom in a woman with abnormal glucose levels.

The presence of glucose in the urine indicated that the level of serum glucose had exceeded approximately 180 mg/dL, the level considered the usual adult renal threshold where the kidneys begin to excrete glucose into the urine. Urine results are not diagnostic but heighten the suspicion for the diagnosis of diabetes. Renal threshold is reduced in children and pregnant women and elevated in the aged. Applying the diagnostic criteria (Table 15.1) to EB's lab results shows that her glucose values are indicative of diabetes.

In the future, it will be important for EB to track her blood glucose values at home. (See the Self-Monitoring section.)

Pharmacologic Interventions

The pathways to controlling blood glucose levels and achieving target goals vary for each person with diabetes. Initially, lifestyle modifications may be sufficient, but as the disease progresses, the pathophysiologic changes diminish insulin sensitivity and beta cell production, requiring medications to reach target goals.

Individualized Plan

The healthcare professional must tailor the medication regimen to the individual and adjust it as necessary to maintain glycemic control. During the first few years of type 2 diabetes, the use of oral medications, usually in a multiple drug regimen, is effective in reaching target goals.

Oral medications (discussed in depth in chapter 18) used for the treatment of diabetes address the various pathophysiologic deficits:

Biguanides (metformin):	Reduce hepatic glucose output
Sulfonylureas (glyburide, glipizide):	Improve insulin secretion
Thiazolidinediones (rosiglitiazone, pioglitazone):	Increase insulin sensitivity
Meglitinides (repaglinide, nateglinide):	Increase circulating insulin levels but have a shorter duration than the sulfonylureas
Alpha-glucosidase inhibitors (miglitol, acarbose):	Act within the intestinal wall to prevent/delay the breakdown of certain carbohydrates

Dipeptidyl peptidase 4 (DPP-4) inhibitors (sitagliptin, saxagliptin):	Act within the gut to inhibit the breakdown of GLP-1, an incretin hormone that improves insulin secretion, reduces hepatic glucose production, and slows gastric emptying
SGLT2 inhibitors (canagliflozin, dapagliflozin):	Lower blood sugar by blocking reabsorption of glucose and increasing its excretion in urine
GLP-1 agonists (exenatide, liraglutide):	Enhance glucose-dependent insulin secretion by the pancreatic beta cell, suppress inappropriately elevated glucagon secretion, and slow gastric emptying
Bile acid sequestrants (colesevelam):	Bind bile acids in the intestine, impeding their reabsorption. However, the exact mechanism by which Welchol improves glycemic control is unknown
Dopamine agonists (bromocriptine):	Inhibit excessive sympathetic tone within the central nervous system (CNS), resulting in a reduction in postmeal plasma glucose levels due to enhanced suppression of hepatic glucose production

As diabetes progresses, oral agents may need to be supplemented with additional medications. Injectable exenatide or liraglutide (glucagon-like peptide-1 [GLP-1] receptor agonists) may be added to the regimen, or insulin therapy may be initiated. (See chapter 18 for more information on medications.) With increasing duration of the disease, many people with type 2 diabetes require insulin therapy to remain in a healthy glycemic range. Both the person with diabetes and the healthcare professional need to determine when to add or convert to insulin therapy.

The decision to start an injectable therapy, particularly insulin, can be a difficult one. Fear of needles or injections, myths and fallacies about insulin therapy, concerns about hypoglycemia when using insulin, and alterations in lifestyle due to the use of injectable therapies all can present barriers to initiation of this therapy. (See chapters 8 and 9 for more information on anxieties and diabetes-specific fears.) Those who did not adhere to their diabetes regimen

may have been threatened with the prospect of insulin therapy, further compounding their reluctance to switch to this therapy when the time was appropriate. Coercion of this type increases fear and resistance to using this safe and effective drug.

There are many different types of insulin and various delivery devices. Patient education is a critical component of management of type 2 diabetes with insulin therapy. Not only must the individual with diabetes and the ancillary caregivers understand how to administer the insulin; they must also learn about the type, timing, and action of insulin. Chapters 6 and 18 provide detailed information.

Case—Part 2: Implementing a Treatment Plan for an Adult

Although EB had stated her reservations about attempting lifestyle changes, the individualized approach to nutrition, presented in a stepwise manner, addressed these concerns so that the necessary adjustment could be made.

Nutrition Plan

Medical nutrition therapy involves a thorough assessment of the person's current lifestyle; eating patterns; and ethnic, cultural, or traditional food preferences; as well as nutritional requirements for stages of growth and development. Medical nutrition therapy also incorporates nutritional changes necessary to prevent or treat other health conditions, such as dyslipidemia or osteoporosis. EB's nutrition plan incorporates the following key elements:

- She can eat the traditional foods she loves but is encouraged to limit portion sizes where appropriate to enhance weight loss.

- During early phases of treatment, carbohydrates such as juices and concentrated sweets will be reduced in order to lower the glycemic load, which will help reduce insulin resistance from glucose toxicity, a condition where pancreatic beta cells are inactive as a result of chronic exposure to high concentrations of glucose.

Physical Activity Plan

EB's life was very active, but she was doing little to improve her cardiovascular system or increase her metabolism to burn calories and contribute to weight loss. An increase in aerobic exercise would address both of these

concerns. In addition, weight loss and exercise might improve her lipid values—raising HDL and lowering triglycerides. Exercise would also provide a healthy outlet for the stress EB experiences in her role as caregiver. Although beginning an exercise program can be daunting, helping EB identify an activity she enjoys will increase the likelihood that she will adhere to her exercise program. Most patients find a walking program an easy and effective way to increase aerobic activity. Planning brief, 10- to 15-minute periods of time to walk throughout the day helps improve insulin sensitivity, reduce weight, and improve cardiovascular fitness. For some patients, the use of a pedometer that records the number of steps taken in a day promotes an increase in physical activity.

Blood Glucose Control

A significant part of EB's treatment plan focused on obtaining and maintaining blood glucose ranges in accordance with target goals established by the ADA.[1] The role of maintaining glycemic control in reducing microvascular complications was an important and empowering message for EB, who feared blindness and renal disease.

Monitoring

To monitor changes in blood glucose levels and the response to treatment, EB needed to learn to check her glucose at home. EB had been checking her mother's glucose level at home sporadically. She had never self-tested. She told the diabetes educator she felt confident using the brand of meter she used for her mother and did not feel the need for further instructions. EB demonstrated proper techniques in the use of her glucose meter and agreed to test before breakfast and again before supper.

(continued)

Training her daughter in use of the meter and the medications will be critical in EB's success, as the daughter can help reinforce the training and provide support to her mother when she is on her own at home.

EB was given an instruction sheet written in Spanish that delineated the steps needed to periodically check the accuracy of the meter. The instructions include the toll-free help-line number for the meter manufacturer, which is available 24/7 with interpreters if needed. EB may need help filling out the warranty card that came with her meter and sending it in. Registering her meter will make it easier for the manufacturer to pull up her information should she need to call the help line.

Medication

Because of her elevated glucose levels, EB needed not only MNT but also medication. She was started on metformin (Glucophage®, Bristol-Myers Squibb Co). She received all written instructions and materials in both Spanish and English.

After receiving a prescription to treat the UTI, a sample of metformin, and instructions to increase her fluid intake while on the antibiotics, EB was scheduled for a follow-up appointment the next week. She was asked to bring her glucose test results diary for discussion and to participate in further dietary instruction. EB's blood pressure and cholesterol should be regularly monitored to decrease her risk of macrovascular complications.

Health Literacy and Numeracy

In chronic disease management, the patient becomes a partner in care and is responsible for day-to-day management of the disease. Patient education, the cornerstone of self-management, requires the dissemination of information, most of which occurs by the written word.

Health literacy, the ability to perform basic reading and numerical tasks required to function in a health environment, significantly impacts diabetes self-management: the ability to read medication labels, appointment cards, and medical nutrition plans. Problems with health literacy are more common among immigrants, older patients, those with disrupted schooling, and those for whom English is not their primary language. However, low literacy can affect anyone. It is not limited to the inability to read but includes comprehension and synthesis of new information. Low health literacy is common among those with diabetes and has been associated with having less knowledge about diabetes and worse glycemic control.[17]

Low numeracy skills, or the inability to use numbers, is a significant part of health literacy. Understanding measurements, time, and multistep operations is important in assessing portion sizes, understanding insulin action curves, and performing capillary glucose testing and other basic diabetes self-care management.

Written instructions and educational literature in Spanish may still present a challenge for EB. It can be difficult to assess health literacy in a person whose primary language is not English, as poor comprehension may be attributed solely to a language barrier. Despite the fact that EB's daughter accompanies her to visits and is willing to interpret, using interpreter services can give a fuller picture of EB's ability to not only read Spanish but interpret the information into an action plan. Family members can be protective and conceal problems with literacy, both the patient's issues and their own. Using an interpreter who is familiar with medical terms and can accurately convey the dialogue between patient and healthcare provider is important in ensuring the patient has been provided with the correct translation. To ascertain understanding of the information, the provider must present the patient with simple tasks that involve the use of information taught, such as selecting the correct insulin dosage from a blood glucose–based algorithm or demonstrating the use of an insulin pen. The educational literature given to EB should have large colorful pictures with simple explanations that provide clear instructions. For example, the use of the plate method for MNT gives an excellent visual representation of the distribution of food type and portion for a meal that is readily understood with limited explanation.

At the follow-up visit, the provider will need to assess blood glucose logs and food and activity diaries not only for issues of blood glucose control but for signs that suggest low health literacy or numeracy problems.

Type 2 Diabetes in Older Adults

The prevalence of diabetes among US adults aged 65 years and older varies from 22% to 33%, depending on the diagnostic criteria used.[18] Postprandial hyperglycemia is a prominent characteristic of type 2 diabetes in older adults,[19–21] contributing to observed differences in prevalence depending on which diagnostic test is used.[20] Using the hemoglobin A1C (A1C) or fasting plasma glucose (FPG) diagnostic criteria, as is currently done for national surveillance, one third of older adults with diabetes are undiagnosed.[5] The epidemic of type 2 diabetes is clearly linked to increasing rates of overweight and obesity in the US population, but projections by the CDC suggest that even if diabetes incidence rates level off, the prevalence of diabetes will double in the next 20 years, in part due to the aging of the population.[22] Other projections suggest that the number of cases of diagnosed diabetes in those aged 65 years and older will increase by more than fourfold (compared to threefold in the total population) between 2005 and 2050.[23]

Physiologic changes in fuel regulation combined with genetic, behavioral, and environmental interactions place this population at risk for diabetes. The elderly metabolism has alterations in glucose counterregulation affecting glucagon, epinephrine, and growth hormone. Declines in adiponectin, leptin, and GLP-1 also affect glucose regulation.[19,20]

Screening and Diagnosis of Older Adults

Diagnostic criteria for diabetes do not alter or become less stringent for older adults. The same set of criteria is applied to the nonpregnant adult regardless of age. Only in the case of pregnancy do guidelines for screening and diagnosing gestational diabetes change, relying on an oral glucose tolerance test (OGTT) to determine the diabetes state.

In the physiology of aging, glucose tolerance declines, with fasting plasma glucose levels increasing by 1 to 2 mg/dL per decade after age 30. Postprandial glucose levels increase by approximately 15 mg/dL per decade. While there is a loss of first-phase insulin response, second-phase insulin release that is glucose induced may be normal. A reduced frequency and amplitude of pulsatile insulin release results in disruption in hepatic glucose inhibition.[21]

Clinical Presentation

As in the younger adult population, type 2 diabetes is more common than type 1 diabetes in older adults. Older adults with diabetes rarely present with the typical symptoms of hyperglycemia.[18] Physiologic changes associated with aging may diminish thirst and increase dehydration. Glycosuria at the usual levels may not be seen, because of the advance in renal threshold associated with aging.

Lean, Older Patients Lean, older adults may exhibit signs of autoimmune changes like those usually seen in type 1 diabetes. Latent autoimmune diabetes of adults (LADA) does occur, presenting in older adults who are not obese. Often, this presentation creates a confusing clinical picture of acute hyperglycemia because this population normally is diagnosed with type 2 diabetes. To be well controlled, LADA requires insulin treatment to preserve beta cell function and promote euglycemia. Although the rates of occurrence are small, the healthcare professional must be aware of the possibility of this diagnosis in lean, older patients. A laboratory blood test to measure antiglutamic acid decarboxylase (anti-GAD) or islet cell antibodies (ICAs) can confirm the autoimmune state and improve treatment of the person with LADA.[18]

Other Presentations Others may present with glucose elevations due to an acute illness, a transient medical condition, or the introduction of a certain medication (steroids, antihypertensives, cardiac medications). This increase in plasma glucose levels may reveal previously undiagnosed diabetes, IGT, or IFG and present an opportunity for further assessment and treatment.[18,24,25]

Care With Older Adults

Interventions must carefully consider nutrition and exercise limitations and medication side effects pertinent to the older adult's situation.

Considerations Regarding Older Adults

Older adults are a heterogeneous group; some may be active and functional, providing their own self-care, while others may suffer from multiple comorbidities and require assistance or total care. The following factors must be carefully considered in planning education and care for the unique needs of individuals in this age group:

- Medical complications
- Physical limitations
- Other prescribed medications
- Effects of aging
- Greater risk of hypoglycemia

Complications

Older persons with type 2 diabetes may have a long duration of diabetes with an increase in complications, both macrovascular and microvascular. The UKPDS showed that macrovascular complications of diabetes are 1.5 to 2 times more prevalent in the older diabetic populations than in the nondiabetic population.[25,26] From the diabetes mortality and morbidity rates collected from Medicare claims data on the elderly population in the United States, the following conclusions have been drawn[26]:

- Leading causes of morbidity are ischemic heart disease and stroke.
- Gangrene, amputation, and lower extremity infection make up the next cohort of diseases associated with morbidity.
- Acute complications (hypoglycemia, ketoacidosis, hyperosmolar syndrome) make up the last group.

Physical Limitations

Older adults with diabetes are about 1.5 times more likely to have physical limitations and alterations in daily living activities than those without diabetes.[27,28] Disabilities may be directly linked to eye disease, stroke, cardiovascular disease, neuropathies, and peripheral vascular disease. Older persons with diabetes may also respond more symptomatically to both hyperglycemia and hypoglycemia. Coupled with additional comorbidities, the long tenure of diabetes may contribute to frailty. Physical limitations necessitate adjustments in management goals and interventions.

Polypharmacy

Older adults with diabetes may also be on multiple medications for a variety of ailments. This can lead not only to dosing and timing errors but also the heightened possibility of drug interactions. The healthcare professional must use caution when prescribing certain diabetes medications for older adults.

Aging

Physiologic changes in aging affect signs and symptoms associated with diabetes and its complications.

Below are facets of normal aging that can significantly impact diabetes care:

- Diminished taste and olfactory sense
- Reduced metabolic rate that alters digestion
- Decreased renal clearance
- Altered pain perception

Cautions With Diabetes Medication in Older Adults[18]

- *Metformin.* In patients >80 years of age, evaluate renal function with creatinine clearance; if <60 mg/dL, do not administer drug. Serum creatinine is a poor correlate of renal health because of the low muscle mass characteristic of the elderly person.
- *Thiazolidinediones.* Contraindicated in Class 3 and Class 4 congestive heart failure (CHF); avoid if CHF is present, determine benefit versus risk.
- *Sulfonylureas.* Beware of long half-life and propensity for hypoglycemia; caution in liver and renal dysfunction. Glyburide also decreases pre-ischemic conditioning and, therefore, should not be used in the elderly.
- *Insulin.* Risk of severe hypoglycemia increases with age.

Higher Risk for Hypoglycemia

Slowed counterregulation of hormones, erratic food intake, certain medications (beta-blockers), and slowed intestinal absorption place the older adult at higher risk for hypoglycemia. The adrenergic response to low blood glucose levels may be diminished or absent. Instead, the initial symptoms, such as lack of motor skills or confusion, represent a neuroglycopenia that may be misdiagnosed or pose a safety risk to the individual.

In light of all the changes in the older adult's health, close attention must be paid to nutrition and exercise interventions and medication side effects. The healthcare professional must keep in mind the individual's preferences and physiologic alterations. The ADA goals for glycemic control in many adults is an A1C <7%, but less stringent goals are recommended for elderly persons with limited life expectancy, advanced diabetes complications, or extensive comorbid conditions.[1]

Factors Influencing Education Strategies

For those with diabetes who are still hardy, diabetes self-care and management goals must reflect their capabilities. Despite the fact that age can affect the processing of information, the capacity to learn and integrate new information remains intact throughout the life cycle. In the educational process, accommodations should be made for the following:

- ◆ Hearing changes
- ◆ Visual changes
- ◆ Cognitive status

Paced Learning and Feedback   Like all adult learners, older persons with diabetes benefit from a stepwise approach to education that recognizes their past experience and builds on it. In addition, several studies have demonstrated that some older adults with type 2 diabetes may experience some mental slowing that affects the ability to perform diabetes self-care behaviors.[27,28] The diabetes educator must assess older patients for comprehension and memory through both verbal and skills feedback.

Equipment Difficulties   Self-care devices that require technical skill and manipulation, such as those for self-monitoring of glucose and insulin administration, have become much easier for the older adult with diabetes to use.

- ◆ *Self-monitoring of glucose.* Glucose meters have larger display screens, audible beeping prompts, reduced sample size, and ergonomically designed easy-to-grip bodies to facilitate ease of use. Some meters have test strips in drums or cartridges that are easier for arthritic hands to maneuver.
- ◆ *Insulin administration.* Insulin pens have made self-administration of insulin safer for the older person with diabetes. Since it is easier to read dosage marks on insulin pens than on syringes, dosing is more accurate. These devices reduce dosage errors and do not require the manual dexterity of the vial

and syringe method. However, the diabetes educator must assess the patient's ability to push hard enough on the end of the pen to adequately deliver the entire dose. The patient also needs enough hand strength to be able to screw the pen needle on and off.

Since some third-party payers do not routinely reimburse for some of these devices, the diabetes educator must endeavor to educate third-party payers regarding the need for these devices and to advocate in behalf of the patient.

Other Barriers   In an older, retired population, financial concerns, insurance issues, and transportation difficulties can become staggering problems, confounding the delivery of health care and health maintenance. For the person with type 2 diabetes, expenses can be a concern—both the expense of medication for diabetes and its comorbidities and the cost of coverage for multiple medical visits plus podiatric, dental, and eye care. The healthcare provider must be aware of these issues and seek to ameliorate them whenever possible. For example, prescribing medications that are preferred and offer maximal reimbursement or coverage whenever possible reduces the financial burden of the person with diabetes.

Institutional Settings   Many older adults live in long-term care facilities, and a large proportion of these individuals have diabetes. In addition to all the usual therapeutic considerations for type 2 diabetes, skin care takes on heightened importance in this population so that infections, ulcerations, and amputations can be avoided. Reduced circulation, neurological impairment, diminished range of motion, and compromised nutritional status contribute to the fragility of the skin. People with diabetes who are no longer capable of self-care depend on healthcare providers to develop effective care strategies to maintain glycemic control and prevent or reduce health-altering consequences. The diabetes educator can help establish strategies to ensure the following:

- ◆ Glucose levels are appropriately monitored and acted upon.
- ◆ Acute complications of hypoglycemia and hyperglycemia are avoided when possible and treated if present.

- Insulin and other diabetes medications are given accurately and in a timely manner; other medications are checked for potential negative interactions.
- Nutrition intervention supplies sufficient calories and is delivered in a manner that best suits the patient's needs and preferences.
- Skin and foot care become an integral part of the daily care regimen to promote circulation and avoid breakdown.

Type 2 Diabetes in Children and Adolescents

Type 2 diabetes represents 8% to 45% of all diabetes reported among children and adolescents.[29] Of this group, 94% belonged to minority groups.

Diagnosis of Type 2 Diabetes in Children and Teens

Risk Factors

Type 2 diabetes in children and adolescents has increased as the frequency of obesity has risen in the United States. At diagnosis, 85% of children with type 2 diabetes are overweight or obese.[29] Nearly all children diagnosed have a positive family history of type 2 diabetes, with 74% to 100% having a first- or second-degree relative with type 2 diabetes and 45% to 80% having a parent with diabetes. Many of these children are of non-European descent (eg, African American, Hispanic, or Native American).

Clinical Presentation

In general, children and adolescents diagnosed with type 2 diabetes have glycosuria without ketonuria, mild thirst, some increase in urination, and little-to-no weight loss; however, up to 33% will have ketonuria at diagnosis, with 5% to 25% having keto-acidosis unrelated to stress, illness, or infection.[30] Polycystic ovarian syndrome (PCOS) and acanthosis nigricans, disorders associated with insulin resistance, are commonly seen,[30,31] as well as lipid disorders and hypertension. At onset 10% to 32% have hypertension, 14% to 22% have microalbuminuria, 10% have retinopathy, and 18% to 83% have dyslipidemia.[30,31] There are ethnic differences in lipids, lipoproteins, and blood pressure with further indications of the metabolic syndrome in this high-risk population. Other clinical problems that arise in this population are sleep apnea associated with obesity, hepatic steatosis, orthopedic complications, and psychosocial concerns.[32–34]

As obesity in this age group rises, the clinical picture of the child with diabetes can be confusing, making it difficult to differentiate type 1 diabetes from type 2 diabetes without laboratory studies. A variation on the presentation of type 2 diabetes occurs in children with a positive family history of early-onset diabetes. Although the child presents in diabetic ketoacidosis, which is usually seen in type 1 diabetes, the antibody tests are negative (both anti-GAD and ICA), and insulin is not required once the acute episode is resolved. These children have elevated C-peptide levels, which indicates a hyperinsulinemia as opposed to reduced insulin levels found in type 1 diabetes. Many of these children are of African-American descent.[32–34]

Due to the difficulty of establishing the type of diabetes in children by presentation alone, in an ideal situation, type 1 diabetes would be confirmed by a test for autoantibodies, while type 2 diabetes would use a test for insulin resistance such as the fasting C-peptide.[35]

Insulin Resistance   The pattern for development of type 2 diabetes in children appears to follow the insidious pathway seen in type 2 diabetes in adults. Insulin levels may be normal or elevated, but first-phase insulin release is not sufficient to compensate for insulin resistance, which leads to hyperglycemia. Just as in adults with type 2 diabetes, obesity and a lack of physical activity promote overt diabetes. Both of these lifestyle factors promote insulin resistance. The onset of type 2 diabetes frequently occurs around the time of puberty, a time when insulin sensitivity declines. This evidence further supports the importance of insulin resistance in the pathogenesis of the disease.[30,32–34]

Intrauterine Environment   The intrauterine environment, specifically birth weight and maternal hyperglycemia, may have links to type 2 diabetes in children. Low birth weight predicts type 2 diabetes in middle age.[35] Low birth weight has also been associated with the development of diabetes in teens and adolescents. Higher levels of amniotic fluid insulin at 33 to 38 weeks' gestation were a strong predictor of later IGT.[36] Children born to mothers with gestational diabetes also appear to have a higher risk of developing type 2 diabetes.[36,37]

Diagnostic Criteria

With the current explosion in the number of new cases of diabetes and the importance of screening, controversies concerning the criteria and the most effective method for screening for diabetes, particularly type 2 diabetes in children, abound. At present, the same diagnostic criteria that are applied to adults are applied to children; however, whether these established cut points are valid in a younger population is not known.

Public Health Interventions The advent of type 2 diabetes in children and adolescents carries with it a significant public health problem. The onset of the disease in younger populations leads to earlier onset of complications, both macrovascular and microvascular. The estimated financial costs and loss of productivity resulting from these health problems represent a significant economic burden. Earlier diagnosis and aggressive treatment may help in preventing or delaying these costly complications, making a strong case for screening. In 2000, the ADA outlined recommendations for testing children at substantial risk for type 2 diabetes. See Table 15.2.

Considerations Regarding Children and Teens

Once a child or adolescent learns he or she has type 2 diabetes, the approach to care must incorporate the youth's developmental needs and psychosocial concerns. Since many of the children and teens diagnosed with type 2 diabetes are overweight or obese, they may have already faced issues that separate them from their peers. Personal appearance (issues of both style and size), participating in competitive athletics, and congregating at fast-food restaurants or malls are often integral aspects of growing up in the United States. Lifestyle adjustments that help reduce weight and control diabetes can seem to run counter to the norm and become problematic. Striving for independence and developing a sense of self are important developmental tasks that are made more difficult in the presence of diabetes. While parental support and

TABLE 15.2 **Diagnosing Type 2 Diabetes in Children**
Criteria for Considering Screening for Diabetes*:
Overweight (BMI 85th percentile for age and sex; weight for height 85th percentile; or weight 120% of ideal for height)
Plus any 2 of the following risk factors:
• Family history of type 2 diabetes in first- or second-degree relative
• Race/ethnicity (American Indian, African American, Hispanic, Asian/Pacific Islander)
• Signs of insulin resistance or conditions associated with insulin resistance (acanthosis nigricans, hypertension, dyslipidemia, PCOS)
Age of Initiation: Age 10, or at onset of puberty if puberty occurs at a younger age
Testing Frequency: Every 2 years
Test: Fasting plasma glucose preferred

*Clinical judgment should be used to test for diabetes in high-risk subjects who do not meet these criteria.

Source: Data from the American Diabetes Association, "Type 2 diabetes in children and adolescents (consensus statement)," *Diabetes Care* 23, no. 3 (2000): 381-9.

guidance are a necessary part of dealing with a medical condition such as diabetes, at this time of life, the adolescent desires less parental involvement.

For adolescents and children with type 2 diabetes, the goals of therapy are the same as for any person with diabetes:

◇ To achieve physical and psychological well-being while maintaining long-term glycemic control and to avoid microvascular and macrovascular complications[31,37]

Lifestyle Interventions[37,38]

Medical nutrition therapy and increased physical activity are the cornerstone of therapy for all age groups; however, weight management in children and adolescents must consider healthy growth and development needs. Thus, aggressive weight-loss programs are not recommended for these age groups. The approach must be one of substitution and reduction, rather than elimination. The following important dietary adjustments still leave room for the adolescent lifestyle:

◆ Learning to make healthy choices at fast-food restaurants
◆ Eating fewer fatty, calorie-dense foods
◆ Drinking less sugary beverages
◆ Choosing healthy snacks

Obese youth may lack the stamina and athletic prowess to compete in sports. Therefore, physical activities can be a source of self-degradation and ridicule by peers and can contribute to low self-esteem. In the treatment of type 2 diabetes, physical activity lowers insulin resistance and helps maintain weight loss. The challenge is to make this important therapy agreeable to an audience that usually eschews it.

The child should be encouraged to improve fitness through individual activities such as rollerblading, biking, or dancing rather than through competitive activities.[37,38] Also, replacing television and computer time with any type of physical movement has benefits.

Pharmacologic Interventions

Many children with type 2 diabetes will require medication in addition to lifestyle modification to achieve glucose goals. Some will need medication at diagnosis. However, the compendium of medications available for use is limited due to lack of pharmacologic clinical trials in this age group. The US Food and Drug Administration (FDA) has approved 2 pharmacologic agents for use in children and adolescents:

◆ Metformin (an oral agent)
◆ Insulin (injectable formulations)

Metformin The oral agent metformin (Glucophage®, Bristol-Myers Squibb Co), a biguanide, has been approved for use in children 10 to 16 years of age with type 2 diabetes. In controlled trials in subjects aged 8 to 16 years with type 2 diabetes, metformin significantly decreased fasting plasma glucose and A1C levels when compared with placebo.[39,40] The drug has 2 common adverse effects:

◆ Diarrhea
◆ Nausea

To minimize adverse effects, metformin should be taken with food and the dosage titrated slowly, starting with one 500-mg tablet per day until the effective dosage is achieved. The extended-release preparation of metformin may lessen or minimize the adverse effects. For children, the maximum dosage is 2000 mg (in adults it is 2550 mg).

In girls with type 2 diabetes and PCOS, use of metformin may normalize ovulatory abnormalities and increase the risk of unplanned pregnancy; therefore, girls of childbearing age using this therapy should be counseled regarding this risk.[38,40] See also the section on teens in chapter 24, on pregnancy with diabetes.

Insulin Insulin therapy has a long history of usage in the pediatric population. Healthcare professionals prescribe insulin for children with type 1 diabetes or type 2 diabetes who present with diabetic ketoacidosis, hyperosmolar hyperglycemic state, moderate ketosis, or symptomatic glycemic levels. The need for insulin in the hyperglycemic state complicated by insulin resistance may persist for weeks after diagnosis. However, once glycemic levels decrease and lifestyle measures are in place, some children are able to maintain euglycemic levels with metformin.

Insulin therapy should be used if oral agents are not effective or when the disease worsens and clinical goals are no longer met with oral agents alone. Insulin can be used as monotherapy or in combination with metformin.

Some children have been able to meet target goals with 1 injection of a long-acting insulin per day, such as insulin glargine (Lantus®, Sanofi-Aventis US, LLC) or detemir (Levemir®, Novo Nordisk), while others have needed multiple daily injections (MDIs) using a basal/bolus regimen. Insulin therapy must be tailored to the physical as well as psychosocial needs of the person with diabetes. Despite the flexibility of an MDI regimen, adolescents may at times feel encumbered by it and switch to prefilled mixed insulin pens to maximize convenience and have a respite from the demands of self-care.[37] In the presence of insulin resistance in type 2 diabetes, larger amounts of insulin are necessary to adequately control glycemic levels. This is also true in children and particularly in adolescents who have type 2 diabetes. During puberty and growth spurts, insulin resistance increases, necessitating compensatory dosing of insulin. Irrespective of ethnicity, insulin sensitivity is reduced while fasting levels are increased in both obese and nonobese children during Tanner stages II through IV of pubertal development.[30,32]

Other Medications Sulfonylureas, glucosidase inhibitors, and meglitinides may be effective in treating type 2 diabetes in children, but more research must be conducted to determine the risks of using these drugs in this population. In particular, researchers must explore whether insulin secretagogues such as sulfonylureas accelerate beta cell demise in this group, especially in the presence of autoimmunity.[32,33]

Social Support

No matter the therapy selected, patient education and family support are vital components of diabetes management in children and teens. For children and adolescents at risk, healthcare professionals can encourage, support, and educate the entire family to make lifestyle changes that may delay or lower the risk for the onset of type 2 diabetes. Studies show that parents are particularly important as role models, encouragers, and facilitators of physical activity and healthy nutrition in children and adolescents.[41,42] Their roles include everything from buying sports equipment, to taking kids to practice, to doling out praise. Other important factors in raising active children include paternal activity levels and positive reinforcement, maternal participation, sibling involvement, time spent outdoors, and family income. Helping families find ways to utilize the resources that are available in their community is vital to sustaining healthy lifestyle behaviors.[43]

Ideally, a diabetes care team will be able to assess, treat, evaluate, and support the youth and family during the initial stages of the disease. Not all communities have access to such services. In many cases, school counselors and nurses, coaches, teachers, family friends, and peers can assist in providing information, supporting dietary changes, encouraging physical activity, and becoming a sounding board for the frustrations and concerns of the young person with diabetes.

Self-Care Behaviors

The AADE7 Self-Care Behaviors™ are applicable throughout the life span for those with type 2 diabetes. Each behavior is critical in attaining self-sufficiency in the management of diabetes. However, each behavior must be modified to incorporate the particular developmental needs of the person with diabetes to reflect the individual's physical capabilities and self-care responsibilities. Strategies pertinent to each behavior are covered more fully in chapters 4 through 10 of this book.

Being Active

All persons with type 2 diabetes need to maintain a program of physical fitness, the definition of which will vary according to age and ability. Creating a program that is sustainable and integrating it into a daily routine may be quite different for a child compared with a nursing home resident; yet for both, exercise is an integral factor in reducing insulin resistance and improving cardiovascular health.

Healthy Eating

Nutritional management skills such as knowing what, when, and how much to eat are the basis of self-care in diabetes. Modifications for age, caloric requirements, and activity level individualize this therapy.

Adults and Older Adults

Adults with diabetes must learn to replace harmful dietary habits with healthy ones. Selecting nutritious foods that are easy to chew and digest and that are also appetizing may pose a problem for some older adults. The elderly adult may also experience social isolation and have a reduced appetite. Financial limitations can also affect healthy eating behaviors.

Teens

Learning how to cope with the typical diet of their peers while maintaining glycemic control is a daunting task for teens. Alcohol consumption and eating disorders, particularly overeating, may also prove a threat (see chapters 4 and 9).

Taking Medication

Polypharmacy in adults and older persons with diabetes can create problems in accuracy and adherence. Issues of vision and manual dexterity complicate this task. For children, medications can be dispensed by a responsible adult or taken under supervision. Despite this, the child needs an age-appropriate understanding of the importance of the medication regimen and the ability to recognize and treat possible side effects such as hypoglycemia.

Monitoring

Learning to accurately monitor glucose levels is a basic skill that is integral to self-managing diabetes, regardless of age. Both the young and the old experience lifestyle changes that can radically alter glucose levels. In such cases, SMBG is an important safety tool for avoiding critically low or high levels.

Problem Solving

Understanding glucose data or interpreting signs and symptoms of acute complications and being able to make appropriate therapeutic adjustments are complex skills that require education and mentoring. Caregivers for those who are homebound or in nursing facilities may assume this task when the person with diabetes is unable to make these decisions alone. In these situations, diabetes healthcare professionals need to educate and support ancillary care providers to ensure that standards of diabetes care are upheld.

Reducing Risks

For the young, much of self-care education focuses on improving glycemic control to prevent future complications. Risk reduction for CVD is of paramount importance in obese children with type 2 diabetes. Smoking abstinence or cessation and control of lipids and blood pressure are also important in reducing risk. Diabetes educators have the task of informing communities of the lifestyle modifications necessary to prevent and treat diabetes in youth. For older persons with diabetes, vigilance in screening is important to delay or prevent complications. Eye exams, prophylactic foot care, flu and pneumonia vaccines, and dental care all help maintain functional status among elderly adults.

Healthy Coping

Psychosocial adaptations are required. Living with a chronic disease requires support, creative coping skills, and a certain hardiness. Remaining motivated in the face of a somewhat capricious disease such as diabetes can be very difficult.

The life stressors present for young and old add considerable burden, and it is not uncommon for persons with diabetes to become depressed. Healthcare providers must help patients learn a variety of coping skills to meet the challenges of life with diabetes, and be ready to appropriately screen for and treat depression. Chapter 9 provides more information on depression.

Summary

Type 2 diabetes is a major problem affecting all ages. With the incidence and prevalence of this disease rising to epidemic proportions, the healthcare professional must address the factors that contribute to the development of diabetes as well as those that contribute to the development of diabetic complications. Obesity, genes, and family history are the prime risk factors; however, attention to interpersonal, intrapersonal, community, and societal issues can help promote healthy lifestyles for those with diabetes.

- ◆ To prevent type 2 diabetes, interventions at the individual, family, and community levels are crucial to reduce the levels of obesity in Western society.
- ◆ Important steps to improve diabetes care include community awareness of lifestyle modifications necessary to reduce risk, appropriate screening for diabetes among those at highest risk, and promotion of and adherence to diabetes standards of care.
- ◆ To be effective, education and medical management must be tailored to the individual, taking into consideration age, socioeconomic status, and cultural and religious affiliations.

By recognizing the needs of individuals with type 2 diabetes throughout the life span, the health professional is better prepared to offer appropriate treatment and guidance.

Focus on Education

Teaching Strategies

⊘ **Be sensitive to issues of age and culture.**   Type 2 diabetes affects a wide range of age groups. Give simple, clear information and messages in a step-wise approach. Tailor content to the specific concerns of that age group. Seek out questions that need to be answered first. Become familiar with various cultural norms and incorporate them into teaching as appropriate. Ask about food staples in the diet and forms of preparation. What is the hierarchy of the family? A child may be cared for by a relative other than the parents.

⊘ **Establish a relationship in order to determine a patient's knowledge, find out the patient's agenda, find out what he or she already knows, and then offer information and handouts.**   Being a guide and partner in diabetes care is an important component in individualizing care. Patients must be able to openly discuss their concerns to create a successful plan of care.

⊘ **Create a milieu.**   Think about a wide range of ages, previous experience with diabetes in the family or with friends, and how to deliver content with more than a single approach. For example, teens and adults who drink soft drinks benefit from measuring teaspoons of sugar that equal the amount of sugar found in a "real" soft drink. This gives a visual of the calorie and glycemic value of a commonly consumed beverage. Adults and teens also respond to seeing test tubes filled with fat that equal the amount of fat in food products such as hamburger, steak, and chicken.

⊘ **Identify polypharmacy problems.**   Polypharmacy may be a problem for persons with diabetes, particularly in older adults. Routinely review all medications the person is taking, including over-the-counter products and dietary supplements. Discuss use and misuse (for example, use in combination with other medicines and street drugs).

⊘ **Recognize psychological concerns.**   Changes in self-esteem, for example, are a concern for all age groups. Accepting diabetes as a chronic disease may be especially difficult for younger individuals, but belief in the chronicity and care needed is of concern to all age groups. As an elderly person's medical and mental status changes, the person may be placed at risk for adverse events. Family involvement is advised for support.

⊘ **Patient-centered pedagogy versus andragogy.** When working with patients throughout their life span, the diabetes educator should consider his or her teaching style and people's learning style. The pedagogical approach happens when a learner is dependent on the instructor for all learning; the experience of the instructor is most influential; students are told what they have to learn in order to advance; learning is a process of acquiring prescribed content; and motivation is based on external pressures, competition for grades, and the consequences of failure.

The andragogical approach happens when the learner is self-directed, experience becomes the source of self-identity, and change is likely to trigger a readiness to learn. Learning must have relevance to real-life tasks, and students are internally motivated via self-esteem, recognition, better quality of life, self-confidence, and self-actualization.

In summary, pedagogy is when diabetes educators believe that they know what the patient needs to know and what to do about it. It is a very conservative strategy of education by providing lecture with the information patients need to know. On the other hand, andragogy is a more liberal approach to education. In an andragogical approach, diabetes educators provide learning opportunities that are organized around life/work situations rather than content.

⊘ **What can patients teach diabetes educators?** Each patient education visit should be an opportunity for diabetes educators to learn from patients. Only when they learn from a patient can they effectively provide accurate teaching. By carefully listening to patients, diabetes educators can assess gaps between where they are now and where they need to be.

⊘ **Patient-centered education.** The theory of multiple intelligences was developed in 1983 by Dr. Howard Gardner and suggests that the traditional interpretation of being smart, based on IQ testing, is not indicative of one's capacity to learn and utilize the knowledge. Diabetes educators can utilize multiple theories of learning and approaches to deliver effective education. There is no one formula for empowering, influencing, and moving one from wanting to learn to actually learning and doing something with the information. Diabetes educators can use words, logic, pictures, music, self-reflection, physical activities, and social interactions to convey information effectively to people with diabetes. The common denominator is to focus on the learner

and his or her needs and desires and consequently deliver a patient-centered education.

Messages for Patients

⊘ **Screening visits protect health longer.** Schedule health visits for screening and then schedule any needed follow-up appointments without delay. Doing so will help you know what you are most at risk for, avoid or delay complications related to having diabetes, and improve the chances for effective treatment.

⊘ **Physical activity helps at every age.** All age groups should engage in fitness. Although competitive sports may be culturally encouraged, fitness and endurance are the true primary focus. Walking and workout programs are examples.

⊘ **Involve family.** Involving family and/or significant others at all levels of self-care diabetes management is encouraged.

Focus on Practice

⊘ **Multidimensional strategies for a multidimensional problem.** Multiple factors within type 2 diabetes management require special attention: ethnic background, family history, obesity, and a sedentary lifestyle. Population-specific education strategies, clinical interventions, public health policies, and media influences are among many factors that impact how an individual internalizes and approaches diabetes care. Diabetes care specialists need to be involved in all aspects of diabetes care, spectrums of delivery, and dimensions of information dissemination.

⊘ **Quality improvement needs to be an easy and welcoming process.** It takes a long time to change systems and the way that diabetes care is practiced. Later, it takes a while to realize that things do not work anymore. Once it is realized that things do not work, it takes a long time to change them. As a result, diabetes educators are often stuck implementing unnecessary processes

and practices that do not produce optimal outcomes. Diabetes educators need to question what they do and ask those involved in diabetes self-management education (DSME), "What does not work?" and "What needs to be done to fix it?"

⊘ **Evidence-based DSME does not always need to be based on randomized clinical trials.** Consider exploratory investigations to identify problems and corresponding solutions, constructive research to develop solutions to a problem, and empirical research to test the feasibility of a solution. Each DSME practice needs to look at the program deliverables: Are you achieving the desired metabolic markers? Are you cost-effective? Are your patients choosing your center as a preferred method of care? Share your successes and challenges with others, allow others to learn from your experience and model you, and adapt strategies that work.

References

1. American Diabetes Association. Standards of medical care in diabetes (position statement). Diabetes Care. 2014;37 Suppl 1:S14-80.

2. Kahn SE. The relative contributions of insulin resistance and beta cell dysfunction to the pathophysiology of type 2 diabetes. Diabetologia. 2003;46:3-19.

3. Nathan DM. Insulin treatment of type 2 diabetes mellitus. In: Inzucchi S, ed. The Diabetes Mellitus Manual: A Primary Care Companion to Ellenberg and Rifkin's. 6th ed. New York: McGraw-Hill; 2005:138-49.

4. Danaei G, Finucane MM, Lu Y, et al. National, regional, and global trends in fasting plasma glucose and diabetes prevalence since 1980: systematic analysis of health examination surveys and epidemiological studies with 370 country-years and 2.7 million participants. Lancet. 2011;378(9785):31-40.

5. Centers for Disease Control and Prevention. National diabetes fact sheet: general information and national estimates on diabetes in the United States, 2011. Atlanta, Ga: US Department of Health and Human Services, Centers for Disease Control and Prevention; 2011.

6. National Diabetes Education Program. Overview of diabetes in children and adolescents. Jun 2011 (cited 2013 Jun 10). On the Internet at: http://ndep.nih.gov/media/youth_factsheet.pdf.

7. The SEARCH for Diabetes in Youth Study Group. The many faces of diabetes in American youth: type 1 and type 2 diabetes in five race and ethnic populations. Diabetes Care. 2009;32 Suppl 2:S99-147.

8. Pociot F, Akolkar B, Concannon P, et al. Genetics of type 1 diabetes: what's next? Diabetes. 2010;59:1561-71.

9. Lyssenko V, Jonsson A, Almgren P, et al. Clinical risk factors, DNA variants, and the development of type 2 diabetes. N Engl J Med. 2008;359:2220-32.

10. Despres JP, Lemieux I. Abdominal obesity and metabolic syndrome. Nature. 2006;444:881-7.

11. Joen CY, Lokken RP, Hu FB, van Dam RM. Physical activity of moderate intensity and risk of type 2 diabetes: a systematic review. Diabetes Care. 2007;30:744-52.

12. Haskell WL, Lee IM, Pate RR, et al. Physical activity and public health: updated recommendation for adults from the American College of Sports Medicine and the American Heart Association. Med Sci Sports Exerc. 2007;39:1423-34.

13. Danish RK, West BB. Rapid progression from prediabetes to severely ill diabetes while under "expert care": suggestions for improving screening for disease progression. Diabetes Spectr. 2005;18(4):229-39.

14. The DCCT Research Group. The effect of intensive treatment of diabetes on the development and progression of long-term complications in insulin-dependent diabetes mellitus. N Engl J Med. 1993;329:977-86.

15. UK Prospective Diabetes Study Group. Intensive blood glucose control with sulphonylureas or insulin compared with conventional treatment and risk complications in patients with type 2 diabetes (UKPD 33). Lancet. 1998;352:837-53.

16. Ranjit Unnikrishnan I, Anjana RM, Mohan V. Importance of controlling diabetes early—the concept of metabolic memory, legacy effect and the case for early insulinisation. J Assoc Physicians India. 2011 Apr;59 Suppl:8-12.

17. Schillinger D, Grumbach K, Piette J, et al. Association of health literacy with diabetes outcomes. Diabetes Care. 2009;32:2149-55.

18. Kirkman SM, Briscoe VJ, Clark N, Florez H, Haas LB, Halter JB. Diabetes in older adults: a consensus report. J Am Geriatr Soc. 2012 Dec;60(12):2342-56

19. Gambert SR, Pinkstaff S. Emerging epidemic: diabetes in older adults: demography, economic impact, and pathophysiology. Diabetes Spectr. 2006;19:221-8.

20. Szoke E, Shrayyef MZ, Messing S, et al. Effect of aging on glucose homeostasis: accelerated deterioration of beta-cell function in individuals with impaired glucose tolerance. Diabetes Care. 2008;31:539-43.

21. Chang AM, Halter JB. Aging and insulin secretion. Am J Physiol Endocrinol Metab. 2003;284:E7-12.

22. Boyle JP, Thompson TJ, Gregg EW, et al. Projection of the year 2050 burden of diabetes in the US adult population: dynamic modeling of incidence, mortality, and prediabetes prevalence. Popul Health Metr. 2010;8:29.

23. Narayan KM, Boyle JP, Geiss LS, et al. Impact of recent increase in incidence on future diabetes burden: US, 2005–2050. Diabetes Care. 2006;29:2114-6.

24. Stratton IM, Adler AI, Neil HA, et al. Association of glycaemia with macrovascular and microvascular complications of type 2 diabetes (UKPDS 35): prospective observational study. BMJ. 2000;321(7258):405-12.

25. Bertoni AG, Krop JS, Anderson GF, Brancati FL. Diabetes-related morbidity and mortality in a national sample of US elders. Diabetes Care. 2002;25(3):471-5.

26. Huang ES. Appropriate application of evidence to the care of elderly patients with diabetes. Curr Diabetes Rev. 2007;3(4):260-3.

27. Sommerfield AJ, Deary IF, Grier BM. Acute hyperglycemia alters mood and impairs cognitive performance in people with type 2 diabetes. Diabetes Care. 2004;27:2335-40.

28. McCrimmon RJ, Ryan CM, Frier BM. Diabetes and cognitive dysfunction. Lancet. 2012;379(9833):2291-9.

29. American Diabetes Association. Type 2 diabetes in children and adolescents (consensus statement). Diabetes Care. 2000;23(3):381-9.

30. Copeland KC, Silverstein J, Moore KR, et al; American Academy of Pediatrics. Management of newly diagnosed type 2 diabetes mellitus (T2DM) in children and adolescents. Pediatrics. 2013;131(2):364-82.

31. Springer SC, Silverstein J, Copeland K, et al; American Academy of Pediatrics. Management of type 2 diabetes in children and adolescents. Pediatrics. 2013;131(2):e648-64.

32. Pinhas-Hamiel O, Zeitler P. Acute and chronic complications of type 2 diabetes mellitus in children and adolescents. Lancet. 2007;369:1823-31.

33. Sinha R, Fisch G, Teague B, et al. Prevalence of glucose tolerance among children and adolescents with marked obesity. N Engl J Med. 2002;346:802-10.

34. Alberti G, Zimmet P, Shaw J, Bloomgarden Z, Kaufman F, Silink M. Type 2 diabetes in the young: the evolving epidemic. Diabetes Care. 2004;27:1798-811.

35. Phillips DI. Birthweight and the future development of diabetes: a review of the evidence. Diabetes Care. 1998; 21 Suppl 2:B150-5.

36. Silverman BL, Metzger BE, Cho NH, Loeb CA. Impaired glucose tolerance in adolescent offspring of diabetic mothers: relationship of fetal hyperinsulinism. Diabetes Care. 1995;18:611-7.

37. Vivian EM. Type 2 diabetes in children and adolescents—the next epidemic? Curr Med Res Opin. 2006;22(2): 297-306.

38. Schreiner B. Promoting lifestyle and behavior change in overweight children and adolescents with type 2 diabetes. Diabetes Spectr. 2005;18(1):9-12.

39. Jones KL, Arslanian S, Peterokova VA, et al. Effect of metformin in pediatric patients with type 2 diabetes: a randomized controlled trial. Diabetes Care. 2002;25:89-94.

40. Kendall D, Vail A, Amin R, et al. Metformin in obese children and adolescents: the MOCA trial. J Clin Endocrinol Metab. 2013;98(1):322-9.

41. Giles-Corti B, Donovan RJ. The relative influence of individual, social, and physical environment determinants of physical activity. Soc Sci Med. 2002;54(12):1793-812.

42. Bradshaw B. The role of the family in managing therapy in minority children with type 2 diabetes mellitus. J Pediatr Endocrinol Metab. 2002;Suppl 1:547-51.

43. Duclos M, Oppert JM, Verges B, et al; SFD Diabetes and Physical Activity Working Group. Physical activity and type 2 diabetes. Recommendations of the SFD (Francophone Diabetes Society) Diabetes and Physical Activity Working Group. Diabetes Metab. 2013;39(3):205-16.

CHAPTER 16

Nutrition Therapy

Janine Freeman, RDN, LD, CDE, CDTP
Marion J. Franz, MS, RDN, LD, CDE

Key Concepts

♦ Nutrition therapy for persons with diabetes should be individualized on the basis of the person's metabolic needs, preferences, and willingness and ability to make lifestyle changes.

♦ Optimal nutrition through healthy eating remains an important goal for all persons with diabetes and should not be compromised to improve glycemia, lipids, or blood pressure control.

♦ Clinical trials and outcome studies have shown that medical nutrition therapy (MNT) can reduce A1C levels by an average of 1% to 2% (ranging from 0.25% to 2.9%).

— In persons with type 2 diabetes, A1C levels can be decreased by 1% to 2%, depending on the duration of the disease and the level of glycemic control.

— In persons with type 1 diabetes, A1C levels can be decreased by ~1% by adjusting mealtime insulin doses to planned carbohydrate intake.

♦ Choosing nutrient-dense, high-fiber foods in appropriate portion sizes instead of processed foods with added sodium, fat, and sugars; avoiding sugar-sweetened beverages; selecting leaner protein sources and meat alternatives;

and substituting foods higher in unsaturated fat for foods high in saturated or *trans* fats are key nutrition therapy strategies for all people with diabetes.

♦ Monitoring the amount of carbohydrate eaten and consistency in food intake are key strategies in achieving glycemic control in persons with type 1 diabetes or type 2 diabetes.

♦ Reducing intake of saturated fat, *trans* fat, dietary cholesterol, and sodium; increasing physical activity; and losing weight (if needed) are lifestyle modifications that can improve lipids and blood pressure and reduce cardiovascular disease (CVD) risk.

♦ Reducing energy intake and increasing physical activity is an important strategy in overweight or obese persons with or at risk for type 2 diabetes. In the absence of contraindications, physical activity should be encouraged in all persons with diabetes to improve glycemic control, assist with weight maintenance, and reduce the risk of CVD.

♦ Diabetes nutrition therapy, self-management education, and support are essential components of diabetes care and essential for improved outcomes in all people with diabetes.

Introduction

Nutrition therapy has been essential in the treatment of diabetes since diabetes was first discovered to be the "sweet urine" disease centuries ago. Nutrition recommendations have changed over the years based on theories of the era. Today, nutrition guidelines are based on available scientific evidence, which has dispelled many of the nutrition myths and misinformation of earlier times. Nutrition therapy, like medicine, remains an ever-changing field as researchers and clinicians learn more about the human body and how various components and combinations of foods and nutrients affect disease risk and management. The Academy of Nutrition and Dietetics published Type 1 and Type 2 Diabetes Evidence-Based Nutrition Practice Guidelines for Adults,[1,2] the American Diabetes Association (ADA) updated its nutrition therapy position statement[3] and annually updates nutrition recommendations to provide healthcare providers and persons with diabetes with the latest information on beneficial nutrition therapies and outcomes,[4] and an American Association of Diabetes Educators (AADE) position statement emphasizes the importance of healthy eating practices as a cornerstone of self-management care that leads to improved quality of life in persons with diabetes.[5]

Medical nutrition therapy (MNT) is defined as an evidence-based application of the Nutrition Care Process provided by the registered dietitian/nutritionist (RDN) and is the legal definition of nutrition counseling by an RDN in the United States.[3] According to the Institute of Medicine (IOM), nutrition therapy is the treatment of a disease or condition through the modification of nutrient or whole-food intake and does not specify that nutrition therapy must be provided by an RDN.[6] The American Association of Diabetes Educators recommends that all members of the healthcare team (ie, nurses, pharmacists, exercise physiologists, etc) be knowledgeable about diabetes nutrition therapy, as they may participate in the delivery of nutrition information in group classes as part of diabetes self-management education and support (DSME/S) or collaborate in the development of an individualized eating plan and support its implementation.[5] Both MNT and nutrition therapy should involve nutrition assessment, nutrition diagnosis, nutrition intervention, and nutrition monitoring and evaluation.[1–3]

Once thought of as a complex set of rigid calculations, nutrition therapy focuses on the individual needs and preferences of the person with diabetes. This focus sets the stage for the adoption of small, incremental lifestyle changes that include food/nutrition and physical activity to improve overall health, reduce the risk of diabetes complications, and manage complications if necessary. Evidence from clinical trials and observational studies supports the effectiveness of nutrition therapy in the primary, secondary, and tertiary prevention of diabetes (ie, preventing or delaying the development of diabetes, and preventing or controlling the complications of diabetes).[1–4] Unfortunately, national data in the United States indicate that only about half of persons with diabetes receive diabetes education and even fewer see an RDN.[7] One study of over 18,000 people with diabetes revealed that only 9.1% had at least 1 nutrition visit within a 9-year time period.[8]

This chapter discusses the role of nutrition therapy in the following areas: diabetes management and prevention; glycemic control, weight management, and prevention and treatment of cardiovascular disease (including hypertension and dyslipidemia) and diabetic kidney disease; nutritional management of complications; and intervention strategies to achieve nutrition therapy goals for youth and adults with diabetes. Evidence-based systematic reviews of diabetes nutrition therapy are the basis for the majority of the recommendations cited in this chapter.[1–3,9]

Goals of Diabetes Nutrition Therapy

Persons with diabetes and those at risk for diabetes should receive individualized nutrition therapy as needed, preferably provided by an RDN familiar with the components of diabetes MNT, to achieve treatment goals.[4] The person with diabetes should be involved in the decision-making process.

Goal of Nutrition Therapy for Persons at Risk for Diabetes[4]:

◆ Decrease the risk for type 2 diabetes and CVD by promoting healthy food choices and physical activity leading to moderate weight loss that is maintained

Goals of Nutrition Therapy for All Persons With Diabetes[3]:

◆ Promote and support healthy eating patterns, emphasizing a variety of nutrient-dense foods in appropriate portion sizes, for the individual with diabetes to promote overall health and to
—Achieve and maintain blood glucose, lipid, and blood pressure goals as recommended by the ADA
—Achieve and maintain body weight goals
—Delay or prevent complications of diabetes

◆ Address individual nutritional needs, taking into consideration personal and cultural preferences, health literacy and numeracy, access to healthy food choices, lifestyle, and willingness and ability to make behavioral changes, as well as barriers to change

◆ Maintain the pleasure of eating by providing positive messages about food choices while limiting food choices only when indicated by scientific evidence

A Healthy Eating Pattern

With the emphasis on glycemic control and the immediate feedback provided through self-monitoring of blood glucose, healthcare providers and individuals with diabetes often focus on normalizing glycemia with little regard to nutritional needs. Optimal nutrition through healthy food choices remains the underlying principle of diabetes nutrition recommendations.[1–5]

Case: Type 2 Diabetes Treated With Glucose-Lowering Medications

LW, a 51-year-old woman with type 2 diabetes of 5 years' duration, was referred for diabetes education.

Nutrition Assessment

- Height: 64 in
- Weight: 175 lb
- Body mass index (BMI): 31 kg/m²

Medical Diagnosis

- Type 2 diabetes, obesity, hypertension, dyslipidemia

Lab Data

- A1C: 8.1%
- LDL-C: 160 mg/dL (8.879 mmol/L)
- HDL-C: 43 mg/dL (2.39 mmol/L)
- TG: 234 mg/dL (12.99 mmol/L)
- Blood pressure: 148/88 mm Hg

Medications

- Glimepiride (Amaryl®, Sanofi Aventis) 4 mg daily, for diabetes; metformin (Glucophage®, Bristol-Myers Squibb) 1000 mg bid, for diabetes
- Simvastatin (Zocor®, Merck) 20 mg daily, for dyslipidemia
- Quinapril (Accupril®, Pfizer) 20 mg daily, for hypertension

Nutrition History

LW stated that she either skips breakfast or eats a light breakfast in her car, eats lunch primarily at fast-food restaurants, and eats out for dinner about half of the time. She occasionally snacks on chips or other salty snacks in the afternoon and usually eats a bowl of sugar-free ice cream in the evening. She does not drink alcoholic beverages. A brief evaluation of LW's usual food/nutrition history reveals that her diet is high in total and saturated fat, is high in sodium, contains few fruits and vegetables, and appears low in fiber and calcium. LW asked if a low-carbohydrate, high-protein diet would help her lose weight and improve her glucose control. LW's job is sedentary. She said she does not have the time or energy to go to the gym after work.

Nutrition Diagnosis

Excessive intake of calories, sodium, and saturated fat related to eating frequently in restaurants and lack of portion control; low energy expenditure due to sedentary job and lack of regular physical activity.

Assessment of LW's metabolic status reveals that she exhibits characteristics common in type 2 diabetes. Markers of LW's increased cardiovascular risk are a pattern of dyslipidemia that includes elevated LDL cholesterol (LDL-C), low HDL cholesterol (HDL-C), and hypertriglyceridemia along with hypertension and obesity (BMI ≥30 kg/m²).

As the chapter progresses, readers will gain insight into the following regarding LW's case: What initial lifestyle changes can be suggested to improve her glycemic control? What aspects of nutrition therapy can reduce her cardiovascular risk? What are the risks and benefits of using a low-carbohydrate diet to achieve her goals?

A healthy eating pattern for all Americans emphasizes nutrient-dense foods and beverages—vegetables, fruits, whole grains, fat-free or low-fat milk and milk products, seafood, lean meats and poultry, eggs, legumes, and nuts and seeds—and limits intake of sodium, solid fats, added sugars, and refined grains.[10]

The ADA reviewed research studies on persons with diabetes on recommended eating patterns, including Mediterranean style, vegetarian and vegan, low-fat, low-carbohydrate, and DASH (Dietary Approaches to Stop Hypertension). It concluded that a variety of eating patterns are acceptable for the management of diabetes.[3] Personal preferences (eg, tradition, culture, religion, health beliefs and goals, economics) and metabolic goals should be considered when implementing one eating pattern over another.

> With nutrition therapy and increased physical activity, the effect on blood glucose level is evident almost immediately.

Nutrition Therapy and Glycemic Control

A primary goal in the management of diabetes is the regulation of blood glucose to achieve individualized blood glucose goals. With changes in lifestyle, the effect on blood glucose levels is evident almost immediately. Clinical trials and outcome studies of diabetes MNT have reported decreases in A1C levels at 3 to 6 months ranging from 0.25% to 2.9% (average 1%-2%), depending on the type and duration of diabetes and level of glycemia.[11] Multiple studies have demonstrated sustained improvements in A1C at 12 months and longer when an RDN provided follow-up encounters ranging from monthly sessions to 3 sessions per year.[1,3,11] Evaluation of the effectiveness of MNT on glucose should be done between 6 weeks and 3 months.[1,3] During this time it can be determined whether target goals can be achieved by implementation of MNT alone or whether medication(s) will need to be combined with MNT.

> Clinical trials and outcome studies of diabetes MNT have reported decreases in A1C levels at 3 to 6 months ranging from 0.25% to 2.9% (average 1%-2%), depending on the type and duration of diabetes and level of glycemia.

Attempts are often made to identify one approach to diabetes nutrition therapy; however, a single approach does not exist, just as there is no one medication or insulin regimen that applies to all persons with diabetes. A variety of interventions—such as reduced energy/fat intake, carbohydrate counting, simplified meal plans, healthy food choices, low-fat vegan diets, individualized meal-planning strategies, exchange choices, insulin-to-carbohydrate ratios, physical activity, and behavioral strategies—are all reported to be effective when implemented appropriately.[1,3,11] In reviewing consistent themes for nutrition interventions, it appears that, for individuals with type 2 diabetes, reducing the energy content of usual food intake is central to successful outcomes. For individuals with type 1 diabetes, adjusting insulin doses for planned carbohydrate intake is of primary importance.[11] Appropriate implementation of nutrition therapy is similar to other therapies which require regular follow-up and evaluation of effect, ease of implementation, adherence, and need for adjustment in therapy. Due to the need for daily adherence, continuous intervention to increase support and maintenance is also an essential component of nutrition care. The number and duration of nutrition encounters may need to be greater if the patient has language, ethnic, or cultural concerns or if the patient's medications have changed (such as the addition of glucose-lowering medications or insulin therapy in type 2 diabetes, or changes in insulin regimens in type 1 diabetes or type 2 diabetes).[1]

Macronutrients

Because all 3 macronutrients (carbohydrate, protein, and fat) require insulin for metabolism and influence the attaining of nutrition therapy goals, including healthy eating, they must be addressed. In the United States, the majority of persons with type 1 diabetes or type 2 diabetes report eating moderate amounts of carbohydrate (~45% of total energy intake) and getting ~35% to 40% of energy intake from fat, with the remainder (~16%-18%) from protein.[12] Generally, as carbohydrate intake decreases, total fat (usually saturated fats) increases. A number of studies have reported on differing percentages of carbohydrate intake in adults with diabetes. The Strong Health Study reported that a lower intake of carbohydrate and higher consumption of total and saturated fats were associated with poorer glycemic control.[13] Similarly, in subjects receiving intensive treatment in the Diabetes Control and Complications Trial (DCCT), diets lower in carbohydrate and higher in total and saturated fats were associated with worse glycemic control, independent of exercise and BMI.[14] However, in clinical trials, both high- and low-carbohydrate diets led to similar changes in body weight and A1C.[15] It appears likely that the total energy intake outweighs the amount of carbohydrate in the eating pattern. Higher carbohydrate diets, which are generally low in fat, tend to have beneficial effects on LDL-C and total cholesterol, whereas lower carbohydrate diets tend to have beneficial effects on triglycerides and HDL-C.[15] Evidence suggests that there is not an ideal percentage of calories from carbohydrate, protein, and fat for all persons with diabetes.[1-4] Therefore, because of the benefits and/or similarities in outcomes, it would seem prudent to recommend an eating pattern that has moderate amounts of carbohydrate and includes healthy sources of carbohydrate in appropriate amounts and portion sizes. The dietary reference intakes (DRIs) from the Food and Nutrition Board of the IOM provide guidance for macronutrient distribution in healthy adults and recommend 45% to 65% of calories from carbohydrate, 10% to 35% from protein, and 20% to 35% from fat.[16] The IOM also recommends not restricting carbohydrate to less than 130 g (minimum of 8-9 carbohydrate servings) per day for adults and children due to the absolute need for glucose as an energy source in the brain and central nervous system.[16]

Carbohydrate and Glycemia

Historically, it was a commonly held belief that sugars, such as sucrose, must be restricted on the assumption that they are more rapidly digested and absorbed than starches and thus aggravate hyperglycemia. However, scientific evidence does not support restricting sucrose based on this belief. Research consistently reports that the total amount of carbohydrate consumed at meals, regardless of the type or source (sucrose or starch), is the primary determinant of postprandial glucose levels. In approximately 20 studies in which sucrose was substituted for equal

amounts of other carbohydrate (starches), the glucose response was nearly identical.[17] Monitoring total grams of carbohydrate, whether by carbohydrate counting or experience-based estimation, is a key strategy in achieving glycemic control.[1-4] Day-to-day consistency in the amount of carbohydrate consumed at breakfast, lunch, and dinner and in snacks can also improve glycemic control, particularly in persons on nutrition therapy alone, glucose-lowering medications, or fixed insulin doses.[1-3]

For persons using multiple daily insulin doses or insulin pumps, adjusting the prandial insulin dose to match planned carbohydrate intake results in improved glucose control.[18] Insulin-to-carbohydrate ratios indicate how many grams of carbohydrate are "covered" or "matched" with 1 unit of prandial insulin. A glucose correction factor (insulin sensitivity factor [ISF]) is the estimated drop in blood glucose (mg/dL) expected from the administration of 1 unit of rapid- or short-acting insulin. The ISF is also related to the individual's insulin sensitivity and body size. A typical ISF for a normal weight adult with type 1 diabetes is 1:50 mg/dL (1 unit of rapid-acting insulin is expected to drop the blood glucose level 50 mg/dL). An overweight/insulin-resistant individual may have an ISF of 1:20 (1 unit of rapid-acting insulin is expected to drop the blood glucose level 20 mg/dL).[18]

After reviewing the evidence, the Academy of Nutrition and Dietetics Evidence-Based Nutrition Practice Guidelines (EBNPG) for Diabetes made the following recommendations regarding carbohydrate intake[1,2]:

- In persons on nutrition therapy alone, glucose-lowering medications, or fixed insulin doses, meal and snack carbohydrate intake should be kept consistent on a day-to-day basis.
- In persons with type 1 diabetes or type 2 diabetes who adjust their mealtime insulin doses or who are on insulin pump therapy, insulin doses should be adjusted to match carbohydrate intake (insulin-to-carbohydrate ratio). This can be accomplished by comprehensive nutrition education and counseling on interpretation of blood glucose patterns, nutrition-related medication management, and collaboration with the healthcare team.

Achieving Glycemic Control

Monitoring total grams of carbohydrate intake is a key strategy in achieving glycemic control. Day-to-day consistency in the amount of carbohydrate consumed can also improve glycemic control.

Sugars

Sugars include glucose, fructose, sucrose (table sugar), and lactose (milk sugar). When consumed separately, glucose causes the highest glycemic peak response compared with other sugars. This is because sugars such as sucrose and lactose are metabolized into only 50% glucose and the other 50% into fructose or galactose. Fructose and galactose are metabolized by the liver into glucose, glycogen, and/or triglycerides (in the case of fructose), but very little, if any, of the glucose enters into the general circulation.[19]

A recent review of studies conducted in persons with diabetes shows that naturally occurring fructose, such as that in fruit, may result in better glycemic control compared with isocaloric intake of sucrose or starch and is not likely to have detrimental effects on triglycerides (ie, if it is not consumed in excess amounts: >12% of total energy).[3,20,21] Excessive consumption of products marketed to individuals with diabetes that contain large amounts of naturally occurring fructose, such as agave nectar, is not recommended.[3]

Starches

The digestive tract is very efficient in breaking down starches to glucose. It is the ability of digestive enzymes to break down the starch, rather than the size of the starch molecule, that determines the glycemic effect of a particular starch. It also depends on the structure of the starch, the source of the starch, and the types of processing and cooking used. Starches composed of higher proportions of amylopectin, such as potatoes, have a greater effect on blood glucose levels than starchy foods that contain more amylose, such as certain types of rice.

Glycemic Index

The glycemic index (GI) is a system of ranking carbohydrate foods according to their effect on postprandial glycemia.[22] The glycemic effect (measured as the area under the curve) of 50 g of digestible carbohydrate from a single food is measured over a 2-hour period. The food is then assigned a percentage value compared with the response of a reference food (glucose or bread). For example, if the area under the curve for a food is three fourths of that of the reference food, it has a GI of 75, or 75%. Diet books and health professionals often claim that the GI measures how rapidly blood glucose levels increase after eating carbohydrate foods, implying that high-GI foods peak rapidly and low-GI foods have a more gradual peak response. However, although the area under the curve for various foods may differ, the general curve shape, including the peak response, is similar within each food category.[22] Therefore, it is incorrect to state that a high-GI food peaks very rapidly and a low-GI food peaks more gradually.

The GI was first developed in 1981 and has been controversial since that time. The variability of the GI responses within and among individuals is a concern. For example, Australian potatoes are reported to have a high GI, whereas potatoes in the United States and Canada have moderate GIs.[23] The mean glycemic response and standard deviation of 50 g of carbohydrate from white bread tested in 23 subjects was 78 ± 73 with an interindividual coefficient of variation (CV) of 94%. The GI values obtained for bread were broad, ranging from 44 to 132 for the mean of 3 tests with a CV of 30%, although the average GI was 71%, nearly identical to the mean value used for reference purposes.[24]

Two trials, each 1 year in duration, reported no significant differences in A1C levels from low-GI versus high-GI diets[25] or ADA diets[26] at study end. Wolever et al noted that their results do not agree with previous meta-analyses showing that low-GI diets reduce A1C levels.[25] However, previous meta-analyses were based largely on studies lasting less than 3 months, and in their study a trend toward lower A1C levels at 3 months was also observed but was not sustained for 1 year.

The GI is not always an indicator of healthy food or meal choices. Very early, Wolever et al noted that one of the strongest correlates of overall diet GI is the intake of simple sugars—low-GI diets are associated with significantly higher sugar intakes than high-GI diets.[27] Many high-sugar foods fall into the moderate- or low-GI categories. For example, Coke (GI = 58), a Snickers bar (GI = 56), and ice cream (GI = 36-80) have moderate GI values, whereas premium ice cream (GI = 37) has a low GI value.[28] Sugars have moderate to low GI values because they are only 50% glucose (the other 50% being fructose or lactose, depending on the sugar), while starches have higher GIs because they are polymers of glucose and have the potential to be metabolized to 100% glucose. Wolever further reports that whole wheat, brown rice, and brown spaghetti have the same GI values as their refined white versions, and whereas fruits generally have a low GI, whole fruits and juice have the same GI.[29]

The glucose response to a food is influenced not only by the glycemic response but also by the amount of carbohydrate in the food. The glycemic load (GL) of foods (or meals) takes into account both the quantity of food consumed and the GI value of the food. The GL is determined by multiplying the GI of the food by the grams of carbohydrate in a serving of food (or for meals by totaling the values for all foods in the meal). For example, GIs for carrots and watermelon are 92 and 72, respectively, but a half cup of carrots has a GL of 5 (.92 × 5 g = 5) and 1 cup of watermelon has a GL of 9 (.72 × 12 g = 9). So although they have a relatively high GI value, their GL is low. In contrast, pizza has a GI of 60, and a 10-oz serving has a GL of 42 (.60 × 70 g = 42). Therefore, carrots and watermelon would be expected to have minimal effect on glucose response compared with pizza, which has a higher GL even though it has a lower GI.

The Academy of Nutrition and Dietetics EBNPG states that studies comparing the GIs of meals, ranging from 2 to 12 weeks and longer (1 year), report mixed effects on A1C levels.[1,2] These studies are complicated by differing definitions of "high GI" and "low GI" diets or quartiles. Although GI results are commonly interpreted as low GI <55, moderate GI 56 to 69, and high GI >70, these categories have not been used consistently in research studies. GIs in the low-GI diets range from 38% to 77% and in the high-GI diets from 63% to 98%.

The ADA systematic review of macronutrients concluded that, in general, there is little difference in glycemic control and CVD risk factors between low-GI and high-GI or other diets.[30] A slight improvement in glycemia may result from a lower GI diet; however, this is confounded by a higher fiber intake. It also notes the need to standardize definitions of low, moderate, and high GIs.

Fiber

The average amount of fiber a person in the United States consumes (10-20 g per day) does not appear to affect glycemia. Fiber studies that have shown improved glycemia included diets containing ~44 to 50 g of fiber per day,[1-3] an amount that may be difficult for many Americans to consume due to the palatability and gastrointestinal side effects. It is recommended that persons with diabetes include foods containing 25 to 38 g of fiber per day, which is the amount recommended for the general public (14 g/1000 calories).[3,16] An emphasis on soluble fiber sources (7-13 g) is recommended.[1,2] Fiber-containing foods are encouraged because they provide vitamins, minerals, and other nutrients important for good health.

Of interest is how to account for the fiber in carbohydrate for carbohydrate counting, as it is incompletely digested, absorbed, and metabolized. In deriving energy values for food labeling, the dietary fiber portion of carbohydrate is calculated as having about half the energy (2 kcal/g) of most other carbohydrates (4 kcal/g).[31] Adjustment in total carbohydrate is practical only if the amount per serving of dietary fiber is >5 g. In that case, subtract half of the fiber grams from the total carbohydrate and only for individuals who are using insulin-to-carbohydrate ratios for managing their diabetes.[31]

Sugar-Sweetened Beverages

The 2013 ADA nutrition recommendations, for the first time, advise avoiding sugar-sweetened beverages (soft drinks, fruit drinks, and energy and vitamin water drinks containing sucrose, high-fructose corn syrup, and/or fruit juice concentrates).[3] Large quantities of sugar-sweetened beverages should be avoided to reduce the risk of worsening the cardiometabolic risk profile and to prevent weight gain.[3,32,33] The ADA also recommends that individuals at risk for type 2 diabetes be encouraged to limit their intake of sugar-sweetened beverages.[4] In a meta-analysis of cohort studies, individuals in the highest versus lowest quartile of sugar-sweetened beverage intake had a 26% greater risk of developing diabetes.[34]

Nonnutritive and Hypocaloric Sweeteners

The Food and Drug Administration (FDA) has approved the use of acesulfame potassium, aspartame, neotame, saccharin, and sucralose as food additives; stevia is approved as "generally recognized as safe" (GRAS). The FDA also determines an acceptable daily intake (ADI) for each nonnutritive sweetener. The ADI is the amount that can be safely consumed on a daily basis over a person's lifetime without adverse effects and generally includes a hundredfold safety factor. It should be noted that many food products containing nonnutritive sweeteners may also contain energy and carbohydrate from other sources that need to be accounted for.[1,3]

A scientific statement from the American Heart Association and the ADA concluded that when used judiciously, nonnutritive sweeteners could facilitate reductions in added sugars intake, thereby resulting in decreased total energy and weight loss/weight control, and promoting beneficial effects on related metabolic parameters. They noted, however, that potential benefits will not be achieved if there is a compensatory increase in energy intake from other sources.[35]

Food products that contain sugar alcohols do impact glycemia. Studies have shown that most sugar alcohols—including erythritol, hydrogenated starch hydrolysates, isomalt, lactitol, maltitol, mannitol, sorbitol, and xylitol—produce a smaller rise in blood glucose. However, there is no evidence that sugar alcohols in amounts likely to be consumed improve long-term glycemia, energy intake, or weight, and although safe to use, they may cause diarrhea, especially in children.[1]

Protein and Glycemia

Although 50% to 60% of ingested protein undergoes gluconeogenesis in the liver, studies have demonstrated that glucose produced from protein does not increase blood glucose concentrations.[1-3] Ingestion of protein results in an acute stimulation of insulin secretion similar to that of carbohydrate but has no long-term effect on insulin requirements. Because it stimulates the release of insulin, protein should not be used to treat or prevent hypoglycemia.[3,4] For persons with diabetes, there is insufficient evidence to suggest that usual protein intake (15%-20% of energy) be changed. For individuals with diabetic kidney disease with either micro- or macroalbuminuria, reducing the amount of protein does not alter

the course of glomerular filtration rate, glycemic measures, or CVD risk measures[3,30] and therefore is not recommended.

Fat and Glycemia

It is also a widely held belief that dietary fat alters the predicted postprandial response to a carbohydrate-containing meal. Dietary fats are said to slow glucose absorption and delay the peak glycemic response to the ingestion of carbohydrate foods. However, evidence to support this belief is difficult to find. Studies show that fat ingested with a carbohydrate meal had minimal postprandial effects on glucose and had either no effect on insulin levels or a slightly greater insulin response.[36] In an early study in subjects with type 2 diabetes, 5, 15, 30, or 50 g of fat (butter) was added to 50 g of carbohydrate (potato), resulting in a mean plasma glucose area response that was similar after ingestion of the potato with or without the various amounts of butter.[37] In another study in subjects with type 2 diabetes, 30 ml of olive oil either was ingested 30 minutes before ingesting a potato or was ingested with the potato.[38] The ingestion of fat before the carbohydrate markedly slowed gastric emptying and lowered the postprandial rise in glucose and insulin. However, when the fat was ingested with the carbohydrate, which is how fat is usually consumed, the effect on gastric emptying and glucose and insulin was not significant. In a similar study, the effects of 50 g of carbohydrate alone (control) or with 100 g of butter or 80 g of olive oil were compared.[36] Again, the addition of both added fats had no effect on glucose or insulin postprandial responses and does not support a commonly heard statement that adding fat to carbohydrates slows the glycemic response.

In subjects with type 1 diabetes, an early study reported that the addition of 200 kcal from fat (20 g of fat) to a standard meal did not increase the glucose response or insulin requirements.[39] A more recent small study utilizing continuous glucose sensor technology reported that when 50 g of fat was added to a dinner with identical amounts of carbohydrate and protein, the high-fat dinner required 3 more units of bolus insulin and, despite the extra insulin, caused more hyperglycemia after the meal.[40] This would suggest that when persons with type 1 diabetes eat a meal with an unusually high amount of fat, they may need to make adjustments in their bolus insulin. However, most persons tend to keep the protein and fat content of their meals fairly consistent. Their need for insulin is likely covered by the basal insulin dose, as the bolus insulin dose covers the carbohydrate content of the meal. But when excessive amounts of fat (and protein) are eaten, extra bolus insulin may be needed to supplement the basal dose.

Epidemiological data and clinical trials implicate chronic intake of higher levels of total dietary fat, especially saturated fats, in the development of insulin resistance.[41,42] Studies suggest that reduced intake of fat, particularly saturated fat, may improve insulin sensitivity independent of energy restriction.[42,43] In addition, unsaturated fats may have a beneficial effect on insulin action.

Vitamin and Mineral Supplementation and Glycemia

Nutrition therapy should include education on how to acquire adequate amounts of vitamins and minerals from food sources. There is no clear evidence of benefits from vitamin and mineral supplementation in individuals with diabetes who do not have underlying deficiencies.[3] For select groups of individuals, such as the elderly, pregnant or lactating women, vegetarians, and those on energy-restricted diets, a multivitamin supplement may be necessary. Supplementation above the tolerable upper intake level (UL) established by the IOM increases the risk of adverse effects and should be considered only after review of safety and efficacy determined by controlled clinical trials.[44] Routine supplementation of antioxidants such as vitamins C and E and beta-carotene is not advised due to possible adverse effects and the lack of efficacy shown in large placebo-controlled clinical trials.[3]

Recent attention on the prevalence of vitamin D deficiency has raised questions about intake recommendations and supplemental needs. In addition, questions have been raised about its possible role in diabetes.[45] A meta-analysis of observational studies assessing the association between blood levels of 25(OH)D and risk of type 2 diabetes reported an inverse and significant association.[46] However, a randomized controlled trial (RCT) in persons with prediabetes and hypovitaminosis D using high doses

of vitamin D for 1 year reported no effect of the supplement on insulin secretion, insulin sensitivity, or the development of diabetes compared with the placebo.[47] Chromium supplementation has been studied for its potential influence on glycemia, insulin resistance, and body weight. Current studies have not conclusively demonstrated efficacy.[48] Evidence is lacking to support the routine use of micronutrients and other herbs/supplements for the treatment of diabetes.

For information on the use of herbal preparations, see chapter 20, on biological complementary therapies in diabetes.

Physical Activity and Glycemia

Physical activity and nutrition therapy should be considered complementary therapies that together promote optimal glycemic control and reduced risk for chronic diseases. In persons with type 2 diabetes, studies have reported improvements in glucose control and insulin sensitivity, reduced cardiovascular risk, assistance with weight management, and improved well-being from regular physical activity.[1,4] In persons with type 1 diabetes, physical activity confers significant health benefits such as improving insulin sensitivity, increasing cardiovascular fitness, and improving muscle strength.[4] However, it also has potential negative effects related to hypo- and hyperglycemic excursions unless variations in activity are carefully monitored and planned for. In individuals at risk for diabetes, a combination of regular physical activity and weight loss significantly reduces the risk of developing diabetes.[49] In overweight and sedentary persons and in persons with type 2 diabetes, both exercise and energy restriction independently and additively reduce glucose and insulin levels.[50]

In persons with type 2 diabetes, 150 minutes of accumulated moderate-intensity aerobic physical activity per week as well as resistance training 3 times per week is recommended.[1,4,49] Both improve glycemic control, independent of weight loss. Individuals with type 1 diabetes are also encouraged to engage in regular physical activity for the overall health benefits, even though exercise may not improve glycemic control. To accommodate physical activity, safety guidelines to prevent hypoglycemia are important. These include frequent glucose monitoring, possible adjustments in insulin dose or carbohydrate intake, and carrying carbohydrate while exercising.

See chapters 5 and 17, on the self-care behaviors related to being active and exercise prescription, for more information.

When to Expect Results

Evaluation of the effectiveness of nutrition therapy on glucose should be done between 6 weeks and 3 months. During this time it can be determined whether target goals have been achieved by implementation of nutrition therapy or whether medication(s) will need to be combined with nutrition therapy.

Alcohol and Glycemia

Moderate amounts of alcohol (1 drink or less per day for adult women and 2 drinks or less per day for adult men) ingested with food have minimal, if any, effect on glucose and insulin concentrations.[3,51] The type of alcohol-containing beverage consumed does not appear to make a difference. One alcohol-containing beverage is defined as 12 oz beer, 5 oz wine, or 1.5 oz distilled spirits. Each contains approximately 15 g of alcohol. Excessive amounts of alcohol (3 or more drinks per day) on a consistent basis can contribute to hyperglycemia.[51] Individuals using insulin or insulin secretagogues should consume food with alcohol to avoid hypoglycemia. Blood glucose testing should be used to determine whether extra carbohydrate and/ or a reduction in insulin will be needed to reduce the risk of hypoglycemia during the night or the next morning following consumption of alcohol the previous evening.[52]

There is a U-shaped relationship between alcohol consumption and risk for diabetes.[53] Compared with nondrinkers, moderate drinkers have a lower risk for diabetes, while those who consume more than 3 drinks daily have a greater risk for diabetes. People with a history of alcohol abuse or dependence, women who are pregnant, and people with medical problems such as liver disease, pancreatitis, advanced neuropathy, or severe hypertriglyceridemia should abstain from alcohol.

Case—Part 2: Improving Glycemic Control

Nutrition Intervention

One of LW's initial short-term goals is to improve glycemic control. In evaluating her usual meals and food choices, she can make a few small changes that may make a significant difference in her blood glucose control. LW appears to be consuming the bulk of her calories and carbohydrate later in the day, often skipping breakfast, eating a light lunch, and eating a heavier dinner. Studies show that eating fairly consistent amounts of carbohydrate spaced throughout the day can improve glycemia. Despite selecting sugar-free ice cream, LW has been ingesting a significant amount of carbohydrate and calories after dinner.

LW can begin with a basic carbohydrate-counting meal-planning approach with carbohydrate spaced throughout the day. Monitoring her blood glucose levels 2 hours after meals will reinforce the effect of varying amounts of carbohydrates on her blood glucose levels. (Chapter 4, on healthy eating, provides a basic explanation of carbohydrate counting.)

LW is also encouraged to begin some type of physical activity, such as brisk walking, to further improve her glycemic control. She is instructed to begin slowly and work toward a goal of accumulating 150 minutes of physical activity per week. A pedometer is recommended as a motivational tool to encourage LW to take more steps in a day. She is also encouraged to add muscle-strengthening activities. Her glycemic control will be evaluated initially with blood glucose records, but after she has implemented her lifestyle changes an A1C test will be done (in ~6-10 weeks) to determine whether she needs to make any changes in her glucose-lowering medication(s).

Nutrition Goals

Follow carbohydrate-counting plan to include limiting carbohydrate to 45 g per meal and 15 g for evening snack; record food/carbohydrate intake and exercise performed for 7 days prior to return visit; walk briskly for at least 30 minutes 4 days per week; and monitor blood glucose twice a day, alternating before and 2 hours after breakfast, lunch, and dinner.

Monitoring and Evaluation

Follow up in 3 weeks to assess glycemic control via blood glucose records, review food and activity records, and monitor weight change.

Nutrition Therapy and Weight Management

A major challenge in diabetes care is the high incidence of overweight and obesity in persons with or at risk for type 2 diabetes. Weight loss is an important goal for overweight or obese persons at risk for diabetes, as it prevents or delays the onset of diabetes. In persons with diabetes, the role of weight loss is controversial. Providers need to be alert to any weight increases and intervene early to assist their patients in weight management.

Weight Loss Effectiveness

A moderate weight loss of 5% to 10% can reduce the risk of developing type 2 diabetes and improve glycemia, primarily in individuals who are insulin resistant, including those with prediabetes and early-onset type 2 diabetes.[4,54,55] However, as the disease progresses and individuals become more insulin deficient, weight loss may or may not significantly improve glycemia.[3,56] With insulin deficiency, additional glucose-lowering medications combined with nutrition therapy are necessary, and prevention of weight gain rather than weight loss becomes the priority.

A review of randomized clinical trials of weight loss interventions from January 1, 2000, to February 1, 2013, with a duration of 12 months and 70% completion rate reported mixed benefits from weight loss in persons with diabetes.[56] Eleven trials met the study criteria. Weight losses from interventions ranged from 1.9 to 8.4 kg at 12 months; however, 9 of the studies reported weight losses ranging from 2.4 to 4.8 kg. A Mediterranean-style diet (MED) implemented in subjects with newly diagnosed diabetes and the Look AHEAD (Action for Health in Diabetes) intensive lifestyle intervention (ILI) reported the largest weight loss at 1 year, 6.2 kg and 8.4 kg, respectively,[57,58] and a low-carbohydrate intervention the smallest, 1.9 kg.[59] Five of the studies reported improvements in A1C at 12 months from a weight loss intervention; however, 6 studies reported nonsignificant changes in A1C from weight loss interventions. The most consistently positive change in lipids was in HDL-C; however, all but the ILI and MED reported nonsignificant changes in various lipids as a result of weight loss. Five studies reported positive blood pressure changes, and 3 studies reported no changes. It appears likely that many persons with type 2 diabetes, unless they are newly diagnosed or receive an intensive intervention as provided in the Look AHEAD trial, find it difficult to lose sufficient weight at 1 year to experience improvements in A1C values, lipids, and blood pressure.

Of the 11 studies, 5 compared weight loss interventions with differing macronutrient percentages (high monounsaturated fat vs. high carbohydrate,[60] low carbohydrate vs. low fat,[59,61] and high protein vs. high carbohydrate[62,63]). All 5 reported that weight changes at 1 year did not differ statistically between groups, and weight losses ranged from 1.9 to 4.0 kg. Furthermore, 4 studies reported nonsignificant changes in A1C from baseline to study end,[59–61,63] and only 1 reported significant but modest changes in A1C in both study groups.[62]

Because of its size and duration, the Look AHEAD trial is of importance. It was conducted in 16 centers across the United States in an attempt to determine the effectiveness of intentional weight loss interventions in reducing rates of heart disease, stroke, and CVD deaths in overweight and obese persons with type 2 diabetes.[58] Half of the 5145 participants randomized to the ILI received meal replacements or structured food plans, were encouraged to achieve 175 minutes of physical activity a week, and attended 3 to 4 education/counseling sessions per month. The other half, the control group, received a general program of diabetes support and education. The trial was stopped early on the basis of a futility analysis with a median follow-up of 9.6 years.[64] The ILI resulted in greater weight loss at study end (6.0% vs. 3.5%) as well as greater improvements in fitness and all CVD risk factors, except for LDL-C. However, the ILI intervention did not reduce the rate of CVD events in the participants.

In general, weight loss intervention (WLI) studies report that individuals lose, on average, 5% to 10% of their starting weight by 6 months, at which time weight loss reaches a plateau.[65] Adaptive mechanisms occur with a reduced energy intake (eg, hormonal regulation, adaptive thermogenesis leading to a decrease in energy expenditure, and decline in basal energy requirement), and, at this point, maintenance of the weight loss should become the focus of the ongoing care and intervention. In studies extending to 48 months, a 3% to 6% weight loss from starting weight was maintained.[65]

The studies reviewed above show a pattern of weight loss that is similar for persons with diabetes, but in the majority of the studies, weight loss was less than 5% between 6 and 12 months in persons with diabetes.[56] Therefore, energy restriction, with or without weight loss, and healthy eating should be the focus of nutrition therapy interventions for persons with type 2 diabetes.

Nutrition Therapy for Weight Management

Nutrition therapy interventions that use a behavioral approach, combine a reduction in energy intake with an increase in physical activity, and provide ongoing counseling and support are needed for beneficial outcomes. Evidence supports the fact that weight loss is primarily associated with energy deficit, diet adherence, and enthusiasm of the counselor, but not with nutrient composition.[66,67] Advice for reducing energy intake should be individualized to account for food preferences and the individual's preferred approach for reducing energy intake.

Nutrition interventions shown to be effective in weight management programs include the following: (1) an individualized reduced-energy diet, (2) total energy intake distributed throughout the day, with the consumption of 4 to 5 meals/snacks per day, including breakfast, (3) portion control emphasized, and (4) meal replacements (eg, liquid meals, meal bars, calorie-controlled packaged meals) for persons who have difficulty with self-selection and/or portion control.[68] In addition, a variety of behavioral strategies that have shown to be helpful can be employed (eg, self-monitoring, stress management, stimulus control, problem solving, contingency management, cognitive restructuring, and social support).[68]

Energy Restriction

Energy restriction, with or without weight loss, and healthy eating should be the focus of nutrition therapy interventions for persons with type 2 diabetes.

Physical Activity and Weight Management

Physical activity is a key component of a comprehensive weight management program. Physical activity and exercise, by themselves, have only a modest weight loss effect. They are to be encouraged because they improve insulin sensitivity independent of weight loss, acutely lower blood glucose, and greatly improve the prospects for long-term weight maintenance.[69] Guidelines for physical activity should take into account a person's ability, safety, willingness, age, previous physical activity level, and conditions that might contraindicate certain types of exercise or predispose the person to injury.[4,49] Individuals should gradually increase duration and frequency of moderate-intensity aerobic physical activity to 150 minutes per week and resistance training to 3 times per week, when possible. Longer activity levels of at least 1 to 1½ hours per day of moderate activity may be needed to achieve successful long-term weight loss and maintenance.

Chapters 5 and 17, on the self-management behaviors related to being active and exercise prescription, provide more information.

Challenges With Pharmacologic Therapy

Diabetes pharmacotherapy often presents an additional challenge to the diabetes care team—in that weight gain often accompanies glucose-lowering pharmacologic therapy, hampering the individual's efforts at weight loss. Diabetes medications that can increase weight include sulfonylureas, thiazolidinediones, meglitinides, and insulin. GLP-1 agonists (exenatide, liraglutide) and pramlintide can result in weight loss, and metformin, alpha-glucosidase inhibitors, DPP-4 inhibitors, and canagliflozin are weight neutral.[70] Decisions are often made to accept some weight gain in exchange for improved glycemic control.

Some clinicians assume that weight gain with the addition of insulin therapy is inevitable. For this reason, clinicians and patients are often reluctant to initiate insulin or intensify treatment despite the need shown by elevated A1C levels. This delay in starting insulin can cause a greater increase in weight gain once insulin is initiated than if insulin was initiated in a timely manner.[71] The weight gain is largely due to a return to previous body weight prior to weight loss due to inadequate insulin and not additional weight gain beyond the person's previous established weight. Engaging patients in nutrition therapy can help them avoid or minimize weight gain so that glycemic control is optimized, long-term complications are minimized, and quality of life is maintained.[72]

Weight Loss Medications and Bariatric Surgery

Weight loss medications currently approved by the FDA are orlistat (Xenical® and Alli®, Hoffman La Roche Ltd), Belviq® (lorcaserin hydrochloride, Arena Pharmaceuticals), and Qsymia™ (phentermine and controlled-release topiramate, Vivus, Inc). Contrave® (bupropion and naltrexone, Orexigen Therapeutics, Inc) is under investigation. Only orlistat has been well studied in persons with diabetes.

Gastric reduction surgery—either gastric banding or procedures that bypass, transpose, or resect sections of the small intestine—when part of a comprehensive team approach, has been shown to be an effective treatment for severe obesity.[4] A recent multisite study of long-term remission and relapse in persons with type 2 diabetes following gastric bypass reported that the gastric bypass surgery was associated with durable remission of type 2 diabetes in many but not all persons; about one third experienced a relapse within 5 years of initial remission.[73] Predictors of relapse were poor glycemic control prior to surgery, insulin use, and longer diabetes duration. The ADA recommends that bariatric surgery be considered for adults with a BMI ≥35 kg/m² and type 2 diabetes, especially if the diabetes or associated comorbidities are difficult to control with nutrition therapy and pharmacologic therapy.[4] These patients will need lifelong lifestyle support and medical monitoring. The ADA cautions, however, that there is currently insufficient evidence

to generally recommend surgery in patients with a BMI <35 kg/m² outside a research protocol.

Nutrition Therapy and the Prevention and Treatment of CVD

Persons with diabetes are at a three- to fourfold increased risk of CVD, which is particularly evident in younger age groups and in women. They have the equivalent CVD risk of persons with preexisting CVD and no diabetes.[74] Closely linked to prediabetes and type 2 diabetes is the metabolic syndrome, the clustering of risk factors including abdominal obesity, physical inactivity, hypertension, atherogenic dyslipidemia, a prothrombotic state, and glucose intolerance. Nutrition therapy and aerobic physical activity are integral to the prevention and treatment of CVD in diabetes. Both glycemic control and cardioprotective nutrition interventions improve the lipid profile and blood pressure and should be addressed in counseling all individuals with prediabetes or type 2 diabetes.

Nutrition Therapy and Dyslipidemia

In persons with prediabetes or diabetes, triglycerides are often elevated, HDL-C is generally decreased, and LDL-C may be elevated, borderline, or normal. LDL particles are small and dense, resulting in more LDL particles for any cholesterol concentration. In addition, these small, dense particles are more atherogenic, as they may be more readily oxidized and glycated. The primary goal in persons with diabetes or prediabetes is to achieve LDL-C goals to reduce cardiovascular risk.[4]

Primary goals of cardioprotective nutrition therapy are to maintain the pleasure of eating with a healthy eating pattern while focusing on major strategies such as reducing saturated and *trans* fatty acids, and dietary cholesterol. Beneficial effects of fiber, phytostanols/phytosterols, omega-3 fatty acids, a Mediterranean-style eating pattern, and other plant-based approaches on atherogenic potential are reported.[75] In persons without diabetes, these nutrition therapy interventions improve the lipid profile, even in the absence of weight loss. Although fewer

---

Case—Part 3: Weight Loss

LW's weight puts her at risk for CVD and other comorbidities. Cutting her daily caloric intake by 500 calories is recommended, even though the weight loss might not significantly improve LW's blood glucose levels, due to the duration of her diabetes and any significant beta cell dysfunction she may have. The diabetes care team might consider the use of antidiabetic medications that can result in weight loss, the GLP-1 agonists (exenatide, liraglutide), in place of the sulfonylurea (glimepiride) that LW is currently taking that can increase weight.

---

studies examining these benefits have been conducted in persons with diabetes, since the 2 groups have equivalent CVD risks, the nutrition therapy recommendations for persons with diabetes are the same as for individuals with preexisting CVD and the general public.

Dietary Fat and Cholesterol

There is insufficient evidence to support the recommendation of a specific amount of total fat intake for people with diabetes; therefore, the goals should be individualized.[3,4] Data suggest that quality of fat is more important than quantity in attaining metabolic goals and reducing the risk of CVD.[3,76] Saturated and *trans* fats are the major components in the diet that increase LDL-C levels. Dietary cholesterol can also raise LDL-C. Due to limited research regarding optimal dietary saturated fat, cholesterol, and *trans* fat in persons with diabetes, recommendations are the same as for the general population. Saturated fat should be reduced to <10% of total energy intake, dietary cholesterol to <300 mg per day, and *trans* fat limited as much as possible.[3,4]

Unsaturated fats, including both monounsaturated (MUFA) and polyunsaturated fatty acids, have been shown to improve blood lipid levels.[3,75] Evidence from large prospective cohort studies, clinical trials, and a systematic review of RCTs reports that high-MUFA diets are associated with improved glycemic control and CVD risk.[30,76,77] Replacing calories from saturated fats with unsaturated fats has been shown to lower LDL-C.[78]

Dietary intake of omega-3 fatty acids from both plant sources (alpha-linolenic acid) and marine sources (eicosapentaenoic [EPA] and docasahexanoic [DHA] acids) is recommended; however, evidence does not support recommending omega-3 supplements.[3] Also recommended is 2 or more servings of fish per week (with the exception of commercially fried fish filets), particularly fatty fish (ie, salmon, herring, and mackerel), along with food sources of alpha-linolenic acid (ie, canola and soybean oil, flaxseed, and English walnuts [the type most commonly sold in the United States]).[79]

Fiber

The addition of fiber, especially soluble fiber, can further reduce LDL-C levels. A fat-modified diet that provides 25 to 30 g of total dietary fiber, including at least 7 to 13 g of soluble fiber (such as oatmeal or oat bran, apples, pears, psyllium, barley, and legumes), is recommended.[79]

Plant Stanols/Plant Sterols

Plant stanols and sterols and their esters come from different plant sources but are all cholesterol-reducing food ingredients that lower LDL-C in a similar way. Because of their similarity to cholesterol, they interfere with dietary and biliary cholesterol absorption in the intestinal tract and thus lower LDL-C levels.[3,79] The amounts naturally present in foods are small, and therefore stanol- or sterol-fortified foods or supplements are necessary. Use of fortified food products that provide ~2 g per day of plant stanols or sterols has been shown to reduce LDL-C and total cholesterol levels.[80] Individuals with hypercholesterolemia can consume 2 to 3 g of plant sterols or stanols to improve LDL-C and total cholesterol levels. Two to four servings of various foods fortified with plant stanols/sterols such as spreads, orange juice, cheese, or yogurt are needed to provide 2 g per day. Calories from these foods need to be considered in the overall food plan.

Mediterranean-Style Eating Pattern

In a large, prospective cohort study, adherence to a Mediterranean diet was associated with a lower risk of diabetes.[81] In a randomized clinical trial, after 4 years patients who were assigned to a Mediterranean-style eating pattern had better glycemic control and were less likely to need antidiabetic medications than patients assigned to a low-fat diet.[57] A Mediterranean-style, monounsaturated fat–rich eating pattern can be recommended in place of a low-fat, higher carbohydrate eating plan.[3] Characteristics of a Mediterranean eating pattern are a high ratio of monounsaturated fats (mainly olive oil) to saturated fats; moderate alcohol consumption; high consumption of legumes, fruits, vegetables, and nonrefined cereals, including bread; low consumption of meat and meat products; and moderate consumption of milk and dairy products.[82]

Alcohol and Dyslipidemia/CVD Risk

In persons with type 2 diabetes, studies show that mild to moderate alcohol consumption (≤1 to 2 drinks per day) is associated with a reduced risk of coronary heart disease and reduced total mortality rates from coronary heart disease and total mortality rates,[83] likely related to improved insulin sensitivity.[84] Moderate amounts of alcohol have not been shown to have a detrimental effect on triglyceride levels and may even have a beneficial effect.[85,86] However, it is recommended that individuals with severe hypertriglyceridemia abstain from alcohol.[3] The available evidence does not support recommending alcohol consumption in persons who do not currently drink. However, for the majority of people who choose to drink alcohol in moderation, alcohol consumption does not need to be discouraged.

Physical Activity and Dyslipidemia/CVD Risk

Strong evidence supports the role of exercise and physical activity in reducing the risk factors for CVD in adults without diabetes. In persons with diabetes, physical activity improves insulin sensitivity and decreases risk for CVD and all-cause mortality.[87,88] Fitness attenuates, but does not completely eliminate, risk, underscoring the importance of promoting regular physical activity, following a cardioprotective eating pattern, and maintaining a healthy weight. A review of the effects of aerobic exercise in participants without diabetes reported increases in HDL-C and reductions in triglycerides, LDL-C, and total cholesterol.[89] However, in a meta-analysis examining the effects of aerobic exercise on lipids and lipoproteins in adults with type 2 diabetes, the authors concluded that exercise lowers LDL-C by about 5%, but no significant improvements were found on other lipid values.[90]

Macrovascular disease prevention and treatment are further discussed in chapter 25. Pharmacotherapy for dyslipidemia and hypertension is the topic of chapter 19.

Nutrition Therapy and the Prevention and Treatment of Hypertension

Randomized controlled trials have demonstrated that lowering blood pressure to <140 mm Hg systolic and <80 mm Hg diastolic can reduce the risk of microvascular and macrovascular complications in persons with diabetes.[4,91,92] Management of hypertension has been demonstrated to reduce the rate and progression of diabetic nephropathy and to reduce complications of hypertensive nephropathy, CVD, and cerebrovascular disease.[74] Adoption of healthy lifestyle strategies is critical for the prevention of high blood pressure and is an indispensable part of the management of high blood pressure for those with hypertension.[91]

Lifestyle modifications effective in preventing and managing hypertension include weight loss, the DASH eating plan, high potassium intake, reduced sodium intake, moderate alcohol intake, and physical activity.[4,92–94] Several studies have demonstrated the additive effects of combining lifestyle interventions.[95–98]

Weight Loss and Hypertension

Obesity and overweight, particularly abdominal obesity, have consistently correlated closely with increased blood pressure independent of other risk factors for hypertension.[99] In almost all weight-reduction studies in the general population, systemic blood pressure was reduced, even if the degree of weight loss was small.[99,100] The JNC 7 (Joint National Committee) summary reports that a 5- to 10-mm Hg reduction in systolic blood pressure is possible per 10 kg of weight loss.[91] However, in persons with diabetes, there is variability in the blood pressure response to weight loss.[56]

DASH Eating Plan

The DASH Trial showed that a diet high in fruits, vegetables, and low-fat dairy foods and low in total fat, saturated fat, and cholesterol significantly reduced blood pressure in the absence of weight change and at sodium intakes typical of those living in the United States.[101] The beneficial effect on blood pressure from the DASH eating plan is likely due to a combination of factors, none of which can be specifically identified from this study. In a small study in people with type 2 diabetes, the DASH eating plan, which included a sodium restriction of 2300 mg per day, improved A1C, blood pressure, and other CVD risk factors.[94]

Sodium and Hypertension

Moderate sodium restriction (~2300 mg per day) has been shown to be an effective strategy in the prevention and treatment of hypertension among the general population, not specifically those with diabetes,[91] and is recommended for the general public. Several studies have demonstrated that reducing sodium intake significantly reduces blood pressure in hypertensive and normotensive individuals, independent of other risk factors for hypertension.[95,96] The DASH-Sodium Trial showed that lower sodium intakes resulted in greater reductions in blood pressure. Combining sodium restriction and the DASH eating plan had the greatest effect on blood pressure.[101] Sodium restriction is likely to be of greater benefit in people with diabetes, as they are reported to have a greater sensitivity to sodium causing hypertension as compared with people without diabetes.[92] However, in both persons with type 2 diabetes and persons with type 1 diabetes, a lower 24-hour urinary sodium excretion (suggesting a lower sodium intake) was associated with increased all-cause and cardiovascular mortality or end-stage renal disease.[92] Although associations do not demonstrate causality, these findings suggest that recommendations for a lower sodium intake in people with diabetes should be individualized and made with caution.[3]

Physical Activity and Hypertension

Physical activity is an important strategy for the prevention and treatment of high blood pressure. Persons who are less active and less fit have a greater risk for high blood pressure. Clinical trials have demonstrated that regular aerobic activity reduces blood pressure in hypertensive and normotensive persons, independent of weight loss.[102] The underlying mechanisms responsible for an exercise-induced reduction in blood pressure are unclear. Insulin resistance and hyperinsulinemia may contribute to the pathogenesis of hypertension, and physical activity reduces insulin resistance and insulin levels in individuals with hypertension.

Alcohol and Hypertension

Although chronic, excessive alcohol intake is associated with an increased risk of hypertension, light to moderate alcohol consumption is associated with reductions in blood pressure.[103,104] However, chronic, excessive alcohol intake (3 or more drinks per day) appears to increase blood pressure in both men and women.[104]

Hypertension is also discussed in chapter 25, on macrovascular disease, and pharmacotherapy for hypertension is the focus of chapter 19.

Case—Part 4: CVD

LW's hyperglycemia, dyslipidemia, and uncontrolled hypertension put her at considerable risk for CVD. Her food history and 24-hour recall revealed that her usual diet is high in total fat and saturated fat (2 factors that increase LDL-C) and high in sodium.

The next goal is to help LW reduce her risk of CVD by improving her blood lipids and blood pressure. A major focus is on reducing her LDL-C to <100 mg/dL. In addition to her walking program and moderate caloric restriction, she may be able to lower her blood pressure by reducing her sodium intake and adopting an eating plan similar to the DASH eating plan that incorporates more fruits, vegetables, and low-fat dairy foods and reduces the total fat, saturated fat, and *trans* fats. This, along with adding at least 2 servings of fish each week to provide omega-3 fatty acids, can also help improve her lipid profile. Adding a margarine-type spread containing a plant sterol/stanol might further reduce her LDL-C.

Since LW does not currently drink alcoholic beverages, she is not encouraged to start, despite the reported benefits of light to moderate alcohol on blood pressure and CVD risk. Alcoholic beverages add calories and may result in less attention to diabetes self-care management.

An initial strategy to help LW achieve her goals is for her to choose what she is willing and able to try: eat out less frequently, eat less when eating out, or make more healthful food choices. The RDN can discuss organizational techniques to help LW with the time constraints involved in preparing more meals at home and taking lunch to work. This would allow her more low-fat, lower sodium options and more availability of fruits and vegetables.

Regular physical activity is encouraged at each of LW's visits to improve lipids, blood pressure, and glycemia. LW is encouraged to perform resistance exercises 3 times a week (she had no contraindications). She was also taught to keep a record of her physical activity along with her blood glucose values to observe the effect on glycemia.

LW was instructed to self-monitor her blood pressure, in addition to blood pressure checks on follow-up visits, to assess the effect of her lifestyle changes and any need for medication additions or changes. The RDN told her that the impact of lifestyle changes on blood lipids could be observed in a lipid profile in just 6 to 12 weeks.

Nutrition Therapy and the Prevention and Treatment of Diabetic Kidney Disease

Glycemic control and effective treatment of hypertension have been shown to delay the onset and progression of diabetic kidney disease (DKD).[4,105,106] In general, every 1% drop in A1C can reduce the risk of microvascular complications such as kidney disease by 40%, and lowering blood pressure can reduce the decline in kidney function by 30% to 70%.[107] Therefore, strictly controlling blood glucose levels and blood pressure is recommended.[4,106]

Although low-protein diets have traditionally been recommended for persons with diabetes and DKD, adherence to them is poor and malnutrition is a reported concern.[106] In people with diabetes, a meta-analysis of low-protein diets (prescribed 0.6-0.8 g/kg per day; actual intake of 0.9 g/kg per day) was compared with normal-protein diets (1.3 g/kg per day).[108] The low-protein diets were not significantly associated with a change in glomerular filtration rates (GFRs) or creatinine clearance rate, but they did result in a decline in urinary protein excretion. The ADA macronutrient systematic review concluded that for individuals with DKD and either micro- or macroalbuminuria, reducing the amount of protein from normal levels does not appear to alter glycemic measures, CVD risk measures, or the course of GFR.[30] Therefore, reducing the amount of protein for people with diabetes and DKD (either micro- or macroalbuminuria) is not recommended.[3]

For further information on DKD, see chapter 27.

Nutrition Therapy in Youth

Nutrition goals for youth with diabetes focus on optimal glycemic goals, lipid and blood pressure goals, and normal growth and development.[109] Children and adolescents with diabetes have nutritional needs similar to those without diabetes. Energy needs can be estimated based on DRIs[16] and a history of the child's or adolescent's usual food intake. Growth and weight gain should be evaluated on a regular basis by recording height and weight on a pediatric growth chart. As energy requirements change with age, physical activity, and growth rate, an evaluation of height, weight, BMI, and the nutrition therapy plan is recommended at least every year.[109] The meal plan must be individualized based on food preferences, cultural practices, family schedules and eating patterns, age, weight, activity level, and insulin action. Macronutrient composition of the meal plan should be based on blood glucose, lipids, and requirements for growth and development. Education in problem solving based on blood glucose monitoring results is important for all youth with diabetes.

Youth With Type 1 Diabetes

Blood glucose goals for children and adolescents with type 1 diabetes are accomplished by balancing food intake, insulin, and physical activity and should emphasize achieving glycemic goals without excessive hypoglycemia. Withholding food to prevent hyperglycemia or having a child eat without an appetite to avoid hypoglycemia should be discouraged. A flexible insulin regimen with long-acting basal and rapid-acting boluses or insulin pump therapy precludes the need for a rigid meal plan, allowing the child or adolescent more flexibility in food choices and timing of meals and snacks. Carbohydrate counting using insulin-to-carbohydrate ratios is a meal-planning approach often used with youths with type 1 diabetes on physiological insulin regimens because it offers more flexibility than matching carbohydrate to a set insulin dose.[110]

For more information on carbohydrate counting, see chapter 4, on healthy eating.

Youth With Type 2 Diabetes

The goals for youth with type 2 diabetes are to facilitate appropriate changes in eating and physical activity habits, as many are overweight or obese.[111] Since these behaviors are generally family behaviors, family involvement in the behavior-change process is encouraged. A number of meal-planning approaches can be used to facilitate the selection of a variety of healthy foods in appropriate portions. Emphasis on carbohydrate consistency can improve blood glucose levels. Successful nutrition therapy is defined as the cessation of excessive weight gain with normal linear growth and near-normal fasting blood glucose and A1C values.[111]

Nutrition Therapy in Pregnancy

See chapter 24, on pregnancy with preexisting diabetes and gestational diabetes.

Nutrition Therapy in Older Adults

Nutrition therapy in older adults with diabetes presents unique challenges. Barriers to the consumption of a healthy eating pattern can be attributed to changes in taste and smell, changes in appetite, difficulty chewing and swallowing, physical disabilities, food availability, difficulty preparing food, changes in mental ability, and side effects from medications.[112,113] In addition, changes in body composition or function in older adults can directly influence nutrient requirements. Reductions in muscle mass, bone density, nutrient absorption, and metabolism make it difficult for older adults to meet nutrition requirements, especially when energy needs are reduced.[114] The Mini-Nutritional Assessment is a widely used, validated screening tool specifically designed for assessing the nutritional status of older adults.[114,115] A thorough nutrition history and an assessment of psychosocial needs are necessary to determine the appropriate nutrition interventions.[3] Nutrition therapy must address adequacy of nutritional needs, glycemic control, and nutrition-related cardiovascular risk factors that are common in this age group. Weight change is the most reliable indicator of poor nutritional status in older adults.[113] Weight loss, both intentional and unintentional, has been associated with an increase in mortality.[116] Overweight and obesity are prevalent in older adults. Older persons can be overweight or obese due to increased fat mass, yet still be malnourished.[113] Body mass index may not be an accurate predictor of the degree of adiposity in some older adults due to changes in body composition with aging.[116] Most studies have reported a U-shaped relationship with increased mortality at lower and higher BMI levels.[117] Aggressive caloric restriction in older adults can potentially worsen sarcopenia, bone mineral

density, and nutrition deficits.[115,116,118,119] A modest calorie reduction with an emphasis on nutrient-dense foods may be beneficial along with physical activity to reduce the loss of muscle mass while improving physical function and reducing cardiometabolic risk.[115,118]

Although energy needs decrease for older adults due to loss of lean body mass and less physical activity, requirements for other nutrients remain the same or increase with age.[119] Data suggest that dietary protein intake declines with age and, due to the contribution of protein undernutrition to sarcopenia and morbidity, older adults may need to be encouraged to consume more foods containing high-quality protein.[117] Meeting micronutrient needs with lower calorie intake is challenging as vitamin and mineral needs often remain constant or may increase, resulting in an increased risk for deficiencies in older adults with diabetes.[115] Recent evidence on dietary trends indicates that older adults are at risk for not meeting the recommended dietary allowance or adequate intake values for calcium; vitamins D, E, and K; potassium; and fiber.[119,120] Nutrient deficiencies can occur with lower than recommended intakes or as a result of malabsorption, such as in vitamin B_{12} malabsorption that occurs in an estimated 6% to 15% of older adults.[119]

When nutrition needs are not met through usual intake, additional interventions may include encouraging smaller, more frequent meals, fortifying usual foods, changing food texture, or adding liquid nutrition supplements (either regular or diabetes-specific formulas) between meals.[115] Adequate intakes of calcium and vitamin D are difficult for older adults to achieve from food alone; therefore, supplements may be necessary to meet recommended amounts.[119] An evidence-based analysis of the literature found that supplementation of vitamin D-3 with calcium resulted in small increases in bone mineral density and reduced fall risk in older adults.[121,122] Either supplementation or food fortification of vitamin B_{12} is recommended for adults older than 50 years due to decreased absorption.[119,123] Nutrition recommendations for older adults include restricting sodium to <2300 mg per day, although this can result in decreased food intake if the taste is undesirable.[3] Physical activity should be encouraged for older adults to minimize the loss of muscle mass, decrease bone loss, decrease central adiposity, improve insulin sensitivity, and improve cardiovascular risk factors.[124] Physical activity improves functional status in older adults with diabetes and is associated with higher self-rated physical health and psychosocial well-being.[115] The care and education of older adults is complicated by their clinical and functional heterogeneity.

Some individuals are limited cognitively or physically with multiple comorbidities, yet others are relatively healthy, physically active, and active learners. A thorough assessment followed by an individualized plan for supporting personal, social, and cultural needs, along with respecting his or her vision of quality of life, is key to successful outcomes in older adults.

Focus on Education

Teaching Strategies

- **Modest weight loss.** Overweight and obese persons benefit from weight loss and increases in physical activity for the prevention or delay of type 2 diabetes. Weight loss also assists with decreasing cardiovascular risk factors and is likely to improve glycemia in individuals with newly diagnosed type 2 diabetes who are primarily insulin resistant. Glycemia is less likely to be reduced through weight loss in individuals with long-standing diabetes who are insulin deficient. It appears that weight loss is more difficult to achieve in persons with diabetes compared with persons without diabetes. Studies report less weight loss from similar weight loss interventions in persons with diabetes compared with persons without diabetes.

- **Monitoring.** Encourage the use of premeal and postmeal blood glucose results to reinforce understanding of the glycemic effect of carbohydrate-containing foods. This can be especially helpful for persons with type 1 diabetes, but it can also help persons with type 2 diabetes if they have questions about certain foods. Additionally, it can help reinforce positive behavior related to portion control and physical activity. Monitoring blood pressure and lipid levels is as important as monitoring blood glucose.

- **Involvement.** Set and prioritize nutrition therapy goals involving each person, and family member if appropriate, to individualize meal plans. Encourage use of food records to evaluate actual food and beverage intake and eating patterns, and determine the individual's understanding of meal-planning principles and food-group choices. Understanding portion sizes is critical for both carbohydrate and calorie counting. Measure progress in behavior changes related to more healthful choices, amount of food/beverage intake, and timing of meals/snacks. Have participants use food models to portray a dinner meal and give them feedback about their choices. Teaching the principle of eating from all the food groups for healthy eating and good nutrition is important. Demonstrating meal planning, preparing menus, and selecting meals from restaurant menus during a teaching event are useful in role-playing the selection of healthy food choices and identifying potential barriers and facilitators to implementing the individual's meal plan. Ask persons with diabetes what their questions, concerns, priorities, and goals are and focus on these to capture their interest and promote continued involvement and success.

Messages for Patients

- **Healthy food choices.** Instead of focusing on weight loss, collaborate with an RDN or other healthcare professional to set short-term goals that include healthier food choices in place of highly processed foods with added fat, sugar, and/or sodium. Involve a friend or family member to assist in reviewing menus, labels, and food products.

- **Carbohydrate.** Planning which foods and meals to eat is effective for improving blood glucose, lipids (cholesterol), and blood pressure. Understanding which foods are carbohydrates, average portion sizes, and how many portions to select for meals or snacks and having consistency in eating have proven to be helpful for many individuals with diabetes.

> **Blood glucose.** Blood glucose values before and after meals can be checked to observe blood glucose response to the type and amount of carbohydrate in a meal. Avoid choosing foods solely on the basis of their effect on blood glucose; food selection to optimize glycemia should not compromise healthy eating. Diabetes medications frequently need to be combined with a food plan to achieve glucose goals. This is not "diet failure" but failure of the beta cells of the pancreas to produce adequate insulin to maintain normal blood glucose levels.

> **Physical activity.** Take energy expenditure as seriously as food (nutritional) intake. Use a pedometer to keep track of the number of steps taken in a day. The baseline and progressive steps provide a goal and motivation. If it has been a long time since you have been physically active, ask your healthcare provider for a referral to a physical therapist or exercise physiologist to develop a personal plan.

> **Goal setting and support.** Setting goals and taking ownership for meeting them are important strategies. Encourage patients to let their healthcare team know their questions, concerns, priorities, and goals. Patients need to seek the support they need to make and maintain lifestyle choices that are best for them.

Health Literacy

> **Health literacy is not just about persons with diabetes skills.** Consider the following when examining your skills and your practice approach to health literacy: general health literacy practice strategies, how to recognize people with low literacy, how to improve communication, and factors to consider when creating documents.

> **Use plain language in order for your patient to understand the information (written and verbal).** Some of the techniques include logical organization of the content (ie, long-term goal and how you will accomplish it). Use "you" and other pronouns, use the active voice, use short sentences, use everyday words, and use easy-to-read design materials. *No one technique defines plain language. Rather, plain language is defined by results—it is easy to read, understand, and use.* The following is an example of plain-language conversion:

- Before: "The Dietary Guidelines for Americans recommends a half hour or more of moderate physical activity on most days, preferably every day. The activity can include brisk walking, calisthenics, home care, gardening, moderate sports exercise, and dancing."
- After: "Do at least 30 minutes of physical activity, like brisk walking, most days of the week."[125]

> **Use specific rather than vague suggestions:**
- Instead of "exercise regularly," use "exercise 3 to 5 days per week for 40 minutes"
- Instead of "don't lift anything heavy," use "don't lift anything over 10 pounds"
- Instead of "get adequate rest," use "get at least 7 hours of sleep each night"

> **Use written materials that are easy to understand.** Use short sentences (10-15 words) and simple language (monosyllable words), be consistent with words and terminology, define technical or difficult words, put important concepts first, use bulleted lists instead of blocks of text, use headings and subheadings, use a readable type style, use 12- to 14-point type for text and 16- to 18-point bold type for headings, use uppercase and lowercase for the text (do not use all capitals, as they are harder to read), have a 50/50 blend of white space and type, use dark text against a light background for sharp contrast, use summary techniques, do not justify the right margin, use columns that are 50 to 60 characters wide, and use pictures.

> **Use verbal communication that the patient understands.** State concepts in logical order, one step at a time; define healthcare terms and explain acronyms; verify understanding: rephrase

message and have the patient explain instructions back to you (teach-back method: "How would you explain this to your friends with diabetes?"); adjust to patient needs; allow your patient to talk; pay attention to nonverbal communication; and be positive.

⊘ **Take time to assess health literacy and health numeracy skills.** Multiple health literacy assessment tools are available. An example of a short, quick, and validated assessment is the Newest Vital Sign, in which patients are given a nutrition label from an ice cream container and then asked 6 questions about how they would interpret and act on the information contained on the label.[126]

Focus on Practice

⊘ **Monitor the quality and outcomes of your nutrition therapy.** Examine how your clients' care outcomes compare with nutrition therapy expectations. Demonstrate the effectiveness of your nutrition therapy to providers to increase referrals.

⊘ **Integrate nutrition therapy into the Chronic Care Model.** Allow for ongoing access, assessment, and reassessment of needs. Recognize a possible nutrition therapy relapse and provide services to identify and treat accordingly.

References

1. Academy of Nutrition and Dietetics. Type 1 and type 2 diabetes evidence-based nutrition practice guidelines for adults. 2008 (cited 2014 Mar 31). On the Internet at: http://adaevidencelibrary.com/topic.dfm?cat=3253.

2. Franz MJ, Powers MA, Leontos C, et al. The evidence for medical nutrition therapy for type 1 and type 2 diabetes in adults. J Am Diet Assoc. 2010;110:1852-89.

3. Evert AB, Boucher JL, Cypress M, et al. Nutrition therapy recommendations for the management of adults with diabetes. A position statement of the American Diabetes Association. Diabetes Care. 2013;36:3821-42.

4. American Diabetes Association. Standards of medical care in diabetes—2014. Diabetes Care. 2014;37 Suppl 1: S14-80.

5. American Association of Diabetes Educators. Healthy eating: incorporating nutritional management into lifestyle. Diabetes Educ. 2012;38:124-8.

6. Institute of Medicine. The Role of Nutrition in Maintaining Health in the Nation's Elderly: Evaluating Coverage of Nutrition Services for the Medicare Population. Washington, DC: National Academies Press; 2000.

7. Ali MK, Bullard KM, Saaddine JB, Cowie CC, Imperatore G, Gregg EW. Achievement of goals in US diabetes care. N Engl J Med. 2013;368:1613-24.

8. Robbins JM, Thatcher GE, Webb DA, Valdmanis VG. Nutritionist visits, diabetes classes, and hospitalization rates and charges: the Urban Diabetes Study. Diabetes Care. 2008;31:655-60.

9. Franz MJ, Evert AB, eds. American Diabetes Association Guide to Nutrition Therapy for Diabetes. 2nd ed. Alexandria, Va: American Diabetes Association; 2012.

10. US Department of Agriculture and US Department of Health and Human Services. Dietary Guidelines for Americans, 2010. 7th ed. Washington, DC: US Government Printing Office; 2010. On the Internet at: http://www.dietaryguidelines.gov.

11. Pastors JG, Franz MJ. Effectiveness of medical nutrition therapy in diabetes. In: Franz MJ, Evert AB, eds. American Diabetes Association Guide to Nutrition Therapy for Diabetes. 2nd ed. Alexandria, Va: American Diabetes Association; 2012:1-18.

12. Oza-Frank R, Cheng YJ, Narayan KM, Gregg EW. Trends in nutrient intake among adults with diabetes in the United States: 1988-2004. J Am Diet Assoc. 2009;109:1173-8.

13. Xu J, Eilat-Adar S, Loria CM, et al. Macronutrient intake and glycemic control in a population-based sample of American Indians with diabetes: the Strong Health Study. Am J Clin Nutr. 2007;86:480-7.

14. Delahanty LM, Nathan DM, Lachin JM, et al; for the Diabetes Control and Complications Trial/Epidemiology of Diabetes. Association of diet with glycated hemoglobin during intensive treatment of type 1 diabetes in the Diabetes Control and Complications Trial. Am J Clin Nutr. 2009;89:518-24.

15. Franz MJ. Macronutrients and nutrition therapy for diabetes. In: Franz MJ, Evert AB, eds. American Diabetes

Association Guide to Nutrition Therapy for Diabetes. 2nd ed. Alexandria, Va: American Diabetes Association; 2012:19-39.

16. Institute of Medicine. Dietary Reference Intakes: Energy, Carbohydrate, Fiber, Fat, Fatty Acids, Cholesterol, Protein, and Amino Acids. Washington, DC: National Academies Press; 2002.

17. Franz MJ, Bantle JP, Beebe CA, et al. Evidence-based nutrition principles and recommendations for the treatment and prevention of diabetes and related complications (technical review). Diabetes Care. 2002;25:148-98.

18. Evert AB. Nutrition therapy for adults with type 1 and insulin-requiring type 2 diabetes. In: Franz MJ, Evert AB, eds. American Diabetes Association Guide to Nutrition Therapy for Diabetes. 2nd ed. Alexandria, Va: American Diabetes Association; 2012:95-116.

19. Feinman RD, Fine EJ. Fructose in perspective. Nutr Metab. 2013;10:45-56.

20. Sievenpiper JL, Carleton AJ, Chatha S, et al. Heterogeneous effects of fructose on blood lipids in individuals with type 2 diabetes: systematic review and meta-analysis of experimental trials in humans. Diabetes Care. 2009;32:1930-7.

21. Livesey G, Taylor R. Fructose consumption and consequences for glycation, plasma triacylglycerol, and body weight: meta-analyses and meta-regression models of intervention studies. Am J Clin Nutr. 2008;88:1419-37.

22. Brand-Miller JC, Stockmann K, Atkinson F, et al. Glycemic index, postprandial glycemia, and the shape of the curve in healthy subjects: analysis of a database of more than 1000 foods. Am J Clin Nutr. 2009;89:97-105.

23. Fernandes G, Velangi A, Wolever TMS. Glycemic index of potatoes commonly consumed in North America. J Am Diet Assoc. 2005;105:557-62.

24. Vega-López S, Ausman LM, Griffith JL, Lichtenstein AH. Interindividual variability and intra-individual reproducibility of glycemic index values for commercial white bread. Diabetes Care. 2007;30:1412-7.

25. Wolever TMS, Gibbs AL, Mehling C, et al. The Canadian Trial of Carbohydrates in Diabetes, a 1-y controlled trial of low-glycemic-index dietary carbohydrate in type 2 diabetes: no effect on glycated hemoglobin but reduction in C-reactive protein. Am J Clin Nutr. 2008;87:114-25.

26. Ma Y, Olendzki BC, Merriam PA, et al. A randomized clinical trial comparing low-glycemic index versus ADA dietary education among individuals with type 2 diabetes. Nutrition. 2008;24:45-56.

27. Wolever TMS, Nguyen PM, Chiasson J-L, et al. Determinants of diet glycemic index calculated retrospectively from diet records of 342 individuals with non-insulin-dependent diabetes mellitus. Am J Clin Nutr. 1994;59:1265-9.

28. Atkinson FS, Foster-Powell K, Brand-Miller JC. International tables of glycemic index and glycemic load values: 2008. Diabetes Care. 2008;31:2281-3.

29. Wolever TMS. Physiological mechanisms and observed health impacts related to the glycaemic index: some observations. Int J Obes. 2006;30 Suppl 3:S72-8.

30. Wheeler ML, Dunbar SA, Jaacks LM, et al. Macronutrients, food groups, and eating patterns in the management of diabetes. A systematic review of the literature, 2010. Diabetes Care. 2012;35:434-45.

31. Wheeler ML, Daly A, Evert A, et al. Choose your foods: exchange lists for diabetes, sixth edition, 2008: description and guidelines for use. J Am Diet Assoc. 2008;108:883-8.

32. Stanhope KL, Schwarz JM, Klein NL, et al. Consuming fructose-sweetened beverages, not glucose-sweetened, increases visceral adiposity and lipids and decreases insulin sensitivity in overweight/obese humans. J Clin Invest. 2009;119:1322-34.

33. Schulze MB, Manson JE, Ludwig DS, et al. Sugar-sweetened beverages, weight gain, and incidence of type 2 diabetes in young and middle-aged women. JAMA. 2004; 292:927-34.

34. Malik VS, Popkin BM, Bray GA, Despres JP, Willett WC, Hu FB. Sugar-sweetened beverages and risk of metabolic syndrome and type 2 diabetes: a meta-analysis. Diabetes Care. 2010;33:2477-83.

35. Gardner C, Wylie-Rosett J, Gidding SS, et al; on behalf of the American Heart Association Nutrition Committee of the Council on Nutrition, Physical Activity and Metabolism, Council on Arteriosclerosis, Thrombosis and Vascular Biology, Council on Cardiovascular Disease in the Young, and the American Diabetes Association. Nonnutritive sweeteners: current use and health perspectives. A scientific statement from the American Heart Association and the American Diabetes Association. Diabetes Care. 2012;35:1798-808.

36. Thomsen C, Storm H, Holst JJ, Hermansen K. Differential effects of saturated and monounsaturated fats on postprandial lipemia and glucagon-like peptide 1 responses in patients with type 2 diabetes. Am J Clin Nutr. 2003;77:605-11.

37. Gannon MC, Ercan N, Westphal SA, Nuttall FQ. Effect of added fat on plasma glucose and insulin response to ingested potato in individuals with NIDDM. Diabetes Care. 1993;16:874-80.

38. Gentilcore D, Chaikomin R, Jones KL, et al. Effects of fat on gastric emptying of and the glycemic, insulin, and incretin responses to a carbohydrate meal in type 2 diabetes. J Clin Endocrinol Metab. 2006;91:2062-7.

39. Peters AL, Davidson MB. Protein and fat effects on glucose responses and insulin requirements in subjects with insulin-dependent diabetes mellitus. Am J Clin Nutr. 1993;58:555-60.

40. Wolpert HA, Atakov-Castillo A, Smith SA, Steil GM. Dietary fat acutely increases glucose concentrations and insulin requirement in patients with type 1 diabetes. Diabetes Care. 2013;36:810-6.

41. Galgani JE, Uauy RD, Aguirre CA, Diaz EO. Effect of the dietary fat quality on insulin sensitivity. Br J Nutr. 2008;100:471-9.

42. Vessby B, Unsitupa M, Hermanses K, et al. Substituting dietary saturated for monounsaturated fat impairs insulin sensitivity in healthy men and women: the KANWU Study. Diabetologia. 2001;44:312-9.

43. Rosenfalck AM, Almdal T, Viggers L, et al. A low-fat diet improves peripheral insulin sensitivity in patients with type 1 diabetes. Diabet Med. 2006;23:384-92.

44. Institute of Medicine. Dietary Reference Intakes: Energy, Carbohydrate, Fiber, Fat, Fatty Acids, Cholesterol, Protein, and Amino Acids. Washington, DC: National Academies Press; 2002.

45. Pittas AG, Lau J, Hu FB, Dawson-Hughes B. The role of vitamin D and calcium in type 2 diabetes. A systematic review and meta-analysis. J Clin Endocrinol Metab. 2007; 92:2017-29.

46. Song Y, Wang L, Pittas AG, et al. Blood 25-hydroxy vitamin D levels and incident type 2 diabetes. A meta-analysis of prospective studies. Diabetes Care. 2013;36:1422-8.

47. Davidson MB, Duran P, Lee ML, Friedman TC. High-dose vitamin D supplementation in people with prediabetes and hypovitaminosis D. Diabetes Care. 2013;36: 260-6.

48. Balk EM, Tatsioni A, Lichtenstein AH, Lau J, Pittas AG. Effect of chromium supplementation on glucose metabolism and lipids: a systematic review of randomized controlled trials. Diabetes Care. 2007;30:2154-63.

49. American College of Sports Medicine. Exercise and type 2 diabetes: a joint position statement of the American Diabetes Association and the American College of Sports Medicine. Med Sci Sports Exerc. 2010;42: 2282-303.

50. Duncan GE, Perri MG, Teriaque DW, et al. Exercise training without weight loss increases insulin sensitivity and postheparin plasma lipase activity in previously sedentary adults. Diabetes Care. 2003;26:557-62.

51. Franz MJ. Alcohol and diabetes. In: Franz MJ, Evert AB, eds. American Diabetes Association Guide to Nutrition Therapy for Diabetes. 2nd ed. Alexandria, Va: American Diabetes Association; 2012:69-94.

52. Turner BC, Jenkins E, Kerr D, et al. The effect of evening alcohol consumption on next-morning glucose control in type 1 diabetes. Diabetes Care. 2001;24:1888-93.

53. Howard AA, Amsten JH, Gourevitch MN. Effect of alcohol consumption on diabetes mellitus. A systematic review. Ann Intern Med. 2004;140:211-9.

54. Klein S, Sheard NF, Pi-Sunyer X, et al. Weight management through lifestyle modification for the prevention and management of type 2 diabetes: rationale and strategies. A statement of the American Diabetes Association, the North American Association for the Study of Obesity, and the American Society for Clinical Nutrition. Diabetes Care. 2004;27:2067-73.

55. The Diabetes Prevention Program Research Group. Reduction in the incidence of type 2 diabetes with lifestyle intervention or metformin. N Engl J Med. 2002;346: 393-403.

56. Franz MJ. The obesity paradox and diabetes. Diabetes Spectr. 2013;26:145-51.

57. Esposito K, Maiorino MI, Ciotola M, et al. Effects of a Mediterranean-style diet on the need for antihyperglycemic drug therapy in patients with newly diagnosed type 2 diabetes: a randomized trial. Ann Intern Med. 2009;151: 306-14.

58. The Look AHEAD Research Group. Reduction in weight and cardiovascular disease risk factors in individuals with type 2 diabetes. One-year results of the Look AHEAD trial. Diabetes Care. 2007;30:1374-83.

59. Guldbrand H, Dizdar B, Bunjaku B, et al. In type 2 diabetes, randomization to follow a low-carbohydrate diet transiently improves glycaemic control compared with advice to follow a low-fat diet producing similar weight loss. Diabetologia. 2012;55:2118-27.

60. Brehm BJ, Lattin BL, Summer SS, et al. One-year comparison of a high-monounsaturated fat diet with a high-carbohydrate diet in type 2 diabetes. Diabetes Care. 2009;32:215-20.

61. Davis NJ, Tomuta N, Schechter C, et al. Comparative study of the effects of a 1-year dietary intervention of a low-carbohydrate diet versus a low-fat diet on weight and glycemic control in type 2 diabetes. Diabetes Care. 2009; 32:1147-52.

62. Larsen RN, Mann NJ, Maclean E, Shaw JE. The effect of high-protein, low-carbohydrate diets in the treatment of type 2 diabetes: a 12 month randomised controlled trial. Diabetologia. 2011;54:731-40.

63. Krebs JD, Elley CR, Parry-Strong A, et al. The Diabetes Excess Weight Loss (DEWL) Trial: a randomized controlled trial of high-protein versus high-carbohydrate diets over 2 years in type 2 diabetes. Diabetologia. 2012;55: 905-14.

64. The Look AHEAD Research Group. Cardiovascular effects of intensive lifestyle intervention in type 2 diabetes. N Engl J Med. 2013;369:145-54.

65. Franz MJ, VanWormer JJ, Crain LA, et al. Weight loss outcomes: a systematic review and meta-analysis of weight loss clinical trials with a minimum 1-year follow-up. J Am Diet Assoc. 2007;107:1755-67.

66. Dansinger ML, Gleason JA, Griffith JL, et al. Comparison of the Atkins, Ornish, Weight Watchers, and Zone diets for weight loss and heart disease risk reduction: a randomized trial. JAMA. 2005;293:43-53.

67. Sacks FM, Gray GA, Carey VJ, et al. Comparison of weight-loss diets with different compositions of fat, protein, and carbohydrates. N Engl J Med. 2009;360:859-73.

68. American Dietetic Association. Position of the American Dietetic Association: weight management. J Am Diet Assoc. 2009;109:330-46.

69. Klein S, Burke LE, Bray GA, et al. Clinical implications of obesity with specific focus on cardiovascular disease: a statement for professionals from the American Heart Association Council on Nutrition, Physical Activity, and Metabolism. Circulation. 2004;110:2952-67.

70. Inzucchi SE, Bergenstal RM, Buse JB, et al. Management of hyperglycemia in type 2 diabetes: a patient-centered approach. Position statement of the American Diabetes Association and the European Association for the Study of Diabetes. Diabetes Care. 2012;35:1364-79.

71. Larger E, Rufat P, Dubois-Laforgue D, Ledoux S. Insulin therapy does not itself induce weight gain in patients with type 2 diabetes. Diabetes Care. 2001;24:1849-50.

72. Daly A. Use of insulin and weight gain: optimizing diabetes nutrition therapy. J Am Diet Assoc. 2007;107:1386-93.

73. Arterburn DE, Bogart A, Sherwood NE, et al. A multisite study of long-term remission and relapse of type 2 diabetes mellitus following gastric bypass. Obes Surg. 2013;23:93-102.

74. Buse JB, Ginsberg HN, Bakris GL, et al. Primary prevention of cardiovascular diseases in people with diabetes mellitus. Diabetes Care. 2007;30:162-72.

75. Karmally W, Zimmerman JS. Nutrition therapy for diabetes and lipid disorders. In: Franz MJ, Evert AB, eds. American Diabetes Association Guide to Nutrition Therapy for Diabetes. 2nd ed. Alexandria, Va: American Diabetes Association; 2012:265-94.

76. Schwingshackl L, Strasser B, Joffmann G. Effects of mono-unsaturated fatty acids on glycaemic control in patients with abnormal glucose metabolism: a systematic review and meta-analysis. Ann Nutr Metab. 2011;58:290-6.

77. Itsiopoulos C, Brazionis L, Kaimakamis M, et al. Can the Mediterranean diet lower HbA1c in type 2 diabetes? Results from a randomized cross-over study. Nutr Metab Cardiovasc Dis. 2011;21:740-7.

78. Summers LK, Fielding BA, Bradshaw HA, et al. Substituting dietary saturated fat with polyunsaturated fat changes abdominal fat distribution and improves insulin sensitivity. Diabetologia. 2002;45:369-77.

79. Academy of Nutrition and Dietetics. Disorders of lipid metabolism evidence-based nutrition practice guidelines.

2011 (cited 2014 Mar 31). On the Internet at: http://adaevidencelibrary.com/topic.cfm?cat=4528.

80. Lee YM, Haastert B, Scherbaum W, Hauner H. A phytosterol-enriched spread improves the lipid profile of subjects with type 2 diabetes mellitus—a randomized controlled trial under free-living conditions. Eur J Nutr. 2003;42:111-7.

81. Martinez-Gonzalez MA, de la Fuente-Arrillaga C, Nunez-Cordoba JM, et al. Adherence to Mediterranean diet and risk of developing diabetes: prospective cohort study. BMJ. 2008;336:1348-51.

82. Brill JB. The Mediterranean diet and your health. Am J Lifestyle Med. 2009;3:44-56.

83. Koppes LL, Dekker JM, Hendriks HJ, Bouter LM, Heine RJ. Meta-analysis of the relationship between alcohol consumption and coronary heart disease and mortality in type 2 diabetes. Diabetologia. 2006;49:648-52.

84. Bantle AE, Thomas W, Bantle JP. Metabolic effects of alcohol in the form of wine in persons with type 2 diabetes mellitus. Metabolism. 2008;57:241-5.

85. Pownall HJ, Ballantyne CM, Kimball KT, et al. Effect of moderate alcohol consumption on hypertriglyceridemia. Arch Intern Med. 1999;159:981-7.

86. Nanchahal K, Ashton WD, Wood DA. Alcohol consumption, metabolic cardiovascular risk factors and hypertension in women. Int J Epidemiol. 2000;29:57-64.

87. Wei M, Gibbons LW, Kampert JB, et al. Low cardiorespiratory fitness and physical inactivity in men with type 2 diabetes. Ann Intern Med. 2000;132:605-11.

88. Church TS, Cheng YJ, Earnest CP, et al. Exercise capacity and body composition as predictors of mortality among men with diabetes. Diabetes Care. 2004;27:83-8.

89. Leon AS, Sanchez OA. Response of blood lipids to exercise training alone or combined with dietary intervention. Med Sci Sports Exerc. 2001;33:S502-15.

90. Kelley GA, Kelley KS. Effects of aerobic exercise on lipids and lipoproteins in adults with type 2 diabetes: a meta-analysis of randomized-controlled trials. Public Health. 2007;9:643-55.

91. Chobanian AV, Bakris GL, Black HR, et al. The Seventh Report of the Joint National Committee on Prevention, Detention, Evaluation, and Treatment of High Blood Pressure: the JNC 7 report. JAMA. 2004;289:747-52.

92. Abersold K, Ostrovsky NW, Wylie-Rosett J. Nutrition therapy for diabetes and hypertension. In: Franz MJ, Evert AB, eds. American Diabetes Association Guide to Nutrition Therapy for Diabetes. 2nd ed. Alexandria, Va: American Diabetes Association; 2012:295-317.

93. Harsha DW, Lin PH, Obarzanek E, Karanja NM, Moore TJ, Caballero B; DASH Collaborative Research

Group. Dietary Approaches to Stop Hypertension: a summary of study results. J Am Diet Assoc. 1999;99 Suppl:S35-9.

94. Azadbakht L, Fard NR, Karimi M, et al. Effects of the Dietary Approaches to Stop Hypertension (DASH) eating plan on cardiovascular risks among type 2 diabetic patients: a randomized crossover clinical trial. Diabetes Care. 2011;34:55-7.

95. Sacks FM, Svetkey LP, Vollmer WM, et al. DASH-Sodium Collaborative Research Group: effects on blood pressure of reduced dietary sodium and the Dietary Approaches to Stop Hypertension (DASH) diet. N Engl J Med. 2001;344:3-10.

96. Vollmer WM, Sacks FM, Ard J, et al. Effects of diet and sodium intake on blood pressure. Ann Intern Med. 2001; 135:1019-28.

97. Appel LJ, Champagne CM, Harsha DW, et al; Writing Group of the PREMIER Collaborative Research Group. Effects of comprehensive lifestyle modification on blood pressure control: main results of the PREMIER clinical trial. JAMA. 2003;289:2083-93.

98. Miller ER III, Erlinger TP, Young DR, et al. Results of diet, exercise, and weight loss intervention trial (DEW-IT). Hypertension. 2002;40:612-8.

99. Kaplan NM. Lifestyle modification for prevention and treatment of hypertension. J Clin Hypertens. 2004;6:716-9.

100. Blumenthal JA, Babyak MA, Hinderliter A, et al. Effects of the DASH diet alone and in combination with exercise and weight loss on blood pressure and cardiovascular biomarkers in men and women with high blood pressure: the ENCORE study. Arch Intern Med. 2010;170:126-35.

101. Appel LJ, Moore TJ, Obarzanek E, et al; for the DASH Collaborative Research Group. A clinical trial of the effects of dietary patterns on blood pressure. N Engl J Med. 1997;336:1117-24.

102. Whelton SP, Chin A, Xin X, He J. Effect of aerobic exercise on blood pressure. Ann Intern Med. 2002;136:493-503.

103. Davies MJ, Baer DJ, Judd JT, Brown ED, Campbell WS, Taylor PR. Effects of moderate alcohol intake on fasting insulin and glucose concentrations and insulin sensitivity in postmenopausal women: a randomized controlled trial. JAMA. 2002;287:2559-62.

104. Xin X, He J, Frontini MG, Ogden LG, Motsamai OI, Whelton PK. Effects of alcohol reduction on blood pressure: a meta-analysis of randomized controlled trials. Hypertension. 2001;38:1112-7.

105. National Kidney Foundation Kidney Disease Outcomes Quality Initiative (KDOQI). Clinical practice guidelines for chronic kidney disease: evaluation, classification, and stratification. 2002 (cited 2014 Mar 31). On the Internet at: http://www.kidney.org/professionals/kdoqi/guidelines_commentaries.cfm#guidelines.

106. Wheeler ML. Nutrition therapy for diabetic kidney disease. In: Franz MJ, Evert AB, eds. American Diabetes Association Guide to Nutrition Therapy for Diabetes. 2nd ed. Alexandria, Va: American Diabetes Association; 2012:307-17.

107. Centers for Disease Control and Prevention. National diabetes fact sheet: national estimates and general information on diabetes and prediabetes in the United States, 2011. Atlanta, Ga: US Department of Health and Human Services, Centers for Disease Control and Prevention; 2011.

108. Pan Y, Guo LL, Jin HM. Low-protein diets for diabetic nephropathy: a meta-analysis of randomized controlled trials. Am J Clin Nutr. 2008;88:660-6.

109. Silverstein J, Klingensmith G, Copeland K, et al. Care of children and adolescents with type 1 diabetes. Diabetes Care. 2005;28:186-212.

110. Spiegel G. Nutrition therapy for youth with diabetes. In: Franz MJ, Evert AB, eds. American Diabetes Association Guide to Nutrition Therapy for Diabetes. 2nd ed. Alexandria, Va: American Diabetes Association; 2012:143-68.

111. American Diabetes Association. Type 2 diabetes in children and adolescents (consensus statement). Diabetes Care. 2000;23:381-9.

112. Stanley K. Nutrition therapy for older adults with diabetes. In: Franz MJ, Evert AB, eds. American Diabetes Association Guide to Nutrition Therapy for Diabetes. 2nd ed. Alexandria, Va: American Diabetes Association; 2012:169-80.

113. Academy of Nutrition and Dietetics. Position of the Academy of Nutrition and Dietetics: Food and nutrition for older adults: Promoting health and wellness. J Acad Nutr Diet. 2012;112:1255-77.

114. Well JL, Dumbrell AC. Nutrition and aging: assessment and treatment of compromised nutritional status in frail elderly patients. Clin Interv Aging. 2006;1:67-79.

115. Kirkman MS, Briscoe VJ, Clark N, et al. Diabetes in older adults (consensus report). Diabetes Care. 2012;35:2650-64.

116. Miller SL, Wolfe RR. The danger of weight loss in the elderly. J Nutr Health Aging. 2008;12:487-91.

117. Villareal DT, Banks M, Siener C, Sinacore DR, Klein S. Physical frailty and body composition in obese elderly men and women. Obes Res. 2004;12:913-20.

118. Shapses SA, Riedt CS. Bone, body weight, and weight reduction; what are the concerns? J Nutr. 2006;136:1453-6.

119. Academy of Nutrition and Dietetics. Food and nutrition for older adults promoting health and wellness evidence analysis project. 2012 (cited 2014 Mar 31). On the Internet at: http://www.andevidencelibrary.com/topic.cfm?cat=3987.

120. Lichtenstein AH, Rasmussen H, Winifred Y, Epstein S, Russell R. Modified MyPyramid for older adults. J Nutr. 2008;138:5-11.

121. Academy of Nutrition and Dietetics. Position of the American Dietetic Association: Nutrient supplementation. J Acad Nutr Diet. 2009;109:2073-84.

122. Cranney A, Horsley T, O'Donnell S, et al. Effectiveness and safety of vitamin D in relation to bone health. Evidence Report/Technology Assessment No. 158. Rockville, Md: Agency for Healthcare Research and Quality; 2007. AHRQ Publication No. 07-E013.

123. Institute of Medicine, Food and Nutrition Board. Dietary Reference Intakes: Thiamin, Riboflavin, Niacin, Vitamin B6, Folate, Vitamin B12, Pantothenic Acid, Biotin, and Choline. Washington, DC: National Academy Press; 1998.

124. McLaughlin S. Diabetes in older adults. In: Ross TA, Boucher JL, O'Connell BS, eds. Diabetes Medical Nutrition Therapy and Education. Chicago: American Dietetic Association; 2005:179-88.

125. Public Health Service, Department of Health and Human Services. Losing weight safely (cited 2013 Aug 29). On the Internet at: http://www.plainlanguage.gov/examples/before_after/pub_hhs_losewgt.cfm.

126. Pfizer Health Communication Initiative, Pfizer Inc. Newest Vital Sign (cited 2013 Aug 29). On the Internet at: http://www.pfizerhealthliteracy.com/physicians-providers/newest-vital-sign.html.

CHAPTER 17

Exercise Prescription

Sheri R. Colberg, PhD, FACSM

Key Concepts

◆ Be familiar with current fitness terminology.

◆ Understand the role of physical activity and fitness in type 2 diabetes prevention and treatment of all types of diabetes.

◆ Understand the physiological responses of blood glucose levels during physical activity.

◆ Identify the individual's risks associated with physical activity and apply clinical strategies to minimize those risks.

◆ Recognize 3 distinct stages in adoption and use of an exercise/physical activity plan.

◆ Implement strategies to enable appropriately self-directed fitness plans.

Introduction

A lifestyle that incorporates sufficient physical activity aids in prevention of type 2 diabetes and is extremely beneficial to general health. For people with any type of diabetes, the beneficial health effects of leading a physically active lifestyle have been recognized since ancient times.[1] The discovery of insulin in the twentieth century prompted modern scientific exploration of the therapeutic effects of physical activity on the blood glucose level.[2]

Today, implementing and maintaining a health-related fitness program is regarded as a primary component of diabetes self-management, especially for individuals with type 2 diabetes or women with gestational diabetes who are attempting to reduce their levels of insulin resistance. For individuals with type 1 diabetes, appropriate regimen changes are needed to effectively manage blood glucose levels with the addition of physical activity. However, regular participation provides general health benefits and helps prevent "double diabetes," which can result from increasing insulin resistance related to a sedentary lifestyle and weight gain.[3]

In 2003, the American Association of Diabetes Educators (AADE) published data identifying 7 behaviors common in people with diabetes who are able to achieve better health outcomes; "being active" is one of those behaviors. The AADE7 Self-Care Behaviors™ emphasize that even small changes in physical activity levels are considered beneficial.[4] More detailed information on self-care behaviors related to being active can be found in chapter 5.

To promote physical activity and help individuals implement an exercise prescription, the diabetes educator must recognize how to adjust variables within the diabetes treatment routine, especially when insulin or certain other medications are taken. The following are key aspects to be considered:

◆ Whether the side effect of hypoglycemia exists within the individual's diabetes medication and dietary regimen

◆ When the individual should perform blood glucose measurements relative to physical activity participation

- How to interpret individual blood glucose responses to physical activity
- How to modify fitness guidelines and plans in the face of diabetes complications and other restrictions or limitations
- How to overcome barriers limiting adequate physical activity participation

Learning to overcome barriers that interfere with a more physically active lifestyle is a large part of diabetes self-management education. When diabetes complications like neuropathy, nephropathy, and retinopathy exist, certain physical movements may pose challenges and safety issues. Also, not all individuals with diabetes are capable of participating or willing to participate in a fitness program, regardless of the benefits they can achieve. The diabetes educator's task is to explore all the options and alternatives available for the patient so that a safe, effective, and realistic fitness plan can be designed and successfully implemented. Doing so requires an understanding of a number of topics addressed in this chapter.

Current Physical Fitness Terminology

In recent years, the role of physical activity in people's daily lives has been widely examined. The rapid adaptation to sedentary lifestyles over the last few decades in Western culture and in developing countries has been associated with a growing prevalence of metabolic diseases in this relatively short time span.

Unfortunately, reporting on this topic has led to much confusion in the lay population. An important factor in clarifying the messages provided to the public is for health, physical fitness, and research professionals to use similar, accepted fitness terminology. In 2000, the President's Council on Physical Fitness collected terms and definitions from many respected sources and organized them into an outline intended for common use.[5]

The term "physical fitness" is simply defined as "a set of attributes that people have or achieve relating to their ability to perform physical activity." What complicates physical fitness for the layperson is that there are many reasons to engage in a physically active lifestyle. Table 17.1 organizes the accepted terminology into 4 categories of physical fitness: physiological fitness, health-related fitness, skill-related fitness, and sports.

While none of these categories are mutually exclusive, neither are they dependent on one another. The terminology of fitness is intended to be inclusive rather than athletic in nature when considering what affects an individual's fitness level and health outcomes. However, most laypersons believe they need to possess skill-related talents, participate in sports, or work out at a fitness club to achieve physiological or health-related benefits. This misperception prevents many people from considering or engaging in a physically active lifestyle. A primary goal of the diabetes healthcare professional should be correcting this misperception and encouraging individuals to engage in appropriate physical activities.

TABLE 17.1 Currently Accepted Terminology Related to Physical Fitness			
Physical Fitness			*Skills*
Physiological	*Health-Related*	*Skill-Related*	*Sports*
Metabolic	Body composition	Agility	Team
Morphological	Cardiovascular fitness	Balance	Individual
Bone integrity	Flexibility	Coordination	Lifetime
Other	Muscular endurance	Power	Other
	Muscular strength	Speed	
		Reaction time	
		Other	

Source: President's Council on Physical Fitness, "Definitions: health, fitness, and physical activity," *Research Digest*, 2000.

Physiological Fitness

The physiological fitness category includes terms that have little to do with how an individual performs a physical activity.[5] However, physiological fitness is influenced by the inclusion of habitual physical activity. For example, cholesterol levels do not influence the ability to walk, yet the more a person walks, the more he or she can expect to see a positive impact on these levels.

- *Metabolic fitness:* Status of metabolic systems and variables predictive of the risk for diabetes and cardiovascular disease
- *Morphological fitness:* Status of body compositional factors, such as body circumference, body fat, and regional body fat distribution
- *Bone integrity* (bone strength): Status of bone mineral density and bone strength

Health-Related Physical Fitness

The health-related physical fitness category contains terms that are recognized for their direct relationship to good health.[5] These terms are also most likely to be of interest to the individual engaging in a fitness program. The layperson often measures success, or lack thereof, on changes seen in these areas.

- *Body composition:* Relative amounts of muscle, fat, bone, and other vital parts of the body
- *Cardiovascular fitness:* Ability of the circulatory and respiratory systems to supply oxygen during sustained physical activity
- *Flexibility:* Range of motion around each joint
- *Muscular endurance:* Muscle's ability to continue to perform without fatigue
- *Muscular strength:* Muscle's ability to exert force

Physical Activity Versus Exercise (Training)

- *Physical activity:* Bodily movement produced by the contraction of skeletal muscle that substantially increases energy expenditure
- *Exercise (training):* Subset of physical activity conducted with the intention of developing physical fitness, which includes cardiovascular, strength, balance, and flexibility training options

TABLE 17.2	Subcategories of Physical Activity			
		Physical Activity		
Exercise	Sports	Leisure activities	Dance	Other

The recommendation to use the broader term "physical activity" in place of the narrower term "exercise" has also caused some confusion. The intent, with evidence supported by research, is to recognize that many types of movements can have a positive impact on health-related physical fitness. More than one type of physical activity may be required to yield measurable improvements for each of the components in the health-related fitness category, which includes aerobic (or cardiovascular) fitness and muscular strength and muscular endurance. Table 17.2 provides an overview of some general categories that can be used to identify options for physical activity. This broader term may also be more acceptable to individuals who have a negative viewpoint of "exercise."

Role of Physical Activity in Prevention and Treatment of Type 2 Diabetes

Most benefits of physical activity on diabetes management and prevention of type 2 diabetes are realized through acute and chronic improvements in insulin action.[6-8] The acute effects of a recent bout of exercise account for the majority of these improvements but are short-lived, while regular exercise training generally results in a more lasting effect. Although responses can vary, most persons with type 2 diabetes experience a decrease in their blood glucose levels during mild- and moderate-intensity exercise and for 2 to 72 hours afterward.[6-9] Much research has been focused on understanding these physiological pathways. There are acute and long-term benefits for the individual with or at risk for developing diabetes. However, the beneficial effects of physical activity diminish quickly if the activity is not performed regularly. Individuals with type 1 diabetes can become similarly insulin resistant (and require larger insulin doses) when not engaging in regular physical activity,[3] although physical activity cannot prevent the onset of type 1 diabetes.

To use physical activity to the best advantage, it behooves the diabetes educator to have a basic understanding of these physiological pathways. This knowledge is of value in the prevention and care of type 2 diabetes and in the prevention and management of its complications in all types of diabetes. With this basis of knowledge, the educator can best assist individuals in implementing physical fitness programs.

The role of physical activity in type 2 diabetes prevention in high-risk individuals was examined in both the Finnish Diabetes Prevention Study[10] and the US Diabetes Prevention Program.[11] Data from both studies showed that modest weight loss as a result of physical activity and nutrition strategies reduced the incidence of developing type 2 diabetes by 58% and that these lifestyle changes were more effective in older individuals. While the studies did not determine which aspect of the combined lifestyle intervention was more effective, the inclusion of moderate-intensity exercise for 150 minutes a week undoubtedly contributed to the positive outcome. Moreover, increased physical activity reduced the risk of type 2 diabetes even when weight loss goals of 7% were not achieved during the latter study.[12]

Physical activity activates the release of the catecholamines epinephrine and norepinephrine, which are released in an exaggerated fashion in response to intense exercise in particular, and other hormones that significantly influence how the primary fuel substrates (carbohydrate, protein, and fat) are used for energy production (see Table 17.3).[13] Exercise-induced changes to the secretion of key hormones allow alternate fuels to be made available as energy sources while maintaining glucose homeostasis. Endogenous insulin secretion normally decreases during physical activity, and its suppression is an essential step in allowing hepatic glucose production to maintain the balance of glucose in the blood.

Glycogen stores in the liver and muscle need to be replenished following each bout of physical activity. This demand is met by an increased rate of glucose uptake until the depleted glycogen stores are fully replaced. This activity may take 24 to 48 hours to complete. This extended recovery period is also characterized by enhanced insulin sensitivity and improved fat oxidation.[9] There are many long-term adaptations (see Table 17.4) to habitual physical activity that may prevent or delay the onset of type 2 diabetes.

Promoting Lifestyle Changes Among Family Members of Those Diagnosed With Type 2 Diabetes

Family history has long been accepted as an important determinant of who may develop type 2 diabetes, but whether the ultimate trigger is genetics or environmental factors, type 2 diabetes is occurring more often in all age and ethnic groups.[14] Therefore, the known person with type 2 diabetes has established an increased risk of developing the disease that is relayed to all other family members. The challenge and opportunity for the diabetes educator is to use

TABLE 17.3	Normal Hormonal Responses and the Resultant Acute Metabolic Effects of Physical Activity	
Hormone	*Response During Physical Activity*	*Metabolic Effect of Hormonal Response*
Insulin	Decreases	Facilitates hepatic glucose production and free fatty acid (FFA) release from adipose tissues
Glucagon	Increases	Increases hepatic glucose production via glycogenolysis and gluconeogenesis, thereby increasing glucose supply available in the blood
Epinephrine	Increases	Stimulates muscle glycogen breakdown and FFA production, which provides glycerol as a substrate for gluconeogenesis; may enhance hepatic glucose production during exercise; decreases insulin secretion
Norepinephrine	Increases	Stimulates hepatic glucose production; reduces muscular glucose uptake during physical activity; decreases insulin secretion
Growth Hormone and Cortisol	Increase	Increase lipolysis; decrease insulin-stimulated glucose uptake (ie, heighten insulin resistance); increase supply of glycerol and amino acids to liver for new glucose production; result in primarily delayed effects that are important during prolonged activities

TABLE 17.4   Metabolic Adaptations to Regular Aerobic Activity

Hormone	*Adaptation*	*Metabolic Effect of Adaptation*
Proinsulin[1]	Decreases	Decreased synthesis of insulin in the pancreas
Glucokinase[1]	Decreases	Decreased secretion of insulin from the pancreas
GLUT4[2,3]	Increases	Increases the capacity for insulin-stimulated glucose transport in the muscle, primarily during rest
PI3-Kinase[4,5]	Increases	Increased activity may improve insulin signaling and action
MAP Kinase Pathway[6]	Increases	Increased activity in this pathway may be associated with changes in the muscle that improve glucose storage and disposal
Nonesterified Fatty Acids (NEFAs)[7,8]	Increases	Increased ability to store and mobilize NEFAs as a fuel source; improved muscle capacity to extract NEFAs from the blood and oxidize for energy during and after exercise

Sources:

1. Koranyi LI, Bourey RE, Slentz CA, Hollosky JO. Coordinate reduction of rat pancreatic islet glucokinase and proinsulin mRNA by exercise training. Diabetes. 1991;40:401-4.
2. Christ-Roberts CY, Pratipanawatr T, Pratipanawatr W, et al. Exercise training increases glycogen synthase activity and GLUT4 expression but not insulin signaling in overweight nondiabetic and type 2 diabetic subjects. Metabolism. 2004;53(9):1233-42.
3. O'Gorman DJ, Karlsson HK, McQuaid S, et al. Exercise training increases insulin-stimulated glucose disposal and GLUT4 (SLC2A4) protein content in patients with type 2 diabetes. Diabetologia. 2006;49(12):2983-92.
4. Kirwin JP, del Aguila LF, Hernandez JM, et al. Regular exercise enhances activation of IRS-1-associated PI3-kinase in human skeletal muscle. J Appl Physiol. 2000;88:797-803.
5. Christ-Roberts CY, Pratipanawatr T, Pratipanawatr W, Berria R, Belfort R, Mandarino LJ. Increased insulin receptor signaling and glycogen synthase activity contribute to the synergistic effect of exercise on insulin action. J Appl Physiol. 2003 Dec;95(6):2519-29.
6. Osman A, Hancock J, Hunt DG, Ivy JL, Mandarino LJ. Exercise training increases ERK3 activity in skeletal muscle of obese Zucker rats. J Appl Physiol. 2001;90:454-60.
7. Boon H, Blaak EE, Saris WH, Keizer HA, Wagenmakers AJ, van Loon LJ. Substrate source utilisation in long-term diagnosed type 2 diabetes patients at rest, and during exercise and subsequent recovery. Diabetologia. 2007;50(1):103-12.
8. Goodpaster BH, Katsiaras A, Kelley DE. Enhanced fat oxidation through physical activity is associated with improvements in insulin sensitivity in obesity. Diabetes. 2003;52(9):2191-7.

the research data to assist those family members as well as the person with diabetes in making the recommended lifestyle changes.

Effect of Physical Activity on Diabetes Management

Aerobic (Cardiovascular) Exercise

Type 2 Diabetes

The chronic effects of performing regular aerobic, or cardiovascular, exercise appear to provide a number of benefits to individuals with type 2 diabetes[15-17]:

◆ Reduced A1C level
◆ Improved insulin sensitivity
◆ Assistance in attaining and maintaining desirable body weight
◆ Decreased coronary artery disease (CAD) risk

Several long-term studies have demonstrated a sustained improvement in glucose control when a regular aerobic training program is maintained.[8,16–18] Thus, remaining physically active is an essential component of diabetes self-management behavior for all individuals with type 2 diabetes. In general, many benefits can be expected with improved functioning of the cardiovascular system that results from aerobic training:

◆ Improved strength and physical work capacity
◆ Fewer or moderated risk factors for CAD
◆ Adjunct therapy for controlling hypertension
◆ Reduction in plasma cholesterol, triglycerides, and low-density lipoprotein (LDL) cholesterol
◆ Increase in high-density lipoproteins (HDL)
◆ Increased insulin sensitivity
◆ Enhanced fibrinolysis
◆ Favorable changes in body composition (reduction of body fat and/or weight; gain of muscle mass)

Type 1 Diabetes

Considerable evidence exists for the health benefits of regular physical activity for people with type 1 diabetes, and, therefore, physical activity in the form of both aerobic and resistance exercise should be included as part of their diabetes self-management program.[19] However, since the literature has shown inconsistent A1C results with physical activity in this population, care must be taken to achieve this goal when promoting blood glucose management as an expected outcome. Instead, focusing on the general health benefits listed in the previous section (related to type 2 diabetes) or the role that physical activity plays in the prevention of insulin resistance may be more productive.[9,18] More study is needed to determine how varying a person's workouts acutely affects the management of type 1 diabetes and how best to manage this added glycemic variable. However, throughout life the individual with type 1 diabetes is fully capable of engaging in a physical fitness plan and gains many health benefits from doing so.[20] Moreover, the glycemic response to aerobic exercise has some degree of reproducibility within an individual with type 1 diabetes, as long as many of the variables known to impact glucose homeostasis are held constant, such as the pre-exercise meal, the insulin dose, and the exercise task itself.[21]

Promote an Active Lifestyle

Remaining physically active is an essential part of self-care for all persons with type 2 diabetes. For those with type 1 diabetes, the health benefits of physical activity are also important to emphasize, but additional regimen changes will likely be needed to maintain control over blood glucose levels.

To safely and successfully pursue a physically active lifestyle, the individual with type 1 diabetes needs to develop hypoglycemia prevention strategies, as do many individuals with type 2 diabetes using insulin or taking insulin secretagogues. The success of a workout should not always be gauged by how much blood glucose numbers fall. In fact, large drops in blood glucose are more likely to lead to rapid-onset hypoglycemia and worsened control. The focus instead needs to be on keeping the blood glucose level from interfering with the workout or intended physical activity. Hypoglycemia prevention is discussed later in this chapter.

Resistance Exercise

Resistance exercise includes strength training and core conditioning. It is an important means of preserving and increasing muscular strength (measured using a 1-repetition maximum), muscular endurance (eg, the number of push-ups done in a minute), power (a 50-yd dash), and balance (standing on 1 leg). Resistance exercise has been shown to improve glycemic control, possibly even more so than aerobic training in persons with type 2 diabetes.[16,22,23] Similarly, previously sedentary individuals with type 1 diabetes (ages 13-30) engaging in 12 weeks of either aerobic or resistance exercise training experienced lower insulin requirements and post-training blood glucose levels, although their A1C levels were not significantly improved.[24] An older adult also receives the added advantage of preventing accidental falls and increased mobility with resistance work. This can allow an elderly person to remain more independent and self-sufficient.[25]

Flexibility Exercise

Stretching should be considered an option to include in the fitness plan for individuals with diabetes. While recent studies question whether this type of exercise protects an individual from injury,[26] traditional stretching, as well as exercises like yoga and tai chi, can provide other fitness benefits. Research conducted on individuals who performed tai chi[27] and yoga[28] reported improvements in participants' cardiovascular fitness levels. A recent meta-analysis of yoga studies stated that the limitations characterizing most studies, such as small sample size and varying forms of yoga, preclude drawing firm conclusions about the benefits to diabetes management.[29] However, both of these modalities include basic stretching movements as part of the instruction. Flexibility exercise combined with resistance training can increase joint range-of-motion in individuals with diabetes[30] and allow them to more easily engage in activities that require flexibility. For this reason, flexibility training may be included as part of a physical activity program, although it should not substitute for other training. An older adult who engages in flexibility exercise has the added advantages of preventing accidental falls and increasing joint mobility during resistance work.[31] In addition, flexibility programs are easy to perform and may provide the perfect introduction to a more physically active lifestyle for deconditioned individuals.

Physiological Responses to Physical Activity: Understanding Changes Associated With Blood Glucose Levels

Blood glucose levels can change during and after physical activity. The physiological responses associated with these changes are detailed in the following paragraphs.

As Physical Activity Begins

Regardless of the fuel source, the release of phosphate from adenosine triphosphate (ATP) produces the direct energy necessary for muscle contraction. Some stored energy is readily available in muscles for the first 10 seconds of activity (as depicted in Figure 17.1). Beyond that, muscles must use alternative energy systems to fuel physical activity, which is primarily accomplished via enzymatic pathways that initially break down carbohydrate and later fat and protein. During the first few minutes of physical activity, the majority of energy is derived from intramuscular glycogen, which is broken down without oxygen. This anaerobic pathway provides only a limited amount of energy, peaks at about 30 seconds into an activity, and lasts a maximum of 2 minutes. When activity is intense, this pathway may result in acid by-products that can cause muscular discomfort (a burning sensation) and a reduced exercise capacity. This energy pathway is particularly important at the onset of physical activity when aerobic conversion of

---

Cases: Facilitating Self-management of Physical Activity

Type 2 Diabetes

DK is a 62-year-old mother of 3 children. She was diagnosed with gestational diabetes mellitus during her third pregnancy. She learned then that her risk of developing type 2 diabetes would be higher. She told herself that she would take off the 80 pounds that had accumulated over the 3 pregnancies. But the years went by, and she found that her days were full working as a dental hygienist, being a wife, and raising her children. Instead of losing weight, she actually gained 40 pounds. She was not surprised when she was diagnosed with type 2 diabetes 6 years ago when seeking treatment of recurrent vaginal yeast infections. While she had been happy to lose 20 pounds over the previous year without any effort on her part, she knew her thirst, fatigue, and blurry vision were not good signs. A blood glucose value of 370 mg/dL (20.6 mmol/L) confirmed her suspicions. She was immediately started on metformin (Glucophage®, Bristol-Myers Squibb).

Type 1 Diabetes

HW is a 48-year-old telecommunications manager who is married and a father of 2 boys. Athletic throughout his life, he often included sports or outdoor pursuits as part of his family time. Everyone was shocked when he was told at age 45 that he had diabetes. He was initially treated for type 2 diabetes. Although the addition of medications helped at first, when his blood glucose levels did not improve on oral agents, his wife convinced him to see his healthcare provider. HW then had autoimmunity tests performed and was diagnosed with latent autoimmune diabetes of the adult, a form of type 1 diabetes.

He was somewhat relieved by this news. He had been doing everything he could to control his blood glucose—exercising to the best of his ability and eating almost nothing (particularly avoiding carbohydrates)—but his blood glucose levels continued to rise steadily over time. As exercise became more physically difficult for him, he was ready to accept that hiking, camping, hunting, biking, kayaking, and ice hockey refereeing were all a thing of the past. The diagnosis of type 1 diabetes explained why his blood glucose levels had stayed so high despite his best efforts. HW was started on insulin therapy and gained new hope that he may be able to resume the active lifestyle he and his family enjoyed.

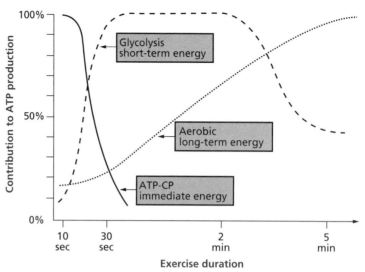

FIGURE 17.1   Energy Systems During Physical Activity

Reprinted with permission from SR Colberg, *Diabetic Athlete's Handbook: Your Guide to Peak Performance* (Champaign, Ill: Human Kinetics, 2009), 27.

energy is too slow to compensate or at any time during a workout when the exercise intensity is increased. As physical activity continues, an adequate supply of energy becomes available through the aerobic breakdown of carbohydrate, fat, and protein, although carbohydrate remains the body's preferred energy source for most activities.[32]

After 5 to 10 Minutes

During sustained movement, carbohydrate, fat, and protein are broken down to continuously provide energy to working muscles. For moderate and intense activity, the primary fuel remains carbohydrate, primarily muscle glycogen with a small amount of blood glucose. After 5 to 10 minutes, circulating glucose arising from glycogen breakdown in the liver (hepatic glycogenolysis) and glucose being synthesized there (hepatic gluconeogenesis) provide additional energy sources for working muscles.[32]

Beyond 20 Minutes

As exercise continues beyond 20 to 30 minutes, muscle glycogen stores may start to become depleted. The rate of glycogen utilization is highly dependent on exercise intensity and duration, with more being used at greater intensities and/or during longer durations.

Whenever glycogen decreases, a shift in the fuel mix is required. During low to moderate exercise intensities, free fatty acids (FFAs) become an increasingly significant source of energy, in addition to blood glucose from hepatic sources. As physical exercise continues, hepatic gluconeogenesis becomes increasingly important for providing the required glucose. The main substrates for hepatic gluconeogenesis are lactate, amino acids (eg, alanine), and glycerol.[32]

Longer Duration Activity

As exercise duration increases further, the contribution of FFA for fuel increases relative to glucose. Exercise of low to moderate intensity relies largely on circulating FFA as the oxidative fuel for muscle, although protein sources may provide 5% to 15% of the total energy. The oxidation of fat-derived substrates cannot completely replace carbohydrate use, given that there is a minimum amount of carbohydrate required for fat to be efficiently used as a fuel. When carbohydrate sources are too limited, fat is not completely oxidized and ketone bodies are formed as a by-product of the incomplete combustion of fat.[32] Ketones are not an efficient source of energy during exercise. Without an adequate supply of carbohydrate available, the exercise intensity cannot be maintained; this may explain exercisers "bonking" or runners "hitting the wall" during long-duration activities like marathons.

Hypoglycemia
Assessing Risk for Hypoglycemia

Being physically active is extremely beneficial to general health, important in the prevention of type 2 diabetes, and an essential health-management behavior for anyone with diabetes. However, due to distinctions in pathophysiology and treatment options, physical activity frequently affects blood glucose levels differently in people with type 1 diabetes or type 2 diabetes. Understanding these differences helps the diabetes educator identify and avoid common blood glucose concerns associated with physical activity.

In type 1 diabetes in particular, a number of factors can increase the risk for exercise-associated hypoglycemia, including the timing, duration, and intensity of the activity. Engaging in a new or unfamiliar activity may also increase the risk, while endurance training may lower it.[33] In addition, individuals with type 1 diabetes have multiple impairments in their counterregulatory hormone response to hypoglycemia and exercise, placing them at high risk for severe hypoglycemia. Both antecedent hypoglycemia and exercise cause reduced neuroendocrine, metabolic, and symptom responses to subsequent hypoglycemia or exercise.[34] After the first few years of the onset of diabetes, the glucagon response to hypoglycemia is typically diminished or lost, although its response to exercise may still be intact.[35,36] Increases in epinephrine are also blunted during both exercise and hypoglycemia.[37] Even if counterregulatory responses to hypoglycemia (and exercise) occur, excessive exogenous insulin dosing can blunt hepatic glucose production and increase peripheral glucose disposal, thereby resulting in rapid hypoglycemia. Other factors like inadequate carbohydrate intake, failure to monitor blood glucose levels, and exercising in the heat may also increase the risk of hypoglycemia. In older individuals with type 2 diabetes, a marked subjective unawareness of hypoglycemia has been reported that does not depend on altered neuroendocrine counterregulation and may contribute to the increased probability of severe hypoglycemia in these individuals.[38]

Medication Impact on Risk for Hypoglycemia

Modern pharmacological regimens for people with diabetes vary greatly based on the individual's needs. Today, the regimens used to treat type 2 diabetes often include combinations of different classes of antihyperglycemic agents. Each class of medication has its own list of potential side effects. Since hypoglycemia is one of the most common concerns associated with physical activity that people with diabetes have, the patient must understand whether the potential of this side effect exists with the medication regimen in use.

Fear of hypoglycemia is the strongest reported barrier to regular physical activity in adults with type 1 diabetes, highlighting the importance of information and support regarding hypoglycemia management for these individuals.[39] Insulin—a part of medication treatment regimens for all individuals with type 1 diabetes and many with type 2 diabetes—is the medication that poses the greatest risk for hypoglycemia. Circulating levels of this hormone are normally reduced by the body naturally during exercise, but injected (or pumped) insulin cannot be regulated as effortlessly without pre-exercise planning. Administration of short- or rapid-acting human insulin or insulin analogs 2 to 3 hours before the onset of physical activity increases hypoglycemia risk, particularly if doses are not adjusted downward in anticipation of being active. Since exercise often occurs in a timeframe of 0 to 4 hours after insulin administration, persons taking regular or rapid-acting insulin analogs are typically exercising when circulating insulin levels are too high, relatively speaking, for aerobic exercise.[37] In these situations, corrections in insulin dosage and/or additional carbohydrates are typically needed.

Basal insulin generally has a lesser acute impact on glycemic balance during most activities, but it may need to be adjusted prior to participation in long-duration events. Moreover, a recent study[40] indicated that hypoglycemia risk may be higher with use of certain basal insulins. Both insulin detemir (Levemir®, Novo Nordisk) and neutral protamine Hagedorn (NPH) were associated with less hypoglycemia than insulin glargine (Lantus™, Sanofi-Aventis) in people with relatively well-controlled type 1 diabetes during and after 30 minutes of exercise undertaken 5 hours after the last mealtime and basal insulin injection.

However, the best indicator of risk is likely the individual's past experiences with physical activity.

By way of contrast, an individual with type 2 diabetes who is not prescribed any diabetes medications has a low risk of experiencing exercise-induced hypoglycemia. Even so, the degree of risk associated with hypoglycemia varies from person to person, based on medication regimen, food intake, and physical activity choices. For example, individuals with a low carbohydrate intake are more likely to deplete muscle glycogen stores rapidly during exercise and increase their risk of exercise-associated hypoglycemia. During assessment, the educator must identify other variables that may contribute to or protect the individual from hypoglycemia (ie, elevated versus near-normal A1C, usual timing of activity, type or duration of diabetes, and food preferences). At times, the best risk indicator for hypoglycemia is the individual's own personal experience. When the risk exists, strategies to prevent it during physical activity need to be reviewed.

Help patients understand their individualized risk for hypoglycemia related to physical activity participation.

When the risk of hypoglycemia does not realistically exist, it is just as important to communicate this information to the patient and family members to eliminate a perceived barrier to a physically active lifestyle. The person with diabetes will no longer harbor fears or have concerns about what he or she has heard about physical activity and hypoglycemia, and will better understand how to prevent unexpected and unwanted decreases in blood glucose levels associated with physical activity.

Table 17.5 can be used as a reference to categorize prescription diabetes medications and identify those that place the user at higher risk for exercise-related hypoglycemia. In addition to the medications listed in the table, diabetes educators and other clinicians must be aware of the possibility of a hypoglycemia side effect from new diabetes medications coming into use and from other medications the person may be taking. Some of the newer medications—such as exenatide, sitagliptin, saxagliptin, pramlintide, and liraglutide—have not been well researched with regard to hypoglycemia risk but appear not to

TABLE 17.5 Risk of Hypoglycemia Side Effects With Various Diabetes Medications	
No or Minimal Risk	*Higher Risk*
Acarbose: Precose®	Glimepiride: Amaryl®
Metformin and combinations with metformin: Glucophage® Avandamet® (metformin/ rosiglitizone)	Glipizide and combinations with glipizide: Glucotrol®, Glucotrol XL® MetaGlip (glipizide/ metformin)
Miglitol: Glyset®	Glyburide and combinations with glyburide: DiaBeta Glynase® PresTab®
Pioglitazone: Actos®	Micronase® Glucovance® (glyburide/ metformin)
Rosiglitizone: Avandia®	Nateglinide: Starlix®
Bromocriptine: Cycloset®	Repaglinide: Prandin®
Exenatide: Byetta® (daily) Bydureon™ (weekly)	Insulin: All types and delivery methods
Liraglutide: Victoza®	
Sitagliptin: Januvia®	
Saxagliptin: Onglyza™	
Pramlintide: Symlin®	
Canagliflozin: Invokana®	
Dapagliflozin: Farxiga®	

Note: Well-known brand names are listed under the generic names. Always consider new diabetes medications that may not be listed and medications prescribed for diabetes complications or other conditions.

confer much risk.[41] However, there are some anecdotal reports of hard-to-treat episodes of hypoglycemia related to physical activity undertaken when exenatide and pramlintide doses were taken close to initiation of activity.[20] Conversely, exenatide has also been shown to cause an exaggerated release of catecholamines and a rise in blood glucose during aerobic exercise in men without diabetes.[42]

Not all hypoglycemic episodes associated with physical activity occur during activity or even immediately afterward. Low blood glucose levels may be biphasic after exercise, both immediately afterward and again 7 to 11 hours later, and occur for up to 24 or more hours after the exercise has stopped.[43] Later onset hypoglycemia becomes a greater concern when carbohydrate stores such as muscle and liver glycogen are depleted during an acute bout of exercise, usually one that is either higher intensity (aerobic or resistance training) or prolonged (usually aerobic). In particular, repeated interval workouts or intense resistance training can result in substantial depletion of muscle glycogen, thereby increasing the risk for later onset hypoglycemia particularly if supplemental insulin or longer lasting sulfonylureas or other insulin secretagogues are taken. [44,45] The consumption of moderate amounts of carbohydrates (5-30 grams, depending on the individual's postexercise blood glucose levels) during and within 30 minutes to 2 hours after exhaustive, glycogen-depleting exercise will lower hypoglycemia risk and allow for more efficient restoration of muscle glycogen.[46]

Other Medication Considerations

Certain diabetes medications must be taken into account when assessing risk of falls or other adverse outcomes potentially associated with physical activity. For example, a recent study[47] assessed whether a link exists between metformin and falls in older persons with type 2 diabetes; while no direct connection was found, an indirect association caused by neuropathy secondary to vitamin B_{12} deficiency (resulting from metformin use) may be of concern. In addition, insulin use has been demonstrated to increase the risk of falls related to hypoglycemia in the elderly, and thiazolidinediones (Actos®, Takeda Pharmaceuticals, and Avandia®, GlaxoSmithKline) increase fracture risk and thus may worsen fall-related outcomes.[47] When creating a physical activity plan, the risk of falls and fall-related complications associated with these medications should not be ignored in certain populations.

Establishing Blood Glucose Goals

Once the individual understands whether he or she is at risk for hypoglycemia, the next step is establishing reasonable blood glucose goals for physical activity. This process engages the individual's problem-solving skills, another of the AADE7 Self-Care Behaviors™.[4] The diabetes educator must tailor the complexity of these steps to the individual's abilities. Additional complications or circumstances that may have an effect must also be considered. For example, steroids and beta-adrenergic blocking agents are two other classes of prescription medications that need to be considered when predicting or interpreting an individual's blood glucose response to physical activity; steroids are likely to result in hyperglycemia, while beta-blockers can cause hypoglycemia. Moreover, beta-blockers also lower the heart rate response to submaximal and maximal exercise and may result in early fatigue. Complications like gastroparesis may already exist, making blood glucose levels erratic at times.[48] If the individual has hypoglycemia unawareness, taking additional blood glucose readings may be helpful.

Nowadays, many active individuals with type 1 diabetes have the option of using continuous glucose monitoring systems to track glucose trends, although rapid changes in blood glucose are still better detected with finger-stick readings. If more blood glucose readings cannot be performed due to finances or the individual's unwillingness to do so, other options should be explored to make sure any risks, including those associated with hypoglycemia, are minimized during and after participation in any physical activity. Modifications may, for example, capitalize on opportunities such as the following: exercising after meals, when blood glucose levels may be higher; making bouts of physical activity shorter but more intense to keep glucose levels higher; exercising at the time of day when blood glucose levels are highest; or exercising in the presence of trained helpers or peers who can watch for symptoms of hypoglycemia.

The individual's personal history can help the educator establish reasonable blood glucose goals for physical activity. These guidelines are a good starting point:

- *Using diabetes medication with hypoglycemia side effect:* Keep blood glucose level above 90 mg/dL during all physical activities.
- *Using insulin:* Keep blood glucose level above 110 mg/dL.
- *With other complications or circumstances:* Keep blood glucose level above 120 mg/dL.

◆ *Using oral agents that do not cause hypoglycemia or not on medication for diabetes:* No minimal threshold is necessary.

Adjusting the Diabetes Regimen to Accommodate Physical Activity

To keep blood glucose levels above the target goal before, during, and after physical activity, most people will need to adjust other aspects of the diabetes regimen. These adjustments are intended to either

◆ *Balance the amount of glucose* available with sufficient blood glucose (through ingestion of carbohydrates), or

◆ *Normalize the amount of insulin* circulating during physical activity (with medication or timing adjustments)

Both strategies may result in the blood glucose level drifting higher for a short period of time. However, once the physical activity begins, this glucose will likely be used to fuel the energy needs of the active muscles. While working out at higher intensities, some individuals may need to make adjustments that lower blood glucose levels rather than working to prevent hypoglycemia.

Questions to Ask

Including questions in the assessment process to determine what persons with diabetes know about their unique exercise responses and what they may have already tried is very helpful. Often, the person understands basic concepts or recognizes patterns but has not implemented regimen adjustments correctly, or the person may know to check blood glucose more often, eat a snack, or adjust the insulin dose, but still may not be seeing the desired blood glucose readings. Below are some appropriate points for discussion.

Troubleshoot hypoglycemia with appropriate questions.

When are the blood glucose readings taken? Frequently the blood glucose reported was taken hours before or after the physical activity was done. The person needs to check within minutes of starting and ending physical activity in order to get more accurate information on the acute effect of exercise. Also,

when later onset hypoglycemia is a concern, individuals may need to monitor more frequently for up to 8 or more hours afterward.[43]

Is hypoglycemia a possibility or concern? If so, ask for an extra reading to be taken during the physical activity to establish usual patterns of response. Sometimes, higher blood glucose readings after the workout are caused by unrecognized hypoglycemia during the workout. If blood glucose levels get too low without being detected, the body may respond with a large increase of glucose-raising catecholamines. If this is the cause, discuss a plan to prevent the possibility of hypoglycemia during the activity.

Was a snack eaten? If so, was it appropriate (in both type and quantity), and was it eaten at the correct time? If not, should a snack be included in the future?

Should a carbohydrate-containing sports drink be recommended to help with both hydration and blood glucose stabilization during exercise? If blood glucose is not a concern, plain water works equally well for hydration and avoids the intake of extra calories.

Why is the blood glucose higher after the physical activity? There are a few possibilities for this blood glucose response:

◆ *How much did blood glucose increase?* Get specifics. If the level went from 105 mg/dL to 117 mg/dL, that still reflects excellent results. If the level went from 209 mg/dL to 277 mg/dL, the person has an A1C of 11% and he or she is trying to avoid insulin, adjustments need to be made so that physical activity can benefit diabetes management, not worsen it.

◆ *Could this be the individual's normal response?* This can be a catch-22 for some people during physical activity. While glucose is in demand as a fuel, it is also being released to keep the supply available. For some people, supply can exceed demand. This is also a normal response to very vigorous types of physical activity. Fortunately, this is usually short-lived and blood glucose usually decreases within an hour or so postexercise. This response does not erase other fitness benefits, but the individual may feel discouraged or be concerned about potentially doing harm. One solution may be to exercise at a lower intensity by using a heart rate monitor to achieve a lower target heart rate (see chapter 5 for details about monitoring exercise intensity). The educator should direct attention to other health outcomes to help the individual recognize the benefits, which include weight loss, lower medication doses, better A1C, and improved lipids. If someone is hyperglycemic and ketotic, though, exercise is best avoided until better metabolic control is achieved.

- ◈ *What role does food have on the blood glucose response?* Sometimes the person does not consider a meal or snack that was eaten before or during the activity, or sometimes the person eats later or eats more food than usual. If this is the cause, the blood glucose reading will probably be better than it would have been if the person had not been physically active. This may not require any changes, only explanations.
- ◈ *Has this happened only once?* A single occurrence may not repeat itself. Just like many blood glucose readings, it may not be useful for clinical consideration. Consider potential confounding variables, such as environmental extremes, time of day that exercise was done, mental stress such as prerace anxiety, physical illness or infection, and hydration status.

Interpreting Hyperglycemia

In some circumstances, extremely high blood glucose readings can be indicative of other medical concerns, such as insulin deficiency. People with type 2 diabetes can have high blood glucose readings resulting from a combination of insulin resistance and inadequate insulin secretion. Extremely elevated glucose with severe dehydration can result in hyperosmolar hyperglycemia (see chapter 22, on hyperglycemia). When hyperosmolar hyperglycemia occurs, it may be aggravated by other extenuating health variables such as dehydration, severe illness, and infections.[49] Individuals with type 2 diabetes typically do not produce ketones; if ketones do exist, it is often termed starvation ketosis, as opposed to insulin deficiency and acidosis.

People with type 1 diabetes are more susceptible to insulin deficiency since they lack the ability to produce any insulin; therefore, they need to receive instruction on why and when to check for ketones. This is especially important if the individual is using an insulin pump. If ketones are present, then the higher blood glucose levels are a result of insulin deficiency, and corrective action should be taken immediately.

Because of this medical concern, most diabetes educators teach people with type 1 diabetes to check

---

Cases—Part 2: Effects of Physical Activity on Blood Glucose

Type 2 Diabetes

When diagnosed with type 2 diabetes, DK decided to start exercising. She was motivated to lose a lot of weight, and the faster she lost it, the better. She remembered when she used to be active and had enjoyed dancing, exercise classes, and playing games with her children. She was not sure how that person got lost, but she was determined to find her again.

DK was cleared to exercise by her healthcare provider, who told her any weight loss would improve her hypertension and hyperlipidemia. A friend told her that a snack was important to eat before exercise to keep her blood glucose from going too low. She remembered that metformin did not cause low blood glucose levels, but she was not sure what to do for exercise.

To be safe, she ate a package of 4 peanut butter crackers before walking a mile around her neighborhood. She became frustrated when she figured out she ate 190 calories but walked off only 100. Also, her blood glucose

readings were a little higher after her walk. This made no sense to her since she remembered being told that exercising should make her blood glucose go down, not up!

Type 1 Diabetes

HW was eager to take care of his diabetes. He was also happy to get back into his fitness routine. He liked to work out in the evenings, the time of day he could most easily get to his fitness club and when he usually refereed hockey games.

He read that hypoglycemia could be prevented by exercising after a meal. Since eating food increases blood glucose and exercise decreases it, he assumed everything would come out even. He took his usual premeal, rapid-acting insulin dose and ate dinner before going to his club. Twenty-five minutes into his moderate aerobic workout, however, HW had to stop and treat a blood glucose of 57 mg/dL (3.2 mmol/L). This was not what he expected!

for ketones when blood glucose levels are consistently above 300 mg/dL.[50] This advice can be followed by the individual with diabetes only when a blood glucose value is measured. Most readings are performed to determine an insulin dose before a meal or snack, when blood glucose levels are usually lower. When the blood glucose is being measured for physical activity, it must be taken at other times of the day as well. Therefore, the individual with diabetes may be seeing what is a normal blood glucose response to a meal but consider it too high for physical activity because it is higher than his or her usual readings. In the absence of moderate or higher levels of urinary or blood ketones, these higher readings are transient and should not pose a medical threat.[51,52] However, some people report headaches, blurry vision, or lack of energy with such elevated blood glucose levels, which may be reason enough to avoid physical activity until the glucose level improves.

Insulin regimens paired with frequent blood glucose measurements greatly diminish the chance of insulin deficiency developing. Therefore, ketones are rarely found when performing blood or urine checks. Hence, in most circumstances, slightly elevated blood glucose levels should not interfere with exercise performance. The individual's problem-solving skills again become important. The educator must consider

the ability of the individual to perform blood glucose and ketone testing and understand the complexity of the information.

On the other hand, physical activity performed at very intense aerobic levels can result in blood glucose levels climbing in individuals with type 1 diabetes.[53] In this circumstance, the catecholamine response to very intense activity results in an exaggerated hepatic production of glucose for fuel. After the activity is stopped, the insulin need can double during the postactivity period. If not met with the correct insulin dosing, this state of hyperglycemia may last for several hours for an individual with type 1 diabetes before returning to the desired level, or it may never return there at all without additional insulin.[54,55] This pattern of hyperglycemia needs to be confirmed and be fairly predictable before suggesting that any action be taken. Those using insulin pump therapy sometimes find it useful to bolus a small amount of insulin to address this physiological need. If the individual is injecting insulin by syringe, an additional injection of short- or rapid-acting insulin can also be administered. The timing and amount of insulin given require careful consideration and monitoring to accomplish the desired blood glucose result. Individuals must take into account any

---

Cases—Part 3: Learning to Make Appropriate Adjustments

Type 2 Diabetes

Snacks and Timing

DK thought about her pre-exercise snack and decided she did not need the peanut butter crackers before walking. However, she was still concerned about hypoglycemia and decided to walk only after she had eaten a meal. Sometimes this worked in her schedule, and sometimes it did not. When she was able to fit in a walk, DK noticed that her blood glucose levels had dropped by the time she finished. She was also glad she could skip all those extra calories. Yet she was sure she would have to walk a lot more to lose weight.

Type 1 Diabetes

Insulin Dose Adjustments

HW remembered being told that he may need to reduce his insulin dose before he exercised. The next time he went to the health club, he took 1 unit less than his normal 10-unit dinner dose. He thought the blood glucose of 154 mg/dL (8.6 mmol/L) before his workout was high enough and hoped to see it go down during exercise. It did drop—but too fast; 15 minutes into his workout he had to stop and treat another low blood glucose, this time 63 mg/dL (3.5 mmol/L). He decided to reduce his insulin by half the next time. He was alarmed, however, when his blood glucose reading the next night was 287 mg/dL (15.9 mmol/L) before his workout. He remembered something about not exercising with a blood glucose over 250 mg/dL (13.9 mmol/L) and ketones. Since he did not have ketone strips with him, he skipped the workout and went home not knowing what to do.

insulin remaining from their last injection or bolus in making subsequent adjustments to insulin doses, as well as factor in the residual effects of the last bout of activity on blood glucose use (ie, postexercise enhancements in insulin action). Regardless of the delivery method, this additional insulin dose can still result in hypoglycemia and may not be advisable in all cases.

Self-Management Strategies for Safe Physical Activity

Adding Carbohydrates

Snacking is the easiest adjustment for laypeople to understand and a strategy that those with diabetes often implement by themselves. Unfortunately, estimating the amount of food needed can be difficult. When the snack is not sufficient, hypoglycemia can still happen. If a snack larger than necessary is eaten, some degree of hyperglycemia may result. When weight loss is a goal of the fitness plan, both of these circumstances can result in more total calories being consumed, and when too many extra calories are consumed, weight gain will result instead of weight loss.

Monitoring

Blood glucose monitoring is useful to determine if and when a snack is required to keep the blood glucose within the established goals.

Encourage frequent blood glucose monitoring for problem solving with regard to physical activity.

Blood glucose readings taken at the *start* and *end* of an exercise session allow the individual to gauge the amount of change happening during physical activity and to determine whether additional carbohydrates are needed.[56] For example, if the blood glucose usually drops 30 to 40 mg/dL during a physical activity and the goal is to stay above 90 mg/dL, a pre-exercise snack should be eaten for readings below 130 mg/dL. For pre-exercise glucose levels between the target starting value and the goal, some—albeit a lesser amount—carbohydrate may still be needed.

A number of factors can influence actual carbohydrate needs, however, including intensity and duration of exercise, starting blood glucose level,

circulating insulin levels, the medication regimen followed, recent food and caloric beverage consumption, and timing of exercise, just to name a few. For example, even in individuals with type 2 diabetes, blood glucose levels are likely to decrease more during physical activity undertaken in the fed state (postmeal) compared with the fasted or premeal state at varying times of day.[57,58]

To prevent hypoglycemia in individuals with a relatively high risk for developing it during exercise, a general guideline is that a snack containing 10 to 30 g of carbohydrate should be consumed for every 30 to 45 minutes of moderate physical activity (see Table 17.6). The actual need will vary from person to person and even among activities done by one individual, making blood glucose monitoring critical for predicting snack requirements to optimize exercise performance and blood glucose control.

Type of Snack

The snack option must meet the fuel needs of the physical activity and the individual. Often, people with diabetes choose to consume juice or glucose tablets at the start of the physical activity because they know these options are used to treat hypoglycemic events and assume they are useful to prevent them as well. These work short-term but may not be the best for long-term prevention of hypoglycemia during extended exercise and afterward.

Snacks to prevent hypoglycemia are not always the same as those used to treat it.

For *preventing* hypoglycemia during exercise, a pre-exercise snack with carbohydrates that are more slowly absorbed or with a small amount of protein

TABLE 17.6 Carbohydrate Requirements During Aerobic Physical Activities		
Intensity	Carbohydrate Replacement	Frequency
Mild	0–10 g	Every 30 minutes
Moderate	5–10 g	Every 15 minutes
High	0–15 g	Every 15 minutes

Source: SR Colberg, *Diabetic Athlete's Handbook: Your Guide to Peak Performance* (Champaign, Ill: Human Kinetics, 2009), 29.

may be a better match for exercise fuel requirements than a rapidly absorbed carbohydrate source like glucose tablets or regular soda (snacks used to *treat* hypoglycemia). People with diabetes report consuming a variety of carbohydrate-based snacks during exercise, including sports bars, gels, and drinks, some of which contain protein (and fat) along with carbohydrate.[20] Carbohydrates that are more slowly absorbed can be found in whole grains, many whole fruits, yogurt, and even many snack bars. The best option is based on the desired blood glucose level throughout the activity, the duration and intensity of the activity, the individual's unique glucose response to exercise and tolerance to foods, and personal preferences.

After a bout of physical activity, additional snacks may be needed to prevent later onset hypoglycemia. The first 30 to 60 minutes after exercise is generally when muscles take up blood glucose to replace glycogen at the fastest rate and with the least insulin needed. Eating a small carbohydrate snack within 30 to 120 minutes postexercise may prevent hypoglycemia during that time. The actual number of carbohydrates required will vary with the type of activity done, the regimen changes implemented for the activity (lower insulin and/or higher carbohydrate intake), and the individual's immediate postexercise blood glucose level.

Hypoglycemia is also common 7 to 11 hours after exercise, and precautions may be needed to prevent its later occurrence, particularly during sleep.[43] The need for and composition of a bedtime snack depend on the blood glucose; for example, no snack may be necessary at levels >180 mg/dL (10 mmol/L), any snack may suffice at levels between 126 and 180 mg/dL (7 and 10 mmol/L), and a standard or protein snack may be needed for levels <126 mg/dL (7 mmol/L).[59] Although research is mixed on the effectiveness of snacking alone (regardless of the fat content) without insulin adjustments,[60,61] postexercise and bedtime snacks for insulin users to prevent late-onset and nighttime lows should likely contain higher relative amounts of fat and protein (such as found in whole milk, chocolate milk, or yogurt), which are metabolized more slowly and keep blood glucose levels more stable over time than carbohydrate alone.[62] A recent study demonstrated that a higher fat dinner meal with the same carbohydrate and protein content as a lower fat one raises insulin resistance and insulin dosing requirements for individuals with type 1 diabetes.[63] Consumption of bedtime carbohydrates that are more slowly digested (eg, uncooked cornstarch) may also prevent nighttime hypoglycemia following daytime exercise.[64]

Timing of Snack

The next consideration is when snacks should be eaten.

  ◆ *If the activity is being performed after a meal or usual snack:* No extra food may be needed. If more food is required, the amount of carbohydrate can be adjusted upward to achieve the desired blood glucose level.
  ◆ *If the activity is being performed more than 2 hours after a meal:* A snack should be eaten within 15 minutes of beginning the physical activity. This gives the glucose sufficient time to be digested and to enter the bloodstream, making fuel available to active muscles.

Fluids and Electrolytes

Maintaining adequate hydration is important during physical activity. Replenishing fluids is especially important if the activity results in excessive perspiration or lasts longer than an hour. If water is being consumed during the activity, additional carbohydrates can be introduced via a sports drink or other beverage.[65] Drinks containing 6% to 8% carbohydrate optimize gastric emptying. However, drinks with a carbohydrate concentration greater than 10% should be avoided during exercise because their high osmolality not only delays gastric emptying but also favors fluid shifts into the gut. Fruit juices and most regular soft drinks contain approximately 12% carbohydrate and can lead to gastrointestinal upset, such as cramps, nausea, vomiting, diarrhea, or bloating and "sloshing" during exercise, if not diluted with water. Since the carbohydrates in sports beverages are quickly absorbed, a few ounces must be consumed every 5 to 10 minutes to provide a consistent supply of fuel to prevent peaks and valleys in blood glucose levels. A 24-oz bottle of a typical sports drink contains about 42 g of CHO, which satisfies the recommended hourly intake for most endurance workouts, along with supplying important electrolytes crucial for fluid and pH balance, electrical impulses of neurons and muscles, and prevention of muscle cramps.

Medication Adjustments

Oral Agents

Meglitinides are the only class of oral antihyperglycemic agents that can be adjusted for physical activity. Since repaglinide (Prandin®, Novo Nordisk) and nateglinide (Starlix®, Novartis) have short durations of action, these medications can be reduced or omitted if physical activity will be performed a few hours after the meal. However, if physical activity is erratic or unpredictable, this may not be the best option. The doses of other oral medications may need to be lowered once a physical activity routine that improves insulin action is established, but not simply in anticipation of a single exercise session.

Insulin Adjustments

When engaging in physical activity, the individual using insulin must focus on the blood glucose level, which is affected by circulating levels of insulin and catecholamine release.

- If the circulating level of insulin is greater than physiological needs, hypoglycemia can occur.
- If the circulating level of insulin is insufficient, hyperglycemia can result.

Problem Solving

Determining the best routine to follow during periods of physical activity takes time—the individual with diabetes must learn, practice, and problem solve. Often, information from multiple workout sessions is needed as well as frequent blood glucose readings and patience. When appropriate, the individual can wear a continuous glucose monitoring (CGM) device. These devices can provide useful information about blood glucose trends before, during, and after physical activity, but the individual should keep in mind that readings from CGM devices are somewhat time-delayed, usually around 15 to 20 minutes, and may not identify hypoglycemia during exercise before it actually occurs. The interpretation of this information—particularly glucose trends during an activity—can lead to a better understanding of the insulin and food adjustments required to support exercise energy needs.

Benefits Gained Can Quickly Diminish

Beneficial effects of physical activity diminish quickly if activity does not occur regularly. Support patients to ensure that both the activity and the benefits continue.

In addition, the educator must consider that the routine will vary from person to person. Each person's blood glucose responses will be different due to the following:

- Type of diabetes
- Type of insulin and delivery method
- Time of day
- Intensity, type (aerobic versus resistance), and duration of physical activity
- Fitness level of individual
- Blood glucose level at start of physical activity
- Many other factors contributing to the blood glucose response to physical activity

As many of these factors can change over time for the individual, at each visit the educator needs to ensure that the routine continues to fit the patient's physiological needs. The following must be regularly considered:

- Seasonal variations
- Weight loss or gain
- Improved or decreased fitness levels
- Changes to medication dosing
- Sleep patterns
- Orthopedic limitations or injury
- Diabetic complications

Many strategies can be considered to effectively prevent hypoglycemia during physical activity:

- *Blood glucose monitoring.* Monitoring before and after a period of physical activity provides crucial feedback for the individual learning to adjust insulin and/or carbohydrate while active. Readings done at the start and end of the activity are the most common to gather, but to identify trends it may be necessary to check within 15 to 45 minutes prior to exercise, in the midst of exercise, or periodically for a few hours after its completion. Individuals using CGM can more easily track blood glucose trends.

- *Adjusting the insulin.* The physiological decrease in circulating insulin levels, which is a typical response to physical activity, does not naturally occur in persons treated with exogenous insulin. These individuals may need to reduce by 20% to 30% their rapid- or short-acting insulin dose administered prior to prolonged exercise of moderate intensity.[66,67] A dose administered within an hour after the activity may also need to be decreased to prevent postexercise hypoglycemia.

- *Proper administration of insulin.* Insulin should be injected into the subcutaneous fat layer. Syringe users should be taught to avoid intramuscular injection of insulin because contractions accelerate the absorption of insulin injected into the muscle into circulation.[68] Changing the injection site (assuming it is subcutaneous) to a part of the body not involved in the activity has not been shown to be helpful in preventing hypoglycemia. If the level of circulating insulin from exogenous sources is elevated, hypoglycemia is likely to occur.

- *Individualized adjustments.* Adjustments should be tailored to each individual's specific response to physical activity (see Table 17.7).

TABLE 17.7 Therapy Adjustments to Prevent Hypoglycemia Associated With Physical Activity
Adjust *insulin* for:
Weight loss (may require less insulin)
Improved control (may require more or less insulin)
Planned, regularly scheduled physical activity (may require less insulin overall)
Adjust with additional *carbohydrate* if:
Pre-exercise blood glucose level is not sufficient to prevent hypoglycemia during activity
Long duration of physical activity is planned
Physical activity is unplanned or erratic
Insulin adjustments are not possible or desired
Oral hypoglycemic medications are prescribed

The choices depend on the individual's goals and may require using a combination of additional carbohydrates and insulin adjustments.

Hypoglycemia often occurs at varying times after physical activity and is a significant concern to the individual treated with insulin. This is the result of acutely increased insulin mobilization and sensitivity, increased glucose utilization, replenishment of glycogen stores, and defective counterregulatory mechanisms.[50] Use these strategies to help individuals minimize future occurrences:

- Educate the patient about the possible causes of hypoglycemia.
- Reduce insulin doses as needed following physical activity.
- Increase the amount of carbohydrate (and protein and fat) consumed after physical activity.
- Make appropriate regimen changes to compensate for physical activity in proximity to bedtime (to prevent overnight hypoglycemia).
- Monitor blood glucose more often following physical activity.

Insulin Pump Therapy

With insulin pump therapy, basal rates and boluses can be adjusted based on the timing, duration, intensity, and type of activity performed. The degree of insulin reduction or carbohydrate supplementation depends on an individual's fitness level and the duration and intensity of the activity. Insulin pump users have these options to prevent hypoglycemia during periods of physical activity:

- Reduce the basal infusion rate (before, during, and/or after physical activity).
- Consume additional carbohydrates.
- Temporarily suspend pump or lower basal rates (before, during, and/or following activity).

As suggested in this chapter, many strategies can be used to prevent hypoglycemia during and following physical activity. Table 17.7 compares the insulin and snack (carbohydrate) adjustment options and suggests when they may be best to use. While one option may be preferred by or for an individual, there will be situations when the opposite or a combination of both of these strategies aids in achieving the desired blood glucose results.

The Exercise Prescription

The exercise prescription is simply the structured physical activity plan a person is to follow to attain physical fitness. The most difficult aspect for the clinician is designing a plan that meets the patient's desired fitness goals. A well-designed exercise prescription is based on technical and evidence-based research. The true artistry of the exercise prescription is found in simplifying its core messages to realistic situations that can be performed as part of everyday life. This requires the educator to understand the 5 components of an exercise prescription:

- Mode
- Intensity
- Frequency
- Duration
- Progression

Educators can additionally access the recommended physical activity guidelines and prescription for adults and older adults through the American College of Sports medicine (http://acsm.org) or the 2008 US federal guidelines (http://health.gov/paguidelines). For a comprehensive, case-study-based resource for exercise prescription that covers the gamut of diabetes types, complications, and other factors, readers are referred to *Exercise and Diabetes: A Clinician's Guide to Prescribing Physical Activity* (American Diabetes Association, 2013).

Determining Appropriate Modes

The type of physical activity chosen by the individual is in many ways less crucial than other components of the exercise prescription. While the mode or modes of physical activity, such as cardiovascular, strength training, or flexibility exercises, are important to consider, any type of increased movement appears to initially improve one's fitness level.[69] Sedentary individuals who begin participating in almost any type of physical activity experience measurable results in their fitness levels.

Accordingly, a wide range of physical activities can be explored and made part of the fitness plan. All opportunities that the individual identifies should be assessed and, if safe to perform, encouraged. As the individual becomes more successful and confident, options can be expanded and other types of physical activities added or substituted. See chapter 5, on being active, for more on strategies in support of this self-management behavior.

Cases—Part 4: Adjusting Workout Duration and Intensity

Type 2 Diabetes

Workout Duration and Progression

DK decided she would just have to walk longer to burn calories and improve her blood glucose level. She decided to walk 60 minutes each day on most days of the week. She was sure this would work—until she tried it. After the first 40 minutes on the first day, she was not even sure she would make it home. When she walked into her house, she felt very shaky and checked her blood glucose. It was 104 mg/dL (5.8 mmol/L)—her lowest number yet. She immediately went to the freezer and pulled out the ice cream. To top off her woes, her right hip was in severe pain for days. She surely was not going to put herself through that again!

Type 1 Diabetes

Workout Intensity and Adjustments

HW decided to try another type of workout with a reduction in his insulin dose: a heavy session of resistance training instead of an aerobic workout. Since his blood glucose had gone too high when he cut his predinner insulin in half, he reduced it by only 25% this time. About 30 minutes into his weight training workout, he started to feel funny so he pulled out his monitor and checked his blood glucose. He was shocked that his reading was even higher than before, reaching 318 mg/dL (17.7 mmol/L). He really had no idea why it had gone higher even with taking more insulin than the previous time, but he knew it was not supposed to get that high. He immediately stopped his workout and again went home not knowing what to do. He woke up in the middle of the night feeling shaky and sweating profusely. His blood glucose was 54 mg/dL (3.0 mmol/L), which was puzzling to him since he had not taken any extra insulin to bring down his high postworkout sugar and it had still been elevated (188 mg/dL [10.4 mmol/L]) at bedtime. Now he was really confused about how to handle his blood glucose and still engage in any type of workout.

Determining Acceptable Intensity

Determining the intensity of the physical activity takes the most care and attention for people with diabetes. This does not mean the harder the workout, the better the results. Rather, the intensity level of the physical activity must be matched to the individual's current fitness capabilities. An activity period that is too easy will not have the intended effect on the fitness level. If the activity period is too hard, the individual will not be able to complete the workout or, worse yet, may become injured or discouraged from exercising. Appropriate measures of intensity, including the "talk test," ratings of perceived exertion (RPEs), and target heart rate based on the heart rate reserve (HRR) method, are detailed in chapter 5.

Determining Acceptable Frequency and Duration

Physical activity sessions can be performed in a variety of combinations of frequency and duration.[69–72]

- ◆ *Frequency.* Most research concludes that physical activity should be performed 3 to 5 days per week to achieve significant health benefits. The latest guidelines for persons with type 2 diabetes suggest that those individuals should undertake at least 150 minutes a week of moderate to vigorous aerobic exercise spread over at least 3 days, with no more than 2 consecutive days without aerobic activity.[73] Adults with type 1 diabetes should aim for 150 minutes a week of moderate activity or 60 to 75 minutes of vigorous activity or a combination thereof.[69–72]
- ◆ *Duration.* The duration of the exercise session has been investigated as well. While 20 minutes has been the minimal recommendation to provide cardiovascular improvements, multiple shorter bouts of 10 minutes, repeated to equal 30 total minutes, have also resulted in measurable improvements.[74] Generally, both the American College of Sports Medicine and the latest federal guidelines suggest that moderate exercise requires a longer duration than more intense exercise to gain the same

cardiovascular benefits.[70–72] Longer bouts of physical activity, lasting 60 minutes or more, may be necessary to achieve weight loss or to prevent weight regain.[70]

While each individual's needs, goals, and circumstances vary, evidence-based research can assist in the design of a program for health-related physical fitness. Special considerations for children, teens, older adults, and pregnant women are discussed below.

Expecting Progress in Appropriate Stages

In the United States, most people lead sedentary lifestyles.[75] Many people do not think about spending, nor do they even think it is possible to spend, the recommended 20 to 30 or more minutes per day doing any type of physical activity. Diabetes educators must, therefore, provide realistic instruction that includes both how to start a fitness program and what to reasonably expect in terms of progress (see Table 17.8). The individual must understand the type, quantity, and rate of progress to expect. Over a period of time averaging at least 4 to 6 months, each individual moves through 3 distinct stages of using a fitness plan:

Initial Stage
in which habits are established

↓

Improvement Stage
in which progress is seen, but habits may weaken

↓

Maintenance Stage
in which extensions are planned

Initial Stage

Most people never make it out of the critical initial stage. They either attempt activities that are too difficult for their fitness level or develop unrealistic expectations of what they will be able to accomplish and when. They quickly become discouraged and stop. The real success from this stage comes from the individual beginning to form physical activity habits that can easily be integrated into his or her lifestyle.

TABLE 17.8 Physical Activity Program Stages and Rates of Progression

Program Stage	Week	Frequency (per week)	Intensity (% HRR)	Duration (minutes)
Initial	1–4	3–4	30%–59%	15–30
Improvement	5–24	3–5	40%–89%	25–40
Maintenance	25+	3–5	40%–89%	20–60

◆ Help the individual understand that measurable changes may not occur during this period. Building fitness habits takes at least 4 weeks, and may take longer in individuals who start with very poor fitness levels.

◆ Sedentary individuals are more likely to form lasting exercise habits when the initial stage starts at a lower intensity and progresses very slowly over time, that is, "start low, go slow."

Improvement Stage

During the improvement stage, the focus shifts from developing habits to improving the fitness level. The individual now has improved stamina and endurance, is able to engage in physical activity for longer amounts of time, and can begin adding to the workload or intensity of the workout. Over the 3 or more months (or longer for deconditioned and older individuals) of this stage, measurable health benefits should start to be observed. However, individuals can interpret this initial success as permanent change, which may sabotage their efforts. The individual may allow other routine parts of everyday life to take priority again and start missing workout sessions.

◆ Identify and seek progress in fitness goals by aiming for moderate (or higher) exercise intensity in this stage.

◆ Once improvements begin to show, help the person avoid becoming complacent or slacking off.

◆ Foster success beyond the first milestone and over the longer term.

Habit Formation: The Initial Goal

In the first 4 weeks or so of a fitness plan, the goal is not to achieve measurable changes in fitness but rather to establish habits and baseline levels of endurance that will make fitness progress possible.

Maintenance Stage

Once an individual has successfully met the major goals originally defined, new goals and a new plan need to be developed (see SMART goal setting in chapter 5). The new goal may be as simple as "preventing weight regain" or as challenging as "training for a competitive event."

◆ Review goals routinely at medical and diabetes education visits.

◆ Reassess for medication changes, new diagnoses, or progression of existing diseases to ensure the fitness routine continues to be safe and effective.

◆ Develop new goals and plans once existing ones are achieved.

◆ Choose appropriate exercise goals with injury prevention and long-term maintenance of activity in mind.

Special Populations
Children and Teens

Physical activity has a direct impact on weight control, cardiovascular risk factors, bone development, and mental health over a lifetime. A sedentary lifestyle in young people is often seen to lead to negative health consequences in the near term and later in life. (See exercise recommendations in chapter 5.)

◆ *Mode.* Care should be taken to identify safe and age-appropriate options for physical activity, which should evolve as the young individual undergoes normal maturation in coordination, motor skills, social development, and personal interests. Athletes with diabetes, especially those youth who participate in sports year-round, may be even more prone to repetitive use, soft tissue injuries that can be avoided with a modified training schedule.

◆ *Frequency and duration.* For the pediatric population, 60 or more minutes of physical activity performed on most days of the week is the general guideline.[76]

◆ *Assigned responsibilities.* Responsibility for diabetes care decisions evolves; teenagers begin to take on more of the responsibility and seek independence from parental supervision. Diabetes counseling should include clear assignment of the expected tasks to be performed and distribution of these care responsibilities.

◆ *Hypoglycemia prevention.* The blood glucose changes that occur during physical activity need to be addressed for anyone at risk of hypoglycemia, including the pediatric population. One research study confirmed lower starting blood glucose levels increased the incidence of hypoglycemia.[77] Hypoglycemia occurred in 86% of subjects performing a 75-minute physical activity session when starting blood glucose values were less than 120 mg/dL, in 13% of subjects when starting glucose was 120 to 180 mg/dL, and in 6% when starting glucose was higher than 180 mg/dL. The study also revealed that a 15-g carbohydrate snack was frequently insufficient to successfully treat a hypoglycemic event. This study reinforces the necessity of beginning at a target blood glucose level and consuming a sufficient amount of carbohydrate to decrease the risk of experiencing a hypoglycemic episode during physical activity. It is also important to teach parents of young exercisers with diabetes not to overreact to postexercise hyperglycemia, which is usually only transient and may need reduced or no insulin to treat effectively for several hours afterward.

◆ *Special concerns.* Disordered eating behaviors are prevalent among teens and young adults, and this behavior has been reported in individuals with type 1 diabetes.[78] Insulin omission and misuse have also been reported in this population. Likewise, exercise patterns can become compulsive in this age group in an attempt to control both blood glucose levels and body weight with excessive physical activity. Educators should be vigilant for signs and symptoms of such behaviors.

Older Adults

Older adults who have been primarily sedentary and may have physical limitations present a challenge for diabetes educators. Older adults who do any kind of physical activity can improve not only their blood glucose control but also their muscle tone, flexibility, balance, and outlook. For perimenopausal and postmenopausal women, physical activity may help reduce the severity of symptoms associated with menopause and result in better health-related quality-of-life measures.[79,80] Physical activity during weight loss also prevents weight regain in this population.[81] Yard work and housework are activities many people feel comfortable doing, but including resistance work to gain strength and retain muscle mass is recommended.

◆ *Frequency and intensity.* It is important that older individuals engage in some physical activity each day.[72] Setting goals that this population can reach is most important. For example, a very sedentary, older person may be able to walk for only 5 minutes 3 days a week and increase that by 1 to 2 minutes per week. Intensity is likely not as important as frequency of activity in this age group.

◆ *Safety.* Safety concerns may preclude someone from walking due to a high risk for falls and subsequent fracture. Options may include using a stationary bicycle, lifting light or moderate weights, or exercising while seated. Exercise videos, classes, and routines that can be done from a chair, rather than standing, may be helpful in this population. Including lower extremity strength and balance training can lower a person's risk of falling.

Pregnant Women

Women with either gestational or preexisting diabetes during pregnancy are encouraged to engage in regular physical activity to help enhance insulin action. In fact, regular exercise may help prevent some cases of gestational diabetes.[82,83] Pregnant women with diabetes can generally follow recommendations made for all pregnant women by the American College of Obstetricians and Gynecologists.[84]

◆ *Frequency and intensity.* Engaging in consistent, regular physical activity makes it easier

Cases—Part 5: Assessing Barriers to Physical Activity

Type 2 Diabetes

Identifying Medical Barriers Related to Prior Exercise

DK called her healthcare provider about the hip pain she had developed from walking. She was sure the type 2 diabetes was now causing some other problems and was afraid she was going to lose her leg. Once her healthcare provider reassured her that was not so, DK was scheduled to have a few medical tests. She learned that diabetes was not the reason for her hip pain; rather, she had some arthritis in her hips that was probably exacerbated by her excess body weight. She was told that while the arthritis would cause some discomfort, weight loss could help decrease the pain, as could regular participation in moderate physical activity. Now exercise was more important for her than ever.

Type 1 Diabetes

Lack of Understanding Leading to Creation of Self-imposed Barriers

HW was frustrated by the large fluctuations in his blood glucose levels caused by his physical activity participation. His healthcare provider had told him he could continue to be physically active, but it just wasn't working out for him. He wanted to call his educator the morning after his post–resistance training hypoglycemia since he desperately wanted to continue being physically active. Instead, he gave up, deciding that he would simply stop working out because it was just too hard to manage his blood glucose levels. He was worried about diabetes-related complications from hyperglycemic episodes. That day he went to work depressed and had a hard time keeping his blood glucose levels low enough to get anywhere near his target level of 100 mg/dL (5.6 mmol/L) before meals.

for pregnant women with any type of diabetes to manage their blood glucose. Exercise intensity should be mild or moderate and should be undertaken for up to 30 minutes at a time; vigorous activities are generally not recommended during pregnancy (unless women have been engaging in them prior to becoming pregnant[85]). Activities to undertake include moderate walking, indoor cycling, swimming and aquatic activities, low-impact aerobics, seated exercise routines, and mild or moderate resistance training.[86]

◆ *Safety.* Safety concerns for pregnant women revolve around prevention of falls, blows to the abdomen, and reduced blood flow through the placenta. Activities to avoid include contact sports, most racquet sports (requiring rapid movements and changes in direction), water and snow skiing, scuba diving, outdoor cycling (later in pregnancy), and running (unless the woman ran before becoming pregnant). Exercises done lying flat on the back or in environmental extremes are also best avoided.[84] Precautions to avoid hypoglycemia or hyperglycemia resulting from exercise are similar for pregnant and nonpregnant women.

Medical Considerations

Pre-activity Medical Exam and Assessment

Individuals diagnosed with diabetes should ideally consult a healthcare provider before beginning any physical fitness program. For individuals who wish to participate in low-intensity activities like walking, physicians and other healthcare providers should use clinical judgment in deciding whether to recommend pre-exercise testing.[51] Conducting exercise stress testing prior to starting a walking program is not routinely necessary as a diagnostic tool and requiring it may create barriers to participation.[73] Consult chapter 5 for more extensive guidelines about which individuals should undergo maximal exercise stress testing.

The medical examination conducted on an individual with diabetes before he or she undertakes a new physical activity or fitness program has a variety of components.[87] Information gathered during this pre-participation exam or chart review of the health information provides the basis for the outcome of this medical consultation. Other comorbidities frequently exist that affect the intended fitness regimen more than the diagnosis of diabetes, such as cardiovascular disease, neuropathy, nephropathy, and retinopathy. Clinicians, therefore, should screen for these conditions to determine whether they exist and, if so, their degree of progression. Factoring in these and other relevant health considerations enhances the medical advice provided and can contribute to a safely designed exercise prescription. Table 17.9 lists the general categories to be considered during this examination.

Cardiovascular Disease

Cardiovascular disease (CVD) is the major cause of morbidity and mortality for people with diabetes. As such, a careful cardiac assessment is warranted prior to initiating any moderate- to vigorous-intensity fitness program. The existence of any cardiac risk factors should be determined, and emphasis should be placed on their management to help prevent or slow CVD. When a fitness program that exceeds the demands of everyday living (ie, more intense than brisk walking) is being considered for a previously sedentary individual, the American Diabetes Association (ADA) has established criteria[73,88] to help determine whether a graded exercise test is warranted (as shown in Table 17.10 and discussed in chapter 5).

Neuropathy

The main forms of diabetic neuropathy present themselves as autonomic neuropathy, gastroparesis, and peripheral neuropathy.[89]

Autonomic Neuropathy

When the autonomic nerves of the cardiac system are affected by the long-term impact of elevated blood glucose levels, it represents a very serious

TABLE 17.9   Components of the Pre-participation Medical Exam
Measurement of
Body weight (body mass index [BMI], waist girth, body composition)
Apical pulse rate and rhythm
Resting blood pressure (seated, supine, standing)
Auscultation of
Lungs, with specific attention to uniformity of breath sounds in all areas (absence of rales, wheezes, and other breathing sounds)
Heart, with specific attention to murmurs, gallops, clicks, rubs
Carotid, abdominal, and femoral arteries
Palpitation of
Cardiac apical impulse, point of maximal impulse (PMI)
Carotid, abdominal, and femoral arteries
Inspection of lower extremities for edema and presence of arterial pulses
Evaluation of
Abdomen, for bowel sounds, masses, visceromegaly, and tenderness
Absence or presence of tendon xanthoma and skin xanthelasma
Tests of neurological function, including reflexes and cognition
Skin, especially lower extremity in patients with diabetes
Follow-up exam related to orthopedic or other medical conditions that would limit exercise

TABLE 17.10   Criteria for Conducting a Graded Exercise Stress Test (ADA)
Age >40 years, with or without CVD risk factors other than diabetes
Age >30 years and
Type 1 diabetes or type 2 diabetes of >10 years' duration
Hypertension
Cigarette smoking
Dyslipidemia
Proliferative or preproliferative retinopathy
Nephropathy, including microalbuminuria
Any of the following, regardless of age
Known or suspected CAD, cerebrovascular disease, and/or peripheral vascular disease
Autonomic neuropathy
Advanced nephropathy with renal failure

Sources: RJ Sigal, GP Kenny, DH Wasserman, C Castaneda-Sceppa, "Physical activity/exercise and type 2 diabetes," *Diabetes Care* 27 (2004): 2518-39; RJ Sigal, GP Kenny, DH Wasserman, et al, "Physical activity/exercise and type 2 diabetes: a consensus statement from the American Diabetes Association," *Diabetes Care* 29, no. 6 (2006): 1433-8; SR Colberg, AL Albright, BJ Blissmer, et al, for American College of Sports Medicine and American Diabetes Association, "Exercise and type 2 diabetes: position stand," *Med Sci Sports Exerc* 42, no. 12 (2010): 2282-303.

complication. The heart rate response is abnormal at rest, when standing, and when performing a Valsalva maneuver.[89,90] The blood pressure response is also abnormal when changing positions or performing isometric exercise, and an exaggerated rise in blood pressure may occur during activity.[91] The individual does not have the physical stamina to perform prolonged periods of activity. Dehydration is a greater concern, as is impaired thermoregulation during exercise in environmental extremes. Cardiac autonomic neuropathy carries a very poor prognosis and greatly increases mortality. Therefore, care must be taken with all components of the exercise prescription.

Gastroparesis

A form of autonomic neuropathy, gastroparesis produces physically uncomfortable and potentially embarrassing episodes for the individual with this complication. Common complaints are nausea, vomiting, feeling "stuffed" after eating, bloating, intestinal pain, alternating bouts of constipation and diarrhea, and lack of appetite.[92] Any of these can make physical activity difficult to perform. Medications and foods must be balanced as part of the exercise prescription to help minimize these symptoms.

Peripheral Neuropathy

Peripheral neuropathy, with an associated decrease in sensation, carries with it an increased risk of injury, along with greater discomfort associated with painful neuropathy during physical activity. The individual with insensate feet may not have the pain sensation needed to recognize that an injury has occurred. A blister or repeated trauma to a bone often goes unnoticed. Also, sensations connected to balance and strength can be diminished. The gait can be altered, contributing to development of orthopedic issues and a greater risk of falling. In fact, individuals with type 2 diabetes without overt peripheral neuropathy exhibit altered and less efficient gait patterns.[93] The individual may become fearful of falling and avoid physical activity. Walking, standing, or getting out of a chair can be difficult. Safety must be the prime consideration of the exercise prescription.

Table 17.11 lists special considerations for physical activity that should accompany each of these forms

TABLE 17.11	Physical Activity Considerations With Neuropathy	
Type of Neuropathy	*Safety Concern Associated With Type of Neuropathy*	*Action to Discuss*
Autonomic	Inability to recognize signs and symptoms of hypoglycemia	Monitor blood glucose during physical activity; set higher blood glucose goals
	Blunted heart rate response to physical activity	Monitor intensity with HRR, RPE, or "talk" test
	Erratic blood pressure response during exercise, increased risk of postural hypotension	Monitor blood pressure during physical activity; determine whether different positions (sitting, standing, reclining, supine) affect results
	Lack of effective thermoregulation for hot and cold environments	Monitor environment; drink fluids to prevent dehydration; wear proper clothing
Gastroparesis	Erratic emptying rate of stomach and digestion of food	Monitor blood glucose as needed; use foods absorbed in the mouth to treat hypoglycemia (eg, glucose tabs, glucose gels, and hard candies); delay injection of rapid-acting insulin until after activity
	Discomfort following consumption of a meal or specific type of food	Determine whether physical activity impedes or promotes food mobility; plan timing of physical activity as symptoms tolerate
Peripheral	Discomfort or pain with physical activity	Limit weight-bearing options based on level of tolerance
	Injury, infection, ulceration	Monitor feet daily for blisters, cuts, scrapes; teach proper hygiene techniques for foot and skin care; choose appropriate footwear (shoes and socks); consider need for orthotics or orthopedic shoes

---

Case Wrap-up: Education Aids Implementation of Exercise Prescription

Type 2 Diabetes

Identifying Activity Options

DK met with a diabetes educator. During her appointment, she learned more about her diabetes medication and how it does not place her at risk of exercise-induced hypoglycemia. She realized she could exercise whenever she could fit it into her day. The diabetes educator also talked about other exercise options. They decided she should add something besides walking because of the pain it caused with her hip. DK has a friend who does water aerobics—something DK might consider trying. The diabetes educator also provided her with information about an exercise program for people with arthritis. She decided that she would look into both of those options.

Working Systematically in Stages

The diabetes educator also helped DK chart a plan for how much time to spend exercising. DK then understood she would need to work on her fitness plan for a few months to get her fitness level to where it should be. She would start with a small amount of exercise and add more as she could tolerate it. She promised she would return to talk to the diabetes educator before she tried to add too much. DK felt she was finally getting her life back!

Type 1 Diabetes

Data Interpretation and Support

HW went to his follow-up appointment with the diabetes educator. He was sure the educator was going to tell him he would have to stop being active. After all, trying to work out was making his blood glucose levels worse. The educator's response surprised him. The educator not only explained how his blood glucose numbers were affected by the type and intensity of training he did, but also encouraged him to keep trying different things until he found what worked best for him. They talked specifically about what he should try and what he should expect to see his blood glucose numbers doing during both aerobic and resistance training activities. He agreed to check and record his blood glucose values before and after exercise, along with the type and duration of exercise, to determine blood glucose patterns. If he had a problem he could not solve on his own, he, much to his relief, was to call the educator right away. He learned that figuring out the right balance of food, insulin, and exercise would take a little time but could be done. He also decided to join an online diabetes forum for athletic individuals to get more ideas about how to better manage his exercise blood glucose levels.

---

of neuropathy. When progression of these symptoms presents safety issues, a clinically supervised exercise setting may be prudent. When this option is not available, self-monitoring is important; the person must be able to make appropriate decisions independently when engaging in physical activity.

Nephropathy

The intensity of the physical activity is the main consideration of the exercise prescription when nephropathy is present, because of the linear association of the blood pressure response to intensity.[94] As the workload being performed increases, the blood pressure response also rises. Light to moderate physical activity, with an acceptable blood pressure response, is generally considered safe and beneficial in those with incipient nephropathy or microalbuminuria (urinary albumin excretion rates of 30-299 mg per day). For those with overt nephropathy or clinical albuminuria (300 mg or greater per day), strenuous physical activity is not prudent due to the exaggerated

blood pressure response in this population. Individuals should keep in mind that while urinary albumin excretion rates can rise proportionally with increasing exercise intensity during the period following the activity, such changes should not be interpreted to mean that exercise is causing additional damage.[95]

The risk of developing specific comorbidities increases as nephropathy progresses. Often, the individual with overt nephropathy has diminished capacity for physical activity, causing a self-limitation of strenuous physical activity. Yet, people at all stages of nephropathy can benefit from staying physically active, and physical activity during dialysis sessions is possible and often recommended to increase functional capacity.[96] Table 17.12 provides information highlighting these considerations for the exercise prescription.

Retinopathy

The presence of retinopathy should be evaluated for all people with diabetes based on established clinical

TABLE 17.12   Physical Activity Considerations With Nephropathy

Increased Risk of	*Physical Activity*	*Points to Consider*
Bone disease	Strength training program	Promotes bone strength; improves balance and gait; reduces risk of falls and fractures
Hypertension or exaggerated blood pressure response to activity	Avoid or modify physical activities that cause extreme increases in systolic blood pressure	Blood pressure should be monitored; medications should be adjusted as needed to keep resting and exercise blood pressure in desired ranges
Edema	As tolerated	Instruction should be provided for dietary and fluid intake to minimize this condition; foot elevation or use of compression stockings may be useful
Anemia	As tolerated	Treat as needed to keep hematocrit levels between 33% and 36%
Loss of independence	Promote physically active lifestyle	Increases ability to maintain activities of daily living, which may limit dependence on others as disease progresses
Depression	Promote physically active lifestyle	Provides a level of protection from depression, hopelessness, and doom

TABLE 17.13   Physical Activity With Retinopathy

Level of Retinopathy	*Physical Activity and Exercise Recommendations*
No diabetic retinopathy	No physical activity/exercise limitations
Mild nonproliferative	No physical activity/exercise limitations
Moderate nonproliferative	Avoid activities that dramatically elevate blood pressure (eg, power lifting)
Severe to very severe nonproliferative	Limit increase in systolic blood pressure (eg, Valsalva maneuver) and avoid activities that jar the head; heart rate should not exceed that which elicits a systolic blood pressure response greater than 170 mm Hg (boxing and intense competitive sports)
Proliferative	Avoid strenuous activity, high-impact activities, Valsalva maneuvers, and activities that jar the head (eg, weight lifting, jogging, high-impact aerobic dance, racquet sports, strenuous trumpet playing, and competitive sports)
	Encourage activities that are low impact and aerobic, and stress cardiovascular conditioning (eg, swimming without diving, walking, low-impact aerobic dance, stationary cycling, and endurance exercising)

guidelines.[97] People without diabetic retinopathy or who have only mild nonproliferative diabetic retinopathy (NPDR) do not have activity limitations. Those with moderate, severe, or very severe NPDR and those with proliferative diabetic retinopathy should be educated on the limitations during exercise and even routine physical activities. Macular edema and glaucoma should be evaluated by an ophthalmologist or optometrist and activity guidelines determined by the results of the examination. More specific information is provided in Table 17.13 for the different levels of retinopathy.

Integrating Exercise Prescription Into the Education Plan

Diabetes educators are charged with providing instruction related to the various components of physical fitness in the prevention and treatment of diabetes.[98] As the individualized assessment is performed, the educator gathers information useful in addressing the role of physical activity in the self-management plan. Physical activity may not be one of the initial goals identified by the diabetes educator or the individual with diabetes to address. Many times, other skills or self-care concepts need to be covered first because they either are health priorities or are more interesting to the person with diabetes (who may already be struggling with the amount of information to master in order to control blood glucose levels). After briefly introducing the importance of physical activity in diabetes management, the diabetes educator works with the patient to choose other goals on which to focus. However, when the time is right, the diabetes educator can redirect the person to goals involving planning, implementing, and assessing the impact of a personalized fitness program.

Questions and Controversies
The Graded Exercise Test

A controversial topic diabetes educators often have to address is the recommendation to have a patient complete a graded exercise test with electrocardiogram (ECG) monitoring prior to exercise participation. Diabetes is an independent risk factor for CVD. The established ADA criteria (listed in Table 17.10) give healthcare providers a broad referral base upon which to determine whether a graded exercise test is warranted. These criteria are more inclusive than exclusive. They can, therefore, be applied to most individuals seen in a diabetes practice. While this offers straightforward access, performing the test may not be the course of action required for each individual, depending on his or her physical activity and fitness goals. The risk of a false-positive result can overshadow the benefits an otherwise healthy individual receives from starting a fitness program. Likewise, a negative test result does not guarantee that the individual is protected from having a cardiovascular event. While careful consideration of the presence of such a disease is important, clinical judgment needs to be included when making the final determination on whether this test is necessary and in evaluating the individual patient's results.

Focus on Education

Teaching Strategies

⊘ **Help the person who hates to exercise.** Many people voice this opposition. When a person makes this statement, the diabetes educator or other clinician has a huge opportunity to ask more questions. Digging deeper, the educator often finds the real root of the problem and can help prevent it from interfering again. Examples include the following:

- *Does not like to sweat.* Promote lighter types of activities such as stretching, pool activities, or leisurely paced walking. The individual may be surprised to find these are options in a fitness plan.
- *Had a bad experience.* Determine what went wrong and prepare a plan that will replace that experience with a positive one.
- *Feels self-conscious in front of others.* May be best to start with "solo" options, such as videos, home-based equipment, or a personal trainer. A group fitness class or specific fitness facility may provide support if the person feels he or she fits in with the other members.

- *Has always "failed" at fitness programs.* Help set reasonable goals, prescribe a fitness program that will meet those goals, and provide positive support to the person through each step whether the person experiences a success or a setback. Build in appropriate progression of exercise.

⊘ **Help the person who underestimates insulin adjustment needs.** Many individuals need reassurance that a large reduction in their insulin dose is the correct action to take. They are willing to take 1 or 2 units off a dose initially but hesitant to do more. With support, they can omit 50% or more of their dose for a given exercise session if that is what is required to achieve acceptable glucose control.

⊘ **Help the person who delays or avoids snacks.** Even when the blood glucose indicates a snack is needed, many individuals will wait to see if they really need a snack. This often results in either hypoglycemia and the need for a larger volume of food to treat the reaction or overtreatment.

Pointing out that a smaller snack at the right time can help them avoid consuming a larger number of calories later to treat a reaction can help.

➔ **Identify support and assistance.** Whether the individual is of school age, a working professional, a parent, or retired, support and assistance from others close to the individual are important. The person may need to ask someone to join him or her in a fitness program to promote consistency or ask someone to take over a chore or responsibility to free up time for recommended physical activity. Financial resources may also need to be allocated so that the individual can buy appropriate clothing and shoes or have access to exercise equipment.

➔ **Be a role model.** Model a lifestyle incorporating physical activity and planned exercise to emphasize that physical activity is a lifestyle priority.

➔ **Help patients establish a healthy relationship with fitness.** Physical activity can be part of an eating disorder or just maladaptive functioning.

Messages for Patients

➔ **Be prepared to troubleshoot your fitness plan.** Determining the best routine to follow to safely and effectively engage in physical activity takes time (eg, frequent blood glucose readings and data from multiple physical activity sessions), patience, and problem solving.

➔ **Monitor levels to gain valuable information.** Recognize the need to measure blood glucose levels before and after exercise to facilitate good decision making in the future. Monitoring provides feedback on decisions about snacks, timing of exercise, and adjustments in medications. The interpretation of observed blood glucose patterns and effects of exercise can be reinforced with this information.

➔ **Time snacks appropriately to help keep calorie counts down.** A smaller snack at the right time can help you avoid consuming a larger number of calories later to treat hypoglycemia. Also, never assume that snacks are needed for all exercise; determine first whether your diabetes medications place you at risk for a decrease in blood glucose levels during any activity.

➔ **Realize that insulin dose adjustments may be larger than you expect.** A large reduction in your insulin dose may be the correct action to take.

➔ **Do not make spontaneous treatment judgments based on just 1 glucose reading.** Determine whether this is a one-time-only situation or a pattern and adjust your therapy accordingly.

➔ **Establish a healthy attitude toward fitness.** Your physical activity routine not only can help you keep glucose under control but can improve overall well-being and empower you to do other great things.

Health Literacy

➔ **Health numeracy.** Numbers can scare people and prevent them from exercising. You might think that pedometers or heart rate monitors are great, but they might be "scary" for your patients with low numeracy skills.

➔ **Effective behavior-change strategies.** Assess importance (why), confidence (how and what), and readiness (when).
- Explore importance by asking, Is it worthwhile? Why should I? How will I benefit? What will change? At what cost? Do I really want to? Will it make a difference?
- Explore confidence by asking, Can I? How will I do it? How will I cope with . . .? Will I succeed if . . .? What change . . .?
- Explore readiness by asking, Should I do it now? How about other priorities?[99]

➔ **Challenge-based learning or situation problem solving.** State a circumstance for a patient and have the patient come up with the solution/strategy. For example, What will you do when you have hypoglycemia during your exercise?

Focus on Practice

⤷ **Fitness facilities/structures and key community resources linked to health care.** Formal partnerships and coalitions formed with community centers are needed to ensure continuity in care, along with a formal fitness referral system to community centers. Physical activity is a clinical intervention and should be treated as such.

⤷ **Communities with access to various fitness channels.** Advocate for healthy communities with sidewalks, bike trails, mall walking, yoga, tai chi, karate, parks, exercise clubs, and fitness centers. Give people choices and opportunities to choose what they like and change the strategy when needed.

⤷ **Medically supervised fitness facilities.** Be part of a system providing evidence-based and medically supervised care. Such systems involve a network of healthcare professionals like physicians, psychologists, dietitians, exercise physiologists, and physical therapists, among others. Communicate with all of the providers, exchange ideas, and advance the practice.

⤷ **Population-based fitness.** Focus on ensuring needed care to all members of a population rather than individual patients (eg, use of registries). Fitness is part of a lifestyle. Quantify its impact.

References

1. Sushruta SCS. Vaidya Jadavaji Trikamji Acharia. Bombay, India: Sagar; 1938.

2. Lawrence RH. The effects of exercise on insulin action in diabetes. BMJ. 1926;1:648-52.

3. Kilpatrick ES, Rigby AS, Atkin SL. Insulin resistance, the metabolic syndrome, and complication risk in type 1 diabetes: "double diabetes" in the Diabetes Control and Complications Trial. Diabetes Care. 2007;30:707-12.

4. Mulcahy K, Maryniuk M, Peeples M, et al. Diabetes self-management education core outcomes. Diabetes Educ. 2003;29(5):768-803.

5. President's Council on Physical Fitness. Definitions: health, fitness, and physical activity. Research Digest; 2000.

6. Boulé NG, Haddad E, Kenny GP, Wells GA, Sigal RJ. Effects of exercise on glycemic control and body mass in type 2 diabetes mellitus: a meta-analysis of controlled clinical trials. JAMA. 2001;286(10):1218-27.

7. Galbo H, Tobin L, van Loon LJ. Responses to acute exercise in type 2 diabetes, with an emphasis on metabolism and interaction with oral hypoglycemic agents and food intake. Appl Physiol Nutr Metab. 2007;32(3):567-75.

8. O'Gorman DJ, Karlsson HK, McQuaid S, et al. Exercise training increases insulin-stimulated glucose disposal and GLUT4 (SLC2A4) protein content in patients with type 2 diabetes. Diabetologia. 2006;49(12):2983-92.

9. Cartee GD, Young DA, Sleeper MD, Zierath J, Wallberg-Henriksson H, Holloszy JO. Prolonged increase in insulin-stimulated glucose transport in muscle after exercise. Am J Physiol. 1989;256(4 Pt 1):E494-9.

10. Tuomilehto J, Lindstrom J, Eriksson JG, et al. Prevention of type 2 diabetes mellitus by changes in lifestyle among subjects with impaired glucose tolerance. N Engl J Med. 2001;344:1343-50.

11. Diabetes Prevention Research Group. Reduction in the incidence of type 2 diabetes with lifestyle intervention or metformin. N Engl J Med. 2002;346(6):393-403.

12. Hamman RF, Wing RR, Edelstein SL, et al. Effect of weight loss with lifestyle intervention on risk of diabetes. Diabetes Care. 2006;29(9):2102-7.

13. Kreisman SH, Halter JB, Vranic M, Marliss EB. Combined infusion of epinephrine and norepinephrine during moderate exercise reproduces the glucoregulatory response of intense exercise. Diabetes. 2003;52(6):1347-54.

14. US Department of Health and Human Services, Centers for Disease Control and Prevention. National diabetes fact sheet: general information and national estimates on diabetes in the United States, 2007. Atlanta: US Department of Health and Human Services, CDC; 2008:5.

15. Zoppini G, Targher G, Zamboni C, et al. Effects of moderate-intensity exercise training on plasma biomarkers of inflammation and endothelial dysfunction in older patients with type 2 diabetes. Nutr Metab Cardiovasc Dis. 2006;16(8):543-9.

16. Holten MK, Zacho M, Gaster M, Juel C, Wojtaszewski JF, Dela F. Strength training increases insulin-mediated glucose uptake, GLUT4 content, and insulin signaling in skeletal muscle in patients with type 2 diabetes. Diabetes. 2004;53(2):294-305.

17. Wang Y, Simar D, Fiatarone Singh MA. Adaptations to exercise training within skeletal muscle in adults with type 2 diabetes or impaired glucose tolerance: a systematic review. Diabetes Metab Res Rev. 2009;25(1):13-40.

18. Christ-Roberts CY, Pratipanawatr T, Pratipanawatr W, et al. Exercise training increases glycogen synthase activity and GLUT4 expression but not insulin signaling in overweight nondiabetic and type 2 diabetic subjects. Metabolism. 2004;53(9):1233-42.

19. Chimen M, Kennedy A, Nirantharakumar K, Pang TT, Andrews R, Narendran P. What are the health benefits of physical activity in type 1 diabetes mellitus? A literature review. Diabetologia. 2012;55:542-51.

20. Colberg SR. Diabetic Athlete's Handbook: Your Guide to Peak Performance. Champaign, Ill: Human Kinetics; 2009.

21. Caron D, Poussier P, Marliss EB, Zinman B. The effect of postprandial exercise on meal-related glucose intolerance in insulin-dependent diabetic individuals. Diabetes Care. 1982;5:364-9.

22. Bweir S, Al-Jarrah M, Almalty AM, et al. Resistance exercise training lowers HbA1c more than aerobic training in adults with type 2 diabetes. Diabetol Metab Syndr. 2009;1:27.

23. Castaneda C, Layne JE, Munoz-Orians L, et al. A randomized controlled trial of resistance exercise training to improve glycemic control in older adults with type 2 diabetes. Diabetes Care. 2002;25(12):2335-41.

24. Ramalho AC, de Lourdes Lima M, Nunes F, et al. The effect of resistance versus aerobic training on metabolic control in patients with type-1 diabetes mellitus. Diabetes Res Clin Pract. 2006;72:271-6.

25. Willey KA, Fiatarone-Singh MA. Battling insulin resistance in elderly obese people with type 2 diabetes: bring on the heavy weights. Diabetes Care. 2003;26:1580-8.

26. Shier I. Stretching before exercise does not reduce the risk of local muscle injury: a critical review of the clinical and basic science literature. Clin J Sport Med. 1999;9:221-7.

27. Lan C, Lai JS, Chen SY. Tai Chi Chuan: an ancient wisdom on exercise and health promotion. Sports Med. 2002;32(4):217-24.

28. Ray US, Sinha B, Tomer OS, Pathak A, Dasgupta T, Selvamurthy W. Aerobic capacity & perceived exertion after practice of hatha yoga exercises. Indian J Med Res. 2001;114:215-21.

29. Innes KE, Vincent HK. The influence of yoga-based programs on risk profiles in adults with type 2 diabetes mellitus: a systematic review. Evid Based Complement Alternat Med. 2007;4(4):469-86.

30. Herriott MT, Colberg SR, Parson HK, Nunnold T, Vinik AI. Effects of 8 weeks of flexibility and resistance training in older adults with type 2 diabetes. Diabetes Care. 2004;27(12): 2988-9.

31. Morrison S, Colberg SR, Mariano M, Parson HK, Vinik AI. Balance training reduces falls risk in older individuals with type 2 diabetes. Diabetes Care. 2010 Jan 22. [Epub ahead of print]

32. Ivy J. Exercise physiology and adaptations to training. In: Ruderman N, Devlin JT, Schneider SH, Kriska A, eds. Handbook of Exercise in Diabetes. Alexandria, Va: American Diabetes Association; 2002.

33. Murillo S, Brugnara L, Novials A. One year follow-up in a group of half-marathon runners with type-1 diabetes treated with insulin analogues. J Sports Med Phys Fitness. 2010;50:506-10.

34. Davis SN, Mann S, Briscoe VJ, Ertl AC, Tate DB. Effects of intensive therapy and antecedent hypoglycemia on counterregulatory responses to hypoglycemia in type 2 diabetes. Diabetes. 2009;58:701-9.

35. Ertl AC, Davis SN. Evidence for a vicious cycle of exercise and hypoglycemia in type 1 diabetes mellitus. Diabetes Metab Res Rev. 2004;20:124-30.

36. Sigal RJ, Fisher SJ, Halter JB, Vranic M, Marliss EB. Glucoregulation during and after intense exercise: effects of beta-adrenergic blockade in subjects with type 1 diabetes mellitus. J Clin Endocrinol Metab. 1999;84:3961-71.

37. Tuominen JA, Karonen SL, Melamies L, Bolli G, Koivisto VA. Exercise-induced hypoglycaemia in IDDM patients treated with a short-acting insulin analogue. Diabetologia. 1995;38:106-11.

38. Bremer JP, Jauch-Chara K, Hallschmid M, Schmid S, Schultes B. Hypoglycemia unawareness in older compared with middle-aged patients with type 2 diabetes. Diabetes Care. 2009;32:1513-7.

39. Brazeau AS, Rabasa-Lhoret R, Strychar I, Mircescu H. Barriers to physical activity among patients with type 1 diabetes. Diabetes Care. 2008;31(11):2108-9.

40. Arutchelvam V, Heise T, Dellweg S, Elbroend B, Minns I, Home PD. Plasma glucose and hypoglycaemia following exercise in people with type 1 diabetes: a comparison of three basal insulins. Diabet Med. 2009;26(10):1027-32.

41. Neumiller JJ, Setter SM. Pharmacologic management of the older patient with type 2 diabetes mellitus. Am J Geriatr Pharmacother. 2009;7(6):324-42.

42. Khoo EY, Wallis J, Tsintzas K, Macdonald IA, Mansell P. Effects of exenatide on circulating glucose, insulin, glucagon, cortisol and catecholamines in healthy volunteers during exercise. Diabetologia. 2010;53(1):139-43.

43. McMahon SK, Ferreira LD, Ratnam N, et al. Glucose requirements to maintain euglycemia after moderate-intensity afternoon exercise in adolescents with type 1 diabetes are increased in a biphasic manner. J Clin Endocrinol Metab. 2007;92(3):963-8.

44. Larsen JJ, Dela F, Madsbad S, Vibe-Petersen J, Galbo H. Interaction of sulfonylureas and exercise on glucose homeostasis in type 2 diabetic patients. Diabetes Care. 1999;22(10):1647-54.

45. Galbo H, Tobin L, van Loon LJ. Responses to acute exercise in type 2 diabetes, with an emphasis on metabolism and interaction with oral hypoglycemic agents and food intake. Appl Physiol Nutr Metab. 2007;32(3):567-75.

46. Jensen J, Rustad PI, Kolnes AJ, Lai YC. The role of skeletal muscle glycogen breakdown for regulation of insulin sensitivity by exercise. Front Physiol. 2011;2:112.

47. Berlie HD, Garwood CL. Diabetes medications related to an increased risk of falls and fall-related morbidity in the elderly. Ann Pharmacother. 2010;44:712-7.

48. Parkman HP, Fass R, Foxx-Orenstein AE. Treatment of patients with diabetic gastroparesis. Gastroenterol Hepatol (N Y). 2010;6:1-16.

49. Manz F. Hydration and disease. J Am Coll Nutr. 2007;26: 535S-41S.

50. American Diabetes Association. Hyperglycemic crises in diabetes (position statement). Diabetes Care. 2004;27 Suppl 1:S94-102.

51. American Diabetes Association. Physical activity/exercise and diabetes. Diabetes Care. 2004;27(90001):S58-62.

52. Sigal RJ, Kenny GP, Wasserman DH, Castaneda-Sceppa C. Physical activity/exercise and type 2 diabetes. Diabetes Care. 2004;27:2518-39.

53. Mitchell TH, Abraham G, Schiffrin A, Leiter A, Marliss EB. Hyperglycemia after intense exercise in IDDM subjects during continuous subcutaneous insulin infusion. Diabetes Care. 1988;11:311-7.

54. Sigal RJ, Fisher SJ, Halter JB, Vranic M, Marliss EB. Glucoregulation during and after intense exercise: effects of beta-adrenergic blockade in subjects with type 1 diabetes mellitus. J Clin Endocrinol Metab. 1999;84(11):3961-71.

55. Purdon C, Brousson M, Nyveen SL, et al. The roles of insulin and catecholamines in the glucoregulatory response during intense exercise and early recovery in insulin-dependent diabetic and control subjects. J Clin Endocrinol Metab. 1993;76:566-73.

56. Biankin SA, Jenkins AB, Campbell LV, Choi KL, Forrest QG, Chisholm DJ. Target-seeking behavior of plasma glucose with exercise in type 1 diabetes. Diabetes Care. 2003;26(2): 297-301.

57. Poirier P, Mawhinney S, Grondin L, et al. Prior meal enhances the plasma glucose lowering effect of exercise in type 2 diabetes. Med Sci Sports Exerc. 2001;33(8): 1259-64.

58. Colberg SR, Zarrabi L, Bennington L, et al. Postprandial walking is better for lowering the glycemic effect of dinner than pre-dinner exercise in type 2 diabetic individuals. J Am Med Dir Assoc. 2009;10(6):394-7.

59. Kalergis M, Schiffrin A, Gougeon R, Jones PJ, Yale JF. Impact of bedtime snack composition on prevention of nocturnal hypoglycemia in adults with type 1 diabetes undergoing intensive insulin management using lispro insulin before meals: a randomized, placebo-controlled, crossover trial. Diabetes Care. 2003;26:9-15.

60. Wilson D, Chase HP, Kollman C, et al. Low-fat vs. high-fat bedtime snacks in children and adolescents with type 1 diabetes. Pediatr Diabetes. 2008;9:320-5.

61. Raju B, Arbelaez AM, Breckenridge SM, Cryer PE. Nocturnal hypoglycemia in type 1 diabetes: an assessment of preventive bedtime treatments. J Clin Endocrinol Metab. 2006;91:2087-92.

62. Hernandez JM, Moccia T, Fluckey JD, Ulbrecht JS, Farrell PA. Fluid snacks to help persons with type 1 diabetes avoid late onset postexercise hypoglycemia. Med Sci Sports Exerc. 2000;32(5):904-10.

63. Wolpert HA, Atakov-Castillo A, Smith SA, Steil GM. Dietary fat acutely increases glucose concentrations and insulin requirements in patients with type 1 diabetes: implications for carbohydrate-based bolus dose calculation and intensive diabetes management. Diabetes Care. 2013;36:810-6.

64. Axelsen M, Wesslau C, Lonnroth P, Arvidsson Lenner R, Smith U. Bedtime uncooked cornstarch supplement prevents nocturnal hypoglycaemia in intensively treated type 1 diabetes subjects. J Intern Med. 1999;245: 229-36.

65. American College of Sports Medicine, Sawka MN, Burke LM, Eichner ER, Maughan RJ, Montain SJ, Stachenfeld NS. American College of Sports Medicine position stand. Exercise and fluid replacement. Med Sci Sports Exerc. 2007;39(2):377-90.

66. Grimm JJ, Ybarra J, Berné C, Muchnick S, Golay A. A new table for prevention of hypoglycaemia during physical activity in type 1 diabetic patients. Diabetes Metab. 2004;30(5):465-70.

67. Guelfi KJ, Jones TW, Fournier PA. New insights into managing the risk of hypoglycaemia associated with intermittent high-intensity exercise in individuals with type 1 diabetes mellitus: implications for existing guidelines. Sports Med. 2007;37(11):937-46.

68. Frid A, Ostman J, Linde B. Hypoglycemia risk during exercise after intramuscular injection of insulin in thigh in IDDM. Diabetes Care. 1990;13:473-7.

69. Garber CE, Blissmer B, Deschenes MR, et al, American College of Sports Medicine. American College of Sports Medicine position stand. Quantity and quality of exercise for developing and maintaining cardiorespiratory, musculoskeletal, and neuromotor fitness in apparently healthy adults: guidance for prescribing exercise. Med Sci Sports Exerc. 2011;43:1334-59.

70. Physical Activity Guidelines Advisory Committee. Physical Activity Guidelines Advisory Committee report, 2008. Washington, DC; 2008.

71. Haskell WL, Lee IM, Pate RR, et al. Physical activity and public health: updated recommendation for adults from the American College of Sports Medicine and the American Heart Association. Med Sci Sports Exerc. 2007;39(8):1423-34.

72. Nelson ME, Rejeski WJ, Blair SN, et al. Physical activity and public health in older adults: recommendation from the American College of Sports Medicine and the American Heart Association. Med Sci Sports Exerc. 2007;39(8):1435-45.

73. Colberg SR, Albright AL, Blissmer BJ, et al, for American College of Sports Medicine and American Diabetes Association. Exercise and type 2 diabetes: position stand. Med Sci Sports Exerc. 2010;42(12):2282-303.

74. Jakicic JM, Wing RR, Butler BA. Prescribing exercise in multiple short bouts versus one continuous bout: effect on adherence, cardiorespiratory fitness, and weight loss in women. Int J Obes Relat Metab Disord. 1995;19:893-901.

75. Chowdhury P, Balluz L, Town M, et al. Surveillance of certain health behaviors and conditions among states and selected local areas—Behavioral Risk Factor Surveillance System, United States, 2007. MMWR Surveill Summ. 2010;59(1):1-220.

76. Janssen I. Physical activity guidelines for children and youth. Can J Public Health. 2007;98 Suppl 2:S109-21.

77. Diabetes Research in Children Network (DirecNet) Study Group. Effects of aerobic exercise on glucose and counterregulatory hormone concentrations in children with type 1 diabetes. Diabetes Care. 2006;29:20-5.

78. Meltzer LJ, Johnson SB, Prine JM, Banks RA, Desrosiers PM, Silverstein JH. Disordered eating, body mass, and glycemic control in adolescents with type 1 diabetes. Diabetes Care. 2001;24(4):678-82.

79. Villaverde-Gutiérrez C, Araújo E, Cruz F, Roa JM, Barbosa W, Ruíz-Villaverde G. Quality of life of rural menopausal women in response to a customized exercise programme. J Adv Nurs. 2006;54(1):11-9.

80. Daley A, Macarthur C, Stokes-Lampard H, McManus R, Wilson S, Mutrie N. Exercise participation, body mass index, and health-related quality of life in women of menopausal age. Br J Gen Pract. 2007;57(535):130-5.

81. Wang X, Lyles MF, You T, Berry MJ, Rejeski WJ, Nicklas BJ. Weight regain is related to decreases in physical activity during weight loss. Med Sci Sports Exerc. 2008;40(10):1781-8.

82. Davenport MH, Mottola MF, McManus R, Gratton R. A walking intervention improves capillary glucose control in women with gestational diabetes mellitus: a pilot study. Appl Physiol Nutr Metab. 2008;33(3):511-7.

83. Ceysens G, Rouiller D, Boulvain M. Exercise for diabetic pregnant women. Cochrane Database Syst Rev. 2006; 3(CD004225).

84. Practice ACO. ACOG Committee opinion. Number 267, January 2002: exercise during pregnancy and the postpartum period. Obstet Gynecol. 2002;99(1):171-3.

85. Zavorsky GS, Longo LD. Exercise guidelines in pregnancy: new perspectives. Sports Med. 2011;41:345-60.

86. Zavorsky GS, Longo LD. Adding strength training, exercise intensity, and caloric expenditure to exercise guidelines in pregnancy. Obstet Gynecol. 2011;117: 1399-402.

87. Bickley LS. Bate's Pocket Guide to Physical Examination and History Taking. 4th ed. Philadelphia: Lippincott, Williams and Wilkins; 2003.

88. Sigal RJ, Kenny GP, Wasserman DH, et al. Physical activity/exercise and type 2 diabetes: a consensus statement from the American Diabetes Association. Diabetes Care. 2006;29(6):1433-8.

89. Vinik AI, Erbas T. Cardiovascular autonomic neuropathy: diagnosis and management. Curr Diab Rep. 2006;6: 424-30.

90. Colberg SR, Swain DP, Vinik AI. Use of heart rate reserve and rating of perceived exertion to prescribe exercise intensity in diabetic autonomic neuropathy. Diabetes Care. 2003;26(4):986-90.

91. Weston KS, Sacre JW, Jellis CL, Coombes JS. Contribution of autonomic dysfunction to abnormal exercise blood pressure in type 2 diabetes mellitus. J Sci Med Sport. 2013;16:8-12.

92. Parkman HP, Fass R, Foxx-Orenstein AE. Treatment of patients with diabetic gastroparesis. Gastroenterol Hepatol (N Y). 2010;6:1-16.

93. Ko SU, Stenholm S, Chia CW, Simonsick EM, Ferrucci L. Gait pattern alterations in older adults associated with type 2 diabetes in the absence of peripheral neuropathy—results from the Baltimore Longitudinal Study of Aging. Gait Posture. 2011;34:548-52.

94. Mogensen CE. Nephropathy: early. In: Ruderman N, Devlin JT, Schneider SH, Kriska A, eds. Handbook of Exercise in Diabetes. Alexandria, Va: American Diabetes Association; 2002.

95. Kornhauser C, Malacara JM, Macias-Cervantes MH, Rivera-Cisneros AE. Effect of exercise intensity on albuminuria in adolescents with type 1 diabetes mellitus. Diabet Med. 2010;29:70-3.

96. Makhlough A, Ilali E, Mohseni R, Shahmohammadi S. Effect of intradialytic aerobic exercise on serum electrolytes levels in hemodialysis patients. Iran J Kidney Dis. 2012;6:119-23.

97. Aiello LP, Wong J, Cavellerano JD, Bursell SE, Aiello LM. Retinopathy. In: Ruderman N, Devlin JT, Schneider SH, Kriska A, eds. Handbook of Exercise in Diabetes. Alexandria, Va: American Diabetes Association; 2002.

98. American Association of Diabetes Educators. The scope of practice, standards of practice, and standards of professional performance for diabetes educators. Diabetes Educ. 2005;31:487-512.

99. Rollnick S, Mason P, Butler C. Health Behavior Change: A Guide for Practitioners. London, England: Elsevier Limited; 1999.

Pharmacotherapy for Glucose Management

Evan M. Sisson, PharmD, MSHA, CDE
Dave L. Dixon, PharmD, BCPS, CDE, CLS

Key Concepts

- The pathophysiology of hyperglycemia helps determine the appropriate therapy for persons with different types of diabetes.

- In the management of hyperglycemia associated with type 2 diabetes, combination therapies that target different aspects of the metabolic abnormality are often employed.

- The goal of insulin therapy, regardless of diabetes type, is to replace lost capacity and mimic normal physiology.

- The various insulin preparations differ in onset, action, and duration after subcutaneous injection.

- The role of the diabetes educator is to help those with diabetes understand the medications they take and to provide guidance for monitoring and effective use of the drug therapies.

Introduction

This chapter primarily reviews pharmacologic therapies for glucose management in type 2 diabetes. Although local preferences determine specific practice patterns, the generally accepted approach to therapy is described in complementary documents: the 2012 consensus statement from the American Diabetes Association (ADA) and the European Association for the Study of Diabetes (EASD), and the 2013 algorithm from the American Association of Clinical Endocrinologists (AACE).[1,2] Both documents emphasize the need to individualize therapy based on patient-specific characteristics.

In the past decade, several new drug therapy choices received approved labeling from the US Food and Drug Administration (FDA) for use in people with diabetes. In addition to oral agents are several peptide substances that mimic endogenous hormones.[1] Insulin administration technology continues to be refined, with the ultimate goal of closely approximating the physiologic action of endogenous insulin. New approaches to improve glycemic control also involve gastrointestinal enzyme alteration and use of products that enhance insulin action.[1,3]

In addition to the expanded armamentarium for managing hyperglycemia, treatment of diabetes often employs medications for the concurrent metabolic disorders related to diabetes. Pharmacologic therapies for hypertension and dyslipidemia in people with diabetes are discussed in Chapter 19. Because diabetes drug regimens can be very complex, the diabetes educator who remains knowledgeable about current standards of care can be extremely valuable to the person with diabetes.

Treatment Goals

The goals of treatment of both type 1 diabetes and type 2 diabetes are to achieve near-normal glucose levels in order to avoid short- and long-term complications. The AACE recommends an A1C goal of <6.5%, whereas the ADA recommends an A1C goal of <7.0%.[2,4] The more aggressive AACE recommendation attempts to overcome clinical inertia among providers, while the ADA recommendation is based on clinical trial evidence of reduced microvascular and macrovascular outcomes. The ADA position statement acknowledges the benefit of more aggressive goals in selected patients, and both guidelines suggest less stringent goals in patients who will not benefit from or may be harmed by lower A1C goals (eg, patients with a history of severe hypoglycemia, limited life expectancy, or advanced microvascular or macrovascular complications).[4]

Case: Type 2 Diabetes

CR is a 52-year-old African-American male with type 2 diabetes. When diagnosed, he had a casual glucose of 226 mg/dL (12.4 mmol/L) and an A1C of 9.3%. He was started on 500 mg of metformin twice daily. Two weeks later, he presented to the clinic with continued, though decreased, polyuria and nocturia. He denied stomach upset or other gastrointestinal disturbance. His blood pressure was 128/82 mm Hg. His fasting glucose was 184 mg/dL (10.2 mmol/L).

Past Medical History

- Hypertension for 3 years
- Hyperlipidemia for 4 months
- Obesity

Family History

- Father: history of cardiovascular disease (CVD)/hypertension; deceased
- Mother: history of type 2 diabetes, hypertension; still living

Social History

- Tobacco: 24 pack-years, currently smokes
- Illicit drug use: none
- Alcohol: occasional/socially

Current Medications

- Metformin (Glucophage®, Bristol-Myers Squibb) 500 mg twice daily
- Pravastatin (Pravachol®, Bristol-Myers Squibb) 40 mg daily
- Metoprolol succinate (Toprol® XL, AstraZeneca) 50 mg twice daily
- Quinapril (Accupril®, Parke-Davis, division of Pfizer) 40 mg daily
- Hydrochlorothiazide (HCTZ) 25 mg daily

Adherence to Drug Therapy

CR picked up his prescription for metformin the day after his appointment 2 weeks ago. He related taking all of his medications as prescribed.

Physical Exam

- Height: 69 in
- Weight: 241 lb
- Body mass index (BMI): 35 kg/m²
- Waist circumference: 42 in

Vitals

- Blood pressure: 128/82 mm Hg
- Heart rate: 72 beats per minute

Lab Data

- Alanine aminotransferase (ALT): 24 international units per liter
- Serum creatinine: 1.4 mg/dL (0.124 mmol/L)
- Fasting blood glucose: 184 mg/dL (10.2 mmol/L)
- A1C: 9.3%
- Total cholesterol: 218 mg/dL (5.6 mmol/L)
- LDL-C: 131 mg/dL (3.4 mmol/L)
- Triglycerides: 162 mg/dL (1.8 mmol/L)
- HDL-C: 37 mg/dL (1 mmol/L)

As this case continues throughout the chapter, the focus will be on pharmacologic interventions to optimize glycemic control.

Management of Type 2 Diabetes

As suggested by the chapter case, type 2 diabetes is a chronic disorder with multiple metabolic abnormalities. Poor glycemic control in type 2 diabetes is associated with 2 defects: insulin resistance (decreased response to insulin action) and diminished insulin secretion (also known as pancreatic beta cell failure). Individuals with type 1 diabetes have only 1 defect resulting in hyperglycemia: lack of insulin production due to pancreatic beta cell destruction. Behavioral interventions (medical nutrition therapy, physical activity, lifestyle changes) are the basis of initial and ongoing treatment of both types of diabetes; however, all individuals with type 1 diabetes also require supplemental insulin beginning at diagnosis. Because worsening hyperglycemia progresses more slowly in type 2 diabetes than in type 1 diabetes, many clinicians choose to begin intensive lifestyle change prior to starting drug therapy to improve glycemic control.[5] However, most individuals with type 2 diabetes require medication by the end of the first year due to progression of the disease.[1]

Approach to Obesity Management

Because obesity and type 2 diabetes are linked, the AACE 2013 algorithm includes a complications-centric model for care of the overweight and obese patient.[2] The first step includes evaluation of complications (presence of cardiometabolic disease and biomechanical problems) and staging of obesity (BMI 25-26.9 kg/m^2, or $\geq$27 kg/m^2). Step 2 includes selection of therapeutic targets, treatment modality, and treatment intensity based on weight loss staging. All patients are enrolled in lifestyle modification, while those with more severe complications are considered for medication therapy and surgical interventions. Addition of drug therapy is generally reserved for patients with either a BMI greater than or equal to 30 kg/m^2 or a BMI greater than 27 kg/m^2 with obesity-related comorbidity (hypertension, dyslipidemia, or diabetes).[6] Step 3 of the algorithm includes intensification of interventions for those patients who fail to meet therapeutic targets or whose complications do not improve.

Approach to Antihyperglycemic Management

Many different pharmacologic treatment options are currently available to treat type 2 diabetes. Recently, 2 evidence-based consensus statements on the management of type 2 diabetes were published. The AACE algorithm recommends pharmacotherapy interventions based on the presenting A1C level (see Figure 18.1).[1,2] The foundation of therapy rests on therapeutic lifestyle change, and metformin is presented as the preferred first agent among the hierarchy of options. For patients with an A1C level less than 7.5%, reasonable alternatives to metformin (depicted with a check mark in the algorithm) include glucagon-like peptide-1 (GLP-1) receptor agonists, dipeptidyl peptidase-4 (DPP-4) inhibitors, and alpha-glucosidase inhibitors. Caution is advised for the use of sodium-glucose co-transporter-2 (SGLT-2) inhibitors, thiazolidinediones, sulfonylureas, and meglitinides (depicted with a "use with caution" triangle in the algorithm). Patients with A1C levels greater than or equal to 7.5% are recommended to start dual or triple drug therapy on top of metformin as the base. Patients with an entry-level A1C greater than 9% plus symptoms are recommended to start insulin in addition to other agents.

The 2012 joint consensus statement from the ADA/EASD built on its 2009 algorithm but shifted away from a proscriptive treatment recommendation in favor of a more patient-centered approach.[1] The domains of consideration when choosing between a more stringent treatment plan and a less stringent one include the following: patient attitude and expected treatment effort, risks potentially associated with hypoglycemia and other adverse events, disease duration, life expectancy, important comorbidities, established vascular complications, and patient resources or support system. As with the AACE algorithm, the foundation of therapy according to ADA/EASD remains healthy eating, weight control, and increased activity; however, metformin is suggested as the single monotherapy option (see Figure 18.2). This recommendation is based on its low cost, low risk of hypoglycemia, and ability to achieve glycemic goals in most patients. Furthermore, data suggest that initiation of metformin within 3 months of diagnosis may preserve

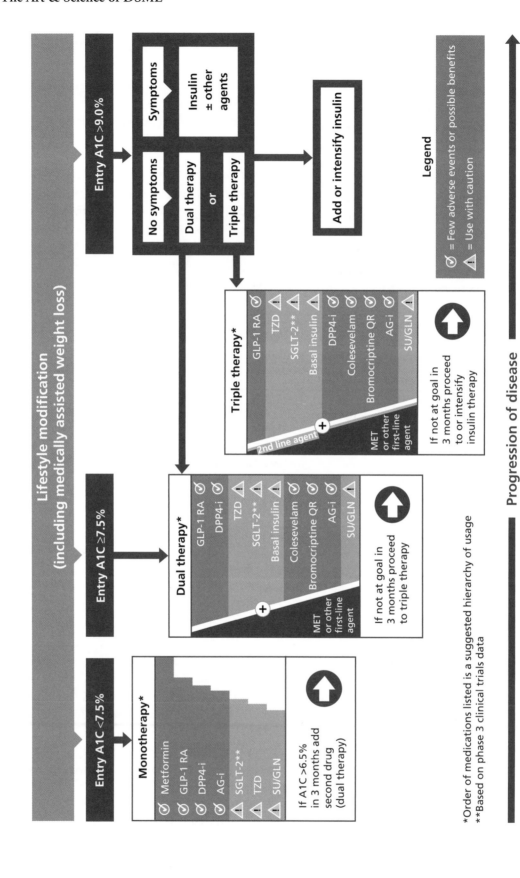

FIGURE 18.1   AACE Algorithm for the Medical Management of Type 2 Diabetes

Source: Reprinted with permission from American Association of Clinical Endocrinologists. AJ Garber, MJ Abrahamson, JI Barzilay, et al, "AACE comprehensive diabetes management algorithm," *Endocr Pract* 19 (2013): 327-36.

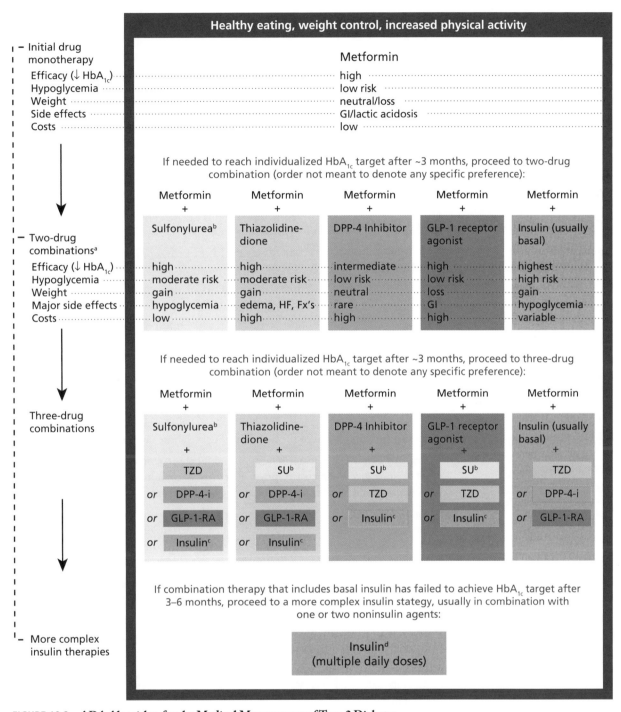

FIGURE 18.2   ADA Algorithm for the Medical Management of Type 2 Diabetes

[a]Consider beginning at this stage in patients with very high HbA1c (e.g., ≥9%).

[b]Consider rapid-acting, nonsulfonylurea secretagogues (meglitinides) in patients with irregular meal schedules or who develop late post-prandial hypoglycemia on sulfonylureas.

[c]Usually a basal insulin (NPH, glargine, detemir) in combination with noninsulin agents.

[d]Certain noninsulin agents may be continued with insulin. Consider beginning at this stage if patient presents with severe hyperglycemia (≥16.7–19.4 mmol/L [≥300–350 mg/dL]; HbA1c ≥10.0–12.0%) with or without catabolic features (weight loss, ketosis, etc.).

Source: SE Inzucchi, RM Bergenstal, JB Buse, et al, American Diabetes Association (ADA), European Association for the Study of Diabetes (EASD), "Management of hyperglycemia in type 2 diabetes: a patient-centered approach: position statement of the American Diabetes Association (ADA) and the European Association for the Study of Diabetes (EASD)," *Diabetes Care* 35, no. 6 (2012): 1364-79, doi: 10.2337/dc12-0413. Epub 2012 Apr 19.

American Association of Diabetes Educators©

pancreatic beta cell function and delay the progression of diabetes.[7] Guideline recommendations for 2- and 3-drug combinations in addition to metformin are based on patient-specific characteristics. Regardless of the drug combinations chosen, it should be noted that all patients with type 2 diabetes eventually arrive at a regimen that includes intensive insulin.

Medications for Obesity Management

Pharmacologic Treatment Options

There are currently 3 classes of orally administered agents used for obesity management (see Table 18.1):

  ◈ Sympathomimetic agents
  ◈ Selective-serotonergic agents
  ◈ Lipase inhibitors

Sympathomimetic Agents

Agents in the sympathomimetic class include phentermine and phentermine with topiramate (PHEN/TPM). The combination product is unique in that both components provide weight reduction benefits; however, both are associated with significant side effects, especially at higher doses. The value of the combination product is achievement of maximum weight loss while using the lowest dose to minimize risk of side effects. The maximum weight loss benefit with PHEN/TPM in clinical trials was 5% to 10% from baseline.[6] The percentage of patients able to achieve 5% weight loss was 44.9% to 75.2% with low-dose PHEN/TPM, compared with 66.7% to 79.3% with high-dose PHEN/TPM. Unfortunately, both components of the combination are associated with significant adverse effects, and weight loss benefits typically reverse upon discontinuation.

TABLE 18.1 Medications for Obesity Management	
Sympathomimetic Agents	
Phentermine • Adipex® (Teva Pharmaceuticals USA)	*Action.* Central nervous system (CNS) effects similar to amphetamines. Reduce appetite by stimulation of the hypothalamus to release norepinephrine. *Expected weight loss.* Phentermine approved for short-term treatment as adjunct to low-calorie diet and increased physical activity. Weight loss amount varies. Patient weight typically returns to baseline after discontinuation. *Contraindications.* History of cardiovascular disease (arrhythmias, heart failure, coronary artery disease, stroke, uncontrolled hypertension), hyperthyroidism, glaucoma, agitated states, history of drug abuse; monoamine oxidase inhibitor (MAOI) therapy; Pregnancy Category X (excreted in breast milk). *Interactions.* Numerous drug-drug interactions related to the stimulatory effects of amphetamines (especially increased blood pressure and heart rate). Alcohol may enhance CNS adverse effects. *Precautions.* Amphetamines may impair the ability to engage in potentially hazardous activities. Discontinue in patients experiencing new-onset chest pain, shortness of breath, or lower extremity edema. May be associated with development of valvular heart disease. Significant abuse potential (C-IV controlled substance).
Phentermine with Topiramate • Qsymia™ (Vivus Inc)	*Action.* Phentermine as above. Topiramate may suppress appetite, but exact mechanism is unknown. *Expected weight loss.* Phentermine with topiramate approved for chronic weight management as adjunct to low-calorie diet and increased physical activity. Patients may lose 5%–10% of baseline weight; 44.9%–75.2% of patients achieve 5% weight loss on low-dose PHEN/TPM; 18.8% to 50.3% of patients lost 10% of weight with low dose PHEN/TPM; 66.7%–79.3% of patients achieve 5% weight loss on high-dose PHEN/TPM. Patient weight typically returns to baseline after discontinuation.

TABLE 18.1 Medications for Obesity Management (continued)	
	Contraindications. Phentermine as above. Topiramate—Pregnancy associated with cleft palate. Phentermine/Topiramate—Pregnancy Category X (excreted in breast milk).
	Interactions. Phentermine as above. Topiramate—Hypokalemia if used with non-potassium-sparing diuretics. Phentermine/Topiramate—May decrease estrogen component of oral contraceptives by 16% and increase the progestin component by 22%.
	Precautions. Cognitive dysfunction and psychiatric disturbances may be related to rapid titration and higher doses. In addition to concerns with phentermine above, the following precautions are related to topiramate use: Associated with acute myopia and glaucoma (typically within 1 month of initiation). Severe hyperthermia may result during strenuous exercise or during exposure to high environmental temperatures. May raise serum creatinine and increase risk of kidney stone formation. Increased seizure risk with abrupt withdrawal; taper doses over at least 1 week. Significant abuse potential (C-IV controlled substance).
Selective-Serotonergic Agents	
Lorcaserin • Belviq® (Arena Pharmaceuticals GmbH)	*Action.* Agonist of selective serotonin (5-HT$_{2c}$) receptors in the hypothalamus resulting in decreased appetite.
	Expected weight loss. Approved for chronic weight management as adjunct to low-calorie diet and increased physical activity. Patients may lose 5% of baseline weight, or 3 kg; 37.5%–47.2% on 10 mg twice daily.
	Contraindications. Pregnancy Category X (unknown if excreted in breast milk).
	Interactions. Use with other serotonergic drugs (selective serotonin reuptake inhibitors [SSRIs], serotonin-norepinephrine reuptake inhibitors [SNRIs], MAOIs) may increase risk of serotonin syndrome. May increase serum concentrations of cytochrome P450 2D6 substrates.
	Precautions. May be associated with development of valvular heart disease. May cause cognitive disturbances (attention or memory, euphoria, dissociation, depression or suicidal thoughts). May cause priapism. Significant abuse potential (C-IV controlled substance).
Lipase Inhibitors	
Orlistat • Xenical® (Genentech USA Inc) • Alli® (GlaxosmithKline Consumer Healthcare)	*Action.* Inhibits gastrointestinal lipases resulting in decreased hydrolysis of dietary fat, a step necessary for absorption.
	Expected weight loss. Patients may lose 2.8% of baseline weight.
	Contraindications. Chronic malabsorption syndrome, cholestasis. Pregnancy Category X (unknown if excreted in breast milk).
	Interactions. Decreased vitamin K absorption may prolong bleeding for patients taking warfarin. Decreased absorption of cyclosporine and levothyroxine (administration of orlistat should be separated by at least 3–4 hours from interacting target drugs).
	Precautions. Gastrointestinal events (spotting, flatus with discharge, fecal urgency, oily stool, fecal incontinence) may increase with high-fat diets (>30% of calories as fat).

American Association of Diabetes Educators©

Sympathomimetic Agents: Dosage Information			
Drug	*Trade Name*	*Common Dose and Available Strengths*	*Common Frequency*
Phentermine	Adipex®	15–37.5 mg daily	Once daily
		Tabs/Capsules: 15 mg, 30 mg, 37.5 mg	
Phentermine with Topiramate	Qsymia™	Initiate at 3.75 mg/23 mg once daily for 14 days	Once daily
		Increase to 7.5 mg/46 mg once daily	
		If 3% weight loss not achieved at 12 weeks, either discontinue therapy or escalate the dose	
		Increase to 11.25 mg/69 mg for 14 days	
		Increase dose to maximum dose of 15 mg/92 mg	
		If 5% weight loss has not been achieved at 12 weeks on the maximum dose then taper drug to discontinuation	
		Capsule: Phentermine 3.75 and topiramate 23 mg	
		PHEN/TPM 7.5/46 mg	
		PHEN/TPM 11.25/69 mg	
		PHEN/TPM 15/92 mg	

Mechanism of Action Phentermine has activity similar to amphetamines and reduces appetite by stimulation of the hypothalamus to release norepinephrine.[6] Topiramate originally received FDA-approved labeling in 1996 as an anticonvulsant. The exact mechanism by which it produces weight loss is unknown. Topiramate is thought to suppress appetite and enhance satiety by a combined effect in the hypothalamus that includes inhibition of carbonic anhydrase.

Dosing Phentermine and PHEN/TPM are classified as C-IV controlled substances. Because of the long list of serious adverse effects associated with PHEN/TPM (especially fetal harm with topiramate), this combination is available only from certified pharmacies according to an FDA risk evaluation and mitigation strategy (REMS). Therapy with PHEN/TPM is usually started at the lowest dose (PHEN/TPM 3.75 mg/23 mg) to avoid cognitive impairment issues associated with the topiramate component. The once-daily dose is taken at any time of the day, without regard to meals, and gradually increased as noted in the table. If weight loss of at least 5% is not achieved by 12 weeks on the maximum dose, PHEN/TPM should be tapered down and discontinued. A slow taper (taking PHEN/TPM every other day for 1 week) is recommended due to the risk of seizures with rapid discontinuation.

Precautions Phentermine can increase resting heart rate, which may exacerbate symptoms in patients with coronary artery disease or hypertension. Concomitant use with alcohol may exacerbate central nervous system effects.

Topiramate is associated with cognitive dysfunction, psychiatric disturbances (mood disorders), and sedation (somnolence or fatigue). Topiramate is also associated with acute myopia and glaucoma that typically occur within 1 month of initiation. Severe hyperthermia due to oligohydrosis may result during strenuous exercise or during exposure to high environmental temperatures. Because topiramate is a weak carbonic anhydrase inhibitor, it may increase the risk of kidney stones by approximately 2 to 4 times that of the untreated population.

Contraindications Phentermine and PHEN/TPM are classified in Pregnancy Category X and are not indicated for use during pregnancy, for breast-feeding women, or for children. Topiramate is also known to cause cleft palate in children of mothers who took the drug during pregnancy. The combination drug may decrease the estrogen component of oral contraceptives by 16% and increase the progestin component by 22%.

Because of its sympathomimetic activity, phentermine should be avoided in patients with a history of cardiovascular disease, including arrhythmias, heart failure, coronary artery disease, stroke, or uncontrolled hypertension. Phentermine is also contraindicated in patients with hyperthyroidism, glaucoma, agitated states, and a history of drug abuse. Concomitant use with MAO inhibitors may exacerbate the hypertensive effect of phentermine. No specific contraindications are listed for topiramate; however, patients should be carefully selected due to the many potential adverse effects.

Monitoring Monitoring parameters for patients on PHEN/TPM include resting heart rate; blood pressure; serum bicarbonate, potassium, and creatinine; suicidal thoughts and mood disorders; visual acuity and symptoms of glaucoma; symptoms of acute acidosis; and weight. Phentermine should be discontinued if weight loss is not observed within the first 4 weeks of therapy. As noted above, the combination drug should be discontinued if weight loss of at least 5% is not achieved by 12 weeks on the maximum dose.

Instructions for Patients Patients should be advised of the side effects related to therapy and encouraged to communicate any changes to their healthcare provider, especially those related to the heart or mood. Because glycemic control may be affected by weight loss, patients should be educated on symptoms of hypoglycemia and its treatment.

Selective-Serotonergic Agents

The neurotransmitter serotonin helps regulate many body functions, including mood, appetite, and sleep. The various responses are determined by which serotonin receptor subtype is activated: 5-HT$_{2A}$ affects mood and may cause hallucinations, 5-HT$_{2B}$ may cause valvulopathy and pulmonary hypertension, and 5-HT$_{2C}$ promotes satiety and weight loss.[6] Lorcaserin is a selective agonist of 5-HT$_{2C}$. In clinical studies, 37.5% to 47.2% of patients taking 10 mg twice daily of lorcaserin lost 5% of weight from baseline; however, patients regained most of their weight upon discontinuation.[6]

Selective-Serotonergic Agents: Dosage Information			
Drug	*Trade Name*	*Common Dose and Available Strengths*	*Common Frequency*
Lorcaserin	Belviq®	10 mg daily *Tabs:* 10 mg	Twice daily

Mechanism of Action Lorcaserin is a selective-serotonin agonist of receptors in the hypothalamus.[8] Activation of these receptors increases satiety and promotes weight loss. Although the drug has a high affinity for the 5-HT$_{2C}$ receptor subtype, it also binds at other 5-HT receptors. The relative selectivity of lorcaserin for 5-HT$_{2C}$ receptors ranges between 8× and 15× that for 5-HT$_{2A}$, and between 45× and 90× that for 5-HT$_{2B}$.[8] This degree of selectivity for 5-HT$_{2C}$ makes off-target activation of 5-HT$_{2A}$ and 5-HT$_{2B}$ unlikely, which is consistent with the observed frequency of corresponding toxicity in clinical trials.

Dosing Lorcaserin is classified as a C-IV controlled substance. The dose of 10 mg twice daily may be taken with or without food. If weight loss of at least 5% is not achieved after 12 weeks, therapy should be discontinued.

Precautions Concomitant administration of lorcaserin with serotonergic agents (eg, selective serotonin reuptake inhibitors [SSRIs], serotonin-norepinephrine reuptake inhibitors [SNRIs], tricyclic antidepressants [TCAs], bupropion, St John's wort, tryptophan), agents that impair metabolism of serotonin (eg, monoamine oxidase inhibitors [MAOIs], dextromethorphan, tramadol, lithium), or antidopaminergic agents (eg, antipsychotics) may increase the risk of serotonin syndrome.[8] Symptoms of serotonin syndrome may include agitation, hallucinations, tachycardia, hyperthermia, nausea, or vomiting.

In clinical trials, valvular regurgitation was observed in 2.4% of patients taking lorcaserin, compared with 2% of patients taking placebo.[8] Lorcaserin has not been studied in patients with heart failure; thus, it should be avoided due to the possible over-expression of 5-HT$_{2B}$ receptors in this population. Routine echocardiogram evaluations are not recommended in the absence of symptoms.

The following rare adverse effects were observed in patients taking lorcaserin: hematologic changes (decreased white blood cell or red blood cell count), increased prolactin, pulmonary hypertension, and priapism. Periodic evaluation of complete blood count (CBC) is likely helpful, but other follow-up laboratory tests and examinations are determined by risk and symptom presentation.

Lorcaserin may cause cognitive impairment (attention and memory), confusion, somnolence, and fatigue.

Patients may also experience euphoria, hallucinations, and dissociation; however, these effects typically occur at doses greater than the recommended 10 mg twice daily.

Contraindications   Lorcaserin is classified in Pregnancy Category X and is not indicated for use during pregnancy, for breastfeeding women, or for children.

Monitoring   Monitoring parameters for patients on lorcaserin include CBC (periodically during use), blood glucose (in individuals with diabetes), and prolactin levels (if galactorrhea, gynecomastia, or other signs and symptoms of hyperprolactinemia arise). Patients should be monitored for signs and symptoms of depression, suicidal thoughts, serotonin syndrome, and valvular heart disease (dyspnea, dependent edema). As noted above, lorcaserin should be discontinued if weight loss of at least 5% is not achieved by 12 weeks on therapy.

Instructions for Patients   Patients should be advised of the side effects related to therapy and encouraged to communicate any changes to their healthcare provider, especially those related to the heart or mood. Because glycemic control may be affected by weight loss, patients should be educated on symptoms of hypoglycemia and its treatment.

Lipase Inhibitors

Originally approved as a prescription-only product, orlistat is available in a lower dose over the counter.[6] Weight loss associated with orlistat is only 2.8% compared with placebo, which is significantly less than other agents. Almost 10% of patients discontinue orlistat due to gastrointestinal complaints related to the inability to absorb dietary fat. Because most of the side effects associated with orlistat are related to dietary indiscretions, the value of orlistat lies in its ability to reinforce positive behavior modification.

Lipase Inhibitors: Dosage Information			
Drug	Trade Name	Common Dose and Available Strengths	Common Frequency
Orlistat	Xenical® Alli®	60–120 mg 3 times daily *Xenical Tabs:* 120 mg *Alli Tabs:* 60 mg	Three times daily

Mechanism of Action   Orlistat is a reversible inhibitor of gastrointestinal lipases resulting in decreased fat absorption from the small intestine.[9] The resulting decrease in caloric intake promotes weight loss.

Dosing   Prescription orlistat (the 120-mg dose) should be given 3 times daily with each main meal containing fat. Doses should be omitted if a meal is missed or if the meal does not contain fat.

Precautions   Concomitant administration of orlistat with lipophilic drugs may reduce serum concentrations by as much as 30%.[9] Patients taking cyclosporine should administer the dose 3 hours after orlistat, while patients taking levothyroxine should separate the dose by at least 4 hours from orlistat administration. Patients taking fat-souble vitamins (A, D, E, and K) should separate the administration time by at least 2 hours before or after the orlistat dose.

The most common complaints with orlistat are associated with its mechanism of action, especially in patients consuming >30% of total daily calories from fat. Gastrointestinal complaints during the first year of treatment include oily spotting (27%), flatus with discharge (24%), fecal urgency (22%), and oily stool (20%). These complaints decreased significantly in patients who continued orlistat into the second year, possibly due to better avoidance of dietary fat.[9]

Rare cases of severe liver injury and increased urinary oxalate have been reported with orlistat.

Contraindications   Orlistat is classified in Pregnancy Category X and is not indicated for use during pregnancy, for breastfeeding women, or for children. It should also be avoided in patients with chronic malabsorption or those with cholestasis.

Monitoring   In addition to weight loss, patients should be monitored for thyroid function if receiving supplementation. Evaluation of liver function should be performed in patients exhibiting symptoms of hepatic dysfunction.

Instructions for Patients   Patients should be advised of the relationship between the mechanism of orlistat, dietary fat, and the side effects. Because orlistat may decrease the absorption of dietary fat-soluble vitamins (A, D, E, and K), patients should take a multivitamin containing fat-soluble vitamins at least 2 hours before or after the orlistat dose. Patients should monitor blood glucose levels while taking orlistat because of its ability to directly inhibit calorie absorption. Patients should be encouraged to communicate any changes to their healthcare provider, especially those related to thyroid therapy or liver injury (severe nausea, inability to eat, discolored urine, or jaundice).

Medications for Antihyperglycemic Management

Pharmacologic Treatment

There are currently 8 classes of orally administered agents used for type 2 diabetes (see Table 18.2):

- Sulfonylureas
- Meglitinides
- Biguanides
- Thiazolidinediones
- Alpha-glucosidase inhibitors
- Dipeptidyl peptidase-4 inhibitors
- Dopamine receptor agonists
- Sodium-glucose co-transporter-2 inhibitors

Generally, monotherapy with any of these agents is associated with a reduction in A1C levels of approximately 0.5% to 2.0%.[1] When combination therapy is used (2 or more oral agents or an oral agent combined with insulin), an additive effect is observed, as demonstrated by a further decrease in the A1C level. Several fixed-dose combination products are available which may improve patient adherence.

TABLE 18.2   Oral Medications for Management of Type 2 Diabetes

Sulfonylureas

Glimepiride • Amaryl® (sanofi-aventis U.S.) Glipizide • Glucotrol® (Roerig, division of Pfizer) • Glucotrol XL® (Roerig, division of Pfizer) Glyburide • Micronase® (Pharmacia and Upjohn Co, division of Pfizer) • Glynase® (Pharmacia and Upjohn Co, division of Pfizer)	*Action.* Reduce glucose by increasing insulin secretion from pancreatic beta cells in patients with residual beta cell function. *Expected decrease in A1C with monotherapy.* 1%–2% *Contraindications.* Documented hypersensitivity; diabetic ketoacidosis (DKA); type 1 diabetes; Pregnancy Category C (positive retrospective data exist with glyburide). *Interactions.* Numerous possible drug interactions, few clinically significant. Sulfonamides may enhance hypoglycemic effect. *Precautions.* Hypoglycemia. Caution in hepatic or renal impairment; risk factors are older age, malnutrition, and irregular eating. May cause rash, sun sensitivity, nausea, vomiting, leukopenia, agranulocytosis, aplastic anemia (rare), intrahepatic cholestasis (rare), disulfiram-like reaction, flushing, headache, and SIADH (syndrome of inappropriate antidiuretic hormone) causing hyponatremia.

Meglitinides

Nateglinide • Starlix® (Novartis Pharmaceuticals Corp) Repaglinide • Prandin® (Novo Nordisk)	*Action.* Short-acting insulin secretagogues; stimulate insulin release from pancreatic beta cells. *Expected decrease in A1C with monotherapy.* 0.5%–1.5% *Contraindications.* Documented hypersensitivity; DKA; type 1 diabetes. *Interactions.* CYP3A4 inhibitors (eg, clarithromycin, ketoconazole, miconazole, erythromycin) decrease metabolism, increasing serum levels and effects. Thiazide diuretics, corticosteroids, estrogens, oral contraceptives, nicotinic acid, calcium channel blockers, phenothiazines, and thyroid products may lower glycemic control. Toxicity increased with highly protein-bound drugs (eg, nonsteroidal anti-inflammatory drugs [NSAIDs], sulfonamides, anticoagulants, hydantoins, salicylates, phenylbutazone). *Precautions.* Hypoglycemia, especially if carbohydrate not eaten after drug. Caution in hepatic impairment.

(continued)

TABLE 18.2　Oral Medications for Management of Type 2 Diabetes (continued)	
Biguanides	
Metformin • Glucophage® (Bristol-Myers Squibb) • Glucophage XR® (Bristol-Myers Squibb)	*Action.* Decrease hepatic gluconeogenesis (primary effect) and increase peripheral insulin sensitivity (secondary effect). Do not increase insulin levels or weight. Monotherapy does not cause hypoglycemia. *Expected decrease in A1C with monotherapy.* 1%–2% *Contraindications.* Serum creatinine level >1.5 mg/dL (men) or >1.4 mg/dL (women) or glomerular filtration rate (GFR) <30 mL/min; hepatic dysfunction; acute or chronic acidosis; local or systemic tissue hypoxia; excessive alcohol intake; drug therapy for congestive heart failure. *Interactions.* Numerous possible drug interactions, few (if any) clinically significant. Can cause gastrointestinal (GI) upset, nausea, and diarrhea; take with food or milk to minimize GI effects. Pregnancy Category B (positive retrospective data exist with metformin). *Precautions.* Fatal lactic acidosis if given with contraindication (rare without contraindication). Discontinue before IV contrast enhancement; do not restart until creatinine level normal. Withhold in acute hypoxia. Check renal function regularly and discontinue if abnormal. Adverse effects, including GI, especially diarrhea (30%), may cause discontinuation (5%).
Alpha-Glucosidase Inhibitors	
Acarbose • Precose® (Bayer HealthCare Pharmaceuticals) Miglitol • Glyset® (Pharmacia and Upjohn Co, a division of Pfizer)	*Action.* Inhibit action of alpha-glucosidase (carbohydrate digestion), delaying and attenuating postprandial blood glucose peaks. Undigested sugars are delivered to the colon, where they are converted into short-chain fatty acids, methane, carbon dioxide, and hydrogen. Do not increase insulin levels or inhibit lactase; major effect is to lower postprandial glucose levels (lesser effect on fasting levels). Do not cause weight gain. May restore ovulation in anovulation due to insulin resistance. *Expected decrease in A1C with monotherapy.* 0.5%–0.8% *Contraindications.* Documented hypersensitivity, DKA, or cirrhosis; inflammatory bowel disease; colonic ulceration; serum creatinine level >2 mg/dL; elevated liver enzyme levels; partial or predisposition to intestinal obstruction. *Interactions.* Hypoglycemia with insulin or sulfonylurea agents (give glucose as dextrose, as absorption of long-chain carbohydrates is delayed). May decrease absorption and bioavailability of digoxin, propranolol, and ranitidine. Digestive enzymes (eg, amylase, pancreatin) may reduce effects. *Precautions.* May cause GI symptoms; not recommended in significant renal dysfunction.
Thiazolidinediones	
Pioglitazone • Actos® (Takeda Pharmaceuticals America) Rosiglitazone • Avandia® (GlaxoSmithKline)	*Action.* Increase peripheral insulin sensitivity by increasing transcription of nuclear proteins that help increase uptake of glucose, probably with effects on free fatty acid levels. About 12–16 weeks to achieve maximal effect. May restore ovulation in anovulation due to insulin resistance. Improve target cell response to insulin without increasing insulin secretion from pancreas. Decrease hepatic glucose output and increase insulin-dependent glucose use in skeletal muscle and possibly liver and adipose tissue. *Expected decrease in A1C with monotherapy.* 0.5%–1.4% *Contraindications.* Documented hypersensitivity; active liver disease; DKA; type 1 diabetes; class III or IV congestive heart failure. *Interactions.* With insulin or oral hypoglycemics (eg, sulfonylureas), may increase risk of hypoglycemia. *Precautions.* Monitor transaminases every 2 months for first year, periodically thereafter; discontinue if alanine aminotransferase is above 3X upper limit of normal. Caution in edema and congestive heart failure. May decrease hemoglobin, hematocrit, and white blood cell (WBC) counts (dilution). Effects on lipids neutral or beneficial (decreased triglyceride, increased HDL levels). May increase fracture risk. Increased risk of cardiovascular events with rosiglitazone.

American Association of Diabetes Educators©

TABLE 18.2 Oral Medications for Management of Type 2 Diabetes (continued)	
Dipeptidyl peptidase-4 inhibitors (DPP-4i)	
Alogliptin • Nesina® (Takeda Pharmaceuticals America) Linagliptin • Tradjenta® (Boehringer Ingelheim Pharmaceuticals) Sitagliptin • Januvia® (Merck Sharp & Dohme Corp, a subsidiary of Merck & Co) Saxagliptin • Onglyza® (Bristol-Myers Squibb)	*Action.* Slows inactivation of incretin hormones (GLP-1) by the enzyme DPP-4. Prolonged action of endogenous GLP-1 increases insulin release and decreases glucagon secretion from pancreatic cells, resulting in lower circulating glucose levels. *Expected decrease in A1C with monotherapy.* 0.5% to 0.8% *Contraindications.* Documented hypersensitivity; history of pancreatitis; DKA or type 1 diabetes. *Interactions.* With insulin secretagogues (eg, sulfonylurea) may increase risk of hypoglycemia; not studied in combination with insulin. Coadministration of saxagliptin with strong CYP3A4/5 inhibitors (eg, ketoconazole) significantly increases saxagliptin concentrations. *Precautions.* Reduced dose recommended with decreased renal function (creatinine clearance <50 mL/min) for all except linagliptin. Postmarketing reports of increased risk of acute pancreatitis (including fatal and nonfatal hemorrhagic or necrotizing pancreatitis) associated with incretin mimetics.
Dopamine Receptor Agonists	
Bromocriptine mesylate • Cycloset®	*Action.* Ergot derivative that is a dopamine receptor agonist improves glycemic control by an unknown mechanism. *Expected decrease in A1C with monotherapy.* 0.1%–0.4% *Contraindications.* Documented hypersensitivity to ergot-related drugs; history of syncopal migraines; nursing women; DKA or type 1 diabetes. *Interactions.* Orthostatic hypotension with antihypertensive medications. May exacerbate psychotic disorders or reduce effectiveness of antipsychotic medications. Interaction with dopamine antagonists such as neuroleptic agents. May increase ergot-related side effects or reduce ergot effectiveness for migraines. Dopamine antagonists (such as metoclopramide) may decrease the effectiveness of bromocriptine. May increase unbound fraction of highly protein-bound therapies, altering their safety and efficacy. Extensively metabolized by CYP3A4. Use caution when coadministered with strong inhibitors, inducers, or substrates for CYP3A4. *Precautions.* May cause somnolence.
Sodium-Glucose Co-Transporter-2 (SGLT-2) Inhibitors	
Canagliflozin • Invokana®	*Action.* Inhibits reabsorption of filtered glucose in the kidney. *Expected decrease in A1C with monotherapy.* 0.8%–1% *Contraindications.* Documented hypersensitivity; severe renal impairment (GFR <45 mL/min), end-stage renal disease, or on dialysis; nursing women. *Interactions.* Use caution when coadministered with UGT inducers (rifampin). Digoxin concentrations may increase. *Precautions.* Hypotension related to hypovolemia especially in patients >65 years old. Hyperkalemia in patients with renal impairment. Increased risk of genital mycotic infections and urinary tract infections; increased urination.

Note: Under each class of orally administered agents, the generic drug is listed, followed by the brand name(s) of that drug.

Insulin is considered first-line therapy for pregnant women; however, metformin or glyburide may also be considered in those women who are unable or unwilling to use insulin.[10–12] Of all the oral medications for type 2 diabetes, only metformin has FDA-approved labeling for use in children.[13] The lack of alternate oral drug therapy options presents a concern with the increased incidence of type 2 diabetes among young people.

Patients should be reminded that any pharmacologic treatment of type 2 diabetes is only a supplement to lifestyle changes. These changes include adherence to a medical nutrition therapy plan, regular appropriate physical activity, and alteration of other specific health habits (eg, smoking cessation). Prior to initiating therapy, the healthcare provider should review the drug mechanism of action, proper dose, daily schedule of when to take each dose, and expected effects. The provider should also review and emphasize the importance of routine self-monitoring of blood glucose. Finally, every patient should be able to identify the signs and symptoms of major side effects and the appropriate action to take when these reactions occur.[14,15]

Sulfonylureas

Sulfonylureas are classified as first- and second-generation oral hypoglycemic agents. The first-generation agents are described as rapid-acting, intermediate-acting, or long-acting products based on their onset and duration.[16] Sulfonylureas are known as hypoglycemic agents because their major pharmacologic action has the potential to reduce blood glucose levels below normal (ie, cause hypoglycemia). Sulfonylurea agents are useful only in patients who still produce endogenous insulin; hence, they are used exclusively in type 2 diabetes.

According to the 2012 ADA/EASD and 2013 AACE treatment algorithms, sulfonylureas may be considered as second-line agents behind metformin in treating type 2 diabetes. A typical candidate for sulfonylurea monotherapy is an individual with type 2 diabetes without dyslipidemia who is not overweight.[1,2] Some individuals will not respond at all to

Sulfonylureas: Dosage Information			
Drug	*Trade Name*	*Common Dose and Available Strengths*	*Common Frequency*
First Generation			
Acetohexamide	Dymelor®	250–1500 mg daily *Tabs:* 250 mg, 500 mg	Daily to twice daily
Chlorpropamide	Diabinese®	100–250 mg to 500 mg daily *Tabs:* 100 mg, 250 mg	Daily
Tolazamide	Tolinase®	100–250 mg to 1.0 g daily *Tabs:* 100 mg, 250 mg, 500 mg	Daily to twice daily
Tolbutamide	Orinase®	500–2000 mg to 3.0 g daily *Tabs:* 500 mg	Three times a day
Second Generation			
Glimepiride	Amaryl®	1–2 mg to 8 mg daily *Tabs:* 1 mg, 2 mg, 4 mg	Daily to twice daily
Glipizide	Glucotrol® Glucotrol XL®	2.5–5 mg to 40 mg daily/max 20 mg with XL daily *Tabs:* 5 mg, 10 mg; XL 2.5 mg, 5 mg, 10 mg	Daily to twice daily
Glyburide Glyburide, micronized	Diabeta® Micronase® Glynase®	2.5–5 mg to 20 mg daily *Tabs:* 1.25 mg, 2.5 mg, 5 mg 1.5–3 mg to 12 mg daily *Tabs:* 1.5 mg, 3 mg, 4.5 mg, 6 mg	Daily to twice daily

sulfonylureas, and most over time will experience treatment failure with sulfonylureas as the disease progresses.

Mechanism of Action/Effects   Sulfonylureas increase the release of insulin from the pancreas, especially at the onset of therapy. These agents close the energy-sensitive potassium channel in the cell membrane of the beta cells. This effect causes an increase in the available insulin for action throughout the body, although these agents may be less effective in those with impaired first-phase insulin release.[17] Absorption of sulfonylureas is generally rapid, fairly complete, and unaffected by food except for short-acting glipizide. Significant variance in metabolism and excretion of these agents helps determine product choice. Most sulfonylureas are metabolized in the liver to active or inactive metabolites. However, chlorpropamide is partially excreted unchanged in the urine. Biliary excretion is significant with glyburide and to a lesser extent with glipizide.[17] Caution must be exercised with liver disease or renal insufficiency.

Dosing   Sulfonylureas should be started at the lowest dose and titrated as needed to reach target blood glucose levels. Outlined in the sulfonylurea chart are the most commonly used dosages. Although first-generation sulfonylureas are rarely used due to their side effect profiles, they are included for completeness.

Precautions   Sulfonylureas are classified in Pregnancy Category C. However, prospective studies with glyburide (Pregnancy Category B) in rats and rabbits revealed no harm to the fetus, and retrospective human data suggest that glyburide may be a suitable option for pregnant women unable or unwilling to use insulin.[1,10–12] Because many drugs are excreted in human milk, sulfonylureas should not be administered to nursing women. Safety and efficacy of sulfonylureas have not been established for children.

People with diabetes can experience a sulfonylurea hypersensitivity reaction. This reaction does not indicate a cross-sensitivity with sulfonamide agents. Rarely, diabetic ketoacidosis (DKA), altered glucose control from a severe infection, surgery, trauma, or other severe metabolic stressors may induce toxicity in patients receiving sulfonylureas.[18] Elderly, debilitated, or malnourished patients and those with adrenal, pituitary, or hepatic insufficiency who are particularly susceptible to the hypoglycemic effects of glucose-lowering agents should be monitored closely when using a sulfonylurea.

Contraindications   Contraindications to sulfonylureas include type 1 diabetes, ketoacidosis, allergy, or documented hypersensitivity to these agents.

Side Effects   Perhaps the most common and most serious adverse reaction is hypoglycemia.[18] An additional complicating factor is a progressive age-related decline in renal function that alters drug clearance and predisposes the person to hypoglycemia. Weight gain probably secondary to increased insulin secretion will occur, and skin rashes can be seen in about 2% of patients using the medication. The skin rashes usually resolve and the sulfonylurea can be continued. Usually mild gastrointestinal disturbances are reported in approximately 5% of users. Metabolic disorders such as a syndrome of inappropriate antidiuretic hormone (SIADH) occur in about 4% of patients treated with chlorpropamide, manifested by hyponatremia and hypervolemia.[19] Blood changes described with tolbutamide and chlorpropamide include abnormal hepatic function tests, thrombocytopenia, agranulocytosis, and hemolytic anemia but are very rare with second-generation sulfonylureas.[20]

Drug Interactions   Sulfonylureas may interact with a variety of medications. These interactions may alter the effect of the sulfonylurea or the other medication or both. It is commonly accepted that more drug-drug interactions occur with the first-generation agents than with the second-generation agents. One of the principal mechanisms of these interactions is a competition for protein-binding sites. As this competition occurs, more sulfonylurea circulates freely in the bloodstream and is capable of exerting its hypoglycemic effect. Altered hepatic enzyme activity may also alter clearance of sulfonylureas.

Monitoring   Baseline renal and hepatic function levels should be documented prior to starting sulfonylurea therapy. People with diabetes who use sulfonylureas should self-monitor their blood glucose daily. They should be able to detect and treat hypoglycemic episodes. The number of tests and timing each day, usually preprandial and at bedtime, should be determined by the goals of therapy and information needs to assess control.

Continued monitoring and follow-up visits should occur to assess the ongoing effectiveness of the agent. Up to 20% of people with diabetes will not respond to sulfonylureas. This is termed a primary failure of therapy. Secondary failure is defined as a significantly diminished or missing response to the sulfonylurea following an initial therapeutic response. People with diabetes who experience this treatment failure should be changed to another class of medication.[14]

Instructions for Patients Sulfonylureas may enhance sensitivity to sunlight, so patients should be advised to use appropriate sun protection. Prevention, recognition, and treatment of hypoglycemia should be included in patient education for people taking these medications (see the section on hypoglycemia in this chapter).

Meglitinides

Meglitinides, which include repaglinide and nateglinide, are similar to sulfonylureas in that they also increase insulin secretion from the pancreas. Although meglitinides share many of the pharmacologic actions and side effects of sulfonylureas, their duration of action is very short.

Meglitinides are often used in combination with other oral agents, especially in patients who experience hypoglycemia on sulfonylureas.[21] Adding meglitinides to concurrent sulfonylurea therapy offers no benefit, and meglitinides should not be used in patients who previously experienced primary or secondary failure on a sulfonylurea. Transition to insulin may be considered when treatment using these medications approaches the maximum dose without achieving target blood glucose levels.

Meglitinides are used as monotherapy in people with type 2 diabetes or in individuals with secondary diabetes with substantial capacity for insulin production. A typical candidate for initial repaglinide monotherapy has type 2 diabetes, without dyslipidemia, with or without renal failure, without being overweight, and with fasting plasma glucose level >20 mg/dL (1.1 mmol/L) above the target concentration.

Nateglinide can be effectively used as monotherapy in people with type 2 diabetes who have a capacity for insulin production, whose hyperglycemia is not adequately controlled by nutrition therapy and physical activity, and who have not been treated long-term with other oral glucose-lowering agents.

Mechanism of Action Meglitinides increase the release of insulin from the pancreas in a glucose-dependent manner and are therefore effective in helping restore first-phase insulin release. Treatment with repaglinide and nateglinide is effective in individuals with well-controlled type 2 diabetes and in those with type 2 diabetes whose control is suboptimal.[22,23] Nateglinide is a D-phenylalanine (amino acid) derivative and a very rapid-acting oral insulin secretagogue that stimulates insulin secretion when needed (postprandial) and then allows insulin concentrations to return to normal basal concentrations.[23]

Patients treated with repaglinide or nateglinide who missed or delayed a meal had less risk of hypoglycemia compared with treatment with longer acting sulfonylurea drugs. Absorption of repaglinide from the gastrointestinal tract is rapid and complete, and food slightly decreases absorption.[24]

Dosing The usual initial and maintenance dose of nateglinide is 120 mg taken just before meals (1-30 minutes before). Titration of dose is usually not necessary. The 60-mg dose may be used in those who are near their A1C goal.[25] Dose adjustment is not needed in the elderly, in patients with mild to severe renal insufficiency, or in those with mild hepatic insufficiency.[25]

Meglitinides: Dosage Information			
Drug	*Trade Name*	*Common Dose and Available Strengths*	*Common Frequency*
Repaglinide	Prandin®	0.5–1.0 mg 3 times per day to 16 mg daily *Tabs:* 0.5 mg, 1 mg, 2 mg	Three times per day before meals
Nateglinide	Starlix®	60–120 mg 3 times per day to 360 mg daily *Tabs:* 60 mg, 120 mg	Three times per day before meals

Repaglinide is initiated at a low, single daily dose, with gradual increases to reach glucose goals, and taken 15 minutes (but no longer than 30 minutes) before each meal. The number of daily doses taken is determined by the number of meals eaten. This type of meal-based dosing frequency may offer advantages for patients who vary the frequency of daily meals. The initial dosage does not need to be adjusted for patients with renal dysfunction, but upward titration should proceed cautiously. The initial dose for those previously treated with glucose-lowering drugs and with an A1C level >8% is usually 1 or 2 mg with each meal. The dose may be adjusted weekly, perhaps doubling each preprandial dose until the desired effect is attained. The maximum dose is 16 mg daily.

Precautions   Repaglinide and nateglinide are classified in Pregnancy Category C and are not indicated for use during pregnancy, for breastfeeding women, or for children.

Repaglinide should be used with caution in patients with impaired hepatic function, with careful monitoring and adjustment of dosing.

Elderly, debilitated, or malnourished patients and those with adrenal, pituitary, or hepatic insufficiency are particularly susceptible to the hypoglycemic effects of repaglinide.

Contraindications   Contraindications to meglitinides include type 1 diabetes, DKA, severe infection, surgery, trauma, or other severe stressors.

Side Effects   Side effects associated with repaglinide include gastrointestinal disturbances in approximately 4% of patients receiving the drug. Upper respiratory infection or congestion problems have been noted along with back pain. Hypoglycemia is the most common serious adverse effect. Different studies document the incidence to be between 16% and 31%.[24] Also, similar to sulfonylurea use, primary or secondary treatment failure occurs when an individual is insensitive to the effects of repaglinide. No clinically significant interactions are noted with nateglinide.

Side effects associated with nateglinide include hypoglycemia, usually mild, in approximately 2.4% of patients in clinical trials. There were no reports of hypoglycemia requiring third-party assistance or nocturnal hypoglycemia in the phase III trials (2400 patients). Dizziness was reported in approximately 3.6% of users with a weight gain of <1 kg from baseline. This weight gain is lowered with concomitant use of metformin.[23]

Monitoring   Blood glucose monitoring should include some premeal and postmeal readings to assess the effectiveness of the medications. The mean time to reach maximum concentrations of nateglinide after oral administration is 0.82 hours. High-fat meals reportedly result in a 12% increase in maximum concentration and a 52% reduction in the time to reach that concentration.[25]

Instructions for Patients   Meglitinides should be taken right before eating. Due to the potential for hypoglycemia, those taking this medication should be advised to monitor blood glucose levels for confirmation and subsequent treatment with fast-acting carbohydrate.

Biguanides

Biguanides are not considered hypoglycemic agents, because their major pharmacologic action does not increase insulin secretion and thus does not increase the risk of hypoglycemia. Currently, only metformin is marketed in the United States. Metformin is indicated for use in type 2 diabetes as a Step 1 drug or adjunct to other therapy. It has proven to be an effective antihyperglycemic agent but requires endogenous insulin production for its effectiveness.[26,27] An ideal candidate for initial metformin monotherapy has type 2 diabetes with dyslipidemia, obesity or genetic factors favoring insulin resistance, and an elevated fasting plasma glucose level.[26]

Mechanism of Action   Metformin improves glycemic control primarily by decreasing hepatic glucose production through reduced gluconeogenesis. Metformin may also decrease intestinal absorption of glucose and improve insulin sensitivity in skeletal muscle.

The oral bioavailability is 50% to 60%, and food decreases the bioavailability with a slight delay in the absorption of metformin. Metformin does not bind to liver or plasma proteins and is primarily excreted by the kidneys, largely unchanged, through an active tubular process.

Biguanides: Dosage Information			
Drug	*Trade Name*	*Common Dose and Available Strengths*	*Common Frequency*
Metformin Metformin extended release	Glucophage® Fortamet® Glucophage XR®	500 mg twice daily to 2550 mg daily (max. effective: 2000 mg daily) *Tabs:* 500 mg, 850 mg, 1 g *XR:* 500 mg, 750 mg, 1 g	Daily to twice daily
Metformin liquid	Riomet®	500 mg twice daily *Solution:* 100 mg/mL	Twice daily

Dosing   Metformin therapy is initiated at a low dose, with gradual increases to obtain desired control. The usual initial dose for the standard formulation is 500 mg or 850 mg daily or twice daily, with doses taken just prior to a meal. The extended-release (XR) formulation dose is usually adjusted every week until the goal is met, while the standard formulation is usually adjusted every 2 weeks. The maximum daily dose is 2550 mg (850 mg twice daily), but the maximal effective dose is achieved with 2000 mg daily. Metformin has FDA-approved labeling for use in children 10 years of age or older.[26] Children's therapy should be started with 250 mg twice daily and titrated slowly until treatment goals are attained.

Precautions   Metformin is classified in Pregnancy Category B. Prospective studies with metformin in rats and rabbits revealed no harm to the fetus, and retrospective human data suggest that metformin may be a suitable option for pregnant women unable or unwilling to use insulin. It is not known whether metformin is excreted in human milk; however, it is excreted unchanged in the milk of lactating rats. Nursing women should either discontinue the drug or discontinue nursing to avoid hypoglycemia in breastfeeding infants.

In acute illness or in any situation that would predispose the individual to acute renal dysfunction or tissue hypoperfusion, metformin should be temporarily withheld. Included in this set of conditions are acute myocardial infarction, acute exacerbation of congestive heart failure, use of iodinated contrast media, and major surgical procedures.[28] People with diabetes using this medication should be instructed to stop the metformin the day of the use of the iodinated contrast media and restart the metformin in 2 days when renal function has returned.[28] Metformin may restore ovulation in women who were previously anovulatory due to insulin resistance.

Contraindications   Metformin is contraindicated in males with serum creatinine levels >1.5 mg/dL (0.133 mmol/L) and in females with levels >1.4 mg/dL (0.124 mmol/L). In 2001, a recommendation was presented to have patients 80 years of age or older undergo a 24-hour creatinine clearance for a more precise assessment of renal function.[13] Because metformin is excreted by the kidneys, it can accumulate in patients with renal dysfunction.

The presence of hepatic dysfunction can predispose patients receiving metformin to lactic acidosis because lactate metabolism is carried out in the liver. Patients with a history of hypoxic conditions (chronic obstructive pulmonary disease or a history of cardiac function decline) are not good candidates due to the potential for lactate accumulation. Patients with a history of alcoholism or binges of alcohol intake are not good candidates for the therapy.

Side Effects   Metformin produces some side effects that can be beneficial for those with diabetes. Frequently, a slight (2-kg to 5-kg) weight loss is seen with metformin therapy, though the mechanistic cause of weight loss is not known. Metformin reduces triglyceride concentrations by approximately 16%, low-density lipoprotein cholesterol (LDL-C) by approximately 8%, and total cholesterol by approximately 5%. Metformin is associated with an increase in high-density lipoprotein cholesterol (HDL-C) by approximately 2%.[29]

Metformin does not directly induce hypoglycemia, though a few patients have reported mild symptoms necessitating dose reductions as their nutrition and physical activity programs became more effective in lowering glucose levels.[30] Patients using metformin in combination with sulfonylureas, meglitinides, or insulin may experience hypoglycemia secondary to the hypoglycemic agent.[30] Gastrointestinal effects such as abdominal bloating, nausea, cramping, feeling of fullness, and diarrhea are experienced in up to 30% of users.[31] A metallic taste in the mouth is also a common complaint. Up to 4% of patients using metformin stop taking the drug due to gastrointestinal effects; however, these effects are usually self-limiting and transient (7-14 days).[30] To minimize gastrointestinal side effects, patients should start with a low dose and slowly titrate the dose upward.

Metformin therapy is associated with a reduction in vitamin B_{12} levels, although no cases of anemia have been reported in the United States. Lactic acidosis can occur with the administration of metformin but is rare (0.03 cases per 1000 patient years).[16] Lactic acidosis is primarily associated with the use of metformin in patients who have contraindications to the drug or in cases of overdose.[32]

Monitoring   Metformin use over the age of 80 is not contraindicated, but due to the deterioration of renal function of the elderly, glomerular filtration rate (GFR) testing should be done at the beginning of therapy and periodically thereafter. Metformin therapy should be monitored with self-monitoring of blood glucose and follow-up visits to achieve target glycemic control. Continual review with the patient who has the potential for the aforementioned renal or hepatic effects should be undertaken, with encouragement concerning the possible gastrointestinal side effects. As with the other oral agents, combination therapy or transition to insulin monotherapy is considered when metformin therapy approaches the maximum effective dose.[30]

Drug interactions with metformin may include the effect that intravenous contrast media have on renal function, enzyme induction in the liver by cimetidine, and alcohol potentiation of lactate production.

Instructions for Patients   Patients should be instructed to take metformin with meals to reduce gastrointestinal side effects. They should also be told that a metallic taste may occur but will subside in time. While metformin itself does not cause

hypoglycemia, combination therapy with sulfonylureas, meglitinides, or insulin can be associated with hypoglycemia. Women of reproductive age should be advised of the risk of pregnancy, as metformin can restore ovulation in anovulation due to insulin resistance.

Thiazolidinediones

Thiazolidinediones (TZDs) are not hypoglycemic agents; the major pharmacologic action does not increase insulin secretion and thus does not increase the risk of hypoglycemia. Currently, the 2 compounds with FDA-approved labeling are pioglitazone and rosiglitazone. These agents may best be described as insulin sensitizers.

Thiazolidinediones: Dosage Information			
Drug	Trade Name	*Common Dose and Available Strengths*	*Common Frequency*
Pioglitazone	Actos®	15–45 mg daily *Tabs:* 15 mg, 30 mg, 45 mg	Once daily
Rosiglitazone	Avandia®	2–8 mg daily *Tabs:* 2 mg, 4 mg, 8 mg	Daily to twice daily

Note: An FDA REMS severely restricts the access and distribution of drugs containing rosiglitazone.

Mechanism of Action   Thiazolidinediones are synthetic ligands for peroxisome proliferator-activated receptor gamma (PPAR-g).[33] Activation of PPAR-g by TZDs alters transcription of genes responsible for carbohydrate and lipid metabolism, resulting in improved insulin sensitivity of peripheral muscle cells. Both rosiglitazone and pioglitazone retain FDA-approved labeling for use as monotherapy or in combination with other agents to treat type 2 diabetes. However, the use of TZDs has declined in recent years due to growing concerns about their safety and efficacy, particularly rosiglitazone. These concerns were so great that the 2009 ADA/EASD consensus group unanimously advised against using rosiglitazone.[16] This recommendation was based on meta-analyses suggesting increased risk of cardiovascular disease with rosiglitazone and the availability of other treatment options. Comprehensive review of these data by the FDA in 2010 led it to restrict the use of rosiglitazone to patients with type 2 diabetes who were unable to achieve glycemic control on other medications.

Dosing   Therapy is usually started at the lowest dose, with gradual increases to reach plasma glucose goals. Thiazolidinediones should be taken with the main meal of the day, or with the 2 primary meals if 2 daily doses are needed. Several weeks (8-12) are necessary to assess the full benefit from a dose level for the medication secondary to its mechanism. The doses may be titrated upward until the desired therapeutic effect is reached. Dose increases are not recommended more frequently than every 4 weeks.

Both of these medications are well absorbed without regard to meals. Pioglitazone is always given once daily, whereas rosiglitazone may need to be given twice daily in many individuals with type 2 diabetes. Both medications are extensively bound (>99%) to serum albumin and are extensively metabolized in the liver. Metabolites and parent compounds are eliminated primarily in the feces with minor amounts in the urine.

Precautions   Thiazolidinediones are classified in Pregnancy Category C and are not indicated for use during pregnancy, for breastfeeding women, or for children. Thiazolidinediones may restore ovulation in women who are anovulatory due to insulin resistance.

Thiazolidinediones cause fluid retention and edema especially when used in combination with insulin, predisposing patients to a twofold increase in the risk of heart failure in those with and without previous history. Due to plasma volume expansion, small reductions in hemoglobin, hematocrit, and neutrophil counts may occur with TZD use. Dose-related weight gain occurs with TZDs alone and in combination with other hypoglycemic agents. The mechanism of weight gain may be related to a combination of fluid retention and subcutaneous fat accumulation.

Small increases in HDL-C and LDL-C may occur with rosiglitazone, while reductions in triglycerides and elevations of HDL-C have been reported

with pioglitazone. The clinical significance of the lipid effects of this class of drugs is unclear.[34]

Several meta-analyses suggest that rosiglitazone may increase the relative risk of myocardial infarction by 30% to 40%. These data differ from studies with pioglitazone, which suggest a beneficial effect on cardiovascular disease risk.[1] In 2011, the FDA announced an REMS that severely restricted access and distribution of drugs containing rosiglitazone. Physicians desiring to prescribe rosiglitazone must be enrolled in the Avandia-Rosiglitazone Medicines Access Program. Patients needed to already be on rosiglitazone or needed to have failed other anti-diabetes drugs and be unwilling to start pioglitazone. The products themselves are only available by mail from participating pharmacies.

A concern specific to pioglitazone is the possible increased risk of bladder cancer. Interim results reported an increased risk of bladder cancer with increasing cumulative dose and duration of therapy, which reached statistical significance after 24 months of patient exposure.[35] Based on these and other data, pioglitazone was withdrawn from use in France in 2011 and no new prescriptions are authorized for patients in Germany.

Increased risk fracture in women and macular edema have also been observed with TZD therapy. Both adipocytes and osteoblasts arise from mesenchymal stem cells. Activation of PPAR-g by TZDs may shift cell differentiation away from osteoblast formation in favor of new adipocytes.

Thiazolidinediones should be used with caution in patients with hepatic dysfunction. Thiazolidinedione therapy can cause elevated hepatic enzymes. Rare cases of severe idiosyncratic hepatocellular injury occurred with troglitazone, prompting its removal from the market; however, pioglitazone and rosiglitazone do not appear to carry the same risk of hepatotoxicity.[33]

Contraindications   Thiazolidinediones are contraindicated in patients with NYHA (New York Heart Association) class III and IV heart failure and active liver disease. Rosiglitazone is metabolized by CYP2C9 and CYP2C8.[34] In vitro studies have suggested that inhibition of these isoenzymes by rosiglitazone does not occur at concentrations usually encountered clinically.[34] The isoenzyme CYP3A4, which is responsible for the metabolism of several drugs, including erythromycin, calcium channel blockers, corticosteroids, and HMG-CoA reductase inhibitors, is also partially responsible for the metabolism of pioglitazone. Therefore, the possibility of altered safety or efficacy should be considered when using these agents with pioglitazone.

Monitoring   Patients who receive either of these medications should perform routine self-monitoring of blood glucose multiple times daily as their condition and glucose control dictate. Serum transaminase levels should be monitored prior to initiating therapy and periodically thereafter per the clinical judgment of the healthcare provider.[13] Liver function studies should also be obtained in the presence of hepatic dysfunction symptoms such as abdominal pain, fatigue, nausea, vomiting, or dark urine. Thiazolidinedione therapy should be discontinued in the presence of jaundice. Edema, shortness of breath, rapid weight gain, and other signs and symptoms of heart failure should be included in assessing TZD therapy.

Instructions for Patients   Thiazolidinediones require several weeks to achieve the maximum benefit from a dosage level, and those taking it should be encouraged to continue the therapy. Patients experiencing edema/swelling, shortness of breath, or muscle aches should contact their healthcare provider for assessment of the side effect. Women should be cautioned regarding the risk of pregnancy, as ovulation may be restored in women who have been anovulatory due to insulin resistance.

Alpha-Glucosidase Inhibitors

Alpha-glucosidase inhibitors are used as monotherapy in type 2 diabetes or secondary diabetes with substantial capacity for insulin production.[36] Good candidates for initial alpha-glucosidase inhibitor monotherapy have type 2 diabetes, dyslipidemia or obesity, and symptoms or blood glucose levels demonstrating significant postprandial hyperglycemia. Due to their limited ability to lower A1C and their side effect profile, these drugs are not commonly used as monotherapy but rather as adjuncts to existing therapy. Individuals demonstrating significant premeal hyperglycemia without a significant premeal-to-postmeal glucose rise would not be

expected to respond optimally to alpha-glucosidase inhibitor monotherapy.

Alpha-Glucosidase Inhibitors: Dosage Information			
Drug	*Trade Name*	*Common Dose and Available Strengths*	*Common Frequency*
Acarbose	Precose®	Start: 25 mg (25 mg to 100 mg) *Tabs:* 25 mg, 50 mg, 100 mg	Three times daily
Miglitol	Glyset®	Start: 25 mg (25 mg to 100 mg) *Tabs:* 25 mg, 50 mg, 100 mg	Three times daily

Mechanism of Action   Alpha-glucosidase inhibitors are not hypoglycemic agents, as their major pharmacologic action does not increase insulin secretion and thus does not increase the risk of hypoglycemia. These agents may best be described as antihyperglycemic agents. They inhibit alpha-glucosidase enzymes in the brush border of the small intestine and pancreatic alpha-amylase, leading to a reduction in carbohydrate-mediated postprandial blood glucose elevation.[37] Alpha-glucosidase enzymes (maltase, isomaltase, glucoamylase, and sucrase) hydrolyze oligosaccharides, trisaccharides, and disaccharides to glucose and other monosaccharides in the brush border of the small intestine. Alpha-amylase enzymes hydrolyze complex starches to oligosaccharides in the lumen of the small intestine. This enzyme inhibition reduces the rate of digestion of starches and the subsequent absorption of glucose.

Dosing   Alpha-glucosidase inhibitor therapy is initiated at low doses to minimize gastrointestinal side effects, with gradual increases to reach glucose goals. The usual initial dose is 25 mg with meals, and each dose should be taken with the first bite of the meal for the drug to be most effective. The dose is increased upward as patient tolerance to the gastrointestinal effects allows, until the desired therapeutic effect is reached. Combination therapy should be considered when the maximum dose is reached.[37]

Precautions   Alpha-glucosidase inhibitors are classified in Pregnancy Category B. Because animal reproduction studies are not always predictive of the human response, this drug should be used during pregnancy only if clearly needed. Because many drugs are excreted in human milk, acarbose should not be administered to nursing women. Safety and efficacy of acarbose have not been established for children.

Alpha-glucosidase inhibitor monotherapy is not associated with hypoglycemia.[37] Patients using combination therapy with insulin or sulfonylureas may experience hypoglycemia secondary to the insulin or sulfonylurea. Hypoglycemia in this situation is best managed with oral glucose (if the person is conscious) or intravenous glucose or glucagon (if the person is unconscious). Alpha-glucosidase inhibitors blunt the digestion of complex sugars to glucose; oral sugar sources other than glucose or lactose (eg, glucose tablets, milk) are unsuitable for rapid correction of hypoglycemia.[37]

Elevation of serum transaminases (AST or ALT) has been observed in clinical trials in patients taking acarbose at a dose of 200 to 300 mg daily.[38] Liver function should be periodically monitored. The effect of alpha-glucosidase inhibitors may be altered by charcoal, and these agents may in turn also decrease the bioavailability of ranitidine, propranolol, and digoxin.

Contraindications   Patients with inflammatory bowel disease, colonic ulceration, obstructive bowel disorders, or chronic intestinal disorders of digestion or absorption should not use these agents.[37] Acarbose is contraindicated in patients with cirrhosis of the liver and not recommended in patients with serum creatinine levels >2.0 mg/dL or a creatinine clearance of <25 mL per minute.

Side Effects   Gastrointestinal effects, occurring primarily at initiation of therapy or when dosage is increased, are abdominal pain, diarrhea, and flatulence (incidence of 19%, 31%, and 75%, respectively) secondary to the drugs' mechanism. These effects are usually self-limiting and transient and can be minimized by starting with a low dose and slow upward titration of dosage. Redistribution of the inhibited enzymes usually occurs after several weeks of therapy, resulting in a mitigation of side effects.[37]

Monitoring   Alpha-glucosidase is often monitored by using 2-hour postprandial glucose measurements. This allows an assessment of the rapid effects and timing of the action of the medication. Serum transaminase levels should be checked every 3 months during the first year and periodically thereafter to monitor for liver toxicity.

Instructions for Patients   Patients using alpha-glucosidase inhibitors should be encouraged to maintain physical movement, especially after a meal, to limit the buildup of gastrointestinal tract gas from the fermenting carbohydrate, as the drug limits carbohydrate absorption. The medication should be taken with the first bite of food at mealtime or with a large snack. While this medication will not induce hypoglycemia, those taking it should be instructed on the products of choice for hypoglycemic episodes if this agent is used in combination with an agent that can induce hypoglycemia (see the section on hypoglycemia near the end of this chapter).

Dopamine Receptor Agonists

Dopamine receptor agonists are used as monotherapy in type 2 diabetes or secondary diabetes with substantial capacity for insulin production.[39] Good candidates for initial dopamine receptor agonist monotherapy have type 2 diabetes with only mildly elevated blood glucose levels. Due to their limited ability to lower A1C and their side effect profile, these drugs are not commonly used as monotherapy but rather as adjuncts to existing therapy.

Dopamine Receptor Agonists: Dosage Information			
Drug	*Trade Name*	*Common Dose and Available Strengths*	*Common Frequency*
Bromocriptine mesylate	Cycloset®	1.6–4.8 mg once daily *Tabs:* 0.8 mg	Once daily within 2 hours after waking

Mechanism of Action   The mechanism by which dopamine receptor agonists improve glycemic control is unknown. Following morning administration of bromocriptine mesylate, postprandial glucose levels improve without increasing plasma insulin concentrations.

Dosing The usual initial dose of bromocriptine mesylate is 0.8 mg taken 2 hours after waking with the first meal of the day. The dose may be increased by 0.8 mg each week until the maximal tolerated daily dose of 1.6 to 4.8 mg is achieved. Dose adjustment is not needed in the elderly, in patients with mild to severe renal insufficiency, or in those with mild hepatic insufficiency.[39]

Precautions Bromocriptine mesylate is classified in Pregnancy Category B. Because animal reproduction studies are not always predictive of the human response, this drug should be used during pregnancy only if clearly needed. Bromocriptine inhibits lactation and should not be administered to nursing women. Safety and efficacy of bromocriptine have not been established for children.

Plasma exposure is increased by 18% to 30% in females compared with males.

Risk of hypotension and syncope may be increased with bromocriptine upon initiation or dose escalation, especially in those patients with a history of orthostasis or those taking antihypertensive medications.

Bromocriptine may exacerbate psychotic disorders or reduce the effectiveness of drugs used to treat psychosis. Dopamine receptor antagonists (eg, clozapine, olanzapine, ziprasidone) may reduce the effectiveness of bromocriptine.

Concomitant use of bromocriptine with other dopamine receptor agonists indicated for the treatment of Parkinson's disease, hyperporlactinemia, restless leg syndrome, acromegaly, and other disorders is not recommended. Combining bromocriptine with ergot-related drugs may increase the risk of ergot-related side effects such as nausea, vomiting, and fatigue; bromocriptine may also decrease the effectiveness of these agents to treat migraine headaches.

Bromocriptine is highly bound to serum proteins and may increase the unbound fraction of other highly protein-bound drugs (eg, salicylates, sulfonamides, chloramphenicol, and probenecid), resulting in altered effectiveness and risk of side effects.

Bromocriptine is extensively metabolized by the liver isoenzyme CYP3A4. Coadministration of bromocriptine with strong inhibitors of CYP3A4, erythromycin, or ketoconazole increases bromocriptine exposure, as measured by area under the curve (AUC), by 2.8-fold.

Contraindications Bromocriptine should not be used to treat type 1 diabetes or DKA. Patients with syncopal migraines should avoid bromocriptine mesylate due to the potential increased risk of hypotension. Nursing women should also avoid this agent due to its ability to inhibit lactation and potential for increased stroke risk in this population while taking bromocriptine. Dopamine receptor agonists are not recommended for patients with severe psychotic disorders.

Side Effects Side effects associated with bromocriptine include somnolence, nausea, fatigue, dizziness, vomiting, and headache.

Monitoring Blood glucose monitoring should include some premeal and postmeal readings to assess the effectiveness of the medication. Patients should also be assessed for signs and symptoms of orthostatic hypotension.[25]

Instructions for Patients Bromocriptine should be taken 2 hours after waking with the first meal of the day. Patients should notify their healthcare provider regarding symptoms of orthostatic hypotension such as dizziness, nausea, or diaphoresis.[39]

Sodium-Glucose Co-Transporter-2 Inhibitors

Approximately 90% of filtered glucose is reabsorbed through the sodium-glucose co-transporter-2 (SGLT-2) transport system in the proximal tubule of the kidney.[40] Normal glucose load in the tubules is approximately 120 mg/min with almost no glucose excreted in the urine. Glucosuria occurs when the plasma glucose concentration rises above 180 mg/dL (10 mmol/L).

Mechanism of Action Canagliflozin blocks the action of SGLT-2, resulting in increased excretion of glucose in the urine. The reduced ability to reabsorb tubular glucose results in lower plasma glucose and potentially excess calories for fat accumulation. In one clinical trial, canagliflozin monotherapy lowered A1C levels by 0.77% with the 100-mg dose and 1.03% with the 300-mg dose.[41] Weight loss in the

Sodium-Glucose Co-Transporter-2 (SGLT-2) Inhibitors: Dosage Information			
Drug	*Trade Name*	*Common Dose and Available Strengths*	*Common Frequency*
Canagliflozin	Invokana®	100–300 mg once daily *Tabs:* 100 mg, 300 mg	Once daily prior to the first meal of the day

study was 2.8 kg and 3.9 kg from baseline for the 100-mg dose and the 300-mg dose, respectively.

Dosing　The initial dose of canagliflozin is 100 mg before the first meal of the day. The dose may be increased to 300 mg daily in patients with normal kidney function, defined as an estimated glomerular filtration rate (eGFR) >60 mL/min/1.73m². The dose should remain at 100 mg daily for patients with impaired kidney function (eGFR between 45 mL/min/1.73m² and 60 mL/min/1.73m²). Patients with poor kidney function (eGFR <45 mL/min/1.73m²) or on hemodialysis should not take canagliflozin.

Precautions　Canagliflozin is classified in Pregnancy Category C. In the absence of adequate trials in humans, this drug should be used during pregnancy only if clearly needed. Canagliflozin should not be administered to nursing women or children.

Risk of hypotension may be increased with canagliflozin in patients with low volume status, especially those patients with a history of orthostasis or renal dysfunction or the elderly. Patients taking diuretics, angiotensin-converting enzyme inhibitors, or angiotensin receptor blockers should be carefully monitored and have their fluid status corrected before starting canagliflozin.

Canagliflozin may cause hyperkalemia, especially in patients with decreased kidney function. Increases in LDL-cholesterol levels have also been observed.

The increased glucose excretion is associated with increased urinary frequency. The high urinary glucose concentration also predisposes patients to genital mycotic infections and urinary tract infections.

Coadministration of canagliflozin with inducers of UDP-Glucuronosyl Transferase (UGT) such as rifampin, phenobarbital, phenytoin, or ritonavir may decrease canagliflozin exposure. Patients with normal kidney function may require a dose increase to 300 mg if continuation of the UGT inducer is required. Canagliflozin itself increases the exposure and peak of digoxin by 20% and 36%, respectively.

Contraindications　Canagliflozin should not be used to treat type 1 diabetes or DKA. Patients with severe kidney disease (eGFR <30 mL/min/1.73m²) or on hemodialysis should not use canagliflozin.

Side Effects　Side effects associated with canagliflozin that occur in greater than 10% of patients include hyperkalemia, mycotic infections, urinary tract infections, and renal insufficiency.

Monitoring　Routine A1C monitoring should be accompanied by potassium and LDL-cholesterol monitoring. Blood pressure and symptoms of mycotic infection should also be checked.

Instructions for Patients　Canagliflozin should be taken with the first meal of the day. Increased urination is expected in about 5% of patients. Patients should notify their healthcare provider regarding symptoms of orthostatic hypotension, dysuria, or urinary retention.[41]

Combination Oral Medications for Type 2 Diabetes

Several fixed-dose combination products of 2 different drug classes are available to treat type 2 diabetes. Many people find it easier to take a single medication as opposed to 2 separate medications, thus improving overall drug adherence and persistence. Fixed-dose combinations are generally started after a patient has failed to reach his or her glycemic goals on 1 drug alone. This stepwise titration is often necessary because the combination products are only available in specific doses (see Table 18.3). In addition, starting combination therapy in drug-naïve patients can create problems determining the specific cause of drug-induced side effects or allergic reactions. In some cases, these combination drug products may cost more than each drug separately; therefore, the provider must weigh the risks and benefits of using combination medications.

TABLE 18.3 Selected Combination Oral Medications for Type 2 Diabetes

Medication (generic)	Available Dosages	Initial Dose
ACTOplus met® (pioglitazone/metformin)	15 mg/500 mg 15 mg/850 mg	*Already on Metformin:* 15 mg/500 mg or 15 mg/850 mg once or twice a day *Already on Pioglitazone:* 15 mg/500 mg twice a day, or 15 mg/850 mg daily *Maximum Dose:* pioglitazone 45 mg/metformin 2550 mg
Avandaryl® (rosiglitazone/glimepiride)	4 mg/1 mg 4 mg/2 mg 4 mg/4 mg	*Already on Rosiglitazone or Glimepiride:* 4 mg/1mg or 4 mg/2 mg daily *Maximum Dose:* rosiglitazone 8 mg/glimepiride 4 mg
Avandamet® (rosiglitazone/metformin)	1 mg/500 mg 2 mg/500 mg 4 mg/500 mg 2 mg/1000 mg 4 mg/1000 mg	*Already on Rosiglitazone:* usual rosiglitazone dose/metformin 1000 mg divided dose twice daily *Already on Metformin:* rosiglitazone 4 mg/usual metformin dose divided dose twice daily *Maximum Dose:* rosiglitazone 8 mg/metformin 2000 mg
Duetact® (pioglitazone/glimepiride)	30 mg/2 mg 30 mg/4 mg	*Already on Glimepiride:* 30 mg/2 mg or 30 mg/4 mg daily *Already on Pioglitazone:* 30 mg/2 mg once daily *Maximum Dose:* pioglitazone 30 mg/glimepiride 4 mg
Glucovance® (glyburide/metformin) generic available	1.25 mg/250 mg 2.5 mg/500 mg 5 mg/500 mg	*As Initial Therapy:* 1.25 mg/250 mg daily or twice daily *As Second-Line Therapy:* 2.5 mg/500 mg or 5 mg/500 mg twice daily *Maximum Dose:* glyburide 20 mg/metformin 2000 mg
Metaglip™ (glipizide/metformin)	2.5 mg/250 mg 2.5 mg/500 mg 5 mg/500 mg	*As Initial Therapy:* 2.5 mg/250 mg daily or twice daily *Maximum for Initial Therapy:* glipizide 10 mg/metformin 2000 mg *As Second-Line Therapy:* 2.5 mg/500 mg or 5 mg/500 mg twice daily *Maximum for Second-Line Therapy:* glipizide 20 mg/metformin 2000 mg
Janumet™ (sitagliptin/metformin)	50 mg/500 mg 50 mg/1000 mg	*As Initial Therapy:* 50 mg/500 mg twice daily *Already on Metformin 850 mg or 1000 mg twice daily:* 50 mg/1000 mg twice daily *Already on Sitagliptin:* 50 mg/500 mg twice daily *Maximum Dose:* sitagliptin 100 mg/metformin 2000 mg

Note: An FDA REMS severely restricts the access and distribution of drugs containing rosiglitazone.

Source: Adapted from "Oral combination products for type 2 diabetes," *Pharmacist's Letter/Prescriber's Letter* 222, no. 2 (2006): 220206.

American Association of Diabetes Educators©

Incretin-Based Therapies

Over the past several years, a great deal of research and attention have been focused on the impact of incretin hormones on glycemic control. Following ingestion of a meal, gut hormones including glucose-dependent insulinotropic peptide (GIP) and glucagon-like peptide-1 (GLP-1) are released into the circulation. Increased GLP-1 levels exert multiple actions that affect plasma glucose. These actions include (1) promotion of satiety in the brain, (2) decreased or slowed gastric emptying rate, (3) increased glucose-dependent insulin release from beta cells, and (4) decreased glucagon release from pancreatic alpha cells. Although naturally occurring GLP-1 is essential in glucose regulation, its utility as a therapeutic target is limited by its rapid inactivation (half-life of 1 to 2 minutes) by the ubiquitous enzyme dipeptidyl peptidase-4 (DPP-4). Recently, 2 different therapeutic approaches emerged which successfully overcome this problem. These new agents to treat type 2 diabetes include glucagon-like peptide-1 receptor (GLP-1R) agonists and dipeptidyl peptidase-4 inhibitors (DPP-4i), which block activity of the DPP-4 enzyme.

GLP-1 Receptor Agonists

Mechanism of Action/Effects

In 2005, the first GLP-1R agonist received FDA-approved labeling for use in people with type 2 diabetes.[42] Exenatide is a synthetic form of a protein found in the saliva of the Gila monster, a lizard that is native to Mexico and the southwestern United States.

Exenatide binds to and activates GLP-1 receptors, resulting in a drop in fasting and postprandial glucose concentrations. Exenatide improves glycemic control in type 2 diabetes through several mechanisms, including increased insulin synthesis and secretion in the presence of elevated glucose concentrations, improvement of first-phase insulin response, reduced glucagon concentrations during hyperglycemic swings, slowed gastric emptying, and reduced food intake.[43]

Concurrent use of insulin, metformin, sulfonylureas, or a combination of these drugs with exenatide is recommended. It is not a substitute or replacement for insulin therapy in type 1 diabetes. Significantly reduced A1C levels have been observed in patients using exenatide, with a reduction in both fasting and postprandial plasma glucose concentrations. A reduction in body weight was also noted in patients who received the higher dose (10 mcg).[44]

In 2010, liraglutide became the second GLP-1R agonist to receive FDA-approved labeling for use in people with type 2 diabetes. Although its effects on glycemic control are similar to exenatide, liraglutide retains several differences. Unlike exenatide, liraglutide possesses an amino acid sequence that is very similar to native GLP-1 (97% homology).[45] Despite this similarity, liraglutide resists DPP-4 inactivation due to the addition of a fatty acid side chain that promotes self-association, delays absorption, and promotes protein binding.

Dosing

Both GLP-1R agonists are administered by subcutaneous injection in the thigh, upper arm, or abdomen. Exenatide should be administered anytime within

GLP-1 Receptor Agonists: Dosage Information			
Drug	*Trade Name*	*Common Dose and Available Forms*	*Common Frequency*
Exenatide	Byetta®	5–10 mcg twice daily *Pen injectors:* 1.2 mL, 2.4 mL	Twice daily
Exenatide LAR	Bydureon®	2 mg once weekly *Pen injector kit:* 2 mg • 1 vial containing 2 mg exenatide • 1 prefilled syringe delivering 0.65 mL diluent • 2 custom needles (23G, 5/16") specific to this delivery system (1 is a spare needle)	Once weekly
Liraglutide	Victoza®	0.6–1.8 mg daily *Pen injectors:* 3 mL (6 mg/mL)	Once daily

the 60 minutes before morning and evening meals. It should not be given after a meal. The initial dose should be 5 mcg twice a day for the first month and then can be increased to 10 mcg twice a day based on the response.[44] If a dose is missed, the treatment should be restarted at the next scheduled dose time.

Liraglutide may be administered once daily at any time of the day.[45] The initial dose of 0.6 mg per day is not effective for glycemic control but should be administered for 1 week to reduce gastrointestinal symptoms. Once the initial dose is tolerated (usually after the first week), it should be increased to 1.2 mg daily. If glycemic goals are not met after 2 to 4 weeks, the dose may be increased to the maximum 1.8 mg per day.

Exenatide is eliminated renally by glomerular filtration with proteolytic degradation. Clearance is only slightly reduced in patients with mild to moderate renal impairment, but exenatide is not recommended in patients with severe renal impairment (creatinine clearance <30 mL per minute).[44] Liraglutide is endogenously metabolized without a specific organ as a major route of elimination.[45] Although no dose adjustments are recommended in patients with impaired renal or hepatic function, caution should be taken in those patients with severe disease.

The extended release formulation of exenatide (Bydureon) is dosed once weekly. The 2 mg of powder must be reconstituted with the included diluent and then mixed and injected subcutaneously. The timing of the injection may be performed without regard to meals.[46]

Precautions

Exenatide and liraglutide are classified in Pregnancy Category C and should be used during pregnancy only if the potential benefit justifies the risk. It is not known whether these drugs are excreted in human milk; however, both are excreted unchanged in the milk of lactating rats. Nursing women should either discontinue the drug or discontinue nursing. Pediatric effectiveness and safety have also not been demonstrated with either agent.

Due to the ability of GLP-1R agonists to slow gastric emptying, the extent and absorption rate of orally administered drugs should be considered. Both exenatide and liraglutide may delay and reduce the peak concentration of digoxin, but exenatide does not affect the overall exposure to digoxin as measured

by the AUC. Both GLP-1R agonists delay the time to peak of lisinopril, and liraglutide also reduces the AUC of lisinopril. Exenatide can reduce the peak concentration and AUC of both lovastatin and acetaminophen.[47] Liraglutide can also reduce the peak concentration of atorvastatin and acetaminophen but does not affect the overall exposure of those agents.

In general, drugs with narrow therapeutic indices should be carefully monitored in patients taking GLP-1R agonists. To avoid acute affects of GLP-1R agonists on gastric emptying, patients may consider taking oral medications that depend on achieving threshold concentrations at least 1 hour before the injection, especially with exenatide.

Exenatide is associated with acute pancreatitis, including fatal and nonfatal hemorrhagic or necrotizing pancreatitis based on postmarketing data. Case reports of pancreatitis also exist for liraglutide.

Liraglutide causes thyroid C-cell tumors in both male and female mice and rats.[45] It is unknown whether liraglutide causes thyroid C-cell tumors in humans; however, the occurrence of tumors in mice and rats was dependent on dose and duration of treatment.

Contraindications

Contraindications to GLP-1R agonists include type 1 diabetes, ketoacidosis, allergy, or documented hypersensitivity to these agents.

GLP-1R agonists should be avoided in patients with severe gastrointestinal disorders, including gastroparesis.[45]

Patients with a personal or family history of medullary thyroid carcinoma (MTC) or multiple endocrine neoplasia syndrome type 2 (MEN 2) should not take liraglutide.[45]

Side Effects

A common side effect is nausea, reported in up to 44% of patients taking exenatide. Vomiting, diarrhea, dizziness, headache, and dyspepsia are also noted, but less frequently. Mild to moderate nausea is reported most often when therapy is started, with frequency and severity decreasing as treatment is continued.

Monitoring

The potential for exenatide and liraglutide to promote antibody formation must be considered in patients whose glycemic control is unresponsive to therapy. Patients who developed these antibodies in clinical trials did not experience a difference in glucose control compared with patients who did not develop measurable antibody levels.

The effectiveness of orally administered medications taken concomitantly with GLP-1R agonists should be carefully monitored, especially medications such as antibiotics, oral contraceptives, and agents with a narrow therapeutic index.[47]

After initiation of therapy or dose increases with GLP-1R agonists, patients should be monitored for signs and symptoms of pancreatitis. Symptoms include persistent severe abdominal pain, sometimes radiating to the back, which may or may not be accompanied by vomiting. If pancreatitis is suspected, GLP-1R agonists and other potentially suspect medications should be promptly discontinued.

For patients taking liraglutide, it is unknown whether routine monitoring of serum calcitonin, a marker for MTC, or thyroid ultrasound decreases the risk of thyroid C-cell tumors. Patients should be counseled regarding the risk of MTC and symptoms of thyroid tumors such as a mass in the neck, dysphagia, dyspnea, or persistent hoarseness.

Instructions for Patients

When used with a hypoglycemic agent, GLP-1R agonists may cause hypoglycemia; therefore, patients should be cautioned to monitor blood glucose levels carefully.

Exenatide is supplied as a sterile solution that contains 250 mcg/mL in a glass cartridge in a pen injector. Two pens, containing 1.2 mL or 2.4 mL, deliver doses of 5 mcg or 10 mcg. Each pen provides 60 doses, to give a 30-day supply. Needles are not included with the pen and are purchased separately. The drug should be stored in the refrigerator and protected from light. The pen should be discarded within 30 days after its first use.[13]

Liraglutide is supplied as a sterile solution that contains 6 mg/mL in a 3-mL glass cartridge in a pen injector. Patients generally require 2 or 3 pens depending on the dose (1.2 mg or 1.8 mg) to provide a 30-day supply. Needles are not included with the pen and are purchased separately. The drug should be stored in the refrigerator and protected from light. The pen should be discarded within 30 days after its first use.[13]

DPP-4 Inhibitors

Mechanism of Action/Effects

In 2006, the first DPP-4i received FDA-approved labeling for use in people with type 2 diabetes.[48] Sitagliptin improves glycemic control by competitive inhibition of the enzyme responsible for GLP-1 inactivation, thus prolonging the effects of endogenous GLP-1. Saxagliptin joined the market in 2009. Both drugs improve glycemic control in type 2 diabetes through prolonged half-life of GLP-1, which increases insulin synthesis and secretion, reduces glucagon concentration, slows gastric emptying, and reduces food intake.[48] The main advantage of DPP-4i drugs over GLP-1R agonists is their oral formulation. However, because DPP-4i drugs depend on endogenous GLP-1 to exert their effect, they produce less weight loss than GLP-1R agonists, which achieve supraphysiologic levels of GLP-1.

Dosing

Both DPP-4i drugs are administered once daily with or without food. The recommended dose of sitagliptin is 100 mg daily, and the recommended dose of saxagliptin is 2.5 mg or 5 mg daily.[48,49] Doses of both drugs should be reduced in the presence of renal impairment. For patients with a creatinine clearance between 30 mL/min and 50 mL/min, 50 mg of sitagliptin is recommended; for patients with a creatinine clearance less than 30 mL/min, 25 mg is recommended.[48] For patients with a creatinine clearance less than 50 mL/min, saxagliptin 2.5 mg is recommended.[49]

Precautions

Sitagliptin and saxagliptin are classified in Pregnancy Category B. Because animal reproduction studies are not always predictive of the human response, DPP-4i drugs should be used during pregnancy only if clearly needed. Both agents are excreted unchanged in the milk of lactating rats. Because many drugs are excreted in human milk, DPP-4i drugs should not be administered to nursing women. Safety and efficacy of DPP-4i drugs have not been established for children.

When DPP-4i drugs are used in combination with sulfonylureas, doses of the sulfonylurea may need to be reduced to avoid hypoglycemia.[48,49]

Sitagliptin is associated with acute pancreatitis, including fatal and nonfatal hemorrhagic or necrotizing pancreatitis based on postmarketing data.

DPP-4 Inhibitors (DPP-4i): Dosage Information

Drug	Trade Name	Common Dose and Available Forms	Common Frequency
Alogliptin	Nesina®	6.25 mg to 25 mg daily Clcr ≥60 mL/minute: No dosage adjustment necessary. Clcr ≥30 to <60 mL/minute: 12.5 mg once daily Clcr ≥15 to <30 mL/minute: 6.25 mg once daily *Tabs:* 25 mg, 12.5 mg, and 6.25 mg	Once daily
Linagliptin	Tradjenta®	2.5 mg to 5 mg daily *Tabs:* 5 mg	Once daily
Saxagliptin	Onglyza™	2.5 mg to 5 mg daily Clcr >50 mL/minute: No dosage adjustment necessary. Clcr ≤50 mL/minute: 2.5 mg once daily *Tabs:* 2.5 mg, 5 mg	Once daily
Sitagliptin	Januvia®	100 mg daily Clcr ≥50 mL/minute: No dosage adjustment necessary. Clcr ≥30 to <50 mL/minute (approximate Scr of >1.7 to ≤3.0 mg/dL [males] or >1.5 to ≤2.5 mg/dL [females]): 50 mg once daily Clcr <30 mL/minute (approximate Scr of >3.0 mg/dL [males] or >2.5 mg/dL [females]): 25 mg once daily *Tabs:* 25 mg, 50 mg, and 100 mg	Once daily

Hypersensitivity reactions (eg, urticaria, facial edema) are reported more commonly with DPP-4i drugs than with placebo. Postmarketing data with sitagliptin include serious allergic reactions such as anaphylaxis, angioedema, and exfoliative skin conditions including Stevens-Johnson syndrome.

Saxagliptin is primarily metabolized by the isoenzyme CYP3A4/5. Coadministration of saxagliptin with inhibitors of CYP3A4/5, diltiazem and ketoconazole, increases saxagliptin peak concentration by 63% and 62%, respectively. Saxagliptin exposure, as measured by AUC, increases by more than twofold with the CYP3A4/5 inhibitors. Saxagliptin does not appear to affect exposure of other concomitantly administered drugs. Sitagliptin may increase the peak concentration and AUC of digoxin.[48]

Contraindications

Contraindications to DPP-4i include type 1 diabetes, ketoacidosis, allergy, or documented hypersensitivity to these agents.

Side Effects

Common side effects in DPP-4i drugs include upper respiratory tract infection and headache; urinary tract infections were also more commonly reported with saxagliptin than with placebo.

Monitoring

In addition to routine measurements of blood glucose and A1C for efficacy, kidney function (serum creatinine) should be monitored to evaluate the need for dose adjustment. After initiation of therapy or dose increases with sitagliptin, patients should be monitored for signs and symptoms of pancreatitis. Symptoms include persistent severe abdominal pain, sometimes radiating to the back, which may or may not be accompanied by vomiting. If pancreatitis is suspected, sitagliptin and other potentially suspect medications should be promptly discontinued.

Instructions for Patients

When used with a hypoglycemic agent (eg, sulfonylurea), DPP-4i drugs may cause hypoglycemia; therefore, patients should be cautioned to monitor blood glucose levels carefully. Patients should be advised of the risks and symptoms of pancreatitis with sitagliptin. Patients should also be advised how to respond in the event of a severe hypersensitivity reaction with either DPP-4i drug.

Case—Part 2: Pharmacologic Intervention

The choice of drug products is generally made by considering the individual's specific characteristics and the agents' actions and effects. Effect on weight, drug interaction potential, required number of daily doses, age-related issues, and cost are also important considerations. Metformin is a good choice for CR because he has good kidney function; metformin monotherapy has a low incidence of hypoglycemia, and it might have favorable effects on his lipids and blood pressure. Although oral agents are easier for patients to start and require much less patient education, insulin and exenatide/liraglutide are also rational choices for therapy. Initiation of insulin should be strongly considered if blood glucose levels are above 300 mg/dL (16.7 mmol/L).

Metformin was initiated concurrently with a nutrition and physical activity plan at diagnosis due to the high blood glucose level and presence of clinical symptoms. Despite CR's adherence to metformin and lifestyle modifications, his glycemic control is not in the recommended target range. Because CR is tolerating metformin without gastrointestinal disturbance, advancement of the dose to 1000 mg twice daily is appropriate.

Amylin Analog

In 1987 amylin was discovered to be produced and co-secreted with insulin from pancreatic beta cells in response to food intake.[50] In people with type 1 diabetes and those with type 2 diabetes who require insulin, secretion of both insulin and amylin is diminished due to pancreatic cell dysfunction or damage. A recombinant form of amylin, pramlintide (Symlin®), is now available for clinical use.[13]

Amylin Analog: Dosage Information

Drug	Trade Name	Common Dose and Available Strengths	Common Frequency
Pramlintide	Symlin®	Type 1 DM: 15 mcg to 60 mcg / Type 2 DM: 60 mcg to 120 mcg	Before meals

Mechanism of Action

Pramlintide affects the rise of postprandial glucose by slowing gastric emptying, suppressing glucagon secretion, and reducing total caloric intake. Some research and discussion of this satiety sensation have led to the possible conclusion of a central effect.[13] Pramlintide is administered subcutaneously just before major meals and is indicated for both type 1 diabetes and type 2 diabetes therapy in people who use mealtime insulin therapy. People with type 2 diabetes who take pramlintide may also take metformin or a sulfonylurea. While always used along with insulin, pramlintide cannot be mixed and must be given as a separate injection.[51]

Dosing

People with type 1 diabetes should receive a starting dose of 15 mcg before major meals titrated in 15-mcg increments to a dose of up to 60 mcg as tolerated with nausea. People with type 2 diabetes using insulin usually receive an initial dose of 60 mcg before major meals. Pending the tolerance to nausea, the dose can be titrated to 120 mcg. Adjustment of the dose occurs to reach the desired glycemic control and tolerance to nausea.[51] The bioavailability of a single subcutaneous dose is approximately 40%, and its half-life is 48 minutes with a 3-hour duration after injection. Pramlintide is primarily metabolized in the kidneys to an active metabolite with a short half-life. Clearance of the drug was not altered in patients with moderate or severe renal impairment.[52]

Precautions

Pramlintide is categorized in Pregnancy Category C and should be used in pregnancy only if the potential benefit justifies the risk. The major concern with pramlintide use is the risk of hypoglycemia; careful monitoring and patient instruction for monitoring this action are mandatory. This effect is not actually due to the pramlintide but rather secondary to the pramlintide, making the insulin more effective, which can induce the blood glucose swing.[52]

Contraindications

Gastroparesis is a contraindication to the use of pramlintide due to its effect in slowing gastric emptying. Further, pramlintide should not be considered for patients taking drugs that alter gastrointestinal motility (eg, anticholinergic agents) or slow absorption of nutrients (eg, alpha-glucosidase inhibitors).[53] Pramlintide can slow the rate of absorption of orally administered medications.

Side Effects

Nausea is the most common side effect noted with use of pramlintide, ranging up to 48% of patients, though the incidence is higher at the start of therapy and decreases with time. Gradual titration to the recommended dose reduces this reaction. Other side effects can include anorexia, vomiting, fatigue, and headache.[52]

Instructions for Patients

Medications that demand a prompt or rapid onset of action should be taken at least 1 hour before or 2 hours after a pramlintide dose.[53] The dose is adjusted to reach the desired glycemic control and tolerance to nausea.[51] Pramlintide vials require refrigeration, though the vial in use can be stored at room temperature at a temperature of less than 77°F. Opened vials must be used within 28 days and then discarded.

Insulin

Physiology of Insulin in Diabetes

Insulin is a hormone produced in the beta cells of the islets of Langerhans in the pancreas; it is formed from a substance called proinsulin. When the pancreas is stimulated, primarily by an elevated blood glucose level, the proinsulin is cleaved at 2 sections of the molecule. When the proinsulin molecule is broken apart, insulin and the connecting peptide (C-peptide) are both secreted and enter the bloodstream in equimolar amounts.[53] Exogenous insulin is manufactured to be chemically identical to human insulin through recombinant DNA technology.[54] Another polypeptide, amylin, is also produced in the pancreas and released with insulin to assist in regulating the effects of insulin and to attenuate the actions of insulin.[55]

Mechanism of Action

The physiologic actions of insulin on body tissues include the following[56]:

- Stimulates entry of amino acids into cells and enhances protein synthesis
- Enhances fat storage (lipogenesis) and prevents mobilization of fat for energy (lipolysis and ketogenesis)
- Stimulates entry of glucose into cells for use as an energy source and promotes the resultant storage of glucose as glycogen (glycogenesis) in muscle and liver cells
- Inhibits production of glucose from liver or muscle glycogen (glycogenolysis)
- Inhibits formation of glucose from noncarbohydrates, such as amino acids (gluconeogenesis)

Several hormones in the body exert antagonistic effects to the hypoglycemic actions of insulin. These hormones are collectively referred to as counterregulatory hormones. The primary counterregulatory hormones include glucagon (produced in the alpha cells of the pancreas), epinephrine, norepinephrine, growth hormone, and cortisol.[57] Blood glucose management in diabetes needs to take into account, and compensate for, the release of 1 or more of these hormones throughout the day in response to a variety of stimuli.

Indications for Use

Insulin is always indicated in people with type 1 diabetes and in many people with type 2 diabetes when other forms of therapy do not effectively achieve glycemic goals. Insulin may also be indicated in those persons with type 2 diabetes who may be well controlled on oral agents but experience periods of physiological stress, such as surgery or infection, which cause severe hyperglycemia that is not responsive to oral agents. Women with gestational diabetes may need insulin if medical nutrition therapy alone does not adequately control blood glucose levels. Patients receiving parenteral nutrition or high-caloric supplements to meet an increased energy need may require exogenous insulin to maintain normal glucose levels during periods of insulin resistance or increased insulin demand. Insulin is necessary in treating DKA and often needed in treating hyperosmolar hyperglycemic state.[58]

Insulin harvested from animal sources is no longer manufactured. Human insulin is less antigenic than beef insulin and slightly less antigenic than pork insulin. Insulin analogs and U-500 insulin all require a prescription, although other insulin preparations are available without a prescription.[13]

The concentrations of insulin currently available in the United States are U-100 and U-500, indicating

100 units/mL and 500 units/mL, respectively.[54] Most patients use U-100 insulin; however, patients requiring large doses of insulin may benefit from the more concentrated U-500 regular insulin.

Insulin products are classified according to onset, peak effect, and duration of action (see Table 18.4). Once absorbed into the bloodstream, all insulin products exert the same effect on insulin receptors. The difference between insulin products depends on the ability of each molecule to dissociate and be absorbed into the bloodstream following subcutaneous administration.

Types of Insulin

Short- or Rapid-Acting Insulin

The currently available rapid-acting insulin products are insulin lispro, insulin aspart, and insulin glulisine.[59] The short-acting agent is regular insulin. Generally, these insulin products are administered into the subcutaneous tissue, although they may also be given intravenously.[13] Regular insulin and the insulin analogs are clear solutions; the other insulin preparations are suspensions. Insulin lispro, aspart, and glulisine, with their very rapid onset and short duration of action, can generally be used in place of regular insulin to provide better coverage of postprandial glycemic excursions with less risk of late-onset hypoglycemia. Several studies show reduced risk of

hypoglycemia in people with type 1 diabetes treated with insulin lispro compared with those treated with regular human insulin.[16] Insulin lispro can be injected immediately prior to eating (generally less than 15 minutes preprandially); injecting insulin lispro 30 to 60 minutes prior to meals may result in profound hypoglycemia. Insulin lispro has also been shown to be suitable for use in insulin pumps. Also, when compared with regular insulin, lispro reduced A1C levels in pump users; however, both products reduced the incidence of hypoglycemia compared with injected insulin.[60]

Insulin aspart improves postprandial glycemic control by reducing hyperglycemic and hypoglycemic reactions when compared with use of regular insulin.[61] Insulin aspart has a glucose-lowering response similar to insulin lispro, and its duration of action is shortest after abdominal subcutaneous injection.[61] Insulin aspart is also reported to be effective when used in insulin pump therapy.[61] Insulin glulisine has a more rapid dissociation rate than regular human insulin, producing a more rapid onset. The pharmacokinetic profile of insulin glulisine is comparable to insulin lispro and insulin aspart. Additionally, insulin glulisine combined with neutral protamine Hagedorn (NPH) insulin produced greater reductions in A1C levels than a regimen of regular and NPH insulin.[54]

TABLE 18.4	Time Action for Insulin Preparations			
Insulin Type	*Preparations (generic)**	*Onset*	*Peak*	*Effective Duration*
Rapid-acting	Humalog® (lispro)	5–15 min	30–90 min	<5 h
	Novalog® (aspart)			
	Apidra® (glulisine)			
Short-acting	Regular, human	30–60 min	2–3 h	5–8 h
Intermediate-acting	NPH, human	2–4 h	4–10 h	10–16 h
Long-acting	Lantus® (glargine)	2–4 h	No peak	20–24 h
	Levemir® (detemir)	3–8 h	No peak	5.7–23.2 h
Fixed combination	70/30 (NPH/regular ratio)	30–60 min	Dual	10–16 h
	50/50 (NPH/regular ratio)	5–15 min	Dual	10–16 h
	75/25 (NPL/lispro ratio)	5–15 min	Dual	10–16 h
	70/30 (NPA/aspart ratio)	5–15 min	Dual	10–16 h

*Most branded products are available via pen delivery systems.

Source: Adapted from *Facts and Comparisons* (St. Louis, Mo: Wolters Kluwer Health, 2005), 287.

Intermediate-Acting Insulin

Neutral protamine Hagedorn (NPH) insulin is an intermediate-acting insulin named for the researcher who derived the formulation. This insulin suspension contains the protein protamine (as well as zinc) and is at a neutral in pH. The zinc/protamine complex prolongs the duration of action. Both protamine and zinc have occasionally been implicated as the causative agents of immunologic reactions such as urticaria or other allergic-type reactions at the injection site. Since protamine is the antidote for heparin toxicity, some have expressed concerns about sensitizing patients to protamine with NPH insulin, but these concerns have not proven to be warranted.

Long-Acting Insulin

Long-acting insulins are the analogs insulin glargine (Lantus®) and insulin detemir (Levemir®). The long-acting analogs provide a peakless pharmacokinetic or drug effect pattern. Interestingly, the 2 agents differ greatly in terms of the biochemical explanation for their extended basal-type action curve.

Insulin glargine is a clear solution prepared in a solution with a pH of 4.0; due to its acidic nature, insulin glargine may cause a mild burning when injected. Following injection, insulin glargine forms a microcrystalline precipitate that results in a depot in the subcutaneous fat. This depot gives the glargine its duration of action. Insulin glargine can be given at bedtime or at any time of the day, but it should be given consistently at the same time each day.[61] Insulin glargine must not be mixed in the same syringe with other insulins. The syringe must not contain any other medicine or residue.[61] Insulin glargine provides only basal insulin coverage, and in most cases it is used in combination with other insulin preparations or oral agents.

Insulin detemir is a clear solution whose protracted action is due to increased self-aggregation and also albumin binding in the plasma and adjacent to the injection site.[61] Initially, a peak effect is reached in 6 to 8 hours; following routine administration, however, a constant rate of insulin detemir is found in the bloodstream. This results in a plateau or basal effect that approaches 24 hours.[61] Insulin detemir must not be diluted or mixed with any other insulin preparations.

Premixed Insulins

Commercially available premixed insulins and insulin analogs (70/30, 50/50, 75/25) are manufactured and stabilized by altered buffering.[61] These products may be appropriate for patients who have difficulty mixing their own insulins or for those in whom these ratios are effective. However, for intensive insulin regimens, these insulins are usually not recommended.

Dosing

The starting dose and schedule of insulin administration are based on several factors, including the type of diabetes; the clinical assessment of insulin deficiency and suspected insulin resistance; and individual patient preferences for eating times, meal composition, physical activity, and waking/sleeping patterns.[16,61] Target blood glucose levels for before meals, after meals, bedtime, and during sleep should be established with the patient. Setting targets enhances acceptance, understanding, and decision making as the patient observes changes in blood glucose levels in relation to changes in food, exercise, stress, or illness. Subsequent adjustments in dose or timing of the insulin are based on self-monitoring of blood glucose results and clinical signs and symptoms of hypoglycemia or hyperglycemia. Other parameters used to refine the insulin dose and schedule include A1C levels, achievement of weight or lipid goals, and variability of lifestyle or activities from day to day.

A goal of contemporary insulin therapy is to mimic, as nearly as possible, the physiologic profile of insulin secretion (basal/bolus).[58] The evolution of insulin management in the United States for people with type 1 diabetes and many with type 2 diabetes has clearly moved from single daily injection therapy to multiple injections with multiple insulin products. Such a pattern was difficult to achieve prior to the era of insulin analogs.[59] To optimize glycemic control, the pharmacology and pharmacokinetics of insulin require that a person with type 1 diabetes receive insulin continuously (basal, also referred to as background insulin), with boluses of insulin before meals and snacks (often called mealtime insulin).[58] Physiologic insulin secretion typically occurs at a rate of 0.5 to 1.0 unit per hour. The metabolic balance among basal insulin, the counterregulatory hormones, hepatic glucose production, and circulating glucose normally provides the body with sufficient glucose to function between meals. Bolus insulin is rapidly released in response to nutrient intake from a meal, and under normal circumstances it reduces postprandial glycemic excursions back to baseline in 60 to 90 minutes.[61]

Insulin requirements for individuals with type 1 diabetes or who are within 20% of ideal body weight are usually 0.5 to 1.0 unit per kilogram of body weight per day. Insulin requirements may be higher (even double) in the presence of intercurrent illness or other metabolic instability. Insulin requirements will be less (0.2 to 0.6 unit per kilogram of body weight per day) during the honeymoon phase, the period of relative remission early in the course of the disease.

Insulin Therapy in Pregnancy

Preexisting Diabetes

Insulin requirements for women with preexisting diabetes during the second and third trimesters of pregnancy gradually increase and can be 0.9 to 1.2 units per kilogram of body weight per day (as much as twice the total daily dosage of insulin needed before pregnancy).[10,11] These increases in plasma insulin are opposed by diminished responsiveness to insulin action due to placental production of counterregulatory hormones. Women with preexisting diabetes should be treated with an intensive insulin regimen, 3 to 4 injections or an insulin pump, to provide the basal/bolus regimen.

Gestational Diabetes Mellitus

Approaches to insulin therapy for gestational diabetes differ greatly. A total dose of 20 to 30 units given before breakfast is commonly used to initiate therapy.[10,11] The total dose is usually divided into two-thirds intermediate-acting insulin and one-third rapid-acting or short-acting insulin. For obese women, a higher starting dose of insulin is usually needed due to insulin resistance. The total initial dosage may be as high as 0.8 to 1.0 unit per kilogram of body weight per day.[10,11]

Insulin Regimens

Insulin regimens vary and should be designed with regard to a person's meals, exercise program, medications, work or activity schedule, and emotional factors. Appropriate alterations can be made in the insulin regimen to accommodate a midnight shift or rotating work schedule or other lifestyle preferences. Figure 18.3 shows some different types of insulin regimens using 2 to 4 or more injections a day. Although the typical split and mixed 2-injection daily regimen is often used, it may not be adequate to reach target ranges.

Multiple injections of insulin (3 or more) are components of the system called flexible or intensive insulin therapy. With 3-injection regimens, insulin is either administered in the morning before breakfast, before the evening meal, and at bedtime or administered before each meal. Before breakfast, a combination of rapid-acting or short-acting and intermediate-acting insulin is often used. Before the evening meal, rapid-acting or short-acting insulin is often used alone. At bedtime, intermediate-acting insulin is often used. This type of therapy can reduce the risk of nocturnal (2-4 AM) hypoglycemia, allow for better insulin coverage for early-morning (5-10 AM) hyperglycemia from the release of cortisol and growth hormone (the dawn phenomenon), and, in some cases, may accommodate sleeping in.[61]

With 4-injection regimens, a long-acting insulin such as insulin glargine or insulin detemir is administered once a day, and a rapid-acting or short-acting insulin is administered at mealtimes. If a snack contains more than 15 g of carbohydrate, an injection of rapid-acting insulin may be needed before the snack. This regimen is illustrated in Figure 18.3. The rapid-acting or short-acting insulin provides postmeal glycemic control, while the long-acting insulin dose ensures a low, steady rate of insulin throughout the day. This type of regimen or use of an insulin pump can best duplicate normal physiologic insulin action.[61] In people with type 1 diabetes, physiologic replacement using basal insulin and a mealtime rapid-acting insulin improves A1C levels and results in fewer episodes of hypoglycemia than previous regimens.[62] This regimen can provide individuals with diabetes the flexibility in insulin doses necessary for busy and active lifestyles.

Pump therapy is a continuous basal amount of insulin (0.5-1.0 unit per hour) that is usually administered in addition to bolus doses given prior to meals.[61] See chapter 21, on intensifying insulin therapy and insulin pump therapy, for more information.

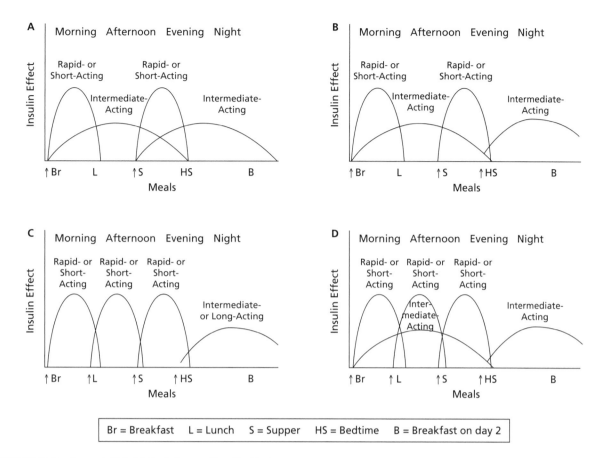

FIGURE 18.3   Potential Multiple-Injection Insulin Regimens

Source: Reprinted with permission from HE Lebovitz, *Therapy for Diabetes Mellitus and Related Disorders*, 5th ed. (Alexandria, Va: American Diabetes Association, 2009), 283.

Insulin Therapy in Type 2 Diabetes

For type 2 diabetes, insulin therapy may be used in 2 ways. First, insulin may be a supplement or additional agent added to 1 or more oral agents. Typically, single daily injections are used, commonly starting at 10 units or 0.2 units per kilogram.[16] Single daily insulin injection regimens for type 2 diabetes are usually administered in the morning or at bedtime. Due to the presence of insulin resistance in type 2 diabetes, the ultimate total daily monotherapy dose of insulin is often very high (0.7-2.5 units per kilogram per day). An intermediate-acting or long-acting insulin is usually used, but this can be combined with a rapid-acting or short-acting insulin product.[63]

Second, type 2 diabetes can also be treated with insulin as the sole pharmacologic agent requiring at least 2 or more injections per day. In 2-injection regimens, insulin is administered in the morning before breakfast and before the evening meal or at bedtime. This regimen may include only intermediate-acting insulin, doses of regular or rapid-acting insulins mixed with long-acting or intermediate-acting insulin, or premixed formulations (ie, mixtures such as Humalog Mix 75/25 or NovoLog Mix 70/30) at 1 or both injection times. Using mixed doses in the morning and before the evening meal is often called a split-mixed regimen and is considered fixed or conventional insulin therapy. Usually two thirds of the total daily dose of insulin is given before breakfast (using a ratio of 1 part rapid-acting or short-acting insulin to 2 parts intermediate-acting insulin), and one third is given before the evening meal (using a ratio of 1:1 or 1:2, rapid-acting or short-acting to intermediate insulin).[63]

Insulin Delivery Devices

Syringe

Disposable insulin syringes for use with U-100 insulin are available in different sizes, chosen according to the dose of insulin to be injected: 0.25 mL (for doses <25 units), 0.3 mL (for doses <30 units), 0.5 mL (for doses <50 units), or 1 mL (for doses 50-100 units). The attached needle length may be 6 mm (15/64-in), 8 mm (5/16-in), or 12.7 mm (1/2-in). The "short needle" (either the 6-mm or the 8-mm length) is appropriate for all patients regardless of BMI. A study of 388 individuals with diabetes divided participants into BMI categories (<25, 25-29.9, and ≥30 kg/m^2) and measured skin thickness at 4 different injection sites.[64] The authors concluded that needle lengths greater than 8 mm were likely to penetrate underlying muscle if inserted perpendicularly. A separate study in 173 patients concluded that a 4-mm (32 gauge) insulin pen needle provided equivalent glycemic control compared with 5-mm and 8-mm (31 gauge) needles.[65] In most situations, patients may safely reuse syringes and needles during a single day; however, reuse may carry an increased risk of infection for some individuals.[54] Advise those patients who choose to reuse syringes that the markings on the syringe may rub off and that the needle becomes dull with repeated use. Instruct patients to safely recap the needle and store at room temperature.

Used insulin syringes should not be discarded in regular trash cans or recycling bins or flushed down the toilet, due to the risk of harming others. The safest way to dispose of used syringes is with a sharps disposal container immediately after use. Sharps disposal containers that are three-quarters full should be closed and discarded according to community guidelines. Patients who do not have access to sharps disposal containers may recap the syringe using a one-handed technique (see the FDA website for details). Alternatively, patients may use needle clippers to make syringes unusable. Note that scissors should not be used to cut insulin syringe needles due to the risk of flying debris.

Pump

Continuous subcutaneous insulin infusion (CSII) pumps became available in 1974. An insulin pump consists of a reservoir filled with insulin, a small battery-operated pump, and a computer chip that allows the user to control the insulin delivery (see chapter 21, on intensifying insulin therapy, for more on insulin pump therapy).

Jet Injector

Jet injectors are a novel, needle-free system that delivers insulin transcutaneously. Jet injectors release a fine stream of insulin at high speed and under high pressure to penetrate the skin.

Pen Device

Pen devices have been a popular insulin delivery option in Europe for years. They were introduced in the United States in 1987. They combine the insulin container and the syringe into a single modular unit that allows for convenient insulin delivery. Insulin pens are available for almost all branded insulin products in a variety of types and styles. Pens are either reusable or prefilled, and both types hold cartridges of insulin. With the reusable pen, the patient must first load an insulin cartridge. This step is eliminated with prefilled pen devices.[66]

Table 18.5 provides information on injectable medications for blood glucose management.

Inhalation Device

An inhalable powdered form of recombinant human insulin (Exubera®) received FDA-approved labeling in January 2006, but its production was halted by the manufacturer in October 2007 due to poor sales.

Future Possibilities

In the future, insulin may be delivered by implantable insulin pumps or transdermal systems. Technical barriers to the market development of implantable insulin pumps include the requirement for surgical placement, relatively short battery life, and occlusion of the insulin delivery catheter.

Insulin Use

Monitoring

Self-monitoring of blood glucose and periodic A1C levels (every 3 months until goal level is attained, then every 6 months) should be the primary long-term monitors for insulin therapy, although blood glucose readings can be valuable in day-to-day blood glucose management. Inquiries about hypoglycemic episode severity and frequency should also be included

TABLE 18.5   Injectable Medications for Blood Glucose Management

Type of Insulin	Onset	Peak Effect	Duration	Available Forms
Humalog (Lispro)	0–15 min	30–90 min	3–6.5 hr	Vial Disposable pen Cartridge
NovoLog (Aspart)	0–15 min	60–120 min	3–5 hr	Vial Disposable pen Cartridge
Apidra (Glulisine)	0–15 min	60–120 min	3–4 hr	Vial Disposable pen Cartridge
Regular (Humulin)	30–60 min	2–3 hr	3–6 hr	Vial
Regular (Novolin)	30–60 min	2–3 hr	3–6 hr	Vial Cartridge
NPH (Lilly)	90 min–4 hr	4–12 hr	12–18 hr	Vial Disposable pen
NPH (NovoLog)	90 min–4 hr	4–12 hr	12–18 hr	Vial Cartridge
Lantus (Glargine)	1–2 hr	flat	24 hr	Vial Disposable pen
Levemir (Detemir)	0.8–2 hr	3.2–9.3 (dose dependent)	Up to 24 hr	Vial Disposable pen
Humulin or Novolin 70/30	70% Isophane suspension 30% Regular			Vial Disposable pen
Humulin 50/50	50% Isophane suspension 50% Regular			Vial
Humalog Mix 50/50	50% Lispro Protamine Suspension (NPL) (intermediate acting) 50% Humalog			Vial Disposable pen
Humalog Mix 75/25	75% Lispro Protamine Suspension (NPL) (intermediate acting) 25% Humalog			Vial Disposable pen Cartridge
NovoLog Mix 70/30	70% Aspart Protamine Suspension (intermediate acting) 30% NovoLog			Vial Disposable pen Cartridge

Source: AACE Diabetes Mellitus Clinical Practice Guidelines Task Force, "American Association of Clinical Endocrinologists medical guidelines for clinical practice for the management of diabetes mellitus," *Endocr Pract* 13 (2007): 3-68.

in the assessment. Normal daily insulin secretion in a healthy, nonpregnant adult who is not obese is approximately 0.5 to 0.7 units of insulin per kilogram of body weight. Since insulin and C-peptide are jointly secreted, a measurement of C-peptide level is used as a clinical monitor of endogenous insulin production and can be used to determine type of diabetes. Direct measurement of insulin secretion is difficult, except under controlled or research conditions, because insulin is rapidly removed from the blood as it exerts its pharmacologic action.[67] Because insulin and C-peptide have different biologic durations, a measurement of C-peptide level may not accurately reflect the endogenous insulin level at that period of time.

Precautions

Insulin is the drug treatment of choice for glycemic control during pregnancy. The major adverse effect of insulin therapy is hypoglycemia. Virtually all patients who inject insulin will experience hypoglycemia at some time. Common causes of hypoglycemia include excessive doses of insulin; delayed, missed, or insufficient food intake; or too much (unplanned) physical activity.[56]

Contraindications

Evaluate drug allergies to avoid acute allergic reaction to some of the preparations.

Side Effects

Various problems or complications may arise from insulin characteristics. Insulin impurity can cause lipodystrophies (atrophy and/or hypertrophy). Atrophy, which is a concavity or pitting of the fatty tissue, is an immune phenomenon that occurs in a small number of patients and is related to species/source or purity. Use of highly purified insulins such as human insulin or purified pork insulin reduces the occurrence of atrophy. Patients who develop this problem may benefit from injecting human or highly purified insulin around the periphery of the atrophied areas.[68] Many clinicians recommend a review of the person's insulin dose and injection technique when lipodystrophy occurs. Hypertrophy, which is a fatty thickening of the lipid tissue, is best prevented by rotating injection sites.

Allergies to insulin are possible but rare. Insulin allergy may occur as local reactions (rash, urticarial cutaneous reaction) or systemic reactions (serum sickness, anaphylaxis). Prior to insulin purification, local cutaneous reactions were more common. Zinc or protamine in the insulin, preservatives, and rubber or latex stoppers have all been implicated in inducing allergic reactions. Both local and systemic reactions appear to be immunologically mediated through induction of high titers of IgG and IgE antibodies. If a systemic reaction occurs, desensitization to the insulin will be necessary. If desensitization is needed, the attending physician should be encouraged to contact the insulin manufacturer for the desensitization kit and the procedure to follow.[69]

Instructions for Patients

Insulin mixing standards are based on published data.[54] Varying the time delay for injecting after mixing may result in a different insulin action. As a general rule, the 2 insulins to be mixed should be of the same brand. Rapid-acting or regular insulin is usually drawn up first, followed by the intermediate-acting insulin. This practice limits the potential for contamination, which may result in dose variance.

All insulin mixtures must be thoroughly resuspended immediately prior to an injection or after storage for any time period. Those using these products should be instructed to gently roll the vial or prefilled syringe or pen device between the palms of the hands several times to thoroughly mix the component insulins.

Strategies to reduce the risk of hypoglycemia include performing routine self-monitoring of blood glucose levels and watching for and responding quickly to early symptoms of hypoglycemia. Insulin users are instructed to ingest appropriate quantities and choices of a pre-exercise carbohydrate supplement and apply a consistent food/meal plan and pattern.[57]

Those using insulin should be instructed to take extra supplies when traveling to foreign countries, as some countries may still use U-40 insulins. Insulin users should be taught to store insulin according to the manufacturer's recommendations. Generally, insulin should be refrigerated at 36°F to 46°F (2°C-8°C). Unopened insulin products may be stored under refrigeration until the expiration date noted on the product label. Injecting a cold insulin preparation can produce local irritation and increased pain at the injection site; to bring the insulin to room temperature, the prepared syringe should be rolled between the palms of the hands. Other options include returning the vial of insulin to room temperature before withdrawing the dose, or storing the insulin at room temperature. Opened or unopened vials of insulin may be stored at a controlled room temperature of 59°F to 86°F (15°C-30°C) for 1 month; unused insulin should be discarded after that time.[54] Storage guidelines differ for used (punctured) or unused cartridge insulin and disposable prefilled insulin pens:

- ◆ Used or unused insulin cartridges or regular prefilled insulin pens may be kept unrefrigerated for 28 days (1.5-mL or 3.0-mL cartridges).
- ◆ Humalog Mix 75/25 may be used for 10 days capped at room temperature (72°F) and out of direct sunlight; the unused portion can be stored without refrigeration for 28 days but should be stored in the refrigerator to preserve its effectiveness until the labeled expiration.

- 70/30 insulin cartridges or prefilled insulin pens may be kept and used unrefrigerated for 10 days; unused units should be refrigerated, but if not refrigerated, they should be discarded in 10 days.
- NPH insulin cartridges or prefilled insulin pens may be kept and used unrefrigerated for 14 days; unused units should be refrigerated, but if not refrigerated, they should be discarded in 14 days.

Manually prefilled syringes of either single formulations or mixtures of insulins are to be refrigerated and used within 21 to 30 days.[54] Availability of insulin and supplies may vary; teach patients to carry insulin and supplies when traveling. Due to the variance of temperature, insulin should not be left in a car or checked through in airline baggage. Instruct those using insulin to examine vials for sediment or other visible changes before withdrawing the insulin into the syringe. Cloudiness or discoloration of clear insulin, clumping of insulin suspensions, or flocculation (frosting) of insulin suspensions indicates that the insulin has lost potency and should not be used; it should be returned to the pharmacy for exchange. The incidence of frosting may be minimized if temperature is stabilized through refrigeration and if agitation or shaking of the vial is minimized.

Teach patients using insulin to follow a specific routine for insulin injections, including consistent technique, accurate dosage, and site rotation. The insulin is injected into the subcutaneous tissue. Most individuals are able to lightly grasp a fold of skin and inject at a 90-degree angle. Thin individuals or children may need to pinch the skin and inject at a 45-degree angle to avoid intramuscular injection.[54] Insulin may be injected into the subcutaneous tissue of the upper arm, the anterior and lateral aspects of the thigh, the buttocks, and the abdomen (with the exception of a 2-in radius around the navel).[54] These sites are chosen because of general patient acceptability and accessibility.

Areas for injection must be determined individually, allowing for scar tissue, areas with less subcutaneous fat, and individual preference. Both the person with diabetes and the health professional need to examine injection areas at regular intervals to detect bruising, redness, infection, lipoatrophy, or lipohypertrophy. Teach patients to rotate injection sites to prevent local irritation. Rotating within a single area is recommended (eg, rotating injections systematically within the abdomen) rather than rotating to a different area with each injection. This practice may decrease variability in absorption from day to day.[54] Insulin absorption may vary depending on several parameters. Abdominal injection provides the most rapid absorption, followed by the arms, thighs, and buttocks.[54] However, note that insulin glargine does not display this difference of absorption rates at different sites.[59] Deeper intramuscular injections induce faster absorption and shorter duration of action. High levels of insulin antibodies can also inhibit insulin

Case—Part 3: Combining Agents

CR returned to the diabetes clinic 2 months after his metformin dose was increased to 1000 mg twice daily. His A1C was still elevated at 8.8%, and he continued to have fasting glucose levels over 200 mg/dL (11.1 mmol/L). He lost about 10 lb since diagnosis by increasing his physical activity and paying more attention to his eating habits. He reported some tingling in his hands and feet and wants better control of his diabetes.

Combining agents is a logical next step to provide optimal treatment of CR's type 2 diabetes. Combinations of agents provide up to 1.8% further improvement of A1C than use of a single agent alone.[70] Appropriate monitoring of the individual components is necessary with any combination of products. Adding a sulfonylurea, TZD, insulin, or exenatide/liraglutide are all viable options.

After discussion with the diabetes team, CR decided to add 20 units (0.2 units per kg) of NPH insulin at bedtime to help lower his fasting glucose. Insulin glargine or detemir was also a viable therapeutic option; however, NPH insulin was chosen to minimize out-of-pocket expenses for this patient due to his poor insurance coverage. Weight-based insulin dosing was chosen due to the presence of symptoms and continued significantly elevated blood glucose levels. CR received diabetes education regarding prevention, recognition, and treatment of hypoglycemia; proper injection technique; and proper storage. A plan for the frequency of self-monitoring of blood glucose was agreed upon, and monthly follow-up was scheduled with the diabetes educator. CR's target is to achieve an A1C of <7%.

action following injection. Exercise or massage of the injection site may induce more rapid absorption.

Drug Interactions

Other drugs can interact with medications used for diabetes control. Certain drugs or foods can have an effect on blood glucose levels by altering the action, the effect, or the outcome from a particular drug regimen. These actions are generally categorized as follows:

◆ Drug-drug (or pharmacokinetic) interaction
◆ Drug-disease (or pharmacodynamic) interaction
◆ Drug-food interaction

A drug-drug interaction is said to occur when a medication is added to an individual's regimen that alters the effect of another medication the person is taking. Some of these interactions are listed in Table 18.6. This type of interaction can occur with changes anywhere along the map of drug transport through the body.[71] Specifically, a drug can have its absorption into the body, distribution through the body, metabolism by the body—usually the liver or kidneys—and elimination from the body changed by another agent. The effect may be an increase or decrease in the rate of a particular step or an altered level of protein binding in the bloodstream, resulting in either a decreased or increased net action by the medication. This type of interaction is also termed a pharmacokinetic interaction, since the alteration is on the flow of the drug through its normal kinetic movement through the body.[72]

A drug-disease interaction has an intrinsic physiologic effect, as a particular medication may alter the level of control of a particular disorder. The interaction can either improve or worsen the level of control of a particular problem and is termed a pharmacodynamic interaction.

Drug actions can also be altered by concurrent ingestion of certain foods. A common mechanism of this interaction is to alter the absorption of a medication from the gastrointestinal tract, although other mechanisms of interactions (eg, effect on hepatic enzymes) may also occur.

TABLE 18.6 Drug-Disease and Drug-Drug Interactions

Interacting Drug	Drug-Disease (Intrinsic Effect)	Drug-Drug Interaction*	Net Effect on Blood Glucose	Notes
Allopurinol	No	Sulfonylureas and Meglitinide	↓	Decreased renal tubular secretion of chlorpropamide
Androgens/ anabolic steroids	Yes	—	↓	Mechanism unknown
Anticoagulants, oral (Dicumarol)	No	Sulfonylureas and Meglitinide		Interfere with metabolism of tolbutamide, chlorpropamide
Asparaginase I	Yes	—	↑[1] ↓[2]	1. Hyperglycemia associated with inhibition of insulin synthesis 2. Hypoglycemia reported occasionally
Aspirin	Yes[3]	Sulfonylureas[4] and Meglitinide	↓	3. Large daily doses (~4 g/d): Increase basal and stimulated release of insulin 4. Displace sulfonylurea from protein binding; decrease urinary excretion of sulfonylurea
β-Adrenergic antagonists	Yes	—	↑↓	Both hypoglycemic and hyperglycemic responses have been reported; may alter physiologic response to, and subjective symptoms of, hypoglycemia; may reduce hyperglycemia-induced insulin release or decrease tissue sensitivity to insulin
Calcium channel blockers	Yes	—	↑↓	Hypoglycemia reported with verapamil Hyperglycemia reported with diltiazem, nifedipine

TABLE 18.6 **Drug-Disease and Drug-Drug Interactions (continued)**				
Interacting Drug	*Drug-Disease (Intrinsic Effect)*	*Drug-Drug Interaction**	*Net Effect on Blood Glucose*	*Notes*
Cholestyramine	No	TZD[5] and Acarbose[6]	↑[5] ↓[6]	5. Cholestyramine reduces absorption of coadministered drugs 6. Cholestyramine may enhance effects of acarbose; interactions may be avoided by administering cholestyramine 2 hours apart from other medications
Chloramphenicol	No	Sulfonylureas and Meglitinide		Decreased hepatic metabolism and/or protein binding displacement of tolbutamide, chlorpropamide
Chloroquine	Yes	—	↓	Mechanism unknown
Cimetidine/ possible other H2 antagonists	No	Sulfonylureas,[7] Meglitinide, and Metformin[8]	↓	7. Increased absorption and/or decreased clearance of glipizide, glyburide, tolbutamide 8. Decreased renal tubular secretion of metformin; other drugs excreted via renal tubular transport may similarly interfere with metformin clearance
Clofibrate	Yes[9]	Sulfonylureas[10] and Meglitinide	↓	9. Intrinsic hypoglycemic effect: mechanism unknown 10. Displace certain sulfonylureas from protein binding
Corticosteroid	Yes		↑	Increased gluconeogenesis; transient insulin resistance
Cyclosporine	Yes	—	↑	—
Diazoxide	Yes		↑	Inhibition of insulin secretion
Dicumarol	No	Sulfonylureas and Meglitinide	↓	Inhibits hepatic metabolism of tolbutamide, chlorpropamide
Disopyramide	Yes	—	↑	Most susceptible: elderly or patients with renal or liver impairment
Diuretics	Yes	—	↑	—
Estrogen products	Yes	—	↑	Mechanism unknown
Ethanol	Yes	Sulfonylureas[11] and Meglitinide	↑[12] ↓[13]	11. Disulfiram-like reaction may occur, especially with chlorpropamide; not noted with second-generation sulfonylureas 12. Chronic alcohol ingestion may increase metabolism of sulfonylurea; alcohol ingestion, especially with carbohydrate-based drink (beer, mixed drink), has caloric effect. 13. Intrinsic hypoglycemic effect; impairs gluconeogenesis and increases insulin secretion; effect is potentiated if alcohol consumed without food or in fasting state
Fluconazole	No	Sulfonylureas and Meglitinide	↓	

(continued)

American Association of Diabetes Educators©

TABLE 18.6	Drug-Disease and Drug-Drug Interactions (continued)			
Interacting Drug	Drug-Disease (Intrinsic Effect)	Drug-Drug Interaction*	Net Effect on Blood Glucose	Notes
Fluoxetine	Yes	—	↑↓	Hypoglycemia and hyperglycemia have been reported
Gemfibrozil	Yes	—	↑	Reported interaction with glipizide
Glyburide	Yes	Acarbose and Miglitol[14]	↑	14. Miglitol reduces the area under the curve (AUC) and peak concentration of glyburide
Guanethidine	Yes	Sulfonylureas[15] and Meglitinide	↓[16]	15. Protein-binding displacement of certain sulfonylureas 16. Intrinsic glycemic effect
Isoniazid	Yes	—	↑	Increases glycogenolysis
Ketoconazole	Yes	Pioglitazone	↑	In vitro studies suggest that ketoconazole inhibits the metabolism of pioglitazone
Metformin	No	Alpha-glucosidase inhibitors	↑	Acarbose reduces metformin bioavailability by ~35% when coadministered; separate doses to avoid interaction
Monoamine oxidase inhibitors	Yes[19]	Sulfonylureas[20] and Meglitinide	↓	19. May stimulate insulin secretion (beta-adrenergic stimulation) or may be secondary to hepatotoxicity 20. May interfere with metabolism of sulfonylurea
Nicotinic acid (niacin)	Yes	—	↑	Dose dependent, when lipid-lowering doses are used Insignificant effect at vitamin supplement dose
NSAID (nonsteroidal anti-inflammatory drugs)	Yes[17]	Sulfonylureas[18] and Meglitinide	↑	17. Possible intrinsic hypoglycemic effect 18. Protein-binding displacement (tolbutamide, tolazamide)
Octreotide	Yes	—	↑↓	Hypoglycemia and hyperglycemia have been reported
Oral contraceptives	Yes	Pioglitazone[21] and Rosiglitazone[22]	↑	21. Pioglitazone has not been evaluated; however, caution should be used 22. No clinically significant effect on ethinyl estradiol or norethindrone
Pancrelipase/ pancreatic enzymes	Yes	—	↑	Do not administer these agents concurrently with acarbose
Pentamidine	Yes	—	↑↓	Initially, hypoglycemia; hyperglycemia may occur days or even months after initiation of therapy
Phenothiazines	Yes	—	↑↓	Hypoglycemia observed with some phenothiazines, hyperglycemia with others
Phenytoin	Yes	—		Decreased insulin secretion
Probenecid	Yes[23]	Sulfonylureas[24] and Meglitinide	↓	23. Intrinsic glycemic effect 24. Decrease urinary excretion of chlorpropamide

	TABLE 18.6 Drug-Disease and Drug-Drug Interactions (continued)			
Interacting Drug	*Drug-Disease (Intrinsic Effect)*	*Drug-Drug Interaction**	*Net Effect on Blood Glucose*	*Notes*
Protease inhibitors	Yes	—	↑	—
Rifampin	Yes[25]	Sulfonylureas[26] and Meglitinide	↑[26] ↓[25]	25. Possible intrinsic hypoglycemic effect 26. Increased metabolism of chlorpropamide, glyburide, tolbutamide
Salicylates	Yes[27]	Sulfonylureas[28] and Meglitinide	↓	27. Large daily doses (~4 g/d): Increase basal and stimulated release of insulin 28. Displace sulfonylurea from protein binding; decrease urinary excretion of sulfonylurea
Sulfonamides, highly protein-bound	No	Sulfonylureas and Meglitinide	↓	Various effects upon chlorpropamide, tolbutamide kinetics: displacement from protein binding, decreased urinary excretion, and/or altered metabolism
Tacrolimus	Yes	—	↑	—
Thyroid products	Yes	—	↑	Once euthyroid status is achieved, diabetes medications may need to be adjusted to compensate for glycemic effect of thyroid product
Urinary acidifiers	No	Sulfonylureas and Meglitinide	↓	Interfere with chlorpropamide excretion

*Interactions with sulfonylureas, meglitinide, metformin, pioglitazone, and rosiglitazone (both thiazolidinediones), alpha-glucosidase inhibitors, and insulin are listed.

Note: This listing is not intended to be all inclusive. Before any new medication is initiated, consult the package labeling (insert) or other reference. In general, these interactions are based on moderate to severe clinical significance and/or possible or established documentation.

Source: JR White, RK Campbell, "Pharmacologic therapy of diabetes mellitus," in MJ Franz, ed, *A Core Curriculum for Diabetes Education: Diabetes Management Therapies*, 5th ed. (Chicago, Ill: American Association of Diabetes Educators, 2003), 120-3.

Medication Side Effects: Self-Management Considerations

Certain drug side effects have an impact on diabetes self-management.[72] People with diabetes who are taking medication must be taught to be attentive to particular signs and symptoms that may indicate impending hypoglycemia or hyperglycemia.

In addition, certain procedures and aspects of diabetes care require the person with diabetes to be alert, coordinated, and capable of making self-management decisions. A drug that mimics an individual's usual warning signs of hypoglycemia or hyperglycemia, or one that impairs a person's ability to perform necessary self-care tasks, may adversely affect glycemic control.

Hypoglycemia

Defining hypoglycemia on the basis of a specific plasma glucose level is difficult. Absolute blood glucose levels cannot be used to describe the severity of hypoglycemic episodes, because glycemic thresholds for the onset of symptoms, as well as symptom magnitude, differ greatly among individuals and from episode to episode, depending on various mediating variables. Some individuals remain alert with only a few symptoms at a plasma glucose level less than 70 mg/dL (3.9 mmol/L), while others become stuporous at the same glucose concentration. Even the same person may tolerate low glucose levels differently on different occasions. The American Diabetes Association Workgroup on Hypoglycemia concluded that hypoglycemic events should be reported on the basis of the following definitions:

- *Severe hypoglycemia* is characterized by an inability to self-treat due to mental confusion, lethargy, or unconsciousness. Because the individual is unable to self-treat, others must provide treatment to raise the blood glucose level out of a dangerously low range.
- *Documented symptomatic hypoglycemia* is characterized by a documented blood glucose level less than or equal to 70 mg/dL with symptoms such as sweating, trembling, difficulty concentrating, lightheadedness, and a lack of coordination. These symptoms are usually alleviated quickly by drinking beverages or eating foods containing carbohydrates.
- *Documented asymptomatic hypoglycemia* is characterized by a documented blood glucose less than or equal to 70 mg/dL without symptoms.[73]

Causes of Hypoglycemia

The first step in determining the cause of frequent hypoglycemia is to carefully examine the treatment regimen. Insulin excess and hypoglycemia are more likely to occur at those times of the day when insulin action is peaking. Some of the newer insulin analogs, including rapid-acting insulins (eg, insulin lispro, aspart, or glulisine) and long-acting insulins (glargine or detemir), appear to reduce some of the problems with hypoglycemia but still carry risk.

Hypoglycemia is more of a risk when an individual has taken insulin or a medication that promotes insulin secretion and has not eaten for several hours, or when an individual takes medication and has significantly increased physical activity. Alcohol consumption, without food intake, may also result in hypoglycemia.

Prevention of Hypoglycemia

Prevention is the best intervention. Treatment regimens should be developed that include intake of carbohydrate at peak times of the insulin or medications if necessary and snacks for increased physical activity. In addition, the individual should understand that foods high in fat or protein and very low in carbohydrate will not prevent hypoglycemia.

Treatment of Hypoglycemia

Treatment of hypoglycemia is to eat or drink 10 to 15 g of glucose or any form of carbohydrate that contains glucose, such as the following:

- 3 to 4 glucose tablets
- 8 to 10 Life Savers® candies
- 2 Tb raisins
- 4 to 6 oz nondiet soft drink
- 4 to 6 oz fruit juice
- 1 piece of fruit
- 1 c low-fat or nonfat milk

The challenge is to treat, but not overtreat. Overtreating hypoglycemia is relatively common and causes posttreatment hyperglycemia. Some patients may continue eating until all symptoms disappear. Others may overeat because they are fearful of the symptoms (often feeling as though they are losing control). It is sometimes difficult to prevent people from overtreating hypoglycemia. Using commercially available, portion-controlled glucose products may help individuals avoid overtreatment.

The choice of glucose or carbohydrate-containing product should be based on its ability to raise blood glucose levels quickly. Drinks or foods that are high in fat content slow gastric emptying and absorption of carbohydrate and, therefore, take longer to raise blood glucose levels. Adding protein to the treatment of hypoglycemia does not raise blood glucose levels and does not prevent subsequent hypoglycemia.

If possible, blood glucose levels should be tested before treatment and again 15 to 20 minutes after initiating treatment. If blood glucose levels remain low (less than 70 mg/dL), treatment should be repeated regardless of symptom presence. If a meal or snack is not scheduled within the next hour, patients should be cautioned that their blood glucose level may fall again.

General guidelines for treating hypoglycemia are the following:

- Do not keep eating after the initial treatment; wait 15 to 20 minutes and then test blood glucose level to determine whether further treatment is needed.
- Do not keep eating until symptoms disappear.
- Avoid using high-fat foods for treatment.
- Always carry some type of carbohydrate.

- Keep something at your bedside to treat nocturnal hypoglycemia.
- Keep something in the car at all times to treat episodes of hypoglycemia that might occur while driving.
- Always wear diabetes identification.

Treatment of hypoglycemia may need to be given by others. A person with type 1 diabetes who is experiencing hypoglycemia often has to be treated by others because hypoglycemia may affect the individual's judgment and behavior. Family members and significant others should be taught how to cope with episodes of severe hypoglycemia and what to expect in terms of the person's behavior (eg, stupor or possible resistance). Coworkers, friends, and teachers also need to know how to respond to symptoms of hypoglycemia, which can be a problem if individuals do not want to reveal their diabetes to others. In cases in which others may be too anxious or frightened to treat the hypoglycemia, they should be instructed to call 911.

Severe hypoglycemia occurs when the individual is unable to self-treat. The following basic guidelines are recommended for treating severe hypoglycemia:

- *Able to swallow.* Patients who are able to swallow without risk of aspiration may be coaxed into drinking juice or a soft drink. If this is not possible, place some glucose gel, honey, syrup, or jelly inside the individual's cheek.
- *Unable to swallow.* Patients who are unable to swallow without risk of aspiration can be given glucagon by subcutaneous or intramuscular injection (see Table 18.7). Glucagon is a hormone that stimulates hepatic glucose production. Glucagon will produce substantial hyperglycemia, but its effects are very short lived. As soon as the individual is able to swallow, liquid carbohydrates should be given to maintain normoglycemia.

The person with diabetes and those likely to be involved in treatment need to know that glucagon may cause nausea and vomiting.

Frequent blood glucose monitoring is needed over the next several hours to detect whether blood glucose levels fall again or to detect hyperglycemia due to overtreatment.

TABLE 18.7 Recommended Doses for Glucagon
Adults and children >20 kg:
1 mg SQ (subcutaneously) or IM (intramuscularly)*
Children <20 kg:
0.5 mg SQ or IM, or 20–30 mcg per kilogram (9.1–13.6 mcg per pound) of body weight*

*If necessary, the dose may be repeated after 15 minutes.

Source: Glucagon [package insert], Indianapolis, Ind: Eli Lilly and Company, 2009.

Family and significant others should be taught how and when to administer glucagon. Patients should keep glucagon in their homes at all times. Individuals who may be required to administer the injection need to know how to use the glucagon kit; this may include a teacher, coworker, roommate, friend, or neighbor. Glucagon kits are obtained by prescription. Patients also need to be aware of the expiration date on their glucagon.

Treating Hypoglycemia in Type 2 Diabetes

Individuals with type 2 diabetes who are taking oral glucose-lowering medication also need to be taught about hypoglycemia, even though they appear to be at less risk for severe hypoglycemia.

Patients who are changing from oral medications to insulin may have considerable fears and concerns about hypoglycemia and need to be taught to monitor themselves for warning symptoms, especially at those times of the day when they are most at risk (eg, just before lunch). These patients may also need to increase the frequency of self-monitoring of blood glucose.

Many people with type 2 diabetes are not adequately educated about hypoglycemia and are not aware of the risks that hypoglycemia can impose. Knowledge about hypoglycemia, including warning symptoms, needs to be assessed even in patients who have been taking medication for a long period of time. Hypoglycemia is treated by carbohydrate consumption, following the guidelines prescribed for people with type 1 diabetes.

People with diabetes also need to be educated about the risk of hypoglycemia in other potentially dangerous situations, such as when caring for young children or when using heavy tools (eg, electric saws, lawn mowers).

Summary

Treatment Plan for Diabetes

Diabetes management requires prompt attention to achieve glycemic control in a timely manner. Quick return to optimal blood glucose levels appears to predict more positive long-term outcomes for the person with diabetes.[74] The foundation of an effective treatment plan relies on sound patient education and support for good nutrition and physical activity habits. Each patient's treatment regimen must be individualized based on the history of drug allergies, renal and/or hepatic function, and the cost of medications. Consideration should also be given to the ability and willingness of the individual to actively participate in his or her care. With good understanding of each patient's needs, plans can be developed that maximize glycemic control while limiting any lifestyle intrusions.

Rather than waiting for extended periods of time to evaluate drug regimen effectiveness, clinicians should aggressively advance drug therapy to achieve the desired glycemic goals. The effectiveness of any drug therapy regimen and nutrition/physical activity plan should be assessed at least every 3 months to reduce chronic complications.[16]

Focus on Education

Teaching Strategies

⊘ **Multiple medications.** Emphasize the unique function of each drug—oral agents, injection therapies, and insulin—and the options available for best control. Encourage monitoring of premeal and postmeal blood glucose levels only as necessary to observe changes and determine medication effectiveness.

⊘ **New medicines.** Many new products are available. Know the dosing, side effects, and population-specific issues of each agent in order to individualize drug therapy.

⊘ **Involvement in decision making.** Empowering patients to make good decisions requires patient-appropriate presentation of factual information and honest discussion of the pros and cons for each medication. Shared documentation of results as a team also helps determine the need for medication changes. In addition, prompt attention to achievement of glycemic goals is important to long-term diabetes success.

Messages for Patients

⊘ **Consider lifestyle changes.** Plan for good nutritional intake, portion control, and a wide variety of foods when planning meals. Make scheduled physical activity and modest lifestyle adjustments part of the plan, as these will assist in weight control and blood glucose management.

⊘ **Consider all the options.** Seek information about each medication, including its function and side effects. Ask for specific instructions as to the timing of medications; the effect of the medications on blood glucose, kidneys, and bodily functions; and the timing of blood glucose testing. Knowing this information enables you to judge the effects of taking the medication.

⊘ **Follow the prescribed medication plan.** All medicines have a timed action. Many of them rely on consistency and take time to build up in the system in order to work. Some require laboratory monitoring to make certain they are tolerated by the body. The importance of following "the plan" cannot be stressed enough.

Health Literacy

⊘ **Health literacy impacts medication safety and contributes to medication errors.** One study indicated that approximately half of the patients were unable to read and correctly state 1 or more of the label instructions on 5 common prescriptions. Rates of misunderstanding were higher among patients with marginal and low literacy. Nevertheless, more than one third of patients with adequate literacy skills misunderstood at least 1 of the label instructions.

Even when the instructions were written at a first-grade level—eg, "Take with food"—not all patients (84%) understood them. Only 56% of patients understood the simple instruction, "This medication should be taken with plenty of water."[75]

⊘ **Health literacy is not just about reading level, plain language, and numeracy.** It also relates to the problem-solving and decision-making capacity. A person with adequate health literacy can read, understand, and act appropriately on health information.

You can help your patients understand the medications they take and provide strategies for monitoring and effective use of the drug therapies. Consider the following communication strategies:

1. Ask your patient to explain what he or she understands about the medication, why it needs to be taken, how it is being taken, and when does it not have to be taken. This way you can discover misunderstandings, gaps in knowledge, and misinterpretations.
2. Ask your patient how he or she would like to receive information or learn about a topic: by reading about it, watching a video, attending a class, or getting reminders.
3. Suggest that a support person accompany the patient on appointments. Another person's perspective may provide insight into possible barriers to effective self-care and provide ongoing support as needed.
4. Advise the patient to review medication-taking instructions with a family member or friend.
5. Ask the patient to carry his or her medication list at all times.
6. Troubleshoot existing medication-taking behaviors. Any challenges can become an opportunity to change therapy to increase compliance.
7. Reevaluate the medication-taking strategy on an ongoing basis. As the circumstances of the daily schedule change, so will the medication-taking behaviors. For example: "Now that you have to get up earlier, how will you remember/have time to take your medication?"

⊘ **Successful diabetes care requires two-way communication between healthcare providers and patients.** Diabetes educators need to examine their communication skills and how they impact health literacy. Low-literacy-level literature will not provide adequate education without the educator's verbal support. When communicating with the patient, consider the following:

1. Involve the patient in treatment decisions— explore options for the patient and what is important to the patient.
2. Get true agreement on short- and long-term goal setting; examine whether the patient is stating a goal just to please you or whether the goal really is important to him or her.
3. Assess not just the knowledge but the skills necessary to implement the tasks needed; people with inadequate literacy may lack the skills to accomplish specific tasks and find it difficult to access and understand healthcare information.
4. Identify possible barriers of language, culture, and a healthcare system that is difficult to navigate. State some of the challenges that are common to other patients to minimize a sense of embarrassment by the patient. Nobody wants to admit that this information is impossible to implement; by normalizing the barriers and challenges you can open a trust between you and a patient and work as a team to strategize accordingly.
5. Celebrate the successes of treatment accomplishments and build a foundation for advancement in therapy. Patients are more likely to add additional behaviors and self-care if they have successfully accomplished something in the past. They need to feel that they can do it and that the change is a good thing in diabetes care.

Focus on Practice

⤳ **Medication therapy management (MTM).** MTM is collaboration among the pharmacist, the patient, and other healthcare professionals for effective medication therapy. The goal is to achieve the expected outcomes with all of the elements of medication taking. The Medicare Modernization Act established the requirement that each Medicare Part D plan sponsor offer an MTM program to targeted beneficiaries, including persons with diabetes. Medicare Part D plans are required to measure and report MTM program outcomes to Medicare and Medicaid Services (CMS). MTM-specific Current Procedural Terminology codes have been established for use by pharmacists when billing for MTM services.

⤳ **Medication adherence rates for persons with type 2 diabetes range from 65% to 85% for oral agents and 60% to 80% for insulin.**[76] The barriers include understanding of the treatment regimen, complexity of the treatment regimen, perception of the benefits of treatment, adverse effects, costs of medications, and emotional well-being. Medication adherence should be assessed at every patient care visit.

References

1. Inzucchi SE, Bergenstal RM, Buse JB, et al; American Diabetes Association (ADA); European Association for the Study of Diabetes (EASD). Management of hyperglycemia in type 2 diabetes: a patient-centered approach: position statement of the American Diabetes Association (ADA) and the European Association for the Study of Diabetes (EASD). Diabetes Care. 2012;35(6):1364-79. doi: 10.2337/dc12-0413. Epub 2012 Apr 19.

2. Garber AJ, Abrahamson MJ, Barzilay JI, et al. AACE comprehensive diabetes management algorithm 2013. Endocr Pract. 2013;19(2):327-36.

3. Frias JP, Edelman SV. Incretins and their role in the management of diabetes. Curr Opin Endocrinol Diabetes Obes. 2007;14:269-76.

4. American Diabetes Association. Standards of medical care in diabetes—2013. Diabetes Care. 2013;36:S11-66. doi:10.2337/dc13-S011.

5. Binder C, Brange J. Insulin chemistry and pharmacokinetics. In: Porte D Jr, Sherwin R, eds. Ellenberg's and Rifkin's Diabetes Mellitus. 5th ed. Stamford, Conn: Appleton and Lange; 1997:689.

6. Fleming JW, McClendon KS, Riche DM. New obesity agents: lorcaserin and phentermine/topiramate. Ann Pharmacother. 2013;47:1007-16.

7. Brown JB, Conner C, Nichols GA. Secondary failure of metformin monotherapy in clinical practice. Diabetes Care. 2010;33:501-6.

8. Belviq [package insert]. Zofingen, Switzerland: Arena Pharmaceuticals GmbH; 2012.

9. Xenical [package insert]. San Francisco: Genentech, Inc; 2012.

10. Guideline Development Group. Management of diabetes from preconception to the postnatal period: summary of NICE guidance. BMG. 2008;336(7646):714-7.

11. Serlin DC, Lash RW. Diagnosis and management of gestational diabetes. Am Fam Physician. 2009;80(1):57-62.

12. Langer O, Conway DL, Berkus MD, Xenakis EM, Gonzales O. A comparison of glyburide and insulin in women with gestational diabetes mellitus. N Engl J Med. 2000;343:1134.

13. Facts and Comparisons eAnswers. St. Louis, Mo: Wolters Kluwer Health, Inc; 2010 (cited 2010 Feb 15). On the Internet at: http://www.factsandcomparisons.com/.

14. DeFronzo RA. Pharmacologic therapy for type 2 diabetes mellitus. Ann Intern Med. 1999;131:281.

15. Burden M. Culturally sensitive care: managing diabetes during Ramadan. Br J Community Nurs. 2001;6:581.

16. Nathan DM, Buse JB, Davidson MB, et al. Medical management of hyperglycemia in type 2 diabetes: a consensus algorithm for the initiation and adjustment of therapy. Diabetes Care. 2009;32:193-203.

17. Melander A, Lebovitz HE, Faber OK, et al. Sulfonylureas: why, which, and how? Diabetes Care. 1990;13 Suppl 3:18.

18. Zimmerman BR. Sulfonylureas. Endocrinol Metab Clin North Am. 1997;26:511.

19. Stenman S, Melander A, Groop PH, Groop LC. What is the benefit of increasing the sulfonylurea dose? Ann Intern Med. 1993;118:169.

20. American Diabetes Association. The pharmacological treatment of hyperglycemia in NIDDM. Diabetes Care. 1996;19 Suppl:S54.

21. Kalbag JB, Walter YH, Nedelman JR, McLeod JF. Meal-time glucose regulation with nateglinide in healthy volunteers. Diabetes Care. 2001;24:73.

22. Heinemann L, Sinda K, Weyer C, Loftager M, Hirschberger S, Heise T. Time-action profile of the soluble, fatty acid acylated, long-acting insulin analogue NN304. Diabet Med. 1999;16:332.

23. Dunn CJ, Faulds D. Nateglinide. Drugs. 2000;60:607.

24. Hatorp V. Clinical pharmacokinetics and pharmacodynamics of repaglinide. Clin Pharmacokinet. 2002;41:471.

25. Lebovitz HE. Insulin secretagogues and repaglinide. In: Lebovitz HE, ed. Therapy for Diabetes Mellitus and Related Disorders. 3rd ed. Alexandria, Va: American Diabetes Association; 1998:160.

26. Bailey CJ, Turner RC. Metformin. N Engl J Med. 1996; 334:574.

27. Bell PM, Hadden DR. Metformin. Endocrinol Metab Clin North Am. 1997;26:523.

28. Kirpichnikov D, McFarlane SI, Sowers JR. Metformin: an update. Ann Intern Med. 2002;137:25.

29. UK Prospective Diabetes Study Group. Effect of intensive blood-glucose control with metformin on complications in overweight patients with type 2 diabetes (UKPDS 34). Lancet. 1998;352:854.

30. Klepser TB, Kelly MW. Metformin hydrochloride: an antihyperglycemic agent. Am J Health Syst Pharm. 1997; 54:893.

31. Aviles-Santa L, Sinding J, Raskin P. Effects of metformin in patients with poorly controlled, insulin-treated type 2 diabetes. Ann Intern Med. 1999;131:182.

32. Stacpoole PW. Metformin and lactic acidosis: guilt by association? Diabetes Care. 1998;21:1587.

33. Yale JF, Valiquett TR, Ghazzi MN, et al. The effect of a thiazolidinedione drug, troglitazone, on glycemia in patients with type 2 diabetes mellitus poorly controlled with sulfonylurea and metformin: a multimember, randomized, double-blind, placebo-controlled trial. Ann Intern Med. 2001;134:737.

34. Mudaliar S, Henry RR. New oral therapies for type 2 diabetes mellitus: the glitazones for insulin sensitizers. Annu Rev Med. 2001;52:239.

35. US Food and Drug Administration. FDA drug safety communication: update to ongoing safety review of Actos (pioglitazone) and increased risk of bladder cancer. Last updated 2011 Jun 15 (cited 2013 Dec 4). On the Internet at: http://www.fda.gov/Drugs/DrugSafety/ucm259150.htm.

36. Campbell LK, Baker DE, Campbell RK. Miglitol: assessment of its role in the treatment of patients with diabetes mellitus. Ann Pharmacother. 2000;34:1291.

37. Lebovitz HE. Alpha-glucosidase inhibitors. Endocrinol Metab Clin North Am. 1997;26:539.

38. Yee HS, Fong NT. A review of the safety and efficacy of acarbose in diabetes mellitus. Pharmacotherapy. 1996;16:792.

39. Cycloset [package insert]. Tiverton, RI: Veroscience; 2009.

40. Nisly SA, Kolanczyk DM, Walton AM. Canagliflozin, a new sodium-glucose cotransporter 2 inhibitor, in the treatment of diabetes. Am J Health Syst Pharm. 2013;70:311-9.

41. Invokana [package insert]. Titusville, NJ: Janssen Pharmaceuticals, Inc; 2013.

42. Vilsboll T, Krarup T, Deacon CF, Madsbad S, Holst JJ. Reduced postprandial concentrations of intact biologically active glucagon-like peptide in type 2 diabetic patients. Diabetes. 2001;50:609.

43. Zander M, Madsbad S, Madsen JL, Holst JJ. Effect of 6-week course of glucagon-like peptide 1 on glycaemic control, insulin sensitivity, and beta-cell function in type 2 diabetes: a parallel-group study. Lancet. 2002;359:824.

44. DeFronzo RA, Ratner RE, Han J, Kim DD, Fineman MS, Baron AD. Effects of exenatide (synthetic exendin-4) on glycemic control and weight over 30 weeks in metformin-treated patients with type 2 diabetes. Diabetes Care. 2005; 28:1092.

45. Victoza [package insert]. Princeton, NJ: Novo Nordisk; 2010.

46. Bydureon [package insert]. Princeton, NJ: Bristol-Myers Squibb Company; 2013.

47. Barnett AH. Exenatide. Drugs Today. 2005;41:563.

48. Januvia [package insert]. Whitehouse Station, NJ: Merck & Co Inc; 2009.

49. Onglyza [package insert]. Princeton, NJ: Bristol-Myers Squibb Company; 2009.

50. Nolte MS, Karam JH. Pancreatic hormones and antidiabetic drugs. In: Katzung B, ed. Basic and Clinical Pharmacology. 8th ed. New York: Lange Medical Books/McGraw Hill; 2001:711.

51. Weyer C, Fineman MS, Strobel S, et al. Properties of pramlintide and insulin upon mixing. Am J Health Syst Pharm. 2005;62:816.

52. Schmitz O, Brock B, Rungby J. Amylin agonists: a novel approach in treatment of diabetes. Diabetes. 2004;53 Suppl:S233.

53. Hussar DA. New drugs: exenatide, pramlintide acetate, and micafungin sodium. J Am Pharm Assoc (Washington, DC). 2005;45:524.

54. American Diabetes Association. Insulin administration (position statement). Diabetes Care. 2004;27 Suppl 1:S106.

55. McQueen J. Pramlintide acetate. Am J Health Syst Pharm. 2005;62:2363-72.

56. Guyton AC, Hall JE, eds. Textbook of Medical Physiology. 10th ed. Philadelphia: WB Saunders; 2000:884.

57. American Diabetes Association. Nutrition recommendations and interventions for diabetes. Diabetes Care. 2008; 31 Suppl 1:S61-78.

58. Hirsch IB. Implementation of intensive insulin therapy for IDDM. Diabetes Rev. 1995;3:288.

59. Comparison of insulins. Pharmacist's Letter/Prescriber's Letter. 2006;22(3):220309.

60. Pickup J, Keen H. Continuous subcutaneous insulin infusion at 25 years: evidence base for the expanding use of insulin pump therapy in type 1 diabetes. Diabetes Care. 2002;25:593.

61. Mooradian AD, Bernbaum M, Albert SG. Narrative review: A rational approach to starting insulin therapy. Ann Intern Med. 2006;145:125-34.

62. Ratner RE, Hirsch IB, Neifing JL, Garg SK, Mecca TE, Wilson CA. Less hypoglycemia with insulin glargine in intensive insulin therapy for type 1 diabetes: US study group of insulin glargine in type 1 diabetes. Diabetes Care. 2000;23:639.

63. DeWitt DE, Hirsch IB. Outpatient insulin therapy in type 1 and type 2 diabetes mellitus: scientific review. JAMA. 2003;289:2254-64.

64. Gibney MA, Arce CH, Byron KJ, Hirsch LJ. Skin and subcutaneous adipose layer thickness in adults with diabetes at sites used for insulin injections: implications for needle length recommendations. Curr Med Res Opin. 2010;26:1519-30.

65. Hirsch LJ, Gibney MA, Albanese J, Qu S, Kassler-Taub K. Comparative glycemic control, safety and patient ratings for a new 4 mm × 32G insulin pen needle in adults with diabetes. Curr Med Res Opin. 2010;26:1531-41.

66. Cefalu WT. Evolving strategies for insulin delivery and therapy. Drugs. 2004;64:1149.

67. DeFelippes M, Frank BH, Chance RE, et al. Insulin chemistry and pharmacokinetics. In: Porte DS, Baron A, eds. Ellenberg's and Rifkin's Diabetes Mellitus. 6th ed. New York: McGraw-Hill; 2003:481.

68. Griffin ME, Feder A, Tamborlane WV. Lipoatrophy associated with lispro insulin in insulin pump therapy: an old complication, a new cause? Diabetes Care. 2001;24:174.

69. Bodtger U, Wittrup M. A rational clinical approach to suspected insulin allergy: status after five years and 22 cases. Diabet Med. 2005;22:102.

70. Chipkin SR. How to select and combine oral agents for patients with type 2 diabetes mellitus. Am J Med. 2002; 118:4S.

71. Gibaldi M, Perrier D. Pharmacokinetics. 2nd ed. New York: Marcel Dekker; 1980.

72. Davies D, ed. Textbook of Adverse Drug Reactions. 3rd ed. Oxford, England: Oxford University Press; 1985.

73. Workgroup on Hypoglycemia, American Diabetes Association. Defining and reporting hypoglycemia in diabetes: a report from the American Diabetes Association Workgroup on Hypoglycemia. Diabetes Care. 2005;28:1245-9.

74. Krentz AJ, Bailey CJ. Oral hypoglycemic agents: current role in type 2 diabetes mellitus. Drugs. 2005;65:385.

75. Davis TC, Wolf MS, Bass PF III, et al. Literacy and misunderstanding prescription drug labels. Ann Intern Med. 2006;145(12):887-94.

76. Rubin RR. Adherence to pharmacologic therapy in patients with type 2 diabetes mellitus. Am J Med. 2005;118:27S-34S.

Pharmacotherapy: Dyslipidemia and Hypertension in Persons With Diabetes

Dave L. Dixon, PharmD, BCPS, CDE, CLS
Evan M. Sisson, PharmD, MSHA, CDE

Key Concepts

- Pharmacotherapy for management of dyslipidemia and hypertension in people with diabetes is complex and continually evolving.

- When developing strategies for managing diabetes, equal emphasis should be given to dyslipidemia and hypertension to reduce the burden of cardiovascular disease. These need to be treated as aggressively as hyperglycemia.

- Treatment strategies for diabetic dyslipidemia and hypertension may require combination therapies that provide different mechanisms of action to obtain optimal levels of lipid and blood pressure control.

- Patients on multiple medications should be monitored frequently for adverse events and possible drug or food interactions.

- Patient education should include the importance of medication adherence, medication safety, proper dosing, and timing medications for optimum effect.

Introduction

Cardiovascular disease (CVD) has been identified as the most common cause of morbidity and mortality for people with diabetes. More alarming is that CVD and its effects may be present for many years prior to the diagnosis, particularly in type 2 diabetes.[1]

Diabetes is associated with a two- to fourfold increased risk for CVD and is recognized as a coronary heart disease (CHD) risk equivalent.[2,3] Risk factors for CHD include hypertension, dyslipidemia, obesity, and smoking.

Persons with diabetes who have a myocardial infarction (MI) are likely to have an increased risk of death from that MI. Results from one Finnish study showed that the 1-year mortality rate following an MI was higher in men and women with diabetes (44% and 37%, respectively) compared with those without diabetes (33% and 20%).[4,5] A Swedish study examined patients hospitalized for an MI who had

not been diagnosed with type 2 diabetes and found that one third had prediabetes and one third had newly diagnosed diabetes.[6,7] Additionally, cardiovascular complications are the most significant cause of healthcare expenditures in people with diabetes.

Therefore, prioritizing and treating CVD risk factors in people with diabetes is crucial. When developing strategies for managing diabetes, equal emphasis must be given to dyslipidemia and hypertension, and they should be treated as aggressively as hyperglycemia.

Diabetic Dyslipidemia

Triglycerides (TGs) and cholesterol are water-insoluble lipids derived from dietary sources (exogenous system) and hepatic synthesis (endogenous system). Lipoproteins, other than TGs and cholesterol, are involved in these systems and include very low-density lipoproteins (VLDL), low-density lipoproteins (LDL-C), and high-density lipoproteins (HDL-C).[8–10] Figure 19.1 depicts the exogenous and endogenous lipid transport system.

Diabetic dyslipidemia is typically composed of elevated TGs and decreased HDL-C, with LDL-C elevations comparable to those of persons without diabetes. However, the particle size of the LDL-C in persons with diabetes tends to be smaller and denser, which can increase atherogenicity.[11–13]

> The small, dense LDL-C particles often seen with diabetes raise the risk for heart disease.

The abnormalities in the small, dense LDL-C composition are partially due to hypertriglyceridemia and are associated with a threefold increased risk of CHD.[12]

This increased risk is caused by the particles' ability to enter blood vessel walls more easily than the normal, large, and less dense LDL-C particles; thus, endothelial function is impaired and susceptibility to thrombosis increases.[13]

> Elevated TGs are a key contributor to low HDL-C.

Elevated TG levels can result from 2 abnormalities: overproduction of VLDL and impaired lipolysis of TGs. Persons with type 2 diabetes overproduce TG-rich VLDL, a result of elevated free fatty acid levels, hyperglycemia, obesity, and insulin resistance.[14] Impaired lipolysis of VLDL TGs is thought to be due to a reduction in lipoprotein lipase activity.[3]

HDL-C is the major lipoprotein responsible for removing excess cholesterol from peripheral tissues, which is known as reverse cholesterol transport. Therefore, suboptimal levels of HDL-C can result in increases in TGs, VLDL, and LDL-C.[8,9]

Cardiovascular Risk Assessment[15]

The aim of conducting an accurate cardiovascular risk assessment is to identify those individuals with accelerated atherosclerosis who are at high risk for MI. As previously stated, diabetes is associated with a high degree of CHD risk which is due to more than hyperglycemia alone. The total risk borne by a patient results from the combination of metabolic risk factors (eg, hypertension, low HDL-C, high TGs,

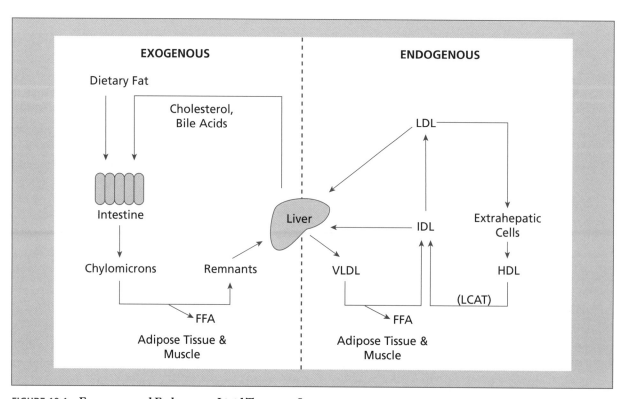

FIGURE 19.1   Exogenous and Endogenous Lipid Transport System

obesity) and degree of hyperglycemia. It is therefore necessary to assess a person's individual cardiovascular risk in order to establish appropriate treatment goals for dyslipidemia.

The Framingham Risk Score algorithm determines a person's 10-year risk of developing CHD by using the person's age, gender, total cholesterol (TC), HDL-C, smoking status, systolic blood pressure, and diagnosis of diabetes. The result categorizes patients as low to moderate risk (10-year risk <10%), moderate to high risk (10-year risk 10%-20%), or high risk (10-year risk >20%). Because diabetes is a CHD risk equivalent, a person with diabetes is categorized as high risk. Despite this, persons with diabetes who are female, younger, and/or lack other major risk factors may not calculate out to a >20% risk. Such is a limitation of the Framingham Risk Score. However, the projected lifetime risk for these individuals will exceed 20% and still warrants intensive risk reduction early on. An online Framingham calculator is available at http://cvdrisk.nhlbi.nih.gov/calculator.asp.

Another tool for determining CVD risk is the Reynolds Risk Score, which assesses a person's risk based on smoking status, systolic blood pressure, TC, HDL-C, family history of a heart attack before age 60, and high-sensitivity C-reactive protein (hsCRP). The Reynolds Risk Score predicts risk in women better than the Framingham. Furthermore, the Reynolds Risk Score includes hsCRP, a blood test that measures the degree of inflammation in the body. High hsCRP levels (>3.0 mg/L) are associated with a higher risk of developing heart disease. The Justification for the Use of Statins in Primary Prevention: An Intervention Trial Evaluating Rosuvastatin (JUPITER) study randomized 17,802 patients who did not have heart disease but did have elevated hsCRP levels to placebo or rosuvastatin.[16] The study was stopped after a median follow-up of 1.9 years because of a 44% risk reduction in the composite of major adverse cardiac events. The hsCRP test is not, however, routine in clinical settings and remains controversial because medications, pregnancy, inflammatory diseases, and other factors may affect hsCRP levels. Debate continues regarding how best to use hsCRP in stratifying CVD risk. An online Reynolds calculator is available at http://www.reynoldsriskscore.org/.

In summary, current guidelines emphasize assessing individual cardiovascular risk rather than relying on proscriptive population norms. The Framingham Risk Score is routinely included in treatment algorithms to assess risk, but the Reynolds Risk Score may be especially useful in women or young adults who have had hsCRP testing performed.

Treatment Goals: Diabetic Dyslipidemia

Dyslipidemia is often exacerbated by chronic hyperglycemia, specifically the postprandial glucose elevations and duration. In some cases, improved glycemic control may reduce dyslipidemia. Some glucose-lowering agents have been shown to improve TG and HDL levels. For example, the Carotid Intima-Media Thickness in Atherosclerosis Using Pioglitazone (CHICAGO) study randomized 462 individuals with type 2 diabetes mellitus to compare the effects of pioglitazone with glimepiride on carotid intima-media thickness (CIMT),[17] as studies have shown that a thicker intima-medial artery puts a patient at increased relative risk for MI and stroke.[18] Results showed that patients receiving pioglitazone had a –0.001-mm change in artery thickness compared with an increase of 0.012 mm in those taking glimepiride. No cardiac events were observed in the pioglitazone group; TG levels decreased by 13.5%, and HDL increased by 12.8%.[17]

In a similar study—the Comparison of Pioglitazone versus Glimepiride on Progression of Coronary Atherosclerosis in Patients With Type 2 Diabetes: The PERISCOPE Randomized Controlled Trial—543 people with type 2 diabetes and coronary artery disease were randomized to receive either pioglitazone or glimepiride to determine the progression to coronary artherosclerosis.[19] Results showed an increase in HDL-C (+5.7 mg/dL) and a decrease in TGs (–16.3 mg/dL) in the pioglitazone group.[19]

Studies are currently being conducted on several of the newer blood glucose–lowering agents to assess their effectiveness on CVD risk factors. For example, data from a 3.5-year follow-up study of exenatide on CVD risk factors showed a 24% increase in HDL-C and a 6% decrease in LDL-C.[20]

Though the lipid improvements with some of the blood glucose–lowering agents are beneficial, achieving lipid goals through euglycemia is very challenging and usually warrants the addition of lipid-lowering agents.

Case: An African American With Type 2 Diabetes

DC is a 64-year-old African-American male who was diagnosed with type 2 diabetes 2 years ago. He presented at the clinic one day for a follow-up visit (from his appointment 2 weeks earlier) to recheck his blood pressure and obtain the results of his recent lab work. At his last visit, his blood pressure was 150/86 mm Hg.

Past Medical History

- Seasonal allergic rhinitis
- Obesity
- Type 2 diabetes

Family History

- Father: history of CVD, MI, deceased
- Mother: history of type 2 diabetes, hypertension, deceased

Social History

- (+) tobacco
- (–) illicit drug use
- (+) alcohol (socially)

Vital Signs

- Blood pressure: 146/88 mm Hg
- Heart rate: 76
- Respiratory rate: 14

Physical Exam

- Height: 70 in
- Weight: 235 lb
- Body mass index: 34 kg/m²
- Waist circumference: 43 in

Current Medications

- Metformin (Glucophage®, Bristol-Myers Squibb) 2000 mg daily
- Pioglitazone (Actos®, Takeda Pharmaceuticals) 15 mg daily
- Multivitamin daily
- Aspirin 81 mg daily
- Fexofenadine (Allegra®, Sanofi) 60 mg twice daily as needed

Adherence to Pharmacologic Therapy

DC picks up most of his medications every 30 days at his pharmacy. However, pharmacy records indicate he purchases his metformin every 45 days. Initially, DC denied missing doses, but upon further interviewing, he admitted to forgetting occasional doses of medications because he "does not like to take too many pills."

Laboratory Data

- TC: 235 mg/dL
- LDL-C: 143 mg/dL
- TGs: 287 mg/dL
- HDL-C: 35 mg/dL
- Fasting blood glucose: 160 mg/dL
- A1C: 7.2%
- Liver function test:
  — Aspartate aminotransferase (AST): 16 U/L (reference range: 10–42)
  — Alanine aminotransferase (ALT): 12 U/L (reference range: 10–40)

Diagnosis

DC was diagnosed with both diabetic dyslipidemia and hypertension. His LDL-C level is above the target of less than 70 mg/dL, his HDL-C level is below the target of greater than 40 mg/dL, and his TG level is above the target of less than 150 mg/dL. An LDL goal of less than 70 mg/dL is most appropriate for DC due to the presence of diabetes plus metabolic syndrome, uncontrolled hypertension, family history, and smoking (see Table 19.1). DC's past and current blood pressure readings indicate his blood pressure is also above the target goal of less than 140/80 mm Hg for a person with diabetes. Since 2 readings have been obtained from 2 separate clinic visits and DC was seated for more than 5 minutes prior to having his blood pressure taken, he has stage 1 hypertension.

The case study progresses throughout the chapter. Considerations for the risk of CVD need to be addressed as well as appropriate treatment options for dyslipidemia and hypertension with diabetes.

When treating persons with diabetes and dyslipidemia it is necessary to review their entire lipid panel (LDL-C, TGs, HDL-C). Treatment strategies may require combination therapy that targets different mechanisms and lipoproteins to achieve treatment goals.

Both the American Diabetes Association (ADA) and the National Cholesterol Education Program (NCEP) Expert Panel on Detection, Evaluation, and Treatment of High Blood Cholesterol in Adults (Adult Treatment Panel III [ATP III]) recommend LDL-C as the primary treatment target.[15,21,22] The only exception to this recommendation is in patients with TGs ≥500 mg/dL because of the increased risk of pancreatitis. Although LDL-C levels are similar between people with diabetes and people without diabetes, the purpose of targeting LDL-C first is to reduce the burden of small, dense LDL particles. Secondary lipid targets may include raising HDL-C and lowering TGs.

Another secondary target is non-HDL cholesterol, which is determined by subtracting HDL-C from TC using a standard lipid panel. The advantage of non-HDL cholesterol is that it is unaffected by the non-fasting state and appears to be a better predictor of CVD risk than LDL-C alone.[23] The NCEP ATP III guidelines recommend non-HDL cholesterol as a secondary target in patients with TGs >200 mg/dL. The treatment goal for non-HDL cholesterol is set at 30 mg/dL higher than the LDL-C goal. For example, a person with diabetes and an LDL-C goal of <100 mg/dL would have a non-HDL cholesterol goal of <130 mg/dL. The American Association of Clinical Endocrinologists (AACE) algorithm and the ADA Standards of Care do not provide a TG cutoff level to advise when to target non-HDL cholesterol. Consequently, non-HDL should be routinely calculated in patients with diabetes and may be considered a co-primary target of therapy especially in patients with TGs >200 mg/dL.

Another option is to measure apolipoprotein (apo) B100, which includes all atherogenic lipoproteins and reflects particle number. ApoB100 is the protein responsible for transporting lipoproteins in the bloodstream and to the tissue. A recent meta-analysis suggests that ApoB100 is a better predictor of CVD risk than non-HDL cholesterol and LDL-C.[24] Despite its advantages, it remains unclear whether ApoB100 testing would be appropriate for all patients or just a subgroup, and whether the additional expense would be cost-effective. Thus, the clinical role of ApoB100 testing remains uncertain.

Both the AACE and the ADA provide treatment guidelines for managing dyslipidemia in persons with diabetes. The AACE algorithm categorizes those with diabetes and multiple major risk factors as high risk and assigns an LDL-C goal of <70 mg/dL, while the ADA Standards of Care establish an LDL goal of <70 mg/dL only for those with diabetes *and* established CVD. Furthermore, the AACE algorithm provides goals for non-HDL cholesterol and ApoB100, while the ADA Standards of Care only briefly mention these measurements and provide no further recommendations. While the AACE guidelines and the ADA guidelines specifically target people with diabetes, resolution of the discrepancies between the guidelines may not be easily determined. Previously, NCEP served as a universal standard regarding the treatment of dyslipidemia; however, an update to ATP-III will not be forthcoming. In the absence of a national benchmark guideline, stakeholder associations such as the National Lipid Association and the American Heart Association will contribute to the conversation regarding best practices for persons with diabetes. Table 19.1 lists these treatment goals.

Lifestyle modification, including medical nutrition therapy (MNT), physical activity, and smoking cessation, should always be a standard treatment of dyslipidemia in addition to pharmacotherapy.

Standard Treatment

Dyslipidemia—Lifestyle modification, including MNT, physical activity, and smoking cessation, should always be a standard treatment of dyslipidemia in addition to pharmacotherapy.

Children and Adolescents

Children with diabetes should be screened and monitored for dyslipidemia; see the ADA Standards of Care for specific recommendations. The initial management approach should consist of optimizing MNT, but statin therapy may be initiated in children ≥10 years of age who have either an LDL-C level >160 or an LDL-C level >130 plus at least 1 CVD risk factor. The LDL-C goal in children with diabetes is <100.[25]

TABLE 19.1   Dyslipidemia Treatment Goals

Lipid	AACE Algorithm[1]		ADA Standards of Care[2]	
	Moderate risk (diabetes with no major risk factors* and/or <40 years of age) Goal (mg/dL)	High risk (diabetes with major risk factors* or CVD) Goal (mg/dL)	Diabetes but without overt CVD Goal (mg/dL)	Diabetes with overt CVD Goal (mg/dL)
LDL-C	<100	<70	<100	<70
Non-HDL cholesterol	<130	<100	—	—
HDL-C	>40 (men) >50 (women)	>40 (men) >50 (women)	>40 (men) >50 (women)	>40 (men) >50 (women)
TG	≤150	<150	≤150	<150
ApoB100	<90	<80	—	—

*Major risk factors include hypertension, family history, low HDL-C, and smoking.

Sources:

1. American Association of Clinical Endocrinologists. AACE comprehensive diabetes management algorithm. Endocr Pract. 2013; 19(2):327-36.
2. American Diabetes Association. Standards of care in diabetes. Diabetes Care. 2013;36 Suppl 1:S11-66.

Pharmacotherapy: Diabetic Dyslipidemia

There are currently 6 classes of lipid-lowering agents prescribed in the treatment of dyslipidemia:

- HMG-CoA reductase inhibitors (statins)
- Selective intestinal absorption inhibitors
- Fibric acid derivatives (fibrates)
- Bile acid resins
- Niacin
- Omega-3 fatty acids

Plant stanols and sterols, although not considered pharmacotherapy, play a role in the management of dyslipidemia as well; see chapter 16, on nutrition therapy, for more information.

HMG-CoA Reductase Inhibitors (Statins)

HMG-CoA reductase inhibitors, commonly referred to as statins, are the most widely used lipid-lowering agent and often the first choice for treatment of diabetic dyslipidemia.[22,26] Their primary lipoprotein effect is in lowering LDL-C, with secondary beneficial effects of decreased TGs and increased HDL-C. Additionally, statins may increase the buoyancy or particle size of LDL-C, thereby reducing the amount of small, dense LDL-C in circulation.[12,13]

HMG-CoA Reductase Inhibitors (Statins): Dosage Information

Drug	Trade Name	Common Dose	Common Frequency
Atorvastatin	Lipitor®	10–80 mg	Once daily
Fluvastatin	Lescol®	20–40 mg	Once to twice daily
	Lescol® XL	80 mg	Once daily
Lovastatin	Mevacor®	10–40 mg	Once to twice daily
	Altoprev®	10–60 mg extended-release	Once daily
Pitavastatin	Livalo®	1–4 mg	Once daily
Pravastatin	Pravachol®	10–80 mg	Once daily
Rosuvastin	Crestor®	5–40 mg	Once daily
Simvastatin	Zocor®	10–80 mg	Once daily

Mechanism of Action

Statins primarily reduce LDL-C by competitively inhibiting HMG-CoA reductase, the enzyme that converts HMG-CoA to melvalonate in the hepatic synthesis of cholesterol, resulting in reduced endogenous cholesterol.

Statins will reduce but not totally block cholesterol synthesis. The decreased endogenous cholesterol production activates LDL-C receptor synthesis, resulting in enhanced clearance of circulating LDL-C particles.[9,26,27]

Dosing

Statins are generally administered once daily, often in the evening since cholesterol synthesis occurs at night. The dosage is dependent on the percentage of lipid lowering needed to achieve target goals. However, initial therapy commonly starts with a low dose and can be titrated up every 4 to 6 weeks as needed to reach the necessary or maximum dosage and to minimize adverse effects.[27–29]

Table 19.2 allows comparison of the lipid-lowering agents and their effects on the various lipoproteins.

TABLE 19.2 Lipid-Lowering Comparison of Various Agents					
		Effect on Lipoprotein (% Change From Baseline)			
Drug	*Daily Dose*	*TC*	*LDL-C*	*TGs*	*HDL-C*
Atorvastatin (Lipitor®)	10 mg	−29	−39	−19	6
	20 mg	−33	−43	−26	9
	40 mg	−37	−50	−29	6
	80 mg	−45	−60	−37	5
Fluvastatin (Lescol®)	20 mg	−17	−22	−12	3
	40 mg	−19	−25	−14	4
	40 mg bid	−27	−36	−18	6
	XL 80 mg	−25	−35	−19	7
Lovastatin (Mevacor®)	10 mg	−16	−21	−10	5
	20 mg	−17	−24	−10	6
	40 mg	−22	−30	−14	7
	40 mg bid	−29	−40	−19	9
Pitavastatin (Livalo®)	1 mg	−23	−32	−15	8
	2 mg	−26	−36	−19	7
	4 mg	−31	−43	−18	5
Pravastatin (Pravachol®)	10 mg	−16	−22	−11	7
	20 mg	−24	−32	−15	12
	40 mg	−25	−34	−20	15
	80 mg	−27	−37	−19	3
Rosuvastin (Crestor®)	5 mg	−33	−45	−35	13
	10 mg	−36	−52	−10	14
	20 mg	−40	−55	−28	8
	40 mg	−46	−63	−28	10
Simvastatin (Zocor®)	5 mg	−19	−26	−12	10
	10 mg	−23	−30	−15	12
	20 mg	−28	−38	−19	8
	40 mg	−31	−41	−18	9
	80 mg	−36	−47	−24	8

(continued)

TABLE 19.2 Lipid-Lowering Comparison of Various Agents (continued)					
		Effect on Lipoprotein (% Change From Baseline)			
Drug	*Daily Dose*	*TC*	*LDL-C*	*TGs*	*HDL-C*
Fenofibrate (Tricor®)	145 mg	–18	–20	–29	11
Gemfibrozil (Lopid®)	600 mg bid	–10	±10	–20 to 50	10–15
Niacin 500-mg tablet	1 g/d		–6		
	1.5 g/d		–12		
	2 g/d		–16		
Extended-release niacin (Niaspan®)	500 mg	–2	–3	–5	10
	1000 mg	–5	–9	–11	15
	1500 mg	–11	–14	–28	22
	2000 mg	–12	–17	–35	26
Colesevelam (Welchol®)	3.8 g (6 tablets)	–7	–15	10	3
Cholestyramine (Questran®) 4 g/9 g powder 4 g/5 g powder	4–8 g bid max 24 g/d		–15 to 30	5–10	3–5
Colestipol (Colestid®) 5 g/7.5 g powder 1-g tablets	max 30 g/d max 16 g/d		–15 to 30	5–10	3–5
Ezetimibe (Zetia®)	10 mg	–13	–18	–8	+1
Omega-3-acid ethyl esters 90 (Lovaza®)	4 g		+45	–45	9
Icosapent ethyl (Vascepa®)	4 g		–5	–27	–4
Plant Stanols (Benecol®)	3 servings daily	–10	–14		
Plant Sterols (Take Control®)	2 servings daily		–17		

Key: HDL-C = high-density lipoprotein cholesterol; LDL-C = low-density lipoprotein cholesterol; TC = total cholesterol; TGs = triglycerides

Note: Generic names of drugs are listed first; brand names are in parentheses for reader convenience.

Sources: Lexicomp, Version 2.0.1(165) (Hudson, Ohio: Lexi-Comp, Inc, 2013); CR Worz, M Bottorff, "Treating dyslipidemic patients with lipid-modifying and combination therapies," *Pharmacotherapy* 23 (2003): 625-37; P Jones, S Kafonek, I Laurora, et al, "Comparative dose efficacy study of atorvastatin versus simvastatin, pravastatin, lovastatin, and fluvastatin in patients with hypercholesterolemia (the CURVES study)," *Am J Cardiol* 81 (1998): 582-7; "Antilipidemic Agents," in *Monthly Prescribing Guide: November* (Montvale, NJ: Thompson PDR, 2005): 89-95; "Cardiovascular System: Hyperlipoproteinemias," in *Monthly Prescribing Reference: November* (cited 2010 Feb 17), on the Internet at: http://www.empr.com.

Pregnancy, Precautions, and Contraindications

Statins are contraindicated in pregnancy and in women who are breastfeeding; they should be used cautiously in those with impaired renal or hepatic function.[27,30,31]

Adverse Effects

Overall, statins are well tolerated with minimal side effects, especially if monitored appropriately. Common adverse reactions include headache, nonspecific muscle and joint pain, and gastrointestinal complaints, such as nausea, diarrhea, constipation, flatulence, and abdominal pain.[27,30,31]

Significant elevations of liver enzymes can occur. There have been reports of hepatic toxicity associated with statins: from 0.1% to 0.4% in persons on usual daily doses and up to 2% in persons on maximum doses.[27] Discontinue treatment when liver enzymes are greater than 3 times the upper limit of normal.[30] The frequency of monitoring at baseline and during therapy varies with each drug in the statin family; see package inserts for the most current monitoring guidelines for each compound.

Myopathy (a disease of the muscle) and rhabdomyolysis (the breakdown of striated muscle) have been reported in 1% to 5% of patients and in 1 in 2000 patients, respectively. Therefore, instruct patients to report any experience of muscle weakness, tenderness, pain, or fever. Laboratory testing of serum creatinine kinase can confirm or rule out rhabdomyolysis.[30] An increase in creatinine kinase to 3 to 10 times the upper limits of normal (450 to >1000) can be observed in myopathy and myositis (an inflammation of the voluntary muscles), respectively. The degree of muscle pain associated with myopathy and myositis can vary among individuals. Rhabdomyolysis, a more severe adverse effect, typically presents with additional signs and symptoms that include weight gain from fluid retention, fever, nausea, tachycardia, and dark or colored urine.

Statins have also been associated with causing new-onset diabetes (JUPITER Study). However, a post-hoc analysis of this finding found that new-onset diabetes developed only in those individuals enrolled in the trial who had at least 1 risk factor for diabetes.

Furthermore, the benefits of statin therapy exceeded the diabetes risk in those at high risk of developing diabetes.[32] It appears that there is merely an "association" but no definitive evidence that statins "cause" diabetes.

Drug Interactions

Most statins are metabolized through the cytochrome P-450 3A4 pathway in the liver. Concurrent medications and foods that are also metabolized through this system (such as grapefruit juice) should be used cautiously and patients should be monitored for increased levels and adverse reactions.[27,33]

Statins typically are the drug that is affected by inhibitors or inducers of the CYP-450 pathway, thereby delaying or enhancing their elimination from the body and resulting in increased or decreased statin serum concentration. Monitoring adverse effects and lipid profiles can help identify potential drug interactions and reduce the risk of toxicity, myopathy, and/or rhabdomyolysis. Table 19.3 lists common drugs that interact with statins.

Monitoring

A baseline lipid profile, creatinine phosphokinase (CPK) enzyme, liver function, and renal function tests should be conducted prior to initiating statin therapy. Monitor lipid profiles and liver function tests every 12 weeks in the first 6 months of treatment and periodically thereafter. Creatinine phosphokinase levels should be monitored if the individual complains of muscle pain or discomfort.[27,30,31]

Instructions

Statins are best dosed in the evening, either with supper or at bedtime. They can be taken with or without food in most cases. Monitoring for cholesterol reduction and liver enzyme elevation should be done every 12 weeks within the first 6 months of initial treatment and periodically thereafter. Educate patients on the signs and symptoms of myopathy, such as persistent muscle or joint pain. Patients should disclose all medications, prescribed and over the counter, to their healthcare provider to reduce the risk of potential drug interactions with statins. Caution patients on consuming large amounts of grapefruit juice (more than 8 oz per day).

American Association of Diabetes Educators©

TABLE 19.3	Statin Use: Selected Interactions Between Cytochrome P-450 Isoenzymes and Common Drugs		
Isoenzyme	*Substrate*	*Inhibitor*	*Inducer*
CYP3A4	Amlodipine (Norvasc®)	Clarithromycin (Biaxin®)	Carbamazepine (Tegretol®)
	Atorvastatin (Lipitor®)	Diltiazem (Cardizem®)	Dexamethasone (Decadron®)
	Diltiazem (Cardizem®)	Erythromycin	
	Felodipine (Plendil®)	Fluconazole (Diflucan®)	Phenytoin (Dilantin®)
	Fluvastatin (Lescol®)	Fluoxetine (Prozac®)	Primidone (Mysoline®)
	Glyburide (DiaBeta®; Micronase®; Glynase®)*	Grapefruit juice	Rifampin
		Ketoconazole (Nizoral®)	Pioglitazone (Actos®)*
	Lovastatin (Mevacor®)	Miconazole	
	Nifedipine (Procardia)	Norfloxin (Noroxin®)	
	Pravastatin (Pravachol®)	Verapemil (Calan®)	
	Repaglinide (Prandin®)*	Zafirlukast (Accolate®)	
	Simvastatin (Zocor®)		
	Verapamil (Calan®)		
	R-Warfarin (Coumadin®)		
CYP2C9	Glimepiride (Amaryl®)*	Amiodarone (Cordarone®)	Carbamazepine (Tegretol®)
	Losartan (Cozaar®)	Cimetidine (Tagamet®)	Phenytoin (Dilantin®)
	S-Warfarin (Coumadin®)	Fluconazole (Diflucan®)	Pioglitazone (Actos®)*
		Fluoxetine (Prozac®)	Rifampin
		Fluvastatin (Lescol®)	Rosiglitazone (Avandia®)
		Isoniazid	
		Ketoconazole (Nizoral®)	
		Metronidazole (Flagyl®)	
		Nateglitinide (Starlix®)*	
		Omeprazole (Prilosec®)	
		Sertraline (Zoloft®)	
		Sulfonamides	
		Zafirlukast (Accolate®)	

Note: Drugs in bold are statins. Drugs marked with an asterisk (*) are common oral glucose-lowering medications.

Sources: Lexicomp, Version 2.0.1(165) (Hudson, Ohio: Lexi-Comp, Inc, 2013); "Antilipidemic Agents," in *Monthly Prescribing Guide: November* (Montvale, NJ: Thompson PDR, 2005), 89-95; Monthly Prescribing Reference, "Cardiovascular system: hyperlipoproteinemias" (cited 2010 Nov 30), on the Internet at: http://www.empr.com.

Bile Acid Resins

The primary lipoprotein affected by bile acid resins is LDL-C, with a secondary effect of a modest increase in HDL-C. Bile acid resins are not commonly prescribed in the treatment of diabetic dyslipidemia. They can often increase TGs, which are often elevated in persons with diabetes; thus, bile acid resins should not be used as monotherapy in cases with high TGs (>250). However, in the early stage of type 2 diabetes when gastrointestinal motility is increased, some bile acid resins may improve or slow gastrointestinal motility, thereby reducing postprandial excursions.

Mechanism of Action

Bile acid resins bind to bile acids in the intestinal lumen, thereby decreasing cholesterol production.

They also inhibit enterohepatic circulation of bile acids and increase elimination of fecal acidic steroids, resulting in a decrease in LDL-C.[9,27]

Bile Acid Resins: Dosage Information			
Drug	*Trade Name*	*Common Dose*	*Preparation*
Cholestyramine	Questran®	4–16 g per day	1-g tablets, powder (1 scoop = 4 g)
Colesevelam	Welchol®	3.8–4.5 g per day	625-mg tablets
Colestipol	Colestid®	2–16 g per day	1-g tablets, powder (1 scoop = 5 g)

Bile acid resins may increase TGs due to increased production of VLDL from the upregulation of cholesterol synthesis.

Dosing

Bile acid resins are available as a tablet and as a powder for dilution. Dosing can be once to twice daily. A low dose is recommended for initial therapy and can be titrated up every 4 to 8 weeks as necessary to reach optimal or maximum dose.[27,30,31]

Pregnancy, Precautions, and Contraindications

The safety of bile acid resins in pregnancy varies with the different agents. Colesevelam is listed as category B, indicating no evidence of risk in humans, whereas cholestyramine and colestipol are listed as category C, indicating risk cannot be ruled out.[27,30]

Bile acid resins are contraindicated when the TG level is >400 mg/dL and in primary biliary cirrhosis. As noted above, they should not be used as monotherapy when the TG level is above 250 mg/dL.

Caution should be used in persons with renal insufficiency, volume depletion, and chronic constipation. Bowel and biliary obstructions are contraindications.[30,31]

Adverse Effects

The adverse effects reported with bile acid resins are mostly gastrointestinal in nature, due to the lack of systemic absorption. The most common complaints are headache, unpalatable taste, nausea, bloating, flatulence, and constipation.[30,31]

Drug Interactions

Bile acid resins can bind to other medications, resulting in decreased absorption and clinically significant drug interactions. Therefore, it is recommended to separate bile acid resins from other medications by administering the other medications 1 hour before or 4 hours after the bile acid resins.[27,33]

Prolonged use of bile acid resins may result in decreased absorption of fat-soluble vitamins and folic acid.[9,27]

Monitoring

A baseline lipid profile with a follow-up at 4 to 6 weeks for efficacy is recommended for bile acid resins. This medication is not systemically absorbed and is considered safe overall, except, as noted above, in cases of high TGs. Electrolytes should be routinely checked, as imbalances have been reported. Prolonged use of bile acid resins may produce hyperchloremic acidosis.[27,30,31] Due to the gastrointestinal discomfort associated with bile acid resins, patient compliance should be reviewed at each visit.

Instructions

Tablets should be swallowed whole and taken with plenty of liquid. Powder packets must be thoroughly diluted in liquid prior to consuming. Bile acid resins should be taken separately from other medications, either 1 hour after or 4 hours before.

Selective Intestinal Absorption Inhibitors

The primary effect of selective intestinal absorption inhibitors is observed in the reduction of LDL-C; however, slight decreases in TGs and increases in HDL-C may also be noticed. Selective intestinal absorption inhibitors have often been prescribed in combination with statins for persons with diabetic dyslipidemia to enhance the lowering of LDL-C. However, new studies suggest niacin added to statin therapy may do a better job of reducing CIMT than the addition of selective intestinal absorption inhibitors.[34]

Mechanism of Action

Selective intestinal absorption inhibitors reduce cholesterol by selectively inhibiting its absorption from the small intestine. This results in a decreased delivery of cholesterol to the liver and a reduction of hepatic cholesterol stores, with an overall lowering of cholesterol, primarily LDL-C.[27]

Selective Intestinal Absorption Inhibitors: Dosage Information			
Drug	*Trade Name*	*Common Dose*	*Common Frequency*
Ezetimibe	Zetia®	10 mg	Once daily

Dosing

Initial and maintenance dosage is 10 mg once daily and may be used in conjunction with statins or bile acid resins.[27,30,31]

Pregnancy, Precautions, and Contraindications

Ezetimibe (Zetia®, Merck) is listed as category C for pregnancy and should be avoided to reduce risks. Caution should be used in persons with hepatic dysfunction.[27,30]

Adverse Effects

Ezetimibe is generally well tolerated with minimal adverse effects. Common complaints are gastrointestinal issues, such as diarrhea and abdominal pain, as well as back pain, arthralgia, and sinusitis.[27,30]

Drug Interactions

Bile acid resins may interfere with absorption. Therefore, ezetimibe should be administered 1 hour before or 4 hours after the bile acid resins if used concurrently. Fibrates can increase cholesterol excretion into the bile; concurrent use is not recommended. International normalized ratios (INRs) should be monitored in those on warfarin.[27,30,33]

Monitoring

A baseline lipid profile and liver function tests should be conducted prior to initiating therapy. When used concurrently with statins, liver enzymes should be monitored prior to initiating statin therapy and every 12 weeks in the first 6 months of treatment and periodically thereafter.[27,30]

Instructions

Tablets can be taken with or without food. Statins can be taken at the same time as ezetimibe; however, bile acid resins must be separated, either 1 hour after or 4 hours before ezetimibe.

Fibric Acid Derivatives (Fibrates)

Fibrates exert their lipoprotein-lowering effects on TGs, with an additional benefit of increasing HDL-C. These agents are more commonly prescribed when elevations in TGs are present. They are also useful in combination with statins to cover the entire spectrum of lipoprotein abnormalities in diabetic dyslipidemia. However, close monitoring is warranted with combination therapy.

Mechanism of Action

Fibrates are most effective for decreasing VLDL and TG levels while raising HDL-C levels.[9,27] Although the mechanism of action is not clear, these agents can increase lipoprotein lipase, resulting in the breakdown of VLDL. Fibrates also decrease hepatic VLDL synthesis while enhancing the removal of TG-rich lipoproteins.[9]

Fibrates: Dosage Information			
Drug	*Trade Name*	*Common Dose*	*Common Frequency*
Fenofibrate	Tricor® Antara® Fenoglide® Lipofen® Lofibra® Triglide®	48–145 mg	Once daily
Gemfibrozil	Lopid®	600 mg	Twice daily

Dosing

Fibrates are generally administered once to twice daily, often prior to or with a meal. The dosage depends on the percentage of lipid lowering needed to achieve target goals. However, initial therapy commonly starts with a low dose and can be titrated up every 4 to 8 weeks as necessary to reach the optimal or maximum dosage and to minimize adverse effects.[27,30,31]

Pregnancy, Precautions, and Contraindications

Fibrates are listed as category C for pregnancy and should be avoided to reduce risks.[27,30]

Caution and lower dosages should be used for patients with renal dysfunction and for the elderly.

Preexisting gallbladder disease, hepatic dysfunction, and severe renal dysfunction are contraindications.[30,31]

Adverse Effects

Fibrates are generally well tolerated with minimal adverse reactions. Common adverse effects are gastrointestinal and include indigestion, nausea, diarrhea, flatulence, and abdominal pain. Rare side effects that have been reported are rash, fever, weight gain, muscle weakness, drowsiness, decreased potassium levels, anemia, and low white blood cell count.[27,30] Myopathy and rhabdomyolysis have been seen in monotherapy but are more common in conjunction with HMG-CoA reductase inhibitors.[27,31]

Drug Interactions

Fibrates are highly protein bound and can increase the adverse reactions of medications that are also highly protein bound. Common protein-bound medications include warfarin, sulfonylureas, and meglitinides.[27,33]

Bile acid resins may impair absorption. Fibrates should be administered 1 hour before or 4 hours after the bile acid resins.

Monitoring

Triglyceride and cholesterol levels should be measured prior to initiating fibrate therapy and at 3- to 6-month intervals. Liver function tests and complete blood cell counts should also be monitored at baseline and 6-month intervals. Discontinue treatment when liver enzymes are greater than 3 times the upper limit of normal. Monitor for hematologic changes such as decreased hemoglobin and hematocrit, thrombocytopenia, and neutropenia.[9,27,30]

If concurrent therapy includes statins, sulfonylureas, warfarin, or bile acid resins, close monitoring for enhanced adverse reactions is warranted, especially for hypoglycemia and increased INR.

Instructions

Gemfibrozil (Lopid®, Pfizer) should be taken 30 minutes prior to a meal. Fenofibrate (Tricor®, AbbVie, Inc) can be administered with or without regard to meals. Patients should be educated on the signs and symptoms of myopathy, such as persistent muscle or joint pain, especially if they are concurrently on an HMG-CoA reductase inhibitor.

Niacin

The primary lipoprotein effect of niacin is an increase in HDL-C, with a modest reduction in TGs and LDL-C. Although niacin can be useful in increasing HDL-C levels, it can also increase blood glucose levels, especially in prediabetes or newly diagnosed patients.

Mechanism of Action

Niacin reduces the catabolism of HDL and selectively decreases the excretion of HDL apo-A-1, stimulating reverse cholesterol transport in hepatic cells.[9,27] Additionally, niacin reduces hepatic VLDL production, resulting in a reduction of LDL-C, thereby lowering TG and LDL-C levels.[9]

Niacin: Dosage Information			
Drug	*Trade Name*	*Common Dose*	*Common Frequency*
Niacin sustained release	Niaspan®	500–1000 mg	Once daily
Nicotinic acid immediate release	Niacin®	100–1000 mg	1–3 times daily
Nicotinic acid sustained release	Slo-Niacin®	250 mg	Once to twice daily

Dosing

Niacin is available in immediate-release, sustained-release, and extended-release doses; these formulations should not be interchanged.

Immediate-release nicotinic acid is often preferred over sustained release for initial treatment, due to unfavorable adverse drug effects. Therapy should be started with small doses and titrated up as necessary and tolerable. Doses as low as 100 mg 3 times daily can be gradually increased to the maximum dose of 3 g per day in divided doses.[27,30,31]

Sustained-release nicotinic acid can be initiated at 250 mg twice daily and titrated up as tolerated to a maximum dose of 2 g per day, administered in a single or divided dose. Single doses can be given at bedtime with a low-fat snack.[27,30,31,35]

Pregnancy, Precautions, and Contraindications

Niacin is listed as category C for pregnancy and should be avoided to reduce risks.[30]

Caution should be used in persons with preexisting gout, heavy alcohol use, or renal dysfunction.

Liver dysfunction, active peptic ulcer disease, and arterial bleeding are contraindications.[27,30]

Adverse Effects

The adverse effects of niacin can be a drawback. Common effects include headache; hypotension; and gastrointestinal discomfort, such as nausea, vomiting, and diarrhea; as well as the more notorious dermatological reactions of flushing, pruritis, and rash.[9,27,30,35] Flushing typically decreases with continuous use and can be reduced by taking niacin with meals. Aspirin taken once daily, 30 minutes prior to the niacin dose, can also minimize flushing.[27]

Patients on large doses of niacin, greater than 2 g per day, may be at increased risk of hepatotoxic effects. Significant elevation of liver enzymes can occur. Discontinue treatment when liver enzymes are greater than 3 times the upper limit of normal.[27,30]

Drug Interactions

Niacin is known to inhibit the release of insulin from the beta cell, resulting in hyperglycemia. This is especially notable in those newly diagnosed with type 2 diabetes and in those with prediabetes, in whom beta-cell production of insulin has not been diminished or exhausted. The benefits of increasing HDL-C levels must outweigh the risks of increased blood glucose levels with niacin therapy.

Alcohol and hot drinks can increase flushing and pruritis effects. Rhabdomyolysis may occur when used in combination with HMG-CoA reductase inhibitors.[27,30]

Monitoring

A baseline lipid profile, liver function, uric acid, and blood glucose levels should be performed prior to initiating niacin therapy and repeated at 6-week intervals while adjusting the dosage. Lipid profiles should be reviewed at 3- to 6-month intervals. Blood glucose levels should be monitored regularly, especially in those newly diagnosed or with prediabetes. Liver enzymes should also be monitored at 12-week intervals during the first year of treatment.[27,30,35]

Instructions

Niacin should be taken 30 minutes after an aspirin or with a low-fat snack to minimize flushing effects. Advise patients to avoid taking niacin with hot beverages or alcohol. Blood glucose levels need to be monitored to identify glycemic elevations. Educate patients on the signs and symptoms of myopathy, such as persistent muscle or joint pain, especially if they are concurrently on an HMG-CoA reductase inhibitor.

Omega-3 Fatty Acids

Lower TGs is the primary effect observed with omega-3 fatty acids, which include eicosapentaenoic acid (EPA) and docosahexaenoic acid (DHA). Increasing HDL-C is a secondary benefit; however, this occurs only when higher doses are used. LDL-C levels tend to increase, and the increase is dose related. However, one formulation of omega-3 fatty acids, icosapent ethyl (Vascepa®, Amarin Pharma Inc), contains only EPA and does not appear to increase LDL-C.

Mechanism of Action

Omega-3 fatty acids are effective at lowering elevated TGs through a reduction in hepatic VLDL production. Omega-3 fatty acids reduce the quantity of free fatty acids available for TG synthesis, subsequently lowering VLDL synthesis and increasing lipoprotein lipase activity, which results in TG clearance.[27,36-38]

Omega-3 Fatty Acids: Dosage Information			
Drug	*Trade Name*	*Common Dose*	*Common Frequency*
Omega-3-acid ethyl esters 90	Lovaza®	4000 mg	Once daily
Icosapent ethyl	Vascepa®	4000 mg	Once daily

Dosing

The daily dose of omega-3 fatty acids, such as omega-3-acid ethyl esters (Lovaza®, GlaxoSmithKline) and icosapent ethyl, is four 1000-mg capsules, which can also be given as two 1000-mg capsules twice daily. Omega-3-acid ethyl esters and icosapent ethyl should be taken with food to minimize gastrointestinal adverse effects.[27,36,37]

Pregnancy, Precautions, and Contraindications

There are no adequate studies with pregnant women; therefore, omega-3 fatty acids should be avoided during pregnancy. Caution should be used in persons with renal or hepatic dysfunction, elderly patients, and those at high risk of hemorrhage.[27]

Adverse Effects

Common adverse effects are dizziness and gastrointestinal effects, such as dyspepsia, nausea, and abdominal pain. Rare adverse effects of headache, pruritis, and hyperglycemia have been reported.[27,36-38]

Drug Interactions

Omega-3 fatty acids may decrease the production of thromboxane A_2, resulting in an increase in bleeding time. International normalized ratios can increase in concurrent use with warfarin. Limited studies have been done with other lipid-lowering therapies and other medications.[27,36–38]

Monitoring

A baseline lipid profile and liver function tests should be performed prior to initiating omega-3 fatty acids therapy and repeated at regular intervals, especially while adjusting dosage. Patients on anticoagulant therapy should have their INR monitored for increases in bleeding time.[36–38]

Instructions

Omega-3 fatty acids should be taken with food to minimize adverse effects.

Combination Therapies

When designing treatment strategies in diabetes management, multiple agents are often necessary to achieve desired blood glucose goals. The same holds true for designing a treatment strategy for diabetic dyslipidemia. Since multiple lipoprotein abnormalities are common in patients with diabetic dyslipidemia, multiple agents may be necessary to reach optimal lipid levels. Additionally, combination therapies are useful to achieve LDL-C goals in patients on maximum tolerated statin therapy who are not at their LDL-C goal. Combination therapies also minimize pill burden and may help improve medication adherence.

Available combination therapies include (1) Vytorin® (Merck), which contains ezetimibe (a selective intestinal absorption inhibitor) and simvastatin (an HMG-CoA reductase inhibitor); (2) Liptruzet® (Merck), which contains ezetimibe and atorvastatin (an HMG-CoA reductase inhibitor); (3) Advicor® (AbbVie, Inc), which contains lovastatin (an HMG-CoA reductase inhibitor) and niacin; and (4) Simcor® (Abbott), which contains simvastatin and niacin.[27,30]

Considerations in Diabetic Dyslipidemia Therapy

Treatment goals and strategies for diabetic dyslipidemia must be given equal emphasis and be as aggressive as those developed for hyperglycemia.

Primary Target

The primary lipoprotein target is the LDL-C; however, TGs, HDL-C, and particle size of the LDL-C must be

acknowledged in the treatment plan. Once the role of targeting non-HDL cholesterol and ApoB100 is fully elucidated, future guidelines may emphasize these targets over LDL-C. Combinations of lipid-lowering agents may be necessary to achieve LDL-C and other lipoprotein goals, especially in very high-risk patients and those who are intolerant of high-dose statin therapy.

Adding a medication to an existing regimen requires behavior change by the patient. Thus, the person's readiness to change, conviction, and confidence levels require assessment. The use of combined medications can be beneficial for persons who are reluctant to take more medication.

First-Line Therapy

Statins are traditionally the initial drug of choice in diabetic dyslipidemia. However, the addition of a selective intestinal absorption inhibitor can enhance the LDL-C lowering, a fibrate can reduce TG levels and raise HDL-C, and niacin can increase HDL-C and decrease TGs and LDL-C. Two or more lipid-lowering agents may be necessary for some patients.

Lipid profiles, liver enzymes, and adverse effects as well as patient adherence must be routinely monitored.

Hypertension

Blood pressure is the product of cardiac output (CO) and total peripheral resistance (TPR), where CO is the result of stroke volume and heart rate. The pathophysiology of hypertension in most people is a multifactorial process that occurs due to the body's inability to maintain the homeostasis between CO and TPR.[39]

Two important systems exist that work to maintain normal blood pressure: the autonomic nervous system and the renin-angiotensin-aldosterone system (RAAS).[39] Evidence suggests that the RAAS is part of the multifactorial progression of diabetes, CVD, and renal disease. Through RAAS inhibition, blood pressure is reduced and albuminuria can be reversed. Studies have also shown that RAAS inhibition can decrease CVD and slow progression of diabetes.[40,41]

Renin-Angiotensin-Aldosterone System

Understanding of the RAAS has evolved over the decades and continues to do so. The RAAS regulates the balance of fluid volume, electrolytes, and blood volume in the body. Changes in the RAAS result in changes in vascular tone and sympathetic nervous system activity.

Stimulation of the RAAS leads to vasoconstriction, sodium retention, smooth muscle proliferation, and increased antidiuretic hormone in the vasculature.[42-44] In the kidney, activation of the RAAS is associated with intraglomerular hypertension, a precursor of proteinuria. Endothelial cells line the glomerulus as well as the blood vessels and function as the gatekeeper for cardiovascular and renal systems.[43,44] Abnormal RAAS activity can impair endothelium-dependent vasodilation in persons with type 2 diabetes, resulting in decreased acetylcholine stimulation and enhanced oxidative stress.[43,44] These changes lead to insulin resistance, endothelial dysfunction, and microalbuminuria.

To briefly review, the RAAS begins with a release of renin, an enzyme synthesized in the kidney, in response to changes within or outside the kidney. Renin then acts on angiotensinogen, a hepatic peptide, to create angiotensin-I (AT-I). Angiotensin-converting enzyme (ACE), located in the pulmonary and vascular endothelium, converts AT-I to angiotensin-II (AT-II).[42-44] Angiotensin-converting enzyme converts approximately 30% of circulating AT-I to AT-II. Other enzymes, such as chymase, tonin, and cathepsin-G, are responsible for the remaining 70% of AT-II production.[44,45] This peptide, AT-II, binds to AT-I receptors, which are primarily in vascular and myocardial tissue, to increase vasoconstriction, sympathetic activity, and aldosterone secretion. These increases result in peripheral vascular resistance, vasoconstriction and increased heart rate, and fluid retention, respectively, which contribute to the development of hypertension.[43-45] Figure 19.2 summarizes this process.

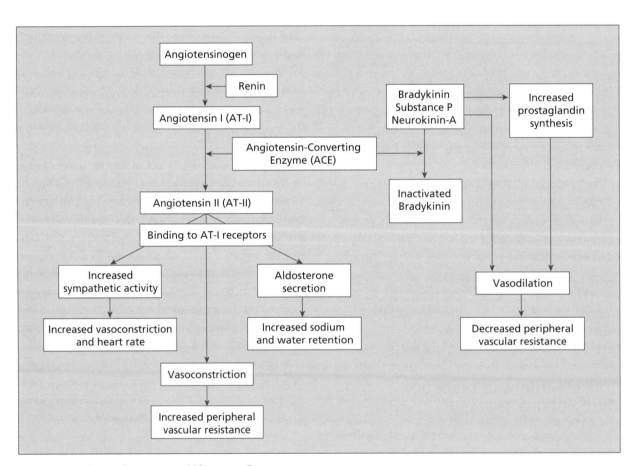

FIGURE 19.2   Renin-Angiotensin-Aldosterone System

Sources: BL Carter, JJ Saseen, "Hypertension," in JT Dipiro, RL Talbert, GC Yee, GR Matzke, BG Wells, LM Posey, eds, *Pharmacotherapy: A Pathophysiologic Approach*, 6th ed. (New York: McGraw-Hill, 2005), 185-218; BL Carter, "Management of Essential Hypertension," in *Pharmacotherapy Self-Assessment Program Book 1: Cardiovascular I*, 4th ed. (Kansas City, Mo: American College of Clinical Pharmacy, 2001), 1-39; EJ Jacobsen, "Hypertension: update on use of angiotensin II receptor blockers," *Geriatrics* 56, no. 2 (2001): 25-8.

Diagnosis: Hypertension

The Seventh Report of the Joint National Committee on Prevention, Detection, Evaluation, and Treatment of High Blood Pressure (JNC 7 Report) identifies evidence-based treatment strategies for the management of hypertension.[46]

Blood pressure has been classified into 4 stages: normal, prehypertension, stage 1 hypertension, and stage 2 hypertension.[46] Table 19.4 lists the criteria for each stage. Diagnosis and classification of hypertension is determined from the average of 2 blood pressure readings obtained from 2 separate clinic visits; it is measured with the person in a seated position, after a 5- to 10-minute rest.

TABLE 19.4 Classification of Hypertension in Adults		
Stage	Systolic Pressure (mm Hg)	Diastolic Pressure (mm Hg)
Normal	<120 *and*	<80
Prehypertension	120–139 *or*	80–89
Stage 1 hypertension	140–159 *or*	90–99
Stage 2 hypertension	≥160 *or*	≥100

Source: AV Chobanian, GL Bakris, HR Black, et al, "The Seventh Report of the Joint National Committee on Prevention, Detection, Evaluation, and Treatment of High Blood Pressure: the JNC 7 report," *JAMA* 289 (2003): 2560-72.

Hypertension Goal

In adults with diabetes, the blood pressure goal is <140 mm Hg systolic and <80 mm Hg diastolic; a lower goal of <130 mm Hg systolic and <80 mm Hg diastolic may be appropriate in certain individuals, such as younger patients, if achievable without causing harm.[25,46-48] The systolic blood pressure goal of <140 mm Hg is higher than previously recommended and reflects findings from the Action to Control Cardiovascular Risk in Diabetes (ACCORD) trial.[49] The blood pressure arm of ACCORD failed to observe significant cardiovascular benefits in patients with a systolic blood pressure goal <120 mm Hg compared with a goal of <140 mm Hg. These findings and others led expert consensus panels in Europe and the United States to relax goal recommendations for systolic blood pressure.

Case—Part 2: What Pharmacotherapy for Dyslipidemia, If Any, Is Appropriate?

Provided DC's CPK levels and renal and hepatic function are within normal limits, a statin could be added to his medications. Statins are the first-line treatment option in diabetic dyslipidemia. Choice of statin should be based on the percentage of LDL-C lowering needed to obtain his lipoprotein goals.

Dosage

The initial dosage of the statin should be on the low end and titrated up if necessary and tolerated. DC's liver enzymes should be checked 12 weeks after the start of therapy, and his lipid profile should be reviewed in 3 months.

Three-Month Follow-up

If in 3 months DC has not reached optimal lipoprotein levels, increasing the dosage of his current therapy or adding a second lipid-lowering agent may be warranted.

Pharmacotherapy Options

Options for DC at that point would include increasing his current statin dose or using a precombined lipid-lowering agent, such as Vytorin® or Simcor.®(Simcor® contains a statin plus niacin, whereas Vytorin® has a statin plus a selective intestinal absorption inhibitor.) Since DC was diagnosed with type 2 diabetes 2 years ago, the functioning of his pancreatic beta cells must be considered. Adding niacin may inhibit the release of insulin, resulting in elevated blood glucose levels. Therefore, Vytorin® may be the preferred choice for DC at this time.

A bile acid resin would not be preferred, since it may worsen DC's TGs.

DC's readiness to change, conviction, and confidence in regard to adding another medicine should be assessed. Because DC may have a problem with adhering to his metformin, adding another medication may not be the best therapy plan. If adherence to pharmacologic therapy is not determined to be a problem, adding a fibrate would be an acceptable option.

Patient empowerment, education, close monitoring, and follow-up are needed to obtain and maintain the lipoprotein levels necessary to reduce this man's risk of CVD and cardiac events.

Treatment strategies for hypertension often require combination therapy that targets different mechanisms to obtain optimal levels in blood pressure.

Children and Adolescents

The 2013 ADA Standards of Medical Care in Diabetes recommend that blood pressure should be measured at every routine visit, and those children noted to have high-normal blood pressure or hypertension should have their blood pressure repeated and confirmed on a separate day.[2] Hypertension in childhood is defined as an average systolic or diastolic blood pressure ≥95th percentile for age, sex, and height percentile or if the blood pressure is consistently >130/80 mm Hg (if 95% exceeds that value). "High-normal" blood pressure is defined as an average systolic or diastolic blood pressure ≥90th but <95th percentile for age, sex, and height percentile. Normal blood pressure levels for age, sex, and height and appropriate methods for determinations are available online at http://www.nhlbi.nih.gov/health/prof/heart/hbp/hbp_ped.pdf.

Treatment in Children and Adolescents

Lifestyle Intervention   Treatment of high-normal blood pressure (systolic or diastolic blood pressure consistently above the 90th percentile for age, sex, and height) should include dietary intervention and exercise, aimed at weight control and increased physical activity, if appropriate.

Pharmacotherapy   If target blood pressure is not reached within 3 to 6 months of lifestyle intervention, pharmacologic treatment should be initiated. Pharmacologic treatment of hypertension should be initiated as soon as the diagnosis is confirmed. Angiotensin-converting enzyme inhibitors should be considered for the initial treatment of hypertension. Reproduction counseling may also be necessary in females of childbearing age because of teratogenicity associated with ACE inhibitors. These pharmacotherapy recommendations from the ADA are based on expert consensus or clinical experience.

Pharmacotherapy: Hypertension

Lifestyle modification should always be a standard treatment of hypertension in addition to pharmacotherapy. Medical nutrition therapy, increased activity, moderation of alcohol consumption, and modest weight reduction can have beneficial effects on blood pressure.[47,48] See chapter 16's discussion of the role of nutrition therapy in hypertension prevention and management.

Classes of Antihypertensive Agents

Many classes of antihypertensive agents target different mechanisms in the treatment of hypertension (see Table 19.5).[50] However, several classes are preferred and traditionally used as first-line therapy because of their blood pressure–lowering and renal-protection effects in people with diabetes.[40,41] Medications that target the RAAS and can delay the progression of microalbuminuria to macroalbuminuria include ACE inhibitors, angiotensin II receptor blockers (ARBs), and

TABLE 19.5   Classes of Antihypertensive Medications
Angiotensin-converting enzyme inhibitors
Angiotensin II receptor blockers
α1-Receptor blockers
β-Blockers
Combined α- and β-receptor blockers
Calcium channel blockers
Central-acting α-adrenergic agonists
Direct Renin Inhibitors
Diuretics
Thiazide
Loop
Potassium sparing
Carbonic anhydrase inhibitors
Vasodilators

Note: Classes listed in bold are preferred in persons with diabetes.

direct renin inhibitors (DRIs). Thiazide diuretics are commonly used as adjunct therapy because of their synergistic effect with ACE inhibitors and ARBs.[47,51] It is common that 2 or more medications from different classes are needed to attain blood pressure treatment goals. Other classes of antihypertensive agents can be used in people with diabetes provided their adjunct benefits outweigh the risks.

Standard Treatment

Hypertension—Standard treatment of hypertension includes pharmacotherapy plus lifestyle modifications: MNT, increased activity, moderation of alcohol consumption, and modest weight reduction.

Any of these classes can be used as monotherapy or in combination for the treatment of hypertension. Figure 19.3 outlines pharmacologic treatment of hypertension.

Diuretics

Diuretics are clinically classified based on their mechanism and/or site of action. There are 4 types: thiazide-type, loop, potassium-sparing, and carbonic anhydrase inhibitors; carbonic anhydrase inhibitors, however, are not used in the treatment of essential hypertension. Baseline renal function and serum potassium are important factors in determining the initial choice of diuretic. Typically, diuretics are not the first-line therapy for hypertension in persons with diabetes.[47] However, thiazide diuretics are often used

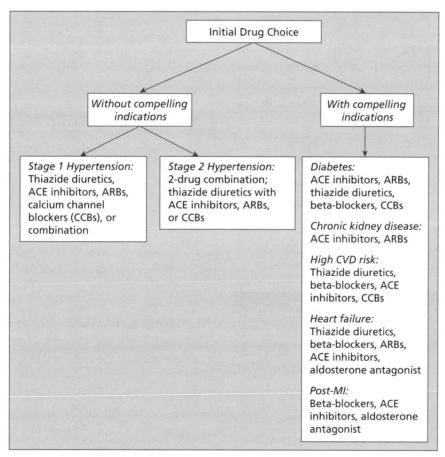

FIGURE 19.3 Hypertension: Pharmacotherapy Recommendations

Sources: AV Chobanian, GL Bakris, HR Black, et al, "The seventh report of the Joint National Committee on Prevention, Detection, Evaluation, and Treatment of High Blood Pressure: the JNC 7 report," *JAMA* 289 (2003): 2560-72; American Diabetes Association position statement, "Standards of medical care in diabetes-2013," *Diabetes Care* 36 Suppl 1 (2013): S11-66; "Cardiovascular System: Antihypertensives," in *Monthly Prescribing Reference: November* (cited 2010 Nov 28), on the Internet at: http://www.empr.com; HR Black, "The evolution of low-dose diuretic therapy: the lessons from clinical trials," *Am J Med* 101, no. 3A (1996): 47S-52S.

for their additive effects with other preferred antihypertensive agents when treating hypertension in those with diabetes.[46]

Thiazide-Type Diuretics

The JNC 7 Report recommends thiazide-type diuretics as first-line therapy for uncomplicated hypertensive patients.[46] Hydrochlorothiazide (HCTZ) is the most frequently prescribed diuretic for the treatment of hypertension alone. In fact, many hypertensive drugs have HCTZ coformulations, in which HCTZ is combined with a drug from the same or another class, such as an ACE inhibitor or an ARB. Some examples of coformulations include Hyzaar® (ARB with HCTZ; Merck), Prinizide® (ACE inhibitor with HCTZ), and Aldactazide® (potassium-sparing diuretic with HCTZ).

Chlorthalidone is another thiazide-type diuretic that has been used more in recent years. In fact, a combination product, Edarbyclor® (Takeda), is now available that includes an ARB (azilsartan) and chlorthalidone. The reason for this change is that several landmark clinical trials used chlorthalidone-based regimens instead of HCTZ. Chlorthalidone is also more potent than HCTZ and provides better 24-hour blood pressure control. However, these characteristics of chlorthalidone increase the potential for electrolyte abnormalities, especially hypokalemia.

Thiazide diuretics are also used when treating hypertension with compelling indications. They can be used as monotherapy and in combination in the management of heart failure, recurrent stroke prevention, and diabetes and in individuals at high CVD risk.[46]

Thiazide-Type Diuretics: Dosage Information

Drug	Trade Name	Common Dose	Common Frequency
Hydrochlorothiazide	HydroDIURIL® Microzide®	12.5–50 mg	Once daily
Chlorthalidone	Clorpres®	12.5–25 mg	Once daily
Metolazone	Zaroxolyn®	2.5–5 mg	Once daily
Indapamide	Lozol®	1.25–2.5 mg	Once daily

Loop Diuretics

Loop diuretics are often employed when the person's glomerular filtration rate (GFR) falls below 30 mL per minute or the person needs greater diuresis due to another disease state (eg, heart failure). Thiazide-type diuretics (except metolazone) are relatively ineffective when GFR falls below 30 mL per minute. Reduced GFR allows more opportunity for sodium and water reabsorption to occur.[39]

Loop Diuretics: Dosage Information

Drug	Trade Name	Common Dose	Common Frequency
Furosemide	Lasix®	20–40 mg	Once to twice daily
Torsemide	Demadex®	5–10 mg	Once daily
Bumetanide	Bumex®	0.5–2 mg	Once to twice daily

Potassium-Sparing Diuretics

As their name implies, potassium-sparing diuretics are the only diuretics that increase serum potassium; other diuretics lower it. Potassium-sparing diuretics are combined with a thiazide-type diuretic to balance serum potassium.[39] Individually, they do little to lower blood pressure.

Potassium-Sparing Diuretics: Dosage Information

Drug	Trade Name	Common Dose	Common Frequency
Amiloride	Midamor®	5–10 mg	Once daily
Triamterene	Dyrenium®	37.5–75 mg	Once daily
Spironolactone	Aldactone®	25–50 mg	Once to twice daily
Eplerenone	Inspra®	50 mg	Once to twice daily

Mechanisms of Action

The various types of diuretics exert their effects on different areas of the kidney. Thiazide-type diuretics inhibit the Na^+/Cl^- symporter on the distal convoluted tubule of the nephron, whereas loop diuretics inhibit the $Na^+/K^+/2Cl^-$ symporter on the ascending limb of the loop of Henle.[39,42] These inhibitions increase the urinary excretion of sodium, chloride, potassium, and water. Initially, the drop in blood pressure from diuretics is due to a decreased cardiac output as a result of decreased blood volume. With chronic use, the blood pressure reduction is not a result of diuresis. Cardiac output normalizes and the blood pressure reduction becomes a result of decreased peripheral vascular resistance.[39,42]

The mechanism of potassium-sparing diuretics is more complicated. Potassium-sparing diuretics inhibit the absorption of Na^+ and the excretion of K^+ in the principal cells of the late distal tubule and collecting duct.[39] Amiloride and triamterene inhibit the luminal Na^+ channels of the principal cell. Spironolactone and eplerenone are antagonists at aldosterone receptors on the principal cell.[39]

Dosing

Diuretics are generally taken once daily in the morning. The rationale for morning dosing is that people prefer to deal with the increased frequency of urination from diuretics during the day rather than during the night. Some potassium-sparing and loop diuretics may be dosed up to twice daily to increase diuresis for conditions other than hypertension.[50,52] A low dose is recommended for the initial therapy and can be titrated up if necessary. When solely treating hypertension, high doses have not shown any additional benefit of further decreasing blood pressure when compared with low doses.[46,53]

Pregnancy, Precautions, and Contraindications

Diuretic safety in pregnancy varies with the different agents. Most are category C, where risk cannot be ruled out; however, HCTZ, torsemide, eplerenone, indapamide, and metolazone are listed as category B, indicating there is no evidence of risk in humans. Reference to the packet insert of the individual diuretic is always recommended.[50,52]

Caution should be used when treating persons with preexisting gout or uric acid stone disease, severe renal impairment, hepatic dysfunction, and/or electrolyte imbalances.[52]

Thiazide-type diuretics (except metolazone) are contraindicated in persons with a known hypersensitivity to sulfonamides. The absolute risk of cross-sensitivity in a sulfa-allergic patient is not well established. However, extreme caution is advised in patients with a documented allergic reaction.[50,54]

Adverse Effects

Adverse effects associated with diuretics are often associated with changes in serum electrolytes, such as hypokalemia, hypomagnesemia, hyperuricemia, hyperglycemia, hyperlipidemia, and hyper/hypocalcemia. Signs and symptoms of these imbalances are muscle cramps, fatigue, dizziness, and cardiac arrhythmias.[27,50,52] Other common adverse effects include headache, photosensitivity, dry mouth, taste alterations, nausea, vomiting, impotence, and orthostatic hypotension.[46]

Drug Interactions

Since diuretics increase the excretion of sodium and potassium, many drug interactions stem from changes in electrolytes. Significant interactions include nonsteroidal anti-inflammatory drugs (NSAIDs), which can decrease the antihypertensive efficacy of diuretics. Evidence suggests that this might occur more often with ibuprofen and indomethacin.[52] Diuretics can substantially increase lithium levels by decreasing lithium's elimination; therefore, lithium levels should be monitored 5 to 7 days after starting or discontinuing a diuretic.[33] Also, high sodium intake can decrease the effectiveness of diuretics.

Thiazide diuretics are known to inhibit the release of insulin from the beta cell, resulting in hyperglycemia. This is especially notable in persons newly diagnosed with type 2 diabetes or with prediabetes, where beta-cell production of insulin has not been diminished or exhausted. In general, this disease interaction is clinically insignificant at lower doses, such as less than 25 mg of HCTZ daily.[51,55]

Monitoring

Baseline blood pressure, serum electrolytes, uric acid, glucose, and lipids should be measured prior to initiating therapy and periodically thereafter. A regimen with diuretic therapy is often supplemented with potassium and magnesium.[50,52] When diuretics are combined with other antihypertensive agents, monitoring for hypotension is warranted.

Instructions

Diuretics should be taken in the morning, with or without food. Intake of foods high in potassium, such as bananas or strawberries, can help maintain adequate potassium levels. Blood pressure must be monitored daily to identify elevations and patterns. Blood glucose levels need to be monitored to identify possible glycemic elevations from the diuretic.

Patients should be educated on signs and symptoms of hypokalemia, such as muscle cramps and fatigue. To avoid episodes of orthostatic hypotension, patients should be reminded to rise slowly from lying or seated positions.

Angiotensin-Converting Enzyme Inhibitors

An ACE inhibitor or an ARB is traditionally used as first-line or preferred therapy for hypertension and renal protection in persons with diabetes.[40,42,44] An ACE inhibitor can delay the progression of microalbuminuria to macroalbuminuria.

Angiotensin-converting enzyme inhibitors are also beneficial in the treatment of hypertension with compelling indications, such as heart failure, post-MI, recurrent stroke prevention, and chronic kidney disease.[40]

Angiotensin-Converting Enzyme Inhibitors: Dosage Information

Drug	Trade Name	Common Dose	Common Frequency
Benazepril	Lotensin®	10–40 mg	Once daily
Captopril	Capoten®	12.5–50 mg	2–3 times daily
Enalapril	Vasotec®	2.5–20 mg	Once to twice daily
Fosinopril	Monopril®	10–40 mg	Once daily
Lisinopril	Prinivil® Zestril®	10–40 mg	Once daily
Moexipril	Univasc®	7.5–30 mg	Once daily
Perindopril	Aceon®	4–8 mg	Once daily
Quinapril	Accupril®	10–80 mg	Once daily
Ramipril	Altace®	2.5–20 mg	Once daily
Trandolapril	Mavik®	1–4 mg	Once daily

Mechanism of Action

Angiotensin-converting enzyme inhibitors inhibit the formation of AT-II by blocking the conversion of AT-I to AT-II. Additionally, ACE inhibitors block the action of kininase, the enzyme that converts bradykinin, substance P, and neurokinin-A to inactive ingredients, thereby increasing their concentrations. The increase in bradykinin stimulates the release of nitric oxide, a vasodilator.[40,42,44]

Dosing

Angiotensin-converting enzyme inhibitors are generally administered 1 to 3 times daily with or without food. Once-daily dosing can be in the morning or evening, based on patient preference and adverse effects such as drowsiness. However, taking the medication at the same time every day is important. The presence of food may affect the absorption of captopril and moexipril, and dosing prior to a meal may be warranted. The effects of blood pressure lowering can be seen within 1 hour of administration, with maximum effects after 6 to 8 hours. Initial therapy often starts with a low dose and can be titrated up as tolerated.[50,52] Adding a thiazide diuretic is usually more beneficial at lowering blood pressure than increasing the dosage of the ACE inhibitor. Angiotensin-converting enzyme inhibitors are often coformulated with low-dose HCTZ (6.25-25 mg) to enhance blood pressure reduction and improve patient adherence in taking medication.

Pregnancy, Precautions, and Contraindications

Angiotensin-converting enzyme inhibitors are contraindicated during pregnancy. Use in the second or third trimester can lead to fetal injury or death.

Angiotensin-converting enzyme inhibitors are also contraindicated in persons with bilateral renal artery stenosis or unilateral stenosis of a single, functional kidney. They cause dilation of the efferent arteriole in the renal circulation, which can substantially reduce GFR and result in acute renal failure.

Caution should be used in patients with a history of renal and/or hepatic dysfunction, angioedema, heart failure, and hyperkalemia.[52]

In African-American patients, ACE inhibitors are often less effective at lowering blood pressure due to low renin levels common to this ethnic group.[52,56] Coadministration of thiazide diuretics is often sufficient to overcome the low renin levels and return observed blood pressure lowering with ACE inhibitors to that of the general population. African Americans are also more likely to experience angioedema and should be appropriately counseled prior to initiating therapy.

Adverse Effects

Overall, ACE inhibitors are well tolerated with few side effects, especially if monitored appropriately. The most common adverse effect, and often the reason for discontinuation of ACE inhibitors, is cough. This adverse effect is primarily due to the increase in bradykinin activity that increases prostaglandin synthesis. An estimated 10% to 20% of persons taking ACE inhibitors will develop a cough.[27,52]

Other adverse effects commonly associated with ACE inhibitors include fatigue, headache, dizziness, drowsiness, hyperkalemia, acute hypotension, and gastrointestinal problems, such as diarrhea, nausea, and vomiting. Skin rash, taste disturbances, angioedema, and hematologic effects, such as neutropenia and agranulocytosis, have also been reported.[50,52]

Drug Interactions
Concurrent use of NSAIDs, potassium-sparing diuretics, and potassium supplements may increase potassium levels significantly. Angiotensin-converting enzyme inhibitors can increase lithium levels, due to decreased fluid volume and loss of sodium ions; therefore, close monitoring of lithium levels is recommended.[33]

Monitoring
Blood pressure, serum electrolytes, and renal function should be measured at baseline and periodically throughout treatment. Potassium levels should be monitored within the first month of initial therapy and periodically thereafter due to the rapid onset of hyperkalemia.[52]

Changes in renal function can occur with the use of ACE inhibitors; this is more common in patients with preexisting renal dysfunction. Kidney function should be closely monitored throughout treatment and especially during dose titration. Discontinuation of the ACE inhibitor is not always necessary, provided the patient is being monitored and assessed closely.[52]

Instructions
Angiotensin-converting enzyme inhibitors should be taken at the same time daily. If the patient experiences drowsiness or dizziness, taking the medication in the evening can minimize these effects when the patient is awake. Monitor blood pressure daily to identify elevations and patterns. Patients who develop a persistent cough within the first few months of initial therapy should discuss this with their healthcare provider at their next clinic visit. To avoid episodes of orthostatic hypotension, patients should be reminded to rise slowly from lying or seated positions.

Angiotensin Receptor Blockers

Angiotensin receptor blockers can be beneficial for persons with diabetes because these medications lower blood pressure and have renoprotective ability. Angiotensin receptor blockers are traditionally prescribed when ACE inhibitor therapies are not tolerated. However, they have been used as first-line therapy in some cases and are preferred over other antihypertensive agents for persons with diabetes. Additional compelling indications for which ARBs are used as monotherapy or in combination include heart failure and chronic kidney disease.[40,45]

Angiotensin receptor blockers and ACE inhibitors lower blood pressure and protect kidneys due to their renoprotective ability. They are preferred over other antihypertensive agents for persons with diabetes.

Mechanism of Action
Angiotensin receptor blockers inhibit AT-II release by blocking the AT-I receptor. This leads to a reduction in aldosterone secretion, vasoconstriction, and sympathetic activity.[39,44]

Angiotensin Receptor Blockers: Dosage Information			
Drug	*Trade Name*	*Common Dose*	*Common Frequency*
Azilsartan	Edarbi®	40–80 mg	Once daily
Candesartan	Atacand®	8–32 mg	Once daily
Eprosartan	Teveten®	600 mg	Once daily
Irbesartan	Avapro®	150–300 mg	Once daily
Losartan	Cozaar®	25–100 mg	Once daily
Olmesartan	Benicar®	20–40 mg	Once daily
Telmisartan	Micardis®	20–80 mg	Once daily
Valsartan	Diovan®	80–320 mg	Once daily*

*Dose divided and given 2 times daily if patient also has heart failure

Dosing
Angiotensin receptor blockers are generally administered once daily and can be dosed in the morning or evening, based on patient preference and adverse

effects such as drowsiness. However, taking the medication at the same time every day is important. Fluid volume or sodium depletion must be corrected prior to initiating therapy with ARBs.[50,52] Initial therapy often starts with a low dose and can be titrated up as tolerated. Adding a thiazide diuretic is usually more beneficial at lowering blood pressure than increasing the dosage of ARBs.

Angiotensin receptor blockers are often coformulated with low-dose HCTZ (6.25-25 mg) to enhance blood pressure reduction and improve patient adherence in taking medication.

Pregnancy, Precautions, and Contraindications

Angiotensin receptor blockers are listed as category C for the first trimester of pregnancy and category D for the second and third trimesters; therefore, ARBs should be avoided in pregnancy.

They are also contraindicated in persons with bilateral renal artery stenosis or unilateral stenosis of a single functional kidney.[52]

Caution should be used in persons with renal and/or hepatic dysfunction, angioedema, and/or heart failure. Severe hypotension can occur in patients with heart failure.[50,52]

Adverse Effects

Angiotensin receptor blockers are generally well tolerated with minimal side effects. Common adverse effects associated with this class of antihypertensive agents include dizziness, drowsiness, diarrhea, dyspepsia, hyperkalemia, headache, and upper respiratory complaints, such as infection, pharyngitis, rhinitis, and cough. However, the frequency of cough associated with ARBs is significantly less than that with ACE inhibitors.[27,50,52]

Drug Interactions

Concurrent use of potassium-sparing diuretics, potassium supplements, or salt substitutes may increase serum potassium levels significantly. Increases in serum creatinine in persons with heart failure have also been reported. Use of ACE inhibitors and/or beta-adrenergic blocking agents with ARBs should be avoided in patients with heart failure.[33] Angiotensin receptor blockers can increase lithium levels due to decreased fluid volume and loss of sodium

ions; therefore, close monitoring of lithium levels is recommended.[33]

Monitoring

As with ACE inhibitors, blood pressure, serum electrolytes, and renal function should be measured at baseline and periodically throughout treatment. Potassium levels should be monitored within the first month of initial therapy and periodically thereafter due to the rapid onset of hyperkalemia.[50,52]

Changes in renal function can occur with use of ARBs and tend to be more common in persons with preexisting renal dysfunction. Renal impairment can occur soon after initiating therapy. Kidney function should be closely monitored throughout treatment and especially during dose titration.[27,52]

Instructions

Angiotensin receptor blockers should be taken at the same time daily. If the patient experiences drowsiness or dizziness, taking the medication in the evening can minimize these effects when the patient is awake. Blood pressure needs to be monitored daily to identify elevations and patterns. To avoid episodes of orthostatic hypotension, patients should be reminded to rise slowly from lying or seated positions.

Direct Renin Inhibitors

Direct renin inhibitors are a newer class of medications that lower blood pressure and have renal-protective benefits in people with diabetes. Despite these benefits, their place in therapy remains unclear following publication of results from the Aliskiren Trial in Type 2 Diabetes Using Cardiovascular and Renal Disease Endpoints Including 12 Month Safety Follow-up Off-treatment (ALTITUDE).[57] This study compared the effects of aliskiren versus placebo when added to ARBs or ACE inhibitors. The trial was stopped prematurely due to lack of benefit with the aliskiren combination and an increase in adverse events that included nonfatal stroke, renal complications, hyperkalemia, and hypotension. The FDA-approved labeling for aliskiren was subsequently changed in 2012 to warn against using aliskiren in combination with ARBs or ACE inhibitors for people with diabetes or decreased kidney function.

Mechanism of Action

Direct renin inhibitors block RAAS at the point of activation to inhibit the conversion of angiotensinogen to AT-1, thereby reducing plasma renin activity and lowering blood pressure.[27,58]

Direct Renin Inhibitors: Dosage Information			
Drug	Trade Name	Common Dose	Common Frequency
Aliskiren	Tekturna®	150–300 mg	Once daily

Dosing

Direct renin inhibitors are taken once daily, and though they can be taken with or without food, high-fat meals may decrease absorption. Initial therapy often starts with a low dose and can be titrated up as tolerated. The addition of an ARB or thiazide diuretic has been shown to be beneficial in lowering blood pressure. Direct renin inhibitors are coformulated with HCTZ (12.5-25 mg), amlodipine, and valsartan to enhance blood pressure reduction and improve patient adherence in taking medication.[27,58]

Pregnancy, Precautions, and Contraindications

Direct renin inhibitors are contraindicated during pregnancy and should be discontinued as soon as pregnancy is detected. Use in the first, second, or third trimester can lead to fetal injury, as DRIs act directly on the RAAS.[27,58]

Caution should be used in patients with moderate to severe renal dysfunction or with a history of or currently on dialysis. Additionally, volume and sodium depletion should be reviewed and corrected prior to starting therapy and closely monitored if needed. Coadministration with potassium-sparing diuretics or potassium supplements should be avoided if possible.[27,58]

Use of DRIs (alone or in combination with ACE inhibitors or ARBs) in people with diabetes has been associated with increased risk of renal impairment, hypotension, and hyperkalemia. Furthermore, DRIs are contraindicated in people with diabetes who are also taking an ACE inhibitor or ARB.[27,58]

Adverse Effects

Direct renin inhibitors are well tolerated and have minimal adverse effects. They may produce a cough because of the increase in bradykinin, but it is notably less frequent than that produced by ACE inhibitors. Diarrhea, dizziness, drowsiness, headache, rash, edema, elevated uric acid levels, and hypotension have been reported.[27,58]

Drug Interactions

Aliskiren is metabolized in the liver by the cytochrome P-450 3A4 isoenzyme. Concurrent medications that are also metabolized through this system should be used cautiously, and aliskiren should be monitored for increased or decreased levels and risk of adverse reactions. Agents that have demonstrated notable increases in aliskiren include atorvastatin, ketoconazole, cyclosporine, and verapamil. Decreases in aliskiren levels were noted with irbesartan.[27,58]

Monitoring

As with other RAAS blood pressure–lowering agents, blood pressure, serum electrolytes, and renal function should be measured at baseline and periodically throughout DRI treatment.

Instructions

Direct renin inhibitors should be taken daily and as close to the same time as possible. Though DRIs can be taken with or without food, they should not be taken with a high-fat meal. If drowsiness occurs, aliskiren can be taken in the evening. Patients should monitor their blood pressure regularly. For the most part, DRIs are well tolerated in terms of adverse effects; however, patients should immediately report any swelling of the face, lips, tongue, throat, arms, or legs, or of the whole body, as angioedema is a rare adverse effect that can happen at any time while taking aliskiren.[27,58]

Beta-Blockers

Beta-blockers are commonly prescribed as an addition to an existing hypertension treatment plan for persons with diabetes. They are traditionally not first-line or preferred treatment for persons with diabetes, but they may be a second or third option. Beta-blockers are beneficial for persons with CVD. In addition to reducing hypertension, beta-blockers are indicated for persons at high risk of coronary disease and for prevention of a second MI and heart failure.

Beta 1–Selective Receptor Blockers: Dosage Information

Drug	Trade Name	Common Dose	Common Frequency	Lipid Solubility
Acebutolol*	Sectral®*	200–400 mg	Twice daily	Low
Atenolol	Tenormin®	25–100 mg	Once daily	Low
Betaxolol	Kerlone®	5–20 mg	Once daily	Low
Bisoprolol	Zebeta®	2.5–10 mg	Once daily	Low
Metoprolol tartrate	Lopressor®	25–50 mg	Once to twice daily	Moderate
Metoprolol succinate	Toprol XL®	25–100 mg	Once daily	Moderate
Nebivolol	Bystolic®	2.5–40 mg	Once daily	High

*Agents with intrinsic sympathomimetic activity

Nonselective Beta-Receptor Blockers: Dosage Information

Drug	Trade Name	Common Dose	Common Frequency	Lipid Solubility
Nadolol	Corgard®	40–120 mg	Once daily	Low
Penbutolol*	Levatol®*	20 mg	Once daily	High
Pindolol*	Visken®*	5–20 mg	Twice daily	Low
Propanolol	Inderal®	40–120 mg	Twice daily	High
Propanolol extended release	Inderal LA®	80–160 mg	Once daily	High
Timolol	Blocadren®	10–30 mg	Twice daily	Low to moderate

*Agents with intrinsic sympathomimetic activity

Combined Alpha- and Beta-Receptor Blockers: Dosage Information

Drug	Trade Name	Common Dose	Common Frequency
Carvedilol	Coreg®	6.25–25 mg	Twice daily
Labetalol	Normodyne®	100–300 mg	Twice daily

Mechanism of Action

There are 2 main types of beta-receptors in human physiology: beta 1 and beta 2. Receptors are located on the heart, where activation causes an increase in heart rate, contractility, and conduction velocity. Blockade of these receptors reduces cardiac output.[59]

Beta-receptors also have a wide range of functions in the body outside the heart. Activation of beta 1 receptors located in the juxtoglomerular cells of the kidney affect the RAAS by stimulating the release of renin.[27] Activation of beta 2 receptors in the liver increases hepatic-mediated glucose output.[60] Activation of beta 2 receptors in the lungs induces bronchodilation.[59] Beta 2–receptor activation also causes an increase in intraocular pressure and relaxation of skeletal muscle vessels.[27] Beta-receptor blockade opposes all these effects. In some of these cases, beta-receptor blockade is beneficial, and in others it is not.

As for differences with beta-blocker drugs, some are beta 1–receptor selective and preferentially inhibit the beta 1 receptor. Others are nonselective and inhibit both beta 1 and beta 2 receptors with equal affinity. It is important to remember that when higher doses of a beta 1–selective blocker are given, selectivity diminishes.[59] Beta-receptor blockers also differ in lipid solubility. Highly lipid-soluble beta-receptor blockers cross the blood brain barrier (BBB) readily and increase the risk of adverse effects to the central nervous system (CNS). Some beta-blockers also have intrinsic sympathomimetic activity (ISA). Intrinsic sympathomimetic activity beta-blockers act as a partial agonist at beta-receptors while blocking physiological beta-agonists such as epinephrine. The net effect is some preservation of beta-receptor function and a potential decrease in side effects.[59] These agents are used infrequently, however, due to inferior clinical trial data in post-MI patients.[61]

Dosing

Beta-blockers are administered once to twice daily and given without regard to meals. If drowsiness is experienced, daily doses can be given in the evening to minimize this adverse effect when the patient is awake. However, administration should occur at a consistent time. Initial therapy often starts with a low dose and can be titrated up as tolerated.

Pregnancy, Precautions, and Contraindications

Most beta-blockers are classified as pregnancy category C. Atenolol is classified as pregnancy category D. Atenolol crosses the placental barrier and has resulted in the birth of infants small for their gestational age. Beta-blockers should be used with caution in pregnancy, if at all, and used only if the benefit clearly outweighs the risk.[59]

Beta-blockers are contraindicated in persons with sinus bradycardia.[59] Nonselective beta-blockers are contraindicated in persons with asthma, due to the blockade of beta 2–mediated bronchodilation.[59]

Beta 1–selective agents should be used cautiously and with the lowest possible dose.[62] Additionally, beta-blockers must be used with caution in older adults who have preexisting ventricular dysfunction.[59]

Persons with diabetes must also exercise caution when using beta-blockers. Beta-blockers may inhibit the release of insulin from the pancreas, resulting in increased blood glucose levels in persons with type 2 diabetes. Additionally, all beta-blockers have the potential to mask hypoglycemic-induced tachycardia, which can decrease the individual's awareness of hypoglycemia.[59,60] Dizziness and sweating induced by hypoglycemia are typically unaffected by beta-blockers.[59] Nonselective beta-blockers can reduce beta 2–mediated hepatic glucose output.[60] Normally, this would be a beneficial effect, but during an episode of hypoglycemia it may delay the body's ability to return to normoglycemia.[63]

Adverse Effects

Common adverse effects associated with this class of antihypertensive agents are CNS-related, such as sedation, dizziness, drowsiness, lightheadedness, fatigue, and headache. Other notable adverse effects include bradycardia, hypotension, depression, and sexual dysfunction, especially in older adults. Gastrointestinal effects of constipation, diarrhea, and nausea are reported but less frequent.[59]

Drug Interactions

Beta-blockers have additive effects with nondihydropyridine calcium channel blockers (CCBs) (diltiazem and verapamil), amiodarone, and digoxin.[59] Concurrent use of these agents may cause heart block; therefore, extreme caution should be used when combining these agents. Typically, persons taking beta-blockers need to be tapered off the drug and should not abruptly discontinue.[59] Diphenhydramine and hydrochloroquine may increase the plasma concentrations of some beta-blockers through inhibition of the cytochrome P-450 isoenzyme CYP2D6, resulting in enhanced adverse effects including hypotension.[59] Nonsteroidal anti-inflammatory drugs may decrease the antihypertensive effects of beta-blockers.[59]

Monitoring

Baseline blood pressure, heart rate, lipid profile, and blood glucose levels should be conducted. Since beta-blockers can decrease heart rate, patients should have their heart rate assessed at each clinician visit.[59] Generally, the beta-blocker dose is adjusted if the heart rate falls below 50 beats per minute. Beta-blockers also have the potential to increase total cholesterol, LDL-C, and TGs and decrease HDL-C, although these effects are transient and usually of little clinical significance.[64] Nevertheless, serum lipids should be monitored regularly, especially when coadministered with other agents that increase serum lipids, such as thiazide diuretics.[59] Blood glucose levels should be monitored regularly, especially in those newly diagnosed with diabetes or with prediabetes.

Instructions

Educate patients not to stop beta-blockers abruptly, unless directed by their healthcare provider. Abrupt withdrawal could lead to increased blood pressure and worsening of preexisting angina and possibly lead to MI. Monitor blood pressure and heart rate daily to identify changes, elevations, and patterns. Encourage people with diabetes to monitor their blood glucose levels more frequently. Educate patients on the signs and symptoms of hypotension and worsening heart failure, such as edema and difficulty in breathing during activity.

Calcium Channel Blockers

Calcium channel blockers are usually not used as first-line therapy for lowering blood pressure in persons with diabetes. These agents are commonly a second or third option since they have less of an impact on CVD risk when compared with other antihypertensive agents, such as ACE inhibitors, ARBs, diuretics, and beta-blockers. Consider non-dihydropyridine CCBs for people who do not tolerate ACE inhibitors or ARB therapy. Non-dihydropyridine CCBs may have anti-proteinuric effects.[65-68]

Non-dihydropyridine CCBs: Dosage Information

Drug	Trade Name	Common Dose	Common Frequency
Diltiazem sustained release	Cardizem SR®	60–180 mg	Twice daily
Diltiazem extended release	Cardizem CD® Tiazac® Cardizem LA®	120–360 mg	Once daily
Verapamil immediate release	Calan®	40–80 mg	Three times daily
Verapamil sustained release	Calan SR®	120–360 mg	Once daily
Verapamil extended release	Covera-HS® Verelan PM®	120–360 mg 100–300 mg	Once daily

Mechanism of Action

Calcium channel blockers are classified into non-dihydropyridine or dihydropyridine, based on their chemical structure. Calcium channel blockers block the L-type calcium channel, which results in vasodilation. Non-dihydropyridine CCBs primarily cause vasodilation within coronary vessels and have a more depressive effect on cardiac conduction. Thus, blood pressure reduction is due to decreased CO.[69,70] Dihydropyridine CCBs primarily cause vasodilation in the vascular smooth muscle. Thus, blood pressure reduction is due to decreased TPR.[69]

Dosing

Calcium channel blockers are dosed 1 to 3 times daily and can be taken with food to minimize adverse effects. Dose initially at the low range and titrate up every 2 weeks based on patient tolerance, blood pressure, and heart rate. The immediate-release dosage forms are rarely used for treating hypertension. Once-daily formulations are dosed in the morning, except verapamil extended-release products, which are dosed at bedtime.[69]

Dihydropyridine CCBs: Dosage Information

Drug	Trade Name	Common Dose	Common Frequency
Amlodipine	Norvasc®	2.5–10 mg	Once daily
Felodipine	Plendil®	2.5–20 mg	Once daily
Isradipine controlled release	DynaCirc CR®	5–10 mg	Once daily
Nicardipine sustained release	Cardene SR®	30–60 mg	Twice daily
Nifedipine long-acting	Adalat® CC Procardia XL®	30–60 mg	Once daily
Nisoldipine	Sular®	10–40 mg	Once daily

Dihydropyridine CCBs are dosed once daily and can be given without regard to time of day. However, administration should be at a consistent time. Dose initially at the low range and titrate up gradually based on patient tolerance, blood pressure, and heart rate.[69]

Pregnancy, Precautions, and Contraindications

All CCBs are pregnancy category C and should be avoided unless the benefit outweighs the risk.

Calcium channel blockers are also contraindicated in persons with sick sinus syndrome or a heart block, without a pacemaker. Non-dihydropyridine CCBs, specifically, are contraindicated in persons with heart failure.

Caution should be used in persons with renal and/or hepatic dysfunction.[69]

Adverse Effects

Calcium channel blockers have a wide range of adverse effects, which can include headache, dizziness, nausea, dyspepsia, flushing, and constipation. Non-dihydropyridine CCBs are associated with cardiac adverse effects including cardiac conduction abnormalities and bradycardia, which are typically found in persons with preexisting cardiac conditions. Dihydropyridine CCBs have adverse effects related to their relaxing of vascular tone. Peripheral edema occurs more frequently with these agents; however, all CCBs have the potential to cause peripheral edema.[69]

Drug Interactions

Most CCB drug interactions stem from the cytochrome P-450 enzyme system. All inducers and inhibitors of the CYP3A4 isoenzyme affect the metabolism of CCBs, thereby delaying or enhancing their elimination from the body and resulting in increased or decreased CCB concentration.[69] Concurrent medications and foods that are also metabolized through this system (such as grapefruit juice) should be used cautiously and patients should be monitored for increased levels and adverse reactions. Additionally, diltiazem and verapamil can inhibit other CYP3A4 substrates, such as statins and theophylline.[69] Monitoring adverse effects and blood pressure can help identify potential drug interactions and reduce the risk of toxicity. See Table 19.3 for a list of common drugs that interact with CCBs.

Calcium channel blockers may also inhibit platelet function, resulting in an increased risk of bleeding if used concurrently with anticoagulants, such as warfarin or aspirin. Although this interaction is usually not clinically significant, caution is warranted.[69] Concurrent use of diuretics, beta-blockers, and ACE inhibitors may increase risk of hypotension. Additive effects may occur with agents that affect cardiac contractility.[69]

Monitoring

Blood pressure, heart rate, liver enzymes, and cardiac function should be measured at baseline and periodically throughout treatment, especially when titrating doses of CCBs and/or other medications metabolized by the cytochrome P-450 system.[69] Monitor for heart failure, edema, angina, and changes in heart rate. For patients on warfarin therapy, more frequent monitoring of the international normalized ratio (INR) may be warranted.

Instructions

Calcium channel blockers should be taken at the same time daily. For once-daily dosed CCBs, patients can take the medication in the evening if they experience drowsiness or dizziness. Taking CCBs with meals can minimize gastrointestinal adverse effects and can often increase adherence. Monitor blood pressure daily to identify changes, elevations, and patterns. Educate patients on the signs and symptoms of heart failure, such as edema and shortness of breath at rest or during activity.

Alpha 1–Receptor Blockers

Although indicated for the treatment of hypertension, alpha 1–receptor blockers are infrequently prescribed for this indication, especially in persons with diabetes. They are most beneficial in persons with benign prostatic hyperplasia (BPH). Alpha-receptor blockers can be a treatment option for persons with both diabetes and BPH.

Mechanism of Action

The alpha 1–receptor blockers inhibit the binding of norepinephrine to vascular alpha 1 receptors. Activation of the alpha 1 receptor by norepinephrine leads to vasoconstriction, resulting in an increase in TPR. In addition, inhibition of the alpha 1 receptor in the prostate causes a decrease in urethral resistance and improvement in symptoms in persons with BPH.[71]

Dosing

The alpha 1–receptor blockers are preferably dosed at bedtime to minimize the risk of postural hypertension often observed within hours after administration. Initial therapy often starts with a low dose and can be titrated up as tolerated.[71]

Alpha 1–Receptor Blockers: Dosage Information			
Drug	Trade Name	Common Dose	Common Frequency
Doxazosin	Cardura®	1–16 mg	Once daily
Prazosin	Minipress®	1–5 mg	2–3 times daily
Terazosin	Hytrin®	1–10 mg	Once to twice daily

Pregnancy, Precautions, and Contraindications

All alpha 1 blockers are classified as pregnancy category C and should be avoided unless the benefit outweighs the risk. Animal studies indicated possible risk, and no human studies exist.

The alpha 1–receptor blockers also cause a mild decrease in neutrophils and white blood cell counts. In most persons, the decrease is clinically insignificant, but caution is advised in immunocompromised patients.[71]

Adverse Effects

Adverse effects commonly associated with alpha 1–receptor blockers include fatigue, malaise, dizziness, shortness of breath, hypotension, edema, and weight gain. Blurred vision, palpitations, and sexual dysfunction have also been reported. Thrombocytopenia has been observed in patients on terazosin.[71]

Drug Interactions

The alpha 1–receptor blockers have relatively few drug interactions. Alcohol increases the risk of hypotension with these agents, and coadministration of verapamil increases the serum concentrations of prazosin and terazosin. Concurrent use of other antihypertensive agents with alpha 1 blockers may increase the risk of hypotension.[71]

Monitoring

Monitor blood pressure and heart rate at baseline and frequently after initiating treatment. If antihypertensive agents are added, assess the patient for first-dose syncope and postural hypotension.[71] Syncope is managed by having the patient lie down, rest, and receive supportive care as necessary. Syncope may be prevented by starting with a low dose and increasing slowly. Dizziness and lightheadedness are more common than loss of consciousness.[71] Interruptions in therapy increase the risk; thus, nonadherent patients are poor candidates for this drug.

Instructions

Educate patients that alpha 1–receptor blockers have the potential to cause syncope and postural hypotension. Alcohol, exercise, long periods of standing, and hot weather can increase the risk.[71] Educate patients and their families on the management of syncope in case it occurs. Advise patients to avoid driving or operating machinery after the first dose, an increase in dose, or the addition of another antihypertensive agent until they can tolerate treatment. Lastly, advise male patients to go immediately to the emergency room if they experience a prolonged erection lasting 4 hours or more.

Central-Acting Alpha-Adrenergic Agonists

Although indicated for the treatment of hypertension, central-acting alpha-adrenergic agonists are rarely prescribed for this indication, especially in persons with diabetes.

Mechanism of Action

Central-acting alpha-adrenergic agonists stimulate alpha 2 receptors in the brain, inhibiting the production of serotonin, dopamine, norepinephrine, and epinephrine. This inhibition results in a decrease in heart rate and TPR.[72]

Central-Acting Alpha-Adrenergic Agonists: Dosage Information			
Drug	Trade Name	Common Dose	Common Frequency
Clonidine tablets	Catapres®	0.1–0.8 mg	Twice daily
Clonidine patch	Catapres-TTS®	0.1- to .3-mg per day patch	Once weekly
Methyldopa	Aldomet®	250–1000 mg	2–3 times daily

Dosing

Central-acting alpha-adrenergic agonists are available in either tablets or a transdermal patch. Tablets are taken in daily divided doses, preferably at consistent times. Patches are applied once weekly.[73] When methyldopa is administered with any other antihypertensive agent, other than thiazide-type diuretics, limit the initial dose to no more than 500 mg per day in divided doses.[72]

Pregnancy, Precautions, and Contraindications

Clonidine is classified as pregnancy category C and should be avoided.[73] Methyldopa is pregnancy category B and therefore can be used in pregnancy. It is converted to alpha-methylnorepinephrine, a natural by-product of catecholamine breakdown. There are no documented fetal adverse effects despite wide use, and it does not reduce maternal cardiac or fetal blood flow.[74] Although it can be used during pregnancy, methyldopa presents with many adverse effects to the mother that often lead to discontinuation (see adverse effects below).

The use of a monoamine oxidase inhibitor (MAOI) is contraindicated in persons taking methyldopa. Although the mechanism is unknown, there are numerous reports of hypertensive crisis in persons taking both medications.[72]

Central-acting alpha-adrenergic agonists are contraindicated in persons with severe coronary insufficiency, recent MI, cerebrovascular disease, and renal or hepatic dysfunction.[72-74]

Adverse Effects

Although methyldopa can be used in pregnancy, it presents with many adverse effects to the mother and to the general patient. Some of these include nausea, vomiting, constipation, dry mouth, and CNS-related effects, such as sedation, weakness, nervousness, dizziness, and drowsiness. Hypotension, blood dyscrasia, sexual dysfunction, and hair thinning or loss have also been reported.[72]

Drug Interactions

The use of an MAOI is contraindicated in persons taking methyldopa. Although the mechanism is unknown, there are numerous reports of hypertensive crisis in persons taking both medications.[72]

Iron can decrease the absorption of methyldopa by up to 66%. Therefore, iron should be separated by at least 2 hours from methyldopa administration.[72] Methyldopa also increases the risk of lithium toxicity, even in the presence of normal lithium levels. Monitor for signs and symptoms of lithium toxicity, such as lethargy and muscle weakness.[74] Patients should also exercise caution when taking entacapone (Comtan®, Novartis) and methyldopa. Entacapone is a catechol-O-methyltransferase (COMT) inhibitor, and methyldopa is metabolized by COMT.[74]

The over-the-counter drug products pseudoephedrine and ma huang (ephedra, ephedrine) can increase blood pressure. This is greatly enhanced for persons taking methyldopa and clonidine.[72-74] Tricyclic antidepressants—eg, amitriptyline (Elavil®) and imipramine (Janimine®, Tofranil®)—may antagonize central alpha 2 receptors. Use clonidine and methyldopa with caution when combined with beta-blockers, since withdrawal of these agents has led to life-threatening increases in blood pressure.[72-74]

Case—Part 3: What Pharmacologic Treatment for Hypertension, If Any, Is Appropriate?

Provided that DC's electrolytes, primarily potassium, and renal and hepatic function are within normal limits and that he has no signs or symptoms of heart failure, DC may be prescribed ACE inhibitors or ARBs. Angiotensin-converting enzyme inhibitors or ARBs are the first-line treatment option in hypertension for persons with diabetes.

Dosage

Dose initially at the low end and titrate up if necessary and tolerated. Monitor blood pressure, electrolytes, and renal function within the first month of initiating ARB therapy.

Three-Month Follow-up

If after 3 months of therapy DC has not reached optimal blood pressure goals, increasing his current therapy dose or adding a second antihypertensive agent may be warranted.

Pharmacotherapy Options

Options for DC at this point include increasing his current ARB dose or using a precombined ARB with a low-dose HCTZ agent.

Behavior Change Considerations

DC's readiness to change, conviction, and confidence in regard to adding another medicine should be assessed. As mentioned earlier, DC may have a possible adherence problem with his medications; therefore, adding another medication may not be the best therapy plan.

Patient empowerment, education, close monitoring, and follow-up with the patient are necessary to ensure that optimal blood lipids and blood pressure goals are met and to decrease CVD risks and events.

Monitoring

Monitor blood pressure and heart rate at baseline and frequently after initiating treatment. Monitor patients for signs of depression at follow-up visits. Clinicians who wish to discontinue a central-acting alpha-adrenergic agonist should taper the dose gradually over 2 to 4 days to prevent withdrawal.[72–74] Monitor for tachycardia, rebound hypertension, nausea, vomiting, and flushing. Patients on methyldopa should also undergo liver function testing at periodic intervals.[72]

Instructions

Educate patients to never abruptly discontinue their medication and to review the signs and symptoms of withdrawal. Since these agents affect catecholamine and aldosterone levels, remind persons with diabetes to monitor blood glucose levels more frequently, as greater fluctuation can occur.[72–74] Drowsiness is common, so until the medication is tolerated, patients should exercise caution when driving or operating heavy machinery.[72] Dry mouth can occur during the first 2 weeks of therapy. Ice chips, hard candy, or chewing gum can minimize problems with dry mouth.[72] The clonidine patch should be applied every 7 days on a hairless part of the upper arm or torso. Educate patients to apply the adhesive overlay over the system for proper adhesion. Advise patients taking methyldopa that their urine may darken in color after exposure to air.[72]

Considerations in Hypertension Therapy in Persons With Diabetes

Treatment goals and strategies for hypertension in persons with diabetes must be given equal emphasis and treated as aggressively as hyperglycemia. Most likely, 2 or more antihypertensive agents will be necessary to lower and maintain blood pressure to the goal of 140/80 mm Hg (or <130/80 mm Hg in select patients).[2,46]

When using combination therapy for hypertension in persons with diabetes, medication adherence must be reviewed at each patient visit. Adding medication to existing regimens requires behavior change on the part of the patient; thus, the person's readiness to change, conviction, and confidence levels require assessment. Use of precombined medications can be beneficial for individuals who are reluctant to take more medication.

Angiotensin-converting enzyme inhibitors and ARBs are traditionally the initial drug of choice for hypertension in persons with diabetes. The addition of a thiazide diuretic can enhance the blood pressure–lowering effects of ACE inhibitors and ARBs. However, monitoring for hypotension and electrolyte changes, especially potassium, must be conducted routinely.

Focus on Education

Teaching Strategies

⟳ **Patient education should include medication safety, proper dosing, and timing medications for optimum effect.**

⟳ **Acknowledge the need for lifestyle change.** Lifestyle modification, including MNT, physical activity, and smoking cessation, should always be a standard treatment of dyslipidemia in addition to pharmacotherapy.

⟳ **Dosing starts small and builds.** Initiation of medication therapy is an important change in treatment and health management. Titration of medications to achieve targets is essential for effective and comprehensive diabetes care management.

⟳ **Combining medications.** Combination therapy with medications possessing different mechanisms of action is often necessary to treat dyslipidemia and hypertension. Achieving optimal levels of LDL-C, TGs, and HDL-C should be considered when choosing drug therapy. Describe each medication's unique function and effect.

⟳ **Resisting medications.** Adding medication to existing regimens is a behavior change. Readiness to change, conviction, and confidence levels affect adherence to the regimen. Discuss and plan for accommodation into existing lifestyle. Identify and help diminish barriers to effective pharmacotherapy.

Messages for Patients

↻ **Treatment goals.** Identify target goals for dyslipidemia and hypertension, and be as aggressive with these goals as you are with your blood glucose goals. Be certain you are aware of the target blood levels your healthcare team identifies for lipids, blood pressure, and blood glucose.

↻ **Consistency.** Work with the healthcare team and pharmacist to keep them informed of all the medications you are taking (prescription and over the counter). Always carry a list of current medications and know their interactions and side effects. Never abruptly discontinue a medication; be aware of the signs and symptoms of withdrawal. Have a list of resources to call if you have any questions.

↻ **Therapeutic lifestyle changes.** Healthy eating, physical activity, and stress management are part of your cardiovascular well-being and will help you manage your hypertension and blood lipids.

Health Literacy

↻ **Numerous barriers may exist to prevent patients from properly using their medications.** They might include financial constraints, cultural beliefs, and limited educational attainment. Asking probing questions can help you explore those possibilities and address them accordingly.

↻ **Inadequate health literacy may lead to an increase in medication errors.** Medication error is considered to be the most common medical mistake. Two thirds of US adults 60 years of age or older have inadequate or marginal literacy skills. Eighty-one percent of patients 60 years of age or older at a public hospital could not read or understand basic materials such as prescription labels.[75]

↻ **Patients with low literacy may misunderstand the warning labels on their medication.** One of many studies indicated that patients with low literacy skills demonstrated a lower rate of correct interpretation of the 8 most commonly used prescription drug warning labels than did those with higher literacy skills. Multiple-step instructions, reading difficulty of text, the use of icons, the use of color, and the lack of message clarity were common causes of label misinterpretation.[76]

↻ **The design and layout of medication handouts can make navigation problematic.** Consider the following when developing or using medication handouts:

- Use short, familiar words.
- Use short sentences.
- Use short headings that stand out.
- Use a large type size.
- Use capital and lowercase letters rather than all capital letters.
- Bold, highlight, or enlarge font of content most important to the patient.
- Do not use abbreviations that are not easily referenced.
- Leave plenty of white space.
- Use bullet points to organize lists.
- Use a 3-step rule; multistep instructions are rarely understood.
- Involve your patients in the design of reference/teaching materials.
- Clarify the purpose of the handout as the information for decision making.

↻ **Health numeracy can negatively impact medication taking.** Health numeracy is defined as "the degree to which individuals have the capacity to access, process, interpret, communicate, and act on numerical, quantitative, graphical, biostatistical, and probabilistic health information needed to make effective health decisions."[77] Even the most knowledgeable person is at risk of misusing/misinterpreting the numbers and consequently not taking his or her medications as intended. Ask your patients to bring their medications to the office, and ask what kind of system they have in place to know when and how to take those medications. Ask your patients to answer the following questions in their own words: "What is this medication for?" "Why do you need to take this medication?" "How do you remind yourself to take this medication?" "How often do you skip doses of this medication?" Normalize some predicted non-adherence behaviors by asking patients whether they are exemplifying them. Address the difference between trade names and generic names, as this can be confusing for many.

⊘ **Provide patients with some useful strategies to accurately track medication-taking behaviors.** Strategies could include keeping medicine bottles in the same container with color-coded tops, using colors/rubber bands to mark their medications, or using medication dispensers with daily compartments, among others. Support your patients in establishing good communication with their pharmacist. Explain that the pharmacist is part of their diabetes care team and can educate them not only about medications but on how to take them and what to do if they cannot take them.

Focus on Practice

⊘ **Simple solutions to complicated problems.** A good example is the public health impact of reduced salt intake. If Americans reduced their salt intake by 3 g per day, or approximately one third of a teaspoon, there would be about 100,000 fewer heart attacks each year, about 92,000 fewer deaths each year, and about 66,000 fewer strokes each year. Additionally, it would reduce healthcare costs each year by between $10 billion and $24 billion.[78]

⊘ **Dyslipidemia and hypertension management are part of the chronic care model.** Patients with chronic conditions like dyslipidemia and hypertension need support, as well as information, to become effective managers of their health. An effective decision support mechanism, a delivery system design, a clinical information system, organization of health care, and community support are part of delivering effective care.

⊘ **Quality assurance.** To improve the quality of care, its structure, process, and outcomes need to be evaluated. Follow evidence-based guidelines to optimize resource utilization as well as improve the management and outcome of care for patients with diabetes and hypertension/dyslipidemia. Advance clinicians' knowledge and adherence to current evidence-based pharmacotherapy guidelines and delivery systems.

⊘ **Create a system for effective behavioral interventions.** Strategies include developing prompts and reminder systems, identifying a potential relapse into old behavior, setting appropriate and realistic goals, simplifying regimens to once or twice daily, using opportunities to model behavior, and reinforcing positive behaviors.

References

1. Haffner SM. Dyslipidemia management in patients with diabetes and the metabolic syndrome. Fam Pract. 2005;27: 49-64.

2. American Diabetes Association. Standards of medical care in diabetes. Diabetes Care. 2010;33 Suppl:S4-61.

3. Bierman EL. Atherogenesis in diabetes. Arterioscler Thromb. 1992;12:647-56.

4. Miettinen H, Lehto S, Salomaa V, et al; for the FINMON-ICA Myocardial Register Study Group. Impact of diabetes on mortality after the first myocardial infarction. Diabetes Care. 1998;21:69-75.

5. Kannel WB, McGee DL. Diabetes and cardiovascular disease: The Framingham Study. JAMA. 1979;241:2035-8.

6. Haffner SM, Lehto S, Ronnemaa T, et al. Mortality from coronary heart disease in subjects with type 2 diabetes and in nondiabetic subjects with and without prior myocardial infarction. N Engl J Med. 1998;339:229-34.

7. Norhammar A, Tenerz A, Nilsson G, et al. Glucose metabolism in patients with acute myocardial infarction and no previous diagnosis of diabetes mellitus: a prospective study. Lancet. 2002;359:2140-4.

8. Ganong WF. Review of Medical Physiology. 17th ed. Norwalk, Conn: Appleton & Lange; 1995:277-81, 436-8.

9. Sisson EM, Tisdel KA. Hyperlipidemias. In: Pharmacotherapy Self-Assessment Program Book 1: Cardiovascular I. 4th ed. Kansas City, Mo: American College of Clinical Pharmacy; 2001:45-83.

10. Luscher TF. Endothelial dysfunction in atherosclerosis. J Myocardial Ischemia. 1995;7 Suppl:15-20.

11. Ginsberg HN. Lipoprotein physiology in nondiabetic and diabetic states: relationship to atherogenesis. Diabetes Care. 1991;14:839-55.

12. Lamarche B, Lemieux I, Despres JP, et al. The small, dense LDL phenotype and the risk of coronary heart disease: epidemiology, pathophysiology and therapeutic aspects. Diabetes Metab. 1999;25:199-211.

13. Tribble DL, Holl LG, Wodd PD, et al. Variations in oxidative susceptibility among six low density lipoprotein subfractions of differing density and particle size. Atherosclerosis. 1992;93:189-99.

14. Garg A, Grundy SM. Management of dyslipidemia in NIDDM. Diabetes Care. 1990;13:153-69.

15. Expert Panel on Detection, Evaluation, and Treatment of High Blood Cholesterol in Adults. Executive summary of the third report of the National Cholesterol Education Program (NCEP) Expert Panel on Detection, Evaluation, and Treatment of High Blood Cholesterol in Adults (Adult Treatment Panel III). JAMA. 2001;285:2486-97.

16. Ridker PM, Danielson E, Fonseca FA, et al. Rosuvastatin to prevent vascular events in men and women with elevated C-reactive protein. N Engl J Med. 2008;359:2195-207.

17. Mazzone T, Meyer PM, Feinstein SB, et al. Effect of pioglitazone compared with glimepiride on carotid intima-media cardiovascular system thickness in type 2 diabetes: a randomized trial. JAMA. 2006;296:2572-81.

18. de Groot E, Hovingh K, Wiegman A, et al. Measurement of arterial wall thickness as a surrogate marker for atherosclerosis. Circulation. 2004;109 Suppl 3:33-8.

19. Nissen SE, Nicholls SJ, Wolski K, et al; for the PERISCOPE Investigators. Comparison of pioglitazone vs glimepiride on progression of coronary atherosclerosis in patients with type 2 diabetes: the PERISCOPE randomized controlled trial. JAMA. 2008;299(13):1561-73.

20. Blonde L, Klein EJ, Han J, et al. Interim analysis of the effects of exenatide treatment on A1C, weight and cardiovascular risk factors over 82 weeks in 314 overweight patients with type 2 diabetes. Diabetes Obes Metab. 2006 Jul;8(4):436-47.

21. Grundy SM, Cleeman JI, Merz CN, et al; for the Coordinating Committee of the Recent Clinical Trials for the National Cholesterol Education Program. Adult Treatment Panel III Guidelines. Circulation. 2004;110:227-39.

22. American Diabetes Association. Management of dyslipidemia in adults with diabetes. Diabetes Care. 2003;26 Suppl:S83-6.

23. Liu J, Sempos CT, Donahue RP, et al. Non-high density lipoprotein and very-low-density lipoprotein cholesterol and their risk predictive value in coronary heart disease. Am J Cardiol. 2006;98:1363-8.

24. Sniderman AD, Williams K, Contois JH, et al. A meta-analysis of low-density lipoprotein cholesterol, non-high-density lipoprotein cholesterol, and apolipo-protein B as markers of cardiovascular risk. Circ Cardiovasc Qual Outcomes. 2011;4:337-45.

25. American Diabetes Association Position Statement. Standards of medical care in diabetes—2013. Diabetes Care. 2013; 36 Suppl 1:S11-66.

26. Jones PH. A clinical overview of dyslipidemias: treatment strategies. Am J Med. 1992;93:187-98.

27. Lexi-Comp. Drug Information Handbook ODA Medical Software. Hudson, Ohio: Lexi-Comp, Inc; 2009.

28. Worz CR, Bottorff M. Treating dyslipidemic patients with lipid-modifying and combination therapies. Pharmacotherapy. 2003;23:625-37.

29. Jones P, Kafonek S, Laurora I, et al. Comparative dose efficacy study of atorvastatin versus simvastatin, pravastatin, lovastatin, and fluvastatin in patients with hypercholesterolemia (the CURVES study). Am J Cardiol. 1998;81:582-7.

30. Antilipidemic agents. In: Monthly Prescribing Guide: November. Montvale, NJ: Thompson PDR; 2005:89-95.

31. Monthly Prescribing Reference. Cardiovascular system: hyperlipoproteinemias. Feb 2010. (cited 2010 Feb 17). On the Internet at: http://www.empr.com/.

32. Ridker PM, Pradhan A, MacFadyen JG, et al. Cardiovascular benefits and diabetes risks of statin therapy in primary prevention: an analysis from the JUPITER trial. Lancet. 2012;380(9841):565-71.

33. Lexi-Interact Platinum for Palm OS. Hudson, Ohio: Lexi-Comp, Inc; 2004 (cited 2010 Nov 15).

34. Taylor AJ, Villines TC, Stanek EJ, et al. Extended-release niacin or ezetimibe and carotid intima-media thickness. N Engl J Med. 2009 Nov;361(22):2113-22.

35. McKenney JM, Proctin JD, Harris S, et al. A comparison of the efficacy and toxic effects of sustained versus immediate release niacin in hypercholesterolemia patients. JAMA. 1994;271:672-7.

36. Oh R. Practical applications of fish oil (omega-3 fatty acids) in primary care. J Am Board Fam Pract. 2005;18:28-36.

37. Studer M, Briel M, Leimenstoll B, et al. Effect of different antilipidemic agents and diets on mortality: a systematic review. Arch Intern Med. 2005;165:725-30.

38. Brown M. Do vitamin E and fish oil protect against ischaemic heart disease? Lancet. 1999;354:441-2.

39. Talbert RL. Hyperlipidemia. In: Dipiro JT, Talbert RL, Yee GC, Matzke GR, Wells BG, Posey LM, eds. Pharmacotherapy: A Pathophysiologic Approach. 7th ed. New York: McGraw Hill; 2008:385-407.

40. Sowers JR, Haffner SM. Treatment of cardiovascular and renal risk factors in the diabetic hypertensive. Hypertension. 2002;40:781-8.

41. Higashi Y, Sasaki S, Nakagawa K, et al. Endothelial function and oxidative stress in renovascular hypertension. N Engl J Med. 2002;346:1954-62.

42. Carter BL. Management of essential hypertension. In: Pharmacotherapy Self-Assessment Program Book 1: Cardiovascular I. 4th ed. Kansas City, Mo: American College of Clinical Pharmacy; 2001:1-39.

43. Jacobsen EJ. Hypertension: update on use of angiotensin II receptor blockers. Geriatrics. 2001;56(2):25-8.

44. Ramahi TM. Expanded role for ARBs in cardiovascular and renal disease. Postgrad Med. 2001;109(4):115-22.

45. Willenheimer R, Dahlof B, Rydberg E, et al. AT-1 receptor blockers in hypertension and heart failure: clinical experience and future directions. Eur Heart J. 1999;20(14):997-1008.

46. Chobanian AV, Bakris GL, Black HR, et al. The Seventh Report of the Joint National Committee on Prevention, Detection, Evaluation, and Treatment of High Blood Pressure: the JNC 7 report. JAMA. 2003;289:2560-72.

47. American Diabetes Association. Treatment of hypertension in adults with diabetes. Diabetes Care. 2003;26 Suppl:S80-2.

48. Kidney Disease Outcomes Quality Initiative (K/DOQI). K/DOQI clinical practice guidelines: hypertension and antihypertensive agents in chronic kidney disease. Am J Kidney Dis. 2004;435 Suppl 1:S1-290.

49. The ACCORD Study Group. Effects of intensive blood-pressure control in type 2 diabetes mellitus. N Engl J Med. 2010;362:1575-85.

50. Monthly Prescribing Reference. Cardiovascular system: antihypertensives. Feb 2010. (cited 2010 Feb 17). On the Internet at: http://www.prescribingReference.com.

51. Fries ED. The efficacy and safety of diuretics in treating hypertension. Ann Intern Med. 1995;122(3):223-6.

52. Hypertension/heart failure agents. In: Monthly Prescribing Guide: November. Montvale, NJ: Thompson PDR; 2005:99-126.

53. Black HR. The evolution of low-dose diuretic therapy: the lessons from clinical trials. Am J Med. 1996;101(3A):47S-52S.

54. Sullivan TJ. Cross-reactions among furosemide, hydrochlorothiazide, and sulfonamides. JAMA. 1991;265(1):120-1.

55. Siegel D, Saliba P, Haffner S. Glucose and insulin levels during diuretic therapy in hypertensive men. Hypertension. 1994;236 pt 1:688-94.

56. ALLHAT Officers and Coordinators for the ALLHAT Collaborative Research Group. The Antihypertensive and Lipid-Lowering Treatment to Prevent Heart Attack Trial. Major outcomes in high-risk hypertensive patients randomized to angiotensin-converting enzyme inhibitor or calcium channel blocker vs diuretic: the Antihypertensive and Lipid-Lowering Treatment to Prevent Heart Attack Trial (ALLHAT). JAMA. 2002;288(23):2981-97.

57. Parving HH, Brenner BM, McMurray JJ, et al; for the ALTITUDE Investigators. Cardiorenal end points in a trial of aliskiren for type 2 diabetes. N Engl J Med. 2012;367:2204-13.

58. Tekturna [package insert]. East Hanover, NJ: Novartis Pharmaceuticals Corporation; 2007.

59. Facts and Comparisons. Beta-adrenergic blocking agents. Wolters Kluwer Health, Inc; 2010 (cited 2010 Nov 15). On the Internet at: http://www.factsandcomparisons.com/.

60. Verschoor L, Wolffenbuttel BH, Weber RF. Beta-blockade and carbohydrate metabolism: theoretical aspects and clinical implications. J Cardiovasc Pharmacol. 1986;8 Suppl 11:S92-5.

61. Freemantle N, Cleland J, Young P, et al. Beta blockade after myocardial infarction: systematic review and meta regression analysis. BMJ. 1999;318(7200):1730-7.

62. Salpeter S, Ormiston T, Salpeter E. Cardioselective beta-blockers for reversible airway disease. Cochrane Database Syst Rev. 2002;(1):CD002992.

63. Kleinbaum J, Shamoon H. Effect of Propranolol on delayed glucose recovery after insulin-induced hypoglycemia in normal and diabetic subjects. Diabetes Care. 1984;7(2):155-62.

64. Lakshman MR, Reda DJ, Materson BJ, et al. Diuretics and beta-blockers do not have adverse effects at 1 year on plasma lipid and lipoprotein profiles in men with hypertension. Department of Veterans Affairs Cooperative Study Group on Antihypertensive Agents. Arch Intern Med. 1999;159(6):551-8.

65. Ruggenenti P, Fassi A, Bergamo Nephrologic Diabetes Complications Trial (BENEDICT) Investigators. Preventing microalbuminuria in type 2 diabetes. N Engl J Med. 2004;351(19):1941-51.

66. Smith AC, Toto R, Bakris GL. Differential effects of calcium channel blockers on size selectivity of proteinuria in diabetic glomerulopathy. Kidney Int. 1998;54(3):889-96.

67. Bakris GL, Mangrum A, Copley JB, et al. Effect of calcium channel or beta-blockade on the progression of diabetic nephropathy in African Americans. Hypertension. 1997; 29(3):744-50.

68. Hemmelder MH, de Zeeuw D, de Jong PE. Antiproteinuric efficacy of verapamil in comparison to trandolapril in non-diabetic renal disease. Nephrol Dial Transplant. 1999;14(1):98-104.

69. Facts and Comparisons. Calcium channel blocking agents. Wolters Kluwer Health, Inc; 2010 (cited 2010 Feb 17). On the Internet at: http://www.factsandcomparisons.com/.

70. Diltiazem (drug monograph). In: Klasco RK, ed. DRUG-DEX® System (electronic version). Greenwood Village, Colo: Truven Health Analytics (cited 2010 Feb 17). On the Internet at: http://www.micromedex.com.

71. Facts and Comparisons. Alpha-1-adrenergic blockers. Wolters Kluwer Health, Inc; 2010 (cited 2010 Feb 17). On the Internet at: http://www.factsandcomparisons.com/.

72. Facts and Comparisons. Methyldopa (monograph). Wolters Kluwer Health, Inc; 2010 (cited 2010 Feb 17). On the Internet at: http://www.factsandcomparisons.com/.

73. Clonidine (drug monograph). In: Klasco RK, ed. DRUG-DEX® System (electronic version). Greenwood Village, Colo: Truven Health Analytics (cited 2010 Feb 17). On the Internet at: http://www.micromedex.com.

74. Methyldopa (drug monograph). In: Klasco RK, ed. DRUGDEX® System (electronic version). Greenwood Village, Colo: Truven Health Analytics (cited 2010 Feb 17). On the Internet at: http://www.micromedex.com.

75. Williams MV, Parker RM, Baker DW, et al. Inadequate functional health literacy among patients at two public hospitals. JAMA. 1995;274(21):1677-82.

76. Wolf MS, Davis TC, Tilson HH, Bass III PF, Parker RM. Misunderstanding of prescription drug warning labels among patients with low literacy. Am J Health Syst Pharm. 2006;63(11):1048-55.

77. Golbeck AL, Ahlers-Schmidt CR, Paschal AM, et al. A definition and operational framework for health numeracy. Am J Prev Med. 2005;29(4):375-6.

78. Bibbins-Domingo K, Chertow GM, Coxson PG, et al. Projected effect of dietary salt reductions on future cardiovascular disease. N Engl J Med. 2010;362:590-9.

CHAPTER 20

Biologically Based Practices: A Focus on Dietary Supplements for Diabetes

Laura Shane-McWhorter, PharmD, BCPS, BC-ADM, CDE, FASCP, FAADE

Key Concepts

- Biologically based practices included in complementary and alternative medicine (CAM) use different substances such as different herbs or foods and include dietary supplements. Dietary supplements may include botanical, nonbotanical, and other products.

- The Dietary Supplement Health and Education Act (DSHEA) of 1994 provides a specific definition of dietary supplements.

- Many persons with diabetes use dietary supplements to lower blood glucose or treat diabetes-related comorbidities or complications.

- There are several reasons for concern with the use of CAM and dietary supplements.

- Dietary supplements contain various pharmacologically active ingredients with varying theorized mechanisms of action.

- Dietary supplements may produce side effects and drug interactions.

- Diabetes educators need a clear understanding of dietary supplements to provide unbiased, nonjudgmental information to persons with diabetes.

- Evidence-based references should be used to answer questions about dietary supplements.

Introduction

This chapter reviews information about dietary supplements, a part of biologically based practices that individuals may use to treat diabetes, its comorbidities, or complications. The ever-increasing number of persons with diabetes precipitates a continual interest in different therapeutic modalities. Along with traditional medications, individuals have turned to the use of nontraditional treatments, including biologically based practices, a subset of CAM. The National Institutes of Health (NIH) states there are 4 categories of CAM[1]:

- Natural products (such as dietary supplements or probiotics)
- Mind and body medicine (such as meditation, yoga, or acupuncture)

- Manipulative and body-based practices (spinal manipulation, massage therapy)
- Other practices (movement therapies, traditional healers in Native American culture, energy field manipulation, and whole medical systems such as Ayurvedic and traditional Chinese medicine)

According to NIH, complementary medicine is used along with conventional medicine, and alternative medicine is used instead of conventional medicine (replaces conventional medicine).

The National Health Statistics Report, published by the Centers for Disease Control and Prevention, indicated that Americans spend $34 billion annually on CAM treatment.[2] A total of $14.8 billion was

---

Case: Patient Inquires About Dietary Supplements

TP, a 59-year-old woman with type 2 diabetes, hypertension, hyperlipidemia, atrial fibrillation, and depression, is seen for diabetes education.

- TP is taking a combination of glipizide and metformin (Metaglip®, Bristol-Myers Squibb) for diabetes; a combination of losartan and HCTZ for hypertension (Hyzaar®, Merck); simvastatin (Zocor®, Merck) for hyperlipidemia; digoxin (Lanoxin®, Glaxo SmithKline) for rate control in atrial fibrillation; warfarin (Coumadin®, Bristol-Myers Squibb), a blood thinner, to prevent thromboembolic events associated with atrial fibrillation; and sertraline (Zoloft®, Pfizer) for depression.

- She has heard that some dietary supplements may be useful for diabetes and for her other diseases. These include gymnema sylvestre, cinnamon, fenugreek, ginseng, and chromium. She has also heard that garlic may be useful for hypertension and hyperlipidemia, and St John's wort may be useful for

depression. She is experienceing muscle aches with the simvastatin and is wondering if a supplement may help alleviate the pain.

TP is also concerned about taking so many prescription products. She is hopeful that she may be able to discontinue some of these drugs and substitute them with "natural" products that have no side effects and are more holistic. She asks her diabetes educator to help select some products that may be better alternatives to all the drugs she has to take.

- What products mentioned by TP may be useful? Which ones should be avoided?

- What other "natural" products may TP or another patient consider taking for diabetes or diabetes-related conditions?

- What sources of information may be useful for a diabetes educator to answer the questions TP has raised?

This chapter will help diabetes educators answer some of the questions raised in this case. Diabetes educators must be knowledgeable about products that individuals may consider for diabetes or related conditions.

---

spent on nonvitamin, nonmineral dietary supplements. The DSHEA defines "dietary supplement" as "a product taken by mouth that contains a 'dietary ingredient' intended to supplement the diet."[3] The ingredients may include herbs or other botanical ingredients, vitamins, minerals, amino acids, and other substances. In DSHEA, dietary supplements are considered "foods" rather than "drugs." Biologically based practices include dietary supplements.

Dietary Supplement Health and Education Act of 1994

Dietary supplement use is part of biologically based practices. Prior to 1994, these products were classified as either foods or drugs. In 1994, Congress passed the DSHEA. This legislation created a separate category for botanicals and other products that classifies them as dietary supplements.[3] Hence, supplements are considered foods and are excluded from the same stringent approval process required for drugs. Under DSHEA, supplements do not require proof of safety and effectiveness.

Standards of "purity and potency" are the responsibility of manufacturers. Problems with adulteration and contaminants have posed serious threats.[4] A possible solution is to use standardized products since standardization guarantees that each dose provides a consistent level of the active ingredient. However, standardized extracts may not contain all of the therapeutic ingredients found in the natural product.

When enacted, DSHEA required that good manufacturing practices (GMPs) be established. In 2007, the Food and Drug Administration (FDA) issued a final rule on proposed changes to GMP dietary supplement standards.[5] This rule mandates that products be manufactured without adulterants or impurities and be labeled accurately. These changes are expected to improve manufacturing practices.

Dietary supplement manufacturers must comply with certain labeling requirements.[6] Labels must list the following: product name as well as the word "supplement"; net content quantity; manufacturer's, packer's, or distributor's name and place of business; and directions for use. The label must also include a "supplement facts panel" that lists the serving size, dietary ingredients, amount per serving size, and percent daily value (if established). Products fall under 1 of 3 types of product claims: health claims, nutrient content claims, or structure and function claims. This allows dietary supplement manufacturers to make claims regarding the ability to maintain "structure and function" of the body, but not regarding diagnosis, treatment, cure, or prevention of disease. For instance, a manufacturer may claim that a product "maintains a healthy prostate" but may not state that the product "treats benign prostatic hyperplasia."[7] If a manufacturer makes a claim stating that the product affects body structure or function, the label must include the following statement: "This statement has not been evaluated by the Food and Drug Administration (FDA). This product is not intended to diagnose, treat, cure, or prevent any disease."

An important change in the supplement industry is the Dietary Supplement and Non-Prescription Drug Consumer Protection Act (Public Law 109-462).[7,8] This legislation requires reporting of serious adverse events to the FDA based on specific information received from the public. Individuals and clinicians are encouraged to report supplement-related adverse outcomes through the FDA MedWatch program.[9] **Since patients and healthcare providers are not required to report these events, there may be underreporting of adverse outcomes.** Nevertheless, over half of Class 1 drug recalls (those that may result in serious harm or even death) from 2004 to 2012 were of supplements.[10] The September 2012 issue of *Consumer Reports* on vitamins and supplements stated that more than 6300 serious adverse events were reported to the FDA between 2007 and 2012, and 115 deaths occurred.[11]

Testing of Dietary Supplements

Resources are now available that enable consumers and healthcare professionals to verify the accuracy and purity of ingredients listed on the label of a dietary supplement. However, no available resources evaluate product efficacy.

Some organizations have established certification programs for dietary supplements. US Pharmacopeia (USP) has a program called the Dietary Supplement Verification Program (DSVP).[12] A product showing the "USP-verified" mark on the label indicates the label's product ingredients are accurate, the product is pure and will dissolve properly, and the product has been manufactured using GMPs. The USP Web site lists manufacturers that have gone through the evaluation process. National Sanitation Foundation (NSF) International also verifies products for label and content accuracy, checks the product for purity and for contaminants, and audits the manufacturing process for GMP compliance.[13] Consumer Lab (CL) also tests supplements for accuracy of ingredient identity, content, and purity.[14] The CL seal of approval is licensed for manufactured products that pass the review. Product names that have failed the review are available only to subscribers. The Natural Products Association (formerly National Nutritional Foods Association) also has a GMP program.[15]

Evaluating Claims Made by Manufacturers of Dietary Supplements

Diabetes educators need to be aware of deceptive marketing tactics used by manufacturers to promote their products. Educators may instruct individuals to check the FDA's MedWatch Web site[9] for information regarding products that may contain adulterants, such as steroids. For example, numerous weight-loss products have been found to contain prescription weight-loss drugs. An excellent handout called FDA 101: Health Fraud Awareness is found online, and diabetes educators may refer individuals to this site since one of the categories mentioned is "diabetes fraud," with claims such as "drop your blood sugar 50 points in 30 days" and "eliminate insulin resistance."[16]

Examples of phrases with misleading claims listed in the *Handbook of Nonprescription Drugs* include the following[17]:

◆ Lists disease states or hints that the product may be used to treat conditions normally treated with prescriptions
◆ States that the product has similar efficacy to (or may be used as an alternative) prescription or nonprescription drugs
◆ Lists a wide variety of unrelated clinical conditions ("works for everything") that the product may treat

- States only benefits of the product (and not harmful side effects)
- Neglects to provide information on the label such as expiration date, lot number, or contact information for the manufacturing company
- Uses "pseudo-medical" terminology such as "detoxify," "purify," or "breakthrough treatment"
- Uses terms such as "revolutionary therapy" or "miraculous discovery" or other statements that indicate the product is superior to prescriptions
- Suggests the product is more expensive because it works so well

Resources

A beneficial reference for diabetes educators is Natural Standard, a database that "grades" the efficacy of different supplements for a specific indication according to available evidence.[18] The different evidence grades include the following:

A: Strong scientific evidence
B: Positive scientific evidence
C: Unclear scientific evidence
D: Negative scientific evidence
F: Strong negative scientific evidence

The FDA Center for Food Safety and Applied Nutrition Web site helps individuals evaluate information about dietary supplements. Healthcare professionals can read and direct persons to the center's articles on supplements.[19,20] The Web site includes points to consider, such as these:

- Check with a healthcare provider before using a supplement.
- Understand that some supplements may interact with prescription or over-the-counter medicines.
- Be aware that supplements can have unwanted effects during surgery.
- Know how to report adverse effects of dietary supplements.
- Know how to search the World Wide Web for information on dietary supplements, such as finding out who operates the site, the purpose of the site, information source and references, and whether the information is current.

The following information is helpful when counseling people on the use of dietary supplements[17]:

- Purchase products that have a quality seal on the label, such as the USP's DSVP or that of NSF International, or products that comply with content claims assessed by CL.
- Purchase products from reputable companies that have a reputation to uphold. Manufacturers that also produce prescription or nonprescription medications are more likely to have GMPs in place. Some examples are American Home Products or drugstore chain store brands.
- Continue to use the same brand and formulation. Consider that variability may exist between different product lots. Read the label carefully and do not exceed the recommended dose; do not select a product that lacks dosing recommendations, lot numbers, expiration dates, or contact information for the manufacturer. Do not share the product with others.
- Be cautious about product use in children, pregnant or lactating women, and the elderly.
- Do not combine a supplement with alcohol or drugs that have sedative properties.
- Consider that the product may result in side effects or interact with other medications or supplements. Be especially wary of combining a supplement with blood-thinning drugs.
- Due to possible adverse events or drug interactions, discontinue a supplement 2 weeks before surgery.
- Do not substitute a dietary supplement for a prescription drug.
- Consider that the term "natural" does not mean devoid of side effects or other potential problems.
- Do not expect unrealistic results—if it sounds too good to be true, it probably is.
- Do not substitute the product for a healthy diet, physical activity, or proper rest.
- Use a diary to track the effectiveness of the product and continue to monitor blood glucose, A1C, blood pressure, and lipids.

Reasons for Concern Regarding Use of CAM

No large survey currently available evaluates how many persons with diabetes use CAM, but the educator must be aware that many individuals do use CAM and there are numerous surveys describing CAM use. One survey indicated that persons with diabetes are 1.6 times more likely than persons without diabetes to use CAM.[21] Some surveys have reported that about one third of individuals with diabetes use CAM.[22,23]

The National Health Interview Survey reported that almost half of individuals with diabetes use some type of CAM treatment and 22% use herbal products.[24] In a survey of adults with diabetes, 67% were using some type of vitamin or supplement.[25] A different survey found that herbs and vitamins were used by 81.9% of persons with diabetes, and that product use varied among different ethnic groups. For example, Hispanics used herbs such as nopal or aloe vera, and Asians used products such as ginkgo biloba.[26] A review of medication histories of 459 individuals with diabetes indicated that 55% use a supplement on a daily basis.[27] Children have also used CAM. A survey of parents found that 18% were administering CAM to their children with type 1 diabetes, and modalities included homeopathy, modified diet, and supplements such as aloe vera and cinnamon.[28]

There is no reliable source of information that explains why patients take supplements, but perhaps increased medication and provider visit costs may prompt individuals to seek more easily accessible products.[27] Other factors may include a desire to avoid adverse effects of conventional medications since supplements are viewed as "natural"; the limited efficacy of traditional medications to "cure" diseases; and the ever-powerful influence of friends, coworkers, and possibly the media that suggests supplement use.[29] Diabetes severity and duration may influence supplement use. The National Health Interview Survey (2002 and 2007) suggested that persons with more severe diabetes had nearly twice the odds of using CAM. Severity was based on count of measures of severity, such as 5 or more years since diagnosis, use of insulin or oral hypoglycemic agents, and at least 1 functional limitation secondary to the diabetes

as well as 3 known diabetes complications.[30] Those with diabetes duration greater than 10 years had a 66% higher CAM use compared with those whose diabetes duration was less than 10 years.[30] Hundreds of natural product ingredients have been used to treat diabetes and its comorbidities.[31]

Summarized below are reasons for concern regarding CAM use. There are a number of reasons for concern with dietary supplement use that educators need to convey to persons with diabetes. Table 20.1 summarizes these concerns, with details provided in the paragraphs that follow.

Side Effects and Drug Interactions

Potential side effects and drug interactions of dietary supplements are 2 critical issues that must be considered. Since only 33.4% of patients tell their healthcare provider they are using herbal products or dietary supplements,[24] it may be difficult to determine whether there are any drug interactions. An individual may experience a side effect that the provider attributes to another medication. Since persons with diabetes take several medications, concomitant use of dietary supplements may result in toxicity secondary to exaggerated or subtherapeutic effects of medications. Individuals may concomitantly take several different supplements, and the potential for interactions with conventional medications may dramatically increase. For instance, a person may be taking garlic along with fenugreek, and the potential for bleeding reactions secondary to the intrinsic

TABLE 20.1   Reasons for Concern With Dietary Supplement Use
• Potential side effects
• Drug interactions
• Lack of proven effectiveness
• Product variability
• Lack of product standardization
• Possibility of contamination
• Possibility of misidentification
• Delay in using more effective interventions
• Additional costs for medical care

antiplatelet activity of these agents may provide an additive danger to the individual.

Product Variability

Product variability is another reason for concern. Products are available as capsules, tablets, powders, or liquid forms that are water or alcohol based. The quality of botanical products may depend on what part of the plant was used, how it was grown and stored, length of storage, processing technique, and how the extract was prepared.[32] There may also be variability in doses and consistency of reported ingredients.[33] Lead contamination in some products has been reported.[34]

Lack of Standardization

Standardization should guarantee consistency between different lots as well as stability of the active ingredients. However, standardization is not a simple process, because the active constituents are unknown for many agents. A product that is standardized for certain markers may show consistency, but the marker may not be the active ingredient. Pharmacologic action may be due to additive or synergistic effects of several ingredients, but individual ingredients found separately may not have the same activity as the whole plant.[35] Active constituents in extracts or dried botanicals may vary due to differences in geographic location or soil, exposure to sunlight or rainfall, harvest time, and methods of drying, storage, and processing. These variables may affect pharmacologic activity.[36]

"Other Ingredient" Concerns

Other cautions involve potential misidentification, mislabeling, possible addition of unnatural toxic substances such as heavy metals and steroids, or contamination with microbes, pesticides, fumigants, and radioactive products.[36] For example, a dietary supplement for diabetes was found to contain an unlabeled ingredient, glyburide, a prescription sulfonylurea.[37]

Increased Costs

Another concern is possible increased indirect costs because individuals may substitute proven medications

with ineffective therapies or delay treatment and thus have needless problems. Costs may include hospitalizations, acute problems (ketoacidosis, acute hyperglycemia), or complications such as retinopathy.[38] Other costs include decreased work productivity or ability to function in social or occupational settings.

Points for Education

Discuss with interested individuals how dietary supplements are subject to variability, may or may not have standardized ingredients, or may be vulnerable to product contamination or substitution with unwanted ingredients. All of these factors make the individual vulnerable to potential side effects, drug interactions, and possible increased costs.

Review of Dietary Supplements

Persons with diabetes may inquire most often about products to achieve 2 main goals: lowering blood glucose and decreasing the complications of diabetes. Not all products proposed for these uses can be recommended as safe supplements, therapies, or food, as this part of the chapter will show. The sections that follow describe characteristics of (1) botanical and nonbotanical products used to lower blood glucose and (2) botanical and nonbotanical products to treat diabetes complications. Tables 20.2 and 20.3 provide specific information regarding each entity's name, evidence grade (if available through the Natural Standard grading system), chemical constituents, mechanism of action, side effects, and drug interactions. In several cases the evidence grade assigned by Natural Standard may be lower than expected from study results—possibly because the design and other details of the study may not have warranted a higher evidence grade.

Botanical and Nonbotanical Products to Lower Blood Glucose

Patients may have heard about the following products for use in lowering blood glucose. Not all are safe or effective. Each is discussed in detail in the paragraphs that follow. The educator should note that these are only a few agents and that many other products have been reputed to lower blood glucose levels.

- Aloe
- Berberine
- Bitter melon
- Chromium
- Cinnamon
- Fenugreek
- Ginseng
- Gymnema
- Milk thistle
- Nopal
- Probiotics

Botanical and Nonbotanical Products to Decrease Diabetes Complications

Patients may also inquire about the following products for use in decreasing diabetes complications. Again, not all are safe or effective, and only a few products have been highlighted, although numerous other products are available that patients may use. Each is discussed separately in the paragraphs that follow.

- Alpha-lipoic acid
- Benfotiamine
- Coenzyme Q10
- Fish oil
- Garlic
- St John's wort
- Vitamin D

Botanical and Nonbotanical Products Used to Lower Blood Glucose

Aloe, berberine, bitter melon, chromium, cinnamon, fenugreek, ginseng, gymnema, milk thistle, nopal, and probiotics are among the different products persons with diabetes may use to lower blood glucose levels. Information regarding chemical constituents, mechanism of action, side effects, and drug interactions for each of these products is found in Table 20.2. Each of these 11 products is reviewed separately following Table 20.2.

Aloe

Aloe (*Aloe vera L*) is a desert plant with a cactus-like appearance that belongs to the family *Liliaceae*.[39–41] Aloe gel is the clear substance extracted from the leaf core after the main stalk has been removed. Aloe gel is used topically for burns, sunburn, wound healing, moisturizing, and other skin problems, including psoriasis and seborrhea. Orally, it has also been used to enhance the immune system and to treat asthma and diabetes. While aloe is mostly a benign agent, there are some instances of questionable safety.[39–42] Another plant component, dried aloe leaf juice, was a former ingredient in nonprescription laxative formulations.[39,41]

Evidence

In a small, uncontrolled study in 5 persons with type 1 diabetes, improvements in fasting blood glucose and A1C levels were reported when aloe was given for 4 to 14 weeks.[43] In a 6-week study of 40 persons with newly diagnosed type 2 diabetes, aloe decreased fasting glucose and triglycerides ($P = .01$).[40] Another study showed that aloe added to glibenclamide (a sulfonylurea) resulted in a decline in fasting glucose and triglycerides, without hypoglycemia.[44] A 2-month randomized controlled study compared aloe gel in 30 persons with type 2 diabetes on oral medications (sulfonylureas and metformin) with placebo in another 30 persons with type 2 diabetes.[45] A1C declined by 0.7% in the aloe group compared with a 0.5% increase in the placebo group ($P = .036$). Fasting glucose and low-density lipoprotein (LDL) declined significantly in the aloe group compared with placebo ($P = .036$ for fasting glucose; $P = .004$ for LDL). Although triglycerides decreased, the results were not significant.

Summary

Doses of aloe are variable, ranging from 50 to 600 mg per day of aloe gel.[39,45] In 2 studies, 15 mL twice daily of aloe leaf gel was used.[40,44] Aloe gel contains glucomannan, a polysaccharide that is high in fiber and may slow or prevent glucose absorption. However, aloe juice contains cathartics, and there is concern that there may be inadvertent inclusion of these components in aloe products. Aloe is used as capsules, tablets, or liquids. It is highly used by Hispanics

TABLE 20.2	Botanical and Nonbotanical Products Used to Lower Blood Glucose		
Product	*Chemical Constituents*	*Mechanism of Action*	*Side Effects & Drug Interactions*
Aloe Evidence grade C	Various ingredients[39,40] • Aloe gel contains glucomannan (polysaccharide similar to guar gum and glycoprotein)	Fiber may delay or prevent glucose absorption[39,40]	*Side effects:* Acute hepatitis, thyroid dysfunction[41] *Drug interactions:* • Possible hypoglycemia if combined with secretagogues • Intraoperative blood loss in surgery patients where sevoflurane was used[42]
Berberine Evidence grade C	• Isoquinoline alkaloid[39,46–50]	Various mechanisms[47,48] • Enhances glucose-stimulated insulin secretion • GLUT4 translocation • Alpha-glucosidase inhibition • Enhanced AMPK • Upregulates LDL receptors	*Side effects[39,46]:* • Abdominal upset, constipation • Kernicterus *Drug interactions[39,50]:* • Increased levels of drugs metabolized by CYP3A4 (cyclosporine, certain statins, and calcium channel blockers) • May be involved in CYP2D6 metabolism • Additive hypoglycemia if combined with secretagogues
Bitter melon Evidence grade C	Various ingredients[39,51] • Momordin • Charantin • Polypeptide-P • Vicine[39,51]	Various mechanisms[39,51–53] • Hypoglycemic action • Tissue glucose uptake; glycogen synthesis • Inhibition of enzymes involved in glucose production • Enhanced glucose oxidation of Glucose-6-phosphate-dehydrogenase (G6PDH) pathway • AMPK pathway activation • Alpha-glucosidase inhibition	*Side effects[39,51]:* • Gastrointestinal (GI) discomfort • Hypoglycemic coma • Favism • Hemolytic anemia in persons with G6PDH deficiency • Contains known abortifacients (a and b momorcharin) • Seeds have produced vomiting, death in children *Drug interactions[39,54]:* • Hypoglycemia when used with sulfonylureas
Chromium Evidence grade C	Trivalent chromium[39,61,62]	Various mechanisms[39,61,62] • May enhance cellular effects of insulin • May ↑ number of insulin receptors • May ↑ insulin binding or insulin activation • Lipid metabolism modulation in peripheral tissues	*Side effects[39,61]:* • Related to excessive intake and include renal toxicity *Drug interactions[39,61]:* • May decrease blood glucose if used with secretagogues

TABLE 20.2 Botanical and Nonbotanical Products Used to Lower Blood Glucose (continued)			
Product	*Chemical Constituents*	*Mechanism of Action*	*Side Effects & Drug Interactions*
Cinnamon Evidence grade D	Procyanidin type-A polymers[39,71]	Various mechanisms[39,71-76] • Increased insulin sensitivity and action • Increased insulin receptor phosphorylation and improved insulin signaling • Increased cell/tissue glucose uptake • Promotes glycogen synthesis • Alpha-glucosidase inhibition • Peroxisome proliferator-activated receptor activation • May help delay gastric emptying and reduce excess postprandial glucose and triglyceride levels	*Side effects[39]:* • No side effects reported; may cause irritation or dermatitis if used topically • High coumarin content may result in hepatotoxicity, per animal models *Drug interactions[39,71]:* • May decrease blood glucose if used with secretagogues • Due to a coumarin ingredient, it may theoretically result in bleeding if combined with anticoagulants • Prolonged use of large amounts may theoretically result in hepatotoxicity in persons susceptible to or with preexisting liver disease

Fenugreek
 	
Evidence grade C for type 1 diabetes, grade B for type 2 diabetes
	Various ingredients[39,82,83]
	
	• Saponins
	
	• Glycosides
	
	• Seeds contain:
	  –alkaloids
	  –4-hydroxyisoleucine
	  –fenugreekine
		Various mechanisms[39,82,83]
		
		• Delayed gastric emptying
		
		• Slowed carbohydrate absorption
		
		• Glucose transport inhibition
		
		• ↑ insulin receptors
		
		• Improved peripheral glucose utilization
		
		• Possible stimulation of insulin secretion
			Side effects[39,84]:
			
			• Diarrhea, gas
			
			• Uterine contractions
			
			• Allergic reactions
			
			Drug interactions[39,85]:
			
			• May ↑ anticoagulant effects of warfarin or herbs with anticoagulant activity (boldo, garlic, ginger)

Ginseng Evidence grade C for type 2 diabetes	Ginsenosides[39]	Various mechanisms[39,91-96] • May decrease carbohydrate absorption in portal circulation • May decrease glucose transport and uptake • Modulation of insulin secretion	*Side effects[39,91]:* • Insomnia, headache, restlessness • Increased blood pressure or heart rate • Mastalgia • Mood changes, nervousness *Drug interactions[39,91]:* • Decreased warfarin, diuretic effectiveness Additive estrogenic effects • Possible increased effects of certain analgesics and antidepressants • Possible additive hypoglycemia with secretagogues

(continued)

TABLE 20.2	Botanical and Nonbotanical Products Used to Lower Blood Glucose (continued)		
Product	*Chemical Constituents*	*Mechanism of Action*	*Side Effects & Drug Interactions*
Gymnema Evidence grade B for type 1 diabetes and type 2 diabetes	Various ingredients[39,104,105] • Gymnemosides • Saponins • Stigmasterol • Amino acid derivatives –betaine –choline –trimethylamine	Various mechanisms[39,104–109] • Impairs ability to discriminate "sweet" taste • ↑ enzymes promoting glucose uptake • May stimulate beta cells • May increase beta cell numbers • May stimulate insulin release	*Side effects*[39,110]: • May cause hypoglycemia • Hepatitis *Drug interactions*[39]: • Possible hypoglycemia if combined with secretagogues
Milk thistle Evidence grade C (persons with diabetes mellitus and cirrhosis)	Various ingredients[115,116] • Silymarin, containing silybin, silychristine, and silidianin	Various mechanisms[39,115,116] • Decreased insulin resistance • Reduced oxidative stress on pancreatic beta cells • Other anti-inflammatory and immunomodulating effects	*Side effects*[39,115]: • Diarrhea, weakness, sweating • Possible allergic reactions if also allergic to ragweed, marigolds, daisies, chrysanthemums • May have estrogenic effects, so women with breast or uterine cancer should avoid its use *Drug interactions*[39,115]: • May increase warfarin concentrations and decrease levels of exogenously administered estrogens • Beneficial interactions with hepatotoxic agents such as acetaminophen, antipsychotics, alcohol
Nopal Evidence grade C	Various ingredients[39] • Mucopolysaccharide fibers • Pectin	Various mechanisms[39,123] • Slows carbohydrate absorption • Decreases lipid absorption • Possibly increases insulin sensitivity	*Side effects*[39,123,124]: • Diarrhea, nausea, abdominal fullness • Increased stool volume *Drug interactions*[39,125]: • Potential hypoglycemia when combined with oral glucose-lowering agents
Probiotics No evidence grade assigned	Numerous species[130,131] Examples: • Lactobacillus species • Bifidobacterium species • Streptococcus thermophilus • Saccharomyces boulardii	Theoretical[130–133]: • Release of beneficial organic and free fatty acids that act against pathogenic microbes • Possible enhanced incretin action • Decreased inflammation • Decreased insulin resistance	*Side effects*[130]: • GI upset • Constipation • Possible systemic infections *Drug interactions*[130]: • Antibiotics, antifungals: Decreased probiotic effects • Immunosuppressants (cyclosporine, methotrexate, etc): Weakened state may lead to infections due to probiotic microbes

(the Spanish word for aloe is *sábila*) in shakes and smoothies. A case report of prolonged bleeding when used with the anesthetic agent sevoflurane warrants discontinuation 2 weeks before surgery.[42] Cases of acute hepatitis and thyroid dysfunction have been reported.[41] There is insufficient evidence for use of aloe as an oral product in diabetes. Short-term use has decreased fasting glucose, triglycerides, LDL, and A1C. However, supplementation is not recommended, especially due to the potential contamination with cathartic ingredients and problems with fluid and electrolyte disturbances.

Berberine

Berberine (*Coptis chinensis [Huanglian or French]*) is an isoquinoline alkaloid extracted from many different plants, such as the Chinese herb, *Coptis chinensis [Huanglian or French]*, goldenseal, tree tumeric, European barberry, and others. It was found to lower glucose when it was used to treat bacterial diarrhea in persons with diabetes.[46–50] It also has been shown to have lipid-lowering and weight-loss effects.[47]

Evidence

Berberine was compared with placebo in a 3-month study in 116 persons with newly diagnosed type 2 diabetes mellitus (T2DM) and hyperlipidemia.[47] There was a significant decrease in A1C, fasting, and postprandial glucose in the berberine group compared with placebo ($P < .0001$ for each parameter). A1C decreased from 7.5% to 6.6% in the berberine group and 7.6% to 7.3% in the placebo group. There were also significant decreases favoring berberine in LDL cholesterol ($P < .0001$), weight ($P = .034$), and systolic blood pressure ($P = .038$).

A different randomized study evaluated 97 persons with T2DM for 2 months.[48] Of these, 50 were randomized to berberine, 26 to metformin, and 21 to rosiglitazone. Fasting glucose and A1C decreased significantly from baseline in all 3 groups ($P < .001$ for berberine and metformin; $P < .01$ for rosiglitazone). A1C decreased from 8.3% to 6.8% in the berberine group, 9.4% to 7.2% in the metformin group, and 8.3% to 6.8% in the rosiglitazone group. Triglycerides decreased significantly only in the berberine group ($P < .01$).

Another randomized controlled trial evaluated 2 groups with T2DM—one group was newly diagnosed and the other was poorly controlled.[49] The newly diagnosed group took berberine or metformin for 3 months. In both groups there was a significant decline from baseline in A1C, fasting glucose, and postprandial glucose ($P < .01$ compared with baseline). A1C decreased from 9.5% to 7.5% in the berberine group and from 9.2% to 7.7% in the metformin group. Fasting glucose also decreased in both groups. The authors did not provide a statistical analysis of the comparison between berberine and metformin, but the numbers were very similar. Patients in the poorly controlled group continued their medications (oral agents or insulin), and berberine was added for 3 months. A1C decreased from 8.1% to 7.3%, and fasting and postprandial glucose also decreased. The decreases were all statistically significant ($P < .001$ for all 3 parameters).

Summary

Berberine may work in a variety of ways. It may increase or enhance glucose-stimulated insulin secretion, facilitate GLUT4 translocation, exert alpha-glucosidase inhibitor activity, enhance adenosine monophosphate activated protein kinase (AMPK), increase insulin receptor expression, and possibly upregulate LDL receptors.[47,48] The main side effects are abdominal upset and constipation.[46] However, it should not be used by pregnant or lactating women or in infants, because it may result in fatal kernicterus.[39] Caution is warranted when used with other agents because berberine may inhibit certain Cytochrome P 450 enzymes (CYP3A4) and thus increase levels of drugs metabolized by this system (cyclosporine, certain statins, some calcium channel blockers).[39] It may also be involved in CYP2D6 metabolism.[50] In a meta-analysis comprising 14 randomized controlled trials and 1068 persons, berberine was significantly more effective than placebo, as effective as metformin or sulfonylureas or glitazones, and was also effective when combined with glucose-lowering agents.[46] Doses used in studies have been 500 mg 2 to 3 times daily.

Bitter Melon

Bitter melon (*Momordica charantia*) is also known by other names, such as bitter gourd, bitter apple, bitter cucumber, karolla, and karela. It is a vegetable cultivated in tropical areas, including India, Asia, South America, and Africa. A member of the melon family, bitter melon is yellow-orange, resembles a gherkin, and is bitter but edible.[39] Bitter melon has been used for a variety of reasons, including diabetes, cancer, HIV, and psoriasis.[39–54] Women have used it to help induce menstruation and as an abortifacient.[51]

Evidence

Most studies of bitter melon in humans involve few patients, are of short duration, and provide only vague details of the study design, including blinding and randomization. Studies have been done primarily in individuals with type 2 diabetes,[55] although a small study used injectable polypeptide-P (an insulin-like polypeptide isolated from bitter melon) and included both persons with type 1 diabetes and persons with type 2 diabetes.[56] Results from various studies have shown that there are responders as well as nonresponders. The first randomized, double-blind, placebo-controlled study was conducted in 40 adults with newly diagnosed or poorly controlled type 2 diabetes, and there was a slight nonsignificant decrease in A1C in both groups.[57] A 4-week randomized, double-blind, active-control trial compared 3 different doses of bitter melon with metformin in 123 persons with newly diagnosed type 2 diabetes.[58] Metformin and the highest dose of bitter melon decreased fructosamine significantly, although metformin showed a greater lowering. The difference between treatments was not significant. Contrary to previous studies, bitter melon did not decrease 2-hour glucose levels after an oral glucose tolerance test (OGTT) challenge. A Cochrane Review of randomized controlled trials comparing bitter melon with placebo or other controls reported that there is insufficient evidence to support its use.[59]

Summary

Dosage forms include juice, powder, vegetable pulp suspensions, injections, and now capsules.[60] Manufacturers have stated the recommended dose is 3 g per day.[60] Some sources recommend eating 1 small unripe melon daily or drinking 50 to 100 mL of fresh juice daily with food.[51] Bitter melon contains a variety of ingredients that may produce hypoglycemic effects and affect glucose uptake.[39,51] Bitter melon may inhibit enzymes involved in glucose production and glucose oxidation, which may be of importance in persons of Mediterranean ancestry.[39,51] Adenosine monophosphate activated protein kinase activation[52] and alpha-glucosidase inhibition are other mechanisms.[53] Medical supervision is always necessary when using bitter melon, due to the possibility of adverse effects, especially in certain populations, such as those of Mediterranean ancestry, women of childbearing age, or those with melon allergies. As a food, bitter melon is a safe agent; as a supplement, it may not be safe. A well-designed study reported that a capsule form was not as effective as previously thought.[57]

Chromium

Chromium is a trace element found in certain foods such as brewer's yeast, oysters, mushrooms, liver, potatoes, beef, cheese, and fresh vegetables.[39] Chromium has been used for weight loss and to improve lipid and glycemic control.[39,61,62] Increased chromium levels with supplementation is not the factor that improves hyperglycemia. The concept of chromium responders versus nonresponders has been suggested.[62] Responders are more likely to have higher baseline fasting glucose and A1C, and be more insulin resistant than nonresponders.

Chromium deficiency may occur if a person is on total parenteral nutrition (TPN); during pregnancy; or if the person has a poor diet, high glucose intake, or poor glucose control.[39,61] Currently, no evidence shows that chromium deficiency rates in persons with diabetes are different from those of the general population. The Food and Nutrition Board of the Institute of Medicine (IOM) determined there was not sufficient evidence to set an estimated average requirement for chromium.[63] An adequate intake was set based on estimated mean intakes. The adequate intake for young men is 35 mcg per day (30 mcg per day for age 51 and older) and 25 mcg per day for young women (20 mcg per day for age 51 and older). Because few serious adverse effects are reported from excess intake of chromium from food, no tolerable upper level was established. Since there is no accurate assay for body chromium stores, it is difficult to determine when an individual has chromium deficiency and the efficacy of supplementation.

Evidence

Positive effects of chromium have been shown in persons with type 1 diabetes or type 2 diabetes, gestational diabetes, and impaired glucose tolerance.[39,64–67]

Studies have shown variable benefits for diabetes and hyperlipidemia. Studies have demonstrated the safety of large doses of chromium.[64]

In a randomized, double-blind, placebo-controlled trial in 180 Chinese persons, fasting blood glucose and A1C levels decreased significantly in the group taking 1000 mcg per day of chromium picolinate compared with the group taking 500 mcg per day and the placebo group.[64] However, these individuals may have significantly different dietary chromium intake compared with the US population and may be leaner than many obese persons with type 2 diabetes in the United States. A meta-analysis of randomized controlled trials evaluated the impact of chromium supplementation on insulin and glucose and concluded the data were inconclusive.[68]

Chromium picolinate has been combined with biotin, a water-soluble B vitamin that plays a role in carbohydrate and lipid metabolism and enhances the effect of chromium on glucose disposal and lipid metabolism.[69] A 90-day randomized, double-blind, placebo-controlled study demonstrated improved glycemic control with a combination of chromium and biotin in people with type 2 diabetes.[69] Mean A1C declined by 0.54% from a baseline of 8.73% in the chromium group and by 0.34% from a baseline of 8.46% in the placebo group (*P* = .03 vs. placebo). Mean fasting glucose also decreased significantly in the chromium group.

In 40 persons with newly diagnosed T2DM, half were randomized to 9 g of a brewer's yeast extract containing 42 mcg of chromium, and the other half were randomized to placebo.[70] After 3 months, A1C decreased from 9.5% to 6.86% in the chromium group (*P* < .001), fasting glucose and LDL declined significantly (*P* < .001), and triglycerides also decreased significantly. The placebo group had slight, nonsignificant decreases in these clinical values.

Summary

Although higher doses of chromium have been studied and shown to be effective, a typical dose is 200 mcg per day.[39] Short-term, dose-related responses have been shown, and doses up to 1000 mcg per day for 64 months have not shown adverse effects.[61] However, more study is needed. Results from chromium research are not conclusive, particularly in light of the lack of information regarding the most appropriate

biomarkers for chromium or the most appropriate formulation. If used, the picolinate salt appears to be the most appropriate form. Supplements containing chromium picolinate in combination with biotin have shown promising results.

Cinnamon

Cinnamon (*Cinnamomum cassia*) comes from an evergreen tree that grows in tropical climates, and the aromatic bark is removed in short lengths and dried.[39] Cinnamon has been used in both type 1 diabetes and type 2 diabetes and for gastrointestinal (GI) complaints such as dyspepsia and flatulence. Cinnamon is a popular flavoring agent in different foods and beverages.[39,71–76]

Evidence

A meta-analysis of 5 randomized controlled trials in 282 persons found that A1C does not decrease, although potential benefits in individual studies included decreases in fasting glucose and lipids.[77] A recent 90-day study in 102 individuals found that using 1 g daily showed a significant A1C decrease of 0.83% from baseline, while the control group had a 0.37% A1C reduction.[78] A smaller study in 58 persons with type 2 diabetes showed that 2 g daily decreased A1C by only 0.36%, but this was significant.[79] The Cochrane Database evaluated 10 randomized controlled studies of 577 persons and reported that evidence to support cinnamon use is insufficient.[80] A different meta-analysis of 10 clinical trials of 543 individuals reported that cinnamon does significantly improve fasting glucose by 24.6 mg/dL (1.36 mmol/L), improves fasting lipids, and slightly although nonsignificantly decreases A1C in short-term studies.[81]

Summary

Cinnamon is thought to enhance insulin sensitivity and action, increase insulin receptor phosphorylation and signaling, inhibit alpha-glucosidases, activate peroxisome proliferator-activated receptors, and reduce postprandial glucose levels.[39,71–76] Cinnamon has been found to decrease fasting glucose, total cholesterol, LDL, and triglycerides. Doses used have ranged from 1 to 6 g per day in divided doses.[39] It is unknown whether the most appropriate form is the whole powdered spice (possibly a combination of different types of cinnamon) or an aqueous extract.[75] Overall, cinnamon used as a food is safe.

Fenugreek

Fenugreek (*Trigonella foenum-graecum*) is a member of the *Leguminosae* family, along with other plants such as chickpeas, peanuts, and green peas. The plant grows in India, Egypt, and other parts of the Middle East and has been used for centuries as a cooking spice and flavoring agent and for various other purposes.[39,82–85] The seed has been used medicinally to treat diabetes, constipation, and hyperlipidemia. Fenugreek has also been used postpartum with a substance called jaggery to promote lactation, although there are no studies to verify its efficacy for this use.

Evidence

There are few human studies on fenugreek. Most are short-term involving few patients and do not adequately report details. A 10-day study in 10 persons with type 1 diabetes reported a decrease in fasting glucose and lipids.[86] A 6-month trial evaluated 60 persons with inadequately controlled type 2 diabetes.[87] Twice-daily fenugreek powder decreased fasting and postprandial glucose, and A1C decreased from 9.6% to 8.4% after 8 weeks.[87] In a different 2-month study in 25 persons with newly diagnosed type 2 diabetes, a hydroalcoholic fenugreek seed extract improved "area under the curve" blood glucose, insulin levels, hypertriglyceridemia, and high-density lipoprotein (HDL) cholesterol.[88] Fenugreek, at a dose of 6.3 g daily, in combination with sulfonylureas, has been shown to decrease A1C from a baseline of 8.02% to 6.56% after 12 weeks of use in 69 persons with type 2 diabetes.[89] Another small trial showed that when 10 g per day of powdered fenugreek seeds were first soaked in hot water and then later consumed, fasting glucose and triglycerides decreased significantly.[90]

Summary

Although fenugreek has been categorized by the FDA as generally recognized as safe (GRAS), the quality of studies evaluating this agent is suboptimal. Fenugreek contains a variety of alkaloids, coumarin-like ingredients, and other components that may affect carbohydrate absorption and glucose transport.[39,82–83] Most side effects are uncomfortable GI effects.[39] Pregnant women should avoid fenugreek since uterine contractions may occur.[39] Fenugreek has been used as a galactogogue, and since it may appear in breast milk, it could potentially adversely affect the breastfeeding infant. Individuals taking antiplatelet agents should avoid fenugreek. Hence, fenugreek has limited overall safety. The recommended dose is variable, although a typical dose is 10 to 15 g per day (as a single dose or divided with meals) or 1 g per day of a hydroalcoholic extract.[39,88] Medical supervision is warranted with fenugreek use.

Ginseng

Two main ginseng products are used in diabetes: Asian or Korean ginseng (*Panax ginseng* CA *Meyer*) and American ginseng (*Panax quinquefolius* L). The root is the part used.[39,91] Korean and American ginseng belong to the plant family *Araliaceae* and the genus *Panax*. Ginseng has been described as an adaptogen, an agent that may increase resistance to adverse influences such as infection and stress.[39,91] Individuals use ginseng to enhance physical or psychomotor performance and cognitive function and for immunomodulation, infections, sexual dysfunction, and diabetes.[39,91] Overall, ginseng is a popular product used for diabetes and other purposes because of a variety of pharmacologic effects.[39,91–97]

Evidence

Ginseng has been studied extensively for a variety of uses, and several studies focus on diabetes.[91–98] In persons with newly diagnosed type 2 diabetes, ginseng 100 mg or 200 mg daily was compared with placebo. Although baseline values for glucose and A1C levels were not stated, lower endpoint A1C values were reported.[98] The endpoint A1C level in the 200-mg ginseng group was 6%, and A1C was 6.5% in both the 100-mg and placebo groups. Hence, there may have been an issue with the accuracy of diagnosis or the study population. In 2 other studies, American ginseng was reported to acutely lower postprandial glucose levels when patients were given a 25-g OGTT.[92,93] In a double-blind crossover trial, Korean red ginseng improved erectile dysfunction, which may be of importance to men with diabetes.[39]

One double-blind, randomized, placebo-controlled crossover study in 19 persons with type 2 diabetes found that 6 g per day of Korean red ginseng for 12 weeks did not decrease A1C but the patients were at target A1C at baseline.[99] However, some OGTT indices improved, such as peak plasma glucose and peak plasma insulin. Also, fasting insulin sensitivity increased significantly. A different randomized, placebo-controlled, double-blind crossover study evaluated 2.2 g per day of Panax ginseng given for 4 weeks to 20 persons with type 2 diabetes.[100] Fasting glucose decreased slightly, but significantly, and insulin resistance also improved. A different study in 15 overweight or obese subjects (with impaired glucose tolerance or newly diagnosed type 2 diabetes) found that administration for 30 days of ginseng root extract 8 g per day, ginsenoside Re, or placebo did not improve beta cell function or insulin sensitivity.[101] A systematic review evaluated Panax ginseng for various medical disorders and found that results are promising for glucose metabolism and immune response moderation but that further studies are needed.[102] This review emphasized that studies use a variety of preparations, and this may be problematic.

Summary

Ginseng is a complex product that contains several ginsenosides with varying effects on blood pressure and the central nervous system.[39] Some estimates indicate that 6 million Americans use ginseng regularly for a variety of therapeutic reasons, including increased energy.[39] Although ginseng is used for a variety of reasons, it has been studied in type 2 diabetes. Ginseng may affect glucose transport and insulin secretion.[39,91–97] The 2 main types of ginseng used for diabetes are Asian and American; hence, doses may vary. Asian ginseng is dosed at 200 mg per day.[39,98] American ginseng is dosed at 3 g per day, right before and up to 2 hours before a meal.[39,92,93] Other forms of ginseng used range from fresh and dried roots to extracts, solutions, sodas, teas, and cosmetics. Length of use should be limited to 3 months, due to concerns about hormone-like effects.[39] There has been inconsistency between the actual amount of active ginsenosides contained in ginseng products and the amount stated on the label.[103] Although ginseng may provide some benefits to persons with diabetes, it is difficult to know the appropriate form and dose, and there are a variety of side effects and drug interactions.

Gymnema

A member of the milkweed family, gymnema (*Gymnema sylvestre* R.Br.) is a woody climbing plant that is found in the tropical forests of India (where it is known as *gurmar*) and also in Africa.[39] Gymnema leaf has been used for centuries to treat diabetes and has a unique history of research and use.[104–114]

Evidence

There are only a few human studies. Trials conducted in persons with type 1 diabetes and in persons with type 2 diabetes reported decreases in levels of A1C, fasting blood glucose, and lipids.[111,112] However, these studies did not report important details of study design, such as blinding and randomization. In a study in type 1 diabetes, 27 subjects were followed for 6 to 30 months.[111] A1C declined from 12.8% at baseline to 9.5% after 6 to 8 months ($P < .001$). At the end of 30 months, only 6 individuals remained, and mean A1C was 8.2% (P values not reported).[111] In a study of 22 individuals with type 2 diabetes, A1C declined from 11.9% to 8.5% ($P < .001$) after 18 to 20 months. Fasting glucose and lipids also decreased.[112]

An open-label study evaluated 500 mg per day of gymnema or placebo for 3 months in 58 persons with type 2 diabetes.[113] A total of 39 took gymnema and 19 took either placebo or no supplement. A1C decreased approximately 1% in the gymnema group (9.6% to 8.6%; exact P not provided, but the authors stated it was significant). Fasting glucose also decreased significantly ($P < .005$). Postmeal glucose also declined (exact P not provided, but authors stated it was significant). There was even a small decrease in systolic blood pressure ($P < .005$).[113] Another article reported that 500 mg twice daily of an aqueous extract of gymnema leaf for 60 days in 11 patients reduced mean fasting glucose ($P < .005$) and postprandial glucose ($P < .02$).[114]

Summary

Gymnema has limited efficacy data in humans, although there are ongoing studies. Gymnema has been studied for up to 2 years in type 1 diabetes and type 2 diabetes. The gymnemosides may help stimulate glucose uptake and utilization as well as stimulate beta cell function.[39,104–109] Some have speculated that gymnema may help treat obesity since it binds to the same taste buds where sugar binds and thus may help curb sugar craving.[104] Typical doses are 400 mg per day, standardized to contain 24% gymnemic acids, although new aqueous extract forms are emerging.[39,114]

The product should not be used without medical supervision, because of potential hypoglycemia and a case report of hepatitis.[110] Doses of secretagogues may have to be adjusted if gymnema is used. Safety of gymnema may be a concern when combined with other diabetes medications.

Milk Thistle

Milk thistle (*Silybum marianum*) is a member of the aster family (*Asteraceae* or *Compositae*), which also includes daisies and thistles.[39,115] Milk thistle has been used extensively for various hepatic disorders and for nonalcoholic steatohepatitis.[116,117] It is used for uterine complaints and stimulating menstrual flow. In Europe, it is also used as a vegetable. Chemical constituents are found in the fruit, seeds, and leaves of the plant.

Evidence

Several studies have evaluated effects of milk thistle on hepatic disease with inconclusive results.[116] Studies in persons with type 2 diabetes have included those on insulin or oral agents. In a randomized open-label trial in a small number of persons with type 2 diabetes and cirrhosis, a number of benefits were reported, including improved glucose and liver function and lower insulin requirements.[118] In another small study of persons with cirrhosis, 10 persons on silymarin plus insulin treatment were compared with 10 persons on insulin plus L-ornithine and L-aspartate.[119] Certain liver function tests improved and mean random glucose decreased significantly in the silymarin group ($P < .001$).[119] A unique emerging role is decreased proteinuria when added to angiotensin-converting enzyme (ACE) inhibitors in persons with diabetes. A 3-month randomized, double-blind, placebo-controlled trial of 60 persons with proteinuria and at maximum doses of renin angiotensin system inhibitors evaluated the impact on proteinuria and inflammatory markers.[120] Half were assigned to 420 mg per day of silymarin and half to placebo. Urinary albumin to creatinine ratio (UACR) decreased significantly in the silymarin group. Serum malondialdehyde levels (a marker for oxidative stress) and urinary tumor necrosis factor-α (TNF-α) also decreased significantly.[120] The theorized protective mechanism is that silymarin decreases oxidative stress and inflammation.

In a more traditional 4-month double-blind small trial in persons on oral agents, A1C declined significantly from 7.8% at baseline to 6.8%.[121] A different study showed that milk thistle added to oral agents also resulted in a decreased A1C from 8.9% at baseline to 7.45%.[122]

Summary

Use of milk thistle has been proposed in diabetes to diminish insulin resistance.[118] Side effects include GI upset and possible allergies to members of the daisy family.[39,115] Milk thistle may have estrogenic effects, so women with breast or uterine cancer should avoid its use.[39] However, milk thistle may increase the clearance of exogenously administered estrogens.[39] Milk thistle may inhibit certain isoenzymes and thus increase serum concentrations of warfarin.[39] Beneficial drug interactions include the attenuation of hepatotoxicity of liver toxic drugs.[115] The typical dose of milk thistle for liver disease is 200 mg 3 times daily. Milk thistle is often standardized to contain 70% silymarin (140 mg of silymarin). Since phosphatidylcholine enhances oral absorption, preparations containing this ingredient may be dosed at 100 mg per day.[115] Doses differ from those used in clinical studies, which ranged from 280 to 800 mg per day. Overall, milk thistle may be safe to use and more information is emerging.

Nopal

Nopal (*Opuntia streptacantha*), also known as prickly pear, is a member of the cactus family.[39] Multiple species are known as *Opuntia*, including *Opuntia megacantha*, *Opuntia ficus indica*, and *Opuntia fuliginosa*. Research has focused on *Opuntia streptacantha Lemaire* to lower blood glucose. Nopal originated as a food source in Mexico; the stems, flowers, and fruit are used. Leaves and stems are also used to treat diabetes and hyperlipidemia.[39] Many publications regarding its use are emerging.[39,123–129]

Evidence

Most trials with nopal have been small and published in Spanish only, although abstracts are available in English. In 2 small trials in persons with type 2 diabetes, the acute glucose response of nopal, water, and zucchini or nopal and water were compared.[123,126] A decrease in the postprandial glucose response from nopal was noted. One small study showed that when added to traditional Mexican breakfasts (chilaquiles, burritos, quesadillas), nopal significantly decreased the area under the curve for blood glucose response.[127]

A 200-mg capsule consisting of a mixture of the cladode and fruit skin extract has been studied in a randomized placebo-controlled trial in 29 persons with prediabetes.[128] Patients underwent 2 different OGTT challenges—one without nopal to determine baseline values and one administered 30 minutes after 2 capsules were administered. Glucose values decreased significantly (*P* < .05) when the nopal was administered acutely before the OGTT. Half of the patients also took 1 capsule daily of the supplement and half took placebo for 16 weeks. Glucose declined in both groups, but there was no difference in results between the supplement and placebo.[128]

Summary

Nopal may help lower blood glucose when cooked or taken as a supplement.[39] Used by many Hispanics in smoothies or shakes, nopal is a very popular food. Nopal may decrease carbohydrate absorption due to the soluble fiber and pectin content.[39,123] There is speculation that high concentrations of trivalent chromium in the cactus pad may be responsible for improved glucose metabolism.[129] Major side effects relate to GI upset.[39,124] A possible side effect is hypoglycemia when taken in combination with sulfonylureas and metformin, based on a case report.[125]

The dose used is 100 to 500 g of broiled nopal stems taken with meals.[39] However, ideal doses and the optimal preparation have not been established, and standardized capsule forms are emerging. Nopal is a high-fiber, low-calorie functional food that may be useful for diabetes and hyperlipidemia, and patients should be cautioned regarding hypoglycemia if they are on a secretagogue.

Probiotics

Millions of microbes in the gut constitute what is known as the human microbiota.[130–133] The role of the human microbiota is being researched and evaluated in different disease states such as obesity,[134,135] insulin resistance, and diabetes.[136] Altered gut microbiota may correlate with suppression of beneficial incretins such as glucagon-like peptide-1 (GLP-1), increased inflammation, increased triglyceride production,[137]

inhibition of insulin signaling, and energy changes.[133] Thus, changes in microbiota may be associated with inflammation, obesity, and possibly diabetes.

Evidence

Most available evidence suggests changes in microbiota in diabetes. Recently, a study found that gut microbiota changes may help identify persons who are at risk for diabetes.[138] An evaluation of 36 individuals with and without T2DM found that certain gram-negative bacteria are found in persons with diabetes.[139] In one small 4-week study, 45 males with type 2 diabetes and either impaired glucose tolerance or normal glucose tolerance were randomized to receive treatment with a probiotic or placebo; after 4 weeks, probiotics enhanced insulin sensitivity.[140] Another study in 238 pregnant women randomized to intensive dietary counseling plus probiotics, intensive dietary counseling plus placebo, or standardized dietary counseling found that probiotic use resulted in fewer gestational diabetes cases.[141]

Summary

Studies suggest that persons with diabetes have an altered microbiome, and this may start with changes that are correlated with obesity and insulin resistance. The theoretical mechanisms are that probiotics release beneficial organic and free fatty acids that act against pathogenic microbes associated with obesity and insulin resistance, and also probiotics may enhance incretin effects, decrease inflammation, and enhance insulin sensitivity.[130–133] However, probiotic supplementation is not without adverse effects, and problems may occur. For example, increased mortality in persons with pancreatitis who were given probiotics has been reported.[142] Other effects have included GI upset, constipation, possible microbe migration from the digestive tract into the bloodstream, and transfer of antibiotic resistance to pathogenic bacteria.[130] In immunocompromised patients, infections may occur.[130] Drug interactions may occur with different agents. With antibiotics or antifungals the probiotic benefit may be diminished.[130] Antibiotics should be administered separately from probiotics, at least by 2 hours.[130] Caution should be exercised in persons on immunosuppressants since the probiotic may cause an infection.[130] There are many unknowns, such as what is the most appropriate probiotic or combination of probiotics to use for specific diseases. Another unknown is the most appropriate form since they are available in various formulations (yogurt, powders, supplements, etc). Also, should prebiotics be used instead—these are nondigestible food constituents that help the host organism stimulate growth or activity of gut bacteria[143] and have been shown to enhance incretin secretion in animals.[144] It is important for individuals to learn how to read a probiotic label for information such as the strain, expiration dates, dosing, and storage information.[145] It's also important to know that testing of some products found that product content often varies from what is stated on the label, per the testing laboratory CL.[32] Studies that research the impact of probiotics in persons with diabetes are emerging, and studies that find an improvement are not definitive. More research is needed, and evidence of long-term benefit on morbidity and mortality is absent.

Botanical and Nonbotanical Products Used to Treat Diabetes Complications

Complications of diabetes may be devastating and disrupting to individuals' lives. Many use supplements to try to prevent or treat complications. Alpha-lipoic acid, benfotiamine, Coenzyme Q10, fish oil, garlic, St John's wort, and vitamin D are some of the CAM products individuals may use to reduce the complications of diabetes. Information regarding chemical constituents, mechanism of action, side effects, and drug interactions for these products is found in Table 20.3. Each of these 7 products is reviewed separately following Table 20.3.

Alpha-Lipoic Acid

Alpha-lipoic acid (ALA), a vitamin-like substance also known as thioctic acid, is a disulfide compound that is synthesized in the liver. Foods containing ALA include greens such as spinach and broccoli, potatoes, yams, carrots, and red and organ meat.[39] Alpha-lipoic acid functions as a cofactor in enzyme complexes such as pyruvate dehydrogenase and assists in the conversion of pyruvic acid to acetyl-coenzyme A in oxidative glucose metabolism.[146] Alpha-lipoic acid is readily converted to the reduced form, dihydrolipoic acid (DHLA). Both ALA and DHLA are potent antioxidants.[39] Alpha-lipoic acid may increase insulin sensitivity.[147] Since ALA may decrease oxidative stress (caused by increased blood glucose), it may potentially help minimize symptoms of neuropathy.[39] Alpha-lipoic acid has been much studied for diabetes.[146–148]

Evidence

Alpha-lipoic acid has been studied in the Alpha-Lipoic Acid in Diabetic Neuropathy (ALADIN) trials.[149–151] The first trial in persons with type 2 diabetes with

TABLE 20.3 Botanical and Nonbotanical Products Used to Treat Diabetes Complications			
Product	*Chemical Constituents*	*Mechanism of Action*	*Side Effects & Drug Interactions*
Alpha-lipoic acid Evidence grade A for type 2 diabetes and neuropathy	Disulfide compound synthesized in the liver[146,147]	Various mechanisms[39,146,147] • Increased insulin sensitivity • Functions as antioxidant to: –scavenge free radicals –regenerate endogenous antioxidants (vitamins C and E, glutathione) • Has metal chelating activity • May stimulate glucose transporter systems	*Side effects*[39,148]: • May cause GI upset • Possible skin allergies • Decreased triiodothyronine levels • Possible heart rate and rhythm disturbances *Drug interactions*[39]: • Toxicity with high doses in persons with thiamine deficiency • May be bound by antacids if given at the same time • Possible hypoglycemia if combined with secretagogues

TABLE 20.3	Botanical and Nonbotanical Products Used to Treat Diabetes Complications (continued)		
Product	*Chemical Constituents*	*Mechanism of Action*	*Side Effects & Drug Interactions*
Benfotiamine

No evidence grade available; grade C for parent drug thiamine | Fat-soluble form of thiamine[155] | Various mechanisms[155,156]

• Enhances transketolase activity and may thus inhibit 3 pathways involved in vascular damage:
  – Diacylglycerol-protein kinase C pathway
  – Advanced glycation end product formation pathway
  – Hexosamine pathway | *Side effects*[155]:
• Possible skin rashes

Drug interactions[39]:
• Several drugs may deplete thiamine body stores (metformin, antibiotics, oral contraceptives, diuretics, phenytoin, some chemotherapy agents)
• Some supplements may decrease thiamine activity or deplete thiamine (betel nuts, horsetail) |
| CoQ10

Evidence grade:

Hypertension–B
Heart failure–C
Adjunct to statins–C
Diabetes mellitus (DM)–D | 10-carbon side chain with structure similar to vitamin K[39,167] | Various mechanisms[39,167,168]

• Antioxidant
• Membrane stabilizer
• Cofactor in metabolism in adenosine triphosphate production and oxidative respiration
• Increased glycerol-3-phosphate dehydrogenase activity, thus improving glucose-stimulated insulin secretion | *Side effects*[39,169]:
• GI upset
• No serious effects with long-term use

Drug interactions[39]:
• Theoretical additive hypoglycemia if combined with secretagogues
• May antagonize effects of warfarin and decrease international normalized ratio
• Statins may lower CoQ10 levels
• Theoretical additive hypotension with antihypertensives
• Decreased doxorubicin cardiotoxicity (CoQ10 may also decrease effectiveness of doxorubicin) |
| Fish oil

Evidence grade:

High triglycerides–A
Coronary heart disease–A
DM–D | Omega-3 fatty acids[39,185,186]

Eicosapentaenoic acid (EPA)

Docosahexaenoic acid (DHA) | Various mechanisms[39,185,186]

• Antithrombotic
• Anti-inflammatory due to arachidonic acid cascade inhibition
• Inhibits interleukin-1 and tumor necrosis factor-alpha
• Decreases secretion and increases clearance of very low-density lipoproteins (VLDL)
• Alters metabolism of adhesion molecules (vascular cell adhesion molecule-1, e-selectin, intercellular adhesion molecule-1) | *Side effects*[39,185,186]:
• Fishy aftertaste
• GI upset
• Halitosis
• Increases mercury or polychlorinated biphenyls
• Doses >3 g per day *may* increase glucose
• High doses may increase nonatherogenic LDL particles

Drug interactions[39,185,186]:
• Bleeding if high doses taken with antiplatelet agents
• Possible hypoglycemia if combined with secretagogues
• Possible additive effects with antihypertensives or statins
• Decreases hypertensive effects of cyclosporine |

(continued)

American Association of Diabetes Educators©

TABLE 20.3	Botanical and Nonbotanical Products Used to Treat Diabetes Complications (continued)		
Product	*Chemical Constituents*	*Mechanism of Action*	*Side Effects & Drug Interactions*
Garlic Evidence grade: Hypertension and lipids–A Type 2 diabetes mellitus (T2DM)–C	Various ingredients[39,196,197] • Alliin –Must be converted to allicin (active form) by the enzyme alliinase • Ajoene (formed by acid-catalyzed reaction from 2 allicin molecules) • Allylpropyl disulfide	Various mechanisms[39,196,197] • Antioxidant activity • Allicin may increase levels of catylase and glutathione peroxidase activity • Ajoene decreases the activity of factors needed for lipid synthesis by reducing the thiol group in coenzyme A and HMG CoA reductase and by oxidizing NADPH • Ajoene has antiplatelet activity and interferes with thromboxane synthesis and decreases platelet activity • Allopropyl disulfide may decrease blood glucose and increase insulin • Increased serum insulin and improved hepatic glycogen storage	*Side effects[39,196,197]:* • Increases GI upset • Bleeding reactions *Drug interactions[39,196,197]:* • Additive antiplatelet effects when combined with drugs or complementary products having antiplatelet properties • May induce CYP450 3A4, thus decreasing serum concentrations of many drugs (oral contraceptives, certain calcium channel blockers, angiotensin receptor blockers, certain statins, macrolides, certain anticonvulsants, and cyclosporine) • May increase concentrations of acetaminophen, ethanol, and other drugs
St John's wort Evidence grade A for mild/moderate depression	Various ingredients[39] • Hypericin • Hyperforin	Serotonergic activity as well as possible effects on other neurotransmitters[39]	*Side effects[39]:* • Phototoxicity • Gastrointestinal upset, anxiety • Increased thyroid-stimulating hormone • Withdrawal symptoms when discontinued abruptly *Drug interactions[39]:* • Induces metabolism of certain drugs metabolized by CYP3A4, thereby decreasing their serum concentrations (certain antihypertensives, certain statins, oral contraceptives, cyclosporine, protease inhibitors); also induces CYP2C9, thereby decreasing serum concentrations of warfarin • Glycoprotein modulation, thereby decreasing serum concentrations of digoxin • Serotonin syndrome if combined with serotonergic drugs such as paroxetine or fluoxetine

TABLE 20.3 Botanical and Nonbotanical Products Used to Treat Diabetes Complications (continued)			
Product	*Chemical Constituents*	*Mechanism of Action*	*Side Effects & Drug Interactions*

Vitamin D
 	
Evidence grade:
Cardiovascular disease–C
T1DM and T2DM–C
	Various ingredients[39]
	
	• Ergocalciferol (vitamin D_2)
	
	• Cholecalciferol (vitamin D_3)
		Various mechanisms for diabetes[210–213]
		
		• Must undergo 2 hydroxylations for activation to 25-hydroxyvitamin D [25(OH)D] or calcidiol and to 1,25-dihydroxyvitamin D [1,25(OH)2D] or calcitriol and is essential for calcium absorption in the digestive tract
		
		• Improved pancreatic ß-cell function
		   – Direct, indirect effects on insulin secretion
		
		• Improved insulin action
		   – Direct, indirect effects on insulin action
		
		• Increased calcium concentrations may improve effect on insulin action
		
		• Improved inflammation
		   – Interferes with cytokine generation and action
		   – May down regulate activation of pro-inflammatory markers (nf-kappa ß)
			Side effects[39,211,213]:
			
			• Occur in toxic concentrations ([25(OH)D] >150 ng/mL[165]) and include nausea, vomiting, poor appetite, weight loss, constipation, weakness
			
			• May cause hypercalcemia resulting in confusion, tinnitus, ataxia, arrhythmias, deposition of calcium phosphate in soft tissues
			
			Drug interactions[39,213]:
			
			• Some anticonvulsants decrease vitamin D levels, including phenytoin and phenobarbital
			
			• Rifampin may decrease vitamin D levels
			
			• Certain HIV drugs may decrease vitamin D levels
			
			• Steroids impair calcium absorption and vitamin D metabolism
			
			• Orlistat and cholestyramine may impair vitamin D absorption
			
			• Hypermagnesemia if taken with certain magnesium-containing antacids
			
			• Digoxin if patient has hypercalcemia, because arrhythmias may occur

symptomatic peripheral neuropathy reported improvements in symptoms of neuropathy after 3 weeks of intravenous (IV) ALA.[149] ALADIN II was a trial in persons with type 1 diabetes or type 2 diabetes with polyneuropathy symptoms.[150] Alpha-lipoic acid was administered intravenously for 5 days and then orally for 2 years. Improvements were again noted in symptoms of neuropathy. ALADIN III was a trial in persons with type 1 diabetes.[151] Both IV and oral ALA were studied: IV treatment for 3 weeks, then oral treatment for 6 months. Improvements in symptoms were significant after only 19 days.

The NATHAN I (Neurological Assessment of Thioctic Acid in Neuropathy) trial was a 4-year multicenter trial in North America and Europe that assessed the role of ALA given orally in prevention and treatment of diabetic neuropathy.[148] The study showed there was no significant change in the main outcome—a combination neuropathy symptom and nerve conduction evaluation. However, there were improvements in certain neuropathic impairment symptoms, and fewer patients showed progression of neuropathic impairment symptoms.[148] The NATHAN II trial (still unpublished) was a 3-week study of ALA administered intravenously, which resulted in improved symptoms, but this is certainly not a readily available patient option. The SYDNEY trial[152] was a randomized controlled trial in 120 patients in which ALA or placebo was given intravenously 5 days a week for 14 treatments. Total symptom scores declined significantly.[152] A meta-analysis of 1258 persons in trials who used IV ALA or placebo (ALADIN I and III trials, the NATHAN II and SYDNEY trials) found that 52.7% of patients on ALA versus 36.9% on placebo had improved total symptom scores.[153] The 5-week multicenter Sydney 2 trial was a randomized, double-blind, placebo-controlled trial in 181 subjects and evaluated 3 different doses of ALA (600 mg, 1200 mg, 1800 mg).[154] Total symptom scores declined significantly in the ALA groups compared with placebo ($P < .05$).

Summary

Alpha-lipoic acid is a much-studied agent that may potentially help with peripheral neuropathy. No serious side effects have been reported, even though it has been used intravenously and in long-term trials. The Sydney 2 trial showed that although pain improved significantly, paresthesias and numbness did not.[154] Decreases in A1C levels have not been significant.[149–151] Typical doses of oral ALA are 600 to 1200 mg per day.[39] Although ALA has been used for decades in Germany, long-term trials are necessary to determine whether ALA slows the progression of neuropathy versus only improving the neuropathy symptoms. Overall, studies have confirmed that ALA may improve numbness, pain, burning, and prickly sensations to the feet and legs. The NATHAN I study reported adverse effects related to changes in heart rate or rhythm disturbances in the ALA group versus placebo ($P = .047$), but the authors reported that ALA was well tolerated.[148] Although the American Diabetes Association (ADA) does not recommend use of unproven therapies, ALA has a long track record of proven benefit and is a relatively safe agent to use.

Benfotiamine

Persons with neuropathy may have thiamine deficiency. Different neurological disorders, including diabetes and alcohol-related neuropathy, have been treated with vitamin B_1 (thiamine). However, thiamine is not well absorbed, and high doses are needed for successful treatment. Benfotiamine, a fat-soluble form of thiamine, provides much higher blood and tissue levels and may thus be a more effective form.[155] Benfotiamine may be useful in persons with microvascular complications.[155,156] Another name for these vitamins is allithiamines, because they are found in the *Allium* vegetable family (which includes garlic, onions, shallots, and leeks). Other foods containing thiamine include whole grain cereals and breads and certain meats.[155]

Evidence

Several clinical trials have evaluated benfotiamine for microvascular complications. Some studies are open-label, and others are randomized controlled trials. One open-label 6-week study in 36 persons with T1DM or T2DM with painful neuropathy looked at different doses of benfotiamine in combination with B vitamins.[157] Although all groups had beneficial effects, the best results were reported in those patients taking the highest dose ($P < .01$ for all parameters compared with baseline). A different 3-month open-label study in persons with type 1 diabetes or type 2 diabetes evaluated benfotiamine plus other B vitamins or only B vitamins.[158] The benfotiamine group had better results for neuropathic pain ($P < .001$), and vibration perception threshold also improved.

A 3-week randomized pilot study in 40 persons with type 1 diabetes or type 2 diabetes evaluated benfotiamine or placebo 4 times daily for neuropathy.[159] Painful neuropathy symptoms improved significantly ($P < .05$). A 6-week randomized controlled trial evaluated 133 persons with type 1 diabetes or type 2 diabetes. Neuropathy symptom scores improved in the benfotiamine group.[160] A 12-week randomized, double-blind, placebo-controlled trial evaluated varying doses of benfotiamine plus vitamins B_6 and B_{12} in 24 persons with type 1 diabetes or type 2 diabetes.[161] The benfotiamine group had improved vibration perception threshold scores in the metacarpal and metatarsal nerves (although the results were not significant) and improved nerve conduction velocity scores in the peroneal nerve ($P = .006$) but not the median nerve.

Results are not always positive. A 24-month randomized trial in 67 persons with T1DM found no benefit with benfotiamine for peripheral nerve function.[162] However, the results of this study have been questioned by other researchers.[163]

Summary

Benfotiamine is a promising fat-soluble form of vitamin B_1 for diabetes complications and has been evaluated in both type 1 diabetes and type 2 diabetes.

Although highly studied for neuropathy, it has also been studied for retinopathy[164] and nephropathy.[165,166] It enhances activity of certain enzymes that may inhibit major pathways involved in vascular damage.[155] It may also block hyperglycemia-induced activation of pro-inflammatory transcription factors.[156] It may even diminish or correct cell damage by normalizing cell division rates and decreasing apoptosis.[155] Several medications deplete thiamine levels, including metformin.[39] The dose used for diabetes is 300 to 600 mg daily, administered in divided doses (eg, 100 or 150 mg 3 times a day).[157-161] Benfotiamine is also found in combination with other B vitamins and ALA. Its role in treating diabetes microvascular complications is promising, and overall it is a safe agent to use.

Coenzyme Q10

Coenzyme Q10 (CoQ10) is also known as ubiquinone because it is found in almost all human cells.[167-172] CoQ10 is a lipid-soluble vitamin-like substance that is thought to be deficient in many diseases, including diabetes.[171,173] Humans synthesize CoQ10, and it is highly concentrated in the heart, brain, liver, kidneys, and pancreas.[39,167] Dietary sources include beef, poultry, and broccoli, and dietary supplements are manufactured via beet and sugarcane fermentation.[39,170] Human CoQ10 levels decline with age and with certain cardiovascular diseases (heart failure, hypertension, and other diseases such as Parkinson's).[171] CoQ10 has been used to treat a variety of cardiovascular diseases which are common in persons with diabetes, although there is evidence that it may also help improve glucose.[172] It is widely used to offset the body's decreased CoQ10 levels secondary to statin use.[39] It has been used for a variety of cardiovascular diseases (including hypertension, angina, and heart failure) and for statin-induced myopathy, as well as other disease states, such as Parkinson's disease.[167,171,174]

Evidence

CoQ10 has been evaluated extensively. Two studies of CoQ10 use demonstrated a significant decrease in blood pressure, although the blood pressure was still higher than the target goals in persons with diabetes.[175,176] In one of the hypertension studies, the subjects were thought to have insulin resistance, and

mean baseline glucose decreased in the CoQ10 group after 8 weeks (*P* < .05).[176]

In a randomized, double-blind, placebo-controlled trial in 34 persons with T1DM, there was a nonsignificant decline in fasting glucose and A1C (8.04% to 7.86%).[177] A different 6-month trial in persons with type 2 diabetes showed no improvement in diabetes control, and in fact there was an increase in A1C in the CoQ10 group.[178] Another study in 74 persons with type 2 diabetes and dyslipidemia reported an improvement in A1C in a group with a combination of CoQ10 and the triglyceride-lowering agent fenofibrate.[179] In the same study, both systolic and diastolic pressure decreased slightly but significantly with CoQ10 supplementation.[179] Another small study in 9 persons with T2DM showed that CoQ10 decreased A1C from 7.1% to 6.8% (*P* = .03).[180]

A recent meta-analysis in heart failure showed improved ejection fraction and a slight improvement in New York Heart Association (NYHA) functional class.[181] However, there were few studies, and many trials were older publications where patients were not on agents that are now commonly used to treat heart failure. In combination with selenium, CoQ10 has shown decreased cardiovascular mortality.[182]

Summary

CoQ10 is a highly used product, both by persons with diabetes and by persons without diabetes. One unique reason for use is that statins decrease serum CoQ10 concentrations, and it has been theorized that myopathy may then ensue. However, this benefit has not been conclusively shown.[167] One of the biggest concerns is use by persons who are on the anticoagulant warfarin, since CoQ10 has a structure similar to vitamin K and may thus result in breakthrough thromboembolism.[167] CoQ10 has been used for a variety of disorders, and although blood pressure may decrease significantly, endpoint values are still higher than advocated for persons with diabetes. In persons with type 1 diabetes or type 2 diabetes, CoQ10 supplementation has shown neutral to slightly improved effects on fasting glucose and A1C. Recent information has indicated that CoQ10 supplementation may attenuate hyperglycemia due to reduced GLUT4 protein levels caused by some statins.[183] One of the main reasons it is used in diabetes is because of its improved endothelial dysfunction.[184] The doses are variable, and for hypertension and other cardiovascular diseases, the dose has ranged from 100 to 225 mg daily, although up to 600 mg daily has been used. The dose for diabetes has ranged from 100 to 200 mg daily.[176–179] Although there is much enthusiasm for CoQ10 and long-term use has not shown harm, further studies are needed to determine its place in treatment.

Fish Oil (Omega-3 Fatty Acids)

Omega-3 fatty acids are found in certain plants and fish oil.[39] Plant oils contain alpha-linolenic acid, and sources include flaxseed, walnut, canola, olive, soybean, and chia.[39] Examples of omega-3-containing fish include salmon, lake trout, mackerel, sturgeon, herring, tuna, and sardines.[39,185] Fish oil is primarily used for cardiovascular disease protection and treatment of hypertriglyceridemia, and it may also help decrease oxidative stress.[185] Another benefit is that it may help reduce the risk of type 2 diabetes.[186]

Evidence

Numerous studies have assessed fish oil for cardiovascular disease. A large study evaluated fish oil for secondary prevention in 11,324 persons with a history of myocardial infarction (MI).[187] Patients were randomized to daily 1-g doses of fish oil, vitamin E, a fish oil/vitamin E combination, or placebo. In the 2-way analysis comparing fish oil with placebo, there was a 10% decrease in the primary endpoint of death, nonfatal MI, or nonfatal stroke for the fish oil group ($P = .048$). Risk of cardiovascular death decreased significantly by 17% in the 2-way analysis.

A review of 23 randomized placebo-controlled trials included persons with diabetes.[188] Mean triglyceride levels significantly decreased by approximately 40 mg/dL (0.45 mmol/L; $P < .00001$) in 969 participants in the 18 trials that collected triglyceride data. No benefit was noted in fasting glucose or A1C.

In 2012 two different analyses cast doubt on the cardiovascular protective effect of fish oil since there were no decreases in adverse cardiovascular outcomes. The ORIGIN trial studied 1 g per day of fish oil for 6 years in 12,000 persons with type 2 diabetes or at risk for developing diabetes.[189] The primary outcome, death from cardiovascular cause, was not decreased. A different meta-analysis evaluating approximately

70,000 persons found that there were no benefits from primary or secondary prevention for 1.51 g per day of omega-3 fatty acids (fish oil).[190] An explanation is that 1 study used only 1 g per day, the other only 1.51 g per day. Another explanation is that both reports indicated that fish oil did not impact outcomes to a great extent, possibly because nowadays many more patients take heart-protective medications such as statins, blood pressure medications, and antiplatelets (to inhibit clot formation).

In 2013, a randomized controlled 5-year follow-up trial showed that in 6244 patients randomized to n-3 fatty acids (fish oil) and 6269 assigned to placebo, there was no reduction in cardiovascular morbidity and mortality.[191] Another 2013 publication that looked only at plasma concentrations (not supplementation) of eicosapentaenoic acid (EPA) and docosahexaenoic acid (DHA) found that individuals with the highest concentrations had a 27% reduced risk of all-cause death.[192] A different 2013 publication found that fish oil supplements increase adiponectin levels, and this may be associated with lower risk of type 2 diabetes.[193]

Summary

Fish oil has a variety of therapeutic effects that benefit cardiovascular disease, including antithrombotic, anti-inflammatory effects and cardiac cell membrane stabilization. Fish oil contains EPA and DHA. The Agency for Health Care Research and Quality reviewed studies assessing fish oil in a variety of diseases, including diabetes.[194] The report stated that baseline dietary consumption should be addressed, and although fish oil may decrease triglycerides, other lipid parameters and glucose control may not benefit. However, many persons with diabetes have uncontrolled triglycerides and fish oil may be of benefit.

Many clinicians are unclear as to the amount of EPA and DHA that dietary supplements should contain. One prescription product, 1 g of Lovaza® (GlaxoSmithKline), contains the necessary amount of EPA and DHA (465 mg and 375 mg, respectively) per capsule and is dosed at 1 to 4 capsules daily, depending on triglyceride level.[195] Most supplements contain 200 to 400 mg of EPA plus DHA per capsule, and thus patients may need to take as many as 12 to 16 capsules daily to obtain the amount equivalent to the prescription product. Newer dietary supplements are more concentrated. Persons taking supplements should look for the total amount of EPA and DHA, not just total fish oil. The American Heart Association (AHA) recommends 1 g daily of EPA plus DHA for persons with heart disease and 2 to 4 g daily for persons with very high triglycerides.[185] Although recent research shows conflicting evidence regarding supplementation with fish oil, it's important to note that perhaps the benefit of fish oil was not seen because patients were already taking medications that lower risk, such as statins, ACE inhibitors, and aspirin. It's also important to remember that the AHA and the ADA recommend 2 weekly servings of fatty fish, such as salmon or mackerel.[39,185]

Garlic

Garlic (*Allium sativum*), a member of the lily family, has been used in cooking for thousands of years.[39] Garlic is used for hyperlipidemia, hypertension, cancer prevention, and antibacterial activity.[39,196,197] The name *Allium* is derived from the Celtic word "all," which means "burning." Highly valued in ancient Egypt and ancient Chinese medicine, garlic has a rich history of thousands of years of medicinal use.[196] Garlic has been reported to be helpful for diabetes.

Evidence

Several studies have evaluated the impact of garlic on blood pressure and lipids. A meta-analysis reviewed garlic for cardiovascular risk factors.[198] In this review, systolic pressure was significantly reduced in only 1 trial, and diastolic pressure decreased significantly in 3 trials; blood glucose was lowered significantly in only 1 trial, in persons without diabetes.[198] The same trial reported beneficial effects on lipids that were not maintained after a few months. A meta-analysis of 8 trials evaluated the effect of garlic on mild hypertension.[199] Results showed a modest decrease in systolic blood pressure (7.7 mm Hg) and diastolic blood pressure (5 mm Hg) compared with placebo.[199] However, only 3 trials included hypertensive patients. Another systematic review and meta-analysis separated results for hypertensive and non-hypertensive subjects.[200] The review reported that, compared with placebo, garlic lowered systolic pressure by 8.4 mm Hg ($P < .001$) and diastolic blood pressure by 7.3 mm Hg ($P < .001$) in hypertensive persons.

An older meta-analysis of 13 randomized, double-blind, placebo-controlled trials reported that garlic reduced total cholesterol modestly by 15.7 mg/dL (0.41 mmol/L).[201] However, in the trials with better methodology, there was no difference between garlic and placebo.

More recent meta-analyses have shown varying effects, with some showing a benefit on lipids[202] and others showing no benefit.[203]

A 12-week single-blind, placebo-controlled trial evaluated garlic use in 70 persons with type 2 diabetes and newly diagnosed hyperlipidemia.[204] Several lipid values decreased significantly. Total cholesterol and LDL decreased, and HDL increased.[204] The same group of researchers conducted a 24-week randomized, single-blind, placebo-controlled study that compared a combination of garlic plus metformin in 30 persons with type 2 diabetes with only metformin in 30 patients.[205] Fasting glucose decreased in the combination group ($P < .005$). LDL cholesterol and triglycerides decreased slightly ($P < .005$ for both).[205]

Garlic was recently studied in an open-label 12-week study in combination with metformin in 30 persons with type 2 diabetes and compared with 30 patients who took only metformin.[206] Although A1C decreased slightly from 7.48% to 7.05%, the change was not significant. However, fasting blood glucose, postmeal glucose, and cholesterol decreases were significant in the garlic plus metformin group ($P < .001$ for fasting and postprandial; $P < .05$ for LDL).[206]

Summary

Garlic contains the sulfur-based chemical constituent alliin, which must be converted to the active form, allicin, by the enzyme alliinase. This reaction occurs when the garlic bulb is chewed or crushed.[39] Commercial preparations of garlic usually contain alliin, not allicin or ajoene. Conversion requires alliinase, which is unstable in stomach acids. Dried garlic preparations may be effective if the product is enteric-coated to prevent gastric acid breakdown and permit release in the small intestine. Thus, dried garlic preparations should be enteric-coated to prevent breakdown by stomach acids.

Although historically garlic has been used to improve glucose, only recently have studies been published regarding this effect. Researchers have noted that garlic may increase serum insulin and improve hepatic glycogen storage.[197] Garlic may also inhibit formation of the advanced glycation end products that contribute to microvascular disease.[207] In hyperlipidemia and hypertension studies, garlic extracts (600 to 1200 mg per day in divided doses) have been used. For diabetes, 500 to 900 mg daily has been used. Fresh garlic is effective, and the appropriate amount is approximately 1 clove daily (containing approximately 1% alliin).[39] Garlic demonstrates one of the important controversies regarding supplements—varying results are shown in different studies, and the most appropriate dose and form are not known. Garlic is a very popular product, and it is estimated that up to half of patients with hypertension may take garlic in varying forms.[208] A Cochrane Review that evaluated the impact of garlic in hypertensive patients reported that garlic decreases blood pressure, but there is insufficient evidence to determine the effect on reducing cardiovascular morbidity and mortality.[208] It is important that educators instruct individuals that antiplatelet activity is a serious potential problem and that the person may experience bleeding reactions, especially if using drugs or CAM therapies with antiplatelet properties. As a food, garlic is safe; however, when used as a supplement, very close monitoring is required due to the potential for bleeding reactions.

St John's Wort

St John's wort (*Hypericum perforatum*) is a perennial that grows throughout the United States, Canada, and Europe. The bright yellow flowers bloom in late June, and the flowering top is used in the product.[39] St John's wort (SJW) has been used for many different disorders as well as to treat a variety of psychiatric disorders, including depression and anxiety. Many persons with diabetes have depression, and some clinicians consider this a complication of diabetes.

Evidence

Many published studies have evaluated SJW for depression, and it has been compared with placebo and conventional antidepressants, with varying results. The Cochrane Review assessed randomized controlled studies evaluating SJW for major depression.[209] A total of 5489 persons were assessed in 29 studies. Results indicated that SJW is equivalent to conventional antidepressants and superior to placebo. A unique finding is that SJW has fewer side effects than conventional antidepressants. The review found that trials performed in German-speaking countries found more favorable results.

Summary

St John's wort is a unique botanical product that has been used for centuries to treat depression, although studies show it may be useful only for mild to moderate depression. Two of the chemical constituents, hypericin and hyperforin, have been used as standardized extracts, but some researchers believe the constituents most likely to produce antidepressant effects are hyperforin, adhyperforin, and other related compounds.[39] These compounds modulate different neurotransmitters including serotonin, norepinephrine, and dopamine. The serotonergic effects may be the major antidepressant activity. St John's wort use may have significant consequences because of the potential for serious drug interactions. It is a CYP450 enzyme inducer of important drugs that persons with diabetes may be using, such as certain statins, calcium channel blockers, angiotensin receptor blockers, oral contraceptives, warfarin, and cyclosporine. It may also reduce serum concentrations of digoxin and interact adversely with serotonergic drugs (such as fluoxetine, sertraline, or paroxetine) or narcotics, and result in toxicity. Doses used are 300 to 600 mg 3 times daily.[39] Standardized extracts used in studies include 0.3% hypericin and the hyperforin-stabilized version of this extract. Patients should always inform their healthcare providers if they are taking SJW, particularly because of the potential for drug interactions with medications they may be using. Patients should be informed that SJW may reduce serum concentrations of certain drugs to subtherapeutic levels. Conversely, patients should also be informed that abrupt discontinuation may result in dangerously increased serum concentrations of drugs that normally have lower concentrations during coadministration. Use of SJW has been banned in certain countries, due to the potential for drug interactions. St John's wort may not be considered a safe agent to use in diabetes because of the potential harm if it lowers serum concentrations of medications critical for diabetes or its comorbidities. Moreover, if a person is depressed, use of a traditional antidepressant should be encouraged.

Vitamin D

Vitamin D has emerged as a critical nutrient that may benefit individuals with diabetes. It is a fat-soluble vitamin and is considered a hormone because the active form is produced in one part of the body (kidneys) but its effects are exerted throughout the body.[39,210–213] Vitamin D is found in certain foods, as a dietary supplement, and is also synthesized by humans. Two major forms include ergocalciferol, or vitamin D_2, and cholecalciferol, or vitamin D_3.[39,210–213] Vitamin D_2 is synthesized by plants, and vitamin D_3 is produced in the skin as a result of exposure to ultraviolet B rays from sunlight, and is also present in many foods. Both vitamin D_2 and vitamin D_3 are present in supplements, although D_2 is considered one third as potent as D_3. Foods containing higher amounts of vitamin D include salmon, sardines, cod liver oil, egg yolks, and fortified foods such as milk and orange juice.[39,210–213] Vitamin D is involved in many metabolic processes and disease states and tends to be deficient in persons who live in northern latitudes and thus do not have adequate access to sunshine, persons who are dark skinned, or persons who are obese. Vitamin D is also correlated with cardiovascular health, including hypertension and both type 1 diabetes and type 2 diabetes.

Evidence

There is a large body of published information evaluating the role of vitamin D in different disease states, including rickets and osteoporosis.[211] Vitamin D deficiency may result in muscle weakness and precipitate falls and is also associated with certain cancers such as pancreatic, colon, prostate, ovarian, breast, and Hodgkin's lymphoma.[211] Supplementation may benefit certain autoimmune diseases, such as multiple sclerosis, because it acts as an important immunomodulator.[211]

However, in diabetes, most of the information has been observational data and there are few prospective trials.[39,210–216] In Finnish children, vitamin D_3 supplementation during the first year of life reduced type 1 diabetes risk by 78%.[214] Another 20-year observational study in women found that daily intake of vitamin D and calcium reduced type 2 diabetes risk by 33%.[215] Another study indicated that metabolic syndrome was more prevalent in a vitamin D

deficiency state.[216] A different study evaluating vitamin D levels determined that deficiency is more prevalent in type 2 diabetes than in type 1 diabetes.[217] However, in a recent study of nearly 2000 individuals, vitamin D levels lower than 50 ng/mL were correlated with type 1 diabetes.[218]

Prospective studies of vitamin D supplementation in diabetes have been very short-term, or have been post hoc analyses, or have not measured appropriate serum concentrations. Thus, definitive conclusions regarding the role of vitamin D in diabetes have been questioned.[210] A meta-analysis of 21 prospective studies of 76,220 individuals found that the highest 25-hydroxy vitamin D levels were associated with a lower relative risk for type 2 diabetes of 0.62 (95% confidence interval 0.54 to 0.70).[219] The review also noted a trend analysis that for each 4 ng/mL (10 nmol/L) increase in 25(OH)D levels, there was a 4% lower risk of type 2 diabetes (95% confidence interval 3-6; *P* for linear trend < .0001). Reviews of the correlation between cardiovascular disease and vitamin D deficiency have determined there is a relationship such as higher prevalence of hypertension, myocardial infarction, heart failure, or stroke, but prospective trials need to be done.[212,220] Interestingly, myalgias in persons taking statins may be caused by vitamin D deficiency.[221]

Summary

Vitamin D is an important nutrient implicated in many disease states. It is estimated that many individuals are vitamin D deficient, and this may play a role in cardiovascular disease and diabetes.[212,213] Vitamin D undergoes an initial hydroxylation in the liver to form 25-hydroxy vitamin D [25(OH)D] and a second hydroxylation in the kidney to form 1,25-dihydroxy vitamin D [1,25(OH)$_2$D].[210–213] The form measured to assess vitamin D status is [25(OH)D].[210–213] The IOM states that almost all persons are sufficient at a [25(OH)D] serum level of >20 ng/mL.[213] Vitamin D deficiency may occur at levels <12 ng/mL. Currently, the Food and Nutrition Board at the IOM recommends 400 international units for babies 0 to 12 months, 600 international units for individuals aged 1 to 70 years, and 800 international units for individuals over 70 years of age.[222] However, recent guidelines from the US Endocrine Society suggest 400 to 1000 international units daily in children under

1 year, 600 to 1000 international units if aged 1 year or more, and 1500 to 2000 international units per day for adults over 19 years of age.[223] The American Geriatrics Society has recently recommended that much higher intake (4000 international units daily from all sources including food, supplements, and sun exposure) may be necessary to prevent falls.[224] Most supplements contain vitamin D_3 (cholecalciferol), although a prescription form contains vitamin D_2 (ergocalciferol) that is found in high doses (50,000 international units) and administered only once weekly for 8 weeks if a person is found highly deficient.[39] After serum levels normalize, the individual may be changed to a maintenance dose. A Cochrane Review found that cholecalciferol (vitamin D_3) reduced mortality in adults, whereas other vitamin D forms do not.[225] It is imperative that educators assess vitamin D levels and recommend supplementation, if necessary, to improve the overall health of individuals with diabetes. Educators should also consider that myalgias thought to be secondary to statin use may actually be a sign of vitamin D deficiency, and perhaps repletion may help resolve the muscle aches.[212]

Other Products: More Information

There are hundreds of other products that have been used for diabetes or its complications. Books for both clinicians[8] and consumers[226] provide brief summaries of many products.

The diabetes educator is directed to the statement by the ADA on unproven therapies that acknowledges the widespread use of alternative therapies and the need for cautious evaluation of these products.[227] Educators who want more information in this area can check the FDA's Web site for consumer tips on using supplements,[19,20] the Natural Standard Web site, and the Natural Medicines Comprehensive Database.[39] Major research is under way on CAM therapies. Educators can keep current by checking the NIH Web site for information on different studies.[1,6]

Self-Care Implications

Persons with diabetes need to be made aware that if dietary supplements are used, self-care behaviors should include the following:

- Consider that the dietary supplement may have no impact whatsoever on blood glucose or A1C levels; seek to evaluate results in a defined time period.
- Inform healthcare provider of products used so appropriate monitoring will be done.
- Closely monitor products' effect(s) on blood glucose and A1C levels.

Case Wrap-up

All of the dietary supplements (biologically based practices) that TP has heard about—cinnamon, gymnema, fenugreek, ginseng, and chromium—may have an effect on lowering blood glucose.

Regarding the specific products, these comments can be made:

- TP may be advised that cinnamon may be used in her foods (for instance, in cereal or oatmeal), or if she prefers, as an aqueous extract.

- The other products, particularly gymnema and fenugreek, may produce side effects such as hypoglycemia and interact with the sulfonylurea that she is taking, which may further increase her risk of hypoglycemia. However, gymnema may be useful if she has a sweet tooth and the sulfonylurea dose is reduced. Fenugreek also may produce allergic reactions and adverse GI effects.

- Chromium may be a relatively benign agent and may help as an insulin sensitizer, although there are still unknown consequences with long-term use.

- Ginseng may cause edema, increase blood pressure, and produce anxiety.

- Fenugreek, ginseng, and garlic may interact with warfarin, with the possible resultant effect of increased bleeding.

- Since she experienced myalgias with simvastatin, vitamin D levels should be assessed to determine whether deficiency is the cause.

- St John's wort may lower serum concentrations of the statin, digoxin, and warfarin and result in subtherapeutic effects of these drugs. In combination with the antidepressant, St John's wort may result in serotonin syndrome.

The educator needs to make the patient aware of the AADE7 Self-Care Behaviors™ and remind the patient of the following:

- ◆ Healthy eating—Learn about foods that affect blood glucose, blood pressure, or lipids and remember that supplements do not replace healthy foods.

- ◆ Physical activity—Persons should continue to maintain a regimen of regularly scheduled physical activity.

- ◆ Monitoring—To assess the impact of supplements on blood glucose, it is important to check glucose levels. Other monitoring that is important is the impact of supplements on blood pressure or lipids.

- ◆ Taking medication—It's important that supplements not be used in place of regularly scheduled medications for diabetes, blood pressure, or lipids or for other conditions, such as depression.

- ◆ Problem solving—If a person does not feel well, it may be because of adverse effects caused by supplements. Or if a person's blood glucose levels or other clinical endpoints change (blood pressure or lipids), it's important to consider that supplements may not only be of benefit but may adversely affect these parameters, and it's important to troubleshoot what is occurring.

- ◆ Healthy coping—Learning how to adapt to difficult situations, including the ups and downs of diabetes, is an important lesson for everyone with diabetes. It's important to remember that supplements will not replace creative coping skills or cure depression or anxiety.

- ◆ Reducing risks—Regardless of how beneficial a supplement may be, it's important to remember that evidence-based information resulting from long-term clinical trials has indicated that the best way to reduce risks is to control blood glucose levels, blood pressure, and lipids.

Implications for Special Populations

Certain groups should be closely monitored if the decision is made to try supplements. These groups include vulnerable individuals such as children, the elderly, and pregnant or lactating women. Certain ethnic groups may also be more likely to use supplements—these include Hispanic, Asian, and Native American populations. Individuals who also have other serious diseases, such as lupus, multiple sclerosis, or cancer, are especially vulnerable, and supplements should only be used in consultation with the person's medical provider.

Other Products

There are many other products that persons with diabetes may be tempted to use. For instance, many persons are treated for depression with selective serotonin reuptake inhibitors (SSRIs), such as fluoxetine and sertraline, which may cause them to have difficulty sleeping. Agents such as valerian or kava may sometimes be used to address this problem. There are intrinsic problems in that these agents may interact with prescription sedative-hypnotic medications or with alcohol. Furthermore, kava has the potential for hepatotoxicity and may interact with agents such as statins or glitazones and result in additive toxicity.

Summary

Dietary supplements are not approved for treatment of diabetes, but they may contain biologically active ingredients that may have a benefit in diabetes treatment. However, it is important to note that many have side effects or may interact in adverse ways with other concurrent disease states or with prescription products the individual is taking. For instance, although ginseng may benefit postprandial glucose values, it may also increase blood pressure and attenuate the antihypertensive effects of blood pressure medications the person is taking. Another equally important issue is that some of the products may have contaminants or subtherapeutic or supratherapeutic amounts of the active ingredients. But strides are being made in this area with different verification programs and with use of standardized extracts.

Those working on the diabetes care team must bear in mind that persons with diabetes are more prone to use biologically based practices, including dietary supplements, than other persons. Those involved in diabetes care and education should not turn their backs on the use of these products. The healthcare beliefs of patients must be acknowledged and respected if they decide to use these products. Educators must collaborate with patients so that all aspects of their care may be improved.

Focus on Education

Teaching Strategies

⊘ **Biologically based products (herbs, vitamins, foods, and dietary supplements) are frequently used among people with diabetes in an attempt to control metabolic markers and symptoms.** People might use biologically based therapies as complementary medicine, which is used along with the conventional medicine. In some cases it is used as a stand-alone approach and considered alternative medicine.

⊘ **Be respectful of people's alternative or supplemental medicine choices and preferences.** The diabetes educator's initial reaction to a patient using herbs, vitamins, or dietary supplements can either make or break the whole perception on conventional medicine and the educator's credibility. That person might not come back to see the educator or may choose to withhold sharing this information with the educator and others in the future. That is why it is important for the educator to examine his or her professional CAM health belief system first. How the educator reacts and what he or she says can influence the effectiveness of recommendations and subsequent treatment. Discrediting someone's beliefs may negatively impact the relationship.

⊘ **Support patients' efforts at self-care.** Individuals who use dietary supplements are likely to be very actively involved in their own health care—congratulate them for their initiative. Be aware, however, that many individuals are reluctant to inform their healthcare providers of dietary supplement use. Educators should (1) work in partnership with patients to encourage open communication about biologically based practices, (2) provide safety and efficacy information about supplements, and (3) discourage use of dangerous or ineffective products and those for which there is little evidence of efficacy. Evaluate health literacy by assessing patients' analytical and decision-making skills, along with the ability to apply these skills to health situations. Asking the right questions will allow you to accurately assess people's motivation for taking the supplements.

⊘ **Ask the right questions to assess the patient's use of supplements and belief system.** The right questions will reflect genuine interest in the patient's life and treatment, and will not sound offensive. If you notice resistance in the patient's answer, you may not have asked the right question:

- What supplements or medications do you take that your doctor did not give you a prescription for?
- What do you hope to achieve using this supplement? How does this medication/supplement help you?
- How do you monitor the effects of this medication so you know it does what it is supposed to do?

⊘ **Explore the individual's conviction level in taking supplements or alternative medicine. You can ask the following:**

- On a scale from 1 to 10, how confident are you that this medication will do better than the one recommended to you?
- On a scale from 1 to 10, how willing are you to explore other options?
- What can I do to help you explore other (safer, more effective . . .) options?

⊘ **Be a knowledgeable resource.** Remain nonjudgmental and provide evidence-based information. Examine evidence on what herbs, vitamins, foods, and dietary supplements work versus those that do not work and those that are still under investigation. This will help patients incorporate what works into their treatment regimen.

- Document the use of specific products and why taken (beliefs, financial reasons, knowledge, attitude, etc), along with the patient's willingness to modify and progress in making changes.
- Respect individuals' choices for doing what they believe is right.
- Provide other options to achieve the desired outcomes that are safer, more effective, or more appropriate.
- Allow the individual to examine the options and decide if willing to change or modify.
- Use evidence-based approaches in medical care (use biologically based therapies with strong efficacy) and in counseling.

⊘ **Follow up with the usage and therapeutic impact of the biologically based practices.** Identify the patient's goals. A key role of educators is to keep records of the effects and evaluate the impact on diabetes care. Assess a patient's attitude to change or modify or eliminate its usage (if needed).

⊘ **Help patients share information about their use of supplements with other providers.** Use a multidisciplinary team approach. Explain why and how a doctor, pharmacist, dietitian, and other providers can assist a patient in achieving his or her biologically based therapeutic goals. For example, a pharmacist can help the patient keep a medication history, check for drug interactions, and provide information on supplement potency/quality and expectations. A dietitian can review the meal plan to incorporate therapeutic foods that will positively impact the metabolic goals. The physician can evaluate the effectiveness of the therapy and adjust accordingly.

Messages for Patients

⊘ **Consider the following when using biologically based products:**

- Healthcare professional's knowledge about biologically based practices
- Safety
- Glucose-lowering capacity
- Better options
- Risks of not getting glucose under control by delaying appropriate therapy
- Starting with 1 new product at a time and monitoring outcomes
- Evaluating the effect
- Sharing information with healthcare team

⊘ **Consider the financial implications of supplement use.** Many individuals may decide to stop filling their prescriptions and opt to use supplements, thinking they may be safer, be less expensive, and have more benefits. Hence, all of the issues concerning documentation of use become extremely critical.

References

1. National Center for Complementary and Alternative Medicine, National Institutes of Health. What is complementary and alternative medicine? 2008 Oct (last updated 2013 May; cited 2014 Mar 19). On the Internet at: http://nccam.nih.gov/health/whatiscam.

2. Nathin RL, Barnes PM, Stussman BJ, Bloom B. Costs of complementary and alternative medicine (CAM) and frequency of visits to CAM practitioners: United States, 2007. National Health Statistics Reports; no 18. Hyattsville, Md: National Center for Health Statistics; 2009.

3. Food and Drug Administration. Dietary supplements. Last updated 2014 Feb 26 (cited 2014 Mar 19). On the Internet at: http://www.fda.gov/Food/DietarySupplements/default.htm.

4. Larimore WL, O'Mathuna DP. Quality assessment programs for dietary supplements. Ann Pharmacother. 2003; 37:893-8.

5. US Food and Drug Administration. Current good manufacturing practice in manufacturing, packaging, labeling, or holding operations for dietary supplements. Final rule. Fed Regist. 2007 (cited 2014 Mar 19);72:34752-958. On the Internet at: http://www.fda.gov/ohrms/dockets/98fr/cf0441.pdf.

6. National Institutes of Health, Office of Dietary Supplements. Dietary supplements: background information. Last reviewed 2011 Jun 24 (cited 2014 Mar 19). On the Internet at: http://dietary-supplements.info.nih.gov/factsheets/dietarysupplements.asp.

7. Dietary Supplement and Non-Prescription Drug Consumer Protection Act. Pub L. No. 109-462. 109th Congress. 2006 Dec 22 (cited 2014 Mar 19). On the Internet at: http://www.fda.gov/downloads/AboutFDA/CentersOffices/CDER/ucm102797.pdf.

8. Shane-McWhorter L. Complementary & Alternative Medicine (CAM) Supplement Use in People With Diabetes: A Clinician's Guide. Washington, DC: American Diabetes Association; 2007.

9. US Food and Drug Administration. MedWatch (cited 2014 Mar 19). On the Internet at: http://www.fda.gov/medwatch.

10. Harel Z, Harel S, Waid R, Mamdani M, Bell CM. The frequency and characteristics of dietary supplement recalls in the United States. JAMA Intern Med. 2013 Apr 15:1-3. doi: 10.1001/jamainternmed.2013.379.

11. Ten surprising dangers of vitamins and supplements. Consumer Reports. 2012 Sep (cited 2014 Mar 19). On the Internet at: http://www.consumerreports.org/cro/magazine/2012/09/10-surprising-dangers-of-vitamins-and-supplements/index.htm.

12. US Pharmacopeial. USP's Dietary Supplement Verification Program overview. 2014 (cited 2014 Mar 19). On the Internet at: http://www.usp.org/USPVerified.

13. NSF International. NSF Consumer Information. The importance of dietary supplement certification (cited 2014 Mar 19). On the Internet at: http://www.nsf.org/services/by-industry/dietary-supplements/dietary-supplement-certification.

14. ConsumerLab.com. 2014 (cited 2014 Mar 19). On the Internet at: http://www.consumerlab.com.

15. Natural Products Association. NPA GMP certification program (cited 2014 Mar 19). On the Internet at: http://www.npainfo.org/npa/educationcertification/npagmpcertificationprogram.aspx.

16. FDA Consumer Health Information. FDA 101: health fraud awareness. 2009 May (cited 2014 Mar 19). On the Internet at: http://www.fda.gov/downloads/ForConsumers/ProtectYourself/HealthFraud/UCM167504.pdf.

17. Tsourounis C, Dennehy C. Introduction to dietary supplements. In: Krinsky DL, et al. Handbook of Nonprescription Drugs. 17th ed. Washington, DC: American Pharmacists Association; 2012.

18. Natural Standard Database Evidence Grading System. 2013 (cited 2014 Mar 19). On the Internet at: http://www.naturalstandard.com.

19. US Food and Drug Administration. Tips for dietary supplement users: making informed decisions and evaluating information. 2002 Jan (last updated 2013 Sep 20; cited 2014 Mar 19). On the Internet at: http://www.fda.gov/Food/DietarySupplements/UsingDietarySupplements/ucm110567.htm.

20. US Food and Drug Administration. Tips for older dietary supplement users. Last updated 2013 Oct 31 (cited 2014 Mar 19). On the Internet at: http://www.fda.gov/Food/DietarySupplements/UsingDietarySupplements/ucm110493.htm.

21. Egede LE, Ye X, Zeng D, Silverstein MD. The prevalence and pattern of complementary and alternative medicine use in individuals with diabetes. Diabetes Care. 2002;25:324-9.

22. Ryan EA, Pick ME, Marceau C. Use of alternative medicines in diabetes mellitus. Diabet Med. 2001;18:242-5.

23. Yeh GY, Eisenberg DM, Davis RB, Phillips RS. Use of complementary and alternative medicine among persons with diabetes mellitus: results of a national survey. Am J Public Health. 2002;92:1468-652.

24. Kennedy J. Herb and supplement use in the U.S. adult population. Clin Ther. 2005;27:1847-58.

25. Garrow D, Egede LE. Association between complementary and alternative medicine use, preventive care practices, and use of conventional medical services among adults with diabetes. Diabetes Care. 2006;29:15-9.

26. Villa-Caballero L, Morello CM, Chynoweth ME, et al. Ethnic differences in complementary and alternative medicine use among patients with diabetes. Complement Ther Med. 2010;18:241-8.

27. Odegard PS, Janci MM, Foeppel MP, et al. Prevalence and correlates of dietary supplement use in individuals with diabetes mellitus at an academic diabetes care clinic. Diabetes Educ. 2011;37:419-25.

28. Dannemann K, Hecker W, Haberland H, et al. Use of complementary and alternative medicine in children with type 1 diabetes mellitus—prevalence, patterns of use, and costs. Pediatr Diabetes. 2008;9:228-35.

29. Palinkas LB, Kabongo ML, San Diego Unified Practice Research in Family Medicine Network. The use of complementary and alternative medicine by primary care patients: a SURF*NET study. J Fam Pract. 2000;49:1121-30.

30. Nahin RL, Byrd-Clark D, Stussman BJ, Kalyanaraman N. Disease severity is associated with the use of complementary medicine to treat or manage type-2 diabetes: data from the 2002 and 2007 National Health Interview Survey. BMC Complement Altern Med. 2012;12:193.

31. Chang CLT, LinLin Y, Bartolome AP, et al. Herbal therapies for type 2 diabetes mellitus: chemistry, biology, and potential application of selected plants and compounds. Evid Based Complement Alternat Med. 2013;article ID 378657. Epub 2013 Apr 4. doi: 10.1155/2013/378657.

32. Boullata JI, Nace AM. Safety issues with herbal medicine. Pharmacotherapy. 2000;20:257-69.

33. Garrard J, Harms S, Eberly LE, Matiak A. Variations in product choices of frequently purchased herbs. Arch Intern Med. 2003;163:2290-5.

34. Beigel Y, Ostfeld I, Schoenfeld N. Clinical problem-solving: a leading question. N Engl J Med. 1998;339:827-30.

35. Bonati A. How and why should we standardize phytopharmaceutical drugs for clinical validation? J Ethnopharmacol. 1991;32:195-7.

36. Grant KL. Patient education and herbal dietary supplements. Am J Health Syst Pharm. 2000;57:1997-2003.

37. US Food and Drug Administration. Liqiang 4 Dietary Supplement Capsules. Last updated 2013 Aug 21 (cited 2014 Mar 19). On the Internet at: http://www.fda.gov/Safety/MedWatch/SafetyInformation/SafetyAlertsforHumanMedicalProducts/ucm150476.htm.

38. Gill GV, Redmond S, Garratt F, Paisey R. Diabetes and alternative medicine: cause for concern. Diabet Med. 1994;11:210-3.

39. Jellin JM, Gregory PJ, et al. Pharmacist's Letter/Prescriber's Letter Natural Medicines Comprehensive Database. 13th ed. Stockton, Calif: Therapeutic Research Faculty; 2013.

40. Yongchaiyudha S, Rungpitarangsi V, Bunyapraphatsara N, Chokechaijaroenporn O. Antidiabetic activity of Aloe vera L juice I. Clinical trial in new cases of diabetes mellitus. Phytomedicine. 1996;3:241-3.

41. Ngo MQ, Nguyen NN, Shah SA. Oral aloe vera for treatment of diabetes mellitus and dyslipidemia. Am J Health Syst Pharm. 2010;67:1804-11.

42. Lee A, Chui PT, Aun CST, Jin T, Lau AS. Possible interaction between sevoflurane and Aloe vera. Ann Pharmacother. 2004;38:1651-4.

43. Ghannam N. The antidiabetic activity of aloes: preliminary clinical and experimental observations. Horm Res. 1986;24:288-94.

44. Bunyapraphatsara N, Yongchaiyudha S, Rungpitarangsi V, Chokechaijaroenporn O. Antidiabetic activity of Aloe vera L juice II. Clinical trial in diabetes mellitus patients in combination with glibenclamide. Phytomedicine. 1996;3:245-8.

45. Husseini HF, Kianbakht S, Hajiaghaee R, Dabaghian FH. Anti-hyperglycemic and anti-hypercholesterolemic effects of *Aloe vera* leaf gel in hyperlipidemic type 2 diabetic patients: a randomized double-blind placebo-controlled clinical trial. Planta Med. 2012;78:311-6.

46. Dong H, Wang N, Zhao L, Lu F. Berberine in the treatment of type 2 diabetes mellitus: a systematic review and meta-analysis. Evid Based Complement Alternat Med. 2012; article ID 591654. doi:10.1155/2012/591654.

47. Zhang Y, Li X, Zou D, et al. Treatment of type 2 diabetes and dyslipidemia with the natural plant alkaloid berberine. J Clin Endocrinol Metab. 2008;93:2559-65.

48. Zhang H, Wei J, Xue R, et al. Berberine lowers blood glucose in type 2 diabetes mellitus patients through increasing insulin receptor expression. Metabolism. 2010;59:285-92.

49. Yin J, Xing H, Ye J. Efficacy of berberine in patients with type 2 diabetes mellitus. Metabolism. 2008;57:712-7.

50. Guo Y, Li F, Ma X, et al. CYP2D plays a major role in berberine metabolism in liver of mice and humans. Xenobiotica. 2011;41:996-1005.

51. Basch E, Gabardi S, Ulbricht C. Bitter melon (Momordica charantia): a review of efficacy and safety. Am J Health Syst Pharm. 2003;60:356-9.

52. Tan MJ, Ye JM, Turner N, et al. Antidiabetic activities of triterpenoids isolated from bitter melon associated with activation of the AMPK pathway. Chem Biol. 2008;15:263-73.

53. Nhiem NX, Kiem PV, Minh CV, et al. Alpha-Glucosidase inhibition properties of cucurbitane-type triterpene glycosides from the fruits of Momordica charantia. Chem Pharm Bull (Tokyo). 2010;58:720-4.

54. Aslam M, Stockley IH. Interaction between curry ingredient (karela) and drug (chlorpropamide) (Letter). Lancet. 1979;1:607.

55. Ahmad N, Hassan MR, Halder H, Bennoor KS. Effect of momordica charantia (karolla) extracts on fasting and postprandial serum glucose levels in NIDDM patients. Bangladesh Med Res Counc Bull. 1999;25:11-3.

56. Khanna P, Jain SC, Panagariya A, Dixit VP. Hypoglycemic activity of polypeptide-p from a plant source. J Nat Prod. 1981;44:648-55.

57. Dans AML, Villarruz MVC, Jimeno CA, et al. The effect of Momordica charantia capsule preparation on glycemic control in type 2 diabetes mellitus needs further studies. J Clin Epidemiol. 2007;60:554-9.

58. Fuangchan A, Sonthisombat P, Seubnukarn T, et al. Hypoglycemic effect of bitter melon compared with metformin in newly diagnosed type 2 diabetes patients. J Ethnopharmacol. 2011;134:422-8.

59. Ooi CP, Yassin Z, Hamid TA. Momordica charantia for type 2 diabetes mellitus. Cochrane Database Syst Rev. 2012 Aug 15;8:CD007845. doi: 10.1002/14651858.CD007845.pub3.

60. Charantia [product information]. Las Pinas City, Philippines: Herbcare Corporation; 2004.

61. Cefalu WT, Hu FB. Role of chromium in human health and in diabetes. Diabetes Care. 2004;27:2741-51.

62. Cefalu WT, Rood J, Pinsonat P, et al. Characterization of the metabolic and physiologic response to chromium supplementation in subjects with type 2 diabetes mellitus. Metabolism. 2010;59:755-62.

63. Food and Nutrition Board, Institute of Medicine. Dietary Reference Intakes for Vitamin A, Vitamin K, Arsenic, Boron, Chromium, Copper, Iodine, Iron, Manganese, Molybdenum, Nickel, Silicon, Vanadium, and Zinc.

Washington, DC: National Academies Press; 2005 (cited 2014 Mar 19). On the Internet at: http://www.nap.edu/openbook.php?record_id=10026&page=197.

64. Anderson R, Polansky M, Bryden N, Canary J. Supplemental chromium effects on glucose, insulin, glucagon, and urinary chromium losses in subjects consuming controlled low-chromium diets. Am J Clin Nutr. 1991;54:909-16.

65. Anderson RA, Cheng N, Bryden NA, et al. Elevated intakes of supplemental chromium improves glucose and insulin variables in individuals with type 2 diabetes. Diabetes. 1997;46:1786-91.

66. Cefalu WT, Bell-Farrow AD, Stegner J, et al. Effect of chromium picolinate on insulin sensitivity in vivo. J Trace Elem Exp Med. 1999;12:71-83.

67. Jovanovic L, Gutierrez M, Peterson CM. Chromium supplementation for women with gestational diabetes mellitus. J Trace Elem Exp Med. 1999;12:91-107.

68. Althuis MD, Jordan NE, Ludington EA, Wittes JT. Glucose and insulin responses to dietary chromium supplements: a meta analysis. Am J Clin Nutr. 2002;76:148-55.

69. Albarracon CA, Fuqua BC, Evans JL, Goldfine ID. Chromium picolinate and biotin combination improves glucose metabolism in treated, uncontrolled overweight to obese patients with type 2 diabetes. Diabetes Metab Res Rev. 2008;24:41-51.

70. Sharma S, Agrawal RP, Choudhary M, et al. Beneficial effect of chromium supplementation on glucose, HbA1C and lipid variables in individuals with newly onset type-2 diabetes. J Trace Elemen Med Biol. 2011;25:149-53.

71. Chase CK, McQueen CE. Cinnamon in diabetes mellitus. Am J Health Syst Pharm. 2007;64:1033-5.

72. Kirkham S, Akilen R, Sharma S, Tsiami A. The potential of cinnamon to reduce blood glucose levels in patients with type 2 diabetes and insulin resistance. Diabetes Obes Metab. 2009;11:1100-13.

73. Anderson RA, Broadhurst CL, Polansky MM, et al. Isolation and characterization of polyphenol type-A polymers from cinnamon with insulin-like biological activity. J Agric Food Chem. 2004;52:65-70.

74. Kim SH, Huyn SH, Choung SY. Anti-diabetic effect of cinnamon extract on blood glucose in db/db mice. J Ethnopharmacol. 2006;104:119-23.

75. Rafehi H, Ververis K, Karagiannis TC. Controversies surrounding the clinical potential of cinnamon for the management of diabetes. Diabetes Obes Metab. 2012;14:493-9.

76. Hlebowicz J, Darwiche G, Bjorgell O, Almer L-O. Effect of cinnamon on post-prandial blood glucose, gastric emptying, and satiety in healthy subjects. Am J Clin Nutr. 2007;85:1552-6.

77. Baker WL, Gutierrez-Williams G, White CM, Kluger J, Coleman CI. Effect of cinnamon on glucose control and lipid parameters. Diabetes Care. 2008;31:41-3.

78. Crawford P. Effectiveness of cinnamon for lowering hemoglobin A1C in patients with type 2 diabetes: a randomized, controlled trial. J Am Board Fam Med. 2009;22:507-12.

79. Akilen R, Tsiami A, Devendra D, Robinson N. Glycated haemoglobin and blood-pressure lowering effect of cinnamon in multi-ethnic type 2 diabetic patients in the UK: a randomized, placebo-controlled, double-blind clinical trial. Diabet Med. 2010;27:1159-67.

80. Leach MJ, Kumar S. Cinnamon for diabetes mellitus. Cochrane Database Syst Rev. 2012;9:CD007170. doi:10.1002/14651858.CD007170.pub2.

81. Allen RW, Schwartzman E, Baker WL, et al. Cinnamon use in type 2 diabetes: an updated systematic review and meta-analysis. Ann Fam Med. 2013;11:452-9.

82. Madar Z. Fenugreek (trigonella foenum-graecum) as a means of reducing postprandial glucose levels in diabetic rats. Nutr Rep Int. 1984;23:1267-73.

83. Raghuram TC, Sharma R, Sivakumar D, Sahay BK. Effect of fenugreek seeds on intravenous glucose disposition in non-insulin dependent diabetic patients. Phytother Res. 1994;8:83-6.

84. Patil SP, Niphadkar PV, Bapat MM. Allergy to fenugreek (trigonella foenum graecum). Ann Allergy Asthma Immunol. 1997;78:297-300.

85. Lambert J, Cormier J. Potential interaction between warfarin and boldo-fenugreek. Pharmacotherapy. 2001;21:509-12.

86. Sharma RD, Raghuram TC, Sudhakar Rao N. Effect of fenugreek seeds on blood glucose and serum lipids in type 1 diabetes. Eur J Clin Nutr. 1990;44:301-6.

87. Sharma RD, Sarkar A, Hazra DK, et al. Use of fenugreek seed powder in the management of non-insulin-dependent diabetes mellitus. Nutr Res. 1996;16:1331-9.

88. Gupta A, Gupta R, Lal B. Effect of Trigonella foenum-graecum (fenugreek) seeds on glycaemic control and insulin resistance in type 2 diabetes mellitus: a double blind placebo controlled study. J Assoc Physicians India. 2001;49:1057-61.

89. Lu F, Shen L, Qin Y, et al. Clinical observation on trigonella foenum-graecum L. total saponins in combination with sulfonylureas in the treatment of type 2 diabetes mellitus. Chin J Integr Med. 2008;14:56-60.

90. Kassaian N, Azadbakht L, Forghani V, Amini M. Effect of fenugreek seeds on blood glucose and lipid profiles in type 2 diabetic patients. Int J Vitam Nutr Res. 2009;79:34-9.

91. Kiefer D, Pantuso T. Panax ginseng. Am Fam Physician. 2003;68:1539-42.

92. Vuksan V, Sievenpiper JL, Koo VYY, et al. American ginseng (Panax quinquefolius L.) reduces postprandial glycemia in nondiabetic subjects and subjects with type 2 diabetes mellitus. Arch Intern Med. 2000;160:1009-13.

93. Vuksan V, Stavro MP, Sievenpiper JL, et al. Similar postprandial glycemic reductions with escalation of dose and administration time of American ginseng in type 2 diabetes. Diabetes Care. 2000;23:1221-6.

94. Yuan CS, Wu JA, Lowell T, Gu M. Gut and brain effects of American ginseng root on brain-stem neuronal activities in rats. Am J Chin Med. 1998;26:47-55.

95. Ohnishi Y, Takagi S, Miura T, et al. Effect of ginseng radix on GLUT2 protein content in mouse liver in normal and epinephrine-induced hyperglycemic mice. Biol Pharm Bull. 1996;19:1238-40.

96. Kimura M, Waki I, Chujo T, et al. Effects of hypoglycemic components in ginseng radix on blood insulin level in alloxan diabetic mice and on insulin release from perfused rat pancreas. J Pharmacobiodyn. 1981;4:410-7.

97. Yuan H-D, Kim JT, Kim SH, Chung SH. Ginseng and diabetes: the evidence from in vitro, animal and human studies. J Ginseng Res. 2012;36:27-39.

98. Sotaniemi EA, Haapakoski E, Rautio A. Ginseng therapy in non-insulin dependent diabetic patients. Diabetes Care. 1995;18:1373-5.

99. Vuksan V, Sung MK, Sievenpiper JL, et al. Korean red ginseng (Panax ginseng) improves glucose and insulin regulation in well-controlled, type 2 diabetes: results of a randomized, double-blind, placebo-controlled study of efficacy and safety. Nutr Metab Cardiovasc Dis. 2008; 18:46-56.

100. Ma SW, Benzie IFF, Chu TTW, et al. Effects of Panax ginseng supplementation on biomarkers of glucose tolerance, antioxidant status and oxidative stress in type 2 diabetic subjects: results of a placebo-controlled human intervention trial. Diabetes Obes Metab. 2008;10: 1125-7.

101. Reeds DN, Patterson BW, Okunade A, et al. Ginseng and ginsenoside Re do not improve β-cell function or insulin sensitivity in overweight and obese subjects with impaired glucose tolerance or diabetes. Diabetes Care. 2011;35:1071-6.

102. Shergis JL, Zhang AL, Zhou W, Xue CC. Panax ginseng in randomized controlled trials: a systematic review. Phytother Res. 2013;27(7):949-65. Epub 2012 Sep 12. doi: 10.1002/ptr.4832.

103. Harkey MR, Henderson GL, Gershwin ME, Stern JS, Hacman RM. Variability in commercial ginseng products: an analysis of 25 preparations. Am J Clin Nutr. 2001;73:1101-6.

104. Kanetkar P, Singhal R, Kamat M. *Gymnema sylvestre*: a memoir. J Clin Biochem Nutr. 2007;41:77-81.

105. Anonymous. Gymnema sylvestre. Altern Med Rev. 1999; 4:46-7.

106. Yoshikawa M, Murakami T, Kadoya M, et al. Medicinal foodstuffs. IX. The inhibitors of glucose absorption from the leaves of Gymnema sylvestre R. Br. (Asclepiadaceae): structures of gymnemosides a and b. Chem Pharm Bull. 1997;45:1671-6.

107. Shanmugasundaram ER, Panneerselvam C, Samudram P, Shanmugasundaram ERB. Enzyme changes and glucose utilization in diabetic rabbits: the effect of gymnema sylvestre. J Ethnopharmacol. 1983;7:205-34.

108. Persaud SJ, Al-Majed H, Raman A, Jones PM. Gymnema sylvestre stimulates insulin release in vitro by increased membrane permeability. J Endocrinol. 1999;163:207-12.

109. Shanmugasundaram ERB, Gopinath KL, Shanmugasundaram KR, Rajendran VM. Possible regeneration of the islets of Langerhans in streptozotocin-diabetic rats given Gymnema sylvestre leaf extracts. J Ethnopharmacol. 1990;30:265-79.

110. Shiyovich A, Sztarkier I, Nesher L. Toxic hepatitis induced by Gymnema sylvestre, a natural remedy for type 2 diabetes mellitus. Am J Med Sci. 2010;340:514-7.

111. Shangmugasundaram ERB, Rajeswari G, Baskaran K, Rajesh Kumar BR, Shangmugasundaram KR, Ahmath RK. Use of gymnema sylvestre leaf extract in the control of blood glucose in insulin-dependent diabetes mellitus. J Ethnopharmacol. 1990;30:281-94.

112. Baskaran K, Kizar B, Ahamath K, Shangmugasundaram KR, Shangmugasundaram ERB. Antidiabetic effect of a leaf extract from Gymnema sylvestre in non-insulin-dependent diabetes mellitus patients. J Ethnopharmacol. 1990;30:295-306.

113. Kumar SN, Mani UV, Mani I. An open label study on the supplementation of Gymnema sylvestre in type 2 diabetics. J Diet Suppl. 2010;7:273-82.

114. Al-Romaiyan A, Liu B, Asare-Anane H, et al. A novel gymnema sylvestre extract stimulates insulin secretion from human islets in vivo and in vitro. Phytother Res. 2010;24(9):1370-6.

115. Pepping J. Alternative therapies: milk thistle: *Silybum marianum*. Am J Health Syst Pharm. 1999;56:1195-7.

116. Flora K, Hahn M, Rosen H, Benner K. Milk thistle (silybum marianum) for the therapy of liver disease. Am J Gastroenterol. 1998;93:139-43.

117. Medina J, Fernandez-Salazar LI, Garcia-Buey L, Moreno-Otero R. Approach to the pathogenesis and treatment of nonalcoholic steatohepatitis. Diabetes Care. 2004;27:2057-66.

118. Velussi M, Cernigoi AM, De Monte A, Dapas F, Caffau C, Zilli M. Long-term (12 months) treatment with an antioxidant drug (silymarin) is effective on hyperinsulinemia, exogenous insulin need and malondialdehyde levels in cirrhotic diabetic patients. J Hepatol. 1997;26:871-9.

119. Jose MA, Abraham A, Narmadha MP. Effect of silymarin in diabetes mellitus patients with liver disease. J Pharmacol Pharmacother. 2011;2:287-9.

120. Fallahzadeh MK, Dormanesh B, Sagheb MM, et al. Effect of addition of silymarin to renin-angiotensin system inhibitors on proteinuria in type 2 diabetic patients with overt nephropathy: a randomized, double-blind, placebo-controlled trial. Am J Kidney Dis. 2012;60: 896-903.

121. Huseini HF, Larijani B, Heshmat R, et al. The efficacy of *Silybum marianum* (L.) Gaertn. (silymarin) in the treatment of type II diabetes: a randomized, double blind, placebo-controlled, clinical trial. Phytother Res. 2006;20:1036-9.

122. Hussain SA-R. Silymarin as an adjunct to glibenclamide therapy improves long-term and postprandial glycemic control and body mass index in type 2 diabetes. J Med Food. 2007;10:543-7.

123. Frati-Munari AC, Gordillo BE, Altamirano P, Ariza CR. Hypoglycemic effect of opuntia streptacantha lemaire in NIDDM. Diabetes Care. 1998;11:63-6.

124. Rayburn K, Martinez R, Escobedo M, Wright F, Farias M. Glycemic effects of various species of nopal (Opuntia sp) in type 2 diabetes mellitus. Texas J Rural Health. 1998; 26:68-76.

125. Sobieraj DM, Freyer CW. Probable hypoglycemic adverse drug reaction associated with prickly pear cactus, glipizide, and metformin in a patient with type 2 diabetes mellitus. Ann Pharmacother. 2010;44:1334-7.

126. Frati AC, Gordillo BE, Altamirano P, Ariza CR, Cortes-Franco R, Chavez-Negrete A. Acute hypoglycemic effect of opuntia streptacantha lemaire in NIDDM (Letter). Diabetes Care. 1990;13:45-6.

127. Bacardi-Gascon M, Dueñas-Mena D, Jimenez-Cruz A. Lowering effect on postprandial glycemic response of nopales added to Mexican breakfasts. Diabetes Care. 2007;30:1264-5.

128. Godard MP, Ewing BA, Pischel I, et al. Acute blood glucose lowering effects and long-term safety of Opun-Dia™ supplementation in pre-diabetic males and females. J Ethnopharmacol. 2010;130:631-4.

129. Diaz-Medina EM, Martin-Herrera D, Rodriguez-Rodriguez EM, Diaz-Romero C. Chromium (III) in cactus pad and its possible role in the antihyperglycemic activity. J Funct Foods. 2012;4:311-4.

130. Williams NT. Probiotics. Am J Health Syst Pharm. 2010; 67:449-58.

131. Diamant M, Blaak EE, deVos WM, et al. Do nutrient-gut-microbiota interactions play a role in human obesity, insulin resistance and type 2 diabetes? Obes Rev. 2011; 12:272-81.

132. Musso G, Gambino R, Cassader M. Obesity, diabetes, and gut microbiota: the hygiene hypothesis expanded? Diabetes Care. 2010;33:2277-84.

133. Cani PD, Possemiers S, Van de Wiele T, et al. Changes in gut microbiota control inflammation in obese mice through a mechanism involving GLP-2-driven improvement of gut permeability. Gut. 2009;58:1091-3.

134. Turnbaugh PJ, Ley RE, Mahowald MA, et al. An obesity-associated gut microbiome with increased capacity for energy harvest. Nature. 2006;444:1027-31.

135. Turnbaugh PJ, Hamady M, Yatsunenko T, et al. A core gut microbiome in obese and lean twins. Nature. 2009; 457:480-4.

136. Qin J, Cai Z, Li S, et al. A metagenome-wide association of gut microbiota in type 2 diabetes. Nature. 2012;490: 55-60.

137. Baggio LL, Drucker DJ. Biology of incretins: GLP-1 and GIP. Gastroenterology. 2007;132:2131-57.

138. Karlsson FH, Tremaroli V, Nookaew I, et al. Gut metagenome in European women with normal, impaired and diabetic glucose control. Nature. 2013;498:99-103.

139. Larsen N, Vogensen FK, van den Berg FWJ, et al. Gut microbiota in human adults with type 2 diabetes differs from non-diabetic adults. PLoS One. 2010;5:e9085.

140. Andreason AS, Larsen N, Pedersen-Skovsgaard T, et al. Effects of Lactobacillus acidophilus NCFM on insulin sensitivity and the systemic inflammatory response in human subjects. Br J Nutr. 2010;104:1831-8.

141. Luoto R, Laitinen K, Nermes M, Isolauri E. Impact of maternal probiotic-supplemented dietary counseling on pregnancy outcome and prenatal and postnatal growth: a double-blind, placebo-controlled study. Br J Nutr. 2010;103:1792-9.

142. Besselink MG, van Santvoort HC, Buskens E, et al. Probiotic prophylaxis in predicted severe acute pancreatitis: a randomized, double-blind, placebo-controlled trial. Lancet. 2008;371:651-9.

143. Gibson GR, Roberfroid MB. Dietary modulation of the human colonic microbiota: introducing the concept of prebiotics. J Nutr. 1995;125:1401-2.

144. Cani PD, Dewever C, Delzenne NM. Inulin-type fructans modulate gastrointestinal peptides involved in appetite regulation (glucagon-like peptide-1 and ghrelin) in rats. Br J Nutr. 2004;92:521-6.

145. International Scientific Association for Probiotics and Prebiotics. The P's and Q's of probiotics: a consumer guide for making smart choices. 2001 (cited 2014 Mar 19). On the Internet at: http://www.bifantis.com/pdf/Ps_and_Qs_of_probiotics.pdf.

146. Nichols TW. Alpha-lipoic acid: biological effects and clinical implications. Altern Med Rev. 1997;2:177-83.

147. Evans JL, Goldfine ID. Alpha-lipoic acid: a multi-functional antioxidant that improves insulin sensitivity

in patients with type 2 diabetes. Diabetes Technol Ther. 2000;2:401-13.

148. Ziegler D, Low PA, Litchy WJ, et al. Efficacy and safety of antioxidant treatment with α–lipoic acid over 4 years in diabetic polyneuropathy: the NATHAN 1 trial. Diabetes Care. 2011;34:2054-60.

149. Ziegler D, Hanefeld M, Ruhnau K-J, et al. ALADIN Study Group. Treatment of symptomatic diabetic peripheral neuropathy with the anti-oxidant alpha-lipoic acid: a 3-week multicentre randomized controlled trial (ALADIN Study I). Diabetologia. 1995;38:1425-33.

150. Reljanovic M, Reichel G, Rett K, et al. ALADIN II Study Group. Treatment of diabetic polyneuropathy with the antioxidant thioctic acid (alpha-lipoic acid): a two year multicenter randomized double-blind placebo controlled trial (ALADIN II): Alpha Lipoic Acid in Diabetic Neuropathy. Free Radic Biol Med. 1999;31:171-9.

151. Ziegler D, Hanefeld M, Ruhnau K-J, et al. ALADIN III Study Group. Treatment of symptomatic diabetic polyneuropathy with the antioxidant α-lipoic acid: a 7-month multicenter randomized controlled trial (ALADIN III Study). Diabetes Care. 1999;22:1296-1301.

152. The SYDNEY Trial Study Group. The sensory symptoms of diabetic polyneuropathy are improved with lipoic acid. Diabetes Care. 2003;26:770-6.

153. Ziegler D, Nowak H, Kemplert P, Vargha P, Low PA. Treatment of symptomatic diabetic polyneuropathy with the antioxidant α-lipoic acid: a meta-analysis. Diabet Med. 2004;21:114-21.

154. Ziegler D, Ametov A, Barinov A, et al. Oral treatment with α-lipoic acid improves symptomatic diabetic neuropathy: the SYDNEY 2 trial. Diabetes Care. 2006;29:2365-70.

155. Head KA. Benfotiamine. Altern Med Rev. 2006;11:238-42.

156. Hammes H-P, Du X, Edelstein D, et al. Benfotiamine blocks three major pathways of hyperglycemic damage and prevents experimental diabetic retinopathy. Nature Med. 2003;9:294-9.

157. Winkler G, Pal B, Nagybeganyi E, Ory I, Porochnavec M, Kempler P. Effectiveness of different benfotiamine dosage regimens in the treatment of painful diabetic neuropathy. Arzneimittelforschung. 1999;49:220-4.

158. Simeonov S, Pavlova M, Mitkov M, Mincheva L, Troev D. Therapeutic efficacy of "Milgamma" in patients with painful diabetic neuropathy. Folia Medica. 1997;39:5-10.

159. Haupt E, Ledermann H, Kopcke W. Benfotiamine in the treatment of diabetic polyneuropathy—a three-week randomized, controlled pilot study (BEDIP Study). Int J Clin Pharmacol Ther. 2005;43:71-7.

160. Stracke H, Gaus W, Achenbach U, Federlin K, Bretzel RG. Benfotiamine in diabetic polyneuropathy (BENDIP): results of a randomised, double blind, placebo-controlled clinical study. Exp Clin Endocrinol Diabetes. 2008;116:600-5.

161. Stracke H. A benfotiamine-vitamin B combination in treatment of diabetic polyneuropathy. Exp Clin Endocrinol Diabetes. 1996;104:311-6.

162. Fraser DA, Diep LM, Hovden IA, et al. The effects of long-term oral benfotiamine supplementation on peripheral nerve function and inflammatory markers in patients with type 1 diabetes: a 24-month, double-blind, randomized, placebo-controlled trial. Diabetes Care. 2012;35:1095-7.

163. Ziegler D, Tesfaye S, Kempler P. Comment on: Fraser et al. The effects of long-term long-term oral benfotiamine supplementation on peripheral nerve function and inflammatory markers in patients with type 1 diabetes: a 24-month, double-blind, randomized, placebo-controlled trial. Diabetes Care. 2012;35:1095-7. [Letter] Diabetes Care. 2012;35:e79.

164. Hammes H-P, Du X, Edelstein D, Taguchi T, Matsumura T, Ju Q, et al. Benfotiamine blocks three major pathways of hyperglycemic damage and prevents experimental diabetic retinopathy. Nature Med. 2003;9:294-9.

165. Rabbani N, Alam SS, Riaz S, et al. High-dose thiamine therapy for patients with type 2 diabetes and microalbuminuria: a randomized, double-blind placebo-controlled study. Diabetologia. 2009;52:208-12.

166. Alkhalaf A, Klooster A, van Oeveren W, et al. A double-blind, randomized, placebo-controlled clinical trial on benfotiamine treatment in patients with diabetic nephropathy. Diabetes Care. 2010;33:1598-601.

167. Bonakdar RA, Guarneri E. Coenzyme Q10. Am Fam Physician. 2005;72:1065-70.

168. McCarty MF. Can correction of sub-optimal coenzyme Q status improve α-cell function in type II diabetics? Med Hypotheses. 1999;52:397-400.

169. Langsjoen P, Langsjoen P, Folkers K. Long-term efficacy and safety of coenzyme Q10 therapy for idiopathic dilated cardiomyopathy. Am J Cardiol. 1990;65:521-3.

170. Tran MT, Mitchell TM, Kennedy DT, Giles JT. Role of Coenzyme Q_{10} in chronic heart failure, angina, and hypertension. Pharmacotherapy. 2001;21:797-806.

171. Pepping J. Alternative Therapies—Coenzyme Q10. Am J Health Syst Pharm. 1999;56:519-21.

172. Gaby AR. The role of coenzyme Q10 in clinical medicine: part II. Cardiovascular disease, hypertension, diabetes mellitus and infertility. Alt Med Rev. 1996;1:168-75.

173. Villalba JM, Parrado C, Santos-Gonzalez M, Alcain FJ. Therapeutic use of coenzyme Q10 and coenzyme Q10-related compounds and formulations. Expert Opin Investig Drugs. 2010;19:535-54.

174. Littarru GP, Luca T. Clinical aspects of coenzyme Q10: an update. Nutrition. 2010;26:250-4.

175. Langsjoen P, Langsjoen P, Willis R, Folkers K. Treatment of essential hypertension with coenzyme Q10. Molec Aspects Med. 1994;15(suppl):165-72.

176. Singh RB, Niaz MA, Rastogi SS, Shukla PK, Thakur AS. Effect of hydrosoluble coenzyme Q10 on blood pressures and insulin resistance in hypertensive patients with coronary artery disease. J Hum Hypertens. 1999;13:203-8.

177. Henriksen JE, Andersen CB, Hother-Nielsen O, Vaag A, Aage Mortensen S, Beck-Nielsen H. Impact of ubiquinone (coenzyme Q10) treatment on glycaemic control, insulin requirement and well-being in patients with type 1 diabetes mellitus. Diabetic Med. 1999;16:312-8.

178. Eriksson JG, Forsen TJ, Mortensen SA, Rohde M. The effect of coenzyme Q10 administration on metabolic control in patients with type 2 diabetes mellitus. Biofactors. 1999;9:315-8.

179. Hodgson JM, Watts GF, Playford DA, et al. Coenzyme Q10 improves blood pressure and glycaemic control: a controlled trial in subjects with type 2 diabetes. Eur J Clin Nutr. 2002;56:1137-42.

180. Mezawa M, Takemoto M, Onishi S, et al. The reduced form of coenzyme Q10 improves glycemic control in patients with type 2 diabetes: an open label pilot study. Biofactors. 2012;38:416-21.

181. Fotino AD, Thompson-Paul AM, Bazzano LA. Effect of coenzyme Q_{10} supplementation on heart failure: a meta-analysis. Am J Clin Nutr. 2013;97:268-75.

182. Alehagen U, Johansson P, Bjornstedt M, Rosen A, Dahlstrom U. Cardiovascular mortality and N-terminal-proBNP reduced after combined selenium and coenzyme Q10 supplementation: a 5-year prospective randomized double-blind placebo-controlled trial among elderly Swedish citizens. Int J Cardiol. 2013;167(5):1880-6. Epub 2012 May 23. doi: 10.1016/j.ijcard.2012.04.156.

183. Ganesan S, Ito MK. Coenzyme Q10 ameliorates the reduction in GLUT4 transporter expression induced by simvastatin in 3T3-L1 adipocytes. Metab Syndr Relat Disord. Epub 2013 Mar 15.

184. Hamilton SJ, Chew GT, Watts GF. Coenzyme Q10 improves endothelial dysfunction in statin-treated type 2 diabetic patients. Diabetes Care. 2009;32:810-2.

185. Kris-Etherton PM, Harris WS, Appel LJ, for the Nutrition Committee. Fish consumption, fish oil, omega-3 fatty acids, and cardiovascular disease [published correction appears in Circulation 2003;107:512]. Circulation. 2002;106:2747-57.

186. Nettleton JA, Katz R. N-3 long-chain polyunsaturated fatty acids in type 2 diabetes: a review. J Am Diet Assoc. 2005;105:428-40.

187. Gruppo Italiano per lo Studio della Sopravvivienza nell'Infarto miocardico (GISSI Prevenzione Investigators). Dietary supplementation with n-3 polyunsaturated fatty acids and vitamin E after myocardial infarction: results of the GISSI-Prevenzione trial. Lancet. 1999;354:447-55.

188. Hartweg J, Perera R, Montori V, et al. Omega-3 polyunsaturated fatty acids (PUFA) for type 2 diabetes mellitus. Cochrane Database Syst Rev. 2008;1:CD003205.

189. ORIGIN Trial Investigators. N-3 fatty acids and cardiovascular outcomes in patients with dysglycemia. N Engl J Med. 2012;367:309-18.

190. Rizos EC, Ntzani EE, Bika EE, et al. Association between omega-3 fatty acid supplementation and risk of major cardiovascular disease events: a systematic review and meta-analysis. JAMA. 2012;308:1024-33.

191. Risk and Prevention Study Collaborative Group. N-3 fatty acids in patients with multiple cardiovascular risk factors. N Engl J Med. 2013;368:1800-8.

192. Mozaffarian D, Lemaitre RN, King IB, et al. Plasma phospholipid long-chain omega-3 fatty acids and total and cause-specific mortality in older adults: a cohort study. Ann Intern Med. 2013;158:515-25.

193. Wu JHY, Cahill LE, Mozaffarian D. Effect of fish oil on circulating adiponectin: a systematic review and meta-analysis of randomized controlled trials. J Clin Edocrinol Metab. 2013;98:2451-9.

194. MacLean CH, Mojica WA, Morton SC, et al. Effects of omega-3 fatty acids on lipids and glycemic control in type II diabetes and the metabolic syndrome and on inflammatory bowel disease, rheumatoid arthritis, renal disease, systemic lupus erythematosus, and osteoporosis. Evid Rep Technol Assess (Summ). 2004;(89):1-4. (Prepared by the Southern California/RAND Evidence-Based Practice Center, Los Angeles, Calif) AHRQ Publication No. 04-E012-1. Rockville, Md, Agency for Healthcare Research and Quality.

195. Lovaza [product information]. Research Triangle Park, NC: GlaxoSmithKline Pharmaceuticals; 2012.

196. Tattelman E. Health effects of garlic. Am Fam Physician. 2005;72:103-6.

197. Pareddy SR, Rosenberg JM. Does garlic have useful medicinal purposes? Hosp Pharm Rep. 1993;8:27.

198. Ackermann RT, Mulrow CD, Ramirez G, Gardner CD, Morbidoni L, Lawrence VA. Garlic shows promise for improving some cardiovascular risk factors. Arch Intern Med. 2001;161:813-4.

199. Silagy CA, Neil HA. A meta-analysis of the effect of garlic on blood pressure. J Hypertens. 1994;12:463-8.

200. Ried K, Frank OR, Stocks NP, Fakler P, Sullivan T. Effect of garlic on blood pressure: a systematic review and meta-analysis. BMC Cardiovasc Disord. 2008;8(13):1-12. doi: 10.1186/1471-2261-8-13.

201. Stevinson C, Pittler MH, Ernst E. Garlic for treating hypercholesterolemia: a meta-analysis of randomized clinical trials. Ann Intern Med. 2000;133:420-9.

202. Reinhart KM, Talati R, White CM, Coleman CI. The impact of garlic on lipid parameters: a systematic review and meta-analysis. Nutr Res Rev. 2009;22:39-48.

203. Khoo YS, Aziz Z. Garlic supplementation and serum cholesterol: a meta-analysis. J Clin Pharm Ther. 2009;34:133-45.

204. Ashraf R, Aamir K, Shaikh AR, Ahmed T. Effects of garlic on dyslipidemia in patients with type 2 diabetes. J Ayub Med Coll Abbottabad. 2005;17:60-4.

205. Ashraf R, Khan RA, Ashraf I. Garlic (allium sativum) supplementation with standard antidiabetic agent provides better diabetic control in type 2 diabetes patients. Pak J Pharm Sci. 2011;24:565-70.

206. Kumar R, Chhatwal S, Arora S, et al. Antihyperglycemic, antihyperlipidemic, anti-inflammatory and adenosine deaminase-lowering effects of garlic in patients with type 2 diabetes mellitus with obesity. Diabetes Metab Syndr Obes. 2013;6:49-56.

207. Ahmad MS, Ahmed M. Antiglycation properties of aged garlic extract: possible role in prevention of diabetic complications. J Nutr. 2006;136(3 Suppl):796S-9S.

208. Stabler SN, Tejani AM, Huynh F, Fowkes C. Garlic for the prevention of cardiovascular morbidity and mortality in hypertensive patients. Cochrane Database of Systematic Reviews. 2012 Aug 15;8:CD007653. doi: 10.1002/14651858.CD007653.pub2.

209. Linde K, Berner MM, Kriston L. St John's wort for major depression. Cochrane Database of Systematic Reviews. 2008 Oct 8;4:CD000448. doi: 10.1002/14651858. CD000448.pub3.

210. Pittas AG, Lau J, Hu FB, Dawson-Hughes B. The role of vitamin D and calcium in type 2 diabetes: a systematic review and meta analysis. J Clin Endocrinol Metab. 2007;92:2017-29.

211. Holick MF. Vitamin D deficiency. N Engl J Med. 2007; 357:266-81.

212. Lee JH, O'Keefe JH, Bell D, Hensrud DD, Holick MF. Vitamin D deficiency: an important, common, and easily treatable cardiovascular risk factor? J Am Coll Cardiol. 2008;52:1949-56.

213. NIH Office of Dietary Supplements. Dietary supplement fact sheet: vitamin D (cited 2013 Jun 8). On the Internet at: http://ods.od.nih.gov/factsheets/ VitaminD-HealthProfessional/?print=1.

214. Hyponnen E, Laara E, Reunanen A, Jarvelin M-R, Virtanen SM. Intake of vitamin D and risk of type 1 diabetes: a birth-cohort study. Lancet. 2001;35(8):1500-3.

215. Pittas AG, Dawson-Hughes B, Li T, et al. Vitamin D and calcium intake in relation to type 2 diabetes in women. Diabetes Care. 2006;29:650-6.

216. Chiu KC, Chu A, Go VLW, Saad MF. Hypovitaminosis D is associated with insulin resistance and ß cell dysfunction. Am J Clin Nutr. 2004;79:820-5.

217. Di Cesar DJ, Ploutz-Snyder R, Weinstock RS, Moses AM. Vitamin D deficiency is more common in type 2 than in type 1 diabetes. Diabetes Care. 2006;29:174.

218. Gorham ED, Garland CF, Burgi AA, et al. Lower prediagnostic serum 25-hydroxyvitamin D concentration is associated with higher risk of insulin-requiring diabetes: a nested case-control study. Diabetologia. 2012;55:3224-7.

219. Song Y, Wang L, Pittas AG, et al. Blood 25-hydroxy vitamin D levels and incident type 2 diabetes: a meta-analysis of prospective studies. Diabetes Care. 2013;36:1422-8.

220. McGreevy C, Williams D. New insights about vitamin D and cardiovascular disease. Ann Intern Med. 2011;155: 820-6.

221. Waqas A, Khan N, Glueck CJ, et al. Low serum 25 (OH) vitamin D levels (<32 ng/mL) are associated with reversible myositis-myalgia in statin-treated patients. Translational Research. 2009;153:11-6.

222. Institute of Medicine, Food and Nutrition Board. Dietary Reference Intakes for Calcium and Vitamin D. Washington, DC: National Academy Press; 2010.

223. Pramyothin P, Holick MF. Vitamin D supplementation: guidelines and evidence for subclinical deficiency. Curr Opin Gastroenterol. 2012;28:139-50.

224. American Geriatrics Society Workgroup on Vitamin D Supplementation for Older Adults. Recommendations abstracted from the American Geriatrics Society consensus statement on Vitamin D for prevention of falls and their consequences. J Am Geriatr Soc. 2014;62:147-52.

225. Bjelakovic G, Gluud LL, Nikolova D, et al. Vitamin D supplementation for prevention of mortality in adults. Cochrane Database Syst Rev. 2011;7:CD007470.

226. Shane-McWhorter L. The American Diabetes Association Guide to Herbs and Natural Supplements: From Aloe to Zinc. Washington, DC: American Diabetes Association; 2009.

227. American Diabetes Association. Unproven therapies (position statement). Diabetes Care. 2004;27 Suppl 1:S135.

CHAPTER 21

Nonbiologically Based Therapies

Diana W. Guthrie, PhD, APRN, BC-ADM, CDE, FAADE, FAAN, AHN-BC CHTP

Key Concepts

- Nonbiologically based practices included in complementary and alternative medicine (CAM) include alternative medical systems, mind-body interventions, manipulative and body-based methods, and energy therapies.

- An increasing number of persons with diabetes are using CAM practices—many of which could help, but others which could interfere with their diabetes management.

- Care should be taken in relation to type and use of CAM practices and their effect on blood glucose levels, as well as if or when a person chooses to use a modality that is an alternative therapy in place of conventional wisdom.

- Use of alternative therapies without the knowledge of a person's diabetes educator and other healthcare professionals may lead to problems with the person's diabetes management.

- Side effects must be considered when using any therapy that is not supported by evidence-based references.

- Education on integration of the use of CAM practices should lead to greater safety and efficacy of their use.

- Evidence-based references should be used to answer questions about CAM practices.

Introduction

The National Center for Complementary and Alternative Medicine (NCCAM), under the National Institutes of Health (NIH), classifies CAM into 4 categories[1]:

1. Natural products: dietary supplements, probiotics
2. Mind and body medicine: meditation, yoga, acupuncture, deep breathing, guided imagery, hypnotherapy, progressive relaxation, Qigong, and Tai Chi
3. Manipulative and body-based practices: spinal manipulation (chiropractic, osteopathic), massage therapy
4. Other practices: movement therapy; Feldenkrais Method; Alexander Technique; Pilates; Rolfing Structural Integration; Trager Psychophysiologic

Integration; traditional healers; magnet therapy; light therapy; Qigong; Reiki; healing touch (including therapeutic touch); whole body medical systems: Ayurvedic medicine, traditional Chinese medicine (TCM), homeopathy, and naturopathy

Integrative care includes the use of CAM therapies along with allopathic therapies, commonly called "Western medicine."

Surveys continue to note the increasing use of the self-care practices listed above.[2-5] These surveys are classic references for the reader to note the progress made in the use of CAM therapies and the increased out-of-pocket expense for these therapies used over time.

Complementary Versus Alternative Medicine

Complementary generally refers to using a non-mainstream approach **together with** conventional medicine.

Alternative refers to using a nonmainstream approach **in place of** conventional medicine.

True alternative medicine is not common, except in specific cultures where Western medicine or other whole body medical systems are unknown. Most people use nonmainstream approaches along with conventional treatments. The boundaries between complementary and conventional medicine overlap and change with time. For example, guided imagery and massage, both of which were once considered complementary or alternative, are used regularly in some hospitals to help with pain management.

Integrative Medicine

This array of nonmainstream healthcare approaches may also be considered part of integrative medicine or integrative health care.

For example, cancer treatment centers with integrative healthcare programs may offer services such as acupuncture and meditation to help manage symptoms and side effects for patients receiving conventional cancer treatments such as chemotherapy.

Source: National Center for Complementary and Alternative Medicine, National Institutes of Health, US Department of Health and Human Services. Complementary, alternative, or integrative health: what's in a name? 2008 Oct; last updated 2013 May (cited 2014 Feb 26). On the Internet at: http://nccam.nih.gov/health/whatiscam.

Use of CAM Therapies by People With Diabetes

Many CAM therapies increase relaxation and can help individuals cope with managing diabetes. Appropriate breathing and posture lead to supporting the improved health of a variety of conditions. Traditional Chinese medicine, an alternative medical system, dates back more than 2000 years. Within the broad categories of nonbiological CAM there are a multitude of specific practices. CAM practices reported in 2007 by the population surveyed by the National Center for Health Statistics included TCM (2.3 million), natural products (17.7%), deep-breathing exercises (12.7%), meditation (9.4%), chiropractic/osteopathic (8.6%), massage (6.1%), diet-based therapies (3.6%), progressive relaxation (2.9%), guided imagery (2.2%), and homeopathy therapy (1.8%).[6] The National Health Statistics Report of 2011 cited the top 10 modalities in use as acupuncture, aromatherapy, art therapy, guided imagery or relaxation, massage, music therapy, pet therapy, support group therapy, therapeutic touch, and transcutaneous electrical nerve stimulator (TENS).[7]

Reasons for Concern Regarding the Use of Other CAM Modalities

Therapies that are inappropriately used in place of traditional medicine are cause for concern. These concerns include the following[8]:

- Potential impacts on glycemic control
- Modality variability
- Lack of scientific study on effectiveness and safety
- Delay of use of more effective interventions
- Additional costs for medical care

Potential Impacts

Potential impacts to consider when a patient is using a CAM therapy include the following:

- Will the CAM be used in place of conventional therapy?
- Will the CAM delay the use of needed conventional therapy?
- Will the patient experience an increase in the occurrence of hypoglycemia?
  —If the person becomes so relaxed that epinephrine output is decreased, hypoglycemia may occur unless the diabetes medication is appropriately decreased during, before, and/or after the period of relaxation.
  —If the person becomes so relaxed that sleep occurs, he or she will miss consuming a usual snack.

—If the person has taken too large of a dose of medication for the previous meal, symptoms of hypoglycemia might not be noticed when the person is in a relaxed state (not usually the case, but it could happen).

Modality Variability

Modalities need to be adjusted as appropriate for each person. What might be useful and safe in an adult should be carefully thought out when used with a child. For example, therapeutic touch sessions for children should be shorter than sessions for adults. A family, an adult, or a child using CAM should be warned that more or increased length of use is not necessarily better. A woman who is pregnant or breastfeeding should exercise caution in the use of alternative therapies. For example, the effect of magnet therapy on young children and in pregnancies is unknown.

Just as with the use of botanicals (see chapter 20, on biologically based practices), certain populations, such as children, the elderly, and pregnant or lactating women, should be taught to watch for any side effects of using a particular modality. Especially when

---

Case: The Use of Meditation While on Pump Therapy

HT, a male patient who has had type 1 diabetes since childhood, is on an insulin pump with various basal insulin rates throughout the day and self-administers a variety of bolus insulin doses depending on his dietary intake. Lately he has been experiencing afternoon hypoglycemia on some, but not all, days. Varying his afternoon basal insulin only resulted in hyperglycemia one day and hypoglycemia the next day.

His healthcare provider asked about his lifestyle and learned that, with some coaching, HT is participating in meditation practices in the middle of the afternoon.

Is the use of meditation, a mind-body–based therapy, helpful or harmful?

What could be used in its place? Should HT stop his meditation practice or does he just need to decrease his previous bolus of insulin or decrease his basal insulin during this time?

Where could the diabetes educator find answers to questions that might be raised in the use of this practice (or modality)?

---

first starting a program, individuals should use extra care regarding the time of use, the length of time of use, and the intensity of use.

Lack of Scientific Study

Although anecdotes on the use of CAM therapies might be compelling, they are not evidence. This is especially true in regard to the efficacy of CAM therapies for children. Children are not "small adults." Since children are not usually studied or included in most CAM therapy studies, the results of the studies cannot be applied to them. Such modalities might be valuable as complementary therapy, but care must be taken when using a therapy alternatively, for example, using Reiki in place of a specific medication or known physical therapy practice. If the Reiki were used in concert with an evidence-based practice (although Reiki is becoming more evidence based), the person or child would obtain safer care.

Delayed Use

If people choose CAM therapies over Western medicine or are not guided by their CAM provider to seek such help when needed, the problem could become more serious and valuable time lost.

Additional Costs

If a problem becomes more serious, more time and money will be needed to reverse the situation.

Parents' Choice of Using CAM Therapy on Their Children

The 2007 National Health Interview Survey found that 1.2% of children younger than 18 had used some form of CAM during the past year, especially if parents had also used CAM.[9] Parents cited the reason they selected some form of CAM use for their children was that traditional care (also called conventional care) cost more than using CAM.[9] Natural or herbal products were most frequently used: 3.9%. CAM therapies used by parents are listed in descending order of frequency[9]:

- ❖ Natural products
- ❖ Chiropractic or osteopathic therapies

◆ Deep breathing
◆ Yoga
◆ Homeopathic treatment
◆ Traditional healers
◆ Massage
◆ Meditation
◆ Diet-based therapies
◆ Progressive relaxation

The 2007 survey found that over 83 million US adults spent more than $30 billion in out-of-pocket payments for any CAM use, including biologically based therapies, compared with over $260 billion in out-of-pocket expenses on traditional medicine practices.[9] Over $11 billion was spent on CAM practitioners alone.[9] Additionally, $42 billion was spent on massage therapists; over $4.1 billion on classes for yoga, Tai Chi, and Qigong; $3.9 billion on chiropractic or osteopathic manipulation; $3.1 billion on homeopathic practitioners; and $0.2 billion on relaxation techniques.

Points for Education

A patient assessment should include a question about whether the individual is using any type of CAM therapy along with or separate from biological therapies. The diabetes educator may need to list or describe the CAM therapies since a person may not realize that massage, for example, is considered a CAM therapy. The educator should also ask whether the CAM therapy is impacting blood glucose levels, positively or negatively. A further question would be to assess timing of the therapy practice.

The diabetes educator should help the person locate or evaluate a reliable CAM therapist. Credentialing organizations exist for various CAM practices, a process that considers education, experience, and perhaps an exam before the credential can be used. One source to consider is the National Library of Medicine's Directory of Health Organizations (http://dirline.nlm.nih.gov). The patient should be educated to question the type of therapy or the specific practitioner on its use and ask questions about the timing of the therapy and its effect on blood glucose responses. Individuals and healthcare providers can locate certified CAM therapists through

the NCCAM Web site (http://nccam.nih.gov/). Then the following information should be addressed:

◆ Does the practitioner have experience in treating people with diabetes?
◆ Is the practitioner aware of current research done on the modality as it relates to diabetes?
◆ What is the practitioner's philosophy of care?
◆ What is the cost per session? Is there a charge for cancelled appointments?
◆ Will insurance cover any of the costs? Insurance plans in an increasing number of states are covering massage therapy, TCM, and chiropractic therapy.
◆ Will the patient have to spend an extended period of time in the waiting room, such as when experiencing more than 1 therapeutic modality, that might result in a missed meal? Because the patients are people with diabetes, unplanned gaps between meals can be problematic.
◆ How accessible is the CAM practitioner's office to public transportation? Is free or validated parking available?
◆ What should the person expect on the first and subsequent visits?
◆ Most important: Will the therapy interfere with the patient's conventional treatment, and are there any contraindications to use of the therapy (eg, not using magnets on a pregnant woman)?

Working With Patients Who Are Using CAM Therapies

After the first CAM therapy visit, the diabetes educator should ask the patient to be aware of benefits from the therapy, any risks associated with the therapy (eg, most massage therapists give their clients a bottle of water and request that they keep themselves well hydrated over the next 24 hours), and what their blood glucose reading was before and after the therapy. It is also common for massage therapists to forewarn individuals about feeling a cramp or muscle weakness rather than increased strength.

The diabetes educator also needs to know any effect the particular therapy might have on blood pressure. For example, deep breathing practiced 20 minutes a day will result in a slower pulse, lower blood pressure, and the more efficient use of oxygen, as reported by Benson et al.[10]

Patients should be asked to keep a log or journal of their experiences with CAM therapy, whether the practice is done at home on their own or done with a CAM therapist. If the patient cannot keep a continuous log, he or she should at least make notations during the first few weeks of participation. These should include blood glucose monitoring along with blood pressure checks (if appropriate) and any differences in feelings, emotions, or body responses.

Research

Observational studies have found that people who chose non-evidence-based alternative practices over conventional practices had more problems than individuals who used practices that were complementary to evidence-based practices.

There is a concern for persons with diabetes who use alternative medicine. Gill et al, as far back as 1994, noted that some patients stopped their insulin in favor of faith healing, unusual diets, and supplements of vitamins and trace elements.[8] The response, as might be expected, was that people were going into ketoacidosis. (Note that they were using alternative therapy instead of considering what they were doing as complementary therapy.)

In a 2003 article, Remli and Chan wrote about 43 randomly selected people with diabetes who, through patient interviews and questionnaires and chart records, were found to most commonly use herbal therapy, homeopathy, and reflexology as complementary therapies. Whether using complementary therapy or conventional therapy (Western medicine), all these individuals "showed poorly controlled FBS levels." Their conclusion was that the effect of CAM therapies on diabetes outcomes must be assessed over a longer period of time.[11]

From the standpoint of professionals, Hawk et al found that there was a need to train CAM providers in evidence-based health promotion counseling and in effective communication with the patient's primary care provider.[12]

In another article, Miller et al found that patients felt that overall health was improved when using CAM therapy in a complementary way. Thus, the authors advised the "diabetes healthcare team" to ask about such use and oversee its safe use.[13]

In a later study, Miller et al wanted to learn whether CAM use in children with diabetes correlated with healthcare beliefs, psychosocial variables, and religious beliefs of the child's parents or guardian. Seventy-five percent of the parents in the study had tried CAM. The children most commonly used faith healing or prayer while parents did the same and also used chiropractic therapy, massage, and herbal teas. This appeared to lead to children who used CAM having more problems with adhering to their treatment for diabetes (ie, CAM therapies were used in place of some, but not all, conventional treatments). Miller and colleagues concluded that there were no differences in diabetes control, healthcare beliefs, stress, or quality of life between CAM users and nonusers.[14]

In Europe, Dannemann et al found that the use of CAM in children was less well documented than that for adults. They found that the parents in their population did not question the use of insulin but thought that the use of complementary therapy "improved well-being and the quality of life" for their children.[15]

A study in India found that acupressure followed by naturopathy was most beneficial as an alternative therapy, while homeopathy was found to have the least benefit in persons with type 2 diabetes.[16]

Eight CAM therapies—dietary, herbal, chiropractic, yoga, relaxation, vitamins, prayer, and other (acupuncture, Ayurveda, biofeedback, chelation, energy healing or Reiki therapy, hypnosis, massage, naturopathy, and homeopathy)—were studied in a group of 2474 adults with diabetes and a group of 28,625 adults without diabetes. The overall CAM category excluded the use of vitamins and prayer, as these complementary interventions were found to be commonly used by both groups. When analyzing the group with diabetes, in and of itself, it was found the use of specific CAM therapies was less predictable. If a specific modality was chosen by this group, the use of prayer appeared to be the choice rather than those modalities chosen by adults without diabetes.[17]

Bradley et al found that persons with type 2 diabetes were in favor of using naturopathic medicine more frequently only if naturopathic medicine practices were covered by insurance and if they were less satisfied with their present diabetes care.[18]

Review of the above versus other literature indicates that adults will often use CAM therapies when they are not satisfied with their conventional therapy. Eisenberg et al found that people with a higher socioeconomic status were more apt to use CAM therapies than to use conventional therapy, but this finding was not necessarily associated with the person having diabetes mellitus.[2-4]

If a person with diabetes uses any of the CAM therapies available, it is important that he or she carefully monitor blood glucose levels and report any untoward responses to his or her healthcare professional.

Review of Research on CAM Therapies on Various Types of Diabetes

Whole Body Medical Systems

Ayurvedic Medicine   As with many other studies of Ayurvedic intervention, the conclusion of one 2006 study "warranted further research." The population consisted of 60 adults with diabetes with hemoglobin A1C values between 6.0% and 8.0%. The subjects received an Ayurvedic diet (this is usually a meatless diet that is high in fiber and low in sugar), meditation instruction, and an Ayurvedic herbal supplement. The control patients attended the usual standard diabetes education classes. The parameters measured were all less than $P = .05$, indicating the need to reflect on further research.[19]

Homeopathy   Homeopathy was once the major approach to health and care. It eventually lost its place in Western medicine due to the introduction of antibiotics. Although there has been concern in regard to research based on related changes, whether by beliefs or alteration of symptoms, the Food and Drug Administration has not restricted its use, due to few, if any, side effects.. A recent study by Nayak et al used a total of 25 homeopathic medicines that were believed to have an effect on the nerves of the body.[20] After 12 months, their scoring system showed

significant improvement (the way the group in the study was determining nerve responses), but they did consider that further controlled studies should be done to ensure that it was the intervention alone. An earlier study by Pomposelli et al used the quality of life and the short form (SF-36), along with the diabetic neuropathy symptom score, to determine the effectiveness of their intervention, stating that their treatment was altering neuropathic symptoms.[21] Until more thorough and long-term studies can be carried out, care must be taken when such statements are made.

Native American Medicine   In 2000, Griffin et al found that when working with a specific tribe, it was important to assess community activities and beliefs/attitudes about having diabetes.[22] They concluded that unless this approach was followed with a particular tribe, they would get fewer, if any, subjects for a diabetes-related study, and they would get less, if any, cooperation from those subjects in relation to the participation required. The perspectives on healing by Yaquis with diabetes is a good example. The researchers found that for study participants, (1) their belief in God was expressed in prayers for healing; (2) people had to take care of themselves to keep healthy; (3) a foot ulcer is related to modern illness, so it takes time to heal; and (4) support from their community is important to survive.[23] Shiyanbola and Nelson were faced with the same conclusion in their 2011 work among the South Dakota Indian population of women with diabetes.[24] An understanding of sociocultural factors is needed when working with any population and its use of what Anglos would consider CAM practices.

Naturopathy   Oberg et al studied a naturopathic dietary intervention over a 12-week period. They found a P value = 0.02 in changes of hemoglobin A1C to warrant a full study on the use of such an approach in a larger population of subjects.[25] In 2012, Oberg et al then reported their further study using a naturopathic intervention which emphasizes a patient-centered approach, health promotion, and clinical counseling on wellness and prevention to promote behavior change. Study participants were individuals with type 2 diabetes who were studied for 1 year. Three themes were factored out: (1) the program was patient centered, (2) the focus was on holistic health rather than diabetes, (3) the use of collaboration with the healthcare professional. Among other factors, these themes were effective "in promoting self-efficacy and improving clinical outcomes" (p. 488).[26] Bradley et al also reported improvements in what they termed adjunctive naturopathic care (ANC) in Bastyr University's *Journal of the American Association of Naturopathic Physicians*, which interventions appeared quite similar to those used by Oberg. Their concluding remarks indicated that they needed to determine whether ANC by itself or as part of a plan of care was responsible for the significant changes and that the Hawthorne Effect is certainly possible in such studies.[27]

Osteopathic Medicine The osteopathic approach to a person with diabetes is well reviewed by Shubrook and Johnson. They reported that osteopathic physicians see "(1) the person as a unit of body, mind, and spirit, (2) the body is capable of self-regulation, self-healing, and health maintenance, (3) structure and function are reciprocally interrelated, and (4) rational treatment is based upon an understanding of these basic principles" (p. 18). The article goes on to delineate the actions and intensions of osteopathic care for a person with type 2 diabetes, including the forces that can either help or hinder a person's general health.[28] Shubrook and colleagues concluded that although residency programs were improving related to outcome measures for persons with diabetes, better training is needed for better performance in outcomes related to this population.[29]

Traditional Chinese Medicine Traditional Chinese medicine, which dates back more than 2000 years, called diabetes-related symptoms "Xiaoke disease." Although the use of Chinese herbal medicine is and has been an important part of TCM's therapeutic approach, other parts of care are reported, such as the balance of yin (the moist, cooling water element, or so-called female element) and yang (the warm, dry fire element, or so-called male element), and its part in the holistic approach used in TCM, as noted by Tong et al.[30] Diagnosis by use of the pulse observation of the tongue is related to the quality and function of various parts of the body. Zhao et al reported on the use of Chinese medicine and found "serious adverse events including hypoglycemic coma and death, related to 'adulteration' with orthodox

Chinese herbal medicine, errors in substitution, self-medication, overdoses, and improper preparation."[31] The traditional medical approach of TCM, just as with Western medicine, continues to need much monitoring, whether related to medicine usage or the intervention of other modalities.

Traditional Chinese medicine is commonly known for the use of acupuncture. Acupuncture has been used in the treatment of many health- and pain-related conditions. Belivani et al reported on its use with obese patients. They found that acupuncture needs to be used with diet and exercise for both achieving and maintaining weight loss. In this study they used body acupuncture, auricular or ear acupuncture, manual acupuncture, and electro acupuncture. This may potentially become complementary therapy for weight loss.[32]

Mind-Body Interventions

Aromatherapy Aromatherapy has been around for a long time. The appropriate use of oils can be beneficial, but care must be taken to use the right oil for the right purpose in the right strength and for the right period of time. Aromatherapy is included in the training of nurses in the United Kingdom. To effectively use such a variety of oils, certification from qualified individuals must be obtained. In the hand of the novice, the use or choice of oils or in their preparation can result in toxicity that can lead to illness or even death. Dunning discusses the quality use of essential oils to guide future practices on the use of this modality.[33]

Art Therapy Harel and colleagues studied the use of art therapy in youth who had poorly controlled type 1 diabetes. They concluded that intensive, individualized art therapy in such a population may influence and improve glycemic control.[34] A study is needed to determine whether it was the individualized attention or the art therapy itself that resulted in better diabetes control.

Guided Imagery Guided imagery has a number of approaches. One such approach is the Bonny Method, which includes the use of music to guide thoughts (eg, such as galloping music associated with riding a horse), thereby helping patients to find words through the experience they receive when listening to a specific piece of music. No research has exclusively reported on the use of guided imagery and its effect on diabetes. Beebe and Wyatt studied its use on accessing the unconscious,[35] Burns reported on this method being used with cancer patients,[36] and Marr reported this method being used for spiritual growth.[37] In all 3 articles, states of relaxation were achieved (described) such that it is known that relaxation brings about lowered blood glucose levels.

Hypnosis   Hypnosis is a method of education by a therapist qualified to work with an individual or group in a directive or permissive approach. It may be used in harmful ways when a person thinks that he or she is doing something acceptable, but happens to be quite unacceptable in a particular culture. For helpful purposes, it can be learned by an individual to assist with decreasing pain, anxiety, and depression and general desensitization of fears. In the field of diabetes, it can be used as a calming therapy and one that might be able, for that individual, to allow diabetes treatment to be more acceptable. Hypnosis has been found by Xu and Cardena to demonstrate the need for further study. They felt their study demonstrated that hypnosis used as an adjunct (or complementary) to insulin treatments could aid in lowering and stabilizing blood glucose levels and, in the process, decrease peripheral vascular complications.[38]

Laughter   What about laughter? Hayashi et al found that laughter is linked to gene expression. The researchers wanted to know whether laughter regulates gene expression in those persons with type 2 diabetes, which this particular study did not do.[39] Optimism is another piece, but not necessarily a part of laughter. Fournier et al found that such beliefs are dependent on whether the person feels that he or she has a controllable chronic disease.[40] This reinforced the findings of Chernoff et al (2001), who found in their population that the mother has an ability to have a positive impact on raising a child with a chronic illness.[41]

Pet Therapy   Surprisingly, only 1 article discussed the training of dogs to be acutely aware of their owner's state of glycemia. Most likely, such articles are found in literature sites that recognize that dogs with special abilities may be trained to warn their owners about the oncoming hypoglycemic event, just as they are able to warn owners of oncoming epileptic seizures. Animals have been found to be not only companions but also supporters of health, such as reported in an article about the effect of having an animal on a person's hypertension or hypoglycemic condition.[42]

Prayer and Meditation   Prayer has been studied in a variety of cases and for a variety of situations. In a pilot study, Sacco et al studied the use of the Serenity Prayer in people with type 2 diabetes. After 6 weeks of daily statement of the prayer, they had some questionable results: 2 individuals had lowered serum glucose levels, 2 individuals had increased serum glucose levels, and 4 individuals had no change.[43] Because of this unusual outcome, they determined that future research was needed. When Hispanic farmworkers with type 2 diabetes were asked about their religious practices and use of prayer, Bergland and colleagues found that the population studied used prayer daily. They not only prayed for themselves and their family but also prayed specifically for their diabetes.[44] In another study, Mexican Americans with diabetes were found to emphasize conventional treatment and used alternative treatments only as secondary strategies. They revealed that prayer influenced their health by bringing healing power to the medicines they take for diabetes and other health conditions. Spiritual practices and religious beliefs highlighted in this article support the need to include them in clinical practice, especially when there is the need and desire for behavior change.[43,45]

Relaxation   McGinnis et al described their noted outcome that the use of biofeedback enhances relaxation in persons with type 2 diabetes and lasts up to 3 months after training. They found that hemoglobin A1C was significantly decreased in those who participated in daily relaxation practice training from baseline to 3 months later.[46] During the previous year, van Rooijen et al compared the A1Cs of an exercise group with the A1Cs of a relaxation trained group. Both groups showed improved hemoglobin A1C, but the researchers concluded that such a change was due to the "study effect."[47]

Manipulative and Body-Based Methods

Massage   Massage in and of itself has been questioned in regard to improvement in diabetes control, although an article by Wu and Li indicates that it does.[48] A 2012 article found that massage versus relaxation exercises using a CD for adult Swedish-born patients, also $P < 0.05$, had limited effects on the quality of life of people with type 2 diabetes.[49] They queried that massage might be effective if the perceived levels of stress were higher. In 2011, Sajedi et al found that Swedish massage, as part of a daily routine, was an effective intervention to reduce blood glucose levels in children with diabetes; unknown is whether the results were due to the massage or the attention being given to an individual child.[50]

Chiropractic Medicine   In 1998, Kaptchuk and Eisenberg addressed chiropractic medicine as an important component of the US healthcare system. They shared their concerns with the core chiropractic belief that the correction of spinal abnormality is a critical healthcare intervention. Their conclusion was related to the contributions of patient-physician relationships as noted with their more holistic approach to patient care.[51]

Eighty percent of chiropractic physicians give some form of nutritional counseling in their practice, which supports the notion that such physicians are more holistic in nature than perhaps previously thought.[52] In a review article, Wyatt and Ferrance found that chiropractic physicians need to know how to make "appropriate clinical decisions" along with understanding contraindications to the use of their approach to therapy.[53] In replicating a study related to adverse effects of spinal manipulation published in 2007 by Ernst, Tuchin noted that there were a number of problems. He concluded that appropriate use by legislated treatment needs to be considered when reporting on a particular use of a CAM therapy.[54]

Qigong   Qigong is an area of Chinese medicine that is similar to Tai Chi but not the same. Qigong is considered the name of Chinese therapeutic exercises and has been encouraged for the treatment of type 2 diabetes. In their review of the literature, Freire and Alves found that Qigong increased C-peptide and reduced fasting blood glucose levels, along with improving insulin resistance and hemoglobin A1C.[55] Even though these authors saw such a positive outcome, a large randomized clinical trial was still needed to definitively support the use of this modality. In the

study comparing Yi Ren Medical Qigong (YRMQ) with both progressive resistance training (PRT) and standard care, there were not enough subjects and not enough time for participation to make any credible conclusions in regard to the psychological effects of these approaches in people with type 2 diabetes.[56] This is a useful example of a potentially good study that essentially becomes lost due to a variety of factors that decrease its credibility. Chen et al noted that the quality of studies needs to be improved and that spending time and effort on such studies and having questionable outcomes is disturbing, to say the least.[57]

Reflexology   Reflexology, a common practice in many places, has been studied for a range of conditions, including diabetes. Ernst noted that in the analysis of all the available papers, 18 randomized controlled trial reports stated, in effect, that there was no solid evidence that reflexology is an effective treatment for any medical condition.[58]

Tai Chi   Yan and colleagues, in a 2013 meta-analysis of Tai Chi–related effects in type 2 diabetes, reported that there is not sufficient evidence to support the benefits to people with type 2 diabetes and that larger scale studies are needed to determine long-term efficacy in spite of reduced hemoglobin A1C ($P < .00001$), fasting blood glucose ($P = .003$), and triglycerides ($P = .006$). No improvements were noted for total cholesterol, HDL, or other body parameters.[59] Ahn and Song found that Tai Chi improved glucose control, balance, neuropathic symptoms, and quality of life in persons with diabetes who had neuropathy.[60] Other studies suggest that longer term studies are needed, recognizing that even 12 weeks of Tai Chi chuan exercise improves FBS and peripheral nerve conduction velocities.[61]

Yoga   Yoga has been around for a very long time. Bijlani et al's study of this intervention using postures, breathing exercises, relaxation techniques and group support, meditation, and good nutrition concluded that an introduction as a short lifestyle modification, along with stress management education, leads to improvement in metabolic functioning within a period of just 9 days.[62]

Alexander et al found that yoga, as an 8-week intervention, had little effect on physical activity over time.[63] The authors recommended further research to look at behavioral health outcomes and people with type 2 diabetes. Hegde et al found that yoga can be used to reduce oxidative stress in this same population. They also found that when yoga is used in addition to standard care, body mass index (BMI) and glycemic values may be reduced.[64] In a 2009 article, Kosuri and Sridhar reported that 40 days at a yoga camp not only resulted in a reduced BMI but also improved well-being and reduced feelings of anxiety.[65]

Energy Therapies

Biofield Therapies

Reiki   In 2011, Bowden et al reported on a randomized controlled single-blind trial of the effect of Reiki on mood and well-being. This study was carried out on 40 university students, one half of whom had high depression/mood scores and one half of whom had low depression scores. Both groups received Reiki. Those with the high depression/mood scores had significant improvement in mood as compared with the group with low scores. Since many people with diabetes have greater problems with depression, Reiki might become a useful tool to use on their behalf.[66] Another study, completed by Garrow and Egede, studied 2474 adults with diabetes. Reiki was one of 15 modalities being used in this population. Their research demonstrated that the use of various modalities, including Reiki, was correlated with better use of preventive care services, increased emergency department services, and increased primary care visits.[67]

Therapeutic Touch   Therapeutic touch, although not presently listed in the newer CAM categories, has been used in a variety of settings, but not specifically for people with diabetes. More often, it has been used with individuals with some sort of discomfort, such as postoperative pain. In a study by Coakley and Duff, patients who received therapeutic touch reported less pain and had documented lower cortisol levels and natural killer cells (NKCs).[68] In a review article, 5 of the 7 studies, published between 1997 and 2004, were scientifically well grounded enough to conclude that therapeutic touch supported a reported and documented decrease in the sensation of pain.[69] Studies are needed to determine whether this effect is present in persons with diabetes mellitus who have neuropathic pain and whether its use

contributes to lowering blood glucose levels to any significant degree.

Electromagnetic-Based Therapies

Light Therapy   One study of light therapy, reported in *Diabetes Care* by Lavery et al, found that anodyne MIRE (monochromatic infrared photo energy) was not statistically different from "sham" therapy in the treatment of sensory neuropathy.[70] In 2006, Amall et al demonstrated that pulsed infrared light therapy (PILT) did seem to increase peripheral sensation in persons with diabetic peripheral neuropathy.[71] This positive outcome was found to occur in both people with type 1 diabetes and people with type 2 diabetes when they underwent 30-minute treatments 3 times a week for 8 weeks. Although "the exact mechanism of action is not understood," it is believed that such treatment might increase nitric oxide production and thereby improve peripheral neuropathy (p. 320). This indicates that one type of light therapy might be more effective than another type for neuropathic treatment.

Magnet Therapy   Magnets do have their place as a form of therapy but may not be recognized as such. In addition to magnetic resonance imaging (MRI), another magnetic instrument has been introduced, magnetic resonance spectroscopy. Its place in diabetes treatment has yet to be determined. These magnets are given higher field strength and improve delineation, and thus it is likely that their use will lead to more research into the metabolic syndrome and chronic diseases such as diabetes mellitus.[72] A literature review by Colbert et al was conducted regarding magnets applied to acupuncture points as a therapy.[73] Of the 380 papers reviewed, only 50 studies met their inclusion criteria. They deduced that the use of acupuncture with magnet therapy, if properly studied, would yield some useful results in the treatment of certain conditions, such as neuropathy. A 2002 study in Singapore noted that magnets attached to ear acupuncture points on persons with diabetes lowered blood glucose levels.[74] More details of this study are needed.

TENS Units   One paper on the TENS application and its potential in controlling blood glucose levels reported that when the TENS was in place, the pain was decreased but the patient became hypoglycemic. In continued use of the TENS, it was found that the person's insulin dosage was adjusted to half of what it previously had been to prevent hypoglycemic episodes. Khan's conclusion was that "decreased sympathetic stimulation, enhanced insulin sensitivity or altered muscle metabolism due to electrical stimulation" led to decreased blood glucose levels.[75]

Other Related CAM Research

Studies of CAM, in general, have found an increased use of such modalities among all populations, including those with diabetes.[2–5,16] As a side finding, the researchers noted that people with diabetes were more likely to use prayer but, interestingly enough, less likely to use herbs, yoga, or vitamins when compared with people who did not have diabetes.

A number of studies included a combination of modalities with the conclusion that improvement had been achieved. There is confusion in studies where modalities have been combined, especially those which do not consider the size of the population studied or the composition of subjects. Which modality is responsible for the appropriately lowered and stabilized blood glucose levels? Bay and Bay studied the combination of acupressure, hypnotherapy, and transcendental meditation in 20 patients who were provided 60- to 90-minute training sessions over 10 successive days. "Convenience sampling" of persons with type 2 diabetes who received the combination of modalities found that these individuals had lower blood glucose levels than the placebo group.[76]

Kanodia et al performed a national survey to look at the use of CAM for the treatment of back pain.[77]

More commonly used were massage, herbal therapy, yoga, Tai Chi, Qigong, and acupuncture. All were associated with perceived benefit, but the researchers' concluding remarks indicated that further investigation was needed.

Some remember the initial study that determined that the monofilament had the strongest correlation with the vibratory threshold, and it was found to be valid and simple to use.[78] This is a good example of how an alternative methodology became part of conventional care.

In 2008, Hijmans et al studied the use of vibrating insoles to aid in improving standing balance in people with neuropathy.[79] They concluded that, unless the person was distracted by other means, improvement needed to be made for vibrating insoles to be truly effective.

Case Wrap-up

HT was found to be intermittently practicing meditation in the middle of the afternoon. He reported that he felt relaxed by the end of the meditation session. Coincidentally, he was participating in this practice at about the same time of the peak action of his bolus dose of insulin.

HT was educated to either decrease the bolus dose at the time of his previous meal or have a small snack before the time he chooses to meditate. Overall concern should be on safety first and control second, along with his quality of life and having diabetes. His meditation should contribute to an improved quality of life. It is important to ensure that he stays safe by not becoming hypoglycemic.

Focus on Education

Teaching Strategies

↪ **Be respectful of people's preference for and use of alternative or complementary modalities.** An educator's initial reaction to a patient's using herbs or other modalities can either make or break the whole perception of being a caring and capable healthcare professional.

↪ **Be a knowledgeable resource on dietary supplements and other CAM modalities, and ask the right questions.**
- Are you using any supplements or medications or even other modalities that you have not reported to your health professional?
- What do you hope to achieve by using this medication/supplement/modality? How does this medication/supplement/modality help you?
- How do you know that this medication/supplement/modality does what it is supposed to do?

- Encourage open communication about biologically based therapies, alternative medical systems, mind-body interventions, manipulative and body-based methods, energy therapies, and supplements and/or other modalities, and discourage the use of dangerous or ineffective products and modalities.

- Assess and follow up on diabetes-related impacts and issues with CAM therapies.

- Recommend that people start with one new product or modality at a time.

- For additional help, refer patients to the NCCAM Web site: http://www.nccam.nih.gov.

Messages for Patients

- What is noted as natural is not necessarily safe.

- Look for the USP or standardized notation on the bottle to designate that the product has been inspected for consistency.

- A product advertised on the Internet may not always be in the best interest of the user—consult with a knowledgeable person.

- If in doubt, don't use the product, especially if you have a compromised liver or kidneys.

- **Safety first.** Provide a complete list of all medicines, supplements, or herbs you are taking, as well as any complementary or alternative practices you are using, to your diabetes educator so he or she can help you maintain optimal health.

- **One at a time.** Working with your diabetes educator, incorporate one complementary or alternative practice into your regimen to determine its efficacy.

- **Trial period.** Unless you are suffering ill effects or have been told by your healthcare provider to stop, don't abandon your selected complementary or alternative therapy after a few attempts or sessions. It can take a while for the positive effect of a therapy to become evident.

Focus on Practice

- Recognize the potential value of CAM therapies and be prepared to address them when indicated by the patient's use or interest in use.

- Be prepared to help consumers identify practitioners of CAM therapies that will meet their needs and preferences. Use the NCCAM Web site as a resource: http://nccam.nih.gov/health/decisions.

- Document the use of the specific products/modality in the medical record to communicate your findings with the entire diabetes healthcare team.

- Respect consumers' choices regarding use of CAM therapies, while guiding them on their safe use and precautions they need to take.

References

1. National Center for Complementary and Alternative Medicine, National Institutes of Health, US Department of Health and Human Services. Complementary, alternative, or integrative health: what's in a name? 2008 Oct (last updated 2013 May, cited 2014 Feb 26). On the Internet at: http://nccam.nih.gov/health/whatiscam.

2. Eisenberg DM, Kerssler RC, Foster C, Norlock FE, Calkins DR, Delbanco TL. Unconventional medicine in the United States: prevalence, costs and patterns of use. N Engl J Med. 1993;328(4):246-52.

3. Eisenberg DM, Davis RM, Ettner SL, et al. Trends in alternative medicine use in the United States, 1990-1997: results of a follow-up national survey. JAMA. 1998; 280(18):1569-75.

4. Yeh GY, Eisenberg DM, Davis RM, Phillips RS. Use of complementary and alternative medicine among persons with diabetes mellitus: results of a national survey. Am J Public Health. 2002;92(10):1648-52.

5. Tindle HA, Davis RB, Phillips RS, Eisenberg DM. Trends in use of complementary and alternative medicine by US adults: 1997-2002. Altern Ther Health Med. 2005;11(1):42-9.

6. Pearson NJ, Chesney MA. The CAM Education Program of the National Center for Complementary and Alternative Medicine: an overview. Acad Med. 2007;82(10):921-6. doi: 10.1097/ACM.0b013e31814a5014

7. AARP and the National Center for Complementary and Alternative Medicine. Telephone survey report at the National Institutes of Health. Complementary and alternative medicine: what people aged 50 and older discuss with their health care providers. National Center for Health Statistics Reports, No. 33. Hyattsville, Md; April 2011:16.

8. Gill GC, Redmond S, Garratt F, Paisey R. Diabetes and alternative medicine: cause for concern. Diabet Med. 1994; 11(2):210-3.

9. Nahin RL, Barnes PM, Stussman BJ, Bloom B. Costs of complementary and alternative medicine and frequency of visits to CAM practitioners in the United States, 2007. National Health Statistics Reports, No. 18. Hyattsville, Md; July 30, 2009:1-14.

10. Benson H, Shapiro D, Turskyk B, Schwartz GE. Decreased systolic blood pressure through operant conditioning techniques in patients with essential hypertension. Science. 1971;173(3998):740-2.

11. Remli R, Chan SC. Use of complementary medicine amongst diabetic patients in a public primary care clinic in Ipoh. Med J Malaysia. 2003;58(5):688-93.

12. Hawk C, Ndetan H, Evans MW Jr. Potential role of complementary and alternative health care providers in chronic disease prevention and health promotion: an analysis of National Health Interview Survey data. Prev Med. 2012;54(1):18-22.

13. Miller JL, Binns HJ, Brickman WJ. Complementary and alternative medicine use in children with type 1 diabetes: a pilot survey of parents. Explore (NY). 2008;4(5):311-4.

14. Miller JL, Cao D, Miller JG, Lipton RB. Correlates of complementary and alternative medicine (CAM) use in Chicago area children with diabetes (DM). Prim Care Diabetes. 2009;3(37):149-56.

15. Dannemann K, Hecker W, Haberland H, et al. Use of complementary and alternative medicine in children with type 1 diabetes mellitus—prevalence, patterns of use, and costs. Pediatr Diabetes. 2008;9(3):228-35.

16. Mahrotra R, Bajaj S, Kumar D. Use of complementary and alternative medicine by patients with diabetes mellitus. Natl Med J India. 2004;17(5):243-5.

17. Garrow D, Egede LE. National patterns and correlates of complementary and alternative medicine use in adults with diabetes. J Altern Complement Med. 2006;12(9):895-902.

18. Bradley R, Sherman KJ, Catz S, et al. Survey of CAM interest, self-care, and satisfaction with health care for type 2 diabetes at group health cooperative. BMC Complement Altern Med. 2011;11:121.

19. Elder C, Aickin M, Bauer V, Cairns J, Vuckovic N. Randomized trial of a whole-system ayurvedic protocol for type 2 diabetes. Altern Ther Health Med. 2006;12(5): 24-30.

20. Nayak C, Oberai P, Varanasi R, et al. A prospective multi-centric open clinical trial of homeopathy in diabetic distal symmetric polyneuropathy. Homeopathy. 2013;102(2): 130-8.

21. Pomposelli R, Piasere V, Andreoni C, et al. Observational study of homeopathic and conventional therapies in patients with diabetic polyneuropathy. Homeopathy. 2009;98(1):17-25.

22. Griffin JA, Gilliland SS, Perez G, Upson D, Carter JS. Challenges to participating in a lifestyle intervention program: the Native American Diabetes Project. Diabetes Educ. 2000;26(4):681-9.

23. De Vera N. Perspectives on healing foot ulcers by Yaquis with diabetes. J Transcult Nurs. 2003;14(1):39-47.

24. Shiyanbola OO, Nelson J. Illness perceptions, beliefs in medicine and medication non-adherence among South Dakota minority women with diabetes: a pilot study. S D Med. 2011;64(10):365-8.

25. Oberg EB, Bradley RD, Allen J, McCrory MA. CAM: naturopathic dietary interventions for patients with type 2 diabetes. Complement Ther Clin Pract. 2011;17(3): 157-61.

26. Oberg EM, Bradley R, Hsu C, et al. Patient-reported experiences with first-time naturopathic care for type 2 diabetes. PloS One. 2012;7(11):485-9.

27. Bradley R, Sherman KJ, Catz S, et al. Adjunctive naturopathic care for type 2 diabetes: patient-reported and clinical outcomes after one year. BMC Complement Altern Med. 2012;12:44.

28. Shubrook JH Jr, Johnson AW. An osteopathic approach to type 2 diabetes mellitus. J Am Osteopath Assoc. 2011; 111(9):531-7.

29. Shubrook JH Jr, Snow RJ, McGill SL. Effects of repeated use of the American Osteopathic Association's Clinical Assessment Program on measures of care for patients with diabetes mellitus. J Am Osteopath Assoc. 2011;111(1): 13-20.

30. Tong XL, Dong L, Chen L, Zhen Z. Treatment of diabetes using traditional Chinese medicine: past, present and future. Am J Chin Med. 2012;40(5):877-86.

31. Zhao HL, Tong PC, Chan JC. Traditional Chinese medicine in the treatment of diabetes. Nestle Nutr Workshop Ser Clin Perform Programme. 2006;11:15-25.

32. Belivani M, Dimitroula C, Katsiki N, Apostolopoulou M, Cummings M, Hatzitolios AI. Acupuncture in the treatment of obesity: a narrative review of the literature. Acupunct Med. 2013;31(1):88-97.

33. Dunning T. Applying a quality use of medicines framework to using essential oils in nursing practice. Complement Ther Clin Pract. 2005;11(3):172-81.

34. Harel S, Yanai L, Brooks R, et al. The contribution of art therapy in poorly controlled youth with type 1 diabetes mellitus. J Pediatr Endocrinol Metab. 2013;26(7-8): 669-73.

35. Beebe LH, Wyatt TH. Guided imagery and music: using the Bonny Method to evoke emotion and access the unconscious. J Psychosoc Nurs Ment Health Serv. 2009;47(1): 29-33.

36. Burns DS. The effect of the Bonny Method of Guided Imagery and Music on the mood and life quality of cancer patients. J Music Ther. 2001;38(1):51-65.

37. Marr J. The use of the Bonny Method of Guided Imagery and Music in spiritual growth. J Pastoral Care. 2001; 55(4):397-406.

38. Xu Y, Cardena E. Hypnosis as an adjunct therapy in the management of diabetes. Int J Clin Exp Hypn. 2008;56(1): 63-72.

39. Hayashi T, Urayama O, Kawai K, et al. Laughter regulates gene expression in patients with type 2 diabetes. Psychother Psychosom. 2006;75(1):106.

40. Fournier M, De Ridder D, Bensing J. Optimism and adaptation to chronic disease: the role of optimism in relation to self-care options of type 1 diabetes mellitus, rheumatoid arthritis and multiple sclerosis. Br J Health Psychol. 2002; 7(4):409-32.

41. Chernoff RG, List DG, DeVet KA, Ireys Ht. Maternal reports of raising children with chronic illnesses: the prevalence of positive thinking. Ambul Pediatr. 2001;1(2):104-7.

42. Wright JD, Kriz-Silverstein D, Morton DJ, Wingard DL, Barrett-Connor E. Pet ownership and blood pressure in old age. Epidemiology. 2007;18(5):613-8.

43. Sacco LM, Griffin MT, McNulty R, Fitzpatrick JJ. Use of the Serenity Prayer among adults with type 2 diabetes: a pilot study. Holist Nurs Pract. 2011;25(4):192-8.

44. Bergland JE, Heuer L, Lausch C. The use of prayer by Hispanic migrant farm workers with type 2 diabetes. J Cult Divers. 2007;14(4):164-8.

45. Watkins YJ, Quinn LT, Ruggiero L, Quinn MT, Choi YK. Spiritual and religious beliefs and practices and social support's relationships to diabetes self-care activities in African Americans. Diab Educ. 2013;39(2):231-9.

46. McGinnis RA, McGrady A, Cox SA, Grower-Dowling KA. Biofeedback-assisted relaxation in type 2 diabetes. Diabetes Care. 2005;28(8):2145-9.

47. Van Rooijen AJ, Rheeder P, Eales CJ, Becker PJ. Effect of exercise versus relaxation on haemoglobin A1c in Black females with type 2 diabetes mellitus. Q J Med. 2004; 97(6):343-51.

48. Wu W, Li C. Diabetes mellitus treated by massage. J Tradit Chin Med. 1998;18(1):64-5.

49. Wandell PE, Carlsson SC, Gafvels C, Andersoon K, Tomkvist L. Measuring possible effect on health-related quality of life by tactile massage or relaxation in patients with type 2 diabetes. Complement Ther Med. 2012; 20(1-2):8-15.

50. Sajedi F, Kashaninia Z, Hoseinzadeh S, Abedinipoor A. How effective is Swedish massage on blood glucose level in children with diabetes mellitus? Acta Med Iran. 2011; 49(9):592-7.

51. Kaptchuk TJ, Eisenberg DM. Chiropractic: origins, controversies, and contributions. Arch Intern Med. 1998;158(20): 2215-24.

52. Holtman D, Burke J. Nutritional counseling in the chiropractic practice: a survey of New York practitioners. J Chiropr Med. 2007;6(1):27-31.

53. Wyatt LH, Ferrance RJ. The musculoskeletal effects of diabetes mellitus. J Can Chiropr Assoc. 2006;50(1):43-50.

54. Tuchin P. A replication of the study 'Adverse effects of spinal manipulation: a systematic review.' Chiropr Man Therap. 2012;20(1):30.

55. Freire MD, Alves C. Therapeutic Chinese exercises (Qigong) in the treatment of type 2 diabetes mellitus: a systematic review. Diabetes Metab Syndr. 2013;7(1):56-9.

56. Putiri AL, Lovejoy JC, Gilliham S, Sassagawa M, Bradley R, Sun GC. Psychological effects of Yi Ren Medical Qigong and progressive resistance training in adults with type 2 diabetes mellitus: a randomized controlled pilot study. Altern Ther Health Med. 2012;18(1):30-4.

57. Chen KW, Lie T, Zhang H, Lin Z. An analytical review of the Chinese literature on Qigong therapy for diabetes mellitus. Am J Chin Med. 2009;37(3):439-57.

58. Ernst E. Is reflexology an effective intervention? A systematic review of randomized controlled trials. Med J Aust. 2009;191(5):263-6.

59. Yan JH, Gu WJ, Pan L. Lack of evidence on Tai Chi-related effects in patients with type 2 diabetes mellitus: a meta-analysis. Exp Clin Endocrinol Diabetes. 2013; 121(5):266-71. Epub 2013 Feb 28.

60. Ahn S, Song R. Effects of Tai Chi exercise on glucose control, neuropathy scores, balance, and quality of life in patients with type 2 diabetes and neuropathy. J Altern Complement Med. 2012;18(12):1172-8.

61. Hung JW, Liou CW, Wang PW, et al. Effect of 12 week tai chi chuan exercise on peripheral nerve modulation in patients with type 2 diabetes mellitus. J Rehabil Med. 2009;41(1):924-9.

62. Bijlani RL, Vempati RP, Yadav RK, et al. A brief but comprehensive lifestyle education program based on yoga reduces risk factors for cardiovascular disease and diabetes mellitus. J Altern Complement Med. 2005;11(2):267-74.

63. Alexander G, Innes KE, Bourguignon C, Bovbjerg VE, Kulbok P, Taylor AG. Patterns of yoga practice and physical activity following a yoga intervention for adults with or at risk for type 2 diabetes. J Phys Act Health. 2012;9(1): 53-61.

64. Hegde SV, Adhikari P, Kotian S, Pinto VJ, D'Souza S, D'Souza V. Effect of 3-month yoga on oxidative stress in type 2 diabetes with or without complications: a controlled clinical trial. Diabetes Care. 2011;34(10):2208-10.

65. Kosuri M, Sridhar GR. Yoga practice in diabetes improves physical and psychological outcomes. Metab Syndr Relat Disord. 2009;7(6):515-7.

66. Bowden D, Goddard L, Gruzelier J. A randomized controlled single-blind trial of the efficacy of reiki at benefitting moods and well-being. Evid Based Complement Alternat Med. 2011 March 27. [Epub ahead of print]

67. Garrow D, Egede LE. Association between complementary and alternative medicine use, preventive care practices, and use of conventional medical services among adults with diabetes. Diabetes Care. 2006;29(1):15-9.

68. Coakley AB, Duff ME. The effect of therapeutic touch on postoperative patients. J Holist Nurs. 2010;28(3):193-200.

69. Monroe CM. The effects of therapeutic touch on pain. J Holist Nurs. 2009;27(2):85-92.

70. Lavery LA, Murdoch DP, Williams J, Lavery DC. Does anodyne light therapy improve peripheral neuropathy in diabetes? A double-blind, sham-controlled, randomized trial to evaluate monochromatic infrared photoenergy. Diabetes Care. 2008;31(2):316-21.

71. Amall DA, Nelson AG, Lopez L, et al. The restorative effects of pulsed infrared light therapy on significant loss of peripheral protective sensation in patients with long-term type 1 and type 2 diabetes mellitus. Acta Diabetol. 2006; 43(1):26-33.

72. Dagnellie PC, Leij-Halfwerk S. Magnetic resonance spectroscopy to study hepatic metabolism in diffuse liver diseases, diabetes and cancer. World J Gastroenterol. 2010; 16(13):1577-86.

73. Colbert AP, Cleaver J, Brown KA, et al. Magnets applied to acupuncture points as therapy—a literature review. Acupunct Med. 2008;26(3):160-70.

74. Chen Y. Magnets on ears helped diabetics. Am J Chin Med. 2002;30(1):183-5.

75. Khan MU. Is there a role for TENS application in the control of diabetes mellitus in insulin-dependent patients? Singapore Med J. 2012;53(11):249-50.

76. Bay R, Bay F. Combined therapy using acupressure therapy, hypnotherapy, and transcendental meditation versus placebo in type 2 diabetes. J Acupunct Meridian Stud. 2011;4(3):183-6.

77. Kanodia AK, Legedza AT, Davis RB, Eisenberg DM, Phillips RS. Perceived benefit of complementary and alternative medicine (CAM) for back pain: a national survey. J Am Board Fam Med. 2010;23(3):354-62.

78. Rahman M, Griffin SJ, Rathmann W, Wareham NJ. How should peripheral neuropathy be assessed in people with diabetes in primary care? A population-based comparison of four measures. Diabet Med. 2003;20(5):368-74.

79. Hijmans JM, Geertzen JH, Zijlstra W, Hof AL, Postema K. Effects of vibrating insoles on standing balance in diabetic neuropathy. J Rehabil Res Dev. 2008; 45(9):1441-9.

CHAPTER 22

Hyperglycemia

Dace L. Trence, MD, FACE

Key Concepts

- Diabetic ketoacidosis (DKA) occurs when there is so little insulin available to transport glucose into cells that glucose accumulates in the blood, raising levels to 250 mg/dL or greater (mean 475 mg/dL).[1] Diabetic keto-acidosis can evolve quickly (within 24 hours), causing dehydration and ketosis and electrolyte imbalance and acidosis. This condition requires immediate treatment.

- Hyperosmolar hyperglycemic state (HHS) occurs when hyperglycemia and dehydration slowly exacerbate each other until both are extreme. Blood glucose levels rise to greater than 600 mg/dL, though few, if any, ketones are present. Hyperosmolar hyperglycemic state occurs primarily in undiagnosed or older adults with type 2 diabetes. Residents of

long-term care facilities are at risk and should be monitored to prevent HHS. Hyperosmolar hyperglycemic state is even more life threatening than DKA.

- Chronic hyperglycemia is glucose that is persistently elevated. Everyone with diabetes experiences hyperglycemia and, to some extent, chronic hyperglycemia. How high and how often glucose levels rise over the reference range vary greatly. People with high blood glucose may not feel well, but they typically continue with their usual activities and responsibilities. Very high glucose levels are acute and serious and can evolve from chronic hyperglycemia. Complications due to chronic hyperglycemia are addressed in full in other chapters.

State of the Condition

Hyperglycemia is defined as blood glucose that is above normal. In persons with diabetes, significant hyperglycemia is the objective finding of diabetes out of control. A gradual or abrupt decline of insulin production or availability, typically in conjunction with insulin resistance, contributes to elevated blood glucose levels. Stress, whether psychological or metabolic, can exacerbate insulin resistance, which in turn stimulates hepatic glucose production to further elevate blood glucose. People with diabetes may suffer long-term complications from chronic hyperglycemia as well as acute episodes of life-threatening complications with severely high glucose levels. This chapter will help the reader recognize the symptoms of acute hyperglycemia (acute stages of elevated blood

glucose), understand principles of evaluation and treatment, and prevent recurrent episodes in persons with diabetes. For information on ongoing hyperglycemia, see chapters 23 and 25, on chronic complications and cardiovascular disease (CVD).

Diabetic Ketoacidosis
Pathology

Diabetic ketoacidosis occurs more often in people with type 1 diabetes, but it can also be seen in individuals with type 2 diabetes during acute illness and/ or after they have become insulin deficient.[1] Type 1 diabetes is the most frequent endocrine disease in children, with 65,000 children diagnosed worldwide every year. Up to 80% of these children present with DKA.[2] An unexpected finding in the pediatric population has been the frequency of DKA as a presenting clinical picture in those with type 2 diabetes. In one study, DKA was seen in 59.44% of individuals with type 1 diabetes mellitus (T1DM) and 23.91% of individuals with type 2 diabetes mellitus (T2DM). Of those with T2DM, 58.82% had presented in DKA.[3] Diabetic ketoacidosis also appears as an acute presentation of unrecognized T2DM, as a new diagnosis, particularly in certain ethnicities.[4-7] Type 1 diabetes, by definition, is characterized by insulin deficiency. Treatment provides insulin in an amount designed to match the amount required for glucose uptake into the cells. Available insulin and insulin delivery systems have improved tremendously but remain imperfect. Some situations such as illness may quickly and substantially elevate blood glucose even when good blood glucose control has been previously maintained.[8] Other conditions, such as persistent untreated hyperglycemia, newly prescribed medications, or missed insulin, can also disrupt the perfect match. Anything that increases blood glucose and decreases insulin action can contribute to the development of DKA.

Ingested Glucose

Eating more food or more carbohydrates than usual, without changing insulin dosing, elevates blood glucose. This happens frequently to people who take fixed doses of insulin but not fixed quantities of food. Hyperglycemia itself can stimulate hunger, leading to increased food intake. Excessive food intake alone is not sufficient to cause DKA but may cumulatively contribute to it. Two small studies of pediatric patients reported consumption of large volumes of high-calorie beverages before admission for DKA.[9,10] In type 2 diabetes, alcohol has been associated with DKA development.

Monitoring

Evidence from an international survey of over 35,000 pump wearers showed that good glycemic control is correlated to frequency of blood glucose measurements of 4 to 5 or more times per day.[11] Pump users who monitored blood glucose levels 4 or more times a day achieved a lower average A1C level than patients who monitored levels once or twice daily (7.2% versus 8%). Of patients who self-reported that they monitored blood glucose levels 5 or more times a day, 62% had an average A1C level of less than 7%.[12] On average, an individual with type 1 diabetes monitors 2 to 3 times a day, which is inadequate for intensive insulin therapy.[13] The advent of continuous glucose monitoring used with pump technology has further decreased DKA.[14] More recently available technology using a pump system linked to a continuous glucose sensor that, on reaching a low glucose preset threshold, can automatically shut off pump

---

Case: DKA in a Busy Woman With Type 1 Diabetes

GT is a 24-year-old female who has had type 1 diabetes since age 12. She has been using an insulin pump for 8 years and checks her blood glucose 4 to 6 times per day. She does not understand why others she meets do not take their diabetes more seriously. GT is 5 ft 8 in and 160 lb. Her latest A1C was 6.2%, and her daily glucose readings range from 50 to 200 mg/dL. She has not had any complications, and other than having diabetes, she is a healthy young adult. She is a full-time student working toward an MBA and works part-time as an accountant for a gift shop.

Precipitating Events

GT usually eats regularly, matches her premeal insulin dose to her carbohydrate intake, exercises, and sleeps 7 to 8 hours a night. Since mid-November, though, life has been chaotic as extra hours at work, end-of-semester exams, and holiday preparations converged. Some days she skipped meals, grabbed a sandwich, or snacked from the vending machine. She missed most of her scheduled times at the gym. She was tired and began drinking more coffee and diet soda to keep going. Increased commitments had disrupted her routine.

GT was eagerly awaiting her next 3-month shipment of diabetes supplies, which seemed to be delayed in the mass of holiday packages. She began testing her blood glucose less often to conserve strips and hoped the new shipment arrived before her holiday trip to visit with family. At the end of the semester, she was flying to Maine for a quick visit with her grandparents before heading home for Christmas.

insulin delivery has shown even more impact on lessening DKA episodes.[15]

Inadequate Insulin

Glucose levels rise directly from deficient insulin production and/or an inability to effectively use the insulin produced. People with type 1 diabetes—and, to a lesser extent, people with type 2 diabetes requiring insulin—can receive inadequate insulin from poorly designed or poorly followed treatment plans. Inadequate insulin impacts other physiological functions that elevate glucose levels indirectly.

Glucose stored in the liver as glycogen is available to provide fuel between meals and during sleep. Ideally, hepatic glucose offers stored energy as needed to maintain blood glucose levels, support exercise, and provide extra fuel for extraordinary events such as surgery or fighting a grizzly bear. When adequately available, insulin turns off this hepatic feeding function as soon as there is sufficient glucose available to hungry cells.

When there is inadequate insulin, the liver keeps producing glucose, as there is no ability to sense the problem of inadequate insulin availability to promote glucose entry into cells. This process of glycogenolysis and even gluconeogenesis (the production of glucose from amino acids obtained from protein breakdown) floods the bloodstream with unwelcome sugar molecules. Multiple forms of stress (illness, trauma, menses, pregnancy, fear, worry, excitement, and other physical or emotional stressors) and some medications stimulate the counterregulatory and stress hormones. These hormones stimulate hepatic glucose production and, at the same time, interfere with insulin effectiveness and glucose uptake in the peripheral tissues. Glucagon, secreted in response to meal ingestion, is another hormone that stimulates hepatic glucose production and exacerbates an already disruptive situation.

Ketones

A homeostatic mechanism to feed cells when glucose cannot enter cells is to break down fat (lipolysis) into glucose and ketone bodies. As the concentration of ketones increases, the kidneys via osmotic diuresis excrete both glucose and ketones. The increasing amount of water lost in the process causes dehydration. Dehydration concentrates serum glucose and further increases hyperglycemia. Increased hyperglycemia drives further dehydration.

With dehydration and the increasing accumulation of ketones in the serum, sodium and potassium (key electrolytes that impact muscle and other organ functions) are affected. Potassium is involved with regulating the heart rhythm; therefore, loss of potassium may be life threatening. Further, as potassium is imperative to facilitate insulin action, hypokalemia can inhibit the ability of provided insulin to be therapeutic.

When ketone accumulation is excessive, blood becomes too acidic to support life. Diabetic ketoacidosis can be termed mild, moderate, or severe, depending on parameters of blood glucose levels, acidity, and ketone formation.[8] Prompt treatment is essential.

Precipitating Situations

Inadequate Insulin

Numerous factors contribute to inadequate insulin. The onset or acute decompensation of subclinical type 1 diabetes accounts for 30% of DKA cases.[7] Worsening insulin resistance or suboptimal treatment plans are other reasons for inadequate insulin being available. However, in many instances insulin injections may be skipped because of psychosocial reasons, a lack of adequate planning, or a patient's lack of knowledge about adequate self-management. The following are some examples:

- *Insulin omitted to control weight:* Insulin omission can be a form of bulimia. In a study of subjects aged 11 to 25 years, 36% reported insulin misuse to control weight.[16] The Assessing Health and Eating Among Adolescents With Diabetes survey showed 10.3% of females reported skipping insulin, and 7.4% reported taking less insulin to control their weight.[17] Omission of or not taking adequate insulin may be the most important contributor to DKA in urban African Americans with type 2 diabetes.[18] Musey reported in his study that half of patients (50%) stopped insulin because of a reported lack of money to buy insulin from an outside pharmacy or get transportation to the hospital, 21% stopped insulin because of lack of appetite, 14% stopped insulin because of behavioral or psychological reasons, and 14% did so because they did not know how to manage diabetes on sick days.[19]

- *Psychological problems complicated by eating disorders:* May be a factor in 20% of recurrent ketoacidosis.[8]
- *Insulin omitted to avoid hypoglycemia, especially when home alone or during active workdays*[6]: May be seen as a self-initiated safety measure, or may occur during illness due to the mistaken belief that insulin is not needed when eating less.
- *Insulin omitted to avoid the inconvenience or embarrassment of injecting in a public situation:* Many people feel uncomfortable injecting insulin in a restaurant or asking permission to leave their work site to do so.
- *Inadequate or poorly timed insulin due to inadequate organization:* Some people never seem to have all the supplies they need in the right place at the right time.
- *Insulin dose reduced to save money:* Many people are faced with economic challenges and are forced to choose whether they will spend their limited income on housing, food, or medicine.
- *Insulin dose reduced or omitted when ill:* Some believe they need less insulin if they eat less. Because nausea, vomiting, and stomach pain are symptoms of DKA, omitting insulin for gastrointestinal symptoms may only push glucose levels higher and make symptoms worse.
- *Using insulin that is outdated, improperly stored, inaccurately measured, or incorrectly injected:* Can provide a lower dose than planned.

Excess Hepatic Glucose

Stress, whether physical, emotional, or psychological, can dramatically and acutely increase blood glucose levels. All forms of stress increase adrenal glucocorticoid production and catecholamine levels, both of which raise glucose levels through increased hepatic glucose production. This can increase the risk of DKA if there is no intervention to either decrease the instigating stress or provide compensatory insulin adjustment. The following are examples of situations that increase hepatic production and release glucose:

- Infection—the most common precipitating factor
- Pneumonia and urinary tract infections—account for 30% to 50% of DKA
- Gastrointestinal bleeding
- Cerebrovascular accident (CVA)
- Alcohol abuse
- Pancreatitis
- Myocardial infarction
- Trauma
- Pregnancy
- Drugs that affect carbohydrate metabolism (corticosteroids, thiazides, dobutamine, terbutaline, cocaine)[18]

Prevention

Preventing or at least greatly limiting the severity of DKA due to causes other than acute glycemic decompensation is possible. Early recognition of hyperglycemia and appropriate treatment can prevent acute complications and reduce fatalities, which have been reduced to an overall 2% but rise with age and seriousness of concomitant disease.[20] When hyperglycemia is ignored or occurs unexpectedly, coma and even death are possible.

Inadequate Insulin

If an individual intentionally omits or is deprived of insulin for any reason, discussing DKA prevention may be ineffective unless underlying problems are also addressed.

Some people with diabetes purposely avoid insulin during school or work hours, and others omit insulin as a way to lose weight; disadvantaged children are more vulnerable to episodes of DKA.[21] Intentionally omitting insulin for any reason suggests there are other problems that need to be addressed before further discussing DKA prevention. Also recognized is the possible contribution of drug abuse as a risk factor for DKA. Active use of cocaine has been reported as an independent risk factor for recurrent DKA, supporting toxicology screening in patients with recurrent DKA.[22]

Education regarding glucose self-management during illness and stress management are essential to prevent DKA. Patients benefit from having sick-day management information reinforced over and over again during routine appointments (see Table 22.1).

Also provide information about possible causes and how to recognize symptoms of DKA. Identifying the cause or risks for DKA in the individual's specific situation may help prevent the problem. Common contributors to acute hyperglycemia include the following:

◆ Relying on "how you feel" to assess glucose levels

◆ Skipping insulin when not eating

◆ Inadequate monitoring during illness

Other possible causes for acute hyperglycemia include the following:

◆ Use of expired insulin

◆ Increased insulin needs during growth or hormonal spurts

◆ Preoccupation with other priorities and missing (or not learning to recognize) symptoms of escalating glucose levels

The more patients understand how their medications work, the more able they are to use them to their advantage. Learning to supplement with extra insulin for high glucose levels and for ketones prepares them to handle acute situations.

Remaining attentive to the symptoms of hyperglycemia and monitoring glucose in the midst of other priorities could prevent many incidents of DKA. Finding and using resources, including knowing when to contact a physician, can ease the burden of living with diabetes.

Ultimately, information is essential, but to prevent DKA, patients and their families require more than information. The individual must be prepared to effectively employ self-management strategies to prevent severe hyperglycemia and intervene early when at risk.

TABLE 22.1 **Sick-Day Management**		
	Type 1 Diabetes	*Type 2 Diabetes*
Hydration	8 oz fluid per hour Every third hour, consume this 8 oz as a sodium-rich choice such as bouillon	Same
Self-monitoring of blood glucose	Test every 2–4 hours while blood glucose is elevated or until symptoms subside	Same
Ketones	Test every 4 hours or until negative	Determine for the individual
Medication adjustments	Continue as able Adjust insulin doses to correct hyperglycemia, but do not stop or hold insulin if diagnosed as having type 1 diabetes melltus Hold metformin during serious illness Instruct patients to call their healthcare provider for specific instructions if they have not previously received them	Same
Food and beverage selections	Guide patients to consume 150–200 g carbohydrates daily, in divided doses Switch to soft foods or liquids as tolerated Provide patients a list of foods and beverages in portion sizes containing 15 g carbohydrates	Same
Contact healthcare professionals	Provide guidelines on conditions that require the patient to call: • Vomiting more than once • Diarrhea more than 5 times or for longer than 6 hours • Blood glucose levels >300 mg/dL on 2 consecutive measurements that are not responsive to increased insulin and fluids Moderate or large urine ketones or blood ketones >10.8 mg/dL (>0.6 mmol/L)	Same

Assessing Hyperglycemia

Diabetic Ketoacidosis: Signs, Symptoms, and Laboratory Indicators

The symptoms of hyperglycemia may mimic other diseases or conditions. Assessment of the following helps accurately diagnose the problem:

- Hyperglycemia
- Dehydration
- Electrolyte status
- Ketosis
- Acidosis
- Osmolality

The physical signs and symptoms and the laboratory findings consistent with DKA relate physiologically to one of these markers: hyperglycemia, dehydration, electrolyte imbalance, ketosis, or acidosis. Patients can present with a spectrum of low energy to confusion, lethargy to coma, abdominal pain, polyuria, and polydipsia. Table 22.2 summarizes these markers.

Initial Evaluation Findings

- *Blood glucose:* Finger-stick blood glucose of >250 mg/dL if outpatient; serum glucose will be obtained in urgent or acute care settings
- *Urine ketones:* Positive

Confirmation of Diagnosis (either of the following)

- *Arterial pH:* <7.3
- *Serum bicarbonate:* <16 mEq/L

Identification of Precipitating Factors

- *History and full clinical exam:* To identify precipitating etiologies; includes looking for

TABLE 22.2   Markers of DKA

	Hyperglycemia	Dehydration	Electrolyte Imbalance	Ketosis	Acidosis
Physical signs	Polyuria Polydipsia Blurred vision Polyphagia Weight loss if insulin deficiency is present long enough (days to weeks)	Decreased intravascular volume Decreased neck vein filling from below while person is lying absolutely flat Orthostatic hypotension (systolic blood pressure drop of 20 mm Hg after 1 min of standing) Poor skin turgor: seen earlier in children "Soft eyeballs": late sign of profound dehydration in adults		"Fruity" or acetone breath Nausea Vomiting Abdominal pain	Kussmaul respirations (hyperpnea)
Laboratory tests	Glucose >250 mg/dL	Hemoglobin Hematocrit Total protein values are often mildly elevated Creatinine Blood urea nitrogen (BUN)	Sodium: low, normal, or high Potassium: low, normal, or high Phosphorus: normal or high	Positive ketones	Low pH (<7.2) Low HCO_3 (<15 mEq/L) Low PCO (<35 mm Hg)

potential sources of infection, such as perirectal abscess or cellulitis

❖ *Vital signs:* Weight, blood pressure in the supine and upright positions, and pulse rate to assess hydration status

❖ *Laboratory evaluation*[1]: Serum electrolyte values (with calculated anion gap), blood urea nitrogen (BUN)/creatinine levels, beta-hydroxybutyric acid (or serum ketones, if not available), calcium and phosphorus concentrations, serum-osmolality, complete blood cell count with differential, and electrocardiogram (EKG)

❖ *Additional tests, as needed*[18]: Bacterial blood cultures if infection suspected, urine analysis for urinary tract infection, chest X-ray, EKG, A1C (to identify whether DKA was an isolated event or the cumulative result of undiagnosed or poorly controlled diabetes), or pregnancy (if of childbearing age)

Additional Notes on Markers of DKA

Hyperglycemia

Elevated glucose is a marker of DKA but not a good index of the severity. Diabetic ketoacidosis does occur with lower glucose levels, especially in children, pregnant women, and persons who have been vomiting frequently.

Dehydration

Due to dehydration, the lab values listed are likely to be mildly elevated before treatment of DKA and are likely to correct themselves after treatment. Elevated creatinine or BUN after rehydration suggests further assessment for renal problems.

Electrolyte Imbalance

❖ *Sodium.* Dehydration causes a profound loss of total body sodium (Na^+) that serum levels cannot accurately measure. The results of testing serum sodium may appear low, normal, or high, depending on whether the sodium lost was greater than, equal to, or less than the relative amount of water lost.

❖ *Potassium.* Similarly, total body depletion of potassium always occurs with DKA, but lab values of serum potassium (K^+) can test low,

normal, or high. As with sodium, serum potassium reflects the relative amounts of water lost compared with potassium lost. Potassium may be low before treatment or fall as it enters the cells, with glucose and fluids reducing the serum concentration. The status of renal function should be ascertained before any potassium is replaced.

❖ *Phosphate.* Phosphate concentrations are usually high or high-normal initially and decrease with insulin therapy, sometimes markedly, to very low levels over the next day or two. Phosphate replacement remains controversial at this time, as it is believed that with rapid access to oral normal food intake, phosphate can be replaced without the need for parenteral phosphate.[8]

Ketosis

One ketone produced during DKA, acetoacetate, converts to acetone and is excreted by the lungs. Acetone has a fruity odor that may be detectable on the breath of someone in ketosis. Beta-hydroxybutyric acid is the most prevalent ketone in DKA, and measurement of this acid is the most reliable way to measure treatment progress. Beta-hydroxybutyric acid is measured by serum assessment using the nitroprusside method.

Acidosis

Very deep and sometimes rapid breathing unrelated to exertion or the inability to "catch one's breath" is a symptom of acidosis called Kussmaul respiration or hyperpnea. This form of hyperventilation is an effort to correct the metabolic acidosis by blowing off carbon dioxide.

Increased Osmolality

Mental-status changes seem to correlate best with serum osmolality and less so with glucose levels. People with DKA may be alert, obtunded, stuporous, or in frank coma. The changes in mentation, rather than the status itself, offer clues to diagnosis.

Other Significant Symptoms of DKA

❖ *Nonspecific symptoms.* Include weakness, lethargy, malaise, and headache.

◆ *Acute abdomen.* A common condition; marked by tenderness to palpation, diminished bowel sounds, and some muscle guarding, especially in children. A few patients may have more severe signs (absent bowel sounds, rebound tenderness, boardlike abdomen) that suggest a surgical emergency. These signs can be due to profound DKA and disappear after treatment, but can present a challenge to diagnose, as appendicitis or cholecystitis can be a precipitating cause of DKA.

◆ *Hypotonia.* Signs that do not appear until late in the progression of DKA and suggest a poor prognosis are uncoordinated ocular movements and fixed, dilated pupils.

◆ *Hypothermia.* Common during DKA, making the presence of a fever a strong indicator of infection.

Symptoms of DKA That Are Probably Insignificant

◆ Increased amylase alone does not suggest pancreatitis. In DKA, salivary glands, not the pancreas, release most of the amylase.

◆ Increased white blood cells (WBC) with DKA do not indicate infection. The differential count may be helpful with increased immature WBCs (>10% band forms), but clinical exam findings, such as fever, can supersede laboratory findings.[17]

◆ Mildly elevated liver function tests (LFTs) usually do not suggest liver damage and return to normal in several weeks.

◆ Serum creatinine can be elevated at initial evaluation. This needs to be monitored, as often the creatinine will fall as fluid replacement is initiated, but the issue as to when potassium replacement is safe requires that the creatinine be monitored closely.

Although the symptoms of poorly controlled diabetes may be present for several days, the metabolic alterations typical of ketoacidosis usually occur within a short time frame (typically less than 24 hours). Occasionally, DKA may develop more acutely with no prior signs or symptoms.[2]

Treatment of DKA

The first part of this section describes treatment of moderate-to-severe DKA. Mild DKA is covered at the end of this section. Goals of DKA treatment,[1] listed in Table 22.3, are discussed individually below.

Mortality for moderate-to-severe DKA is high.

Hospitalization may be required for appropriate treatment of DKA that is moderate to severe. Mortality remains high, even in teaching institutions. Treatment always requires supplemental fluids (first), followed by additional insulin.

Although hyperglycemia is the cause of osmotic diuresis, which leads to dehydration, the dehydration must be treated first, then the hyperglycemia—particularly when hypotension indicates potential impending circulatory collapse. Eventually, providing additional glucose is necessary to stop cellular starvation and intracerebral swelling. Treatment of DKA would not be complete without providing information and coaching to help prevent future episodes.

Goal 1: Provide Adequate Fluids to Rehydrate

Begin fluid replacement. In all cases, adequate fluid replacement is critical to maintain circulation, expand volume, and restore renal perfusion.[1]

Initial Fluid Replacement
Initiate rapid administration of saline and reduce rate after first hour. Initial fluid replacement uses one-half

TABLE 22.3   Treatment Goals for DKA
1. Provide adequate fluids to rehydrate
2. Provide adequate insulin to restore and maintain normal glucose metabolism
3. Correct electrolyte deficits and acidosis if needed
4. Prevent complications
5. Provide source of glucose when needed
6. Provide patient and family education and follow-up

Source: MB Davidson, S Schwartz, "Hyperglycemia," in MJ Franz, ed, *A Core Curriculum for Diabetes Education: Diabetes and Complications,* 5th ed (Chicago: American Association of Diabetes Educators, 2003), 27-8.

The holiday commitments GT tried to meet that fall were additional stressors, known to stimulate counter-regulatory hormones and hepatic glucose release. With less sleep and poor eating habits, compounded by hyperglycemia from increasingly poorer glycemic control, GT was at risk for an infection.

She began to feel nauseous and noted decreasing energy. While studying for finals with her roommates, GT started to vomit and complained of stomach cramps. Her friends escorted her to the emergency room. The hospital staff suspected DKA when they learned GT had type 1 diabetes and heard about the nausea, vomiting, and abdominal pain, which were signs of ketones in her blood. The result of a finger-stick glucose reading was 350 mg/dL. Urinary ketones were large.

Diagnosis

GT's laboratory work was compatible with DKA diagnosis (see Table 22.4, listing DKA, HHS, and reference range values):

- Serum glucose was 395 mg/dL.
- The test for beta-hydroxybutyric acid confirmed ketosis.
- Low serum bicarbonate and arterial pH confirmed acidosis.

- Previous lab work had suggested slight anemia, but hemoglobin and hematocrit were now both elevated, as were BUN and creatinine—signs of dehydration.
- Increased serum osmolality conveyed the extent to which glucose was elevated and fluids were lost.
- Sodium was slightly low, and potassium was slightly high—dehydration caused the potassium number to look higher than it was. Excess glucose can falsely lower the laboratory-determined sodium in the blood. In addition, high glucoses caused factitious lowering in the sodium level.

Identification of Precipitating Cause

To find the precipitating cause of DKA, cultures were obtained of GT's blood and urine, as was a pregnancy test. GT's blood glucose had probably been running higher than usual for several weeks as she became increasingly less focused on her diabetes self-management. GT had been unknowingly decreasing her fluid intake, and with accompanying diuresis from hyperglycemia, GT's fluid deficit was increasing over time. The hormonal changes of increasing estrogen (accompanying menses) and the stress of incident infection quickly elevated blood glucose and precipitated ketone production.

TABLE 22.4   GT's Lab Values: Comparing DKA and HHS With Reference Range

Test	Reference Range[1]	DKA[2]	HHS[2]
Serum glucose (mg/dL)	70–140	>250	>600
Serum osmolality (mOsm/kg)	275–295	>320	>320
Sodium bicarbonate (mEq/L)	22–26	<15	>15
Arterial pH	7.36–7.44	<7.2	>7.3
Serum beta-hydroxybutyrate (mmol/L)	0.02–0.27	>1.1 mmol/L	
Ketones	absent	moderate to high	absent to small
Increases Due to Dehydration			
BUN (mg/dL)	5–20	32	61
Serum creatinine (mg/dL)	0.7–1.2	1.1	1.4
Losses Often Masked by Dehydration			
Serum potassium (mmol/L)	3.5–5.0	4.5	3.9
Serum sodium (mmol/L)	135–145	varies, but typically low	varies, but typically above normal
Serum phosphorus (mg/dL)	2.3–4.3	varies	varies

Sources:

1. Bakerman S. Bakerman's ABC's of Interpretive Laboratory Data. Scottsdale, Ariz: Interpretive Laboratory Data, Inc; 2002.
2. Nugent BW. Hyperosmolar hyperglycemic state. Emerg Med Clin North Am. 2005;23(3):629-48.

normal (0.45%) or normal (0.9%) saline, depending on serum sodium and state of hydration. Avoid changes in osmolality by more than 3 mOsm per kilogram per hour.

- *For adults.* The average adult requires 1 to 2 L in the first hour, after which the patient's status is reassessed.[1,10,17]
- *For children.* Deliver 10 to 20 mL per kilogram of body weight in the first hour. If no urination occurs, continue giving 20 mL per kilogram of body weight of fluid during the second and third hours.

Subsequent Fluid Replacement

The level of fluid replacement is monitored and adjusted based on maintenance needs, replacement requirements, and ongoing losses. The rate is adjusted to avoid fluid overload for renal and cardiac patients.

- Hyperglycemia will persist (even with appropriate insulin therapy) if fluid replacement is inadequate.
- Hydration status should typically correct within 48 hours. Several hours of hydration may be necessary before some patients are able to produce urine. If there is no urine flow after 4 hours of appropriate hydration, bladder catheterization may be warranted.

Goal 2: Provide Adequate Insulin to Restore and Maintain Normal Glucose Metabolism

All patients with DKA need insulin. Regular insulin by continuous intravenous infusion is the treatment of choice.[2]

- *Insulin type:* Regular or rapid-acting insulin offers relatively fast results in reducing glucose levels.
- *Delivery method:* Insulin delivery via intravenous infusion rather than injections offers these advantages: (1) more predictable decreases in glucose and (2) reduced risk of cerebral edema.
- *Pediatrics:* Rapid-acting insulin delivered via subcutaneous injections may be a cost-effective way to treat DKA in a pediatric population without admission to the hospital.[20] Target decreases in plasma glucose of 50 to 75 mg/dL per hour.

Goal 3: Correct Electrolyte Deficits and Acidosis If Needed

Potassium

Total body potassium depletion is associated with DKA. All patients with urine flow eventually need potassium repletion to avoid hypokalemia. Hypokalemia, if not treated properly, can lead to death. Prolonged hyperglycemia will be persistent in the setting of hypokalemia.

- The patient is closely observed for clinically significant signs of potential hypokalemia, such as cardiac arrhythmias; serum potassium is checked periodically (ie, every 2 to 4 hours until level is stable or glucose is stable).
- Once urine output is documented, depending on the serum potassium level, 20 to 30 mEq of potassium per liter of fluid to be infused is added.[3]

Serum potassium concentration is frequently monitored, as it is essential to guide therapy. Serum potassium concentrations can drop rapidly from the initial results obtained before therapy. With increased hydration, the intravascular volume expands and renal perfusion increases renal excretion of potassium. With insulin administration, more potassium enters the cells, contributing to a drop in serum potassium while restoring total body potassium.

Phosphate

Serum phosphate (PO_4) levels are monitored. Research does not support routine supplementation with phosphate, as oral intake of food can promptly replace deficits.

Acidosis

Adequate insulin is continued to resolve acidosis. Acidosis takes longer to reverse than does hyperglycemia treated with insulin. The time required to resolve acidosis has not been well studied, because the serial pH measurements necessary to measure acidosis have not been done.

Sodium Bicarbonate

Treating acidosis with sodium bicarbonate ($NaHCO_3$) is controversial. It may be appropriate in special circumstances (as with acute cardiorespiratory arrest or hyperkalemia-induced cardiac arrhythmias). Caution is warranted for the following reasons:

- No clinical benefit has been documented.
- Sodium bicarbonate increases risk for hypokalemic-induced arrhythmias because it causes potassium levels to drop so quickly.
- There is some evidence that bicarbonate increases risk for cerebral edema.[17]

Hyperchloremic Acidosis

In hyperchloremic acidosis, bicarbonate levels plateau at approximately 15 to 20 mEq/L (15 to 20 mmol/L), usually between 12 and 24 hours after treatment began. At this time, chloride levels remain elevated, pH has returned to normal, and serum ketone bodies have dropped to low or absent. Expect hyperchloremic acidosis following DKA to be transient and require no treatment.

Goal 4: Provide Source of Glucose When Needed

- When glucose reaches 250 mg/dL, 5% to 10% dextrose is added to the intravenous solution.[18] Starvation perpetuates ketosis. In addition, sudden drops in glucose can be associated with cerebral edema.
- Ketones are monitored. Ketosis is usually reversed in 12 to 24 hours, although occasionally urinary ketone bodies may be present for several days. If ketones persist, evaluation of adequacy of dietary intake is recommended.

Goal 5: Prevent Complications

Hypoglycemia, hypokalemia, and hyperglycemia are frequent complications of, respectively, overzealous treatment with insulin, use of bicarbonate, and inadequate insulin delivery during the transition from intravenous to subcutaneous administration. A 2-hour overlap between infused insulin and initiation of subcutaneous insulin helps avoid gaps in insulin delivery.

A delay in diagnosis and misdiagnosis add to severity.

Identification and treatment of the initial cause of hyperglycemia as well as early intervention substantially improve clinical outcomes following DKA.

Two common errors—a delay in diagnosis and misdiagnosis—delay treatment and make the consequences of DKA worse than they need to be. The longer that treatment is delayed, the more severe the DKA episode and the more complex the treatment. Diabetic ketoacidosis is often misdiagnosed as gastroenteritis or appendicitis. Hypokalemia and cerebral edema may also go unrecognized, causing critical delays in beginning appropriate therapy for these conditions.

Most deaths occur in older patients with medical complications other than DKA.[17] Older age and depth of coma predict mortality risk. Death is usually due to infection, arterial thrombosis, shock, or an unrecognized precipitating event that is not treated adequately. Complications such as aspiration and pulmonary edema may occur even in the most rigorously controlled treatment environment.

Cerebral Edema

Cerebral edema occurs rarely and is more common in children with DKA, yet it accounts for 90% of the deaths associated with DKA in children. Some studies question the significance of osmolality-induced injury, suggesting instead that cerebral hypoperfusion injury may be a predominant cause of cerebral edema that begins even prior to DKA treatment.[23,24] The optimal fluid type and rate of administration to treat pediatric DKA are currently under study. The Pediatric Emergency Care Applied Research Network (PECARN) is gathering data on more than 1500 pediatric patients in DKA using 4 treatment protocols with different types and rates of fluid administration, with mental status assessments during treatment and neurocognitive testing 3 months after DKA.[25] Cerebral edema occurs early in the course of treatment, typically in the first 24 hours and usually in the first 12 hours of treatment. The following help minimize the risks for this complication:

- Assess mental status frequently (every 1 to 2 hours), especially in children, who are more susceptible to cerebral edema than adults.
- Monitor for headache, lethargy, and mental status changes; all are symptoms of cerebral edema.

- Suspect cerebral edema if improvement in lethargy and mental function is followed by deterioration, while metabolic status continues to improve and normalize.
- Avoid rapid drops in blood glucose, which may be a factor in the development of cerebral edema. To moderate the rate of glucose drop, add intravenous glucose to the regimen as the serum glucose level reaches about 250 mg/dL.
- If cerebral edema does occur, include IV osmotic diuretics (mannitol) and possibly high-dose glucocorticoids (dexamethasone) in the treatment.

The earlier the treatment, the better the prognosis. Treatment of cerebral edema at early stages may be beneficial, but it is usually ineffective at later stages. Once clinical symptoms (seizures, incontinence, bradycardia, respiratory arrest) appear, the mortality rate is >70%, with only 7% to 14% recovering completely.[8]

Goal 6: Provide Patient and Family Education and Follow-up

After an episode of DKA, patients and their families may be more receptive to learning how they might avoid a repeat hospitalization. A multidisciplinary team approach, including psychosocial intervention, may be needed to address concerns of patients with recurrent episodes of DKA. See the earlier section on prevention of DKA.

Self-Care Behaviors in the Prevention of Severe Hyperglycemia

The AADE7 Self-Care Behaviors™ provide a framework for prevention of severe hyperglycemia. Table 22.5 demonstrates how these behaviors can be used in the prevention of DKA. More details on fostering specific self-care behaviors are provided in chapters 4 through 10 in section 1 of this book.

Treating Mild DKA

Some milder cases of DKA can be treated at home without hospitalization or an emergency room visit.[26] The following are parameters:

- The patient can still drink and retain oral fluids without difficulty, and
- The patient or patient's family can provide accurate blood glucose values and results of urine ketone tests, and
- A knowledgeable healthcare professional is available to guide therapy over the phone.

TABLE 22.5 Applying Self-Care Behaviors to Prevention of DKA		
AADE7 Self-Care Behaviors™	*Concept*	*Application*
Being Active	Being safely active: Exercising without adequate insulin can dangerously elevate blood glucose (BG). Maintaining hydration is also important.	If glucose before exercise is high (>250 mg/dL), check for ketones. Presence of ketones indicates glucose is high due to inadequate insulin. Do not exercise until ketones are gone. To compensate for fluids lost during physical activity, drink adequately before, during, and after, especially on hot days.
Healthy Eating	Matching premeal insulin and carbohydrate to manage glucose levels. Having a sick-day plan and supplies (food and fluids).	Identify acceptable, easy-to-digest foods for sick days. Avoid an extreme carbohydrate load by limiting volume of sweetened beverages.

TABLE 22.5 Applying Self-Care Behaviors to Prevention of DKA (continued)		
AADE7 Self-Care Behaviors™	*Concept*	*Application*
Taking Medication	Exogenous insulin is essential to life for people with type 1 diabetes. Taking the right insulin in the right amount at the right time helps prevent very high BG. Other drugs may help improve/stabilize glucose.	Inadequate insulin dosing or poor timing of insulin action increases the risk for DKA. Omitting insulin almost guarantees it. To reduce risks for acute hyperglycemia, understand how insulin works and maintain the skills needed to take it appropriately. Everyone with type 1 diabetes needs this understanding.
Monitoring	Monitoring BG and ketone levels provides feedback about the treatment plan and early warning of impending DKA.	Monitor regularly to help identify hyperglycemia before it becomes life threatening and enable early intervention and progress assessment. Increase monitoring frequency when not eating or ill. Do not rely strictly on "how you feel"— this provides an inaccurate measure of BG. Monitor to obtain accurate BG levels. Access to monitoring supplies may be a barrier to self-monitoring of BG. Address issues of concern. Assess problems with monitoring. Resistance to monitoring may have multiple causes.
Problem Solving	Applying information to individual situations so information already learned helps solve problems—avoiding initial events as well as recurrence.	Review the circumstances preceding a DKA episode. Identify precipitating factors to obtain clues to prevent another episode. Questions to reduce risk may relate to delaying exercise, limiting carbohydrate intake, monitoring blood glucose, or adjusting medication. Review factors contributing to DKA and learn to recognize signs and symptoms to prevent recurrence.
Reducing Risks	Reducing the risk as well as the impact of DKA is possible. Unlike most diabetes management decisions, reducing complications from DKA treatment is primarily a provider responsibility.	Delayed treatment, excessive insulin, and inadequate insulin are common errors of treating DKA. Reduce complications with prompt diagnosis, adjusting insulin to glucose response, and beginning injected insulin before stopping IV. Discuss sick days—interventions for nausea, fever, loss of appetite; correction factors for hyperglycemia and further corrections for ketones; when to seek medical care and after-hours procedures.
Healthy Coping	Eating well, taking medications, testing BG, and using results to problem solve are difficult, never-ending aspects of self-management.	Use information, support, and encouragement to help overcome barriers that interfere with optimal prevention of DKA. Acknowledge the inevitable struggle that is part of living with diabetes. Discuss growth and hormonal spurts. Discuss inattention to signs and distractions of life. Identify resources and situations in which to seek medical attention.

American Association of Diabetes Educators©

Attention to physical symptoms, timely monitoring, and ability to adjust insulin all contribute to reducing the incidence and severity of DKA. Treatment at this stage can focus on oral hydration and supplemental insulin. Fluid intake should target 3 to 5 oz of carbohydrate-containing fluids per hour. The amount may be better tolerated if ingested in smaller doses every 20 to 30 minutes (or at every television commercial). If there are no contraindications (congestive heart failure, hypertension), broths containing sodium may be more efficacious than the carbohydrate fluids, as they are not as likely to be voided as "free water."

Adequate Insulin to Restore and Maintain Normal Glucose Metabolism

In addition to usual insulin, provide supplemental insulin to compensate for hyperglycemia and ketosis. The amount needed depends on the patient's known sensitivity to insulin and current level of ketosis.

◆ *For children.* 0.25 to 0.5 units per kilogram of regular insulin every 4 to 6 hours, or rapid-acting insulin every 3 to 4 hours as needed.[1] A range for insulin replacement might be more appropriate.[27]

◆ *For adults.* 4 to 10 units or 10% to 20% of the usual total daily dose. Monitor frequently and adjust insulin for slow drop in glucose and resolution of ketosis.

Treatment of DKA depends on the severity of the episode, the abilities of the person with diabetes, and access to competent support. When someone with diabetes successfully treats mild DKA at home, clinical follow-up is still appropriate to reinforce information and support efforts to prevent DKA.

Problem Solving for Sick Days

Providers and patients should not automatically assume illness or flu-like symptoms are the cause of elevated blood glucoses. Nausea, vomiting, or

---

Case—Part 3: DKA Treatment, Including Education Components

Before the laboratory results were back, the medical staff started an IV of normal saline to replace GT's fluids. Then they added regular insulin at the recommended dose (0.1 units per kilogram per hour) to slowly lower blood glucose. Glucose and insulin doses were routinely entered into a flow sheet in her medical record.

- After 1 hour, glucose was 260 mg/dL. Because this drop exceeded the target rate for lowering glucose, the physician reduced the insulin drip to 0.08 units per kilogram per hour. The following were reassessed: glucose, sodium, potassium, and phosphorus. The results indicated that glucose was down to 248 mg/dL, potassium 3.9 mEq/L, sodium 135 mEq/L, and phosphate 2.5 mg/dL. The rate of IV insulin was maintained. Potassium was already being supplemented, and the lab finding was in the reference range. However, it was anticipated that potassium would drop further as her glucose level fell and potassium moved intracellularly. Additional potassium was added as potassium phosphate.

- After another hour, glucose was 214 mg/dL and urine ketones were moderate. Glucose was added to GT's IV.

- The next day, GT's labs were much improved. Electrolytes were within the reference range, glucose

ranged from 150 to 220 mg/dL, and ketones were small.

As GT talked with her nurse, she began to see what had happened in the days leading up to this DKA episode. In retrospect, she could see how, little by little, meals had become erratic and had been replaced with caffeine to help keep her going, and insulin doses had been missed. GT had not realized that her growing fatigue probably reflected her climbing glucose levels—something she would have known if she had continued to test regularly. The two reviewed sick-day guidelines and reviewed why GT's body required insulin even when she was not eating as much as usual. The diabetes resource nurse provided sample strips to support her blood glucose testing at home until the mail-order strips arrived, and a new prescription for ketone test strips was filled.

Reviewing the sick-day management principles helped GT. If GT checked and found her blood glucose over 250 mg/dL, she would do a urine test for ketones. If ketones were positive, she could take her usual supplemental insulin dose to lower glucose. Because ketones increase insulin resistance, to effectively lower blood glucose, GT would need to take more supplemental insulin than usual. That information made more sense now. The first time she had heard it, GT had believed DKA would never happen to her; she now knew better.

---

dehydration often herald the onset of DKA. Patients always need to address the areas of hydration, self-monitoring of blood glucose, ketones, medication adjustments, and food and beverage selections in the troubleshooting checklist (see Table 22.1) and then decide whether illness is causing the elevated glucoses.

For those on insulin pump therapy, temporary basal rate increases are particularly useful in treating hyperglycemia due to intercurrent illness or use of steroids. During these times, patients often need reminding to maintain adequate fluid intake with salted broth, water, or noncaloric beverages. If liquid carbohydrates are used for fluid replacement, appropriate boluses must be given. Often, bolus ratios need to be temporarily increased, as does the basal rate until the condition is resolved. When blood glucoses are within target range, and nausea and ketones are present, the patient needs to sip on carbohydrate-containing beverages and give appropriate boluses based on insulin-to-carbohydrate ratio to eliminate ketones.[28] Patients are often reluctant to use additional carbohydrates in this situation, but to reverse ketosis both insulin and carbohydrates are necessary.

Special Inpatient Hyperglycemia Concerns

The development of inpatient protocols for insulin delivery was spurred by awareness that previously accepted glycemic targets, the most recent data suggesting above 180 mg/dL, were associated with greater morbidity and mortality than glycemic targets of less than 180 mg/dL.[29] However, there remains some disagreement with absolute glycemic targets, with the American College of Physicians recent recommendation to target a blood glucose level of 140 to 200 mg/dL in SICU/MICU patients, and with avoiding targets <140 mg/dL because hypoglycemia and associated risks are likely to increase with lower blood glucose targets.[30]

Despite several large-scale trials, absolute targets for glucose control remain controversial due to differences in populations studied, comorbidities, and etiologies to admitting illnesses.[31] Successful improvement in the overall care of hyperglycemic patients is not dependent on glycemic-lowering needs alone.

The Society of Hospital Medicine identifies the following essential elements for inpatient hyperglycemia management[32]:

- Institutional support
- A multidisciplinary team or steering committee
- Data collection and reliable metrics
- Specific aims or goals
- Standardized insulin order sets
- Algorithms, policies, and protocols
- Comprehensive education and certification programs

The 2009 American Association of Clinical Endocrinologists/American Diabetes Association (AACE/ADA) consensus statement recommends a blood glucose target of 140 to 180 mg/dL (7.8-10.0 mmol/L) for most critically ill patients. Greater benefit may be realized at the lower end of this range. Although strong evidence is lacking, somewhat lower glucose targets may be appropriate in selected patients, such as the surgical population in units that have shown low rates of hypoglycemia.[33,34] However, targets below 110 mg/dL (6.1 mmol/L) are no longer recommended (see Table 22.6).

TABLE 22.6 Current Glycemic Targets in Hospitalized Patients		
All Critically Ill Patients in Intensive Care Unit Settings	*Non-critically-ill Patients*	*Hypoglycemia*
Blood glucose level 140–180 mg/dL (7.78–10.0 mmol/L)	Premeal: <140 mg/dL (7.78 mmol/L)	Reassess the regimen if blood glucose level is <100 mg/dL (5.56 mmol/L)
Intravenous insulin preferred	Random: <180 mg/dL (10.0 mmol/L)	Modify the regimen if blood glucose level is <70 mg/dL (3.89 mmol/L)
	Scheduled subcutaneous dosing preferred	Sliding-scale insulin discouraged

Source: ES Moghissi, MT Korytkowski, M DiNardo, et al, "American Association of Clinical Endocrinologists/American Diabetes Association consensus statement on inpatient glycemic control," *Endocr Pract* 15, no. 4 (2009): 1-17.

The National Quality Forum has identified "serious reportable events," also called "never events," defined as "errors in medical care that are clearly identifiable, preventable, and serious in their consequences for patients, and that indicate a real problem in the safety and credibility of a health care facility."[35] Third-party payers, including the Centers for Medicare & Medicaid Services (CMS), have begun to withhold payments for care related to these types of events. The CMS categorizes death or serious disability associated with hyperglycemia or hypoglycemia as a "never event."

Hyperosmolar Hyperglycemic Nonketotic Syndrome

A blood glucose level greater than 600 mg/dL without significant ketones characterizes hyperosmolar hyperglycemic state (HHS).[20] Hyperosmolar hyperglycemic state can occur whether or not diabetes medications are part of usual treatment.[20] Elevated blood glucose can escalate for days before it becomes a serious, acute threat.

> In HHS, extreme dehydration is the primary precipitating factor.

Extreme dehydration, more than profound insulin deficiency, is the primary precipitating factor. Profound dehydration, with subsequent hyperosmolarity and electrolyte losses, compounds the seriousness of this acute complication. Hyperosmolar hyperglycemic state occurs most frequently in undiagnosed or older adults with type 2 diabetes, but it also occurs in children and in people with type 1 diabetes. In 30% to 40% of HHS cases, HHS is the initial presentation of type 2 diabetes. While about 25% of new pediatric cases present with DKA, an estimated 4% of newly diagnosed children present with symptoms of HHS.[21]

Because HHS develops slowly (average 12 days) and does not cause the gastrointestinal pain associated with DKA, it is often overlooked or misdiagnosed.[36] Lack of treatment prolongs the osmotic diuresis secondary to hyperglycemia and worsens the clinical outlook. Due to delayed treatment as well as other medical conditions common in an older population, the mortality rate is about 15%, higher than the rate for DKA.

Pathophysiology of HHS

Hyperosmolar hyperglycemic state is similar to DKA except that insulin deficiency is less profound and dehydration plays a much more significant role. When blood glucose levels exceed 180 mg/dL, the kidneys are no longer able to reabsorb glucose. The concomitant renal water loss reduces renal perfusion and further dehydration. The water loss and concomitant inability to make up this water loss with oral intake causes the more extreme levels of hyperglycemia and osmolarity in HHS than those found with DKA. The alterations in consciousness seen with HHS and the risk for morbidity are related to the degree of osmolarity.

Without significant ketone formation, related symptoms typical of DKA, like ketosis, acidosis, gastrointestinal discomfort, and Kussmaul respirations, do not occur. Without the physical discomfort of ketosis, patients and their caregivers do not recognize a problem and the need for medical care. The mutual exacerbation of hyperglycemia and dehydration can begin with either problem (elevated glucose or inadequate fluids) and steadily escalate.

Precipitating Situations

Anything that elevates blood glucose or reduces hydration can contribute to development of HHS.

Elevated Blood Glucose
- New-onset type 2 diabetes
- Infection—a precipitating factor in 60% of cases[36]
- Surgery
- Myocardial infarction
- Gastrointestinal hemorrhage
- Uremia
- Arterial thrombosis
- Pancreatitis
- CVA
- Pulmonary embolism
- Medications that impact carbohydrate metabolism, such as glucocorticoids, thiazides, phenytoin, and beta-blockers

Decreased Water Intake and Access to Fluids

- Osmotic diuresis due to hyperglycemia—this is primary
- Fever
- Severe burns
- Diarrhea
- Peritoneal and hemodialysis
- Diuretic medications
- Hypertonic feeding
- Impaired thirst mechanism
- Inability to replace fluids may initiate dehydration

Particularly vulnerable are elderly people who must depend on others for their daily care and have difficulty communicating. Older people with impaired thirst who live alone may drink little unless prompted in some way. There are many opportunities to disrupt the development of HHS with regular monitoring and attention to those at risk.

Emphasize the importance of fluids to prevent dehydration. Situations that warrant extra care include physical activity, illness, institutionalized care settings (hospital, long-term care), forgetfulness, and aversion to drinking water or other hydrating fluids

such as thickened liquids for those with swallowing difficulties.

Assessing Hyperglycemia

Hyperosmolar Hyperglycemic State: Signs, Symptoms, and Laboratory Indicators

The signs and symptoms of HHS are similar to those of DKA, with some important exceptions.

The primary markers of HHS are the following:

- Severe hyperglycemia
- Profound dehydration
- Neurologic changes
- Absence of significant ketosis

Severe Hyperglycemia

Blood glucose levels in HHS are greater than 600 mg/dL. The reported mean glucose is greater than 1000 mg/dL, with elevations as high as 1500 mg/dL due to the extreme deficit of intravascular fluids.[37]

Profound Dehydration

Profound dehydration is marked by plasma osmolality greater than 320 mOsm per kilogram. Deficits of 20%

Case: HHS in an Elderly Man With Type 2 Diabetes

Early in October, GT's Grandpa Joe had fallen and broken his hip while shopping. GT understood that the surgery had gone smoothly and that Grandpa was making reasonable progress with physical therapy postoperatively, but Grandma said he seemed a bit confused and slept more and more during the day. Before the fall, Grandpa had been active despite a little arthritis. He had managed his type 2 diabetes with a careful eye on what he ate and had kept his A1C less than 6%. After his fall, Joe needed the help of adult day care so he could receive daily physical therapy. His doctor saw no reason for Grandpa to check his own blood glucose daily at home, as his granddaughter GT, who had "the serious kind" of diabetes, needed to do.

GT delayed her trip to visit her grandparents in Maine until after Christmas. When her flight arrived, Grandpa Joe was still in his physical therapy session, so she took a taxi straight there from the airport. Both grandparents welcomed her warmly and wanted to hear more about her DKA episode. As she talked, she noticed Grandpa nodding off or jumping into the conversation with comments about his "'54 Chevy." Grandma was cheery, but

her face signaled her worry about Grandpa's slow recovery. GT took out her glucose meter and checked Grandpa's glucose from a finger-stick.

They were all flabbergasted when the result read "high," meaning the glucose level was too high for the meter to read it. They called the nurse to double-check that number.

Precipitating Events

It is not unusual for the stress of surgery to elevate glucose levels. Grandpa had little appetite after surgery, so his losing a little weight did not alarm anyone. In fact, he had begun to eat a little more with Grandma there with him for most meals. What no one noticed was that Grandpa was not drinking. He ate rather than drank his calories at meals and left containers of water untouched most of the day.

Slowly, Grandpa became more and more dehydrated, concentrating glucose and further increasing hyperglycemia.

to 25% of total body water or 12% to 15% of body weight may be observed. Physical symptoms include dry mucous membranes, poor skin turgor, and sunken eyes. Weakness, anorexia, leg cramps, dizziness, lethargy, and confusion may be signs of worsening hydration status. Coma affects about 20% of cases.[36]

Electrolyte losses of sodium, potassium, phosphorus, and magnesium accompany fluid losses. Sodium and potassium losses usually require supplementation, but due to their concentration from dehydration, laboratory results may initially appear high and do not represent actual status. Blood urea nitrogen, serum creatinine, hematocrit, and many other routine blood chemistry levels may appear high, but will resolve without treatment following hydration. Persistent elevations in BUN signal follow-up evaluation of renal function, and normal hematocrit when dehydrated is likely to indicate anemia. Access to medical history and information regarding usual lab results help the provider focus on the most relevant parameters.

Neurologic Changes

The neurologic changes of decreased mentation (eg, lethargy and mild confusion) are more common in HHS than in DKA and are the result of extreme dehydration. Patients with HHS may have focal neurological signs (hemisensory deficits, hemiparesis, aphasia, and seizures) that mimic a CVA. These signs will reverse completely as biochemical status returns to normal. As in DKA, decreases in mentation best correlate with serum osmolality.

Absence of Significant Ketosis

Ketone bodies are not present in significant quantities. Starvation and dehydration may elevate serum ketones slightly. If present, gastrointestinal symptoms are usually milder than those found in DKA, and Kussmaul respirations are rare. Arterial pH greater than 7.3 mm Hg and bicarbonate level greater than 15 mEq/L are typical of HHS.

Other Tests

Other tests are necessary to determine the precipitating cause of HHS:

- Cultures of blood, urine, and sputum
- Chest X-ray
- EKG

An EKG is used to assess cardiac status in a population at risk for cardiac complications as well as to quickly evaluate potassium status. Serial EKGs can monitor and guide potassium replacement therapy.

Treatment of HHS

Hyperosmolar hyperglycemic state requires hospitalization for appropriate and effective treatment. Treatment goals for HHS, as listed in Table 22.7, are similar to those for DKA. Each goal is discussed separately below.

Goal 1: Provide Adequate Fluids to Rehydrate

The cornerstone of treatment of HHS is to expand intravascular volume and restore renal perfusion. A guideline for fluid replacement is to infuse half of the fluid deficit over the first 12 hours and the remainder during the following 12 to 24 hours. Glucose levels may drop as much as 80 to 200 mg/dL per hour from rehydration alone.[36]

- *Elderly.* Particularly with an elderly person, care must be taken to adjust the hydration rate to the patient's individual needs and consider the person's current hydration, cardiovascular, and renal status.
- *Renal insufficiency.* For people with renal insufficiency, restoring blood flow is critical; but especially for older patients with compromised cardiovascular status, fluid loss must be replaced with saline slowly and cautiously

TABLE 22.7   Treatment Goals for HHS
1. Provide adequate fluids to rehydrate
2. Correct electrolyte deficits
3. Provide adequate insulin to restore and maintain normal glucose metabolism
4. Prevent complications
5. Treat underlying medical condition
6. Provide patient and family education and follow-up

Source: MB Davidson, S Schwartz, "Hyperglycemia," in MJ Franz, ed, *A Core Curriculum for Diabetes Education: Diabetes and Complications,* 5th ed (Chicago: American Association of Diabetes Educators, 2003), 33-6.

to avoid fluid overload and congestive heart failure.

◈ *Cardiovascular disease.* Patients with a history of CVD must be monitored by central venous pressure or Swan-Ganz catheter.

Goal 2: Correct Electrolyte Deficits

Laboratory tests provide critical information to guide replacement decisions for electrolytes.

Potassium

The EKG provides immediate feedback regarding potassium status. Potassium replacement is similar to that required for DKA even though losses tend to be greater. However, insulin therapy needs to be withheld if initial laboratory results are less than 3.3 mEq/L, indicating profound deficiency. Potassium supplementation begins once renal function is known to be normal.

Sodium

Sodium levels can be falsely low in HHS from extreme glucose concentration. The following correction provides a more accurate assessment of hydration status. Note that if the corrected sodium is high, dehydration is extreme.

$$\text{Corrected Na}^+ \text{ (mg/dL)} = \text{Reported Na}^+ \text{ (mg/dL)} + 1.6 \times \text{(glucose mg/dL} - 100)$$

Phosphorus and Magnesium

Phosphorus and magnesium laboratory readings may come back high or normal, indicating some losses with dehydration, but the levels tend to normalize without replacement therapy.

Routine Blood Work

Routine blood work is similarly elevated with dehydration. Monitor and reassess metabolic status after hydration.

Goal 3: Provide Adequate Insulin to Restore and Maintain Normal Glucose Metabolism

Hydration is essential to lower glucose levels. Following hydration, insulin administration is usually but not always required to restore normal glycemia.

◈ *Insulin.* Treatment of acidosis is not part of HHS, so insulin requirements are typically not as high as those for DKA. Infuse insulin separately. Once insulin is started, do not interrupt delivery until hyperglycemia is adequately resolved.

◈ *Serum glucose.* Expect serum glucose to fall 50 to 75 but less than 100 mg/dL per hour. If serum glucose falls less than 50 mg/dL, consider whether to add or increase insulin and increase hydration. When glucose values reach acceptable levels (~300 mg/dL), reduce insulin and add 5% dextrose to infusion.[38] Monitor glucose hourly.

Goal 4: Prevent Complications

Preventing complications is important in treating HHS.

◈ Monitor frequently for blood pressure, fluid, electrolyte, and glucose levels (but hypoglycemia is unlikely).
◈ Watch for complications of underlying atherosclerosis and consider low-dose heparin for at-risk individuals.
◈ Once insulin is started, do not interrupt delivery until euglycemia is ensured.

Goal 5: Treat Underlying Medical Condition

Treatment of the underlying medical condition(s) is critical to resolving HHS. In an elderly population, potential contributors to HHS are multiple and require thorough exploration and follow-up. It is difficult to prevent excessive fluid losses or control hyperglycemia without identifying the source of the problem.

Goal 6: Provide Patient and Family Education and Follow-up

The risks for HHS include inadequate fluid intake, excessive fluid losses, and prolonged hyperglycemia. The tools to prevent or at least moderate the devastating impact of HHS are not complicated, but they require understanding and attention to daily habits. Regularly monitoring blood glucose and promptly treating mild hyperglycemia can interrupt the cycle leading to HHS before it is much of a problem.

Self-Care Behaviors in the Prevention of HHS

The AADE7 Self-Care Behaviors™ provide a framework for prevention of HHS. Table 22.8 demonstrates how these behaviors can be used in the prevention of HHS. For more details on fostering specific self-care behaviors, see chapters 4 through 10 in section 1 of this book. Most essentially, educators can assist individuals in avoiding HHS by encouraging hydration and identifying those at high risk.

Encourage Hydration

Encourage adequate hydration for everyone with diabetes. Many people will need frequent reminders and

TABLE 22.8 Applying Self-Care Behaviors for Prevention of HHS		
AADE7 Self-Care Behaviors™	*Concept*	*Application*
Being Active	Activity continues to lower insulin resistance and improve blood glucose (BG) levels. Be safely active at all ages. Maintain adequate hydration.	To compensate for fluids lost during physical activity, drink adequately before, during, and after physical activity, especially on hot days.
Healthy Eating	Matching timing of food with medication and activity. Having a sick-day plan and supplies (food and fluids).	To avoid high BG, do not consume extra carbohydrate without taking extra insulin. It is easy to consume extra carbohydrate with liquids. A large soft drink at a fast-food restaurant is equal in carbohydrate to 5 slices of bread.
Taking Medication	If glucose goals are not met with activity and meal planning, medication is necessary.	Inadequate levels of diabetes medication, especially reluctance to initiate insulin when needed, significantly contributes to high glucose levels.
Monitoring— Blood Glucose	Monitoring provides feedback about the treatment plan and warning of impending HHS.	Monitor regularly to help identify hyperglycemia before it becomes life threatening; this is true even for those not treated with medication, especially during illness or other stress. Monitoring allows early intervention and progress assessment. Discuss usual monitoring routine and what to do when not eating or ill. Do not rely strictly on "how you feel"—this has been shown to be an inaccurate measure of BG values. Monitor to obtain an accurate BG level. Access to monitoring supplies may present a barrier to self-monitoring of BG. Address issues of concern. Assess problems with monitoring. Resistance to monitoring may have multiple causes.
Problem Solving	Applying information already learned to individual situations helps solve problems.	Review the circumstances preceding the HHS episode to look for clues to prevent another. Would a system for drinking fluids, monitoring blood glucose, or a change in medication have reduced the risk? To prevent recurrence, review signs, symptoms, and treatment.

TABLE 22.8 Applying Self-Care Behaviors for Prevention of HHS (continued)

AADE7 Self-Care Behaviors™	Concept	Application
Reducing Risks	Reducing the risk as well as the impact of HHS is possible. HHS also increases risks for many concomitant conditions.	As HHS usually occurs in an older, more vulnerable population, individualize and carefully monitor therapy for these persons to help prevent complications. Discuss sick days—interventions for nausea, fever, loss of appetite; correction factors for hyperglycemia; when to seek medical care and after-hours procedures.
Healthy Coping	Eating well, taking medications, testing blood glucose, and using the results to problem solve are difficult, never-ending aspects of self-management.	Use information, support, and encouragement for caregivers as well as patients to help prevent HHS. Identify resources and situations in which to seek medical attention.

Note: See also chapters 4–10 on each of these 7 behaviors in section 1 of this book.

suggestions for specific ways to include more fluids before they will be able to do so.

- *Living alone.* Individuals who live alone may require help devising a system for remembering to drink fluids, such as keeping fluids within reach or having someone remind the individual to drink water every 2-4 hours..
- *Dependent on others.* Intake of adequate fluids can be a special challenge when the individual is dependent on others (eg, older adults in a hospital or nursing home and those who cannot communicate a request for water). These individuals depend on the institution to monitor fluid intake, evaluate fluid status, and establish a plan that keeps residents adequately hydrated.

Identify High-Risk Individuals

Identify high-risk individuals and, when dealing with them, put special emphasis on the basics. Examples are (1) the elderly in nursing homes, hospitals, or other settings where dehydration may not be noticed and (2) persons being treated with glucocorticoids or other medications that may precipitate hyperglycemia. Offer information to both the person with diabetes and the person's family and caregivers. Be sure they understand the rationale for and have the supplies necessary to accomplish the following:

- Obtain adequate fluids.
- Monitor blood glucose regularly.
- Manage sick days that may include fever and vomiting.
- Keep sick-day supplies on hand and accessible (eg, thermometer, acceptable and easy-to-eat food and drink, contact numbers for physician and urgent care services).
- Know the signs and symptoms of HHS and the critical need for medical attention should they appear.
- Know how and when to contact his or her healthcare provider.

Identify Vulnerabilities

Help individuals, especially those at high risk, understand the problems that may occur, signs and symptoms, precipitating factors, and appropriate actions. Provide education to help prevent DKA and HHS.

Case—Part 2: HHS Diagnosis and Treatment

Soon after the nurse took another finger-stick blood glucose that was "high," the physician arrived to examine Grandpa. The physician could tell from looking at Grandpa's skin that he was dehydrated. The physician quickly ordered lab work and had the staff start an IV of normal saline, just as someone had done for GT a few weeks ago; however, for Grandpa, the rate was slower. The physician explained that in a person Grandpa's age, the lab results needed to be examined to be sure Grandpa's heart and kidneys could tolerate a higher infusion rate. The physician also did not start insulin, but told GT and Grandma that because Grandpa Joe's blood was so concentrated, just adding fluids could lower his blood glucose.

- Initial lab results were glucose 699 mg/dL, potassium 3.9 mEq/L, phosphorus 3.3 mmol/L, and serum osmolality 340 mOsm/kg.

- An hour later, glucose was 652 mg/dL, potassium 3.8 mEq/L, and serum osmolality 337 mOsm/kg. Serum osmolality had fallen the maximum 3 mOsm/kg, so the normal saline remained at the slower rate. However, as glucose was still quite elevated, insulin infusion was started.

- It was the better part of a week before Grandpa Joe began acting like his old self again. Because the A1C in Grandpa's chart was in the normal range, the hospital staff unfortunately had not monitored his glucose in the hospital.

With a little persuading from his granddaughter, Grandpa was going to self-monitor his blood glucose from now on. A dietitian came in to brainstorm options to increase Grandpa's fluid intake. Knowing he did not like the taste of water, the dietitian brought a list of several calorie-free products with a few samples for him to try. The staff at the nursing home also met to discuss ways to improve how they monitor the fluid intake of their patients. Slowly but surely, Grandpa became more alert and eager to complete therapy so he could return home to his own bed and Grandma's cooking.

Case Wrap-Up: DKA and HHS

- To treat their respective conditions, Grandpa (experiencing HHS) required more fluids, and GT (experiencing DKA) required more insulin.

- GT needed to test ketones when her blood glucose was high; Grandpa did not.

- Both agreed they would put more effort into drinking fluids, regular monitoring, and responding to monitoring results.

- Grandma joined them for a class on sick-day management and learned how to treat a fever, what to eat when they did not feel like eating, and when to call the doctor.

They all left feeling a little more confident they could prevent a repeat of recent experiences.

Key Aspects of Education, Prevention, and Treatment

Education

Education is the key to preventing hyperglycemia, and the diabetes educator needs to work with the person with diabetes, as well as the members of his or her family, caregivers, and other healthcare providers. Following are the topics that should be addressed with each person or group:

For patients:
- ⬥ Sick-day management
- ⬥ When to call a physician
- ⬥ Medication adjustments during illness

- ⬥ Need for no-calorie fluids and carbohydrate-containing fluids

For family, caregivers, and school personnel:
- ⬥ Recognizing symptoms of hyperglycemia
- ⬥ Knowing what to do about hyperglycemia

For primary care providers:
- ⬥ Patient instruction for supplemental insulin during illness
- ⬥ Who benefits from home blood glucose monitoring

For nursing home/hospital staff and caregivers:
- ⬥ How to monitor glucose, hydration, and mentation
- ⬥ How to identify at-risk patients

Case: Preventing Hyperglycemia in an Institutional Care Setting

A skilled-care facility supervisor called for advice regarding a patient with type 2 diabetes of known 16-year duration. JM is an 85-year-old man who came to the skilled nursing facility after a CVA that resulted in some difficulty ambulating unassisted. He appeared fatigued and somewhat lethargic, and the symptoms seemed to have been slowly more perceptible over the past 3 days. There had been no acute change in overall well-being, but the patient just seemed to appear somewhat different from usual. The CVA also left JM with mild dysarthria, which was exacerbated when he was fatigued, making him more difficult to understand. He was seen in his primary care clinic within the last week, and a thiazide was started to target better control of hypertension. The family members who typically visited JM once a week and were very involved with his care had been out of town, so the supervisor was relying on staff reports of patient change. Staff had not been able to speak with the family about their observations. That day, there was concern regarding JM's increasing lethargy, and a finger-stick blood glucose of 390 mg/dL was obtained.

Case Wrap-Up: Preventing Hyperglycemia in an Institutional Care Setting

Applying the principles presented in the text of this chapter, hydration would be imperative, followed by a discussion on the effects of a thiazide, a medication that can potentiate hyperglycemia.[39,40] Many commonly prescribed pharmacologic agents for treatment of diabetes comorbidities such as hypertension and dyslipidemia can potentiate hyperglycemia.[41]

Inadequate access to water or hydrating fluids is a major confounder of hyperglycemia,[42] and neurologic deficits can be a barrier to appropriate fluid intake.[43,44] The recognition of inadequate water intake can be challenging in a skilled care facility.

Additionally, many metabolic disease states common in the older population can be associated with hyperglycemia; in particular, hyperthyroidism,[45] Cushing syndrome,[45] and even hyperparathyroidism[46] can potentiate hyperglycemia that responds to treatment of the specific instigating metabolic problem.[41] Early identification of the hyperosmolar nonketotic state and prompt initiation of treatment are directly associated with survival.[47]

Prevention

The person with diabetes needs knowledge and skills to perform the necessary actions to prevent hyperglycemic episodes.

Monitoring supplies:
- ◈ How to time monitoring when strips are limited

Hydration:
- ◈ Getting fluids when the person is not thirsty and does not like the taste

Treatment

If a person with diabetes has a hyperglycemic episode, the diabetes educator needs to recognize symptoms and respond quickly and appropriately.

Why infuse dextrose when blood glucose is 250 mg/dL?
- ◈ To prevent cerebral edema

Why not give insulin when blood glucose is 600 mg/dL?
- ◈ Fluids alone can significantly decrease hyperglycemia in HHS

How to adjust sodium for elevated glucose:
- ◈ To correct for dilution from glucose when concentration is very high[36]:

$$\text{Corrected Na}^+ \text{ (mg/dL)} = \text{Reported Na}^+ \text{ (mg/dL)} + 1.6\times \text{ (glucose mg/dL} - 100)$$

Testing for ketones:
- ◈ Measure beta-hydroxybutyrate to evaluate DKA and monitor progress[8]

When to consider phosphorus supplementation:
- ◈ To avoid skeletal and cardiac muscle weakness and respiratory depression in patients with cardiac dysfunction, anemia, or respiratory depression if PO_4 <1.0 mg/dL[8]

When to consider bicarbonate supplementation:
- ◈ If pH is <6.9, although no research substantiates benefit[8]

Ketoacidosis without DKA:
- ◈ Starvation and alcoholic ketoacidosis (AKA)

Focus on Education

Teaching Strategies

⊘ **Know signs and symptoms.**   Diabetes educators should be very familiar with signs and symptoms of impending hyperglycemia so they can help patients recognize it and intervene early.

⊘ **Relate monitoring to prevention.**   Teaching the benefits of blood glucose monitoring can often prevent severe hyperglycemia. Monitoring recognizes low as well as high blood glucose. Teach the concept of testing.

⊘ **Show how planning leads to prevention.**   Planning ahead is an important part of preventing hyperglycemia. This includes having proper supplies (blood glucose meter and ketone testing equipment) and not running out of them, testing and treating with insulin, and knowing when to call the healthcare provider.

⊘ **Be alert for issues among adolescents and elderly adults.**   Teenagers or young adults with type 1 diabetes who have recurrent DKA may be purposely omitting insulin for weight loss or attention. In elderly adults, underlying illness, the cause of high blood glucose, dehydration, and medication compliance can be a concern. Assess the patient and family for referral for counseling.

⊘ **Identify high-risk situations.**   Identify potential high-risk situations such as the following: young adults going off to college, teenagers beginning to drive, elderly in nursing homes who may become dehydrated, and persons being treated with glucocorticoids or other medications that may precipitate hyperglycemia.

⊘ **Provide a "when to call" list.**   Give patients a prepared list of situations of when to call the physician. Include contact information for days, nights, and weekends. This reassures patients that it is necessary to call if they have concerns and that calling is not a bother.

⊘ **Prepare family members.**   Educate family members to recognize high-risk situations and intervene early enough to prevent development of severe, life-threatening hyperglycemia.

⊘ **Educate emergency personnel.**   Offer a hyperglycemia refresher course to local emergency rooms, hospital floor nurses, paramedics, school nurses, and others. Bring equipment for hands-on blood testing and ketone testing. Reinforce the need for ketone testing equipment in the home for early detection and intervention. For HHS, urge earlier identification by recognizing dehydration status, underlying illness, and potential causes.

⊘ **Offer telephone care for mild DKA.**   In some cases in which DKA is mild and recognized early, it can be treated with insulin and oral fluids via telephone consults. Know also when this is not appropriate.

⊘ **Evaluate and reeducate.**   Always carefully assess the reasons for a DKA or HHS occurrence so that preventive strategies can be taught and instituted.

⊘ **Use situational problem solving.**   Identify patient-specific circumstances of hyperglycemia and have a patient verbalize what he or she would do. This could involve role playing with the person with diabetes in the setting of what to do when ill, and role playing with the family members/spouse who would be providing care for an individual with diabetes who is ill. An example is a "sick-day readiness box"—what to include in the box and when to call for medical advice.

Messages for Patients

⊘ **Ensure others understand what puts you at high risk.**   Family members and friends need to recognize high-risk situations and be able to respond with early interventions to prevent the development of severe, life-threatening hyperglycemia. Recognizing the underlying cause of high blood glucose, such as illness, bad insulin, or an inadequate insulin amount, is important.

Distribute handouts so others can help you. Provide family, friends, roommates, your workplace or school, and leaders of groups you participate in with informational handouts and contact information for emergency medical care. Invite family and close friends to attend education classes and clinic visits. Teach appropriate people in your life how to test your blood glucose and ketones. Remind these people, especially if you are an older adult, about the importance of getting adequate fluids.

Be reflective and proactive. Review the events that contributed to the hyperglycemia. Come up with a plan to prevent future occurrence.

Health Literacy

The diabetes educator needs to establish a health literacy level in the patient before initiating education. Explore treatment beliefs within the cultural context of illness. Identify specific herbs/teas/potions that the patient may use in treating common illnesses which could impact body temperature and/or hydration status. Some examples of these practices are:

- Comfrey tea, which contains aspirin-like compounds that could impact body temperature
- Inducing sweating for an illness as in certain Hispanic cultures, which potentially could add to dehydration already seen in hyperglycemic states

  Determine whether the person with diabetes has someone who is familiar with obtaining finger-stick glucoses, helping inject insulin, and so on, who could help him or her when ill.[31]

Health literacy is the ability to obtain, process, and understand basic health information and services needed to make appropriate decisions. Consider 3 steps in hyperglycemia management:

- Recognize hyperglycemia. Identify actual blood glucose numbers that are considered over the desirable range. Provide examples of the actual glucose numbers instead of just indicating "above . . ."
- Process the information by identifying specific circumstances of where and how hyperglycemia occurs.
- Put the meaning to the numbers by asking: What will you do when your blood glucose is . . . ?

Ask a patient to teach you about high blood glucose. Consider asking the following questions:

- How do you know you have high blood glucose (higher than you would like it to be)?
- What do you consider "high" blood glucose?
- When do you typically have high blood glucose?
- What do you do when you have high blood glucose?

Health numeracy. Many people, even those who are highly educated and literate, can have trouble understanding numbers. To communicate quantitative information such as blood glucose levels associated with hyperglycemia, focus on just one idea at a time and express it in simple sentences. The following are additional strategies to make sure that patients understand the numbers and what they mean:

- Draw a picture showing what the low versus high level is.
- Use analogies or reference points to explain glucose levels and ranges.
- Show physical representations of glucose density and what happens in a body when hyperglycemia occurs.
- Encourage patients to create their own images.
- Teach with stories to connect high glucose to specific symptoms or events.

Focus on Practice

→ **Examine the system of decision making on hyperglycemia management.** Physicians, nurses, and quality improvement coordinators need to make hyperglycemia management protocols. Use evidence-based strategies to minimize risks and maximize cost savings and productivity.

→ **Educate staff on hyperglycemia management protocols.** Hyperglycemia management might involve exploring some common misconceptions about hyperglycemia and its corresponding interventions. Implement aggressive but achievable standards of care that involve all necessary parties.

→ **Perform a cost-benefit analysis.** Administrators and third-party payers will need to see the cost benefits that can accrue from shorter hospital stays and fewer complications when hyperglycemia is reduced.

→ **Quality ensure your hyperglycemia management.** Monitor systems and processes to ensure that the protocols are implemented within the desirable scope. Adjust practice based on findings.

References

1. Davidson MB. Diabetic ketoacidosis and hyperosmolar nonketotic coma. In: Davidson MB, ed. Diabetes Mellitus: Diagnosis and Treatment. 4th ed. New York: WB Saunders Company; 1998:159-94.

2. Usher-Smith JA, Thompson M, Ercole A, Walter M. Variation between countries in the frequency of diabetic ketoacidosis at first presentation of type 1 diabetes in children: a systematic review. Diabetologia. 2012;55:2878-94.

3. Cakan N, Kizilbash S, Kamat D. Changing spectrum of diabetes mellitus in children: challenges with initial classification. Clin Pediatr (Phila). 2012;51:939-44.

4. Tan KC, Mackay IR, Zimmet PZ, et al. Metabolic and immunologic features of Chinese patients with atypical diabetes mellitus. Diabetes Care. 2000;23(3):335-8.

5. Westphal SA. The occurrence of diabetic ketoacidosis in non-insulin-dependent diabetes and newly diagnosed diabetic adults. Am J Med. 1996;101:19-24.

6. Wilson C, Krakoff J, Gohdes D. Ketoacidosis in Apache Indians with non-insulin-dependent diabetes mellitus. Arch Intern Med. 1997;157(18):2098-100.

7. Balasubramanyam A, Zern JW, Hyman DJ, et al. New profiles of diabetic ketoacidosis: type 1 vs type 2 diabetes and the effect of ethnicity. Arch Intern Med. 1999;159(19):2317-22.

8. American Diabetes Association. Hyperglycemic crises in patients with diabetes mellitus (position statement). Diabetes Care. 2004;24 Suppl 1:S94-102.

9. McDonnell CM, Pedreira CC, Vadamalayan B, et al. Diabetic ketoacidosis, hyperosmolarity and hypernatremia: are high-carbohydrate drinks worsening initial presentation? Pediatr Diabetes. 2005 Jun;6:90-4.

10. Kershaw MJ, Newton T, Barrett TG, et al. Childhood diabetes presenting with hyperosmolar dehydration but without ketoacidosis: a report of three cases. Diabet Med. 2005;22:645-7.

11. Hammond P, Liebl A, Grunder S. International survey of insulin pump users: impact of continuous subcutaneous insulin infusion therapy on glucose control and quality of life. Prim Care Diabetes. 2007;1(3):143-6.

12. Bode BW, Tamborlane WV, Davidson PC. Insulin pump therapy in the 21st century: strategies for successful use in adults, adolescents, and children with diabetes. Postgrad Med. 2002;111(5):69-78.

13. Gonder-Frederick LA, Julian DM, Cox DJ, et al. Self-measurement of blood glucose: accuracy of self-reported data and adherence to recommended regimen. Diabetes Care. 1988;11(7):579-85.

14. Scaramuzza AE, Iafusco D, Rabbone I, et al. Use of integrated real-time continuous glucose monitoring/insulin pump system in children and adolescents with type 1 diabetes: a 3-year follow-up study. Diabetes Technol Ther. 2011;13:99-103.

15. Bergenstal RM, Klonoff DC, Garg SK, et al; ASPIRE In-Home Study Group. Threshold-based insulin-pump interruption for reduction of hypoglycemia. N Engl J Med. 2013;369:224-32.

16. Peveler RC, Bryden KS, Neil HA, et al. The relationship of disordered eating habits and attitudes to clinical outcomes in young adult females with type 1 diabetes. Diabetes Care. 2005;28:84-8.

17. Neumark-Sztainer D, Patterson J, Mellin A, et al. Weight control practices and disordered eating behaviors among

adolescent females and males with type 1 diabetes. Diabetes Care. 2002;25:1289-96.

18. Charfen MA, Fernandez-Frackelton M. Diabetic ketoacidosis. Emerg Med Clin N Am. 2005;23:609-28.

19. Musey VC. Diabetes in urban African-Americans. I. Cessation of insulin therapy is the major precipitating cause of diabetic ketoacidosis. Diabetes Care. 1995;18:483-9.

20. Kitabchi AE, Umpierrez GE, Fischer JN, et al. Thirty years of personal experience with hyperglycemic crises: diabetic ketoacidosis and hyperosmolar state. J Clin Endocrinol Metab. 2008;93:1541-52. Epub 2008 Feb 12.

21. Agus MS, Wolfsdorf JI. Diabetic ketoacidosis in children. Pediatr Clin North Am. 2005;52:1147-63.

22. Nyenwe EA, Loganathan RS, Blum S, et al. Active use of cocaine: an independent risk factor for recurrent diabetic ketoacidosis in a city hospital. Endocr Pract. 2007;13:22-9.

23. Glaser NS, Wootton-Gorges SL, Marcin JP, et al. Mechanism of cerebral edema in children with diabetic ketoacidosis. J Pediatr. 2004;145:164-71.

24. Glaser NS, Marcin JP, Wootton-Gorges SL, et al. Correlation of clinical and biochemical findings with diabetic ketoacidosis-related cerebral edema in children using magnetic resonance diffusion-weighted imaging. J Pediatr. 2008;153:541-6.

25. Glaser NS, Ghetti S, Casper TC, et al. Pediatric diabetic ketoacidosis, fluid therapy, and cerebral injury: the design of a factorial randomized controlled trial. Pediatr Diabetes. 2013;14(6):435-46. Epub 2013 Mar 13.

26. Trachtenbarg DE. Diabetic ketoacidosis. Am Fam Physician. 2005;71(9):1705-14.

27. Al Hanshi S, Shann F. Insulin infused at 0.05 versus 0.1 units/kg/hr in children admitted to intensive care with diabetic ketoacidosis. Pediatr Crit Care Med. 2011;12(2):137-40.

28. Cramer JA. A systematic review of adherence with medication for diabetes. Diabetes Care. 2004;27:1218-24.

29. The NICE-SUGAR Study Investigators. Intensive versus conventional glucose control in critically ill patients. N Engl J Med. 2009;360:1283-97.

30. Qaseem A, Chou R, Humphrey LL, et al. Inpatient glycemic control: best practice advice from the Clinical Guidelines Committee of the American College of Physicians. Am J Med Qual. 2014;29(2):95-8. Epub 2013 Jun 7.

31. Van den Berghe G, Schetz M, Vlasselaers DJ, et al. Clinical review: intensive insulin therapy in critically ill patients: NICE-SUGAR or Leuven blood glucose target? J Clin Endocrinol Metab. 2009;94(9):3163-70. Epub 2009 Jun 16.

32. Schnipper JL, Magee M, Larsen K, Inzucchi SE, Maynard G; Society of Hospital Medicine Glycemic Control Task Force. Society of Hospital Medicine Glycemic Control Task Force summary: practical recommendations for assessing the impact of glycemic control efforts. J Hosp Med. 2008;3 (5 Suppl):66-75.

33. Trence DL, Kelly JL, Hirsch IB. The rationale and management of hyperglycemia for in-patients with cardiovascular disease: time for change. J Clin Endocrinol Metab. 2003;88(6):2430-7.

34. Penfold S, Gouni R, Hamilton P, et al. Immediate in-patient management of hyperglycaemia—confusion rather than consensus? Q J Med. 2008 Feb;101(2):87-90. Epub 2008 Jan 7.

35. Ishikawa H, Takeuchi T, Yano E. Measuring functional, communicative, and critical health literacy among diabetic patients. Diabetes Care. 2008 May;31(5):874-9. Epub 2008 Feb 25.

36. Della MT, Steinmetz L, Campos PR, et al. Subcutaneous use of a fast-acting insulin analog: an alternative treatment for pediatric patients with diabetic ketoacidosis. Diabetes Care. 2005;28:1856-61.

37. Nugent BW. Hyperosmolar hyperglycemic state. Emerg Med Clin N Am. 2005;23:629-48.

38. Kitabchi AE, Umpierrez GE, Murphy MB, et al. Management of hyperglycemic crises in patients with diabetes mellitus (technical review). Diabetes Care. 2001;224:131-53.

39. Bressler P, DeFronzo RA. Drugs and diabetes. Diabetes Rev. 1994;2(1):53-84.

40. Fonseca V, Phear DN. Hyperosmolar non-ketotic diabetic syndrome precipitated by treatment with diuretics. BMJ. 1982;284:36-7.

41. Trence DL, Hirsch IB. Hyperglycemic crises in diabetes mellitus type 2. Endocrinol Metab Clin North Am. 2001;30(4):817-31.

42. Ennis ED, Stahl E JVB, Kreisberg RA. The hyperosmolar hyperglycemic syndrome. Diabetes Rev. 1994;2(1):115-26.

43. Lorber D. Non-ketotic hypertonicity in diabetes mellitus. Med Clin North Am. 1995;79:39-52.

44. Maccario M. Neurologic dysfunction associated with non-ketotic hyperglycemia. Arch Neurol. 1968;19:525-34.

45. Berelowitz M, Go EH. Non-insulin-dependent diabetes mellitus secondary to other endocrine disorders. In: LeRoith D, Taylor SI, Olefsky JM, eds. Diabetes Mellitus. Philadelphia: Lippincott-Raven Publishers; 1996:496-502.

46. Akgun S, Ertel NH. Hyperparathyroidism and coexisting diabetes mellitus: altered carbohydrate metabolism. Arch Intern Med. 1978;138(10):1500-2.

47. Wachtel TJ, Silliman RA, Lamberton P. Predisposing factors for the diabetic hyperosmolar state. Arch Intern Med. 1987;147:499-501.

CHAPTER 23

Chronic Complications

Kim L. Kelly, PharmD, BCPS, FCCP, CDTC, CPC, CEC

Key Concepts

- Be familiar with the proposed mechanisms of complications.

- Be familiar with the common complications and comorbidities.

- Be familiar with the organizations that have established standards of care and the scope of their standards.

- Be able to describe the relationship between glucose control, glucose variability, and diabetes complications.

- Implement strategies to screen for certain complications and comorbidities.

- Be familiar with autoimmune complications and comorbidities.

- Describe a screening method for obstructive sleep apnea.

Individual chapters are dedicated to each of the major categories of chronic complications (nephropathy—chapter 27, retinopathy—chapter 26, and macrovascular complications—chapter 25). Foot problems are addressed in chapter 28.

Introduction

A primary goal of diabetes treatment and self-management education is the prevention of chronic complications. Diabetes-related complications are caused by damage to tissues, often through the blood vessels and nerves serving those tissues. Specifically, it is damage to the endothelial cells lining the blood vessels that causes the abnormalities (eg, microalbuminuria and accelerated atherosclerosis). Changes in nerves involve deterioration of the nerve itself as well as damage to the blood vessels supplying the nerves.[1]

The classic representation of complications is the "-opathies," such as retinopathy and nephropathy. However, the more we learn about diabetes complications and comorbid conditions, the more we realize that many are multifactorial, and in some cases they affect the development or severity of other complications or comorbidities. Some examples of this are sexual dysfunction, which may involve microvascular

and macrovascular changes, as well as depression in some patients. Foot problems may involve macrovascular and microvascular changes as well as peripheral neuropathy. There are many more examples, and some of the well-documented chronic complications and comorbidities are listed in Table 23.1.[2]

The impact of what has been designated as primarily microvascular complications is demonstrated by diabetes being the leading cause of blindness in adults, kidney failure, and nontraumatic amputations in the United States.[3] Macrovascular damage results in diabetes increasing the risk of cardiovascular disease (CVD). Diabetes-related disabilities are caused by both microvascular complications (eg, blindness and kidney failure) and macrovascular complications (eg, heart attacks and stroke). Mortality among persons with diabetes is primarily related to the macrovascular complications. Heart disease is listed as the cause of death on 68% of

TABLE 23.1 **Chronic Complications and Comorbidities of Diabetes**		
• Hypertension	• Neuropathy	• Cognitive impairment
• Coronary artery disease	• Skin problems	• Obstructive sleep apnea
• Cerebrovascular disease	• Healing impairment	• Hearing impairment
• Heart failure	• Foot problems	• Sexual dysfunction
• Retinopathy	• Fatty liver disease	• Periodontal disease
• Diabetic macular edema	• Low testosterone in men	• Gastroparesis/gastric reflux
• Cataracts	• Fractures	• Thyroid disease
• Nephropathy	• Depression	

diabetes-related death certificates, and stroke was noted on 16%.

The impact of chronic complications extracts a high personal and economic toll. The estimated national cost of diabetes in 2012 was $245 billion, of which $176 billion (72%) represents direct healthcare expenditures. Macrovascular disease accounted for 61% of the total cost of treating complications, while treatment of renal complications accounted for 19%, neurologic 13%, and ophthalmic 12%. The costs related to chronic complications will make a significant contribution to the estimated $336 billion in annual spending related to diabetes by 2034.[3]

Chronic complications do not occur as isolated findings. The NHANES 1999 to 2004 data estimate that 57.9% of persons with diabetes have 1 or more chronic complications.[4] The presence of 1 complication may accelerate another (eg, nephropathy is associated with increased rates of macrovascular complications).

Many people with type 2 diabetes already have complications present at the time of diagnosis. The Hoorn Screening Study reported the prevalence of complications in newly diagnosed persons with type 2 diabetes.[5,6] Microvascular complication rates reached 48.3% for impaired foot sensitivity, 26.7% for microalbuminuria, and 7.6% for retinopathy. The prevalence of macrovascular complications reached 39.5% for ischemic heart disease, 13.3% for myocardial infarction, and 10.6% for peripheral arterial disease.

Adolescents with type 2 diabetes also demonstrate significant rates of complications. The prevalence of complications has been reported to be as high as 20% for retinopathy, 28% for microalbuminuria,

36% for hypertension, 27% for peripheral neuropathy, and 61% for autonomic neuropathy.[7] Complications may develop more quickly in adolescents with type 2 diabetes than in those with type 1 diabetes.[8] The reason for these increased rates is not known. In a recent publication regarding the TODAY study of type 2 diabetes in adolescents and youth,[9] more than 1 in 10 adolescents had hypertension at baseline, and by about 4 years, that had increased to 1 in 3. A total of 6.3% of participants had microalbuminuria, which had increased to 16.6% at about 4 years. The percentage of participants with LDL above 130 mg/dL rose from 4.5% to 10.7% over 36 months. With regard to retinopathy, 13.7% of participants developed the non-proliferative form after an average duration of diabetes of about 5 years.[10]

Older persons with diabetes have higher rates of hypertension, coronary heart disease, and stroke than younger persons with diabetes. Rates of microvascular complications are also increased due to the effects of age and the presence of comorbid conditions. Addressing cardiovascular risk factors, especially hypertension, hypercholesterolemia, and tobacco abuse, is important.[2,11,12]

Mechanisms of Tissue Damage

A1C is formed by protein glycation—the attachment of glucose to the amino acids composing that specific hemoglobin protein—and is a surrogate measure of protein glycation that has been associated with diabetes complications. Advanced glycation end products (AGEs) are a heterogeneous group of compounds, formed in a similar fashion to HbA1c. Advanced glycation end products are implicated in the development of macrovascular disease and microvascular complications.[13] Hyperglycemia contributes to the accumulation of AGEs, which along with oxidative damage from reactive oxygen species are largely responsible for diabetes complications.[1]

Advanced glycation end products can become cross-linked, changing their behavior and interfering with the ability of the body to metabolize the altered proteins. The abnormal turnover of proteins causes thickening of capillary basement membranes in the retina, muscles, and kidneys. Changes in the basement membranes of the kidney lead to microalbuminuria; changes in the eye lead to microaneurysms and capillary leakage of lipids and proteins. Advanced glycation end products contribute to macrovascular disease by changing the structure and function of lipoproteins, and reactive oxygen species can oxidize them as well. Glycosylated as well as oxidized LDL is more readily deposited in vessel walls, causing dysfunction of endothelial cells and development and destabilization of atheromatous plaques.[14] Glycosylated HDL does not participate in reverse cholesterol transport, which means that its role in moving cholesterol out of vessel walls is compromised and that it loses its ability to protect against excess lipid accumulation.[15] Advanced glycation end products can result in complications through several mechanisms: cross-linking matrix proteins in various tissues, posttranslational modification of proteins (structure and function), binding to AGE receptors (RAGE) activating many pathways for reactive cytokines, and reactive oxygen species that, collectively, can significantly damage endothelial cells.[1] Levels of AGEs are higher in persons with diabetes than in the general population, and are even higher when diabetes is complicated by microalbuminuria and coronary artery disease.[16] It is possible to reduce AGE levels. Dietary interventions with low-AGE diets have been shown to decrease the accumulation of AGEs.[17,18] Treatment with metformin and pioglitazone has been shown to decrease AGE formation in in vitro studies.[19] Other medicines to inhibit AGE formation or actions are being studied; however, the major method for reducing AGEs is tight glycemic control.

Other mechanisms for the development of complications have been studied, and their relationship to tissue damage from glucose is controversial; however, a significant literature exists that glycemic variability (whether in plasma glucose or in A1C) is a significant contributor to microvascular and macrovascular complications.[20] It is likely that multiple mechanisms operate, perhaps differentially, in individuals and populations.

Standards of Care and Complications

The standards of diabetes care developed by professional organizations are intended to minimize the occurrence and impact of diabetes complications. Some of the standards are directed toward prevention of chronic complications (optimal control of blood glucose, blood pressure, and cholesterol levels). Those standards are based on studies demonstrating the ability of those therapeutic goals to prevent macrovascular and microvascular complications.

Reductions in average glucose values as measured by hemoglobin A1C correlate with reductions in microvascular complications of diabetes. From the results of the Diabetes Control and Complications Trial (DCCT),[21] the Kumamoto Study,[22] and the United Kingdom Prospective Diabetes Study (UKPDS),[23] the Centers for Disease Control and Prevention (CDC) estimates on average a 40% reduction in microvascular complications for each 1% reduction in A1C. Sustained benefit from early intervention in the UKPDS[24] and with intensive therapy in the DCCT[25] was demonstrated at the 10-year follow-up in each of those trials. A "legacy effect" of early therapy was demonstrated to result in sustained reductions in the occurrence of complications years after the studies ended. While the difference in glycemic control between the study groups was lost, there continued to be better outcomes because of the improved control that occurred earlier in the trials.

For a discussion of the roles of blood pressure and lipoproteins on the development of complications, please see chapters 19 and 25.

The anticipated benefits of improved diabetes management are now being demonstrated in the general population of persons with diabetes. Modern diabetes therapy is resulting in a decrease in mortality due to diabetes,[26,27] decreased rates of preventable hospitalizations,[28] and decreased prevalence of diabetic retinopathy, blindness, and overt nephropathy.[29]

Because achieving treatment goals will not prevent all chronic complications, additional standards were developed to identify problems as early as possible (eg, annual eye examinations). The earlier those complications are detected, the greater the opportunity to intervene and prevent their worsening (eg, treating microalbuminuria to prevent chronic renal failure), thus limiting or preventing disability. Contrariwise, there is a point in the natural history of each complication at which the process is no longer reversible (eg, development of clinical-grade proteinuria, numbness in peripheral nerves, autonomic nervous system dysfunction). It is important that complications be identified while they are still potentially reversible.

When chronic complications are identified, therapeutic interventions are used that may prevent progression and potentially reverse the complications (eg, use of angiotensin-converting enzyme [ACE] inhibitors to reverse microalbuminuria and slow the progression of diabetic nephropathy; laser therapy for diabetic retinopathy). Clinical practice recommendations have been developed by the American Diabetes Association (ADA)[2] and the American Association of Clinical Endocrinologists (AACE).[30] Guidelines for the treatment of children and adolescents have been developed by the ADA[2] and the International Society for Pediatric and Adolescent Diabetes.[31] In addition, the ADA and the European Association for the Study of Diabetes have developed a separate position statement on glycemic control,[32] and the AACE has also recently developed a diabetes management algorithm, which for the first time addresses obesity and prediabetes as well as diabetes.[33] While minor differences are found among the recommendations of the professional societies, there is broad consensus on the general principles governing the management of diabetes.

The development of guidelines for the elderly has been difficult due to a lack of a sufficient number of clinical studies. The American Geriatric Society has published comprehensive guidelines.[34] The ADA has recommended that the guidelines for the adult population be appropriate for older individuals who are cognitively intact and have a significant life expectancy.[35] Those older adults with advanced complications, life-limiting comorbid illness, or substantial cognitive or functional impairment should be treated to less rigorous goals that are not specifically defined.[2,12,36]

AADE7 Self-Care Behaviors™

By definition, the AADE7 Self-Care Behaviors™ framework was designed to empower patients to prevent the chronic complications of diabetes. Frequent assessment of patients' success with implementing these behaviors is required to ensure achievement of the prevention strategies. Ongoing, regular evaluation is required to ensure adherence with the practices to prevent complications.

- ◆ Healthy eating
- ◆ Being active
- ◆ Monitoring
- ◆ Taking medication
- ◆ Problem solving
- ◆ Reducing risks
- ◆ Healthy coping

Practice Tips

- ◆ While microvascular complications have traditionally been the focus of prevention efforts, macrovascular complications are the most expensive, the most common cause of death, and the most common need for hospitalization.
- ◆ A1C reflects short-term glucose control and long-term risk of chronic complications. Keep in mind that it is only an average, and therefore self-monitoring of blood glucose is important for detecting glucose variability. It is important for patients to understand that for every 1% lowering of A1C, there is an average reduction in microvascular complications of 40%. It is also important for patients to know about the "legacy effect": Experiencing tight control for a period of time carries long-term benefits even if the patient's control worsens.
- ◆ Control of blood glucose, blood pressure, and blood lipids is central to the prevention of *all* chronic complications.

- Glycemic variability is a likely contributor to microvascular and macrovascular risk, and measuring and working to minimize that variability should be part of the treatment plan.
- Complications compound the deleterious effects of one another.

  Example 1: Foot amputation is related to peripheral neuropathy (insensate foot leads to traumatic damage) plus compromised immune function (decreased ability to fight infection) plus peripheral vascular disease (decreased ability to deliver antibiotics and oxygen).

  Example 2: Heart attack is related to hyperglycemia (causing glycosylation and triglyceride enrichment of lipoproteins that make them more atherogenic) plus hypertension (independent risk factor for CVD) plus renal insufficiency (increasing atherosclerotic process) plus hyperlipidemia (increased LDL and triglyceride levels).

- A thorough evaluation for complications is conducted:
  —In adults: after initial control of diabetes.
  —In children: based on their age and the duration of diabetes.
- It is important to understand the distinctions among standards of care, clinical practice guidelines, and treatment options. The quality and quantity of evidence determine the category in which care practices reside.
  —Standard of care: Care practices that must be followed in virtually all cases (eg, monitoring of A1C, regular foot and eye examinations). The reason for deviating from a standard requires documentation. The health and economic consequences are well known.
  —Clinical practice guidelines: Care practices that should be followed in most cases but for which deviations are justified by circumstance (eg, if the use of ACE inhibitors to reduce proteinuria is not tolerated, other medicines have been identified that may serve the same purpose—angiotensin receptor blockers [ARBs]).
  —Treatment options: Care practices for which there are a number of acceptable options (eg, initial therapy with oral agents in type 2 diabetes).
- With good control of CVD risk factors, screening for early complications, and intervention to prevent disability, people with diabetes should be able to avoid disabling microvascular complications.

Autoimmune-Related Complications

Type 1 diabetes is most often caused by autoimmune destruction of the islet cells in the pancreas. Persons with type 1 diabetes are at increased risk for other autoimmune disorders—most commonly chronic lymphocytic thyroiditis and celiac disease. Hereditary cell surface markers have been identified as risk alleles for type 1 diabetes (HLA-DR3 and HLSDR4) and are also risk alleles for Hashimoto's thyroiditis. Graves' disease and Addison's disease are associated with HLA-DR3, and other risk alleles are associated with celiac disease (HLA-DQ2 and HLA-DQ8).[37] Because of the increased frequency of autoimmune diseases in persons with type 1 diabetes, the ADA recommends screening for thyroid dysfunction and celiac disease based on signs and symptoms. While the effectiveness of periodic screening in asymptomatic individuals is unknown, screening is still recommended.[2]

Autoimmune Thyroid Disease

Autoimmune thyroid disease is the most frequent autoimmune-associated disorder in type 1 diabetes. The risk of thyroid dysfunction is 2 to 3 times higher in persons with diabetes than in the general population.[38] The vast majority of autoimmune thyroid disease cases are hypothyroidism due to Hashimoto's thyroiditis—as evidenced by the presence of antithyroglobulin and antithyroid peroxidase antibodies. However, hyperthyroidism due to Graves' disease (as evidenced by the presence of thyroid-stimulating antibodies) may also occur. Graves' disease may cause worsening of blood glucose control due to more rapid metabolism of insulin.[39]

The rate of clinical disease ranges widely, from 5% up to 30%, and thyroid antibodies have been found in 20% of persons with type 1 diabetes.[40–42] Persons with antithyroid peroxidase antibodies are 18 times more likely to develop hypothyroidism than those without them.[38] Hashimoto's thyroiditis is more common in girls than in boys, and its prevalence increases with age.[43] Significant thyroid antibody titers are detected within the first 3 to 4 years of diabetes in 50% of children.[39] The antibodies may be present for years prior to the onset of clinical disease. Subclinical hypothyroidism (an elevated thyroid-stimulating hormone [TSH] with normal thyroid hormone levels and no overt symptoms of hypothyroidism) is associated with hypoglycemia[44] and reduced growth rates.[45] Hypothyroidism may result in elevations of LDL-cholesterol and triglycerides; these abnormalities resolve with thyroid hormone replacement therapy.

The ADA recommends screening for the presence of antithyroglobulin and antithyroid peroxidase antibodies at the time of diagnosis of type 1 diabetes.[46] After metabolic control is established, the ADA recommends testing the TSH to assess thyroid function. If the TSH is normal, it should be measured every 1 to 2 years; if the TSH is abnormal, a Free T_4 should also be measured. In addition to the screening testing described, the TSH should be tested if there is evidence of an abnormal growth rate or goiter or if symptoms of thyroid dysfunction occur.[2]

Celiac Disease

Celiac disease (gluten-sensitive enteropathy) is a malabsorption condition caused by an immune-mediated inflammation of the small intestine reacting to dietary gluten and related proteins. The presence of celiac disease is indicated by the presence in the blood of immunoglobulin A (IgA) anti-tissue transglutaminase antibodies, which are the recommended screening test for celiac disease, and measurement of IgA anti-endomysial antibodies is nearly 100% specific for active celiac disease.[47] Celiac disease may present at any age. Typical gastrointestinal symptoms of celiac disease include chronic diarrhea, anorexia, abdominal distension and pain, vomiting, and weight loss. Children may also present with failure to thrive. However,

only a minority of children with type 1 diabetes present with gastrointestinal symptoms. Instead, the initial findings include erratic blood glucose values, recurrent hypoglycemia, and growth failure because of inconsistent absorption of nutrients.[48] Nongastroenterologic symptoms in adults may include iron deficiency anemia, osteopenia and osteoporosis, dermatitis herpetiformis, mild transaminase elevations, selective IgA deficiency, infertility, and atrophic glossitis.[49]

Celiac disease occurs in up to 16% of persons with diabetes compared with a rate of only 0.3% to 1.0% in the general population.[50,51] Endomysial antibodies are found in 7% to 10% of persons with type 1 diabetes.[52] Risk factors for celiac disease include female gender, younger age of onset of diabetes, longer duration of diabetes, and the presence of thyroid disease.[53] Treatment of celiac disease is a gluten-free diet. Clinical response to a gluten-free diet in children includes reversal of weight loss, increased growth, and an improvement in A1C.[54]

Vitamin B$_{12}$ Deficiency

Chronic autoimmune gastritis may result in vitamin B_{12} deficiency. While pernicious anemia from B_{12} deficiency occurs in approximately 1% of the general population, that incidence may be increased three- to fivefold in people with type 1 diabetes.[55] In addition to the possibility of autoimmune mediated B_{12} deficiency more often found in persons with type 1 diabetes, there is recent evidence that *non*-autoimmune B_{12} deficiency can occur in patients receiving metformin.[56] Further research is needed to better understand this phenomenon and the role it may play in the cognitive decline seen in some patients with diabetes.

Addison's Disease

Adrenal failure due to autoimmune mediated destruction of the gland is known as Addison's disease. This condition affects less than 1% of children with type 1 diabetes. Antiadrenal antibodies have been identified in about 2% of children with type 1 diabetes.[57] Treatment consists of replacement of the glucocorticoid (eg, hydrocortisone) and mineralocorticoid (eg, fludrocortisone) hormones.

Pertinent AADE7 Self-Care Behaviors™

◆ Healthy eating—Adherence to a gluten-free diet is the primary treatment of celiac disease and requires instruction from a registered dietitian.

◆ Monitoring—Changes in glucose control may be the first sign of thyroid or celiac disease.

◆ Healthy coping—Additional counseling may be helpful in adjusting to the additional dietary restrictions of celiac disease.

Practice Tips

◆ Autoimmune problems frequently occur together (type 1 diabetes, Hashimoto's thyroiditis, Addison's disease, vitamin B_{12} deficiency); therefore, providers need to watch for signs and symptoms of these problems in persons with diabetes.

◆ Abnormal growth is a sign of a number of problems of diabetes in children. Abnormal growth is identified by a decrease in the growth percentile (a young person growing along the 50th percentile curve on a standard growth chart has a slowing in his or her growth so that he or she decreases to the 25th percentile curve). Abnormal growth may indicate poor glucose control, hypothyroidism, and celiac disease. Addressing these problems may restore the child to his or her original growth percentile.

◆ Antibodies may be present in autoimmune disorders for some time before the clinical disease becomes apparent (eg, anti-insulin antibodies are measurable for months to years before the clinical onset of type 1 diabetes; antithyroglobulin and antithyroid peroxidase antibodies may be present for years, indicating Hashimoto's thyroiditis prior to clinical hypothyroidism).

◆ IgA deficiency may be present in persons with celiac disease. Therefore, when screening with anti-endomysial antibodies, a serum IgA level should also be drawn to ensure that a low IgA level is not causing a low endomysial antibody level.

Dermatologic Conditions Associated With Diabetes

Diabetes-related skin conditions develop in up to two thirds of both persons with type 1 diabetes mellitus and persons with type 2 diabetes mellitus. Cutaneous manifestations of diabetes occur because of the microvascular damage in diabetes, impaired wound healing, and other yet undetermined mechanisms.[58-60] The most commonly encountered skin lesions are described herein. The reader is referred to online or print atlases of dermatology to fully understand and recognize these lesions.

Acanthosis nigricans is a poorly defined, brown to black, velvety hyperpigmentation of the skin. It is usually found in body folds, such as the posterior and lateral folds of the neck, the armpits, groin, navel, forehead, and other areas.

Acrochordons (skin tags) are benign, soft, flesh-colored, pedunculated papules that are common in persons with diabetes. They are most common on the eyelid, neck, or axilla and are often found in conjunction with acanthosis nigricans. The association between diabetes and the development of skin tags is well established, and diabetes should be considered in patients with numerous skin tags.[59]

Diabetic dermopathy (shin spots) are the most common cutaneous lesions in diabetes. Up to 40% of persons with diabetes have these lesions.[61] They begin as round to oval atrophic hyperpigmented lesions on the pretibial areas of the lower extremities. They occur bilaterally but have an asymmetrical distribution. The lesions resolve spontaneously but leave scars.[62]

Diabetic thick skin. Ultrasound studies have demonstrated that persons with diabetes have thicker skin than persons without diabetes.[63] Skin thickening may manifest as scleroderma-like changes of the hand associated with stiff joints and limited mobility. Thickened skin is found in up to 50% of persons with type 1 diabetes and is thought to be due to glycosylation of the connective tissue in the skin.[64] This skin lesion has been associated with retinopathy, nephropathy, and neuropathy.

Huntley's Papules (pebbled or rough skin over the interphalangeal joints, particularly the knuckles) has been found in up to 72% of persons with diabetes.[65] The pebbles represent thickening of the skin in those areas.

Diabetic bullae are large blister-like lesions that occur spontaneously (often overnight) without antecedent trauma. They occur most often in elderly males with type 2 diabetes. They typically occur on the hands and feet and usually resolve without scarring. Treatment is directed at protecting the thin skin from trauma and preventing secondary infection in the bullae.[66]

Diabetic cutaneous infections are seen in uncontrolled diabetes and ketosis, but individuals whose diabetes is well controlled are not more susceptible to infections than the general population.[67] Bacterial infections of the skin are usually caused by *Staphylococcus aureus* and beta-hemolytic streptococci, resulting in impetigo, erysipelas, cellulitis, and necrotizing fasciitis. Treatment is with topical and systemic antibiotics.

Erythrasma, caused by *Corynebacteria minutissimum*, occurs in the intertriginous folds of skin and is more frequently found in obese persons with diabetes than in the general population.[68] Candida skin infections are an indicator of undiagnosed diabetes and of poorly controlled diabetes. Increased serum glucose levels cause candidal overgrowth in the mouth and vagina.[69] Genital cutaneous mycotic infections have been found to be increased in both women and uncircumcised men with the newest class of antihyperglycemic agents, sodium-glucose co-transporter 2 (SGLT2) inhibitors. Correction of hyperglycemia and use of topical and systemic antifungal agents are the main modalities of treatment.[70]

Eruptive xanthomas are firm, inflammatory 1- to 4-mm yellow papules with an erythematous base that occur on the extensor surfaces of the arms, legs, and buttocks. These lesions are a manifestation of markedly elevated triglycerides. Clinically, the lesions come in crops during times of triglyceride elevations and resolve over several weeks with lowering of the triglyceride levels.[58] Microscopic examination demonstrates the presence of lipid-laden macrophages, termed "foam cells," along with lymphocytes, neutrophils, and histiocytes. Recent studies have suggested that tumor necrosis factor (TNF-α) antagonists such as etanercept and infliximab have had therapeutic success.[59]

Onychomycosis is a fungal infection of the nail or nails. Several epidemiological studies have reported a higher prevalence of onychomycosis in persons with diabetes than in the general population. The severity of nail disease is correlated with the length of time of infection. Treatment of onychomycosis is important because severe fungal infections of the toenail can contribute to the development of foot ulcers in persons with diabetes who have vascular insufficiency and neuropathy.

Vitiligo is an autoimmune mediated loss of the pigment-producing cells in the skin, creating hypopigmented lesions in about 9% of persons with type 1 diabetes.[71] Patients with these lesions often have a personal or family history of autoimmune diseases such as Addison's disease, Hashimoto's thyroiditis, and pernicious anemia. There is no treatment, and the consequences are solely cosmetic.

Pertinent AADE7 Self-Care Behaviors™

- Healthy eating—Weight loss may improve or resolve acanthosis lesions.
- Monitoring—Inspecting the skin, especially on the feet, each day is an important self-care behavior. Instruct patients to contact their healthcare provider with any changes or lesions noted.

Practice Tips

- Skin and nail problems are common in people with diabetes; look for these problems and institute treatment where appropriate.
- Controlling blood glucose and lipoprotein levels will reduce some skin lesions (acanthosis nigricans, diabetic cutaneous infections, eruptive xanthomas).

Diabetes-Associated Infections

Hyperglycemia adversely affects the immune system in ways that make persons with diabetes more susceptible to infections. Glycosylation of immunoglobulins and complement proteins results in diminished killing of bacteria and viruses.[72] Hyperglycemia also compromises the function of immune cells, resulting in abnormalities of chemotaxisis, adherence, phago-cytosis, and the bactericidal capacity.[73,74] It is not clear from published studies that diabetes represents an independent risk factor for infections, but studies of surgical-site infections support lower rates of infections among persons with better blood glucose control.[75,76] A number of infections appear to occur more commonly in persons with diabetes; these are organized by the areas of the body affected.

Skin

See "Diabetic cutaneous infections" above.

Necrotizing fasciitis is a fulminant infection of the skin and fascia that is caused by a mixture of aerobic and anaerobic organisms. The infection results in extensive tissue destruction, thrombosis of blood vessels, and sepsis. Treatment requires antibiotics and extensive surgical debridement. Mortality rates are high, especially if surgical debridement is delayed. The infections may also involve the head and perineal regions.[77]

Head

Zygomycosis (mucormycosis) is a fungal infection that may occur as a complication of diabetes. Mucormycosis refers to several different diseases caused by infection with fungi in the order of Mucorales. *Rhizopus* species are the most common causative organisms. The infection starts in the nasal passages but may spread rapidly to the orbits of the eyes and the brain. Treatment requires extensive surgical debridement and intravenous fungal therapy[78] (eg, amphotericin B). One series reported a mortality rate of 44% in persons with diabetes.[79]

Malignant external otitis is an invasive infection of the external auditory canal and base of the skull that presents as severe ear pain and drainage. It is caused by *Pseudomonas aeruginosa*. It typically occurs in elderly patients and has a mortality rate of up to 50%.[80]

Dental and Oral Disease

Oral health complications of diabetes include severe periodontitis and subsequent tooth loss, gingivitis,

and dental abscesses. In addition, diabetes increases the risk of xerostomia and soft tissue lesions of the tongue and oral mucosa, such as candidiasis. Other commonly seen oral lesions in individuals with diabetes include lichen planus, angular cheilitis, and burning mouth syndrome.

The elevated glucose levels of diabetes increase the onset, frequency, progression, and severity of oral and periodontal disease.[81] Oral and periodontal infections may worsen blood glucose control, while treatment of periodontal disease has been shown to decrease A1C levels.[82] Regular dental cleanings have also been shown to improve glycemic control in patients with poorly controlled diabetes.[83]

The accumulation of AGEs in the gingival tissues is thought to be responsible for the oral complications of diabetes.[84] As a result, persons with diabetes have a two- to threefold increase in the prevalence of oral lesions and periodontal disease.[85] Oral disease has implications in other chronic complications of diabetes. Severe periodontal disease has been demonstrated to be an independent risk factor for mortality from ischemic heart disease and diabetic nephropathy. Further, subjects with severe periodontal disease had 3.2 times the risk of death from these complications.[86,87]

Children with diabetes do not have higher rates of dental caries than other children. However, they do have more plaque and gingival inflammation and have a greater number of teeth demonstrating gum attachment loss. Periodontal disease begins early in the life of children with diabetes, especially in those between the ages of 12 and 18 years.[88]

Not enough attention is given to the oral health of persons with diabetes. Despite the importance of good dental care, a survey of persons with diabetes showed that only 65.8% had seen a dentist in the preceding 12 months. The rate of dental exams was lower than the rate of visits with medical providers (86.3%) and foot examinations (67.7%). The disparity among rates of dental exams was greater than for any other type of healthcare visits.[84] Data from the Behavioral Risk Factor Surveillance System (BRFSS) surveys for 1999 and 2004 showed similar low rates of dental care as the previous study.[85] Regular dental exams should be used as opportunities for prevention, early detection, and treatment of periodontal disease; moreover, regular dental cleaning improves glycemic control in persons with poorly controlled diabetic conditions.[84]

Pertinent AADE7 Self-Care Behaviors™

- Taking medication—Some medications (diuretics and antidepressants) may contribute to dry mouth, which in turn increases tooth decay and periodontal disease.
- Reducing risks—Proper oral hygiene reduces the risk of oral and dental complications. Encourage regular visits with dentists just as you do annual eye examinations.

Practice Tips

- Ask when the patient's last dental exam was, and realize that the poorer the glucose control the more likely it is that the patient could have periodontal disease.
- Subclinical oral infections may worsen glucose control. In turn, good dental hygiene and treatment can significantly improve glucose control.

Chest

Influenza: Diabetes is associated with an increased rate of hospitalization for influenza and its complications; therefore, immunization is recommended annually for all persons with diabetes over 6 months of age unless the person has an egg allergy.[89] Despite significant efforts by healthcare providers, the influenza vaccination rate is still only about 50%.[90]

Pneumococcal pneumonia: Persons with diabetes have a higher risk for the bacteremic form of pneumonia, which has a mortality rate of up to 50%.[89] Immunization with the polyvalent vaccine is recommended for all persons 2 years of age or older. Repeat vaccination should be given once after 65 years of age. More frequent vaccination (every 5 years) is recommended for persons with chronic lung disease, nephrotic syndrome, chronic renal disease, and other immunocompromised states, such as after transplantation.[2]

Abdomen

Emphysematous cholecystitis is an infection of the gallbladder wall by gas-forming organisms (eg, *Clostridium welchii* and *Escherichia coli*). The gas in the wall of the gallbladder is visible on imaging studies, and it causes crepitus of the overlying skin. The typical symptoms of cholecystitis (abdominal pain, nausea, vomiting, and fever) are also present. This rare infection most commonly affects men in the fifth to seventh decade of life.[91]

Hepatitis: Hepatitis B virus (HBV) causes acute and chronic infection of the liver, leading to substantial morbidity and mortality. Since 1996, 29 outbreaks of HBV infection in one or multiple long-term care facilities in the United States, including nursing homes and assisted-living facilities, were reported to the CDC. An estimate of the risk for HBV infection for adults with diabetes living in long-term care facilities was not available; continuing outbreaks suggest that it might be substantial. Because chronic HBV infection can persist for decades, persons with chronic HBV infection are the reservoir for continuing HBV transmission. Chronic HBV infection is associated with high morbidity and mortality, leading to cirrhosis and liver cancer in more than 15% of affected adults. As a result, the CDC has recommended Hepatitis B vaccination,[92] and this now appears as a recommendation in the ADA Standards of Care.[2]

Feet

See chapter 28 regarding foot care.

Pelvis

Emphysematous urinary tract infections: Gas-forming organisms (usually *Escherichia coli* or *Klebsiella pneumoniae*) can cause severe infections of the kidneys and/or bladder. Most patients are women over the age of 60 years. As with other diabetes-related infections, mortality is high.[93]

Pertinent AADE7 Self-Care Behaviors™

- Monitoring—More frequent monitoring will be required to maintain glucose control during times of illness.

- Taking medication—Clinical symptoms often improve before the recommended course of antibiotics is completed. Emphasize the need to complete the course of medication even if the fever has broken and symptoms have improved.
- Problem solving—Sick-day management skills are critical to improving glucose control. Optimal glucose control will enable the immune system to eliminate the infection.
- Reducing risks—Proper immunizations against influenza, pneumococcal pneumonia, and Hepatitis B are critical to preventing and/or minimizing the impact of these infections.

Practice Tips

- Worsening glucose control may be the first sign of an impending infection. Patients should consider the possibility when they experience sustained glucose elevations in the absence of other explanations. Educators should question patients for possible smoldering infections. For example, "Do you have any sores or boils that are draining?" "Do you have any burning on urination?" "When is the last time you saw a dentist, and do you have bleeding when you brush?"
- Chronic poor glucose control makes patients more susceptible to infections (eg, oral, intertriginous, and vaginal fungal infections).
- Compromised immune function caused by diabetes makes patients more susceptible to infections and less capable of combating them.
- Elderly patients may not develop high fevers to the same extent as younger persons.

Obstructive Sleep Apnea

The overall prevalence of obstructive sleep apnea (OSA) is approximately 71% of people with type 2 diabetes, based on an average of multiple studies.[94]

The prevalence of diabetes in people with OSA is around 30%, with overweight or obesity being a major contributing factor.[95] Obstructive sleep apnea is one form of sleep disordered breathing (SDB) and is diagnosed based on polysomnography (sleep study) recordings of the number and duration of episodes of apnea (cessation of breathing) or hypopnea (overly shallow breathing or abnormally slow respiratory rate). The number of episodes recorded per hour is called the apnea-hypopnea index (AHI) and is used to stage the severity of OSA. An AHI of less than 5 indicates no OSA, 5 to 15 indicates mild OSA, 15 to 30 indicates moderate OSA, and an AHI greater than 30 indicates severe OSA.

Recent studies suggest that OSA and type 2 diabetes not only frequently coexist but also have a bidirectional association wherein each condition exacerbates the other. Treating the patient's breathing problem can improve his or her glycemic control and ease some of the complications of diabetes.[94] Sleep architecture may be altered in adults with type 1 diabetes or type 2 diabetes, and even youth with type 1 diabetes are potential candidates for SDB. In a recent study of 50 youths between 10 and 16 years of age with type 1 diabetes and no other potential risk factors for SDB, 14 subjects met the criteria for SDB, and concomitant continuous glucose monitoring (CGM) recordings in those individuals showed higher CGM glucose levels, indicating that even mild SDB appears to contribute to high glucose levels and longer periods of hyperglycemia.[96]

Treatment of OSA involves a variety of options including surgery (both maxillofacial for obstruction relief and bariatric for weight loss), oral appliances, and continuous positive airways pressure (CPAP), which is the most effective.[97] Treatment with CPAP has been shown to result in a decrease in blood glucose in persons with diabetes, but more importantly CPAP results in a significant decrease in long-term cardiovascular mortality and morbidity.[98]

Screening for OSA is an important part of assessing patients. The Epworth Sleepiness Scale, the Berlin Questionnaire, and the STOP-Bang questionnaire are just a few of the several screening tools available. Good correlation exists between higher scores on the STOP-Bang questionnaire and the presence of significant OSA.[99]

Pertinent AADE7 Self-Care Behaviors™

◆ Monitoring—More frequent monitoring will be required to maintain glucose control, and frequent periods of hyperglycemia should raise suspicion of the potential for SDB.

◆ Reducing risks—OSA is a significant risk for CVD, increased blood pressure, and, in general, cardiovascular morbidity and mortality.

Practice Tips

◆ Screen people with diabetes for the potential of OSA. Questions regarding daytime sleepiness, snoring, and other symptoms should lead to a more formal screening tool.

◆ Obtain a copy of the STOP-Bang questionnaire, learn about its use, and employ it to screen most people with type 2 diabetes, and adults and children with type 1 diabetes if symptoms exist.

Depression and Diabetes

Depression and other psychological problems may interfere with the efforts of persons with diabetes to care for their illness; therefore, detection and treatment of depression are important to achieving other treatment goals.[100] Depression of all degrees of severity (not just major depression) is associated with nonadherence to diabetes self-care, including diet, exercise, medication adherence, and glucose monitoring.[101] Assessment of depression should be part of each regular visit. It should also be performed when self-management practices are poorly implemented and when treatment goals are not being achieved.

Depression is twice as common in persons with diabetes than in the general population. Rates of depression are the same in both type 1 diabetes and type 2 diabetes; however, depression is more common among women (28%) than men (18%). In screening for depression it is important to use a standardized assessment tool, as it is more effective at detecting depression than diagnostic interviews.[102] A variety of instruments have been used to screen for depression. While each tool has been evaluated in clinical studies, the most effective tool will be the one that works well and is easy to use. In that regard, the PHQ-9 and its 2-question simple version (PHQ-2) are both effective and easier to use than the 21-question Beck Depression Inventory or the Hamilton Depression rating scale, both time-honored but more complicated tools.[103]

The lack of treatment or inadequate treatment of depression adversely impacts the medical outcomes of diabetes. The negative impact can be seen in not only increased risk of microvascular complications such as incident retinopathy and macrovascular complications such as coronary artery disease, but also mixed complications such as diabetic foot ulcers.[104] The most often cited significant impact is on cardiovascular and all-cause mortality rates among persons with diabetes and depression.[104,105] Effective treatment of depression does not add to the overall costs of caring for diabetes and may help reduce costs among more severely medically ill patients.[106] In a study of older patients receiving care that included intervention for depression, mortality was lowered by 51% compared with those in usual-care practices.[107]

Rates of depression do not differ among ethnic groups. However, African Americans are less likely than others to receive any depression treatment, antidepressant medications, or treatment from a mental health professional.[108] Depression is more prevalent in older persons with diabetes.

In children with diabetes, depression is strongly associated with diabetes complications. To date, few studies have tested the effectiveness of treatment of depression in children with diabetes.[109] It is important to identify and treat depression in children with diabetes early in the course of their illness, before medical complications develop.[109–111]

The ADA identifies the following as indications for referral to a mental health specialist familiar with diabetes management: gross noncompliance with medical regimen (by self or others), depression, the possibility of self-harm, debilitating anxiety (alone or with depression), findings of an eating disorder, or cognitive functioning that significantly impairs judgment.[112] The ADA encourages providers to use the provider-patient relationship to encourage patients to seek treatment of depression and other psychological problems as an important part of the treatment regimen of diabetes.

Pertinent AADE7 Self-Care Behaviors™

- ◆ Healthy eating—Work with patients to find alternative coping measures other than eating.
- ◆ Being active—Physical activity helps relieve stress, dissipate anxiety, and improve sleep.
- ◆ Monitoring—Monitoring often decreases during depression. The use of motivational interviewing techniques is recommended to empower patients to come up with an action plan of their own around monitoring after

you have discussed the pros and cons with them. Follow-up with the patient is critical to their success in doing their action plan.
- ◆ Healthy coping—Involve appropriate professionals in addressing personal and family issues.

Practice Tips

- ◆ Encourage patients to see mental health problems as being as legitimate as physical health problems.
- ◆ Obtain a copy of the PHQ-9 screening tool, and use it to screen patients with symptoms of depression or diabetes distress.

Focus on Education

Teaching Strategies

↪ **Empower patients to self-care adequately to minimize the possibility of diabetes complications.** A primary goal of diabetes treatment and self-management education is the prevention of chronic complications. The goal is for patients to have control over the long-term diabetes outcomes.

↪ **Use ongoing positive reinforcement to support change.** Using fear by itself to motivate will likely not be effective. People might be motivated by fear when a threat seems immediate and likely (eg, hypoglycemia). However, using fear to get them to take actions to minimize its long-term negative consequences might not work well. Most people know the long-term complications of diabetes. Helping patients achieve small successes in their self-management empowers them to make additional, more difficult changes. Threat and efficacy have been shown empirically to be the 2 major factors of a health-risk message. Threat determines the strength of the response, while efficacy determines the nature of the response.

The self-efficacy assumption is that people will be more inclined to take on a task if they believe they can succeed. Low self-efficacy can lead them to believe tasks are harder than they actually are. People with high self-efficacy in a particular task are more likely to expend more effort and persist longer. They also are generally of the opinion that they are in control of their own lives.

↪ **Focus on adding healthy habits that will eventually replace the unhealthy ones.** Minimizing the possibility of diabetes complications requires modifying existing unhealthy behaviors. Helping patients see the long-term investment they are making by their current hard work can be a challenge. Diabetes long-term care investment is like a retirement investment: some people are not saving and some people are planning well for the future.

The first step in helping your patients invest in future health and well-being is to set a foundation by appropriately connecting with them in the present, setting expectations, observing progress, preparing for challenges, and being available. The second step is actual learning by providing opportunities to learn, giving feedback on accomplishments, asking questions to explore beliefs, and listening reflectively. Action becomes the final stage when a patient feels ready and confident to carry out the action plan. Your role is to provide ongoing support, praise the patient for accomplishing baby steps, help him or her overcome barriers and challenges by listening, and get permission to provide suggestions and needed information.

Messages for Patients

→ **Enjoy your healthy lifestyle.** The lifestyle changes that people with diabetes need to implement are the same as for anybody who is trying to become healthy. Healthy eating, physical activity, progress monitoring, and problem solving are characteristic behaviors of people who are healthy.

→ **Be in tune with your body.** Being healthy makes you feel well. Celebrate the changes that have taken place while you become healthier.

→ **Gradual but ongoing changes lead to improved health.** Think of diabetes as the opportunity to become healthier and improve daily well-being. Daily changes become a routine, and consequently healthy daily habits. With time, healthy daily behaviors will minimize the risks of diabetes complications.

→ **Keep the ABCs (A1C, blood pressure, and cholesterol) under control.** Diabetes-related complications are caused by damage to the blood vessels servicing the affected tissues. Keeping glucose, blood pressure, and cholesterol under control minimizes diabetes-related complications.

→ **Put the AADE7 Self-Care Behaviors™ into action:** Healthy eating, being active, monitoring, taking medication, problem solving, reducing risks, and healthy coping. Diabetes care may seem overwhelming with all that needs to be done. Focusing on one healthy behavior at a time makes it more achievable. The great feeling of accomplishing one task will lead to more motivation to address the next one. One good thing leads to another good thing!

→ **Your body changes and your diabetes changes with time.** Glucose control, blood pressure control, and other clinical symptoms change even if you are generally living a healthy lifestyle. Diabetes is a progressive condition that requires symptom management and appropriate adjustments. Changing medications and increasing doses are necessary to maintain control and should not be looked at as signs of failure. Appropriate screenings and ongoing evaluation of health status are needed. Check for cardiac, autoimmune, and dermatologic infections; dental and psychological conditions; and others.

→ **You are in charge of your diabetes.** Self-care is the cornerstone of diabetes care, as over 90% of managing the condition is self-management. People with diabetes need the knowledge, skills, and motivation to assess the risks, to understand what can be gained from changing their lifestyle, and to act on that understanding by engaging in appropriate behaviors.

The value of diabetes education is evident from the research demonstrating that patients who received diabetes education showed a decreased risk of major complications.[113] Education should be a lifelong process, starting at the point of diagnosis and remaining as an essential component of diabetes care.

Health Literacy

→ **Focus on the patient's agenda first.** Address what is most relevant and most important to the patient first. Use situational problem solving by identifying a potential challenge and coming up with solutions. Poor health literacy is common, so take time to make sure the patient understands the issues or changes, and have him or her repeat back his or her understanding from your discussions.

⊘ **Allow your patient to teach you about his or her diabetes.** This will allow your assessment to more accurately identify actual needs.

⊘ **Measure and celebrate small and big accomplishments.** Each patient has to do a lot of things and often wants to accomplish everything at the same time. Help patients identify their diabetes care vision: goals and benchmarks that align with desirable diabetes care outcomes. Provide ongoing and direct support through coaching, modeling, and observing.

⊘ **Maximize learning:**
- Be reflective.
- Explain your role versus the patient's role.

- Be ready to try new patient-centered strategies.
- Realize the value of education research and utilize it in practice.
- Express aha moments and share them collectively.
- Trust patients' own judgment.
- Believe that patients can learn and that they play a major role in learning.
- Examine the ownership of learning.
- Realize learning is continuous; apply what you know now.
- Keep it simple.
- Listen.
- Ask questions to problem solve.
- Welcome any opportunities to talk with your patients.

Focus on Practice

⊘ **Diabetes self-management education (DSME) is an ongoing process.** Provide opportunities for patients to follow up on the initial DSME. Reassess patient's clinical and behavioral needs on a regular basis.

⊘ **Individualize your clinical and education approaches.** There is no "one size fits all" approach. Evaluate ownership of the decision making: Is it the patient's solution or yours?

⊘ **Integrate AADE7 Self-Care Behaviors™ as the assessment of ongoing diabetes care.** The 7 Self-Care Behaviors allow the person with diabetes to focus on one task at a time, monitor progress, and attain goals. Quantify progress by evaluating clinical markers of success and behavioral indicators.

⊘ **Integrate diabetes education into the Chronic Care Model.** Assess and quality-ensure diabetes

education and its delivery methods among all providers and patients. Make sure that diabetes education is part of the system that monitors outcomes, learns from the best practices, and self-reflects on its growth and development. All practitioners play a role in diabetes education.

⊘ **Learn about screening tools for diabetes complications such as SDB and depression.** Use screening tools to assess your patients and communicate the results to other members of the healthcare team.

⊘ **Practice evidence-based diabetes education.** Evaluate and examine existing evidence on providing effective diabetes education in the same manner as you do for clinical care. Diabetes educators often modify clinical care approaches based on the new research, and they should do the same for diabetes education methods.

References

1. Forbes JM, Cooper ME. Mechanisms of diabetic complications. Physiol Rev. 2013 Jan;93:137-88.

2. American Diabetes Association. Standards of medical care in diabetes—2014. Diabetes Care. 2014;37 Suppl l: S14-80.

3. Centers for Disease Control and Prevention. 2011 national diabetes fact sheet (cited 2014 Mar 27). http://www.cdc.gov/diabetes/pubs/factsheet11.htm.

4. Mitka M. Report quantifies diabetes complications. JAMA. 2007 Jun 6;297(21):2337-8.

5. Spijkerman AM, Henry RM, Dekker JM, et al. Prevalence of macrovascular disease amongst type 2 diabetic patients detected by targeted screening and patients newly diagnosed in general practice: the Hoorn Screening Study. J Intern Med. 2004 Nov;256(5):429-36.

6. Spijkerman AM, Dekker JM, Nijpels G, et al. Microvascular complications at time of diagnosis of type 2 diabetes are similar among diabetic patients detected by targeted screening and patients newly diagnosed in general practice: the Hoorn Screening Study. Diabetes Care. 2003 Sep;26(9): 2604-8.

7. Eppens MC, Craig ME, Cusumano J, et al. Prevalence of diabetes complications in adolescents with type 2 compared with type 1 diabetes. Diabetes Care. 2006 Jun;29(6): 1300-6.

8. Pinhas-Hamiel O, Zeitler P. Acute and chronic complications of type 2 diabetes mellitus in children and adolescents. Lancet. 2007 May 26;369(9575):1823-31.

9. TODAY Study Group. Rapid rise in hypertension and nephropathy in youth with type 2 diabetes. Diabetes Care. 2013;36:1735-41.

10. TODAY Study Group. Retinopathy in youth with type 2 diabetes participating in the TODAY clinical trial. Diabetes Care. 2013;36(6):1772-4.

11. Hermans MP, Ahn SA, Mahadeb YP, Rousseau MF. Sleep apnoea syndrome and 10-year cardiovascular risk in females with type 2 diabetes: relationship with insulin secretion and insulin resistance. Diabetes Metab Res Rev. 2013 Mar;29(3):227-34.

12. Kirkman MS, Briscoe VJ, Clark N. Diabetes in older adults: consensus report. Diabetes Care. 2012;35: 2650-64.

13. Huebschmann AG, Regensteiner JG, Vlassara H, Reusch JE. Diabetes and advanced glycoxidation end products. Diabetes Care. 2006 Jun;29(6):1420-32.

14. Zhou Z, Wang K, Penn MS, et al. Receptor for AGE (RAGE) mediates neointimal formation in response to arterial injury. Circulation. 2003 May 6;107(17):2238-43.

15. Duell PB, Oram JF, Bierman EL. Nonenzymatic glycosylation of HDL and impaired HDL-receptor-mediated cholesterol efflux. Diabetes. 1991 Mar;40(3):377-84.

16. Kilhovd BK, Berg TJ, Birkeland KI, Thorsby P, Hanssen KF. Serum levels of advanced glycation end products are increased in patients with type 2 diabetes and coronary heart disease. Diabetes Care. 1999 Sep;22(9):1543-8.

17. Vlassara H, Cai W, Crandall J, et al. Inflammatory mediators are induced by dietary glycotoxins, a major risk factor for diabetic angiopathy. Proc Natl Acad Sci USA. 2002 Nov 26;99(24):15596-601.

18. Kelly NJ, Savige GS. Dietary advanced glycation end-product restriction for the attenuation of insulin resistance, oxidative stress and endothelial dysfunction: a systematic review. Eur J Clin Nutr. 2013;67:239-48.

19. Rahbar S, Natarajan R, Yerneni K, Scott S, Gonzales N, Nadler JL. Evidence that pioglitazone, metformin and pentoxifylline are inhibitors of glycation. Clin Chim Acta. 2000 Nov;301(1-2):65-77.

20. Ceriello A, Kilpatric ES. Glycemic variability: both sides of the story. Diabetes Care. 2013;36 Suppl 2:S272-5.

21. Diabetes Control and Complications Trial Research Group. The effect of intensive treatment of diabetes on the development and progression of long-term complications in insulin-dependent diabetes mellitus. N Engl J Med. 1993 Sep 30;329(14):977-86.

22. Ohkubo Y, Kishikawa H, Araki E, et al. Intensive insulin therapy prevents the progression of diabetic microvascular complications in Japanese patients with non-insulin-dependent diabetes mellitus: a randomized prospective 6-year study. Diabetes Res Clin Pract. 1995 May;28(2):103-17.

23. UK Prospective Diabetes Study (UKPDS) Group. Intensive blood-glucose control with sulphonylureas or insulin compared with conventional treatment and risk of complications in patients with type 2 diabetes (UKPDS 33). Lancet. 1998 Sep 12;352(9131):837-53.

24. Holman RR, Paul SK, Bethel MA, Matthews DR, Neil HA. 10-year follow-up of intensive glucose control in type 2 diabetes. N Engl J Med. 2008 Oct 9;359(15): 1577-89.

25. Diabetes Control and Complications Trial/Epidemiology of Diabetes Interventions and Complications Research Group. Retinopathy and nephropathy in patients with type 1 diabetes four years after a trial of intensive therapy. N Engl J Med. 2000 Feb 10;342(6):381-9.

26. Gulliford MC, Charlton J. Is relative mortality of type 2 diabetes mellitus decreasing? Am J Epidemiol. 2009 Feb 15;169(4):455-61.

27. Eliasson M, Talbäck M, Rosén M. Improved survival in both men and women with diabetes between 1980 and 2004—a cohort study in Sweden. Cardiovasc Diabetol. 2008 Oct 20;7:32.

28. Wang J, Imai K, Engelgau MM, Geiss LS, Wen C, Zhang P. Secular trends in diabetes-related preventable hospitalizations in the United States, 1998-2006. Diabetes Care. 2009 Jul;32(7):1213-7.

29. Romero-Aroca P, Fernández-Balart J, Baget-Bernaldiz M, et al. Changes in the diabetic retinopathy epidemiology after 14 years in a population of type 1 and 2 diabetic patients after the new diabetes mellitus diagnosis criteria and a more strict control of the patients. J Diabetes Complications. 2009 Jul-Aug;23(4):229-38.

30. American Association of Clinical Endocrinologists. Medical guidelines for clinical practice for developing a diabetes mellitus comprehensive care plan. Endocr Pract. 2011;17 Suppl 2:1-53.

31. International Society for Pediatric and Adolescent Diabetes (ISPAD). Clinical practice consensus guidelines 2009 (cited 2014 Mar 27). On the Internet at: http://www.ispad.org/content/ispad-clinical-practice-consensus-guidelines-2009.

32. Inzucchi SE, Bergenstal RM, Buse JB, et al. Management of hyperglycemia in type 2 diabetes: a patient-centered approach. Diabetes Care. 2012;35:1364-79.

33. American Association of Clinical Endocrinologists. AACE comprehensive diabetes management algorithm 2013. Endocr Pract. 2013;19(2):327-36.

34. Brown AF, Mangione CM, Saliba D, Sarkisian CA; California Healthcare Foundation/American Geriatrics Society Panel on Improving Care for Elders with Diabetes. Guidelines for improving the care of the older person with diabetes mellitus. J Am Geriatr Soc. 2003 May;51(5 Suppl Guidelines):S265-80.

35. American Diabetes Association. Standards of medical care in diabetes—2013. Diabetes Care. 2013;36 Suppl 1: S11-66.

36. Sinclair AJ, Paolisso G, Castro M, et al. European diabetes working party for older people 2011: clinical guidelines for type 2 diabetes mellitus—executive summary. Diabetes Metab. 2011;37:S27-38.

37. Gough SLC, Simmonds MJ. The HLA region and autoimmune disease. Curr Genomics. 2007;8(7):453-65.

38. Umpierrez GE, Latif KA, Murphy MB, et al. Thyroid dysfunction in patients with type 1 diabetes: a longitudinal study. Diabetes Care. 2003 Apr;26(4):1181-5.

39. Kordonouri O, Deiss D, Danne T, Dorow A, Bassir C, Grüters-Kieslich A. Predictivity of thyroid autoantibodies for the development of thyroid disorders in children and adolescents with type 1 diabetes. Diabet Med. 2002 Jun;19(6):518-21.

40. Roldán MB, Alonso M, Barrio R. Thyroid autoimmunity in children and adolescents with type 1 diabetes mellitus. Diabetes Nutr Metab. 1999 Feb;12(1):27-31.

41. Kordonouri O, Klinghammer A, Lang EB, Grüters-Kieslich A, Grabert M, Holl RW. Thyroid autoimmunity in children and adolescents with type 1 diabetes: a multicenter survey. Diabetes Care. 2002 Aug;25(8):1346-50.

42. Kordonouri O, Hartmann R, Deiss D, Wilms M, Grüters-Kieslich A. Natural course of autoimmune thyroiditis in type 1 diabetes: association with gender, age, diabetes duration, and puberty. Arch Dis Child. 2005 Apr;90(4):411-4.

43. Karavanaki K, Kakleas K, Paschali E, et al. Screening for associated autoimmunity in children and adolescents with type 1 diabetes mellitus (T1DM). Horm Res. 2009;71(4): 201-6.

44. Mohn A, Di Michele S, Di Luzio R, Tumini S, Chiarelli F. The effect of subclinical hypothyroidism on metabolic control in children and adolescents with type 1 diabetes mellitus. Diabet Med. 2002 Jan;19(1):70-3.

45. Chase HP, Garg SK, Cockerham RS, Wilcox WD, Walravens PA. Thyroid hormone replacement and growth of children with subclinical hypothyroidism and diabetes. Diabet Med. 1990 May;7(4):299-303.

46. American Diabetes Association. Standards of medical care in diabetes—2013—executive summary. Diabetes Care. 2013;36 Suppl 1:S4-10.

47. Fasano A, Catassi C. Celiac disease. N Engl J Med. 2012 Dec 20;367(25):2419-26.

48. Freemark M, Levitsky LL. Screening for celiac disease in children with type 1 diabetes: two views of the controversy. Diabetes Care. 2003 Jun;26(6):1932-9.

49. AGA Institute. AGA Institute Medical Position Statement on the Diagnosis and Management of Celiac Disease. Gastroenterology. 2006 Dec;131(6):1977-80.

50. Holmes GK. Screening for celiac disease in type 1 diabetes. Arch Dis Child. 2002 Dec;87(6):495-8.

51. Rewers M, Liu E, Simmons J, Redondo MJ, Hoffenberg EJ. Celiac disease associated with type 1 diabetes mellitus. Endocrinol Metab Clin North Am. 2004 Mar;33(1): 197-214, xi.

52. Crone J, Rami B, Huber WD, Granditsch G, Schober E. Prevalence of celiac disease and follow-up of EMA in children and adolescents with type 1 diabetes mellitus. J Pediatr Gastroenterol Nutr. 2003 Jul;37(1):67-71.

53. Cerutti F, Bruno G, Chiarelli F, Lorini R, Meschi F, Sacchetti C; Diabetes Study Group of the Italian Society of Pediatric Endocrinology and Diabetology. Younger age at onset and sex predict celiac disease in children and adolescents with type 1 diabetes: an Italian multicenter study. Diabetes Care. 2004 Jun;27(6):1294-8.

54. Amin R, Murphy N, Edge J, Ahmed ML, Acerini CL, Dunger DB. A longitudinal study of the effects of a gluten-free diet on glycemic control and weight gain in subjects with type 1 diabetes and celiac disease. Diabetes Care. 2002 Jul;25(7):1117-22.

55. Kibirig D, Mwebaze R. Vitamin B12 deficiency among people with diabetes mellitus: is routine screening and supplementation justified? J Diabetes Metab Disord. 2013 May 7;12(1):17.

56. Moore EM, Mander AG, Ames D. Increased risk of cognitive impairment in patients with diabetes is associated with metformin. Diabetes Care. 2013;36(10):2981-7. Epub 2013 Sept 5.

57. Peterson P, Salmi H, Hyöty H, et al. Steroid 21-hydroxylase autoantibodies in insulin-dependent diabetes mellitus. Childhood Diabetes in Finland (DiMe) Study Group. Clin Immunol Immunopathol. 1997 Jan;82(1):37-42.

58. Nern K. Dermatologic conditions associated with diabetes. Curr Diab Rep. 2002 Feb;2(1):53-9.

59. Levy L, Zeichner JA. Dermatologic manifestation of diabetes. J. Diabetes. 2012;4:68-76.

60. Behm B, Schreml S, Lanthaler M, Babilas P. Skin signs in diabetes mellitus. J Eur Acad Dermatol Venereol. 2012; 26:1203-11.

61. Shermer A, Bergman R, Linn S, Kanto Y, Friedman-Birnbaum R. Diabetic dermopathy and internal complications in diabetes mellitus. Int J Dermatol. 1998 Feb;37(2): 113-5.

62. Jelinek JE. Cutaneous manifestations of diabetes mellitus. Int J Dermatol. 1994 Sep;33(9):605-17.

63. Huntley AC, Walter RM Jr. Quantitative determination of skin thickness in diabetes mellitus: relationship to disease parameters. J Med. 1990;21(5):257-64.

64. Brik R, Berant M, Vardi P. The scleroderma-like syndrome of insulin-dependent diabetes mellitus. Diabetes Metab Rev. 1991 Jun;7(2):120-8.

65. Hollister DS, Brodell RT. Finger "pebbles": a dermatologic sign of diabetes mellitus. Postgrad Med. 2000 Mar;107(3): 209-10.

66. Basarab T, Munn SE, McGrath J, Russell Jones R. Bullosis diabeticorum: a case report and literature review. Clin Exp Dermatol. 1995 May;20(3):218-20.

67. Perez MI, Kohn SR. Cutaneous manifestations of diabetes mellitus. J Am Acad Dermatol. 1994 Apr;30(4):519-31.

68. Meurer M, Szeimies RM. Diabetes mellitus and skin diseases. Curr Probl Dermatol. 1991;20:11-23.

69. Knight L, Fletcher J. Growth of Candida albicans in saliva: stimulation by glucose associated with antibiotics, corticosteroids, and diabetes mellitus. J Infect Dis. 1971 Apr;123(4):371-7.

70. Riser Taylor S, Harris KB. The clinical efficacy and safety of sodium glucose cotransporter-2 inhibitors in adults with type 2 diabetes mellitus. Pharmacotherapy. 2013;33(9): 984-99.

71. Romano G, Moretti G, Di Benedetto A, et al. Skin lesions in diabetes mellitus: prevalence and clinical correlations. Diabetes Res Clin Pract. 1998 Feb;39(2):101-6.

72. Bell DS. Inflammation, insulin resistance, infection, diabetes, and atherosclerosis. Endocr Pract. 2000 May-Jun;6(3): 272-6.

73. Delamaire M, Maugendre D, Moreno M, Le Goff MC, Allannic H, Genetet B. Impaired leucocyte functions in diabetic patients. Diabet Med. 1997 Jan;14(1):29-34.

74. Llorente L, De La Fuente H, Richaud-Patin Y, et al. Innate immune response mechanisms in non-insulin dependent diabetes mellitus patients assessed by flow cytoenzymology. Immunol Lett. 2000 Nov 1;74(3):239-44.

75. Latham R, Lancaster AD, Covington JF, Pirolo JS, Thomas CS. The association of diabetes and glucose control with surgical-site infections among cardiothoracic surgery patients. Infect Control Hosp Epidemiol. 2001 Oct;22(10):607-12.

76. Estrada CA, Young JA, Nifong LW, Chitwood WR Jr. Outcomes and perioperative hyperglycemia in patients with or without diabetes mellitus undergoing coronary artery bypass grafting. Ann Thorac Surg. 2003 May;75(5):1392-9.

77. Brook I, Frazier EH. Clinical and microbiological features of necrotizing fasciitis. J Clin Microbiol. 1995 Sep;33(9):2382-7.

78. Kauffman CA, Malani AN. Zygomycosis: an emerging fungal infection with new options for management. Curr Infect Dis Rep. 2007 Nov;9(6):435-40.

79. Roden MM, Zaoutis TE, Buchanan WL, et al. Epidemiology and outcome of zygomycosis: a review of 929 reported cases. Clin Infect Dis. 2005 Sep 1;41(5):634-53.

80. Rubin Grandis J, Branstetter BF IV, Yu VL. The changing face of malignant (necrotising) external otitis: clinical, radiological, and anatomic correlations. Lancet Infect Dis. 2004 Jan;4(1):34-9.

81. Taylor GW, Borgnakke WS. Periodontal disease: associations with diabetes, glycemic control and complications. Oral Dis. 2008 Apr;14(3):191-203.

82. Teeuw WJ, Gerdes VEA, Loos BG. Effect of periodontal treatment on glycemic control of diabetic patients. Diabetes Care. 2010;33:421-7.

83. Centers for Disease Control and Prevention (CDC). Dental visits among dentate adults with diabetes—United States, 1999 and 2004. MMWR Morb Mortal Wkly Rep. 2005 Nov 25;54(46):1181-3.

84. Tomar SL, Lester A. Dental and other health care visits among U.S. adults with diabetes. Diabetes Care. 2000 Oct;23(10):1505-10.

85. Mealey BL, Oates TW, American Academy of Periodontology. Diabetes mellitus and periodontal diseases. J Periodontol. 2006 Aug;77(8):1289-303.

86. Saremi A, Nelson RG, Tulloch-Reid M, et al. Periodontal disease and mortality in type 2 diabetes. Diabetes Care. 2005 Jan;28(1):27-32.

87. Humphrey LL, Fu R, Buckley DI, Freeman M, Helfand M. Periodontal disease and coronary heart disease incidence: a systematic review and meta-analysis. J Gen Intern Med. 2008;23(12):2079-86.

88. Lalla E, Cheng B, Lal S, et al. Periodontal changes in children and adolescents with diabetes: a case-control study. Diabetes Care. 2006 Feb;29(2):295-9.

89. Smith SA, Poland GA, American Diabetes Association. Influenza and pneumococcal immunization in diabetes. Diabetes Care. 2004 Jan;27 Suppl 1:S111-13.

90. Centers for Disease Control and Prevention. Age-adjusted percentage of adults aged 18 years or older with diagnosed diabetes receiving an influenza vaccination in the last year, United States, 1993-2010 (cited 2014 Mar 27). On the Internet at: http://www.cdc.gov/diabetes/statistics/preventive/fZ_flu.htm.

91. Sarmiento RV. Emphysematous cholecystitis: report of four cases and review of the literature. Arch Surg. 1966 Dec;93(6):1009-14.

92. Centers for Disease Control and Prevention. Vaccine recommendations of the Advisory Committee for Immunization Practices. MMWR. 2011 (cited 2014 Mar 27);60:1709. On the Internet at: http://www.cdc.gov/vaccines/hcp/acip-recs/recs-by-date.html.

93. Huang JJ, Tseng CC. Emphysematous pyelonephritis: clinicoradiological classification, management, prognosis, and pathogenesis. Arch Intern Med. 2000 Mar 27;160(6):797-805.

94. Pamidi S, Tasali E. Obstructive sleep apnea and type 2 diabetes: is there a link? Front Neurol. 2012;3:article 126.

95. Mahmood K, Akhter N, Eldeirawi K, et al. Prevalence of type 2 diabetes in patients with obstructive sleep apnea in a multi-ethnic sample. J Clin Sleep Med. 2009;5(3):215-21.

96. Perfect MM, Patel PG, Scott RE, et al. Sleep, glucose and daytime functioning in youth with type 1 diabetes. Sleep. 2012;35(1):81-8.

97. Adult Obstructive Sleep Apnea Task Force of the American Academy of Sleep Medicine. Clinical guideline for the evaluation, management and long-term care of obstructive sleep apnea in adults. J Clin Sleep Med. 2009;5(3):263-76.

98. Marin JM, Carrizo SJ, Vincente E, Agusti AG. Long-term cardiovascular outcomes in men with obstructive sleep apnoea-hypopnoea with or without treatment with continuous positive airway pressure: an observational study. Lancet. 2005;365(9464):1046-53.

99. Chung F, Subramanyam R, Liao P, Saski E, Shapiro C, Sun Y. High STOP-Bang score indicates a high probability of obstructive sleep apnoea. Br J Anaesth. 2012;108(5):768-75.

100. Delahanty LM, Grant RW, Wittenberg E, et al. Association of diabetes-related emotional distress with diabetes treatment in primary care patients with type 2 diabetes. Diabet Med. 2007 Jan;24(1):48-54.

101. Gonzalez JS, Safren SA, Cagliero E, et al. Depression, self-care, and medication adherence in type 2 diabetes: relationships across the full range of symptom severity. Diabetes Care. 2007 Sep;30(9):2222-7.

102. Anderson RJ, Freedland KE, Clouse RE, Lustman PJ. The prevalence of comorbid depression in adults with diabetes: a meta-analysis. Diabetes Care. 2001 Jun;24(6):1069-78.

103. Bell MH. Screening tools for depression. Am Fam Physician. 2008 Jul 15;78:244-6.

104. Pouwer F, Nefs G, Nouwen A. Adverse effects of depression on glycemic control and health outcomes in people with diabetes: a review. Endocrinol Metab Clin North Am. 2013;42:529-42.

105. Egede LE, Nietert PJ, Zheng D. Depression and all-cause and coronary heart disease mortality among adults with and without diabetes. Diabetes Care. 2005 Jun;28(6):1339-45.

106. Katon WJ, Russo JE, Von Korff M, Lin EH, Ludman E, Ciechanowski PS. Long-term effects on medical costs of improving depression outcomes in patients with depression and diabetes. Diabetes Care. 2008 Jun;31(6):1155-9. Epub 2008 Mar 10.

107. Bogner HR, Morales KH, Post EP, Bruce ML. Diabetes, depression, and death: a randomized controlled trial of a depression treatment program for older adults based in primary care (PROSPECT). Diabetes Care. 2007 Dec;30(12):3005-10.

108. de Groot M, Pinkerman B, Wagner J, Hockman E. Depression treatment and satisfaction in a multicultural sample of type 1 and type 2 diabetic patients. Diabetes Care. 2006 Mar;29(3):549-53.

109. Markowitz S, Gonzalez JS, Wilkinson JL, Safren SA. Treating depression in diabetes: emerging findings. Psychosomatics. 2011;52:1-18.

110. Stewart SM, Rao U, White P. Depression and diabetes in children and adolescents. Curr Opin Pediatr. 2005 Oct;17(5):626-31.

111. Springer SC, Silverstein J, Copeland K, et al. Management of type 2 diabetes mellitus in children and adolescents. Pediatrics. 2013;131(2):e648-64.

112. American Diabetes Association. Standards of medical care in diabetes—2014. Diabetes Care. 2014;37 Suppl 1:S49.

113. Stern E, Benbassat CA, Goldfract M. Impact of a two-arm educational program for improving diabetes care in primary care centres. Int J Clin Pract. 2005;59:1126-30.

CHAPTER 24

Pregnancy With Diabetes

Diane M. Reader, RD, CDE
Alyce Thomas, RD

Key Concepts

◆ Higher incidences of maternal and fetal complications are associated with poor glycemic control in preexisting and gestational diabetes.

◆ Optimal blood glucose levels are associated with lower perinatal morbidity and mortality rates.

◆ Preconception counseling should be available to all women with preexisting diabetes and those with previous gestational diabetes and prediabetes to decrease the risk of congenital anomalies and spontaneous abortions.

◆ Strategies to improve outcomes include maternal and fetal testing and self-management skills.

◆ Weight gain goals based on current recommendations from the Institute of Medicine are established at the initial prenatal visit.

◆ Health professionals involved in the care of pregnant women with diabetes should develop an understanding of the pathophysiology of diabetes and pregnancy.

◆ Women who have gestational diabetes mellitus have 7 times the risk of developing type 2 diabetes after delivery. Steps should be taken to prevent diabetes through weight control, food choices, and physical activity.

◆ Unless contraindicated, breastfeeding is recommended for all women with preexisting or gestational diabetes.

Introduction

The most prevalent medical complication in pregnancy is diabetes mellitus. Diabetes in pregnancy is divided into 2 groups:

◆ Women with *preexisting diabetes*, which includes type 1 diabetes and pregnancy (T1DP) and type 2 diabetes and pregnancy (T2DP)

◆ Women with *gestational diabetes mellitus* (GDM), which is defined as any degree of glucose intolerance with onset or first recognition during pregnancy[1]

Approximately 34% of pregnant women with preexisting diabetes have type 1 diabetes. In recent years, intensive insulin therapy and greater attention to diabetes self-management have resulted in better maternal glycemic control. The current perinatal mortality rate in women with preexisting diabetes is 2%, which is comparable to women without diabetes.[2]

The incidence of GDM varies among populations and ethnicities, as well as with the diagnostic criteria used. In the United States, it is estimated that 6% to 7% of pregnancies are complicated by diabetes mellitus and that approximately 90% of these are GDM.[3] The rate of GDM in any community or geographic region will vary depending on multiple factors; the range is quite wide, from as low as 2% to as high as 50%.[4] More importantly, the rate is increasing, likely due to the high rates of overweight and obesity in the population of women in their childbearing years.

Glycemic control is key to decreasing fetal risks and infant morbidity associated with maternal hyperglycemia. The greatest success in maintaining optimal glycemic control throughout pregnancy comes from partnering with a multidisciplinary team and receiving targeted self-management education. Key components of care include antenatal testing and the effective use of self-management skills.

It is important to acknowledge that all pregnancies, including those complicated by diabetes, have the same goal, which is a healthy outcome for both mother and child. This chapter begins by reviewing the normal physiology of pregnancy and then goes on to describe the components of a healthy pregnancy that apply to all women: weight gain based on current recommendations, consuming a nutritious diet, and participating in daily physical activity. An additional goal for pregnancies complicated by diabetes is to achieve glycemic control without sacrificing weight gain, good nutrition, or physical activity.

Normal Pregnancy
Physiology of Pregnancy

The fetus depends on an adequate but not excessive supply of fuel from maternal sources. Glucose, which is transported across the placenta via facilitated diffusion, is the fuel source preferred by the fetus over any other energy-producing nutrient.[5] The first trimester is often characterized by maternal glucose levels that are lower than those of nonpregnant women. Hormonal levels (estrogen, progesterone, human placental lactogen) progressively increase in the second and third trimesters, resulting in increased insulin resistance. Fetal growth accelerates in the third trimester as free fatty acids are mobilized for maternal energy needs. This allows for additional placental transfer of glucose to the developing fetus. The normal response to the increased insulin resistance in pregnancy is progressively increasing insulin secretion, which may be 100% above nonpregnant levels by the third trimester (see Figure 24.1).

Weight Gain

The 2009 guidelines from the Institute of Medicine (IOM) provide the basis for determining appropriate

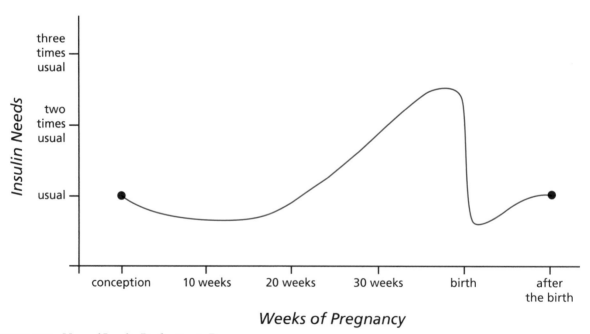

FIGURE 24.1   **Normal Insulin Production in Pregnancy**

Source: Reprinted with permission from *Pregnancy Planning and Care for Women With Diabetes* (Minneapolis, Minn: International Diabetes Center, 2012).

American Association of Diabetes Educators©

weight gain during pregnancy.[6] Weight gain categories are based on the woman's prepregnancy body mass index (BMI) established by the World Health Organization (see Table 24.1). A high BMI increases both maternal and fetal risks, including hypertension, preeclampsia, macrosomia, surgical or difficult delivery, and gestational diabetes. It is interesting to note that over 50% of women in their childbearing years have a BMI of 25 or higher at conception.[7]

The amount of weight gained during pregnancy may affect pregnancy outcomes. Excessive gestational weight gain is associated with heavier infants and greater postpartum weight retention. A key recommendation to all health professionals is to identify women at risk for excessive gestational weight gain early in the pregnancy and intervene to help control their weight gain.

Nutrition During Pregnancy

Most dietary recommendations for pregnant women without diabetes may be followed by women with diabetes. This includes appropriate weight gain and providing adequate nutrients for maternal and fetal health. Table 24.2 provides guidelines for the number of servings of fruit, vegetables, grains, dairy, meat, fats, and additional calories for a normal-weight woman who

TABLE 24.1 Recommended Ranges of Total Weight Gain for Pregnant Women			
Weight-for-Height Category	*Recommended Total Weight Gain (Singleton Gestation)*	*Weekly Weight Gain Rates in the Second and Third Trimesters (Singleton Gestation)*	*Recommended Total Weight Gain (Twin Gestation)*
Underweight (BMI* <18.6)	28–40 lb (12.7–18.2 kg)	1 lb (.5 kg)	
Normal weight (BMI 18.6–24.9)	25–35 lb (11.3–16 kg)	1 lb (.5 kg)	37–54 lb (16.8–24.5 kg)
Overweight (BMI 25.0–29.9)	15–25 lb (6.8–11.3 kg)	⅔ lb (.3 kg)	31–50 lb (14.1–22.7 kg)
Obese (BMI >30)	11–20 lb (4.5–9.0 kg)	½ lb (.25 kg)	25–42 lb (11.3–19.1 kg)

*BMI = weight/height^2

Source: National Academy of Sciences, *Weight Gain During Pregnancy: Reexamining the Guidelines* (Washington, DC: National Academy Press, 2009).

TABLE 24.2 Sample Dietary Guidelines for Pregnancy*				
	First Trimester	*Second Trimester*	*Third Trimester*	*Examples*
Total calories	1800	2200	2400	
Grains	6 servings	7 servings	8 servings	1 slice bread; ½ c potato, rice, pasta
Vegetables	2½ c	3 c	3 c	Carrots, broccoli, onion 2 c greens = 1 c vegetables
Fruits	1½ c	2 c	2 c	Whole fruit, juice
Milk	3 c	3 c	3 c	Milk, yogurt, cheese
Meat and beans	5 oz	6 oz	6½ oz	½ c beans = 1-oz serving of meat
Extras	290 calories	360 calories	410 calories	May come from additional food groups or from higher calorie, higher fat foods
Fats and oils	6 tsp	7 tsp	8 tsp	Oil, butter, nuts

*For a normal-weight woman who exercises less than 30 minutes per week

Source: MJ Franz, AB Evert, *American Diabetes Association Guide to Nutrition Therapy for Diabetes* (Washington, DC: American Diabetes Association, 2012).

exercises less than 30 minutes a week.[8–10] Goals specific to diabetes will be addressed in subsequent sections.

Nutrition Requirements

Energy   The dietary reference intakes (DRIs)[11,12] are used to determine the estimated energy requirements (EERs) in pregnancy, which are based on age, height, weight, and physical activity level. The EERs for pregnancy are as follows:

- ◆ *1st trimester:* Adult EER + 0
- ◆ *2nd trimester:* Adult EER + 160 kcal (8 kcal/wk × 20 wk) + 180 kcal
- ◆ *3rd trimester:* Adult EER + 272 kcal (8 kcal/wk × 34 wk) + 180 kcal

The 8 kcal per week represents the change in total energy expenditure due to pregnancy; the 180 kcal is the mean energy deposition during pregnancy. An example of estimated calorie needs for a 30-year-old woman with a BMI of 24.7 is provided in Table 24.3.

Protein   The recommended dietary allowance (RDA) for protein in the nonpregnant woman is 0.8 g per kilogram per day, or 46 g per day. Protein requirements increase to 1.1 g per kilogram per day, or 25 g extra per day, for a singleton gestation and 50 g extra for twin pregnancies.[12]

Carbohydrate   The DRI for carbohydrate in pregnant women ages 19 to 50 is a minimum of 175 g per day. This amount of carbohydrates provides an adequate source of glucose for fetal growth (approximately 33 g per day) and for the maternal brain.[12]

Vitamins and Minerals   Adequate calcium, iron, folate, vitamin D, and magnesium intakes are especially important in pregnancy. Dietary reference intakes in pregnancy are listed in Table 24.4.

Safe Eating During Pregnancy

Nonnutritive Sweeteners

All nonnutritive sweeteners approved by the Food and Drug Administration (FDA) are approved for use by the general public, which includes pregnant and lactating women.[13] However, the consensus of most registered dietitians and diabetes educators is to limit the use to 3 servings or less during pregnancy and lactation.

Alcohol

Use of all alcoholic beverages during pregnancy is discouraged because of the risks of fetal alcohol spectrum disorders.[14]

Mercury-Contaminated Fish

The FDA has recommended that pregnant women and women of childbearing age avoid eating shark, swordfish, jack mackerel, and tilefish. These fish often contain high levels of methyl-mercury, a potent human neurotoxin, which readily crosses the placenta and has the potential to damage the fetal nervous system.[15] Women should consult their local health department for further fish advisories in their area.

Listeriosis

Food safety is of primary concern in pregnancy. The Centers for Disease Control and Prevention (CDC) estimates a fivefold risk of contracting listeriosis

TABLE 24.3   Example of EERs Before and During Pregnancy for a 30-Year-Old Woman with a BMI of 24.7 kg/m² (65 in [1.65 m] and 150 lb [68.0 kg])

Physical Activity Level	Nonpregnant and First Trimester EER (kcal/d)	Second Trimester EER + 340 kcal*	Third Trimester EER + 450 kcal*
Sedentary	1983	2300	2450
Low active	2203	2550	2650
Active	2479	2800	2950

*Calories rounded to the nearest 50

Source: MJ Franz, AB Evert, *American Diabetes Association Guide to Nutrition Therapy for Diabetes* (Washington, DC: American Diabetes Association, 2012).

Nutrient	Pregnant Woman	Lactating Woman
Protein (g)[1]	+25	+25
Vitamin A (mcg) 14–18 years 19–50 years	750 770	1200 1300
Vitamin D (mcg)[2]	15	15
Vitamin K (mcg) 14–18 years 19–50 years	75 90	75 90
Vitamin C (mg) 14–18 years 19–50 years	80 85	115 120
Thiamin (mg)	1.4	1.4
Riboflavin (mg)	1.4	1.6
Niacin (mg NE)	18	17
Vitamin B$_6$ (mg)	1.9	2.0
Folate (mcg FE)	600	500
Vitamin B$_{12}$ (mcg)	2.6	2.8
Calcium (mg)[2] 14–18 years 19–50 years	1300 1000	1300 1000
Phosphorus (mg) 14–18 years 19–50 years	1250 700	1250 700
Magnesium (mg) 14–18 years 19–30 years 31–50 years	400 350 360	360 310 320
Iron (mg) 14–18 years 19–50 years	27 27	10 9
Zinc (mg) 14–18 years 19–50 years	12 11	13 12
Iodine (mcg)	220	290
Selenium (mcg)	60	70

TABLE 24.4 Dietary Reference Intakes for Pregnant and Lactating Women

Sources:

1. Trumbo P, Schlicker S, Yates AA, Poos M. Dietary reference intakes for energy, carbohydrate, fiber, fat, fatty acids, cholesterol, protein and amino acids. J Am Diet Assoc. 2002;102:1621-30.
2. Institute of Medicine of the National Academies. Dietary Reference Intakes for Calcium and Vitamin D. Washington, DC: The National Academies Press; 2011.

during pregnancy. Approximately one third of all listeriosis cases involve pregnant women. Listeriosis can be transmitted to the fetus via the placenta. The risks of listeriosis are preterm delivery, spontaneous abortions, and other complications. Pregnant women are advised to avoid the following:

- Deli meats, hot dogs, and luncheon meats, unless reheated until steaming hot
- Soft cheeses (such as feta, Brie, Camembert, blue-veined), queso blanco, and queso fresco (hard cheeses and pasteurized cheese are recommended)
- Refrigerated patés and meat spreads (canned and shelf-stable paté and meat spreads can be consumed)
- Refrigerated smoked seafood, unless cooked
- Raw or unpasteurized milk

Physical Activity During Pregnancy

Physical activity guidelines for pregnancy and the postpartum period are as follows[16]:

- Healthy women who are not already highly active or performing vigorous-intensity activity should get at least 150 minutes of moderate-intensity aerobic activity per week during pregnancy and the postpartum period (see Table 24.5).
- Pregnant women who habitually engage in vigorous-intensity aerobic activity or are highly active can continue physical activity during pregnancy and the postpartum period, provided they remain healthy and discuss with their healthcare provider how and when activity should be adjusted over time.

TABLE 24.5 Contraindications for Physical Activity in Pregnancy

- Incompetent cervix/cervical cerclage
- Multiple gestation at risk of preterm labor
- Intrauterine growth retardation
- Persistent second- or third-trimester bleeding
- Placenta previa
- Preeclampsia or pregnancy-induced hypertension
- Premature labor or history of preterm labor
- Premature rupture of membranes

Frequency and Duration of Physical Activity

- *Goal of 30 minutes daily.* In the absence of medical or obstetric complications, pregnant women should participate in 30 minutes or more of moderate-intensity physical activity on most, if not all, days of the week.[16] Active women can continue similar activities during pregnancy.
- *Intervals as short as 10 minutes can be effective.* The physical activity can be short bouts of 10 minutes each, accumulated over the course of the day.
- *Sedentary lifestyle.* Pregnancy generally is not a time for a woman who was previously sedentary to initiate strenuous activity; however, walking is possible for most women, and a 15- to 20-minute walk can lower blood glucose by 20 to 40 mg/dL.

Breastfeeding

The EER for lactation is calculated from total energy expenditure, milk energy output, and energy mobilization from tissue stores.[12] In the first 6 months postpartum, lactating women experience an average weight loss of 0.8 kg per month, which is equivalent to 170 kcal per day. The milk energy output is approximately 500 kcal per day. As the infant is introduced to solid foods, usually at 6 months, the amount of milk produced is reduced and the milk energy output decreases to 400 kcal per day. The EER for lactation is as follows:

- *1st 6 months:* EER + 500 − 170 (milk energy output − weight loss)
- *2nd 6 months:* EER + 400 − 0 (milk energy output − weight loss)
- *RDA for protein:* 1.1 g per kilogram per day, or an additional 25 g per day (same as in pregnancy)[12]
- *RDA for carbohydrate:* 210 g per day[12]

Diabetes in Pregnancy

Preconception Care and Education

Evidence shows that intensive diabetes management can improve perinatal outcome.[17] For women with preexisting diabetes, care should begin before conception, which is sometimes referred to as the "12-month pregnancy."

Case: Type 1 Diabetes—A Pregnancy With Preconception Care

PB is a 33-year-old woman with type 1 diabetes of 18 years' duration who was referred by a diabetes treatment center to a tertiary level center for obstetrical care. At her first prenatal visit, she was confirmed at 7 weeks' gestation. This is her third pregnancy; her previous pregnancies ended in first-trimester spontaneous abortions 4 and 5 years ago (at 8 weeks' and 10 weeks' gestation, respectively). In planning for this pregnancy, PB was instructed by the diabetes center to delay conception until her blood glucose levels were at optimal control.

Preconception Care and Education

PB delayed conception for 6 months using contraception, a low-dose progestin-only oral contraceptive agent, until her A1C was 6.3%. The following protocol was established to achieve optimal diabetes control before PB attempted conception:

- Discuss safe and realistic goals (her husband was included in the decision-making process).

- Assess any vascular complications; include a dilated retinal examination; thyroid function tests; kidney function testing to determine creatinine, creatinine clearance, and microalbumin; and an EKG. She had proliferative retinopathy, for which she received laser photocoagulation therapy 7 years ago; she has a history of diabetic ketoacidosis (DKA), with the last episode occurring 3 years ago; and she began experiencing neuropathy in her feet at age 24.

- Refer for genetic counseling because of the family history of diabetes. PB's father has type 2 diabetes, and a 25-year-old brother was diagnosed with type 1 diabetes at age 9.

- Refer to a registered dietitian for adjustments to her food plan.

- Begin folic acid supplementation of 400 mcg per day.[18]

- Assess her self-management skills, including insulin administration, glucose monitoring, and treatment of hypoglycemic episodes.

- Continue contraception until glucose goals are attained.

Care and Education During Pregnancy

Pathophysiology in Type 1 Diabetes

PB began her pregnancy with planning and implementing efforts to optimize her glycemic control and improve the outcomes.

Diabetes Management During Pregnancy

At her first prenatal visit, PB brought her last laboratory tests, from 10 weeks ago, and blood glucose records. Her A1C was 6.3% and hemoglobin and hematocrit were 13.8 mg/dL and 40.6%, respectively. Her recent assessment of kidney function (24-hour urine for protein and creatinine) was within normal limits. Her BMI was 22.4. Her fasting blood glucose ranged from 75 to 115 mg/dL (4.2 to 6.4 mmol/L), premeal 58 to 132 mg/dL (3.2 to 7.4 mmol/L), and 1 hour postprandial 115 to 145 mg/dL (6.4 to 8.1 mmol/L). PB monitors her blood glucose 7 times a day (fasting, premeal, 1 hour postmeal, and bedtime), and her insulin regimen is 4 injections per day, with rapid-acting insulin before meals and a long-acting insulin analog (detemir) at night.

Complications

Care and education are important to achieve and maintain optimal glycemic control and improve perinatal outcome. PB had proliferative diabetic retinopathy and is at higher risk for progression of the condition during pregnancy. She has also experienced DKA in the past. Since conception was delayed until her glycemic levels were at optimal control, the risk for fetal complications was decreased.

Healthy Coping

Facing some stressful and fearful situations, PB needed support from the diabetes care team and her family. The diabetes center recommended continuous subcutaneous insulin infusion (CSII), which PB had avoided in the past but was now considering because of the pregnancy. She indicated her willingness to comply with all instructions to ensure that this pregnancy was carried to term, but she also expressed cautious optimism because of her past obstetrical history. She was referred to a social worker to discuss her concerns.

Healthy Eating

PB denied use of alcohol and drugs. With early morning nausea, occasional vomiting, and an aversion to cooking odors, her appetite has decreased in the past 2 weeks.

Care Plan

As a result of preparations made early in the pregnancy and even before conception, the following elements of care were planned as optimal management during pregnancy:

- Maternal and fetal surveillance and testing (eg, nuchal translucency, ultrasound, nonstress test, biophysical profile, maternal serum alpha fetal protein, and amniocentesis [PB opted not to have the amniocentesis])

- Referral to an ophthalmologist for a baseline eye exam to detect changes during pregnancy

- Referral to a registered dietitian for medical nutrition therapy (MNT)

- Referrals to other specialists, as necessary

Diabetes Education

The following were identified as topics for which PB required education and/or intervention:

- *Diabetic ketoacidosis prevention:* Teach PB how to prevent DKA

- *Risks:* Discuss with PB and her husband the risks associated with type 1 diabetes and pregnancy

- *Intensity of care:* Explain how prenatal care is more intensive than preconception care and it includes more frequent obstetrical visits and tests

- *Hypoglycemia:* Assess the husband's knowledge of signs and symptoms of hypoglycemia and how to administer glucagon

- *Assessment of social-emotional well-being:* Assess PB's response to feelings, since the 2 earlier pregnancies ended in miscarriage; as needed, refer the couple to a social worker or behavioral health specialist to discuss their feelings regarding this pregnancy

Medical Nutrition Therapy

Medical nutrition therapy was necessary to evaluate PB's eating habits. PB was referred to a registered dietitian, who provided her with information on the following:

- Recommended weight gain and rate of gain according to her prepregnancy BMI

(continued)

Case: Type 1 Diabetes—A Pregnancy With Preconception Care (continued)

- Managing nausea and vomiting to avoid hypoglycemia

- Managing other gastrointestinal discomforts that may occur (eg, heartburn, constipation, ptyalism)

- Use of nonnutritive sweeteners during pregnancy

- Food safety issues

- Physical activity, if no contraindications

- Infant feeding plans

- Keeping food records

To avoid hypoglycemia, PB had to maintain consistency in her meal and snack times and portion sizes. She was told that insulin-to-carbohydrate ratios may be different depending on the meal. For example, the insulin-to-carbohydrate ratio at breakfast may be larger than at other meals because of increased cortisol and growth hormone levels that appear to contribute to morning glucose intolerance. Monitoring of blood glucose levels, blood or urine ketones, appetite, and weight gain guided the registered dietitian in developing an appropriate individualized food plan and in making adjustments to this plan throughout the pregnancy.[19]

Insulin Therapy

Aspects of insulin therapy that needed to be addressed through diabetes education included glucose targets during pregnancy and the need to adjust the insulin regimen as the pregnancy progressed.

- *Glucose targets.* Optimal blood glucose control is necessary to decrease the risk of complications in pregnancy. Treatment of hypoglycemia is necessary if blood glucose levels are below 65 mg/dL (3.6 mmol/L). Changes in blood glucose recommendations for pregnancy were discussed (lower than prepregnancy values). PB's last episode of DKA was 3 years ago. The signs, symptoms, and management of DKA were discussed. More frequent self-monitoring of her blood glucose levels is appropriate, especially if she experiences nocturnal hypoglycemia.

- *Changing insulin requirements.* PB was told that her insulin regimen would change throughout the pregnancy. Her requirements might decrease during the first trimester but increase in the second and even triple her prepregnancy dosage by the third trimester. The benefits of CSII were discussed since this was suggested by the diabetes treatment center.

PB decided to delay switching to the insulin pump until after delivery. She was compliant with her diabetes and pregnancy regimen. She did not miss any appointments with her healthcare provider, diabetes educator, or registered dietitian. Blood glucose records were consistently kept and verified by her memory meter, as were food records, which she e-mailed to the dietitian. The results of both maternal and fetal surveillances were normal, and PB discovered during an ultrasound appointment that she was having a girl! PB and her husband attended childbirth education classes offered at the hospital where she would deliver.

Diabetes Care During Labor and Delivery

PB's blood glucose levels were frequently monitored, and insulin and glucose were administered as necessary. At 39 weeks' gestation and after 6 hours of labor, she vaginally delivered baby Brianna, a 3540-g girl.

Postpartum Care and Education

Lactation

Soon after conceiving, PB had decided she would breastfeed. Brianna spent a day in the neonatal intensive care unit to be assessed for any anomalies or complications. With no complications, she was reunited with her mother. Because PB knew her milk production might be delayed, she began pumping her breasts soon after delivery. She noticed a drop in her glucose level whenever Brianna nursed. PB received a visit from the lactation consultant during her hospital stay, and the diabetes nurse educator called her to discuss postpartum glycemic changes.

Assessment Phone Call

Two weeks after delivery, the diabetes nurse educator phoned PB again to assess how she was adjusting to motherhood. PB told her that breastfeeding was going well and Brianna was gaining weight. PB's insulin requirements had decreased, which necessitated more frequent glucose monitoring. To assess for postpartum depression, the diabetes educator asked PB how she felt emotionally; PB denied any emotional changes.

Office Visit

PB made an appointment with the diabetes educator to discuss changes to her regimen during the postpartum period. The diabetes educator stressed the need to maintain optimal glycemic control for the duration of the breastfeeding period and while weaning. Hypoglycemic

Case: Type 1 Diabetes—A Pregnancy With Preconception Care (continued)

awareness during breastfeeding was also emphasized, which may increase the frequency of glucose self-monitoring. During the appointment, PB informed the diabetes educator that although she was happy being a new mother, she wanted to wait at least 2 years before attempting to conceive again. The educator reviewed contraceptives that were safe while breastfeeding and after weaning, and discussed postpartum depression. After her 6-week postpartum checkup, PB was scheduled to return to the diabetes center for care and to make an appointment with the registered dietitian to discuss weight loss and adjustments to her food plan.

Preconception care, as demonstrated with PB's case, is key to improving outcomes in pregnancies complicated by diabetes. Both the American Diabetes Association (ADA) and the American College of Obstetricians and Gynecologists (ACOG) recommend that diabetes care and education begin before conception.[1,4] Sufficient time must be allowed to evaluate the mother's health status and to normalize or maximize glycemic control, thereby offering the best chance for the fetus.

Case: Type 2 Diabetes—A Pregnancy Requiring Hospitalization

LR is a 27-year-old Hispanic woman who, at 13 weeks' gestation, was referred to a high-risk obstetrical clinic for her first pregnancy. She had fainted at home and was rushed to the emergency room, where the pregnancy was confirmed by ultrasound. She was admitted from the emergency room for glucose control when her random blood glucose level was 210 mg/dL (11.7 mmol/L). At her initial prenatal visit, LR weighed 248 lb.

Preconception Care and Education

LR never received preconception counseling. She was diagnosed with type 2 diabetes 4 years ago and was prescribed glyburide and metformin (Glucophage®, Bristol-Myers Squibb), 500 mg twice a day, but stopped taking them a year ago. When asked why, she replied, "I sometimes forget to take my medication."

Care and Education During Pregnancy

Pathophysiology of Type 2 Diabetes

LR presented for her first visit with many of the challenges of poorly controlled type 2 diabetes; her case was further complicated by an unstable home situation. She needed the help of a comprehensive diabetes care team.

Diabetes Management During Pregnancy

LR was unsure of her prepregnancy weight but weighed 248 lb at her initial prenatal visit (height 64 in, BMI 42.5). Her A1C was 11.0%, and her hemoglobin was 12.5 mg/dL. She complained of recurrent urinary tract infections (UTIs) and is currently taking antibiotics.

Assessment

It is important to assess why LR discontinued the diabetes treatment plan, including her medications. Her family history includes diabetes in both maternal and paternal grandfathers. She has experienced some significant changes in her life, including an unplanned pregnancy and a recent separation; more information is needed about her current living conditions. Referral to a social worker or mental health professional would be helpful in establishing baseline information on her willingness and ability to follow a care plan.

- What is her current relationship with her husband? Is there anyone who could assist her during the pregnancy?

- What is her financial situation? Does she have health insurance? If she does not have health insurance, is she able to purchase diabetes supplies such as insulin and syringes, test strips, and lancets?

- Is she willing to follow an intensive insulin regimen requiring her to self-inject insulin and monitor her blood glucose levels multiple times daily?

Complications

LR has been experiencing frequent UTIs and might be vulnerable to other complications associated with obesity—such as chronic hypertension, obstructive sleep apnea, preeclampsia, higher rate of cesarean sections, and difficult delivery. Careful and comprehensive assessment for complications was required, and appropriate interventions were initiated. At each subsequent visit, LR was screened for UTI.

(continued)

Case: Type 2 Diabetes—A Pregnancy Requiring Hospitalization (continued)

Insulin Therapy

LR was started on an insulin regimen of 4 injections daily: lispro before meals, detemir at night. She monitors her blood glucose levels 4 times daily (fasting and 2-hour postprandial). She was started on insulin immediately to bring her glycemic levels to normal. Because of her BMI, the initial insulin initiation was calculated at 1.5 units per kilogram of actual body weight. She was informed that because insulin resistance increases in the third trimester, the insulin dose may increase to 2.0 units per kilogram.

Medical Nutrition Therapy

LR received MNT when first diagnosed, but she followed the food plan only for about 6 months. She found the food plan given during the current admission difficult to follow at home. Before providing appropriate MNT, the registered dietitian needed to understand LR's lifestyle, eating preferences, and barriers to using a food plan for diabetes management. The original food plan was modified to include LR's food preferences. LR was income-eligible for WIC and Food Stamps and a referral was made to these programs. By the third visit with the dietitian, LR was adhering with the food plan. She had decided to formula-feed the baby.

Diabetes Education

LR needed information about the risks she and her baby may encounter, healthy and reasonable expectations regarding weight gain, mental preparation for the increase in antenatal testing, and support regarding her use of the food plan.

Risks

LR needed assistance in understanding that obese pregnant women with type 2 diabetes are at higher risk for adverse pregnancy outcomes, including macrosomia.

- *Weight.* She received information on weight gain recommendations and the importance of avoiding weight loss to decrease the risk for starvation ketosis and intrauterine growth retardation. She was informed that calorie restriction is not recommended

during pregnancy because of the possible effect of ketonuria or ketonemia on the fetus.

- *Food plan.* She was given information on how women with type 2 diabetes may benefit from a lower calorie food plan of no fewer than 1800 calories a day. Effective implementation of MNT could help LR avoid ketosis and excessive weight gain and provide adequate nutrients.

- *Medical care.* Maternal and fetal testing would begin according to the gestational week. Because of the elevated A1C at conception, in addition to the usual laboratory testing in diabetes and pregnancy, LR would be offered an amniocentesis to assess chromosomal abnormalities. She learned that frequent scanning was necessary to assess fetal well-being.

- *Glycemic control.* She was informed about the value of good glycemic control in the short and long term, for the health of both her unborn child and herself.

LR works as a part-time school bus aide and was able to meet with the diabetes educator between bus runs. She expressed gratitude for the assistance. She met with the social worker and was referred for financial assistance to help with insulin and monitoring supplies. An amniocentesis was performed, and the test results were negative for Down syndrome and neural tube defects. Having learned from the diabetes educator that maternal glycemic levels can affect the fetus, LR complied with the insulin and monitoring schedule.

Postpartum Care and Education

LR delivered a 3630-g baby boy at 38 weeks via cesarean section. Throughout the pregnancy, the diabetes educator emphasized to LR the importance of maintaining postpartum glycemia to levels as near to normal as possible to decrease the risk of complications. Four weeks after delivery, LR resumed taking glyburide and metformin (Glucovance®) as prescribed. She scheduled an appointment with the registered dietitian to discuss weight loss and a new eating plan.

Preconception Counseling for Women With Preexisting Diabetes

Preconception care is a set of preventive and management interventions that identify and modify risk factors that can affect pregnancy outcome.[20] The CDC recommends incorporating preconception

care into the routine health care of all women of childbearing age. However, since more than half of all pregnancies in the United States are unplanned or unintended, most women do not receive preconception care, including those with preexisting diabetes or prediabetes, or women with previous GDM.[20]

The ACOG recommends preconception counseling for women with preexisting diabetes as a beneficial and cost-effective service.[21] Counseling that focuses on achieving euglycemia prior to and during the critical period of organogenesis may help prevent anomalies.

In a study that examined preconception counseling rates in managed care, 52% of the women recalled a discussion on glucose control with their healthcare provider, and only 37% received advice on family planning.[22] Women with type 2 diabetes tend not to be referred for preconception care as often as their type 1 counterparts.[23] An Australian study showed that while 27.8% of women with type 1 diabetes received preconception counseling, only 12% of those with type 2 diabetes received the same services.[24]

Elevated maternal glucose levels during organogenesis are associated with higher rates of congenital anomalies and spontaneous abortions. The risk of complications decreases if the woman with diabetes enters pregnancy in optimal blood glucose control.

If the A1C level is less than 7% at conception, the rate of congenital malformations is similar to the nondiabetic pregnant woman.[1] The ADA recommends that women with diabetes delay conception until their blood glucose levels are in optimal control.[25] An effective method of contraception should be used until the desired glycemic results are achieved (see Table 24.6).

A pregnant woman with preexisting diabetes may or may not have received self-management instructions prior to conception. She may not be aware of the importance of optimal glycemic control and how best to avoid the complications associated with hyperglycemia in pregnancy, such as congenital anomalies and macrosomia. Without preconception counseling, a woman may not be prepared to apply problem-solving and self-management skills to the critical situations that may arise quickly in early pregnancy or in emergency situations that may require hospitalization. Plans for diabetes education during pregnancy must thus factor in whether the woman had preconception care.

TABLE 24.6 Contraceptive Use in Women With Preexisting Diabetes or Prior History of GDM		
Contraceptive Type	*Efficacy*	*Safety*
Barrier methods: diaphragm, condoms, spermicides, cervical caps[1,2,4]	70%–97% depending on method and if used alone or in combination with another method	No contraindications
Intrauterine devices (IUDs)[1,2,4]	98%–99%	Not recommended if high-risk exposure to sexually transmitted diseases
Oral contraceptives (OCs)[1,2,4]	97%–99.5%	Low-dose progestin or combination of lowest progestin/estrogen dose preferred for women without vascular complications or strong family history of myocardial disease Women with prior history of GDM should not use progestin-only OC while breastfeeding
Non-oral hormonal[1–4] contraceptives (eg, implants, injections, transdermal patches)	99%	May affect glucose and lipid levels

Sources:

1. Kitzmiller JL, Jovanovic L, Brown F, Coustan D, Reader DM, eds. Managing Preexisting Diabetes and Pregnancy. Alexandria, Va: American Diabetes Association; 2008.

2. Kim C, Seidel KW, Begier EA, et al. Diabetes and depot medroyprogesterone contraception in Navajo women. Arch Inter Med. 2001;161.

3. Chuang CH, Chase GA, Bensyl DM, Weisman CS. Contraceptive use by diabetic and obese women. Women's Health Issues. 2005;15(4):167-73.

4. Kjos SL, Buchanan TA. Postpartum management, lactation, and contraception. In: Reece EA, Coustan DR, Gabbe SG, eds. Diabetes in Women: Adolescence, Pregnancy, and Menopause. Philadelphia, Pa: Lippincott Williams & Wilkins; 2004:441-9.

Diabetes and pregnancy care have a more reassuring start when the woman has received adequate preconception counseling. During pregnancy, particularly in the first trimester, topics for diabetes education include the following:

- Keeping glycemic levels in optimal control
- Mild to severe hypoglycemia as a result of increased insulin sensitivity
- Increased visits with the diabetes team at the beginning of pregnancy
- Continuation of successful self-management skills

Preconception care for the woman with preexisting diabetes should include self-management education with a multidisciplinary team. The initial preconception visit consists of a comprehensive medical and obstetrical history, physical examination, laboratory evaluation, and management plan. The woman should be referred for evaluations of her renal and retinal status, peripheral and autonomic neuropathy, hypoglycemic risk, peripheral vascular disease, and thyroid.[26] Certain medications, such as statins, angiotensin II receptor blockers (ARBs), and angiotensin converting enzyme (ACE) inhibitors, are contraindicated during pregnancy. Healthcare providers will generally change these medications to those less teratogenic to the fetus. Women with type 2 diabetes or prediabetes on oral glucose-lowering medications will most likely switch to insulin. According to the ADA's position statement on preconception care, the woman should be seen at 1- to 2-month intervals until her A1C results indicate stable glycemic control and the risk and status of her diabetes complications have decreased.[25] When these 2 goals are achieved, contraception can be discontinued; however, preconception care should continue until pregnancy occurs.

There are no specific recommendations for preconception care for women with prediabetes. The ADA recommends lifestyle interventions for persons with prediabetes, which have been shown to lower their risk of developing type 2 diabetes.[1] These interventions include MNT, physical activity, and weight loss, if indicated. The Evidence-Based GDM Nutrition Practice Guidelines of the Academy of Nutrition and Dietetics recommend weight loss after pregnancy in women with previous GDM to prevent the risk of developing type 2 diabetes or GDM in subsequent pregnancies.[27] Women with prediabetes or previous histories of GDM may follow the recommendations for a nonpregnant person with prediabetes to achieve and maintain optimal glycemic levels before conception.

Pathophysiology

Type 1 Diabetes

In the first trimester, women with type 1 diabetes may actually experience a decrease in their insulin requirements as their glycemic levels fall and insulin sensitivity increases.[19,28] As the pregnancy progresses, the absence of maternal pancreatic beta cell function increases the concentration of glucose, fatty acids, ketones, and amino acids transported across the placenta to the fetus. Exogenous insulin requirements may increase two- to threefold over prepregnant amounts to maintain euglycemia and reduce the risk of fetal complications. Pedersen hypothesized that maternal hyperglycemia is the primary reason for fetal hyperinsulinemia resulting from the overstimulation of fetal pancreatic beta cells.[29] Other factors that affect fetal growth include insulin growth factors, leptin, and tumor necrosis factor.[30]

Type 2 Diabetes

Type 2 diabetes is characterized by insufficient insulin receptors in response to a given degree of glycemia. As insulin resistance increases, beta cell function declines and glucose levels rise. Insulin resistance can be substantially greater in women with type 2 diabetes than in women with type 1 diabetes because women with type 2 diabetes are more likely to be obese. If glycemic levels are elevated around conception and organogenesis, the risk of congenital malformations and spontaneous abortions increases. Hyperglycemia is a particular problem in the second and third trimesters, when maternal hormone levels increase. Self-management education should prepare the woman for the expected increase in insulin requirements.

Complications

Maternal

Diabetes can affect the health of the mother and the fetus in T1DP and T2DP. Complications may have predated or may develop during the pregnancy. Specific complications are described below.

Diabetic Retinopathy   Hormones, such as growth hormone and insulin-like growth factor (IGF-1), along with the rise in estrogen, progesterone, and cortisol levels, may accelerate retinopathy.[31,32] Rosenn et al[33] found that pregnancy-induced hypertension or preexisting chronic hypertension was the most important risk factor associated with the progression of retinopathy in pregnancy. Rapid normalization of blood glucose can cause acute progression of retinopathy.[34] Pregnant women with diabetes and no background of mild retinopathy are less likely to have progression than those with advanced retinopathy. In most situations, background retinopathy that occurs during pregnancy regresses after delivery. If the woman has untreated proliferative retinopathy, pregnancy should be delayed until after laser photocoagulation.

Diabetic Nephropathy   Hypertension, increased glomerular filtration rate, increased protein intake and excretion, and poor glycemic control are factors that contribute to the development of diabetic nephropathy. Diabetic nephropathy is associated with poor pregnancy outcome. Optimal maternal hypertensive and glycemic control may improve renal function and slow the progression of nephropathy during and after pregnancy. Angiotensin converting enzyme inhibitors are contraindicated during pregnancy because of potential fetal risks.

Hypertension   Hypertension in pregnancy is classified into 4 categories based on guidelines by the ACOG Task Force in Hypertension in Pregnancy (see Table 24.7).[35] As a result of poor glycemic control, the incidence of hypertensive disorders in pregnancy is higher in women with diabetes.[36]

Diabetic Ketoacidosis   Diabetic ketoacidosis is more common in women with type 1 diabetes than in women with type 2 diabetes. Increased insulin resistance and accelerated starvation ketosis play roles in the higher incidence of DKA in T1DP than in nonpregnant women with type 1 diabetes. In pregnancy, DKA increases the risk of fetal demise. Other factors associated with DKA include hyperemesis, gastroparesis, and treatment with corticosteroids or beta-mimetic, tocolytic medications, such as terbutaline or ritodrine.[21]

Complications Associated With Obesity   Obesity is a risk factor associated with a higher incidence of perinatal mortality and morbidity.[6,37–39] Complications associated with obesity in pregnancy include chronic hypertension, obstructive sleep apnea, preeclampsia, increased UTIs, and higher rates of cesarean and difficult deliveries in the mother.[40]

Another maternal risk that occurs during pregnancy is polyhydramnios (excessive amniotic fluid).

Fetal

Congenital Malformations   Congenital anomalies occur during organogenesis (the first 8 weeks of gestation) and are more common in women with preexisting diabetes.[1] In a large Danish study that compared pregnancy outcomes in T1DP with a nondiabetes population, the perinatal complications in the former group were higher in women with increasing A1C levels and poor self-care.[41] Wren et al found a fivefold increase in the risk of cardiovascular malformations in infants born to women with preexisting diabetes than in women without diabetes.[42] Birth defects associated with preexisting diabetes in pregnancy are listed in Table 24.8.

TABLE 24.7 Hypertensive Disorders in Pregnancy	
Preeclampsia–eclampsia	Hypertension in association with thrombocytopenia, impaired liver function, the new development of renal insufficiency, pulmonary edema, or new-onset cerebral or visual disturbances
Chronic hypertension	Hypertension that predates pregnancy
Preeclampsia superimposed on chronic hypertension	Chronic hypertension in association with preeclampsia
Gestational hypertension	BP elevation after 20 weeks of gestation in the absence of proteinuria

Source: Hypertension in Pregnancy (Washington, DC: The American College of Obstetricians and Gynecologists, 2013).

TABLE 24.8 Congenital Malformations in Infants Born to Women With Preexisting Diabetes

Cardiovascular

Transposition of great vessels

Ventricular septal defect

Atrial septal defect

Hypertrophic cardiomyopathy

Aortic stenosis

Coarctation or interruption of the aortic arch

Hydroplastic left heart syndrome

Truncus arteriosus

Ebstein anomaly

Pulmonary stenosis

Tricuspid valve dysplasia

Double-outlet right ventricle (DORV)

Central nervous and skeletal

Sacral agenesis

Anencephalus

Hydrocephalus

Neural tube defects

Genitourinary

Renal agenesis

Hydronephrosis

Ureteral duplication

Anal/rectal atresia

Gastrointestinal

Duodenal atresia

Anorectal atresia

Sources: C Wren, G Birrell, G Hawthorne, "Cardiovascular malformations in infants of diabetic mothers," *Heart* 89 (2003): 1217-20; T Farrell, L Neale, T Cundy, "Congenital anomalies in the offspring of women with type 1, type 2 and gestational diabetes mellitus," *Diabetes Med* 19 (2002): 322-26; MB Landon, SG Gabbe, "Diabetes mellitus," in WM Barron, MD Lindheimer, JM Davison, eds. *Medical Disorders in Pregnancy* (St. Louis, Mo: Mosby, 2000).

Macrosomia   Macrosomia is defined as infant birth weight greater than 4000 g.[43] Macrosomic infants have trunks and shoulders that are disproportionately larger than the head. A cesarean section is often indicated to prevent birth trauma if the infant birth weight exceeds 4500 g.[44]

The Pedersen hypothesis provides the best explanation for the link between macrosomia and diabetes.[29] As the mother's blood circulates nutrients to her fetus, a high maternal level of glucose results in a high level of glucose in the fetus. Sensing elevated glucose levels, the fetal pancreas begins producing insulin to normalize this high level of glucose. As a growth hormone, insulin stimulates fetal growth. An increase in adipose tissue in the organs, chest, and abdomen means the trunk and shoulders become disproportionately larger than the head, which increases the risk for shoulder dystocia, Erb's palsy, and brachial plexus palsy. Macrosomic infants are also at increased risk for developing glucose intolerance during their lifetime.

Neonatal Hypoglycemia   Neonatal hypoglycemia in the newborn is a blood glucose level less than 35 mg/dL (1.9 mmol/L) and in the preterm infant, less than 25 mg/dL (1.4 mmol/L). Neonatal hypoglycemia may result if the infant continues to produce excessive insulin after delivery when the maternal glucose supply is no longer available. This occurs within the first 12 hours of life and will require oral or intravenous glucose to return glucose levels to normal. The first preventive strategy in neonatal hypoglycemia is optimal maternal blood glucose levels during labor and delivery. The second is the early initiation of oral feeding. Risks associated with neonatal hypoglycemia include seizures, cerebral damage, and death.[45]

Other Fetal Complications   Other problems associated with uncontrolled glucose levels in the infant include respiratory distress syndrome (RDS), hypocalcemia, polycythemia, and hyperbilirubinemia.

AADE Self-Care Behaviors™ During Pregnancy: Preexisting Diabetes

The AADE7 Self-Care Behaviors™ provide a framework to assess and evaluate outcomes throughout pregnancy in women with preexisting or gestational diabetes (see Table 24.9). The following section covers managing women with preexisting diabetes.

TABLE 24.9 AADE7 Self-Care Behaviors™ for Diabetes and Pregnancy*	
Healthy eating	Consume adequate calories to avoid weight loss and ketone production
	Consume adequate nutrients for maternal stores and fetal growth and development; consume adequate intakes of fruit, vegetables, dairy, and protein
	Avoid alcohol and other substances that could be harmful to the fetus
	Avoid foods that can lead to foodborne illnesses
	Minimum carbohydrate intake of 175 g per day
	Control total and per-meal carbohydrate based on food plan and medications
	Match carbohydrate with rapid-acting or bolus insulin using insulin-to-carbohydrate ratio
	Avoid high-carbohydrate, low-nutrient foods, such as sweetened soft drinks
	May need to reduce/restrict high glycemic index foods
Being active	Participate in daily physical activity, if no contraindications
	Carry extra carbohydrate for hypoglycemia prevention, if taking oral glucose-lowering agents or insulin
Monitoring	Monitor blood glucose levels fasting, premeal, and postmeal; frequency and targets determined by healthcare provider
	Test ketones as instructed by healthcare provider
	Keep food and blood glucose records as instructed by healthcare team
	Self-monitoring of blood glucose is used to make therapy adjustments
	Continuous glucose monitoring may be used to assess trends in blood glucose levels
	A1C is not used to determine the need for therapy adjustments
Taking medications	Understand that insulin requirements increase as pregnancy progresses
	Understand that certain oral glucose-lowering agents and other medications for cardiometabolic risk may be discontinued until after delivery
	GDM—Women with GDM may need glucose-lowering medication in addition to MNT
Problem solving	Identify symptoms and treatment of hypoglycemia and hyperglycemia
	Identify criteria for when to contact the healthcare provider
	Schedule follow-up visits with healthcare providers and diabetes educators to review self-management skills
Reducing risks	Identify and treat hypoglycemia for women using insulin or oral glucose-lowering agents
	Understand risk of maternal hyperglycemia on fetal outcome
	Manage weight to decrease long-term health risks
	Understand the importance of fetal surveillance (eg, kick counts, serial ultrasounds)
	GDM—Describe risk of developing type 2 diabetes postpartum; encourage lifestyle changes that lead to diabetes prevention
Healthy coping	Refer to childbirth education
	Understand the necessity of a higher degree of intensive care, including more frequent healthcare visits
	Obtain support and referral, as necessary
	Offer support and referral if needed
	Guide development of a positive and cooperative response to lifestyle changes; emphasize benefits to the baby
	GDM—Acknowledge common emotional reactions to the diagnosis: fear, anger, guilt

*These behaviors apply to all pregnant women with diabetes unless specified.

American Association of Diabetes Educators©

Healthy Eating

An individualized food plan is important to optimize blood glucose control. Medical nutrition therapy for preexisting diabetes in pregnancy has 4 important goals:

◆ Assist in appropriate gestational weight gain
◆ Avoid maternal ketosis
◆ Provide adequate nutrients for maternal and fetal health
◆ Minimize blood glucose excursions

Energy Requirements

Adequate calories are necessary to provide for fetal growth and to avoid ketonemia from either ketoacidosis or accelerated starvation ketosis in all pregnant women.[18,46] Adjustments to the food plan may be necessary to compensate for erratic blood glucose levels caused by fluctuating hormonal levels.

Carbohydrate Guidelines for Preexisting Diabetes

The amount and distribution of calories and carbohydrates are individualized and based on the woman's food preferences, blood glucose records, and physical activity level. Mealtime insulin must match the amount of mealtime carbohydrate to keep glucose levels in the target range before and after eating. Many women use an insulin-to-carbohydrate ratio to determine mealtime insulin. Since insulin requirements increase substantially during pregnancy, the insulin-to-carbohydrate ratio will change frequently during the second half of the pregnancy.

Being Active

The ADA recommends at least 150 minutes of moderate-intensity aerobic physical activity every week for persons with diabetes.[1] Regular exercise has been shown to improve blood glucose control, reduce cardiovascular risk factors, contribute to weight loss, and improve well-being. If there are no contraindications, pregnant women with diabetes are encouraged to participate in regular physical activity. Research indicates that regular physical activity during pregnancy aids in improved glycemic control and reduces the common discomforts of pregnancy, without a negative effect on the maternal or neonatal outcome.[27]

Diabetes, Pregnancy, and Physical Activity Self-Care Instructions

Diabetes education should include the following:

◆ Explain to the woman that, as with any physical activity for persons with diabetes, planning, adjustments, and education for safety are needed.
◆ Instruct the woman using insulin or oral glucose-lowering medications to always carry additional carbohydrate in case of hypoglycemia.
◆ Advise the woman to always carry a medical ID (such as a bracelet) which identifies her as having diabetes.
◆ Advise the woman to test her blood glucose before and after physical activity.
◆ Teach the woman to palpate her uterus during physical activity to detect contractions.
◆ Caution the woman against becoming dehydrated, overheated, tachycardic (heart rate >140 bpm), or dyspneic.
◆ Advise the woman of contraindications for physical activity in pregnancy, which include abnormally high or low blood glucose levels (see Table 24.10).[45]

Monitoring

Although there is a lack of agreement regarding precise glucose thresholds and timings, maintaining normal blood glucose levels remains the ultimate goal in the management of diabetes and pregnancy. Table 24.11 summarizes the range of plasma glucose targets recommended by the ADA, the ACOG, and other experts. Diabetes control is monitored through measurements of glycemic levels, ketones, and A1C as discussed below.[26]

Blood Glucose

Self-monitoring of blood glucose (SMBG) is needed pre- and postprandially in T1DP to evaluate the effectiveness of rapid-acting or short-acting insulin. No studies have specifically compared preprandial with postprandial blood glucose monitoring in T2DP. Studies in women with T1DP and GDM have shown that

TABLE 24.10 Physical Activity Guidelines for Pregnant Women With Preexisting Diabetes

- Discuss with healthcare provider to determine safety, type, and duration of the physical activity

- Get screened for proliferative retinopathy, neuropathy, and cardiovascular disease

- Monitor blood glucose levels before, during, and after physical activity

- Add carbohydrate if the glucose level before physical activity is <100 mg/dL (5.6 mmol/L) and the woman is taking insulin

- Avoid vigorous activity in the presence of ketones. However, physical activity does not need to be postponed if the woman feels well and urine and/or blood ketones are negative

- Be aware of immediate and prolonged hypoglycemia after the physical activity

- Carry a readily available form of glucose at all times to treat hypoglycemia, if necessary

- Avoid injecting insulin into an extremity to be used during exercising

- Avoid physical activity during peak insulin action times

- Learn to palpate uterus to detect contractions

Sources: Adapted from American Diabetes Association, "Standards of medical care in diabetes—2013," *Diabetes Care* 36 (2013): S11-66; JL Kitzmiller, L Jovanovic, F Brown, D Coustan, DM Reader, eds, *Managing Preexisting Diabetes and Pregnancy* (Alexandria, Va: American Diabetes Association, 2008); Academy of Nutrition and Dietetics, "Gestational diabetes mellitus evidence analysis project," Evidence Analysis Library (cited 2013 May 31), on the Internet at: http://www.andevidencelibrary.com; AM Thomas, YM Gutierrez, *American Dietetic Association Guide to Gestational Diabetes Mellitus* (Chicago, Ill: American Dietetic Association, 2005); American College of Obstetricians and Gynecologists: Committee on Obstetric Practice, ACOG Committee Opinion No. 267, "Exercise during pregnancy and the postpartum period," *Obstet Gynecol* 99, no. 1 (2002): 171-3; MW Carpenter, "The role of exercise in pregnant women with diabetes mellitus," *Clin Obstet Gynecol* 43 (2000): 56-64.

TABLE 24.11 Blood Glucose Goals in Normal and Preexisting Diabetes Pregnancy

	Daily Mean Glucose (mg/dL)	*Fasting, Premeal, Nighttime Glucose (mg/dL)*	*1 Hour Postprandial Glucose (mg/dL)*	*2 Hour Postprandial Glucose (mg/dL)*	*A1C (%)*
Normal pregnancy, mean ± SD					
Capillary glucose by meter	82.0 ± 5.8	69.3 ± 5.7	108.4 ± 6.0		5.0 ± 0.4
Continuous interstitial glucose	83.7 ± 18	76.6 ± 11.5	105.3 ± 12		
Preexisting diabetes					
Goals before and during early pregnancy	<125	60–119	100–149		<6.3
Goals during second and third trimesters	<110	60–99	<140	<120	<6.0

Sources: JL Kitzmiller, L Jovanovic, F Brown, D Coustan, DM Reader, eds, *Managing Preexisting Diabetes and Pregnancy* (Alexandria, Va: American Diabetes Association, 2008); American College of Obstetricians and Gynecologists, "Pregestational diabetes mellitus," ACOG Bulletin #60 2005 (reaffirmed 2010), *Obstet Gynecol* 105 (2005): 675-85; American Diabetes Association, "Preconception care of women with diabetes," *Diabetes Care* 26 Suppl 1 (2003): S91-3.

postprandial testing is more closely associated with a lower incidence of maternal and fetal complications. Blood glucose records are verified by the use of memory meters to help identify glucose patterns. Because alternate site testing may not identify rapid changes in blood glucose concentrations characteristic of pregnant women, finger-stick testing is best in pregnancy.[26]

Ketone Testing

Ketone testing is necessary during illness, weight loss, or a reduction in calorie intake caused by nausea and/or vomiting or if the blood glucose level is ≥180 mg/dL. The presence of ketones may indicate impending DKA. The woman should be instructed to contact her healthcare provider immediately if moderate or large ketones are present in her urine. Studies have demonstrated an association between elevated plasma ketone levels and poor glucose control with lower IQ scores in offspring.[47,48] In early pregnancy, a reduction in calorie intake caused by nausea and/or vomiting may be suggestive of starvation ketosis. A registered dietitian will need to evaluate the food plan to determine the appropriate calorie level.

A1C

The goal of A1C during preconception and the first trimester is to be at the lowest level possible without undue risk of hypoglycemia in the mother. Measurements of A1C may be obtained every 2 to 6 weeks, as A1C may significantly decrease within 2 weeks when compared with the baseline elevation.[26] Relatively mild elevations of A1C have been associated with increased fetal morbidity.[1]

Taking Medications

Euglycemia is the goal of a pregnancy complicated by diabetes. Combining medications with a food plan is necessary for the successful management of pregnancy and preexisting diabetes. This section describes medications used during pregnancy and precautions for use. Also see chapter 18, on pharmacologic therapies for glucose management.

Insulin and Insulin Analogs

The use of rapid-acting insulin analogs (lispro, aspart) in pregnancy has yielded results comparable to short-acting insulin.[49-54] In pregnancy, intensive insulin therapy requiring 3 or 4 injections is used to achieve the best glycemic control. One example of an insulin regimen in pregnancy is as follows:

- *Morning:* Intermediate- and rapid-acting or short-acting insulin and intermediate-acting insulin or detemir
- *Lunch:* Rapid-acting insulin
- *Dinner:* Rapid-acting or short-acting insulin
- *Bedtime:* Intermediate-acting insulin or detemir

Table 24.12 lists the FDA categories for drugs used in pregnancy. Long-acting insulin analogs, such as glargine and detemir, are used to provide basal coverage.

- *Glargine* is a long-acting insulin analog that provides a 24-hour peakless basal pattern.
- *Detemir* is another long-acting insulin analog. It is used in combination with short- or rapid-acting insulin and was recently upgraded to Category B. The basis of the upgrade was a trial involving 310 T1DP, of which half were randomized to detemir and the other half to NPH. Both groups achieved similar reductions in A1C, and the perinatal outcomes of the women on detemir were the same as the women on NPH.[55,56]

Insulin Requirements (Daily Dose)

Insulin requirements in pregnancy are based on current weight, gestational age, blood glucose monitoring results, and caloric intake. The total daily dose per kilogram per day has a different range in each trimester (see Table 24.13).

Pump Therapy

Continuous subcutaneous insulin infusion therapy delivers insulin in a pattern similar to the normal physiologic secretion of insulin. Insulin pump therapy lowers the amount of circulating basal insulin, thereby decreasing the incidence of premeal hypoglycemia while efficiently controlling the more dramatic rise in postprandial glucose common during pregnancy.[57] Other advantages of insulin pump therapy during pregnancy include more rapid and predictable insulin absorption, decreased severe hypoglycemia, enhanced lifestyle flexibility, and simplified morning sickness management.[58] Women continuing on insulin pump therapy after delivery

TABLE 24.12 FDA Categories of Glucose-Lowering Medications in Pregnancy

Category	Interpretation	Diabetes Medication
A	Adequate well-controlled studies in pregnant women have not shown an increased risk of abnormalities in any trimester of pregnancy.	
B	Animal studies have revealed no evidence of harm to the fetus; however, there are no adequate well-controlled studies in pregnant women. **OR** Animal studies have shown an adverse effect, but adequate well-controlled studies in pregnant women have failed to demonstrate a risk to the fetus in any trimester.	Lispro Aspart Detemir Regular NPH Glyburide Metformin
C	Animal studies have shown an adverse effect, and there are no adequate well-controlled studies in pregnant women. **OR** No animal studies have been conducted, and there are no adequate well-controlled studies in pregnant women.	Glulisine Glargine
D	Adequate well-controlled or observational studies in pregnant women have demonstrated a risk to the fetus. The benefits of therapy may outweigh the potential risk. For example, the drug may be acceptable if needed in a life-threatening situation or for a serious disease for which safer drugs cannot be used or are ineffective.	
X	Adequate well-controlled or observational studies in animals or pregnant women have demonstrated positive evidence of fetal abnormalities or risks. The use of the product is contraindicated in women who are or may become pregnant.	

TABLE 24.13 Insulin Requirements During Pregnancy

	Insulin (units/kg)
First trimester	0.7–0.8
Second trimester	0.8–1.0
Third trimester	0.9–1.2
With obesity (>150% of desirable body weight)	1.5–2.0, secondary to insulin resistance

Source: American College of Obstetricians and Gynecologists, "Pregestational diabetes mellitus," Practice bulletin No. 60, *Obstet Gynecol* 105 (2005): 680.

postpartum were shown to have significantly lower A1C levels 1 year after delivery compared to women receiving multiple daily injections of insulin.[59]

Pregnant women using insulin pumps must be highly motivated. Complications can arise, such as frequent and severe hyperglycemia, if there is an interruption in the delivery of insulin or an infection at the infusion site.[60]

Oral Glucose-Lowering Agents

Oral glucose-lowering agents are generally not recommended during pregnancy for women with preexisting diabetes. Traditionally, T2DP were switched to insulin for glycemic control. While glyburide and metformin are used in the treatment of GDM, a recent randomized controlled trial which compared the safety of metformin with that of insulin in T2DP showed no difference in glucose measure between the 2 groups, with significantly fewer episodes of hypoglycemia in the metformin group.[61]

Tocolytic Agents

Tocolytic agents such as ritodrine and terbutaline, used to treat premature labor, have been reported to cause deterioration of blood glucose control and ketosis in pregnant women with diabetes.[26] These agents should not be the first line of therapy for women with diabetes; if they are used, blood glucose levels must be carefully monitored.

Problem Solving

Pregnant women with preexisting diabetes who do not receive preconception care will need to learn self-management skills quickly to achieve and maintain euglycemia throughout the remainder of their pregnancies. Specifically, they must develop the flexibility to make adjustments to the care plan if they experience gastrointestinal discomforts during pregnancy. These adjustments include the following:

- Recognizing and treating hypoglycemic episodes
- Consistency in monitoring
- More frequent interactions with the healthcare team, including (1) discussing food plan adjustments with the registered dietitian, (2) follow-up diabetes education visits to assess self-management skills, and (3) when to contact the appropriate healthcare provider to discuss the plan of care

Nausea and vomiting occur more often during the first and early second trimesters and most frequently in the morning ("morning sickness"); however, a woman may experience these symptoms at any time during pregnancy. Hypoglycemia may occur if the woman is experiencing nausea and vomiting and is unable to eat. All pregnant women with diabetes should be instructed on sick-day rules and how to treat hypoglycemia, especially if on insulin or oral glucose-lowering medications. If vomiting occurs after taking a premeal rapid-acting or short-acting insulin dose, glucagon may be administered to help prevent hypoglycemia until the vomiting subsides. The woman should contact her healthcare provider if the vomiting becomes severe.[62]

Hyperemesis gravidarum is a severe and persistent form of nausea and vomiting characterized by weight loss, ketosis, dehydration, nutritional deficiencies, and electrolyte imbalance. Hospitalization for treatment, which could include rehydration, antiemetics, or enteral or parenteral nutrition, may be necessary to control the vomiting.

Reducing Risks of Diabetes Complications

Women with preexisting diabetes have a higher incidence of poor perinatal outcomes than women with GDM. If no preconception care occurs, hospitalization may be necessary to begin intensive diabetes control and education. Indications for hospitalization include the following:

- Hyperemesis
- Maternal hyperglycemia with ketones
- Noncompliance with previous instructions
- Obstetric complications, such as preeclampsia or preterm labor

Self-management skills reinforced or taught for the first time during pregnancy will have long-term benefits for the mother by establishing good habits that continue beyond the postpartum period. As glycemic levels remain within normal ranges, the woman's risk of developing long-term complications associated with diabetes is reduced.

Reducing risks also involves surveillance to assess the well-being of the fetus. The woman may be referred to other testing centers, such as genetics, for fetal assessment (see Table 24.14).

TABLE 24.14   Maternal and Fetal Testing

- Ultrasonography—provides an image of the fetal anatomy and estimates the delivery date.

- Nuchal translucency—an ultrasound that measures the fetal nuchal translucency thickness, which is the skin fold area behind the nape of the neck. This test is performed at 10–14 weeks' gestation and is a risk predictor for chromosomal abnormalities and congenital cardiac defects.

- Maternal serum alpha fetal protein—a test performed early in the second trimester which may indicate neural tube defect or Down syndrome in the fetus.

- Amniocentesis or chorionic villus sampling—invasive tests in which amniotic fluid is extracted for fetal analysis.

- Nonstress testing—measures fetal heart rate acceleration in response to fetal activity.

- Biophysical profile—a noninvasive test that combines an ultrasound with nonstress testing to measure fetal movement, heart rate, breathing rate, muscle tone, and amniotic fluid.

- Fetal kick counts—the mother keeps track of fetal activity by counting the number of kicks or movements within a certain time period.

Healthy Coping

Women with preexisting diabetes may feel overwhelmed and not be prepared for the degree of intensive care associated with pregnancy. This includes the occasional uncomfortableness of a growing fetus, interaction with a new healthcare provider or team (obstetrician and/or perinatal center), and more frequent healthcare visits and testing. Diabetes education will help the woman to emotionally prepare for more intensive care.

- *Changes to insulin regimen.* T1DP will have their insulin regimens changed several times during the pregnancy.
- *Injections.* T2DP may be resistant to more frequent monitoring or switching from oral agents to insulin injections.

A referral for childbirth education classes is helpful for the expectant mother to learn about the physical and emotional changes of pregnancy. The usual topics of discussion in childbirth classes include labor and delivery, relaxation, breathing techniques, and medical interventions.

See chapter 9 for more information on addressing barriers to self-management. If a woman is not able to cope, a referral to a psychologist or social worker who understands diabetes is recommended.

Diabetes Care During Labor and Delivery

The key to successful intrapartum management is to monitor blood glucose levels frequently and administer insulin and glucose as necessary. The following is an example of a regimen used to manage blood glucose levels during labor and delivery:

1. Administer the usual dose of intermediate-acting insulin at bedtime.
2. Withhold the morning dose of insulin and begin an intravenous infusion of normal saline.
3. Once active labor begins or the glucose level decreases to less than 70 mg/dL (3.9 mmol/L), change the infusion to dextrose to keep blood glucose levels below 110 mg/dL (6.1 mmol/L).[21] The rate of dextrose administered is 2.0 to 2.5 mg per kilogram per minute.

4. Measure maternal blood glucose values every hour.
5. Administer insulin by continuous intravenous infusion as necessary to maintain euglycemia and help prevent neonatal hypoglycemia.[19]

Postpartum Care

After the birth of her infant, the mother with diabetes will face new challenges. Her focus and attention will shift from self-care to caring for her baby. Postpartum care and education should begin prior to her hospital discharge. This time can be used to review the self-management skills learned during pregnancy and continued later at home.

After the woman has been at home with her infant for a couple of weeks, a follow-up phone call by a diabetes educator is appropriate. About 6 weeks after delivery, the woman should have a scheduled office visit with both the diabetes educator and the registered dietitian. Topics for education include the following:

- Glycemic control with decreasing insulin requirements
- More frequent SMBG
- Balancing infant care with self-care for the new mother
- Postpartum depression and stress
- Readjusting the insulin regimen or resuming oral glucose-lowering medications
- Readjusting the food plan, whether breastfeeding or not
- Weight loss or weight management
- Family planning and contraception (refer to Table 24.6)

Lactation

Unless contraindicated, breastfeeding should be strongly encouraged in women with diabetes. Women with type 2 diabetes may be switched from insulin to oral glucose-lowering medication. Key education points on lactation and diabetes are the following:

- *Insulin:* Breastfeeding mothers may require less insulin because of the calories expended during nursing. The insulin dosage will vary and may need to be frequently readjusted. A small snack either before or during breastfeeding may help to avoid hypoglycemia and frequent dosage adjustments.

* *Oral glucose-lowering medications:* Glipizide, glyburide, metformin, and acarbose are considered compatible with breastfeeding.[26,63]
* *Monitoring:* Breastfeeding mothers may need more frequent SMBG because of hypoglycemic episodes.

Gestational Diabetes Mellitus

Gestational diabetes mellitus is defined as any degree of glucose intolerance with onset or first recognition during pregnancy.[1] It affects about 7% of all pregnancies.[64] The potential to develop diabetes during pregnancy is associated with risk factors that are similar to the risk of developing type 2 diabetes (see Categories of Increased Risk for Developing GDM).

Gestational diabetes mellitus primarily develops in the second half of pregnancy. Women at high risk for developing GDM should be tested for undiagnosed type 2 diabetes, using the usual testing methods as described in chapter 13 of this book. If diagnosed with type 2 diabetes, they will need immediate treatment to normalize glucose levels, as discussed earlier in this chapter. All women, except those diagnosed with pre-existing diabetes, should be screened for abnormal glucose tolerance between 24 and 28 weeks of pregnancy.

Categories of Increased Risk for Developing GDM

* Women who are older
* Women who are heavier
* Women who have delivered a large-for-gestational-age infant
* Women with a history of glucose intolerance
* Women with a family history of diabetes
* Women with a history of polycystic ovary syndrome

* Women of certain ethnicities (highest risk listed first): Native American, Hispanic, Asian or Chinese descent, African American, Non-Hispanic white.[64]

Risk Assessment

In recent years, the incidence of obesity and diabetes in women of childbearing age has increased, leading to more pregnant women with type 2 diabetes and women entering pregnancy with undiagnosed diabetes. Poor glucose control in the first trimester can lead to congenital anomalies and other complications of pregnancy. To address this issue, the concept of risk assessment at the first prenatal visit was proposed in 1997 at the Fourth International Workshop-Conference on Gestational Diabetes Mellitus.[65] The risk assessment determines who is screened for GDM and at what time during the pregnancy. Table 24.15 shows the risk categories, characteristics, and the timing of glucose testing to be considered at the first prenatal visit.

Recommendations on Screening and Diagnosis of GDM

The diagnosis and screening recommendations for GDM have changed several times since the original criteria were accepted at the First International Conference-Workshop on GDM in 1979. Beginning in 2001, the ADA and the ACOG recommended the 2-step method using the Carpentar-Coustan criteria for all women between 24 and 28 weeks' gestation.

In January 2011, the ADA accepted the recommendations of the International Association of Diabetes and Pregnancy Study Group (IADPSG) to revise the diagnostic criteria for GDM, based on the results of the Hyperglycemia and Adverse Pregnancy Outcome (HAPO) study.[66] In September 2011, the ACOG did not accept the IADPSG recommendations.[67] In March 2013, the National Institutes of Health held the Consensus Conference on the Diagnosis of Gestational Diabetes. The consensus panel concluded there is insufficient evidence to adopt a 1-step approach, such as that proposed by the IADPSG, and recommended the continuation of the 2-step approach.[68]

TABLE 24.15	Risk Assessment at First Prenatal Visit	
Risk Category	*Characteristics*	*Timing of Glucose Testing*
High risk	History of large infant History of glucose intolerance or GDM BMI ≥30 Strong family history of type 2 diabetes High-risk ethnic group Polycystic ovary syndrome (PCOS)	Test for type 2 diabetes using accepted diagnostic criteria at first prenatal visit (see chapter 13) If normal at first prenatal visit, then glucose challenge test (GCT) between 24 and 28 weeks
Normal risk	Does not fit other categories	GCT between 24 and 28 weeks; if positive results then perform 100-g oral glucose tolerance test
Low risk	<25 years of age No history of poor obstetrical outcome No first-degree family history of diabetes Normal weight or underweight Low-risk ethnic group	Not routinely screened Screened based on clinician assessment

Currently in the United States, there are 2 methods to diagnose GDM: the 2-step approach using the 100-g oral glucose tolerance test (OGTT) and the 1-step approach using the 75-g OGTT. The US Preventive Services Task Force (USPSTF) recommends screening for GDM in asymptomatic pregnant women after 24 weeks of gestation.[69]

2-Step Approach: Using 100-g OGTT

The first step is a 50-g glucose challenge test (GCT) given at any time of the day. The cutoff for the 1-hour test is not clear. The ACOG recommends that healthcare providers select either ≥135 or ≥140 mg/dL (7.2 or 7.8 mmol/L) as a single consistent cutoff based on factors such as community prevalence rates.[3] If the result 1 hour later is greater than the cutoff, then the second step, a 100-g OGTT, is scheduled. The woman reports to the lab, having fasted for at least 8 hours and having consumed a normal carbohydrate load of at least 150 g for 3 days. Blood is drawn at fasting and at 1, 2, and 3 hours. The woman cannot smoke, is required to stay seated and resting, and may drink only water, if necessary. The diagnosis of GDM is made when 2 or more of the 4 values are equal to or greater than the criteria in Table 24.16.

TABLE 24.16	Current Methods to Diagnose GDM	
	100-g OGTT 2 abnormal values needed for diagnosis	*75-g OGTT 1 abnormal value needed for diagnosis*
Fasting	≥95 mg/dL (5.3 mmol/L)	≥92 mg/dL (5.1 mmol/L)
1 hour	≥180 mg/dL (10.0 mmol/L)	≥180 mg/dL (10.0 mmol/L)
2 hour	≥155 mg/dL (8.6 mmol/L)	≥153 mg/dL (8.5 mmol/L)
3 hour	≥140 mg/dL (7.8 mmol/L)	

1-Step Approach: Using 75-g OGTT

Following the same criteria for a 2-step OGTT, the woman reports to the lab, having fasted for at least 8 hours and having consumed a normal carbohydrate load of at least 150 g for 3 days. Blood is drawn at fasting and at 1 and 2 hours. The diagnosis of GDM is made when 1 or more of 3 values is equal to or greater than the criteria in Table 24.16.

Case—Part 1: A Pregnancy With GDM

MA had a number of risk factors for GDM:

- She is a member of a high-risk ethnic group.

- She is both older and overweight.

- She has a history of a large-for-gestational-age infant.

- Her mother and grandmother had type 2 diabetes.

At MA's first prenatal appointment, her obstetrician determined she was at high risk for GDM and might have undiagnosed diabetes. After her appointment, MA went to the lab for a 50-g GCT. At 1 hour, a blood glucose level was drawn, which was 123 mg/dL. With a glucose value of less than 140 mg/dL, MA passed the screening test but needed to be rescreened between the 24th and 28th week of pregnancy. MA was concerned and wanted to control her weight gain better during pregnancy.

The GCT was repeated at 26 weeks and the result was 155 mg/dL (8.6 mmol/L), which was abnormal. She returned within a week for the 3-hour, 100-g OGTT. Her results are shown in the table.

Blood Glucose After 100 g of Glucose	Criteria: 2 or More Results Equal to or Greater Than:	MA's Test Results
Fasting	95 mg/dL (5.3 mmol/L)	93 mg/dL (5.2 mmol/L)
1 hour	180 mg/dL (10.0 mmol/L)	210 mg/dL (11.7 mmol/L)
2 hour	155 mg/dL (8.6 mmol/L)	176 mg/dL (9.8 mmol/L)
3 hour	140 mg/dL (7.8 mmol/L)	132 mg/dL (7.3 mmol/L)

MA was diagnosed with GDM because at least 2 of the 4 tests were equal to or greater than the diagnostic criteria. The OGTT determines the diagnosis; however, it is interesting to ask whether the OGTT also predicts her course with GDM. There appears to be a continuous relationship between increasing maternal glycemia and morbidities of pregnancy, so the higher the number the greater the likelihood MA will need insulin therapy.

Case—Part 2: Clinical Outcomes and Initial Therapy

What clinical outcomes needed to be set for MA? Glucose control was primary as blood glucose levels within the normal range help prevent macrosomia and a large-for-gestational-age infant, as MA had in her last pregnancy.

- *Self-monitoring.* MA was taught SMBG and asked to test her fasting and after meals.

- *Weight gain.* MA needed to control weight gain. With a BMI of 27, her weight gain target for the pregnancy was 15 to 25 lb.

- *Ketone testing.* She was asked to test her urine for ketones. She would be eating both fewer

carbohydrates in an attempt to control glucose and fewer calories to control weight gain, yet not so few as to develop starvation ketosis.

- *Records.* She needed to eat a healthy diet, so she was asked to record her food intake as well as blood glucose values; these records would be assessed at a follow-up visit in 1 or 2 weeks.

Because MA's fasting result on the OGTT was less than 95 mg/dL (5.3 mmol/L), initial therapy for GDM was MNT.

Case—Part 3: Self-management Education Begins

MA's healthcare provider referred her to the diabetes education center. Her first appointment was within a week of diagnosis, at 29 weeks' gestation.

The diabetes educator discovered that MA was very motivated to follow through with the protocol. Because

her mother and grandmother had diabetes, she was familiar with blood glucose monitoring, as well as how to inject insulin. MA was surprised that her blood glucose targets were so much lower than the blood glucose values she saw her family members obtain. She was instructed

Case—Part 3: Self-management Education Begins (continued)

to record her blood glucose test results 4 times per day on her food record form and test her urine for ketones every other morning.

- *Healthy eating.* MA was very motivated to change her diet. She stopped drinking regular soda after she was diagnosed with GDM. She readily admitted that she likes to eat but could cut back on the fat in her diet.

- *Being active.* MA was physically active at work. She was busy at home with her family but did not intentionally walk or exercise. MA considered whether a

daily walk after dinner would be beneficial to her glucose control and desire to control weight gain.

- *Behavior-change goals.* MA and her diabetes team set up 3 behavior-change goals at the first visit:

  1. Test blood glucose every morning before breakfast and 1 hour after the start of each meal

  2. Follow the food plan; count carbohydrates and record food intake

  3. Test urine ketones every other morning

Case—Part 4: Focus on the Food Plan

To help MA understand and quickly begin using the food plan, the registered dietitian (RD) worked with her to create a sample 1-day intake that incorporates the changes suggested in this chapter. The RD assessed that MA would be capable of learning carbohydrate counting. The food plan gave a suggested starting range of carbohydrate choices based on the sample food plan they

developed together. MA was instructed to record all of the food and beverages she consumed during the next week and return in 1 week. The chart below shows a typical day's intake for MA on the left and the new food plan and sample menu on the right. Also shown below is a table summarizing the RD's recommendations for modifying MA's food intake.

Typical Day	*Typical Day's Intake*	*New Food Plan*	*Sample Menu*
Breakfast, 9 AM	Cornflakes, whole milk, fruit, coffee	*Breakfast, 9* AM *(2 carb choices)*	Slice of toast with peanut butter, 1 c 1% milk
		Snack, 11 AM *(1–2 carb choices)*	A piece of fruit
Lunch, 1 PM	Hamburger or sandwich, fries or chips, and 20-oz regular soda from a fast-food restaurant near work	*Lunch, 1* PM *(4 carb choices)*	Sandwich, fruit, small container (6-oz.) light yogurt
		Snack, 4 PM *(1–2 carb choices)*	Carrots, ¼ c peanuts
Dinner, 8 PM	Traditional Mexican dinner of 4 tortillas made with rice, beans, chicken	*Dinner, 8* PM *(4–5 carb choices)*	2 rice-and-bean tortillas, chicken strips, salad, 1 c 1% milk
		Bedtime snack, 11 PM *(1–2 carb choices)*	1 tortilla with cheese, ½ c juice

(continued)

American Association of Diabetes Educators©

Case—Part 4: Focus on the Food Plan (continued)

Summary of Dietitian's Recommendations for Modifying MA's Food Intake

Topic	MA's Typical Intake	Recommendations
Number of meals and snacks	3 meals, no snacks More than 12 hours between dinner and breakfast the next morning	Add morning and afternoon snacks Add bedtime snack to avoid so many hours without food
Intake of high-carbohydrate foods	Drinks regular soda Does not eat desserts (eg, cookies, ice cream, pastries, candy) regularly	Discontinue regular soda May have 1–2 diet sodas per day Good she does not have a sweet tooth
Total amount of carbohydrate at each meal and snack	Breakfast about 4 carbs Lunch about 8 carbs Dinner about 8 carbs	Reduce total carbs per meal; try 3–4 carbs per meal and test postmeal; add snacks
Estimate of calorie intake and weight-gain goal	Has gained 10 lb BMI category: overweight	Weight gain seems on track Gain 1/2 lb per week Weight gain goal 15–25 lb
Fat content of diet	Uses whole milk Prepares tortillas and beans with lard	Reduce fat content of milk to 2%, 1%, or skim Cook using monounsaturated oil; use less oil/fat
Anticipation of potential problems	Cornflakes at breakfast Fast foods	Avoid processed cereal at breakfast Avoid fast foods if postmeal reading is too high
Adequate nutrition in all food groups	Fruit: 1 serving per day Milk: on cereal only Protein: 2 servings per day Vegetables: at dinner	Increase fruit intake; add between meals or at lunch Increase milk to 3–4 servings per day; drink milk instead of soda Protein intake adequate Add another serving of vegetables with lunch or between meals

Case—Part 5: Therapy Evolves as Pregnancy Progresses

Medical Nutrition Therapy

At 30 weeks' gestation, MA had her follow-up visit with the diabetes educators, 1 week after her initial visit. The diabetes educators assessed her progress and discussed the following points[14]:

- What her glucose levels were and how often she met her target levels

- How often she was able to follow her meal plan

- Whether she felt confident in her ability to count carbohydrates

- How often she found her hunger satisfied

- How happy she was with her weight gain

- What her urine ketone results had been

Case—Part 5: Therapy Evolves as Pregnancy Progresses (continued)

Most of MA's blood glucose readings were on target. The glucose readings that were too high were explained by errors in counting carbohydrates. She understood the errors and was willing to adjust her food intake. All elevated postmeal glucose readings were after the dinner meal. MA and her educators agreed that adding a daily walk after dinner would help postmeal glucose control. Her weight did not change and all ketone tests were negative. The RD's overall assessment was that the food plan would provide for MA's calorie needs and satisfy her appetite.

Exercise Prescription

The diabetes care team provided MA guidance on implementing a safe physical activity plan that could help her manage her blood glucose level after meals. MA agreed to start with a daily walk after dinner.

Behavior Change

Like other women with gestational diabetes, MA had to learn and implement diabetes self-management in a very short period of time.

Case—Part 6: Achieving Glucose Control

At 33 Weeks

MA returned to her healthcare provider with food, blood glucose, and ketone records. Her weight was 167, up 1 lb. She was comfortable with her food plan, and all blood glucose values were in target range.

At 36 Weeks

MA had her final visit for GDM management. She had done well and was happy with her blood glucose values.

The educator discussed her risk for developing diabetes postpartum and explained the strategies for diabetes prevention. MA had made many changes in her eating and activity habits that she planned to continue after delivery. She saw GDM as an opportunity to make changes that improved the health of her whole family. Now she was looking forward to delivery.

Case Wrap-up

At 39½ weeks, MA delivered an 8 lb 2 oz (3685 grams) baby boy. Baby M's blood glucose was tested at 1 hour, and it was 70 mg/dL (3.9 mmol/L). He started breastfeeding and could stay with his mother in her room. During her hospital stay, MA's fasting blood glucose level was tested the day after delivery. It was in the normal range. When she left the hospital, she was instructed to continue testing her blood glucose levels once a week—fasting and 2 hours after eating—and to return in 6 weeks for an evaluation of glucose control.

At her 6-week postpartum visit, all blood glucose values were within the normal (nonpregnant) range: fasting <100 mg/dL (5.5 mmol/L) and 2 hour <140 mg/dL (7.8 mmol/L). To confirm that she did not have diabetes,

her healthcare provider ordered a 75-g OGTT. MA's test results were in the normal range. She continued with her food plan, walked every evening with her husband, and remained pleased to have lost 6 lb; she was feeling great. Her healthcare provider discussed her risk of getting type 2 diabetes and supported the excellent lifestyle changes she had already made. MA was instructed to return annually for a blood glucose test.

MA was told that if she becomes pregnant again, her risk for developing GDM again is 30% to 65%.[9] She was also made aware of factors that increase her risk: the amount of weight gained between pregnancies, hip-to-waist ratio, and diet composition.

Complications of GDM

Recent research has described a strong continuous association between maternal glucose concentrations and perinatal complications, even at glucose levels below the current diagnosis of GDM.[70] GDM primarily develops in the second half of pregnancy and is not associated with the risk for congenital anomalies that occur with preexisting diabetes. Hyperglycemia in the second trimester is associated with an increased risk for macrosomia, cesarean section, difficult delivery, and neonatal hypoglycemia. Explanations of these complications are found earlier in the chapter.

AADE7™ in GDM

This section highlights the unique guidelines and recommendations for gestational diabetes. The reader should refer to Table 24.9 that describes the goals for all pregnancies.

Healthy Eating for GDM

Carbohydrate Guidelines for Gestational Diabetes The Evidence-Based GDM Nutrition Practice Guidelines of the Academy of Nutrition and Dietetics suggest dividing carbohydrate intake into 3 small-to-moderate meals with 2 to 4 snacks.[27] This eating pattern accommodates the pregnant woman well because the amount of food tolerated at a time decreases as the pregnancy progresses. An initial food plan would suggest the following carbohydrate ranges for each meal and snack:

- ◆ *Breakfast:* 15 to 45 g
- ◆ *Lunch and dinner:* 45 to 75 g each
- ◆ *Snacks:* 15 to 45 g

The most difficult blood glucose level to manage is the postbreakfast value, due to higher hormonal levels in the morning. Consensus is to restrict carbohydrate at breakfast time to 15 to 45 g.[27] Breakfast cereals are often discouraged, as the total amount of carbohydrate is higher than 45 g and postmeal blood glucose levels are higher than with other food choices. The glycemic index may help explain why some foods produce higher postmeal glucose levels. Highly processed breakfast cereals, sweetened beverages, fast foods, and pizza are frequently found to raise postmeal levels higher than less processed, higher fiber foods with the same amount of total carbohydrate. However, the total amount of carbohydrate is more significant than the type of carbohydrate, and controlling the amount of rice, pasta, potato, and other starches is the most important initial message to the patient.[71,72]

As women with GDM learn about controlling their carbohydrate intake to manage their blood glucose levels, they may unintentionally decrease their nutrient-rich carbohydrates such as fruit, dairy, and starches. Diabetes educators and healthcare providers should review the food record and analyze the number of servings of fruit, milk or dairy, and grains to ensure an adequate intake. It is a common practice to shift milk and fruit to snack time so that a more normal portion of starch can be consumed during meals.

Being Active for GDM

Just as physical activity improves glucose tolerance in type 2 diabetes, it also improves glucose control in GDM. If there are no contraindications for physical activity (see Table 24.5), women with GDM should undertake 30 minutes per day of low-impact activity.

Monitoring for GDM

Glucose Monitoring Monitoring fasting and postmeal glycemic levels is recommended for women with GDM. Recommended glucose targets for both 1 hour and 2 hours postmeal are provided in the Table 24.17, but the rationale for choosing 1 hour or 2 hours is not given. Recent research using continuous glucose monitoring indicates that the peak glucose is reached 80 minutes after eating.[73,74] There is no research regarding the frequency of testing. As previously stated, the goal is to achieve euglycemia, and whatever amount of testing is needed to achieve that goal is recommended.

Ketone Testing The presence of ketones with normal or low blood glucose levels is suggestive of starvation ketosis and usually indicates an inadequate food intake. Positive ketone results may help assess whether the woman with GDM is eating insufficient calories to control her postmeal glucose levels.

A1C The A1C test is the standard for overall glucose control, but its role in GDM is not clear. However, the A1C may be used in women diagnosed with GDM in the first trimester.

TABLE 24.17	Target Plasma Glucose in Gestational Diabetes Pregnancy		
Testing Time	*5th International Conference on GDM[1]*	*ADA[2]*	*ACOG[3]*
Fasting	≤95 mg/dL (5.3 mmol/L)	≤95 mg/dL (5.3 mmol/L)	60–90 mg/dL (3.3–5.0 mmol/L)
Before meals			60–105 mg/dL (3.3–5.8 mmol/L)
1 hour	≤140 mg/dL (7.8 mmol/L)	≤140 mg/dL (7.8 mmol/L)	
2 hour	≤120 mg/dL (6.7 mmol/L)	≤120 mg/dL (6.7 mmol/L)	At or below 120 mg/dL (6.7 mmol/L)

Sources:

1. Metzger BE, Coustan DR, eds. Proceedings of the Fifth International Workshop-Conference on Gestational Diabetes Mellitus. Diabetes Care. 2007;30 Suppl 2:S254.
2. American Diabetes Association. Clinical Practice Recommendations 2014. Diabetes Care. 2014;37 Suppl 1:S14-80.
3. Landon MB, Gabbe SG. Gestational diabetes mellitus. Obstet Gynecol. 2011;118:1386.

Taking Medication for GDM

Euglycemia is the goal of a pregnancy complicated by diabetes. Some women with GDM are able to use MNT alone for glucose management. Depending on the population, 10% to 50% of women with GDM will need additional pharmacologic therapy for glucose management.[72] This section describes medications used for managing GDM. Also see the section on taking medications for preexisting diabetes.

Insulin Therapy in GDM

Insulin therapy is still the preferred treatment when endogenous insulin production is inadequate. There is no one insulin regimen that has been shown to be the most effective in managing women with GDM. Rapid-acting insulin analogs and NPH insulin are the most commonly used types of insulin in a GDM pregnancy.[75] See the section Insulin and Insulin Analogs earlier in this chapter.

There is no protocol for starting insulin therapy in GDM; the ADA position statement recommends that SMBG guide the doses and timing of the insulin regimen.[76] Many women who need insulin during pregnancy require basal insulin coverage with NPH insulin twice daily, or 1 injection if using detemir. Insulin resistance continues to increase dramatically during the third trimester, which means insulin doses need to be adjusted weekly until about 36 to 37 weeks of pregnancy. The dose of insulin at delivery is about 1.0 units per kilogram.[77]

Noninsulin Therapies for GDM

Glyburide   Historically, adding insulin was the only option for the woman with GDM. In 2000, the *New England Journal of Medicine* published an article that compared glyburide and insulin in women with gestational diabetes.[78] Langer demonstrated that the oral hypoglycemic agent glyburide is a clinically effective alternative to insulin. Sulfonylurea drugs were not used in pregnancy because of concern about teratogenicity and neonatal hypoglycemia. Glyburide was not detected in the cord serum of any infants in the glyburide group, eliminating worries that the drug would cause fetal problems. Since then, other studies have reported successful management of GDM using glyburide therapy.[79] Glyburide (Diabeta®, Glynase® PresTab®, Micronase®) is a second-generation sulfonylurea that stimulates the pancreas to produce more insulin. Starting doses are 2.5 mg once or twice a day; maximum dose is 20 mg. Many healthcare providers do not use glyburide therapy for women with GDM.

Metformin   Since glyburide has been successfully used in the management of GDM, there has been interest in the use of metformin. One study, the Metformin Versus Insulin for the Treatment of Gestational Diabetes, found that metformin was not associated with an increase in perinatal complications compared with insulin.[80] At this time, the ADA and the ACOG have not yet recommended use of this oral agent in pregnancy.[1,81]

Diabetes medications not recommended during pregnancy include thiazolidinediones, DPP-4 Inhibitors, and GLP-1 Agonists.

Healthy Coping

Although GDM is short-lived, major lifestyle changes during the middle of pregnancy can be stressful and emotional. A number of issues related to diabetes self-management can occur, and the diabetes educator should look for and address these. Some common feelings and issues are listed below:

◆ *Guilt:* Many women feel guilty or embarrassed because they are overweight and know their food habits are not what they should be.
◆ *Anger:* Some women may be angry that they have to change their lifestyle through diet, monitoring, and self-injections.
◆ *Fear:* Many women are fearful of insulin injections and may withhold or manipulate data about elevated blood glucose levels and food intake.

Postpartum Follow-up After GDM

Women with a history of GDM should be screened for diabetes 6 to 12 weeks after delivery using the 75-g OGTT for nonpregnant individuals.[1] If the results are normal, testing should be repeated at 3-year intervals. More frequent testing may be considered depending on the initial results and risk status (see Table 24.18).

The Academy of Nutrition and Dietetics recommends postpartum weight loss in women with previous GDM who are overweight or obese. Research indicates that the risks of recurrent GDM or development of type 2 diabetes can be reduced with weight loss.[27] The prevalence of GDM is higher in women with high BMIs or who have gained weight between pregnancies.

All women should be actively encouraged to breastfeed their infants during the first year of life.[75] Breastfeeding has been associated with decreasing the woman's risk of becoming overweight later in life and developing metabolic syndrome and type 2 diabetes.[82]

TABLE 24.18   Criteria for the Diagnosis of Diabetes
1. A1C ≥6.5% **OR**
2. FPG (fasting plasma glucose) ≥126 mg/dL (7.0 mmol/L) **OR**
3. 2-hour OGTT ≥200mg/dL (11.1 mmol/L) using a 75-g glucose load* **OR**
4. RPG (random plasma glucose) ≥200 mg/dL (11.1 mmol/L)

*In the absence of unequivocal hyperglycemia, criteria 1 should be confirmed by repeat testing.

Source: American Diabetes Association, "Standards of medical care in diabetes, 2013," *Diabetes Care* 36 Suppl 1 (2013): S13.

Focus on Education: Preexisting Diabetes and Pregnancy

Key Points

⟳ **Preconception counseling has become the key for good perinatal outcomes.** An increasing number of women are developing type 2 diabetes during their childbearing years. Growing, too, is the number of women with type 1 diabetes desiring to have children.

⟳ **Encourage the woman to see herself as a vital part of the multidisciplinary team.** The woman's willingness to work together with the other members of the healthcare team before and during her pregnancy can result in an improved outcome.

Teaching Strategies

The diabetes educator has many opportunities to make important contributions during a woman's pregnancy and to assist her in planning for motherhood.

From preconception to postpartum care, the mother and her infant will benefit from the diabetes educator's involvement.

⟳ **Relieve the stress.** Diabetes educators are pivotal in helping coordinate the woman's care to decrease the anxiety and stress of the mother-to-be. Women with preexisting diabetes may be concerned about preterm delivery or their infants having major malformations.

⟳ **Set attainable goals during the pregnancy.** Attending to the immediate issues of glycemic control, pregnancy care, and diabetes self-management, the educator assists the woman in establishing achievable goals for the pregnancy. As the pregnancy progresses, the educator and the woman (family also, if needed) will frequently review the goals and revise if necessary.

⊘ **Develop the opportunity to improve the woman's long-term health.** The educator helps the woman establish goals and habits that can last beyond pregnancy and childbearing—the woman gains knowledge that can be of value in subsequent pregnancies and lowers her risk of long-term complications.

Messages for Patients

Motivation is key to the success of a good outcome in pregnancy.

⊘ **Expect more intense care and monitoring requirements.** In pregnancy complicated by diabetes, additional testing and monitoring may be necessary during the pregnancy. Glycemic control within the optimal range is necessary to decrease the risk of congenital malformations and spontaneous abortions. Periodic adjustments in insulin dosage and food intake may require more frequent SMBG.

⊘ **Pay attention to food plans and weight gain.** Weight gain goals will be established based on the IOM recommendations. Medical nutrition therapy will be based on current eating habits and the DRIs for pregnant women.

⊘ **Expect changes in medication.** Medication therapy changes frequently during pregnancy as hormones impact insulin needs. Therapies also change at delivery and in the postpartum phase.

⊘ **Breastfeed to attain immunological benefits.** Breastfeeding is encouraged because of the immunological benefits to the mother and infant. Lactation may be delayed because of early separation of the infant; however, pumping the breasts soon after delivery can establish a steady milk supply.

Focus on Education: GDM

Teaching Strategies

⊘ **Enable timely initial visits.** See new patients as soon as possible, within 1 week of referral.

⊘ **Involve team in glucose goals.** Achieve target glucose control as quickly as possible, within the context of a healthy pregnancy; get to know team members in obstetrics-gynecology, endocrinology, and family medicine and involve them in agreeing on targets, curriculum handouts, and content.

⊘ **Take action and offer support.** Women with GDM need more support than the person with type 1 diabetes or type 2 diabetes, as there is so much to learn and implement in just a few weeks.

⊘ **Offer hope for a healthy future.** Present the information that implementing lifestyle changes now may lead to diabetes prevention as well as reduce an individual's chances of developing other chronic diseases, including cardiovascular disease.

⊘ **Model the lifestyle.** Consider how you and your team can best model positive approaches to lifestyle changes intended to lead to diabetes prevention and a reduction in obesity, cardiovascular disease, and cancer.

Messages for Patients

⊘ **Use your diabetes team.** Educators, clinicians, and specialty services are available to help you in any way to understand and manage GDM.

⊙ **Manage GDM.** Good control balances glucose control with the goals of a healthy pregnancy.

⊙ **Be comfortable with insulin.** Do not be afraid of adding insulin, as it is a hormone your body makes, not a drug; during the pregnancy, you may need extra insulin, via injection, to keep blood sugar under control.

⊙ **Guard your own health after delivery.** Knowing you had GDM is a clear signal that you are at risk for developing diabetes. Take steps to prevent diabetes by improving your eating and exercise habits and maintaining an appropriate weight after your baby is born. These healthy habits will not only help you but help your whole family.

Health Literacy for Pregnancy with Preexisting Diabetes or GDM

⊙ **Health literacy is defined as the degree to which individuals have the capacity to obtain, process, and understand basic health information and the services needed to make appropriate health decisions.**[83] It includes the ability to interpret health information presented by healthcare providers and to make decisions based on an understanding of the information.[84] If patients lack the necessary skills to understand what is said or written, it could result in a negative impact on their health. The American Medical Association considers poor health literacy as a stronger predictor of a person's health than age, income, employment status, education level, and race.[85]

⊙ **Although health literacy is not necessarily based on reading ability, reading ability is of particular concern in persons with low literacy skills, especially women of childbearing age.** If a woman has difficulty understanding the information or following directions, this may affect either her health or the health of her child. Women with diabetes may be even more vulnerable to poorer outcomes if they are unaware of the health consequences associated with diabetes and pregnancy. Low health literacy in pregnant women with preexisting diabetes may affect birth outcome. In a study of 74 pregnant women with preexisting diabetes, those with low functional literacy were less likely to have received preconception care.[86]

⊙ **The ACOG recommends the following general health literacy guidelines when working with women:**
- Tailor speaking and listening skills to individual patients.
- Tailor the health information to the intended user.
- Develop written materials that keep the message simple.

Focus on Practice

⊙ **When providing education and care for pregnant women with preexisting diabetes or gestational diabetes, be sure to establish good relationships with the obstetrics department.**
- Diabetes educators who work with pregnant women with diabetes are, in most cases, already working with individuals with type 1 diabetes or type 2 diabetes. They probably have good relationships with clinicians who work in primary care, internal medicine, and endocrinology.
- Work together to agree on the referral process, the method of documentation, and the message that communication is important for consistent care for the patient.

⊘ **Include comprehensive preconception, prenatal, postpartum, and interconception self-management education as part of your program.**
- Be prepared to discuss preconception care with your type 1 diabetes or type 2 diabetes patients.
- Consider multicultural concerns for GDM, type 1 diabetes, or being pregnant with type 2 diabetes.

- Provide appropriate care during the postpartum period (ie, breastfeeding and nutritional and insulin management, taking medication); provide referrals for pediatricians, endocrinologists, and other providers involved in preconception, prenatal, postpartum, and interconception care.
- Work with service providers such as WIC or other social services to coordinate appropriate care.

References

1. American Diabetes Association. Standards of medical care in diabetes, 2014. Diabetes Care. 2014;37 Suppl 1:S14-80.

2. Engelgau MM, Herman WH, Smith PJ, et al. The epidemiology of diabetes and pregnancy in the US, 1988. Diabetes Care. 1995;18:1029-33.

3. American College of Obstetricians and Gynecologists. Committee Opinion Number 504. Screening and diagnosis of gestational diabetes mellitus. Obstet Gynecol. 2013;122:406-15.

4. Hartling L, Dryden DM, Guthrie A, et al. Screening and Diagnosing Gestational Diabetes Mellitus. Evidence Report/Technology Assessment No. 210. AHRQ Publication No. 12(13)-E021-EF. Rockville, MD: Agency for Healthcare Research and Quality; 2012.

5. Koos BJ, Moore PJ. Maternal physiology during pregnancy. In: DeCherney AH, Nathan L, eds. Current Obstetric and Gynecologic Diagnosis and Treatment. New York: Lange Medical Books/McGraw-Hill; 2003:154-62.

6. Institute of Medicine. Weight Gain During Pregnancy: Reexamining the Guidelines. Washington, DC: National Academy Press; 2009.

7. American College of Obstetricians and Gynecologists. Committee Opinion Number 549. Obesity in pregnancy. Obstet Gynecol. 2013;121:213-7.

8. Franz MJ, Evert AB. American Diabetes Association Guide to Nutrition Therapy for Diabetes. Washington, DC: American Diabetes Association; 2012.

9. American College of Obstetricians and Gynecologists. Your Pregnancy and Childbirth: Month by Month. 5th ed. Washington, DC: American College of Obstetricians and Gynecologists; 2010.

10. Widen E, Siega-Riz AM. Prenatal nutrition: A practical guide for assessment and counseling. J Midwifery Womens Health. 2010;55:540-9.

11. Institute of Medicine of the National Academies. Dietary Reference Intakes for Calcium and Vitamin D. Washington, DC: The National Academies Press; 2011.

12. Institute of Medicine of the National Academies. Dietary Reference Intakes: Energy, Carbohydrate, Fiber, Fat, Fatty Acids, Cholesterol, Protein, and Amino Acids. Washington, DC: The National Academies Press; 2002.

13. Academy of Nutrition and Dietetics. Position of the Academy of Nutrition and Dietetics: use of nutritive and non-nutritive sweeteners. J Acad Nutr Diet. 2012;112:739-58.

14. Centers for Disease Control and Prevention. Notice to readers: Surgeon General's advisory on alcohol use in pregnancy. MMWR Morb Mortal Wkly Rep. 2005; 54(9):229.

15. Evans EC. The FDA recommendations on fish intake during pregnancy. J Obstet Gynecol Neonatal Nurs. 2002;31:715-20.

16. US Department of Health and Human Services. Physical Activity Guidelines Advisory Committee final report (cited 2013 May 31). On the Internet at: http://www.health.gov/PAGuidelines/Report/Default.aspx.

17. Kitzmiller JL, Jovanovic L, Brown F, Coustan D, Reader DM, eds. Managing Preexisting Diabetes and Pregnancy. Alexandria, Va: American Diabetes Association; 2008.

18. Abrams BF, Laros RK Jr. Prepregnancy weight, weight gain and birth weight. Am J Obstet Gynecol. 1986;154:503-9.

19. Landon MB, Gabbe SG. Diabetes mellitus. In: Barron WM, Lindheimer MD, Davison JM, eds. Medical Disorders in Pregnancy. St. Louis, Mo: Mosby; 2000:71-100.

20. Centers for Disease Control and Prevention. Recommendations to improve preconception health and health care—United States. MMWR Morb Mortal Wkly Rep. 2006;55(RR06):1-23.

21. American College of Obstetricians and Gynecologists. Pregestational diabetes mellitus. Practice bulletin No. 60. Obstet Gynecol. 2005;105:675-85.

22. Kim C, Ferrara A, McEwen LN, Marrero DG, Gerzoff RB, Herman WH, TRIAD Study Group. Preconception care in managed care: the translating research into action for diabetes study. Am J Obstet Gynecol. 2005;192(1):227-32.

23. Dunne F. Type 2 diabetes and pregnancy. Sem Fetal Neonatal Med. 2005;10:333-9.

24. McElduff A, Ross GP, Lagström JA, et al. Pregestational diabetes and pregnancy: an Australian experience. Diabetes Care. 2005;28:1260-1.

25. American Diabetes Association. Preconception care of women with diabetes. Diabetes Care. 2004;27 Suppl 1:S76-8.

26. Kitzmiller JL, Jovanovic L, Brown F, Coustan D, Reader DM, eds. Managing Preexisting Diabetes and Pregnancy. Alexandria, Va: American Diabetes Association; 2008.

27. Academy of Nutrition and Dietetics. Evidence-analysis library. Gestational diabetes (cited 2013 June 6). On the Internet at: http://andevidencelibrary.com/default.cfm?auth=1.

28. Catalano PM, Buchanan TA. Metabolic changes during normal and diabetic pregnancies. In: Reece EA, Coustan DR, Gabbe SG, eds. Diabetes in Women: Adolescence, Pregnancy, and Menopause. Philadelphia: Lippincott Williams & Wilkins; 2004:129-45.

29. Pedersen J. The Pregnant Diabetic and Her Newborn. 2nd ed. Baltimore: Williams & Wilkins; 1977.

30. Eidelman AI, Samueloff A. The pathophysiology of the fetus of the diabetic mother. Sem in Perinatol. 2002;26:232-6.

31. Jovanovic L. Diabetic retinopathy. In: Reece EA, Coustan DR, Gabbe SG, eds. Diabetes in Women: Adolescence, Pregnancy, and Menopause. 3rd ed. Philadelphia: Lippincott Williams & Wilkins; 2004:371-82.

32. Lauszus FF, Klebe JG, Bek T, et al. Increased serum IGF-I during pregnancy is associated with progression of diabetic retinopathy. Diabetes. 2003;52:852-6.

33. Rosenn B, Miodovnik M, Kranias G, et al. Progression of diabetic retinopathy in pregnancy: association with hypertension in pregnancy. Am J Obstet Gynecol. 1992;166:1214-8.

34. Brinchmann-Hansen O, Dahl-Jorgensen K, Hanssen KF, et al. Effects of intensified insulin treatment on various lesions of diabetic retinopathy. Am J Ophthalmol. 1985;100:644-53.

35. Report of the National High Blood Pressure Education Program Working Group on High Blood Pressure in Pregnancy. Am J Obstet Gynecol. 2000;183:S1-22.

36. Hinton AC, Sibai BM. Hypertensive disorders in pregnancy. In: Reece EA, Coustan DR, Gabbe SG, eds. Diabetes in Women: Adolescence, Pregnancy, and Menopause. 3rd ed. Philadelphia: Lippincott Williams & Wilkins; 2004:363-70.

37. Cundy T, Gamble G, Townend K, et al. Perinatal mortality in type 2 diabetes mellitus. Diabet Med. 2000;17:33-9.

38. Ehrenberg HM, Mercer BM, Catalano PM. The influence of obesity and diabetes on the prevalence of macrosomia. Am J Obstet Gynecol. 2004;191:964-8.

39. Clausen TD, Mathiesen E, Ekbom P, et al. Poor pregnancy outcome in women with type 2 diabetes. Diabetes Care. 2005;28:323-8.

40. American Dietetic Association. Position of the American Dietetic Association and American Society for Nutrition: obesity, reproduction and pregnancy outcomes. J Am Diet Assoc. 2009;109:918-27.

41. Jensen DM, Damm P, Moelsted-Pedersen L, et al. Outcomes in type 1 diabetic pregnancies. Diabetes Care. 2004;27:2819-23.

42. Wren C, Birrell G, Hawthorne G. Cardiovascular malformations in infants of diabetic mothers. Heart. 2003;89:1217-20.

43. American College of Obstetricians and Gynecologists. Fetal macrosomia. ACOG Practice Bulletin No. 22. Washington, DC: American College of Obstetricians and Gynecologists; 2000.

44. Coustan DR. Delivery: timing, mode, and management. In: Reece EA, Coustan DR, Gabbe SG, eds. Diabetes in Women: Adolescence, Pregnancy, and Menopause. 3rd ed. Philadelphia: Lippincott Williams & Wilkins; 2004:433-9.

45. Thomas A, Gutierrez YM. American Dietetic Association Guide to Gestational Diabetes Mellitus. Chicago: American Dietetic Association; 2005.

46. Rizzo TA, Dooley SL, Metzger BE, et al. Prenatal and perinatal influences on long-term psychomotor development in offspring of diabetic mothers. Am J Obstet Gynecol. 1995;173:1753-8.

47. Rizzo T, Metzger BE, Burns WJ, et al. Correlations between antepartum maternal metabolism and child intelligence. N Engl J Med. 1991;325:911-6.

48. Churchill JA, Berendes HW. Intelligence of children whose mothers had acetonuria during pregnancy. In: Perinatal Factors Affecting Human Development. Pan American Health Organization Scientific Publication. Washington, DC: Pan American Health Organization; 1969;185:300.

49. Pettit DP, Kolaczynski JW, Ospina P, et al. Comparison of an insulin analog, insulin aspart and regular human insulin with no insulin in gestational diabetes mellitus. Diabetes Care. 2003;26:183-6.

50. Lapolla A, Dalfrà MG, Fedele D. Insulin therapy in pregnancy complicated by diabetes: are insulin analogs a new tool? Diabetes Metab Res Rev. 2005;21:241-52.

51. Gamson K, Chia S, Jovanovic L. The safety and efficacy of insulin analogs in pregnancy. J Matern Fetal Neonatal Med. 2004;15:26-34.

52. Garg SK, Frias JP, Anil S, Gottlieb PA, MacKenzie T, Jackson WE. Insulin lispro therapy in pregnancies complicated by type 1 diabetes: glycemic control and maternal and fetal outcomes. Endocr Pract. 2003;9:187-93.

53. Cypryk K, Sobczak M, Pertyńska-Marczewska M, Zawodniak-Szalapska M, Szyczak W, Wilczyński J, et al. Pregnancy complications and perinatal outcome in diabetic women treated with Humalog (insulin lispro) or regular human insulin during pregnancy. Med Sci Monit. 2004;10:129-32.

54. Hirsch IB. Insulin analogues. N Engl J Med. 2005;352: 174-83.

55. Hod M, Mathiesen ER, Jovanovic L, et al. A randomized trial comparing perinatal outcomes using insulin detemir or neutral protamine Hadedorn in type 1 diabetes. J Matern Fetal Neonatal Med. 2014;27:7-13.

56. Mathiesen ER, Hod M, Ivanisevic M, et al. Maternal efficacy and safety outcomes in a randomized, controlled trial comparing insulin detemir with NPH insulin in 310 pregnant women with type 1 diabetes. Diabetes Care. 2012; 35:2012-17.

57. Rudolf MC, Coustan DR, Sherwin RS, et al. Efficacy of the insulin pump in the home treatment of pregnant diabetics. Diabetes. 1981;30:891-5.

58. Kitzmiller J, Younger D, Hare J, et al. Continuous subcutaneous insulin therapy during early pregnancy. Obstet Gynecol. 1985;66:606-11.

59. Gabbe SG. New concepts and applications in the use of the insulin pump during pregnancy. J Matern Fetal Med. 2000;9:42-5.

60. Radermecker RP, Scheen AJ. Continuous subcutaneous insulin infusion with short-acting insulin analogues or human regular insulin: efficacy, safety, quality of life, and cost-effectiveness. Diabetes Metab Res Rev. 2004;20: 178-88.

61. Hickman MA, McBide R, Boggess KA, Strauss R. Metformin compared with insulin in the treatment of pregnant women with overt diabetes: a randomized controlled trial. Am J Perinatol. 2013;30:483-90.

62. Jovanovic-Peterson L, ed. Medical Management of Pregnancy Complicated by Diabetes. 3rd ed. Alexandria, Va: American Diabetes Association; 2000:7.

63. Feig DS, Briggs GG, Koren G. Oral antidiabetic agents in pregnancy and lactation: a paradigm shift? Ann Pharmacother. 2007;41:1147-80.

64. Getahun D, Nath C, Ananth CV, Chavez MR, Smulian JC. Gestational diabetes in the United States: temporal trends 1989 through 2004. Am J Obstet Gynecol. 2008;198:525. e1-5.

65. Metzger BE, Coustan DR, eds. Proceedings of the Fourth International Workshop-Conference on Gestational Diabetes Mellitus. Diabetes Care. 1998;21 Suppl 2:B1-167.

66. American Diabetes Association. Diagnosis and classification of diabetes mellitus. Diabetes Care. 2011;34 Suppl 1:S62-9.

67. American College of Obstetricians and Gynecologists. Committee Opinion Number 504. Screening and diagnosis of gestational diabetes mellitus. Obstet Gynecol. 2011;118: 751-53.

68. VanDorsten JP, Dodson WC, Espeland MA, et al. National Institutes of Health Consensus Development Conference Statement: diagnosing gestational diabetes mellitus. NIH Consens State Sci Statements. 2013;29(1):1-30.

69. Moyer VA. Screening for gestational diabetes mellitus: U.S. Preventive Task Force recommendation statement. Ann Intern Med. 2014;60(6):414-20.

70. HAPO Study Cooperative Research Group. Hyperglycemia and adverse pregnancy outcomes. N Engl J Med. 2008;358(19):1991-2002.

71. Bantle JP, Wylie-Rosett J, Albright AL, et al. Nutrition recommendations and interventions for diabetes—2006. Diabetes Care. 2009;32:193-203.

72. Moreno-Castilla C, Hernandez M, Bergua M, et al. Low carbohydrate diet for the treatment of gestational diabetes. Diabetes Care. 2013;36:2233-8.

73. Ben-Haroush A, Yogev Y, Rosenn B, Hod M, Langer O. The postprandial glucose profile in the diabetic pregnancy. Am J Obstet Gynecol. 2004;191(2):576-81.

74. Yogev Y, Ben-Haroush A, Chen R, Rosenn B, Hod M, Langer O. Diurnal glycemic profile in obese and normal weight non-diabetic pregnant women. Am J Obstet Gynecol. 2004;191:949-53.

75. Metzger BE, Buchanan TA, Coustan DR. Summary and recommendations of the Fifth International Workshop-Conference on Gestational Diabetes Mellitus. Diabetes Care. 2007;30 Suppl 2:S251-60.

76. American Diabetes Association. Gestational diabetes mellitus (position statement). Diabetes Care. 2004;27 Suppl 1:S88-90.

77. de Veciana M, Major CA, Morgan MA, Asrat T, Toohey JS, et al. Postprandial versus preprandial blood glucose monitoring in women with gestational diabetes mellitus requiring insulin therapy. N Engl J Med. 1995;333:1237-41.

78. Langer O, Conway D, Berkus M, Xenakis EM, Gonzales O. A comparison of glyburide and insulin in women with gestational diabetes mellitus. N Engl J Med. 2000; 343:1134-8.

79. Dhulkotia JS, Ola B, Fraser R, Farrell T. Oral hypoglycemic agents vs insulin in management of gestational diabetes: a systematic review and metaanalysis. Am J Obstet Gynecol. 2010;203:457.e1-9.

80. Rowan JA, Hague WM, Gao W, Battin MR, Moore MP. Metformin versus insulin for the treatment of gestational diabetes. N Engl J Med. 2008;358:2003-15.

81. Landon MB, Gabbe SG. Gestational diabetes mellitus. Obstet Gynecol. 2011;118:1379-93.

82. Gunderson EP, Hedderson MM, Chiang V, et al. Lactation intensity and postpartum maternal glucose tolerance and insulin resistance in women with recent GDM. The SWIFT cohort. Diabetes Care. 2012;35:50-6.

83. United States Department of Health and Human Services. Healthy People 2010—Health Literacy (cited 2010 Feb 10). On the Internet at: http://nnlm.gov/outreach/consumer/hlthlit.html.

84. American College of Obstetrics and Gynecology. ACOG Committee Opinion No. 391. Health literacy. Obstet Gynecol. 2007;110:1489-91.

85. American Medical Association Ad Hoc Committee on Health Literacy for the Council on Scientific Affairs. JAMA. 1999;281:552-7.

86. Endres LK, Sharp LK, Haney E, Dooley SL. Health literacy and pregnancy preparedness in pregestational diabetes. Diabetes Care. 2004;27:331-4.

CHAPTER 25

Cardiovascular Complications of Diabetes

JoAnn Sperl-Hillen, MD

Key Concepts

- Diabetes is a major cause of cardiovascular (CV) events. Despite advances in detection and treatment, heart attacks and strokes continue to be the leading cause of complications, disability, and premature death for people with diabetes.

- Increased effort is needed to identify modifiable risk factors earlier in people with diabetes for intervention with education and preventive treatments.

- Important modifiable risk factors are obesity, hypertension, dyslipidemia, hyperglycemia, tobacco use, and underuse of antiplatelet therapy in high-risk individuals.

- Calculation of CV risk using the American College of Cardiology (ACC)/American Heart Association (AHA) Pooled Cohort Equation can support individualized treatment recommendations and may be a useful tool for patient counseling, education, and shared decision making.

- A multidisciplinary strategy that includes lifestyle and multiple pharmacologic considerations, care coordination, and frequent follow-up is recommended to treat CV risk.

- The prevalence of CV disease differs among sex, racial, and ethnic groups in the United States. Special attention may be warranted for high-risk subgroups.

Introduction

With the dramatic global increase in the number of people with type 2 diabetes mellitus (T2DM), CV complications are particularly significant due to the associated frequency, morbidity, mortality, and economic consequences.[1,2] Data from the Framingham cohort show that the incidence of CV events in both the diabetic and the nondiabetic population has diminished since the 1950s.[3] The reduced mortality rate followed a highly significant improvement in control of blood pressure and cholesterol. However, diabetes is underreported on death certificates and is still the seventh leading reported cause of death in the United States. People with diabetes are at least twice as likely to have heart disease or strokes as people without diabetes, and their risk of death is at least twice that of people of similar age without diabetes. Sixty-five

percent of deaths in people with diabetes are due to either coronary or cerebrovascular events.[4–6]

People with diabetes have 2 to 3 times the risk of stroke, myocardial infarction (MI), and sudden death as those without diabetes.

This chapter begins by describing the importance of recognizing and treating CV risk factors early and aggressively. It discusses methods for quantifying CV risk and clinical considerations helpful in engaging patients in the process of treating modifiable risk. It includes a discussion of issues and challenges for patients related to common CV problems and ends with pearls for practice, a worthwhile to-do list for diabetes educators.

Manifestations of Cardiovascular Disease

Coronary Heart Disease
- Angina
- Myocardial infarction
- Congestive heart failure

Cerebrovascular Disease
- Cerebrovascular accident (stroke)
- Transient ischemic attack

Peripheral Artery Disease
- Lower extremity ischemia

The Relationship Between Diabetes and Cardiovascular Disease

Epidemiology of Diabetes and Cardiovascular Disease

A number of large epidemiologic studies have shown that chronic hyperglycemia, as evaluated by fasting blood glucose or A1C, is an independent risk factor for cardiovascular disease (CVD).[7] For example, in the United Kingdom Prospective Diabetes Study (UKPDS), people with T2DM with A1C in the upper tertile had a 50% increase in CV risk.[8] The EPIC-Norfolk study found that men with diabetes have not only increased CV morbidity and mortality but also a 28% greater risk of CV events for each 1% increase in A1C—even if it is within the normal range.[9] A similar effect was found for peripheral artery disease (PAD).[10] The Atherosclerosis Risk in Communities study demonstrated that increased levels of A1C were correlated with increased carotid intima-media thickness (IMT), a measure of early atherosclerosis.[11] Pooled data from a meta-analysis suggest that a 1% increase in A1C is associated with a 1.2- to 1.3-fold increased risk of CVD, including coronary T2DM events, stroke, and PAD.[12]

People with type 1 diabetes mellitus (T1DM) are at a tenfold increased risk for CV events overall,[13,14] and those who are between the ages of 20 and 39 are at a fivefold increased risk.[15] A number of authorities have outlined treatment implications in response to early evidence of increased risk of CVD in young

people with diabetes. In general, the recommendation is that classic risk factors—particularly dyslipidemia, smoking, and hypertension—should be aggressively addressed in both T1DM and T2DM populations.[16,17]

Why Is the Risk of CV Events Higher in People With Diabetes?

For many years, the assumption was that MI and thrombotic stroke were the result of progressive occlusion of coronary or cerebral vessels. More recent research has shown that a rupture of weakened areas within plaques of partially occluded blood vessels often leads to acute coronary and cerebral thrombosis.[18] This rupture allows the release of highly thrombogenic plaque contents into the vessel lumen. The interaction of these lipid and necrotic substances with platelets and coagulation factors triggers an acute thrombosis. Diabetes, insulin resistance, and glucose intolerance are also associated with a state of enhanced thrombosis by affecting platelets and production of clotting factors, increasing the development of thrombi that cause acute events. In acute coronary events, endothelial function is altered in ways that accelerate atherosclerotic change, including increased vasospasm, enhanced thrombosis, and increased local inflammatory responses.[19]

Factors contributing to cardiometabolic risk are described in Figure 25.1. Factors such as hyperlipoproteinemia, smoking, diabetes, and hypertension disturb endothelial function in a variety of ways. Further, the effects of these factors appear to be synergistic rather than just additive. Increasing evidence suggests that both hyperglycemia and insulin resistance also affect vascular function, and when both are present, the effects are much greater than when either is present alone.[20] Chronic hyperglycemia and insulin resistance may produce vasoconstrictive substances and advanced glycation end products that disturb endothelial function and affect the vessel walls by causing increased stiffness and decreased compliance of the arterial wall.[21] Other risk factors for decreased arterial compliance include advanced age, hypertension, presence of components of the metabolic syndrome, microalbuminuria, central obesity, and low cardiopulmonary fitness.

Many researchers are interested in emerging evidence that suggests that postprandial hyperglycemia

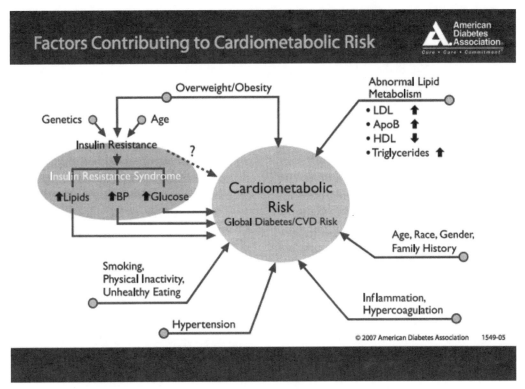

FIGURE 25.1   Factors Contributing to Cardiometabolic Risk in People With Diabetes

Source: Reproduced with permission from the American Diabetes Association, "Factors contributing to cardiometabolic risk" (cited 2014 Mar 14), on the Internet at: http://professional.diabetes.org/UserFiles/File/Resources%20for%20Professionals/CMR_Chart.pdf.

excursions may also play a role in the pathophysiology of microvascular and macrovascular complications of diabetes. Epidemiologic data support the association of postprandial hyperglycemia and increased CV risk.[22,23] A number of epidemiologic studies and glycemic intervention studies suggest that postprandial spikes in blood glucose and triglycerides (TGs) may each play a greater role in CVD than either average or fasting glucose.[23–27] Several interventional studies targeting postprandial hyperglycemia support the hypothesis that reducing postprandial glucose excursions may decrease CV risk in people with prediabetes and diabetes.[28–30]

Can Better Management of Glycemic Control in People With T2DM Prevent CV Events?

Extensive data support the concept that better glycemic control can reduce microvascular complications of diabetes. However, despite the strong observational association between diabetes and macrovascular disease, the evidence is less compelling about whether

and to what extent improved glycemic control can reduce the risk of events, particularly in T2DM.[31] In the UKPDS study, the intensive group, which achieved a median A1C of 7.4%, had 16% fewer MIs than the control group, but this effect missed statistical significance.[32] A secondary analysis of UKPDS data showed a statistically significant 12% decrease in the rate of MI for each 1% reduction in A1C, but the effect of glycemic control was much less than the effect of hypertension or hyperlipidemia control. After the UKPDS study ended, the hemoglobin A1C difference between the intensive and control groups was lost within 1 to 2 years. Nonetheless, a 10-year follow-up found a significant reduction in MI, diabetes-related death, and all-cause mortality in the intensively treated group.[33]

Although epidemiologic data suggest that interventions to lower glucose might reduce the rate of CV events in T2DM, 3 recent large randomized trials failed to show a significant effect of more intensive glycemic control on their primary CV event outcomes. The Action to Control Cardiovascular Risk in Diabetes (ACCORD) study randomly assigned

10,251 people at risk for CVD to a strategy targeting A1C <6.0% versus 7.0% to 7.9%. The enrolled subjects had an A1C of 8.1% at baseline and at least 2 CV risk factors; they had had diabetes for, on average, 10 years, and 35% were taking insulin at baseline.[34] The intensive and control group patients achieved median A1C levels of 6.4% and 7.5%, respectively. The ACCORD study was stopped early due to increased all-cause mortality in the intensively treated group.[35] The study was insufficiently powered to determine the cause of increased mortality; however, despite a lower MI rate trend in the intensive group, a higher rate of fatal MI was observed.

The Action in Diabetes and Vascular Disease: Preterax and Diamicron Modified Release Controlled Evaluation (ADVANCE) study randomly assigned 11,140 people with T2DM to either standard care (A1C based on local guidelines) or an intensive group with target A1C ≤6.5%.[36] Enrolled subjects had an A1C of 7.2% at baseline and had had diabetes for, on average, 8 years; 1.5% were on insulin. The intensive group achieved a median A1C of 6.3%, compared with the standard group A1C of 7.0%. Although microvascular disease (primarily nephropathy) was reduced in the intensively treated group, there was no difference in the rate of vascular events between the 2 groups.[34]

The Veterans Administration Diabetes Trial (VADT) randomly assigned 1791 people with T2DM to intensive therapy, targeting an A1C 1.5% lower than the standard therapy group.[37] Enrolled subjects were 97% male and had had diabetes for 11.5 years and a baseline median A1C of 9.4%. The median A1C achieved in the intensive group was 6.9%, compared with 8.5% in the standard therapy group.[34] Again, there was no significant difference between the 2 groups for the primary endpoint of major CV events or any component of the outcome. There were no observed differences in microvascular complications (except for progression of albuminuria), and rates of hypoglycemia were significantly higher in the intensive therapy group.

So, why did these well-designed interventions fail to show any effect? Are the pathological macrovascular effects of long-term hyperglycemia not substantially reversible? The intervention effects may have been inconsistent among these studies because of the different characteristics of the patients who received interventions in these trials. For example, patients

in the UKPDS study were younger and had a more recent diabetes diagnosis than those in later interventional trials such as ACCORD, in which subjects had had diabetes longer and had a greater degree of preexisting suboptimal glycemic control and insulin use at study entry.

The implication that early intervention is beneficial, whereas later intervention may not be, is supported by further analyses of the VADT, which suggest that duration of diabetes interacts with effects of intensive control; subjects with a shorter duration of diabetes appear to benefit more from intensive management, whereas those with longer duration appear to either receive no benefit or receive an adverse effect. A lesser degree of preexisting CVD, as measured by coronary calcium scores, may also predict greater benefit from intensive control.[34]

> Studies suggest that glycemic control may have greater CV benefits in people with diabetes if started early in the disease process.

What Are the Effects of Specific Drugs on CV Risk?

Rosiglitazone was implicated as a drug that increased CV risk in some studies. A meta-analysis of 42 trials comparing rosiglitazone therapy with either placebo or an active comparator found an increase in the rate of MI in patients treated with rosiglitazone.[38] This analysis precipitated a US Food and Drug Administration (FDA) box warning for the heart-related risks, and rosiglitazone became available only through a restricted distribution process in 2007. However, a randomized trial designed to evaluate CV outcomes in patients treated with rosiglitazone, RECORD, assigned more than 4200 patients to either rosiglitazone or placebo plus metformin or sulfonylurea. These patients were followed for 6 years. There were no significant differences between the 2 groups with regard to total mortality, CV mortality, or nonfatal MI. Rosiglitazone-treated patients had a greater incidence of congestive heart failure (CHF), consistent with known fluid-retaining characteristics of thiazolidinediones (TZDs).[39] These data were later reexamined and confirmed by an independent review group, leading an FDA advisory panel to loosen restrictions on this controversial drug in 2013.

Due to lingering questions related to CV safety of T2DM drugs, the FDA developed regulations requiring larger and more comprehensive phase 2, phase 3, and postapproval CV safety outcome studies in 2011.[40] Currently, multiple large multicenter clinical trials are testing the CV effects of dipeptidyl peptidase-4 inhibitors, glucagon-like peptide-1 agonists, and emerging therapies. Results of 2 of these studies were recently published. The SAVOR-TIMI study reported that saxagliptin did not increase or decrease the rate of ischemic events for patients at risk for CV events. However, there was a statistically significant increase in rates of hospitalization for heart failure in the saxagliptin treated group (3.5% vs. 2.8%).[41] The EXAMINE study reported no increase in cardiac events from alogliptin among patients with T2DM and recent acute coronary syndrome.[42] Additional analysis and results from multiple other ongoing clinical trials will help evaluate the safety and CV effects of these drug classes.

Considerations for T1DM

The major predictor of CVD in people with T1DM appears to be duration of the disease.[43] Several lines of evidence support the long-term effects of glycemic control on macrovascular risk. Pancreas transplantation normalizes glucose and has been shown to reduce increased carotid IMT to normal within 2 years of successful transplantation.[44] In a study of kidney transplant patients who received a subsequent islet transplant, the kidney-islet group had improved cardiac function and stabilization of carotid IMT compared with the kidney-alone group.[45]

Long-term follow-up of the Diabetes Control and Complications Trial (DCCT) cohort has provided interesting data about the impact of intensive control on the development of macrovascular disease in T1DM. After the DCCT ended in 1992, most participants were enrolled in a long-term follow-up study, the Epidemiology of Diabetes Interventions and Complications (EDIC) study. Glycemic control, as determined by A1C, between the 2 groups remained minimally different for 4 years; however, by the fifth year after the DCCT ended, there was no difference between the 2 groups. Carotid IMT was measured from 1994 to 1996 and again 4 years later. Progression of carotid IMT was associated with a number of conventional risk factors, including age, systolic

blood pressure, smoking, the ratio of low-density lipoprotein cholesterol (LDL-C) to high-density lipoprotein cholesterol (HDL-C), and albuminuria. Most important, progression of carotid IMT 6 years after the DCCT ended was closely associated with allocation to the intensive therapy group during the 6.5 years of the DCCT.[46] Subsequent data from the same group found that early intensive control of glycemia reduced all CV events by 42%, and nonfatal MI, cerebrovascular accident, and CV death by 57%. These effects were mediated by glycemic control during the DCCT. Thus, the combined DCCT/EDIC studies proved that early intensive control of T1DM decreases the risk of both microvascular and macrovascular complications.[47]

Assessing CV Risk
Using a CV Risk Calculator

An assessment of cardiometabolic risk gives the educator and the patient a picture of the patient's health and potential risk of CV events. Patients with known coronary heart disease (CHD), regardless of age, are generally considered to have a 10-year CV risk of 20% or higher. In addition, most men with diabetes aged 50 and older and most women aged 60 and older with at least 1 additional major CV risk factor (eg, hypertension, smoking, dyslipidemia, albuminuria, family history of CVD) have a 10-year CV risk of 10% or greater. However, outside of these high-risk generalizations, studies show that clinicians are often inaccurate in their predictions of CV risk without the support of risk model calculations.[48]

The use of validated risk-prediction models can more precisely determine CV risk and guide education and engagement efforts to influence patient behavior.[49] Although data are sparse and more research is needed in this area, 2 systematic reviews support the conclusion that risk assessment plus counseling is associated with favorable changes in patient knowledge and intention to change and with provider prescribing behavior and risk factor control.[50,51]

Many methods of estimating 10-year CV risk, such as the Framingham and Reynolds risk scores, have been recommended.[52] In 2013, the ACC/AHA Guideline on the Treatment of Blood Cholesterol to Reduce Atherosclerotic CV Risk in Adults recommended use of a new risk calculator, the Pooled Cohort Equation.[52] The Pooled Cohort Equation for 10-year risk of atherosclerotic CV disease (ASCVD) has advantages over Framingham CHD risk estimations because it was developed using pooled cohorts that included participants from several large randomized and geographically dispersed cohort studies sponsored by the National Heart, Lung, and Blood Institute (NHLBI).[53] Data needed to use the Pooled Cohort Equation include the following:

- Age
- Sex
- Systolic blood pressure
- Total cholesterol
- HDL cholesterol
- Hypertension treatment (yes/no)
- Diabetes status (yes/no)
- Race (non-Hispanic white or non-Hispanic African American)

One notable gap in the Pooled Cohort Equation is the lack of ethnic-specific risk algorithms for Hispanic-American and Asian-American populations. When compared with that of non-Hispanic whites, the estimated 10-year risk for ASCVD is generally lower in these populations and higher in American-Indian populations. Until better algorithms are developed for these populations, providers may consider using the equations for non-Hispanic whites for these patients. However, it is important to remember that the risks may be overestimated, especially for Hispanic Americans and Asian Americans.[53]

It is also important to keep in mind that some individuals with significant CV risk factors may not have a high 10-year CV risk if they are young. However, extensive epidemiological, pathological, and basic science data indicate that the development of atherosclerosis, the precursor of ASCVD, occurs over decades and is related to long-term and cumulative exposure to causal, modifiable risk factors. Thus, a life course perspective on risk assessment and prevention must be considered, especially among younger individuals. For younger individuals (ie, aged 20-59) free of ASCVD and not at high short-term risk, use of a 30-year or lifetime ASCVD risk assessment can help with counseling on lifestyle and healthy behavior[53,54] (Table 25.1).

TABLE 25.1	Examples of ASCVD Risk Calculations Using the ACC/AHA Pooled Cohort Equation		
	Black Male Age 70	*White Female Age 50*	*White Female Age 48*
Total cholesterol (TC)	230 mg/dL	180 mg/dL	180 mg/dL
HDL-C	35 mg/dL	50 mg/dL	55 mg/dL
Systolic blood pressure (SBP)	159 mm Hg	135 mm Hg	130 mm Hg
Hypertension treatment?	Yes	Yes	No
Diabetes?	Yes	Yes	Yes
Smoker?	Yes	Yes	No
Calculated 10-year ASCVD risk	70%	10%	2%
10-year ASCVD risk with optimal risk factors*	9%	1%	1%
Lifetime ASCVD risk	Not useful in older patients	50% (would be 8% with optimal risk factors*)	39% (would be 8% with optimal risk factors*)
Recommendations to consider	Stop smoking, initiate high-intensity statin therapy, intensify blood pressure therapy, encourage lifestyle modifications	Stop smoking, initiate high-intensity statin therapy, encourage lifestyle modifications	Initiate moderate-intensity statin therapy, encourage lifestyle modifications

Abbreviations: ASCVD, atherosclerotic cardiovascular disease; HDL-C, high-density lipoprotein cholesterol.

*Optimal risk factors include TC 170 mg/dL, HDL-C 50 mg/dL, SBP 110 mm Hg, not taking medications for hypertension, no diabetes.

The ACC/AHA guideline suggests estimation of 10-year and lifetime risk for ASCVD using a Web-based calculator available at http://my.americanheart.org/cvriskcalculator or http://www.cardiosource.org/science-and-quality/practice-guidelines-and-quality-standards/2013-prevention-guideline-tools.aspx. The calculator can also be downloaded to a mobile device as an app from several sources, including iTunes. The calculator is easy to use and requires minimal input of patient data. The calculation can give the clinician a picture of a patient's total risk for CV events in the next 10 years and be used for educational and counseling purposes to influence patient behavior.

Instruction Opportunity—Explaining CV Risk Calculator Results to Patients

It is important to understand the underlying model for the risk calculator you are using. For example, the Framingham 10-year CHD risk equation predicts total CHD events (angina, unstable angina, MI, and CHD death), but the 10-year ACC/AHA Pooled Cohort Equation predicts hard ASCVD events (MI, CHD death, stroke, and fatal stroke). Models and calculators are also available to predict 10-year and 30-year (lifetime) ASCVD risk. Different risk calculators may be more useful, depending on the patient's situation. To give the patient some context for his or her risk, it can be useful to inform him or her what the risk would be for a patient of the same age, gender, and race if the other CV risk factors were optimal.

⬥ For a comprehensive picture of a patient's short-term ASCVD risk (useful in patients over age 40), use a general 10-year ASCVD risk calculator (eg, ACC/AHA Pooled Cohort Equation). Results can be explained to the patient as, "You have an X% chance of having a heart attack or stroke in the next 10 years. A patient of your age, race, and gender who has optimal risk factors has a Y% chance of having a heart attack or stroke in the next 10 years."

⬥ For determining CV risk in younger patients (aged 21-39), it may be more useful to use a 30-year general risk calculator. Results can be explained to the patient as, "You have an X% chance of having a heart attack or stroke in the next 30 years. A person of the same age, gender, and race with optimal CV risk factors has a Y% chance of having a heart attack or stroke in the next 30 years."

Case Example—Using a CV Risk Calculator and Explaining Results to a Patient

MS, a 50-year-old white woman, is seeing you today for diabetes education. She has T2DM and a body mass index (BMI) of 32. She has a history of hypertension that has been well controlled with lisinopril. She is a smoker with no other known significant health issues. Her blood pressure is 135/84 mm Hg. Her most recent labs, as shown in the middle column of Table 25.1, were as follows: A1C 6.6%, total cholesterol 180 mg/dL, HDL-C 50 mg/dL, TGs 140 mg/dL, and LDL-C 102 mg/dL. You want to help MS understand her future risk of heart attack and stroke. You can explain her calculated 10-year CV risk of 10% and lifetime risk of 50% as follows:

MS, your risk of having a stroke or heart attack in the next 10 years is 10%. This means that if you were in a group of 100 persons with the same danger, we would expect about 10 people to have a heart attack or stroke in the next 10 years. If 100 people the same age and gender were to have optimal control of cholesterol, blood pressure, and smoking, we would expect 1 person to have a heart attack or stroke in the next 10 years.

Your risk of having a heart attack or stroke in your lifetime is 50%. This means that in a group of 100 persons with the same danger as you, we would expect 50 of them to have a heart attack or stroke in their lifetime. With optimal control of cardiovascular risk, we would expect 8 to have a heart attack or stroke in their lifetime.

CVD Risk-Reduction Strategy

Understanding and prioritizing modifiable CV risk factors can facilitate earlier intervention with education and treatment. Because many patients have multiple risk factors, it is important to recognize and emphasize the relative priorities of the patient's individualized risk factors when communicating about CV risk reduction. The priority for clinical attention should always be modifiable risk factors.

Nonmodifiable Risk Factors

In the prevention and management of CV events, the emphasis is on CV risk reduction in patients with the potential to reverse (modify) their risk with lifestyle and pharmacologic interventions. Age, sex, family history/genetics, and race/ethnicity are examples of nonreversible risk factors. However, nonmodifiable risk factors can still influence clinical decision making in these ways:

◆ *Family history/genetics.* Genetics plays a role in the development of complications of CVD, but currently, clinically useful gene markers are not available. Family history of premature heart disease (often defined as CHD before age 55 for men or 65 for women in a first-degree relative) is associated with increased risk of future CHD, independent of other established risk factors. Men with a family history of premature heart disease have about a 50% higher lifetime risk of both CHD and CVD mortality than men without a family history.[55] However, adding data related to family history to the risk equation models does not improve the classification of clinically relevant risk for individuals.[53,56] Therefore, family history of premature CHD is useful information and can influence clinical judgment, but the information is not necessary for CV risk calculation.

◆ *Age.* There is a relationship between both age and duration of diabetes and CV risk. The older the individual and the longer he or she has had diabetes, the higher the risk for CV problems. The general health of the patient and long-term prognosis may influence CV risk factor management. Aggressive treatment to prevent long-term complications is not warranted for very elderly patients and others with limited life expectancy.

◆ *Sex.* Before menopause, there is a sex-protective factor for females without diabetes for CVD and CVD events; however, there is no sex-protective advantage for females with diabetes. Females and males with diabetes are at equal risk for CVD.[57] Some experts believe that clinicians may tend to take women's CV complaints less seriously than men's. The CV risks of women with diabetes should be addressed as seriously as those of men.

◆ *Race/ethnicity.* African Americans with diabetes have a higher incidence of macrovascular disease than whites with diabetes,[58] and Mexican Americans with diabetes have an increased risk of peripheral vascular disease.[43] Peripheral artery disease is also prevalent in African Americans and Hispanics with diabetes.

Modifiable Risk Factors

The following are modifiable risk factors targeted for intervention because there is reasonable evidence that treatment can improve CV outcomes. Evidence to support paying attention to each of these factors is described in detail later in the chapter.

◆ Lifestyle (overweight/obesity/physical inactivity)
◆ Tobacco cessation
◆ Statin use
◆ Hypertension
◆ High blood glucose
◆ Aspirin use in appropriately selected patients
◆ Increased urine albumin excretion

Take a Multifactorial Treatment Approach

Taking a multifactorial treatment approach to managing risk factors in people with T2DM improves patient outcomes. The STENO-2 study instituted intensive behavioral and pharmacologic therapy to target hyperglycemia, hypertension, dyslipidemia, and microalbuminuria for 80 people with established T2DM and microalbuminuria. Most patients were also treated with aspirin. Although few patients reached target goals for all interventions, those in the more aggressively treated intervention group had significant reductions in CVD, retinopathy, nephropathy, and autonomic neuropathy and a 20% decrease in all-cause mortality after 13 years of follow-up.[59]

The National Quality Forum, a nonprofit organization that reviews, endorses, and recommends standardized health performance measures to improve patient outcomes, has endorsed a multifactorial measure for optimal diabetes care.[60] While changes have recently been proposed to the measurement definitions for the components of optimal or comprehensive diabetes measurement to make the measures more consistent with the latest ACC/AHA and Eighth Joint

National Committee (JNC8) guidelines, the importance of multifactorial treatment to reduce the risk of ASCVD continues to be highlighted in performance measurement as well. Table 25.2 describes the latest (modified) evidence-based guideline recommendations for the most treatable CV clinical domains.

Instruction Opportunity—Communicating the "Multifactorial" Approach

The "D5" terminology is a way of communicating to patients the importance of a multifactorial approach to CV risk reduction.[61] D5 communicates goals for glycemia, blood pressure, lipids, tobacco, and aspirin

TABLE 25.2 National Guidelines for Treating CV Risk Factors for Adults With Diabetes

Clinical Domain	Subgroup	Achievable Goal	Source	Individual Considerations
Lipids	Age >21 with ASCVD	High-intensity statin	2013 ACC/AHA	Excludes patients with NYHA Class II-IV CHF and renal disease on dialysis. Use moderate-intensity statin for patients at higher risk for adverse effects who would otherwise be candidates for high-intensity statin.
	Age >21 with LDL ≥190 mg/dL	High-intensity statin	2013 ACC/AHA	
	Age 40–75 with ASCVD risk ≥7.5% and LDL 70–189 mg/dL	High-intensity statin	2013 ACC/AHA	
	Age 40–75 with ASCVD risk <7.5% and LDL 70–189 mg/dL	Moderate-intensity statin	2013 ACC/AHA	
	Age <40	Assess 30-year ASCVD risk. Lifestyle modification.	2013 ACC/AHA	Consider statins in patients with significant CV risk
Blood pressure	Adults age 18 or greater	<140/90 mm Hg	2013 JNC8	Antihypertensive recommendations differ by CKD status (ACEI and ARB preferred if CKD) and by race (ACEI and ARB not recommended first line in blacks)
	All adults	<140/80	2014 ADA	Consider <130/80 in younger patients if achievable without difficulty
A1C	Adults	<8%	2014 ADA	Lower A1C goal recommended if achievable without difficulty
Aspirin for secondary prevention	Adults	Low-dose aspirin use	2014 ADA and 2009 USPSTF	Assess and consider GI bleeding risks
Aspirin for primary prevention	Men ≥ age 50 with ≥1 additional CV risk factor	Low-dose aspirin use	2014 ADA	Assess and consider GI bleeding risk
	Women ≥ age 60 with ≥1 additional CV risk factor	Low-dose aspirin use	2014 ADA	Assess and consider GI bleeding risk
	Men ≥ age 45 and women ≥ age 55	Start aspirin if benefit > risk	2009 USPSTF	Use USPSTF table based on age and CHD risk for men and stroke risk for women
Tobacco	All who use tobacco products	Cessation	USPSTF	

Abbreviations: ACC/AHA, American College of Cardiology and the American Heart Association; ADA, American Diabetes Association; USPSTF, United States Preventive Services Task Force; JNC8, Eighth Joint National Committee; LDL, low-density lipoprotein; ASCVD, atherosclerotic cardiovascular disease; NYHA, New York Heart Association; CV, cardiovascular; CHD, coronary heart disease; CKD, chronic kidney disease; ACEI, angiotensin-converting enzyme inhibitor; ARB, angiotensin receptor blocker.

use. It uses a simple message to make it easier for people with diabetes to set and achieve goals to better manage the disease: "When you achieve D5 success, you reduce your risk of complications such as heart attack, stroke, and problems with your kidneys, eyes, and nervous system." While target levels for the components should be individualized to more intensive levels for some patients (and the lipid goal may need to be updated based on new guidelines), attention to all D5 clinical domains is appropriate and beneficial for almost all people with diabetes.

> The D5 message is a simple way to help patients understand the importance of a multifactorial treatment approach to reducing their risk of heart attack and stroke. Figure 25.2 is an example of patient information on the Internet to help communicate the D5 message: "The D5 represents 5 goals you need to achieve to reduce your risk for complications."

For patients with multiple risk factors outside of target/goal range, help them set priorities for treating their risk factors. There are different ways to set priorities, but exploring the following can be helpful:

◈ *Distance from clinical goal.* Treating the risk factors furthest from goal usually has a greater impact on reducing cardiovascular risk than treating risk factors already close to goal.

◈ *Ease of treatment.* Relatively simple adjustment of existing medication can be easier for patients than prescribing a new medication, especially if there are concerns about potential interactions and side effects.

◈ *Patient preference.* Adherence can be improved by learning if the patient strongly prefers or fears a particular treatment.

◈ *Current therapy.* The degree of risk reversibility is dampened if the patient is already on near-maximum pharmacologic treatment. For example, a patient above blood pressure

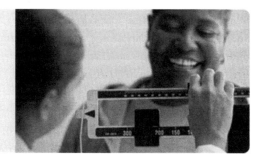

FIVE GOALS. ONE REASON: LIVING WELL.

If you have diabetes, it is important to take steps to manage your conditions. The D5 represents 5 goals you need to achieve to reduce your risk for complications.

Diabetes (dye-uh-BEE-teez) occurs when there is too much glucose (sugar) in the blood and not enough in the cells of your body. This can interfere with your body's ability to convert food into energy needed for daily life.

You achieve the D5 when you meet all five goals:

1. Your blood pressure is less than 140/90 mmHG
2. Your bad cholesterol, LDL, is less than 100 mg/dl
3. Your blood sugar, A1c, is less than 8%
4. You are tobacco-free
5. You take an aspirin as appropriate

The D5 was created to make it easier for people with diabetes to work together and set and achieve goals to better manage the disease. When you achieve D5 success, you reduce your risk for complications such as heart attack, stroke and problems with your kidneys, eyes and nervous system.

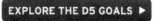

EXPLORE THE D5 GOALS ▶

FIGURE 25.2   **Setting Patient Goals to Achieve the "D5."**

Source: Minnesota Community Measurement (MNCM), http://mncm.org/reports-and-websites/the-d5/.

goal who is already on 3 antihypertensive medications will likely benefit less from intensifying blood pressure therapy than a patient with a similar blood pressure who is on 1 or no blood pressure medications. For patients not at goal on near-maximum pharmacologic treatment, additional assessment for possible barriers to adherence and psychosocial issues should be pursued before further intensifying treatment.

Lifestyle Management (Diet, Physical Activity, and Weight Loss)

Diet

The US population has become more obese as a result of less healthy eating patterns and decreased physical activity. Thus, the benefits of a therapeutic lifestyle change go well beyond reducing CVD in people with diabetes. As a result, the American Diabetes Association (ADA), the AHA, and the American Cancer Society are working together to effect lifestyle changes to reduce rates of diabetes, heart disease, and cancer.[62] The effects of a healthy diet have been shown to include improvement in weight, blood pressure,[63] and dyslipidemia and reduced CV event rates.[64-66]

The diet with the strongest evidence to improve CV outcomes is the Mediterranean diet, which is characterized by high intake of olive oil, fruit, nuts, vegetables, and cereals; moderate intake of fish and poultry; low intake of dairy products, red meat, processed meat, and sweets; and wine in moderation at meals.[66] In the randomized PREDIMED study of persons at high CV risk but without known CVD, a Mediterranean diet supplemented with extra-virgin olive oil or nuts significantly reduced the incidence of major CV events (relative risk reduction of 30%).[66]

The DASH dietary pattern also has strong evidence to support improvement in CV risk factors. The diet is high in vegetables, fruits, low-fat dairy products, whole grains, poultry, fish, and nuts and low in sweets, sugar-sweetened beverages, and red meats. The DASH dietary pattern is low in saturated fat, total fat, and cholesterol. It is rich in potassium, magnesium, calcium, protein, and fiber. Studies demonstrated that the DASH diet, compared with typical American diets of the 1990s, without changes in body weight or sodium intake, can lower blood pressure by about 5 to 6 mm Hg and LDL-C by 11 mg/dL.[54]

Weight Loss

Among overweight and obese adults, analysis of observational data shows that the greater the BMI, the higher the risk of CVD, T2DM, and all-cause mortality in both sexes. The current BMI cutpoints for overweight (BMI ≥25.0 kg/m^2) and obesity (BMI ≥30.0 kg/m^2) compared with normal weight (BMI 18.5 to <25.0 kg/m^2) are associated with elevated risk of fatal CHD. Lifestyle changes that produce even modest, sustained weight loss of 3% to 5% produce clinically meaningful health benefits. Greater weight loss reduces blood pressure, improves LDL-C and HDL-C, and reduces the need for medications to control blood pressure, glucose, and lipids, as well as further reduce TGs and blood glucose. Overweight and obese individuals who would benefit from weight loss should be invited to participate in a comprehensive lifestyle program consisting of a lower calorie diet and increased physical activity through the use of behavioral strategies.[67]

> Overweight and obese individuals who would benefit from weight loss should be invited to participate in a comprehensive lifestyle program consisting of a lower calorie diet and increased physical activity through the use of behavioral strategies.[67]

The Look AHEAD study was designed to examine whether weight loss in overweight persons with T2DM would decrease CV morbidity and mortality. A total of 5145 individuals in 16 study centers were randomly assigned either to intensive lifestyle intervention promoting weight loss and physical activity or to a control group with basic education. More patients in the intervention group experienced weight loss (not a large difference), reduced A1C, and improved fitness and CV risk factors (except LDL). Nevertheless, the study was stopped early after 10 years due to futility (no difference in CV outcome).[68] While this was disappointing to some, many experts believed that the weight loss achieved in the intensive group was too small to see the hypothesized effect. The positive news from this study is that, despite the modest between-group differences, the intervention did result in many other desirable outcomes, such as improvements in kidney disease, eye disease, depression, and quality of life; fewer hospitalizations; enhanced mobility; and reduced medication use.

Bariatric Surgery

In obese adults, bariatric surgery generally results in a more favorable impact on obesity-related comorbid conditions than usual care, conventional medical treatment, lifestyle intervention, or medically supervised weight loss. Among obese persons with diabetes at baseline who achieve a 20% to 35% weight loss 2 to 3 years after bariatric surgery, fasting glucose and insulin are reduced, and diabetes remission is more likely. However, longer term follow-up (10 years) shows that diabetes and hypertension may recur over time in individuals who see improvement in the short term.[67] Evidence is emerging from nonrandomized studies that bariatric surgery may be associated with reduced rates of CV events and deaths in obese adults.[69] Higher baseline insulin concentrations were associated with more favorable CV outcomes[20] and were a better predictor of CV outcomes than baseline weight. Prospective randomized trials are needed to confirm these relationships. Despite encouraging data, safety risks associated with bariatric surgery include surgical complications, vitamin deficiencies, gallstones, and anemia; the risks need to be balanced with potential benefits. Data on the efficacy of bariatric surgery for weight loss and maintenance or CV risk factors for longer than 2 years post-surgery in patients with BMI <35 are insufficient.[67]

> Adults with diabetes and other obesity-related comorbid conditions and a BMI ≥35 who are motivated to lose weight and have not achieved sufficient weight loss after behavioral treatment with or without pharmacotherapy may be candidates for bariatric surgery. Consider offering a referral to an experienced bariatric surgeon for consultation and evaluation.[67]

Physical Activity

A number of prospective epidemiologic studies have shown the benefits of physical activity on reducing CV events.[70] More recent data indicate the same effect is present in people with diabetes. A prospective study of more than 1700 persons with T2DM found that moderate-to-high levels of exercise decreased total and CV mortality. Although smoking and higher levels of blood pressure, BMI, and cholesterol were associated with a higher risk of death from CVD, the effect of exercise was independent of these risk factors.[71] Among men and women, 40 minutes of moderate-to-vigorous aerobic physical activity 3 to 4 times per week decreases systolic and diastolic blood pressure, on average, by 2 to 5 mm Hg and 1 to 4 mm Hg, respectively.[54] When sedentary adults aged 55 to 75 initiate a program of regular supervised physical training, they can experience a significant reduction in metabolic markers of CV risk and a lower rate of abnormal exercise stress test results and angina pectoris.[54,72]

Smoking Cessation

Nearly 20% of deaths from CVD can be directly linked to cigarette smoking. Stopping smoking can reduce the risk of coronary death by 50% within 1 year.[73] A number of randomized clinical trials have shown that brief counseling in smoking cessation is efficacious and cost-effective. For the patient motivated to quit, the combination of pharmacologic therapy such as nicotine replacement and counseling is more effective than either treatment alone.[74]

Three commonly used medications to support smoking cessation are the following:

- Nicotine replacement therapy, which helps by replacing the nicotine from cigarettes. Each type (eg, gum, lozenge, patch, nasal spray, inhaler) comes with different instructions.
- Bupropion, which is a non-nicotine pill that acts on neurotransmitters, "chemical messengers" that carry messages to cells in the brain. This medication should be taken for 1 to 2 weeks before stopping smoking. Possible side effects include abdominal pain, constipation, decreased appetite, dizziness, dry mouth, sweating, nausea or vomiting, trembling or shaking, and trouble sleeping.

◈ Varenicline, which produces nicotine effects to ease withdrawal symptoms and lessens the satisfaction of smoking by blocking the effects of nicotine. This medication should be started 1 week before quitting smoking. Possible side effects include nausea, insomnia, headache, abdominal pain, constipation, and flatulence. Some people have had changes in behavior including hostility, agitation, depression, and suicidal thoughts while on or after stopping varenicline.[75]

Side effects of these medications can lessen or disappear as the body adjusts to treatment. All of these medications should be taken under the direction of a doctor. Strategies addressing the motivational, behavioral, and social aspects of smoking cessation are also very important and should be used in combination with smoking cessation medications. Many free state and national phone and online resources are available to help patients stop smoking (eg, http://smokefree.gov).

Lipid Management

Thirty years have passed since publication of the MRFIT study, which attempted to prove that lowering total cholesterol through diet would reduce CV events.[76] Since then, a plethora of articles have investigated the role of statins for lipid lowering, including the landmark Scandinavian Simvastatin Survival Study (4S) and CARDS Study.[77] Although the studies were not limited to only people with diabetes, most included a large diabetes subgroup. Studies have shown benefits from statin therapy in both secondary prevention in people with established coronary disease[78,79] and primary prevention in people with diabetes with no evidence of preexisting CVD.[79] A meta-analysis of 6 primary prevention studies and 8 secondary prevention studies showed relative risk reductions of 22% and 24%, respectively, through use of statins in people with T2DM.[80] In another meta-analysis of statin therapy for primary prevention with more than 18,000 patients followed for a mean of 4.3 years, all-cause mortality decreased 9% and vascular mortality decreased 13% for each mmol/L (38 mg/dL) reduction in LDL.[81–85] The benefits of statin therapy are also observed in people

with diabetes at lower LDL levels and moderate CVD risk.[79,86] Although statin use increases the risk of developing diabetes, the CV event rate reduction outweighs the risk of incident diabetes.[87,88]

Low levels of HDL and elevated TGs are also commonly observed in people with diabetes. In the Veterans Affairs High-Density Lipoprotein Cholesterol Intervention Trial,[89] gemfibrozil therapy reduced CVD events by 24% in men with diabetes with previous CVD, low HDL, and modestly elevated TGs. In addition, the more recent FIELD trial[90] found that fenofibrate treatment resulted in fewer nonfatal MIs and coronary revascularizations but no significant difference in total coronary mortality. A side benefit to fenofibrate therapy was a decrease in urinary microalbumin and retinopathy requiring laser therapy. However, therapy targeting higher HDL/lower TGs using combinations of statins with other pharmacotherapy such as fibrates and niacin was studied in large clinical trials (ACCORD and Aim High, respectively) and did not reduce CV event rates more than statin therapy alone.[90–92] Moreover, in ACCORD, *reversible* worsening of renal function occurred more often with fenofibrate.[91]

Statins

In the absence of severe hypertriglyceridemia (TGs >1000 mg/dL is associated with risk of acute pancreatitis), the first priority of lipid therapy is statin use. The 2014 ADA Standards of Medical Care recommend statin use and an LDL goal of <100 mg/dL (or <70 mg if CHD is present) for most people with diabetes. The 2013 ACC/AHA guideline, published after completion of the 2014 ADA Standards of Medical Care, emphasizes the importance of statin therapy over particular LDL goals in high-risk patients. It recommends statin therapy for most people with diabetes (excluding those on hemodialysis, those with New York Heart Association [NYHA] class II-IV heart failure, and those who are older than age 75 unless clinical ASCVD is present). Statin therapy, if tolerated, is recommended for all individuals with T1DM or T2DM in the following subgroups:

◈ Older than age 21 with clinical ASCVD (high-dose statins recommended)
◈ Older than age 21 with LDL ≥190 mg/dL (high-dose statins recommended)

◆ Age 40 to 75 with ASCVD risk ≥7.5% and LDL 70 to 189 mg/dL (high-dose statins recommended)

◆ Age 40 to 75 with ASCVD risk <7.5% and LDL 70 to 189 mg/dL (moderate-dose statins recommended)

Examples of high-intensity statin therapy are daily doses of atorvastatin, 40 to 80 mg, or rosuvastatin, 20 to 40 mg. Examples of moderate-intensity therapy are daily doses of atorvastatin, 10 to 20 mg; rosuvastatin, 5 to 10 mg; and simvastatin, 20 to 40 mg.[52] The FDA does not recommend initiation of high-dose simvastatin (80 mg) due to increased risk of myopathy and rhabdomyolysis. In addition, increasing doses of simvastatin beyond 40 mg/d could be harmful. Statins are contraindicated in pregnancy, and extreme caution should be used if considering statin therapy in women of childbearing age.

Statin therapy can be considered for individuals with diabetes who are younger than 40 or older than 75, based on consideration of additional risk factors influencing ASCVD risk, benefits and adverse effects, drug-drug interaction potential, and patient preferences.

The ACC/AHA Expert Panel made no recommendations regarding statin initiation or discontinuation for patients with NYHA class II-IV heart failure (Table 25.2) or on hemodialysis. In the 4 randomized controlled trials reviewed, there was insufficient information on which to base recommendations in patients with these comorbidities; therefore, individualized assessment is needed to evaluate reduction benefit, adverse effects, drug-drug interactions, and other cautions.[52]

Statin Safety

Patients predisposed to adverse effects of statins (eg, those with impaired renal or hepatic function, other serious coexisting conditions, a history of statin intolerance, concomitant use of drugs affecting statin metabolism, or unexplained elevation of alanine aminotransferase [ALT] levels that are 3 times the upper limit of normal; and those who are age >75) should use moderate-intensity statin therapy when high-intensity therapy would otherwise be recommended.[93] Baseline ALT before statin initiation should be checked and monitored at follow-up if symptoms suggest hepatotoxicity (eg, unusual fatigue or weakness, loss of appetite, abdominal pain, dark-colored urine, jaundice). It is also reasonable to measure baseline creatinine kinase (CK) before statin initiation in individuals at risk for adverse muscle events based on personal or family history of statin intolerance or muscle disease or receiving concomitant drug therapy that increases myopathy risk. It is reasonable to discontinue statin therapy for muscle pain or symptoms until the symptoms are fully evaluated. Some patients tolerate a change from one statin to another, so a change in statin therapy can be considered if therapy is stopped and restarted. During therapy, CK measurement can be repeated in patients with muscle symptoms, tenderness, stiffness, cramping, weakness, or generalized fatigue.

Dietary Modification

Lifestyle modification (eg, heart-healthy diet, regular exercise, avoidance of tobacco, maintenance of a healthy weight) is also a critical component of the management of hyperlipoproteinemia.[52,54] Dietary modification, as discussed earlier in detail, can include the following recommendations:

◆ Consume a diet that consists largely of vegetables, fruits, and whole grains; includes low-fat dairy products, poultry, fish, legumes, nontropical vegetable oils, and nuts; and limits intake of sweets, sugar-sweetened beverages, and red meats.

◆ Reduce intake of saturated fat to 5% to 6% of total calories and minimize *trans* fat from partially hydrogenated vegetable oils.

LDL-C Monitoring

The ADA recommends annual screening for lipid abnormalities using a fasting lipid profile in most adults with diabetes. The newer ACC/AHA guidelines also necessitate lipid testing for most patients to determine the recommended intensity of statin therapy. However, because the guideline no longer emphasizes target LDL levels, it eliminates the need for routine assessment of cholesterol levels in patients receiving statin therapy.[93] However, it is reasonable to do follow-up testing after statin initiation to consider a dose reduction if LDL values are consistently lower than 40 mg/dL.

Lipid levels should be measured after an overnight fast, because postprandial TG elevations may interfere with evaluation of the lipid profile. Calculation of LDL-C is often inaccurate with elevated TG, and most laboratories do not report the LDL-C if the TG level is greater than 400 mg/dL. In this case, the direct LDL-C assay may be useful.

Other Lipid Treatments

Hypertriglyceridemia should be addressed with dietary and lifestyle changes. Severe hypertriglyceridemia (≥1000 mg/dL) warrants immediate pharmacologic therapy with a fibrate, niacin, or fish oil to reduce the risk of acute pancreatitis. In the absence of severe hypertriglyceridemia, the evidence does not support pharmacologic intervention with fibrates or niacin, in addition to statin therapy, to achieve HDL and TG goals. However, these drugs may be considered in patients intolerant of statin therapy. Niacin, fenofibrate, ezetimibe, and bile acid sequestrants can all lower LDL cholesterol. Niacin therapy can increase blood glucose at doses required to improve lipids, and intensification of glycemic therapy may be needed.

> The 2013 ACC/AHA guideline emphasizes the importance of statin therapy over particular LDL-C goals in people with diabetes. Most people with diabetes and 10-year ASCVD risk ≥7.5% should receive high-intensity statin therapy. Moderate-intensity statin therapy is recommended for people with diabetes predisposed to adverse statin effects or ASCVD risk <7.5%.

Hypertension Management

Numerous studies have shown that blood pressure reduction in people with diabetes and hypertension can reduce overall CV mortality and, in particular, the incidence of stroke. This effect is shown with even modest reductions in blood pressure; for example, in the UKPDS, the intensive group reached a mean blood pressure of 144/82 mm Hg, compared with the control group's 154/87 mm Hg. Diabetes-related death was reduced by 32% and stroke by 44%.[94] There was a nonsignificant 21% reduction in MI with blood pressure control. Most studies have shown

the same pattern: a dramatic reduction in stroke and total CV mortality and a less dramatic effect on MI.[95]

Blood Pressure Measurement Technique

Blood pressure should be checked at every routine visit, and at least yearly, for all people with diabetes. Blood pressure should be checked accurately with appropriate cuff size and the patient in a seated position, feet on the floor with arm supported at heart level, after 5 minutes of rest. Use of automated blood pressure cuffs can increase the accuracy of blood pressure measurement and eliminate the interpretation bias and digit preference observed in manual auscultatory measurements.[96,97]

Patients with elevated blood pressure should have blood pressure confirmed on a separate day. The educator should stress that patients with an elevated blood pressure reading should return for a repeat blood pressure in a timely fashion. There are no strict guidelines for the time frame for a repeat blood pressure, but a reasonable time frame is within a month if the situation is not urgent and within days if blood pressure is ≥180/110 mm Hg. Too often in many care systems, patients with elevated blood pressure are lost to follow-up for long periods.

Home and ambulatory blood pressure monitoring may help with diagnosis and management of hypertension—especially when there is a discrepancy between office and home readings (eg, "white coat hypertension"). Ambulatory blood pressure measurements correlate with CVD risk better than office measurements. Asleep systolic blood pressure mean and sleep-time relative to systolic blood pressure decline are the most significant predictors of CVD events.[98] Recommended ambulatory blood pressure thresholds for men, without compelling clinical indications for more aggressive treatment, are 135/85 mm Hg for awake and 120/70 mm Hg for asleep systolic blood pressure/diastolic blood pressure means. Recommended thresholds for higher risk persons with diabetes, chronic kidney disease (CKD), or CHD are often 15/10 mm Hg lower. If ambulatory blood pressure monitoring becomes more available and cost-effective, it may permit greater individualization of blood pressure treatment intensification based on higher-risk nocturnal blood pressure patterns.

Blood Pressure Goals

For people without diabetes or CKD, blood pressure control to <140/90 mm Hg is recommended for the general population older than 18 and younger than 60, and <150/90 mm Hg is recommended for those 60 and older to reduce rates of CHD events, stroke, and nephropathy.[99] The JNC8 recommendation for people with diabetes, regardless of age, is blood pressure <140/90 mm Hg. The Hypertension Optimal Treatment Study, a randomized trial published in 1998 which targeted lower diastolic blood pressures for people with diabetes, demonstrated additional CV benefit down to a diastolic blood pressure target of 80 mm Hg.[100] Thus there remains some controversy about whether the diastolic goal should be lower for people with diabetes. However, more recent clinical trials have not demonstrated the benefits of targeting a systolic blood pressure <140 mm Hg.[101] The ACCORD trial, which examined whether a systolic blood pressure <120 mm Hg would provide greater benefit than a systolic blood pressure 130 to 139 mm Hg, found that neither the primary outcome (overall CV event rates) nor microvascular complications were significantly reduced in the more intensively treated group. Although strokes were reduced to a small degree, serious adverse events (eg, syncope, hyperkalemia) occurred at a higher rate in the intensively treated group.[102] Another large trial, ADVANCE, showed reduced mortality rates in the more intensively treated group, but the achieved mean systolic blood pressure was 135 mm Hg.[103] The ADA guidelines suggest that a lower target of <130 mm Hg may be appropriate for certain individuals (eg, younger patients) if it can be reached without undue treatment burden.[104]

Treatment of Hypertension

Evaluation of people with hypertension and diabetes begins by addressing lifestyle factors that may contribute to hypertension and CV risk. This is clearly in the purview of the diabetes educator. Lifestyle modification is a mainstay of treatment for *all* individuals with prehypertension and hypertension. Suggested lifestyle changes may include the following:

- ◆ Weight reduction
- ◆ Adoption of the DASH eating plan
- ◆ Dietary sodium reduction
- ◆ Increased physical activity
- ◆ Moderation of alcohol consumption
- ◆ Avoidance of nonsteroidal anti-inflammatory drugs (NSAIDs)

Numerous clinical trials have explored the benefits of specific antihypertensive pharmacotherapy on CV outcomes. The largest of these was ALLHAT, which compared chlorthalidone (a thiazide diuretic), amlodipine (a dihydropyridine calcium-channel blocker [CCB]), lisinopril (an angiotensin-converting enzyme [ACE] inhibitor), and doxazosin (alpha blocker).[105] The doxazosin arm of the study was discontinued due to increased incidence of heart failure, and the remaining 3 arms of the study showed decreased rates of fatal and nonfatal MI. Chorthalidone was superior to amlodipine and lisinopril in preventing new-onset heart failure, although the benefit may have been due to greater blood pressure lowering observed in the chlorthalidone group.

Angiotensin-converting enzyme inhibitors and angiotensin-receptor blockers (ARBs) may have several advantages in people with diabetes, including relatively low toxicity and additional renal protection. However, many experts conclude from the data that the achieved blood pressure, rather than the specific drug class used, is the primary determinant of benefit. The JNC8 workgroup recommended a thiazide diuretic, CCB, ACE inhibitor, or ARB for initial antihypertensive treatment for the general nonblack population, including those with diabetes. For the general black population, including those with diabetes, initial antihypertensive treatment should include a thiazide diuretic or CCB. In the general population with CKD, regardless of diabetes status, an ACE inhibitor or ARB therapy is recommended for initial or add-on therapy to improve kidney outcomes. The main objective of blood pressure management is to attain and maintain the recommended blood pressure goal by reinforcing medication and lifestyle adherence and intensifying pharmacologic therapy, if indicated. Angiotensin-converting enzyme inhibitors and ARBs should not be used together. Referral to a hypertension specialist may be indicated for patients whose goal blood pressure cannot be attained using the above strategy with 3 or fewer drugs.[99] Full details of medical nutrition therapy, lifestyle modification, and specific pharmacologic treatment (including dosing, contraindications, and side effects) of hypertension are included in chapters 16 and 19.

Instruction Opportunity—Supporting Patients in Achieving Blood Pressure Goals

Most people with T2DM need at least 2 or 3 medications to achieve blood pressure goals (a mean of 2.3 drugs was required in ACCORD patients with a systolic blood pressure goal of 130–139 mm Hg, 3.4 drugs for patients with a goal of <120 mm Hg).[106] Setting this expectation early in the educational process may help. The level of blood pressure achieved is generally considered more important than the choice of drugs used to achieve the goal.

Assess patients routinely for potential barriers to adherence, such as medication adherence, cost of medications, and side effects. Help patients keep track of their medication schedule and adhere to their medication plan with tables of medications, their purpose, and when to take them. Explain that, even if hypertension is asymptomatic, it is very important to continue treatment to prevent heart attacks and strokes.

Pharmacists, nurses, and dietitians, if available in the patient's care system, can facilitate pharmacologic management using medication protocols (if within their practice scope and licensure). For patients with established hypertension, home blood pressure telemonitoring with phone-based case management can result in lower mean blood pressure and a higher percentage of patients achieving recommended blood pressure targets.[107]

Appropriate Use of Aspirin

One of the earliest studies of antiplatelet agents, the Early Treatment Diabetic Retinopathy Study,[108] was designed primarily to determine the effect of aspirin therapy on retinopathy. The study found that aspirin had no significant effect on retinopathy but that it decreased the rate of MI by 28%.[109] Subsequent studies confirmed and expanded understanding of the effect of aspirin on CV risk, as reviewed in the 2010 ADA position statement.[110,111] Thus, for secondary prevention in patients with a history of known CHD, ischemic stroke, transient ischemic attack, and/or

PAD, the benefits of aspirin generally outweigh the risks (for patients untreated with other anticoagulants or other antiplatelet drugs and with no history of gastrointestinal ulcer or bleeding). Aspirin is also recommended for primary prevention of stroke in patients with a history of atrial fibrillation if anticoagulants cannot be used. However, more recent data have questioned the balance between the risks and benefits of aspirin therapy for primary prevention in people with and without diabetes.[112]

A clear benefit of aspirin therapy to reduce CV risk in people with diabetes for primary prevention is unproven.[113] Evidence that the benefits outweigh the risks is less strong but does support a beneficial effect in men with elevated CHD risk and women with elevated stroke risk. The beneficial effects must be weighed against the harm from gastrointestinal bleeding (which has a well-established relationship with increasing age). Therefore, the decision to use aspirin for primary prevention should be individualized based on the balance of risks and benefits. If aspirin is used, clinicians should inform patients about signs and symptoms of gastrointestinal bleeding (eg, dark stools, vomiting blood, bright red blood from the rectum, syncope, lightheadedness).

For primary prevention in people with diabetes, the ADA recommends aspirin for most men older than 50 and most women older than 60 with at least 1 additional major CV risk factor (eg, family history of CVD, hypertension, smoking, dyslipidemia, or albuminuria). Aspirin is not routinely recommended for men younger than 50 or women younger than 60 without other major risk factors. For patients not in these categories (younger individuals with risk factors and older individuals without other risk factors), clinical judgment is required.

Another approach to assessing the benefits of aspirin for primary prevention in patients is to use the US Preventive Services Task Force (USPSTF) tables using patient age and calculated 10-year CHD risk in men and 10-year stroke risk in women. The USPSTF does not recommend aspirin for men younger than 45, women younger than 55, or anyone older than 80. For others, if the patient's general CV risk has been calculated (as detailed previously), the CHD risk for men can be roughly estimated at 73% of the general CV risk, and stroke risk for women at about 24% of the general CV risk (these estimates were validated with Framingham risk calculations and are not published for the ACC/AHA risk calculation).[114] Once the 10-year CHD risk (men) or 10-year stroke risk (women) has been determined, the USPSTF table can be used to make an aspirin recommendation. If the CV risk exceeds the threshold in Table 25.3 for age and sex, aspirin is recommended.

Other considerations in the balance of benefits and harms of aspirin therapy include a strong family history of CHD, a positive test for urinary albumin, and a family history of colon cancer (aspirin may be protective in this situation). Other patient factors can increase the risk of gastrointestinal bleeding and should be considered when balancing the benefits and harms of aspirin therapy. Nonsteroidal anti-inflammatory drugs combined with aspirin roughly quadruples the risk for serious gastrointestinal bleeding compared with aspirin alone. The rate of serious bleeding is 2 to 3 times higher in patients with a history of gastrointestinal ulcer. Enteric-coated or buffered preparations do not clearly reduce aspirin's gastrointestinal effects.

Even though CV risk is very high in elderly patients, the use of aspirin in patients older than 80 is not currently recommended due to concerns over the high risks. If aspirin is used in persons older than 80, it should be limited to those without additional risk factors for gastrointestinal bleeding and those in good enough health to tolerate a serious gastrointestinal bleed. This recommendation may change based on results of a large randomized trial of aspirin use in the elderly that is currently under way.[115]

Aspirin is not usually recommended for patients taking other anticoagulants or antiplatelet agents. Dual antiplatelet therapy with clopidogrel and aspirin may increase risks, but combination therapy is associated with a reduction in the risk of CV events compared with aspirin alone in patients with symptoms of acute coronary syndrome.[116] Antiplatelet therapy is also indicated to reduce the risk of MI, stroke, or vascular death in individuals with PAD. Aspirin in daily doses of 75 to 325 mg is usually recommended for PAD, but clopidogrel (75 mg/d) is an effective alternative. The combination of aspirin and clopidogrel can be considered in patients with symptomatic PAD, including intermittent claudication, limb ischemia, or history of amputation.[116,117] The FDA has approved clopidogrel for the reduction of ischemic events in patients with PAD.

The optimum dose of aspirin for preventing CVD events is not known. Primary prevention trials have demonstrated benefits with various regimens, including dosages of 75 and 100 mg/d and 100 and 325 mg every other day. A dosage of about 75 mg/d seems as effective as higher dosages. The risk of gastrointestinal bleeding may increase with increasing aspirin doses.

TABLE 25.3   Determining Aspirin Recommendations for Primary Cardiovascular Prevention Using USPSTF Guidelines

Men		Women	
Age (Years)	*Threshold for Recommending Aspirin*	*Age (Years)*	*Threshold for Recommending Aspirin*
	10-year CHD risk (%)*		**10-year stroke risk (%)***
45–59	≥4	55–59	≥3
60–69	≥9	60–69	≥8
70–79	≥12	70–79	≥11

Abbreviations: ASCVD, atherosclerotic cardiovascular disease; CHD, coronary heart disease.

*10-year CHD risk for men is approximately 73% of the total general CV risk, and 10-year stroke risk for women is approximately 24% of the total general CV risk using Framingham data.[114] ASCVD risk thresholds in this table were calculated using the calibration thresholds.[114]

Source: "Aspirin for the prevention of cardiovascular disease: US Preventive Services Task Force recommendation statement," *Ann Intern Med* 150, no. 6 (2009): 396-404.

Aspirin Use for Primary Prevention of CV Events

For primary prevention in people with diabetes, the ADA recommends aspirin for most men 50 and older and most women 60 and older with at least 1 additional major CV risk factor (eg, family history of CVD, hypertension, smoking, dyslipidemia, or albuminuria). Aspirin is not recommended for men younger than 50 or women younger than 60 without other major risk factors. For younger patients with risk factors and older patients without risk factors, clinical judgment is required. The USPSTF has published tables to help assess the balance of benefits and harm in individual patients based on age and calculated CVD risk.

Instruction Opportunity—Using Aspirin Appropriately

Aspirin has been heavily marketed for prevention for CV events. Because aspirin is available over the counter, many patients take it without the knowledge or recommendation of their provider. It is important that the patient's providers are aware of aspirin use and that it is documented in the medication list. Patients must understand that aspirin is not without risk and that their risk of gastrointestinal hemorrhage must be balanced with the possible benefits of risk reduction (MI in men and stroke in women). The decision to use aspirin is best individualized using a shared decision-making approach with a fully informed patient. Patients who take aspirin should be advised to avoid NSAIDs and to seek prompt medical attention for signs or symptoms of gastrointestinal bleeding (eg, dark stools, vomiting blood, bright red blood from the rectum, syncope, lightheadedness).

ACE Inhibitors or ARBs for Patients With Increased Urinary Albumin Excretion

Increased urinary albumin excretion (eg, increased urine microalbumin:creatinine ratio) indicates endothelial dysfunction and can help predict CV events. Persons with diabetes and microalbuminuria have 2 to 8 times the risk of CV events than persons with diabetes without microalbuminuria.[118] Both the presence of increased urinary albumin and its progression predict increased coronary mortality in T2DM.[119] Angiotensin-converting enzyme inhibitors or ARBs are recommended for patients with urinary albumin to prevent progression of renal disease[99] and may also significantly reduce the risk of CV events in patients beyond their blood pressure–lowering effect.[120]

Nontraditional and Emerging New CV Risk Factors

Traditional risk factors such as diabetes, hypertension, smoking, and dyslipidemia are generally understood to explain only about 50% to 60% of the variability in CV risk. Thus, the past decade has seen a concerted effort to identify other risk factors to help predict CV events in individuals for more accurate risk assessment. Some nontraditional biomarkers associated with CV risk are high-sensitivity C-reactive protein (hs-CRP), lipoproteins, apolipoproteins A-I and B, CKD testing such as glomerular filtration rate (GFR) and microalbuminuria, fibrinogen, white blood cell count, cystatin C, homocysteine (Hcy), B-type natriuretic peptide (BNP), coronary artery calcification (CAC) scores, ankle-brachial index (ABI), and carotid IMT.[121] The ACC/AHA guideline indicates that assessments of family history of premature CVD, measurement of hs-CRP, CAC scores, and ABI show promise for clinical use based on limited data.[53] However, the ACC/AHA guideline workgroup concluded that evidence is insufficient that these markers can improve the CV risk prediction over the recommended Pooled Cohort Equation. Likewise, the addition of family history of CHD or BMI did not improve discrimination of the model.[53] However, if a risk-based treatment decision is uncertain after quantitative ASCVD risk assessment, assessment of 1 or more of family history, hs-CRP, CAC score, or ABI may help inform treatment decision-making.[93] The USPSTF concluded that "current evidence is insufficient to assess the balance of benefits and harms of using the nontraditional risk factors studied to screen asymptomatic men and women with no history of CHD to prevent CHD events" (p. 474).[122]

Nontraditional Therapies to Lower CV Risk

Supplements with vitamins and antioxidants such as A, C, and E and multivitamins with folic acid have been touted as CV risk-reduction strategies, but evidence does not support their use. In the NORVIT study, vitamin B$_6$ and folate increased the risk of MI by 21%. The SEARCH study revealed that the addition of vitamin E to simvastatin, an HMG-CoA reductase inhibitor, also increased the risk of CV events.[123] An analysis of data from the HOPE and HOPE-TOO studies found that vitamin E supplementation in people with diabetes or CVD did not reduce the rate of major CV events and may have increased the risk of heart failure.[124] Beta carotene supplementation could also be dangerous and should be discouraged.[125] The USPSTF recommends that patients who take vitamins be encouraged to adhere to dosages recommended in the dietary reference intakes (DRIs) of the Institute of Medicine.[126] Inappropriate use of antioxidants and vitamins may not only blunt the protective effects of other therapies but often creates the misperception that "natural" therapies are always better than drugs, diverting the patient from proven therapies.

CV Risk Management Issues Specific to Children and Adolescents

An observed linear increase in T1DM and T2DM in childhood is expected to significantly increase the prevalence of diabetes in youth over the next 40 years (2010 to 2050). The prevalence of T1DM is projected to triple and T2DM to quadruple, with the greatest increase in youth in minority racial/ethnic groups.[127] The prevalence of having at least 2 CVD risk factors is about 21% (roughly 92% of youth with T2DM and 14% of youth with T1DM).[128] The implications of this increase are staggering. A continuation of this increase in the number of young people with T2DM will lead to a massive increase in microvascular and macrovascular disease over the next 3 decades.[129] Strategies for weight, lipid, and blood pressure control in youth with diabetes are needed to prevent or delay the development of CVD as they mature.

> Strategies for weight, lipid, and blood pressure control in youth with diabetes are critical to prevent or delay the development of CVD as they mature.

Blood Pressure Management in Children and Adolescents

Normal blood pressures for age, sex, and height and appropriate methods for determination are available at http://www.nhlbi.nih.gov/health/prof/heart/hbp/hbp_ped.pdf. The 2014 ADA Standards of Medical Care in Diabetes discuss screening for and management of hypertension for children and adolescents with diabetes and make these recommendations[88]: Blood pressure should be measured at all routine visits. The target is a blood pressure consistently <130/80 mm Hg or below the 90th percentile for age, sex, and height (whichever is lower). Treatment including dietary intervention, exercise, and weight control should be initiated in youth with high-normal blood pressure consistently above the 90th percentile. If blood pressure targets are not reached within 3 to 6 months of lifestyle intervention, pharmacologic treatment should be considered. Hypertension in childhood is defined as an average systolic or diastolic blood pressure ≥95th percentile for age, sex, and height percentile confirmed on at least 3 separate days. Pharmacologic treatment for hypertension should be considered as soon as the diagnosis is confirmed. See chapter 19 for details on pharmacologic interventions for hypertension in youth.

Lipid Management for Children and Adolescents

A 2011 NHLBI expert panel recommended universal screening of children ages 9 to 11 with a nonfasting lipid panel, plus targeting screening with 2 fasting lipid profiles of children aged 2 to 8 and 12 to 16. The American Academy of Pediatrics endorsed the recommendations despite controversy created by a lack of evidence for benefit, harm, and cost and reliance on opinions of many experts with industry conflicts of interest. The expert panel recommended starting with lifestyle treatment, with a decision to begin pharmacotherapy based on the average results of 2 fasting lipid profiles obtained 2 weeks to 3 months apart. The 2014 ADA Standards of Medical Care in Diabetes recommend screening children >2 years soon after diagnosis if they have a family history of hypercholesterolemia or CV event before age 55; otherwise, the first lipid screening should be obtained at puberty (age ≥10) or when diabetes is diagnosed after puberty. The recommended goal is LDL <100 mg/dL. If it is higher, repeat screening every 5 years is recommended. If LDL is ≥100 mg/dL, initial therapy may consist of glycemic control and nutritional therapy.

Pharmacotherapy for children younger than 10 is generally not recommended and should be used only under the direction of a pediatric lipid specialist. Pharmacotherapy is advocated for children 10 and older with diabetes if LDL is refractory to nonpharmacotherapy and CV risk factors are present. Pharmacotherapy can be recommended for people with diabetes and LDL ≥160 mg/dL or ≥130 mg/dL if other CV factors (hypertension, smoking, BMI >95th percentile, HDL <40 mg/dL) or high-risk conditions (eg, CKD, heart transplant, Kawasaki disease with coronary aneurysm, chronic inflammatory diseases, HIV, nephritic syndrome) are present. Neither long-term safety nor CV outcome efficacy has been established for statins in children, and they are not approved for children younger than 10. Statins are category X in pregnancy and should be used cautiously in postpubertal girls.[88]

Coronary Artery Disease

How Does Coronary Artery Disease Present?

Coronary artery disease (CAD) most often presents with either angina pectoris or MI. Chest pain is a common symptom that may or may not be angina or MI. Persons with diabetes are at very high risk for CAD and should be educated about the warning signs (Table 25.4).

Autonomic neuropathy, which is common in people with long-standing diabetes, often includes cardiac denervation, which may result in the atypical chest pain of coronary ischemia. Rather than angina pectoris or substernal pain, the patient may experience only weakness, diaphoresis, dyspnea, or nausea with the onset of ischemia or infarction.

Patients who show evidence of autonomic neuropathy should be educated about atypical cardiac symptoms.

Should Patients Be Screened for CAD?

Diagnostic tests are used when there is a clinical indication of disease. The question remains whether additional cardiac testing to screen for CAD in asymptomatic patients improves patient outcomes. Several important questions need to be answered when considering screening for CAD in people with diabetes:

- Who should be screened?
- Why should they be screened?
- How should they be screened?

Some studies suggest that everyone with T2DM should be considered to have CAD.[130] So should everyone with T2DM be screened? Screening the more than 23 million people in the United States with T2DM would be very expensive. So how do clinicians decide who should be screened?

Studies have not demonstrated a reduced CV outcome when asymptomatic people with diabetes underwent cardiac stress testing or screening with adenosine SPECT myocardial perfusion scanning.[131,132] The lack of effect may reflect the general improvement in CV outcomes as a result of more aggressive management of dyslipidemia and hypertension. Intensive medical therapy of CV risk factors is indicated for high-risk patients, regardless of results of screening tests, and seems to provide outcomes equal to those of invasive revascularization.[133,134] Therefore, current evidence does not show cost-effectiveness or benefits to routine cardiac screening of people with diabetes without cardiac symptoms and with a normal EKG.

Noninvasive cardiac screening methods for CAC with computed tomography (CT) and CT angiography are gaining popularity. More research is needed to clarify how to interpret the results of these tests and whether they benefit people with diabetes known to be at CV risk who have started statins, aspirin, and blood pressure control. Routine use of these tests can expose patients to radiation and may lead to unnecessary invasive testing and procedures. Thus, determining whether the benefits of screening for coronary disease in asymptomatic patients relative to the cost and risk of this technology requires further research.

The ADA practice guidelines suggest that patients with typical or atypical cardiac symptoms or abnormal

TABLE 25.4	Warning Signs of CAD	
	Angina	*MI*
Etiology	Coronary ischemia; partial occlusion of coronary artery (may be caused by 70%–80% narrowing of 1 or more coronary vessels); usually gradual onset	Sudden total occlusion of coronary artery; often caused by 40%–50% occlusion; vulnerable soft plaque with thin fibrous caps that rupture and release necrotic, lipid-filled material into the artery that can initiate a thrombus and occlude an artery
Quality	Squeezing, tightness, pressure or heavy weight on the chest; more discomfort than pain	Intense, severe squeezing or crushing pain
Location	Diffuse over chest, radiating to neck, lower jaw, or left arm	Midsternal pain radiating to arms, neck, and jaw; epigastric pain
Timing	Rarely lasts more than 5 minutes; remits when precipitating activity is stopped (may be triggered by exercise, sexual intercourse, cold weather, cocaine use)	30–60 minutes
Associated symptoms	Dyspnea, diaphoresis, cold and clammy skin, fatigue, syncope	Diaphoresis, nausea, vomiting, weakness, dyspnea, sense of impending doom, paleness
Notes	Elderly and those with diabetic autonomic neuropathy may have no pain	Autonomic neuropathy may cause loss of pain sensation; may present with onset of diabetic ketoacidosis in people with T1DM; in patients suspected of having MI, advise chewing a full-strength aspirin and calling 911

resting EKGs are candidates for more cardiac testing. Most often, the initial screening or diagnostic test is a fasting exercise EKG. The EKG leads are placed in the standard locations for a 12-lead EKG. The individual then begins to walk on a level treadmill at a slow pace. The speed and incline of the treadmill are gradually increased until symptoms or EKG abnormalities occur. In another functional test, the stress echocardiogram, the myocardium is imaged by sonography during exercise. Areas of abnormal motion indicate ischemia.

Instruction Opportunity—Preparing Patients for an Exercise Stress Test

Patients usually fast before exercise stress testing. Significant hyperglycemia or hypoglycemia may interfere with the ability to exercise at an appropriate level. Although the stress test is usually limited to 12 to 15 minutes, it may be enough to precipitate hypoglycemia during or shortly after the exercise in people taking long-acting insulin or sulfonylureas.

The educator should discuss hypoglycemia with the patient. This type of hypoglycemia is usually short-lived and can be treated with oral carbohydrate.

Sulfonylureas and short-acting insulins should be held until the first posttest meal.

Treatment of Acute MI

Treatment of acute MI in people with diabetes is similar to that in people without diabetes. Treatment may include thrombolytic agents, coronary angioplasty, stents, and revascularization. Outcomes may be worse for people with diabetes. Despite advances in cardiac care over the past 4 decades, the presence of diabetes still doubles the risk of death after MI.[135] Once the patient is stable, the cardiologist may perform testing to evaluate short-term risk and therapies (eg, exercise stress testing, echocardiogram, coronary angiogram). In some cases, further revascularization may be performed.

Hyperglycemia in a person with MI increases the risk of death and CHF whether or not the person had a diagnosis of diabetes before admission.[136] There is increasing evidence that MI may be the initial presentation of diabetes.[137] The Diabetes Mellitus, Insulin Glucose Infusion in Acute Myocardial Infarction (DIGAMI) trial studied the effect of aggressive diabetes control in the immediate post-MI period with an intravenous insulin-glucose drip and 3 months of a 4-shot regimen. Patients randomly assigned to the intensive protocol had significantly reduced mortality. The risk reduction was greatest in those classified as low risk who were not previously treated with insulin.[138] However, the follow-up DIGAMI 2 study did not confirm the findings of DIGAMI; there was no significant difference in mortality between the intensively and non-intensively treated groups.[139] Thus, current recommendations for the treatment of diabetes in people with acute MI do not differ from those of other hospitalized patients. Insulin is the drug of choice: intravenous insulin for patients in critical care units and subcutaneous insulin for other patients. Long-term diabetes management for these patients does not differ from that of high-risk patients previously described.

Risk-factor management and education begin in the hospital. Diabetes control should be stressed and the patient prepared for post-discharge lifestyle changes and risk-factor reduction. A statin, an ACE inhibitor, a beta blocker, and an antiplatelet agent are often instituted as soon as possible if there are no contraindications.

Instruction Opportunity— Educating Patients After an MI

Persons with an MI undergo a major psychological trauma. They are often discharged from the hospital within 4 or 5 days after an uncomplicated MI, usually with a myriad of unanswered and unasked questions. The following are important education topics:

◆ *Follow-up care.* Schedule appointments with the physician, educator, mental health counselor, and cardiac rehabilitation team, as needed.

◆ *Medications.* Most people with an MI go home with many new medications, including a statin, an ACE inhibitor, a beta blocker, aspirin, and perhaps another antiplatelet agent in addition to their diabetes medication, which may well be new or intensified at this time (see Treatment of Acute MI section above).

◆ *Exercise.* Some people with a recent MI may be afraid to exercise, and some, in the throes of denial, may overdo it. Cardiac rehabilitation programs enable the individual to work

with a trained clinical team to carefully increase exercise in a supervised setting. A cardiac rehabilitation center can be an excellent venue for your diabetes self-management education program as well.

◆ *Therapeutic lifestyle change.* This includes smoking cessation and medical nutrition therapy.

◆ *Psychosocial issues.* Up to one third of people with MI have significant depressive symptoms afterward, and major depression occurs in nearly one fifth.[140] Depression, which is common in people with diabetes, is associated with a twofold to threefold increase in risk of death in the first 6 months after MI.[141] Another study of highly stressed individuals after MI found that home nursing visits were associated with a significant reduction in subsequent fatal and nonfatal cardiac events.[142]

◆ *Sexual activity.* Many patients are concerned about safely resuming sexual activity. Sexual dysfunction may be common, and its treatment should be discussed with the patient.

How Should Patients Be Prepared for Elective Cardiac Catheterization and Angioplasty?

Issues to discuss with the patient and the physician include the following:

◆ *Timing and food consumption.* Whenever possible, elective cardiac catheterization for people taking insulin should be scheduled in the morning. In most cases, the patient fasts after midnight for an early-morning procedure. If the procedure is later in the day, a light meal may be allowed up to 2 to 4 hours before.

◆ *Diabetes medications.* Advise the patient about whether to decrease or withhold certain diabetes medications.

—In general, there is no reason to change evening or bedtime insulin or oral agents if morning self-monitored glucose is acceptable.

—Persons on insulin pumps should continue their normal basal insulin infusion.

—Sulfonylureas, secretagogues, and acarbose should be held on the morning of the procedure and resumed when the person resumes normal eating.

—Metformin is held the morning of the procedure and resumed when creatinine has been rechecked and it is certain that the angiogram dye has caused no adverse renal effects.

—Thiazolidinediones can be held or given because they are long-acting drugs.

◆ *Hyperglycemia and hypoglycemia.* Planning should include addressing hyperglycemia and hypoglycemia before and during the procedure.

◆ *Hydration.* Patients should be instructed to increase fluid intake to enhance excretion of the angiogram dye.

◆ *Steroid pretreatment.* In patients with a history or risk of allergy to the angiogram dye, steroids such as prednisone may be given the day before and the day of the procedure. Most patients note a significant increase in their glucose for 2 to 3 days after beginning an oral steroid. Patients should be adequately prepared for this effect so they can appropriately adjust their medication.

Cerebrovascular Disease

Atherosclerosis affecting the central nervous system presents in 3 characteristic ways:

◆ Transient ischemic attack
◆ Cerebrovascular accident
—*Ischemic:* Thrombotic, embolic, or systemic hypotension
—*Hemorrhagic:* Intracranial or subarachnoid
◆ Vascular dementia

What Causes a Cerebrovascular Accident?

About 80% of strokes are ischemic, and the rest are hemorrhagic. By definition, a cerebrovascular accident (CVA) is tissue death resulting from disruption from either hemorrhage or ischemic infarction. Ischemic CVA may be caused by atherosclerotic disease in intracranial or extracranial arteries. The process may be intrinsic to the affected artery, as in atherosclerotic thrombi, or the result of embolus from either the heart or extracranial arteries. The clinical presentation depends on the area of the brain served by the affected arteries.

Ischemic strokes are more likely to occur at a younger age in African Americans, when hypertension is present, and when there is a history of MI.[58] Most thrombotic and embolic strokes occur in persons older than 40, but this may be less predictive in the future because today's youth with T2DM will reach their forties with a history of almost 30 years of diabetes.

Is a Stroke Preventable?

Hypertension, including isolated systolic hypertension, is the most important risk factor for stroke. Diabetes and smoking also contribute to stroke risk. Smoking increases the prevalence of extracranial occlusive arterial disease and more than doubles the risk of stroke. Diabetes is also associated with a doubling of stroke risk, affecting both small and large arteries. Statin therapy has been shown to decrease the risk of fatal and nonfatal stroke.[143]

Effective antihypertensive therapy, statin therapy, and smoking cessation have been shown to decrease stroke risk.[94,144]

What Is a Transient Ischemic Attack?

Transient ischemic attack (TIA), sometimes called "mini stroke" by lay people, is classically defined as the sudden onset of a neurologic deficit that lasts less than 24 hours and is not associated with a permanent residual defect. Transient ischemic attack is presumably caused by a transient decrease in blood supply, causing focal ischemia in the area of the brain that produces the symptoms.

The syndromes caused by TIA depend on the pathogenesis and location. Transient ischemic attacks may be caused by decreased flow in a large artery, either intracranial or extracranial. Less often, an embolus from a larger artery or the heart results in a TIA. Transient ischemic attack may result from lesions in either the anterior (carotid) or posterior (vertebral) circulation. The symptoms of ischemia differ significantly because these vascular beds supply areas of the brain with markedly different functions.

Initial evaluation of a person with a suspected TIA starts with a carefully taken history. In most cases, the episode has passed by the time the person is seen by a clinician. It is important to differentiate an ischemic event from a metabolic event such as hypoglycemia. Although seizure disorders, syncope, and migraine auras may mimic TIA symptoms, it is important to first rule out TIA. Urgent medical attention and evaluation of patients with TIA symptoms, even if they have disappeared, is important. Risk of CVA in the months after a TIA is very high. From 11% to 20% of patients with a TIA have a CVA in the next 90 days; half of the strokes occurred in the first 2 days.[145,146]

> Transient ischemic attacks occur suddenly, with symptoms that may have passed by the time the patient is seen. They require urgent evaluation and referral due to the high risk of stroke.

Instruction Opportunity—Recognizing Signs of a TIA or Stroke

The AHA promotes the acronym FAST as an easy way to help patients remember the warning signs and symptoms of stroke.[147] According to the AHA's Web site, FAST is described as the following:

- Face drooping—Does one side of the face droop or is it numb? Ask the person to smile. Is the smile uneven?
- Arm weakness—Is one arm weak or numb? Ask the person to raise both arms. Does one arm drift downward?
- Speech difficulty—Is speech slurred? Is the person unable to speak or hard to understand? Ask the person to repeat a simple sentence, like "The sky is blue." Is the sentence repeated correctly?
- Time to call 9-1-1—If someone shows any of these symptoms, even if the symptoms go away, call 9-1-1 and get the person to the hospital immediately. Check the time so you'll know when the first symptoms appeared.

Symptoms of cerebrovascular disease may mimic those of hypoglycemia. See the early-warning symptoms of stroke in Table 25.5. Current therapeutic approaches to thrombotic CVA (the most common form in diabetes) call for early institution of thrombolytic agents.

TABLE 25.5 Early-Warning Symptoms of Stroke
The Stroke Association has publicized these early-warning symptoms of stroke and recommends that the person or witness call 911 if they occur: • Sudden numbness or weakness of the face, arm, or leg, especially on one side of the body • Sudden confusion, trouble speaking or understanding • Sudden trouble seeing in 1 or both eyes • Sudden trouble walking, dizziness, or loss of balance or coordination • Sudden, severe headache with no known cause

Source: Stroke Association, "Learn more stroke warning signs and symptoms" (last reviewed 2013 Apr 3, cited 2014 Apr 3), on the Internet at: http://www.strokeassociation.org/STROKEORG/WarningSigns/Learn-More-Stroke-Warning-Signs-and-Symptoms_UCM_451207_Article.jsp.

Transient ischemic attacks may be an early warning of an impending CVA. Thus, early identification is essential. Educating people with diabetes about the difference between a hypoglycemic episode and a TIA or an early CVA is clearly important. Many of these symptoms are similar to the symptoms of hypoglycemia; there is no perfect way to distinguish them other than to test glucose during an episode.

Peripheral Artery Disease

Peripheral artery disease is the third most important manifestation of atherosclerosis after coronary and cerebral disease. An estimated 12 million people in the United States have PAD, although it is difficult to estimate its prevalence, because more than half of those with PAD are asymptomatic or have atypical symptoms. About one third have classic symptoms of intermittent claudication, and about one sixth have more severe ischemia. Data from the Framingham study suggest that roughly 20% of people with PAD have diabetes; these data are likely to be an underestimate, given the frequency of asymptomatic PAD.[148] A survey of people with diabetes older than 50 found the prevalence of PAD by ABI determination to be almost 30%.[65] People with long-standing diabetes and PAD may have atypical symptoms due to neuropathy and may not present for medical care until a neurogenic or ischemic ulcer or gangrene develops.

The increased risk of PAD in diabetes is likely to be caused by the same etiologic factors as those of other vascular beds, including hypertension, dyslipidemia, tobacco, and endothelial dysfunction. Thus, the clinical diagnosis of PAD should raise concern about other vascular beds, including the coronary arteries, renal arteries, and cerebral vessels. Patients with PAD are at increased risk for CV events, including stroke, renovascular hypertension, MI, and sudden death.

One in three people with diabetes older than 50 likely has PAD.[149]

How Does PAD Present in People With Diabetes?

The pattern of PAD in those whose primary risk factor is diabetes is different from the pattern in those with other risk factors, such as smoking and hypertension. In the presence of diabetes, PAD occurs more often in the distal arteries—those below the knee (femoral-popliteal and tibial). Other risk factors, such as hypertension and smoking, are associated with a more proximal (aortic, iliac, and proximal femoral) arterial distribution.

The effects of PAD are determined by its progression, presence of symptoms, and associated CV risk. Although most patients with PAD remain stable, more than one fourth have progression of symptoms over 5 years, with amputation occurring in about 4%. One fifth have a CV event within 5 years. Severe ischemia carries a greater risk; 30% have an amputation, and fatality rates approach 20% in 6 months.[150] Although these data are from the general population and there have been no long-term follow-up studies of people with diabetes, event rates are likely to be even higher in people with diabetes.

How Is PAD Detected and Diagnosed?

Screening for and diagnosing PAD is important for 2 reasons. First, the presence of PAD indicates that the person is at increased risk for other events, including stroke and MI. Second, PAD contributes to disability, particularly in those with diabetes. Much of the difference between people with PAD with diabetes and those with PAD without diabetes can be explained by peripheral neuropathy.[151] Adverse effects of PAD include diminished walking ability, with slower walking and shorter walking distances. This leads to deconditioning, which contributes to diminished quality of life and progressive disability.

People with diabetes and PAD are more prone to sudden events, including arterial thrombosis, neuroischemic ulceration, and infection. These events lead to critical limb ischemia and increased risk of amputation. By diagnosing PAD in its early stages, preventive measures can be instituted to diminish its progression or arrange for elective revascularization in a threatened limb before amputation is necessary.

Evaluation for PAD begins with a carefully taken history and physical assessment. The classic symptom of PAD is *intermittent claudication*. The patient complains of pain, cramping, or aching in the calves, thighs, or buttocks. This pain recurs with walking and is relieved by rest. This pattern differs from that of diabetic peripheral neuropathy, in which pain is usually exacerbated by rest and relieved by walking. The pain of spinal stenosis also increases with walking and may be confused with claudication. As PAD progresses, it may cause ischemic pain at rest, tissue loss, or gangrene. The combination of PAD and peripheral neuropathy places the person with diabetes at greater risk for lower-limb amputation.

The educator should ask the patient about symptoms of claudication, pain at rest, and limitations to walking. A carefully taken exercise history often uncovers symptoms of claudication; patients often do not volunteer this information, so it is important to seek it. The pattern of the pain will help differentiate PAD from neuropathy. Peripheral artery disease may cause a wide variety of symptoms, ranging from no symptoms to severe leg pain at rest. It is also important to identify patients with risk factors, such as smoking and hypertension, in addition to their diabetes. Because the person with PAD is at increased risk for other vascular events, eliciting a history of chest pain or atypical angina symptoms is important. Unfortunately, a stroke history is usually self-evident, but a history of TIAs may indicate atherosclerosis in the cerebral circulation.

The physical assessment for diabetic foot problems is part of every diabetes visit. "Shoes and socks off" should be the rule. The ischemic foot may be pale or have "dependent rubor," a deep red color when the foot is hanging down but pallor on elevation. There is hair loss on the distal foot and toes; cool, dry, atrophic skin; and dystrophic toenails. The dorsalis pedis and posterior tibial pulses should be palpated; if they are absent, the popliteal pulse should be palpated as well. It is important to note that palpating pulses is a skill that takes practice and has a high rate of false-negative and false-positive results.

Ankle-Brachial Index

The ABI is a ratio of the systolic pressure at the ankle (posterior tibial or dorsalis pedis pulses) and the brachial artery. The ABI has been found to be a reasonably accurate, reproducible measure for the screening and detection of PAD and its severity. The ABI is determined by placing the blood pressure cuff just above the ankle and inflating it to above systolic pressure. A simple handheld Doppler device is used to detect the systolic pulse in the dorsalis pedis and posterior tibial arteries as the cuff is slowly deflated. The same procedure is used in both feet and 1 arm. To obtain a ratio, the systolic pressure in each of the 4 lower limb arteries is divided by the brachial systolic pressure. The higher value in each limb is the ABI for that limb (Table 25.6). The ADA recommends that an ABI be considered part of initial screening, because many patients with PAD are asymptomatic.

An abnormal ABI is indicative of, but not diagnostic of, PAD and necessitates a referral to a vascular

laboratory for more formal testing. In addition, patients with poorly compressible arteries should be considered for formal vascular testing if there is a high degree of suspicion for PAD. Patients with PAD are generally treated with aggressive support for smoking cessation, daily use of antiplatelet agents, and endovascular and open surgical revascularization for critical limb ischemia. Patients with claudication, absent pedal pulses, or abnormal ABI should be referred to a vascular specialist for further evaluation.

Congestive Heart Failure

Congestive heart failure is a major contributor to morbidity and mortality in the United States, affecting an estimated 5 million people. Common treatments of CHF include sodium restriction, diuretics, ACE inhibitors, and beta blockers. Thiazolidinedione treatment should be avoided in patients with symptomatic CHF. Metformin use should be individualized for patients with pharmacologically treated heart failure; it may be used in patients with stable CHF with normal renal function but should be discontinued in unstable or hospitalized patients.[104] Current evidence does not support use of statins in patients with NYHA Class II-IV CHF (Table 25.7).[52]

TABLE 25.6   ABI Diagnostic Criteria

Normal: 1.00–1.40

Borderline: .91–.99

Abnormal: ≤.90

Elevated pressures (>1.40) may indicate poorly compressible arteries and the presence of arterial calcification. If so, the ABI may not represent the true degree of obstruction.

Source: TW Rooke, AT Hirsch, S Misra, et al, "2011 ACCF/AHA Focused Update of the Guideline for the Management of Patients With Peripheral Artery Disease (updating the 2005 guideline): a report of the American College of Cardiology Foundation/ American Heart Association Task Force on Practice Guidelines," *J Am Coll Cardiol* 58, no. 19 (2011): 2020-45.

TABLE 25.7   NYHA Functional Classification of Heart Failure

NYHA Class	*Symptoms*
I	Cardiac disease without symptoms and/ or limitation in ordinary physical activity (eg, shortness of breath when walking or climbing stairs)
II	Mild symptoms (mild shortness of breath and/or angina) and slight limitation during ordinary activity
III	Marked limitation in activity due to symptoms, even during mild activity (eg, walking short distances [20–100 meters]) Comfortable only at rest
IV	Severe limitations. Symptoms experienced even while at rest. Most patients are bedbound.

Focus on Education

Teaching Strategies

⮎ **Stress that management of CV risk factors is as important as glycemic control for people with diabetes.**

⮎ **Help patients understand their personal ASCVD risk.** Calculate ASCVD risk and explain what the numbers mean in terms that patients can understand.

⮎ **Use a multifactorial risk-reduction approach.** Cardiovascular risk reduction requires addressing all of the patient's modifiable risk factors. Cardiovascular risk can be lowered the most by achieving the "D5 goals": controlling hypertension, achieving lipid goals, smoking cessation, blood glucose control, and use of antiplatelet therapy, when appropriate.

⮎ **Individualize the approach with the patient and use shared decision making to help him or her prioritize treatment strategies based on the risk factors furthest from goal, complexity of the treatment recommendations, and current therapy.**

⮎ **Review and individualize instructions.** Educational needs are highly individualized. When preparing for education and care planning, spend time preparing and individualizing the treatment options. Have appropriate descriptive materials, take-home handouts, and media for viewing in the clinical setting and reviewing at home.

⮎ **Information, individualization, shared decision making, skill building, and follow-up are the keys to care.**

Messages for Patients

⮎ **People with diabetes are at higher risk for heart attacks and strokes.**

⮎ **Prevention of heart attacks and strokes requires multiple treatments, such as statin use, blood pressure control, tobacco cessation, blood glucose control, and aspirin use, if appropriate.** Achieving these targets significantly reduces your risk of complications such as heart attack and stroke, as well as problems with your kidneys, eyes, and nervous system.

⮎ **Support is available for smoking cessation.** If you have diabetes, smoking is like adding fuel to a fire. Work with your healthcare team to find the support you need to quit smoking.

⮎ **Heart-healthy eating, physical activity, and stress management benefit all aspects of well-being.** Healthy lifestyle behaviors will benefit not just CV health but your overall quality of life.

⮎ **The AHA recommends statin therapy for most people with diabetes.**

⮎ **Know your numbers.** Monitor how changes in your lifestyle and medication affect your blood pressure and A1C.

Health Literacy

⮎ **Numerous studies have found that CV care outcomes can be improved with targeted patient education and improved clinician communication skills that consider patients' health literacy.** One study found that only half of clinicians took appropriate action to properly communicate with and educate low-literacy patients—even when the clinicians knew about their patients' literacy level.[152]

⮎ **Everyone, regardless of age, income, or education level, is at risk for low health literacy.** Help patients make decisions by describing the nature of the decision, assessing their understanding, eliciting their preferences, and discussing the alternatives, risks and benefits, and related uncertainties.

⮎ **Social and cultural variances among patients create barriers in understanding health care.** Some perceptions can influence the patients' view of and adherence to treatment. Many patients choose treatment options that seem logical based on their interpretation of the conditions; however, patients often misinterpret the conditions. Ask patients what the information means to them or what they will do differently based on what they have learned. Also, normalizing that it is common to feel overwhelmed about this information allows you to ask, "What is most confusing for you about this information?"

⊘ **Evaluate health numeracy, the ability to reason and apply simple numerical concepts.** Innumeracy can cause patients to make poor health-related decisions because of inaccurate perceptions of the information. Basic numeracy involves counting pills or using a calendar to schedule an appropriate date for an appointment. Analytical numeracy enables patients to understand if blood pressure, cholesterol, and blood glucose levels are within normal range and to determine whether screening tests are necessary. Statistical health numeracy enables patients to weigh the risks and benefits of treatment options. Recognizing poor

health numeracy can help the clinician convey the information more appropriately.

⊘ **Numbers can be a powerful motivator for change in cases of "silent" diseases like hypertension and diabetes.** However, patients need to know the meaning of the numbers and track any changes. They need to understand the norm and how their test results deviate from it.

⊘ **Diabetes educators can maximize learning among patients with low health literacy by doing the following:**
- Assess patients' health literacy skills
- Use simple language instead of medical terminology
- Show or draw pictures
- Limit information given at each interaction, and repeat instructions
- Use a "teach back" or "show me" approach to confirm understanding
- Be respectful, caring, sensitive, and interested
- Consider the result: It is not what you know but what your patient knows

Focus on Practice

⊘ **If not readily available, create systems that allow efficient assessment of CV risk factors and 10-year ASCVD risk.**

⊘ **Develop team-based CV care and education protocols for your institution.** Collaborate with all departments, including nutrition, pharmacy, nursing, primary care providers, and specialists.

⊘ **If within the scope of your practice, develop consensus and approval for simple protocol-driven adjustment of statin and blood pressure therapies.**

⊘ **Create systems with reminders, case management, and quality-improvement mechanisms.**

⊘ **Use continuous quality improvement methods, with measurement performance for optimal diabetes care, feedback, and benchmarking.**

⊘ **Select CVD as a quality focus because it is relevant to all health plan populations.** Establish appropriate baseline measurements and performance goals. Identify barriers to quality CV care and prevention.

⊘ **Identify appropriate target population for intervention.** Compare CV performance data with goals. Pay attention to healthcare disparities due to race, ethnicity, or sex.

⊘ **Consider the financial benefits of total CV risk management, which through the prevention of serious complications can reduce the economic burden of diabetes to health plans, employers, patients, and society.**

References

1. American Diabetes Association. Economic costs of diabetes in the U.S. in 2007. Diabetes Care. 2008;31(3):1-20.

2. International Diabetes Federation. IDF Diabetes Atlas. 6th ed. Brussels, Belgium: International Diabetes Federation; 2013.

3. Preis SR, Hwang SJ, Coady S, et al. Trends in all-cause and cardiovascular disease mortality among women and men with and without diabetes mellitus in the Framingham Heart Study, 1950 to 2005. Circulation. 2009;119(13): 1728-35.

4. Gorina Y, Lentzner H. Multiple causes of death in old age. Aging Trends. 2008 Feb(9):1-9.

5. Centers for Disease Control and Prevention. National diabetes fact sheet, 2011 (cited 2014 Mar 3). On the Internet at: http://www.cdc.gov/diabetes/pubs/pdf/ndfs_2011.pdf.

6. National Diabetes Information Clearinghouse. Diabetes, heart disease, and stroke. 2013 Aug (cited 2014 Mar 3). On the Internet at: http://diabetes.niddk.nih.gov/dm/pubs/stroke/.

7. Coutinho M, Gerstein HC, Wang Y, Yusuf S. The relationship between glucose and incident cardiovascular events: a metaregression analysis of published data from 20 studies of 95,783 individuals followed for 12.4 years. Diabetes Care. 1999;22(2):233-40.

8. Turner RC, Millns H, Neil HA, et al. Risk factors for coronary artery disease in non-insulin dependent diabetes mellitus: United Kingdom Prospective Diabetes Study (UKPDS: 23). BMJ. 1998 Mar 14;316(7134):823-8.

9. Khaw KT, Wareham N, Luben R, et al. Glycated haemoglobin, diabetes, and mortality in men in Norfolk cohort of European Prospective Investigation of Cancer and Nutrition (EPIC-Norfolk). BMJ. 2001 Jan 6;322(7277):15-8.

10. Muntner P, Wildman RP, Reynolds K, Desalvo KB, Chen J, Fonseca V. Relationship between HbA1c level and peripheral arterial disease. Diabetes Care. 2005 Aug;28(8):1981-7.

11. Selvin E, Coresh J, Golden SH, Boland LL, Brancati FL, Steffes MW. Glycemic control, atherosclerosis, and risk factors for cardiovascular disease in individuals with diabetes: the atherosclerosis risk in communities study. Diabetes Care. 2005 Aug;28(8):1965-73.

12. Selvin E, Marinopoulos S, Berkenblit G, et al. Meta-analysis: glycosylated hemoglobin and cardiovascular disease in diabetes mellitus. Ann Intern Med. 2004 Sep 21;141(6):421-31.

13. Krolewski AS, Kosinski EJ, Warram JH, et al. Magnitude and determinants of coronary artery disease in juvenile-onset, insulin-dependent diabetes mellitus. Am J Cardiol. 1987 Apr 1;59(8):750-5.

14. Dorman JS, Tajima N, LaPorte RE, et al. The Pittsburgh Insulin-Dependent Diabetes Mellitus (IDDM) Morbidity and Mortality Study: case-control analyses of risk factors for mortality. Diabetes Care. 1985 Sep-Oct;8 Suppl 1:54-60.

15. Miller J, Silverstein J. Risk factors for cardiovascular disease in children with diabetes. Practical Diabetology. 2004;23(2):13-8.

16. American Diabetes Association. Management of dyslipidemia in children and adolescents with diabetes. Diabetes Care. 2003 Jul;26(7):2194-7.

17. Orchard TJ, Forrest KY, Kuller LH, Becker DJ. Lipid and blood pressure treatment goals for type 1 diabetes: 10-year incidence data from the Pittsburgh Epidemiology of Diabetes Complications Study. Diabetes Care. 2001 Jun;24(6):1053-9.

18. Libby P, Ridker PM, Maseri A. Inflammation and atherosclerosis. Circulation. 2002 Mar 5;105(9):1135-43.

19. Davignon J, Ganz P. Role of endothelial dysfunction in atherosclerosis. Circulation. 2004 Jun 15;109(23 Suppl 1): III27-32.

20. Golden SH, Folsom AR, Coresh J, Sharrett AR, Szklo M, Brancati F. Risk factor groupings related to insulin resistance and their synergistic effects on subclinical atherosclerosis: the atherosclerosis risk in communities study. Diabetes. 2002 Oct;51(10):3069-76.

21. Stehouwer C. The many faces of vascular dysfunction in diabetes. Paper presented at: 20th Camillo Golgi Lecture; delivered at European Association for the Study of Diabetes; 2005; Athens, Greece.

22. Bonora E, Muggeo M. Postprandial blood glucose as a risk factor for cardiovascular disease in Type II diabetes: the epidemiological evidence. Diabetologia. 2001 Dec;44(12):2107-14.

23. Ceriello A. Postprandial hyperglycemia and diabetes complications: is it time to treat? Diabetes. 2005 Jan;54(1):1-7.

24. DECODE Study Group, European Diabetes Epidemiology Group. Glucose tolerance and cardiovascular mortality: comparison of fasting and 2-hour diagnostic criteria. Arch Intern Med. 2001 Feb 12;161(3):397-405.

25. Rodriguez BL, Lau N, Burchfiel CM, et al. Glucose intolerance and 23-year risk of coronary heart disease and total mortality: the Honolulu Heart Program. Diabetes Care. 1999 Aug;22(8):1262-5.

26. Bonora E. Postprandial peaks as a risk factor for cardiovascular disease: epidemiological perspectives. Int J Clin Pract Suppl. 2002 Jul;129:5-11.

27. Ceriello A, Taboga C, Tonutti L, et al. Evidence for an independent and cumulative effect of postprandial

hypertriglyceridemia and hyperglycemia on endothelial dysfunction and oxidative stress generation: effects of short- and long-term simvastatin treatment. Circulation. 2002 Sep 3;106(10):1211-8.

28. Chiasson JL, Josse RG, Gomis R, Hanefeld M, Karasik A, Laakso M. Acarbose treatment and the risk of cardiovascular disease and hypertension in patients with impaired glucose tolerance: the STOP-NIDDM trial. JAMA. 2003 Jul 23;290(4):486-94.

29. Hanefeld M, Cagatay M, Petrowitsch T, Neuser D, Petzinna D, Rupp M. Acarbose reduces the risk for myocardial infarction in type 2 diabetic patients: meta-analysis of seven long-term studies. Eur Heart J. 2004 Jan;25(1):10-6.

30. Esposito K, Giugliano D, Nappo F, Marfella R. Regression of carotid atherosclerosis by control of postprandial hyperglycemia in type 2 diabetes mellitus. Circulation. 2004 Jul 13;110(2):214-9.

31. Huang ES, Meigs JB, Singer DE. The effect of interventions to prevent cardiovascular disease in patients with type 2 diabetes mellitus. Am J Med. 2001 Dec 1;111(8): 633-42.

32. Intensive blood-glucose control with sulphonylureas or insulin compared with conventional treatment and risk of complications in patients with type 2 diabetes (UKPDS 33). UK Prospective Diabetes Study (UKPDS) Group. Lancet. 1998 Sep 12;352(9131):837-53.

33. Holman RR, Paul SK, Bethel MA, Matthews DR, Neil HA. 10-year follow-up of intensive glucose control in type 2 diabetes. N Engl J Med. 2008 Oct 9;359(15): 1577-89.

34. Skyler JS, Bergenstal R, Bonow RO, et al. Intensive glycemic control and the prevention of cardiovascular events: implications of the ACCORD, ADVANCE, and VA diabetes trials: a position statement of the American Diabetes Association and a scientific statement of the American College of Cardiology Foundation and the American Heart Association. Diabetes Care. 2009 Jan;32(1): 187-92.

35. Gerstein HC, Miller ME, Byington RP, et al. Effects of intensive glucose lowering in type 2 diabetes. N Engl J Med. 2008 Jun 12;358(24):2545-59.

36. Patel A, MacMahon S, Chalmers J, et al. Intensive blood glucose control and vascular outcomes in patients with type 2 diabetes. N Engl J Med. 2008 Jun 12;358(24): 2560-72.

37. Duckworth W, Abraira C, Moritz T, et al. Glucose control and vascular complications in veterans with type 2 diabetes. N Engl J Med. 2009 Jan 8;360(2):129-39.

38. Nissen SE, Wolski K. Effect of rosiglitazone on the risk of myocardial infarction and death from cardiovascular causes. N Engl J Med. 2007 Jun 14;356(24):2457-71.

39. Komajda M, Curtis P, Hanefeld M, et al. Effect of the addition of rosiglitazone to metformin or sulfonylureas versus metformin/sulfonylurea combination therapy on ambulatory blood pressure in people with type 2 diabetes: a randomized controlled trial (the RECORD study). Cardiovasc Diabetol. 2008;7:10.

40. Hirshberg B, Raz I. Impact of the U.S. Food and Drug Administration cardiovascular assessment requirements on the development of novel antidiabetes drugs. Diabetes Care. 2011 May;34 Suppl 2:S101-6.

41. Scirica BM, Bhatt DL, Braunwald E, et al. Saxagliptin and cardiovascular outcomes in patients with type 2 diabetes mellitus. N Engl J Med. 2013 Oct 3;369(14): 1317-26.

42. White WB, Cannon CP, Heller SR, et al. Alogliptin after acute coronary syndrome in patients with type 2 diabetes. N Engl J Med. 2013 Oct 3;369(14):1327-35.

43. Stern M. Diabetes in Hispanic Americans. In: National Diabetes Data Group, eds. Diabetes in America, 2nd ed., Vol. 95-1468. Bethesda, MD: National Institute of Diabetes and Digestive and Kidney Diseases; 1995:631-60.

44. Larsen JL, Colling CW, Ratanasuwan T, et al. Pancreas transplantation improves vascular disease in patients with type 1 diabetes. Diabetes Care. 2004 Jul;27(7):1706-11.

45. Fiorina P, Gremizzi C, Maffi P, et al. Islet transplantation is associated with an improvement of cardiovascular function in type 1 diabetic kidney transplant patients. Diabetes Care. 2005 Jun;28(6):1358-65.

46. Nathan DM, Lachin J, Cleary P, et al. Intensive diabetes therapy and carotid intima-media thickness in type 1 diabetes mellitus. N Engl J Med. 2003 Jun 5;348(23):2294-303.

47. Nathan DM, Cleary PA, Backlund JY, et al. Intensive diabetes treatment and cardiovascular disease in patients with type 1 diabetes. N Engl J Med. 2005 Dec 22;353(25):2643-53.

48. Pignone M, Phillips CJ, Elasy TA, Fernandez A. Physicians' ability to predict the risk of coronary heart disease. BMC Health Services Research. 2003;3:13.

49. Moons KG, Kengne AP, Woodward M, et al. Risk prediction models: I. Development, internal validation, and assessing the incremental value of a new (bio)marker. Heart. 2012 May;98(9):683-90.

50. Sheridan SL, Crespo E. Does the routine use of global coronary heart disease risk scores translate into clinical benefits or harms? A systematic review of the literature. BMC Health Serv Res. 2008;8:60.

51. Sheridan SL, Viera AJ, Krantz MJ, et al. The effect of giving global coronary risk information to adults: a systematic review. Arch Intern Med. 2010 Feb 8;170(3):230-9.

52. Stone NJ, Robinson J, Lichtenstein AH, et al. 2013 ACC/AHA Guideline on the Treatment of Blood

Cholesterol to Reduce Atherosclerotic Cardiovascular Risk in Adults: a Report of the American College of Cardiology/American Heart Association Task Force on Practice Guidelines. Circulation. Epub 2013 Nov 12.

53. Goff DC Jr., Lloyd-Jones DM, Bennett G, et al. 2013 ACC/AHA Guideline on the Assessment of Cardiovascular Risk: a Report of the American College of Cardiology/American Heart Association Task Force on Practice Guidelines. J Am Coll Cardiol. Epub 2013 Nov 7.

54. Eckel RH, Jakicic JM, Ard JD, et al. 2013 AHA/ACC Guideline on Lifestyle Management to Reduce Cardiovascular Risk: a Report of the American College of Cardiology/American Heart Association Task Force on Practice Guidelines. Circulation. Epub 2013 Nov 12.

55. Bachmann JM, Willis BL, Ayers CR, Khera A, Berry JD. Association between family history and coronary heart disease death across long-term follow-up in men: the Cooper Center Longitudinal Study. Circulation. 2012 Jun 26; 125(25):3092-8.

56. Sivapalaratnam S, Boekholdt SM, Trip MD, et al. Family history of premature coronary heart disease and risk prediction in the EPIC-Norfolk prospective population study. Heart. 2010 Dec;96(24):1985-9.

57. Kuhn FE, Rackley CE. Coronary artery disease in women: risk factors, evaluation, treatment, and prevention. Arch Intern Med. 1993 Dec 13;153(23):2626-36.

58. Tull E, Roseman J. Diabetes in African Americans. In: National Diabetes Data Group, eds. Diabetes in America, 2nd ed., Vol 95-1468. Bethesda, Md: National Institute of Diabetes and Digestive and Kidney Diseases; 1995:613-30.

59. Gaede P, Vedel P, Larsen N, Jensen GV, Parving HH, Pedersen O. Multifactorial intervention and cardiovascular disease in patients with type 2 diabetes. N Engl J Med. 2003 Jan 30;348(5):383-93.

60. National Quality Forum (cited 2014 Mar 3). On the Internet at: http://www.qualityforum.org.

61. MN HealthScores. The D5: five goals for living well with diabetes. 2013. On the Internet at: http://mnhealthscores.org/thed5/.

62. Eyre H, Kahn R, Robertson RM, et al. Preventing cancer, cardiovascular disease, and diabetes: a common agenda for the American Cancer Society, the American Diabetes Association, and the American Heart Association. Stroke. 2004 Aug;35(8):1999-2010.

63. Chobanian AV, Bakris GL, Black HR, et al. The Seventh Report of the Joint National Committee on Prevention, Detection, Evaluation, and Treatment of High Blood Pressure: the JNC 7 report. JAMA. 2003 May 21;289(19):2560-72.

64. Expert Panel on Detection, Evaluation, and Treatment of High Blood Cholesterol in Adults. Executive Summary of the Third Report of the National Cholesterol Education Program (NCEP) Expert Panel on Detection, Evaluation, and Treatment of High Blood Cholesterol in Adults (Adult Treatment Panel III). JAMA. 2001 May 16;285(19):2486-97.

65. Pi-Sunyer X, Blackburn G, Brancati FL, et al. Reduction in weight and cardiovascular disease risk factors in individuals with type 2 diabetes: one-year results of the look AHEAD trial. Diabetes Care. 2007 Jun;30(6):1374-83.

66. Estruch R, Ros E, Salas-Salvado J, et al. Primary prevention of cardiovascular disease with a Mediterranean diet. N Engl J Med. 2013 Apr 4;368(14):1279-90.

67. Jensen MD, Ryan DH, Apovian CM, et al. 2013 AHA/ACC/TOS Guideline for the Management of Overweight and Obesity in Adults: a Report of the American College of Cardiology/American Heart Association Task Force on Practice Guidelines and the Obesity Society. Circulation. 2013 Nov 12.

68. Wing RR, Bolin P, Brancati FL, et al. Cardiovascular effects of intensive lifestyle intervention in type 2 diabetes. N Engl J Med. 2013 Jul 11;369(2):145-54.

69. Sjostrom L, Peltonen M, Jacobson P, et al. Bariatric surgery and long-term cardiovascular events. JAMA. 2012 Jan 4; 307(1):56-65.

70. Sigal RJ, Kenny GP, Wasserman DH, Castaneda-Sceppa C. Physical activity/exercise and type 2 diabetes. Diabetes Care. 2004 Oct;27(10):2518-39.

71. Hu G, Jousilahti P, Barengo NC, Qiao Q, Lakka TA, Tuomilehto J. Physical activity, cardiovascular risk factors, and mortality among Finnish adults with diabetes. Diabetes Care. 2005 Apr;28(4):799-805.

72. Petrella RJ, Lattanzio CN, Demeray A, Varallo V, Blore R. Can adoption of regular exercise later in life prevent metabolic risk for cardiovascular disease? Diabetes Care. 2005 Mar;28(3):694-701.

73. Samet JM. The 1990 Report of the Surgeon General: The Health Benefits of Smoking Cessation. Am Rev Respir Dis. 1990 Nov;142(5):993-4.

74. U.S. Preventive Services Task Force. Counseling and interventions to prevent tobacco use and tobacco-caused disease in adults and pregnant women: U.S. Preventive Services Task Force reaffirmation recommendation statement. Ann Intern Med. 2009 Apr 21;150(8):551-5.

75. Chantix [package insert]. New York: Pfizer (last revised 2012 Dec, cited 2014 Mar 14). On the Internet at: http://labeling.pfizer.com/showlabeling.aspx?id=557.

76. The multiple risk factor intervention trial (MRFIT): a national study of primary prevention of coronary heart disease. JAMA. 1976 Feb 23;235(8):825-7.

77. Randomised trial of cholesterol lowering in 4444 patients with coronary heart disease: the Scandinavian Simvastatin Survival Study (4S). Lancet. 1994 Nov 19;344(8934):1383-9.

78. Pyorala K, Pedersen TR, Kjekshus J, Faergeman O, Olsson AG, Thorgeirsson G. Cholesterol lowering with simvastatin improves prognosis of diabetic patients with coronary heart disease: a subgroup analysis of the Scandinavian Simvastatin Survival Study (4S). Diabetes Care. 1997 Apr;20(4):614-20.

79. Colhoun HM, Betteridge DJ, Durrington PN, et al. Primary prevention of cardiovascular disease with atorvastatin in type 2 diabetes in the Collaborative Atorvastatin Diabetes Study (CARDS): multicentre randomised placebo-controlled trial. Lancet. 2004 Aug 21;364(9435): 685-96.

80. Vijan S, Hayward RA. Pharmacologic lipid-lowering therapy in type 2 diabetes mellitus: background paper for the American College of Physicians. Ann Intern Med. 2004 Apr 20;140(8):650-8.

81. Shepherd J, Barter P, Carmena R, et al. Effect of lowering LDL cholesterol substantially below currently recommended levels in patients with coronary heart disease and diabetes: the Treating to New Targets (TNT) study. Diabetes Care. 2006 Jun;29(6):1220-6.

82. Collins R, Armitage J, Parish S, Sleigh P, Peto R. MRC/BHF Heart Protection Study of cholesterol-lowering with simvastatin in 5963 people with diabetes: a randomised placebo-controlled trial. Lancet. 2003 Jun 14;361(9374):2005-16.

83. Sever PS, Poulter NR, Dahlof B, et al. Reduction in cardiovascular events with atorvastatin in 2,532 patients with type 2 diabetes: Anglo-Scandinavian Cardiac Outcomes Trial—lipid-lowering arm (ASCOT-LLA). Diabetes Care. 2005 May;28(5):1151-7.

84. Taylor F, Ward K, Moore TH, et al. Statins for the primary prevention of cardiovascular disease. Cochrane Database Syst Rev. 2011(1):CD004816.

85. Baigent C, Blackwell L, Emberson J, et al. Efficacy and safety of more intensive lowering of LDL cholesterol: a meta-analysis of data from 170,000 participants in 26 randomised trials. Lancet. 2010 Nov 13;376(9753):1670-81.

86. Kearney PM, Blackwell L, Collins R, et al. Efficacy of cholesterol-lowering therapy in 18,686 people with diabetes in 14 randomised trials of statins: a meta-analysis. Lancet. 2008 Jan 12;371(9607):117-25.

87. Sattar N, Preiss D, Murray HM, et al. Statins and risk of incident diabetes: a collaborative meta-analysis of randomised statin trials. Lancet. 2010 Feb 27;375(9716): 735-42.

88. Amerian Diabetes Association. Standards of medical care in diabetes—2014. Diabetes Care. 2014;37 Suppl 1:S14-80.

89. Rubins HB, Robins SJ, Collins D, et al. Gemfibrozil for the secondary prevention of coronary heart disease in men with low levels of high-density lipoprotein cholesterol: Veterans Affairs High-Density Lipoprotein Cholesterol Intervention Trial Study Group.N Engl J Med. 1999 Aug 5;341(6): 410-8.

90. Keech A, Simes RJ, Barter P, et al. Effects of long-term fenofibrate therapy on cardiovascular events in 9795 people with type 2 diabetes mellitus (the FIELD study): randomised controlled trial. Lancet. 2005 Nov 26; 366(9500):1849-61.

91. Ginsberg HN, Elam MB, Lovato LC, et al. Effects of combination lipid therapy in type 2 diabetes mellitus. N Engl J Med. 2010 Apr 29;362(17):1563-74.

92. Boden WE, Probstfield JL, Anderson T, et al. Niacin in patients with low HDL cholesterol levels receiving intensive statin therapy. N Engl J Med. 2011 Dec 15;365(24): 2255-67.

93. Keaney JF Jr., Curfman GD, Jarcho JA. A pragmatic view of the new cholesterol treatment guidelines. N Engl J Med. 2014 Jan 16;370(3):275-8.

94. Tight blood pressure control and risk of macrovascular and microvascular complications in type 2 diabetes: UKPDS 38. UK Prospective Diabetes Study Group. BMJ. 1998 Sep 12;317(7160):703-13.

95. Sowers J. Treatment of hypertension in patients with diabetes. Arch Intern Med. 2004;164:1850-7.

96. Beevers G, Lip GY, O'Brien E. ABC of hypertension: Blood pressure measurement. Part II—conventional sphygmomanometry: technique of auscultatory blood pressure measurement. BMJ. 2001 Apr 28;322(7293):1043-7.

97. Keary L, Atkins N, Molloy E, Mee F, O'Brien E. Terminal digit preference and heaping in blood pressure measurement. J Hum Hypertens. 1998;12:787-8.

98. Hermida RC, Smolensky MH, Ayala DE, Portaluppi F. 2013 ambulatory blood pressure monitoring recommendations for the diagnosis of adult hypertension, assessment of cardiovascular and other hypertension-associated risk, and attainment of therapeutic goals. Chronobiol Int. 2013 Apr;30(3):355-410.

99. James PA, Oparil S, Carter BL, et al. 2014 evidence-based guideline for the management of high blood pressure in adults: report from the panel members appointed to the Eighth Joint National Committee (JNC 8). JAMA. 2014 Feb 5;311(5):507-20.

100. Hansson L, Zanchetti A, Carruthers SG, et al. Effects of intensive blood-pressure lowering and low-dose aspirin in patients with hypertension: principal results of the Hypertension Optimal Treatment (HOT) randomised trial. HOT Study Group. Lancet. 1998 Jun 13;351(9118): 1755-62.

101. Cooper-DeHoff RM, Gong Y, Handberg EM, et al. Tight blood pressure control and cardiovascular outcomes among hypertensive patients with diabetes and coronary artery disease. JAMA. 2010 Jul 7;304(1):61-8.

102. Cushman WC, Evans GW, Byington RP, et al. Effects of intensive blood-pressure control in type 2 diabetes mellitus. N Engl J Med. 2010 Apr 29;362(17):1575-85.

103. Patel A, MacMahon S, Chalmers J, et al. Effects of a fixed combination of perindopril and indapamide on macrovascular and microvascular outcomes in patients with type 2 diabetes mellitus (the ADVANCE trial): a randomised controlled trial. Lancet. 2007 Sep 8; 370(9590):829-40.

104. American Diabetes Association. Standards of medical care in diabetes—2013. Diabetes Care. 2013 Jan;36 Suppl 1: S11-66.

105. ALLHAT Officers and Coordinators for the ALLHAT Collaborative Research Group. Major outcomes in high-risk hypertensive patients randomized to angiotensin-converting enzyme inhibitor or calcium channel blocker vs diuretic: the Antihypertensive and Lipid-Lowering Treatment to Prevent Heart Attack Trial (ALLHAT). JAMA. 2002 Dec 18;288(23):2981-97.

106. Cushman WC, Evans GW, Byington RP, et al. Effects of intensive blood-pressure control in type 2 diabetes mellitus. N Engl J Med. 2010 Apr 29;362(17):1575-85.

107. Margolis KL, Asche SE, Bergdall AR, et al. Effect of home blood pressure telemonitoring and pharmacist management on blood pressure control: a cluster randomized clinical trial. JAMA. 2013 Jul 3;310(1):46-56.

108. Early Treatment Diabetic Retinopathy Study Research Group. Effects of aspirin treatment on diabetic retinopathy. ETDRS report number 8. Ophthalmology. 1991 May;98(5 Suppl):757-65.

109. ETDRS Investigators. Aspirin effects on mortality and morbidity in patients with diabetes mellitus. Early Treatment Diabetic Retinopathy Study report 14. JAMA. 1992 Sep 9;268(10):1292-300.

110. Antithrombotic Trialists' Collaboration. Collaborative meta-analysis of randomised trials of antiplatelet therapy for prevention of death, myocardial infarction, and stroke in high risk patients. BMJ. 2002 Jan 12; 324(7329):71-86.

111. Pignone M, Alberts MJ, Colwell JA, et al. Aspirin for primary prevention of cardiovascular events in people with diabetes: a position statement of the American Diabetes Association, a scientific statement of the American Heart Association, and an expert consensus document of the American College of Cardiology Foundation. Diabetes Care. 2010 Jun;33(6):1395-402. doi: 10.2337/dc10-0555.

112. US Preventive Services Task Force. Aspirin for the prevention of cardiovascular disease: U.S. Preventive Services Task Force recommendation statement. Ann Intern Med. 2009 Mar 17;150(6):396-404.

113. De Berardis G, Sacco M, Strippoli GF, et al. Aspirin for primary prevention of cardiovascular events in people with diabetes: meta-analysis of randomised controlled trials. BMJ. 2009;339:b4531.

114. D'Agostino RB Sr, Vasan RS, Pencina MJ, et al. General cardiovascular risk profile for use in primary care: the Framingham Heart Study. Circulation. 2008;117: 743-53.

115. US National Institutes of Health. Aspirin in Reducing Events in the Elderly (ASPREE). 2009 Dec 21 (last updated 2013 Oct 18, cited 2014 Mar 12). On the Internet at: http://clinicaltrials.gov/show/NCT01038583.

116. Walker CW, Dawley CA, Fletcher SF. Aspirin combined with clopidogrel (Plavix) decreases cardiovascular events in patients with acute coronary syndrome. Am Fam Physician. 2007 Dec 1;76(11):1643-5.

117. Rooke TW, Hirsch AT, Misra S, et al. 2011 ACCF/AHA Focused Update of the Guideline for the Management of Patients With Peripheral Artery Disease (updating the 2005 guideline): a report of the American College of Cardiology Foundation/American Heart Association Task Force on Practice Guidelines. J Am Coll Cardiol. 2011 Nov 1;58(19):2020-45.

118. Park HY, Schumock GT, Pickard AS, Akhras K. A structured review of the relationship between microalbuminuria and cardiovascular events in patients with diabetes mellitus and hypertension. Pharmacotherapy. 2003 Dec;23(12):1611-6.

119. Spoelstra-de Man AM, Brouwer CB, Stehouwer CD, Smulders YM. Rapid progression of albumin excretion is an independent predictor of cardiovascular mortality in patients with type 2 diabetes and microalbuminuria. Diabetes Care. 2001 Dec;24(12):2097-101.

120. Yusuf S, Sleight P, Pogue J, Bosch J, Davies R, Dagenais G. Effects of an angiotensin-converting-enzyme inhibitor, ramipril, on cardiovascular events in high-risk patients. The Heart Outcomes Prevention Evaluation Study Investigators. N Engl J Med. 2000 Jan 20;342(3):145-53.

121. Myers GL, Christenson RH, Cushman M, et al. National Academy of Clinical Biochemistry Laboratory Medicine Practice guidelines: emerging biomarkers for primary prevention of cardiovascular disease. Clin Chem. 2009 Feb;55(2):378-84.

122. US Preventive Services Task Force. Using nontraditional risk factors in coronary heart disease risk assessment: U.S. Preventive Services Task Force recommendation statement. Ann Intern Med. 2009 Oct 6;151(7):474-82.

123. Brown BG, Cheung MC, Lee AC, Zhao XQ, Chait A. Antioxidant vitamins and lipid therapy: end of a long romance? Arterioscler Thromb Vasc Biol. 2002 Oct 1;22(10):1535-46.

124. Lonn E, Bosch J, Yusuf S, et al. Effects of long-term vitamin E supplementation on cardiovascular events and cancer: a randomized controlled trial. JAMA. 2005 Mar 16; 293(11):1338-47.

125. Omenn GS, Goodman GE, Thornquist MD, et al. Risk factors for lung cancer and for intervention effects in CARET, the Beta-Carotene and Retinol Efficacy Trial. J Natl Cancer Inst. 1996 Nov 6;88(21):1550-9.

126. US Preventive Services Task Force. Routine vitamin supplementation to prevent cancer and cardiovascular disease: recommendations and rationale. Ann Intern Med. 2003 Jul 1;139(1):51-5.

127. Imperatore G, Boyle JP, Thompson TJ, et al. Projections of type 1 and type 2 diabetes burden in the U.S. population aged <20 years through 2050: dynamic modeling of incidence, mortality, and population growth. Diabetes Care. 2012 Dec;35(12):2515-20.

128. Rodriguez BL, Fujimoto WY, Mayer-Davis EJ, et al. Prevalence of cardiovascular disease risk factors in U.S. children and adolescents with diabetes: the SEARCH for diabetes in youth study. Diabetes Care. 2006 Aug;29(8):1891-6.

129. Dean H, Flett B. Natural history of type 2 diabetes diagnosed in childhood: long term follow-up in young adult years. Diabetes. 2002;51(Suppl 2):A24.

130. Haffner SM, Lehto S, Ronnemaa T, Pyorala K, Laakso M. Mortality from coronary heart disease in subjects with type 2 diabetes and in nondiabetic subjects with and without prior myocardial infarction. N Engl J Med. 1998 Jul 23;339(4):229-34.

131. Young LH, Wackers FJ, Chyun DA, et al. Cardiac outcomes after screening for asymptomatic coronary artery disease in patients with type 2 diabetes: the DIAD study: a randomized controlled trial. JAMA. 2009 Apr 15;301(15):1547-55.

132. Wackers FJ, Young LH. Lessons learned from the detection of ischemia in asymptomatic diabetics (DIAD) study. J Nucl Cardiol. 2009 Nov-Dec;16(6):855-9.

133. Frye RL, August P, Brooks MM, et al. A randomized trial of therapies for type 2 diabetes and coronary artery disease. N Engl J Med. 2009 Jun 11;360(24):2503-15.

134. Boden WE, O'Rourke RA, Teo KK, et al. Optimal medical therapy with or without PCI for stable coronary disease. N Engl J Med. 2007 Apr 12;356(15):1503-16.

135. Braunwald E. Shattuck lecture—cardiovascular medicine at the turn of the millennium: triumphs, concerns, and opportunities. N Engl J Med. 1997 Nov 6;337(19):1360-9.

136. Wahab NN, Cowden EA, Pearce NJ, Gardner MJ, Merry H, Cox JL. Is blood glucose an independent predictor of mortality in acute myocardial infarction in the thrombolytic era? J Am Coll Cardiol. 2002 Nov 20;40(10):1748-54.

137. Norhammar A, Tenerz A, Nilsson G, et al. Glucose metabolism in patients with acute myocardial infarction and no previous diagnosis of diabetes mellitus: a prospective study. Lancet. 2002 Jun 22;359(9324):2140-4.

138. Malmberg K. Prospective randomised study of intensive insulin treatment on long term survival after acute myocardial infarction in patients with diabetes mellitus. DIGAMI (Diabetes Mellitus, Insulin Glucose Infusion in Acute Myocardial Infarction) Study Group. BMJ. 1997 May 24;314(7093):1512-5.

139. Mellbin LG, Malmberg K, Norhammar A, Wedel H, Ryden L. The impact of glucose lowering treatment on long-term prognosis in patients with type 2 diabetes and myocardial infarction: a report from the DIGAMI 2 trial. Eur Heart J. 2008 Jan;29(2):166-76.

140. Ziegelstein RC. Depression in patients recovering from a myocardial infarction. JAMA. 2001 Oct 3;286(13):1621-7.

141. Carinci F, Nicolucci A, Ciampi A, et al. Role of interactions between psychological and clinical factors in determining 6-month mortality among patients with acute myocardial infarction. Application of recursive partitioning techniques to the GISSI-2 database. Gruppo Italiano per lo Studio della Sopravvivenza nell' Infarto Miocardico. Eur Heart J. 1997 May;18(5):835-45.

142. Frasure-Smith N. In-hospital symptoms of psychological stress as predictors of long-term outcome after acute myocardial infarction in men. Am J Cardiol. 1991 Jan 15;67(2):121-7.

143. Taylor F, Huffman MD, Macedo AF, et al. Statins for the primary prevention of cardiovascular disease. Cochrane Database Syst Rev. 2013;1:CD004816.

144. Kawachi I, Colditz GA, Stampfer MJ, et al. Smoking cessation and decreased risk of stroke in women. JAMA. 1993 Jan 13;269(2):232-6.

145. Johnston SC, Gress DR, Browner WS, Sidney S. Short-term prognosis after emergency department diagnosis of TIA. JAMA. 2000 Dec 13;284(22):2901-6.

146. Streifler JY, Eliasziw M, Benavente OR, et al. The risk of stroke in patients with first-ever retinal vs hemispheric transient ischemic attacks and high-grade carotid stenosis. North American Symptomatic Carotid Endarterectomy Trial. Arch Neurol. 1995 Mar;52(3):246-9.

147. American Heart Association/American Stroke Association. Spot a stroke. Stroke warning signs and symptoms (cited 2014 Mar 12). On the Internet at: http://www.strokeassociation.org/STROKEORG/WarningSigns/Stroke-Warning-Signs-and-Symptoms_UCM_308528_SubHomePage.jsp.

148. Murabito JM, D'Agostino RB, Silbershatz H, Wilson WF. Intermittent claudication: a risk profile from the Framingham Heart Study. Circulation. 1997;96:44–9.

149. US Department of Health and Human Services, National Institutes of Health, National Heart, Lung, and Blood Institute. Facts about peripheral arterial disease (P.A.D.). 2006 Aug (cited 2014 Mar 14). On the Internet at: https://www.nhlbi.nih.gov/health/public/heart/pad/docs/pad_extfctsht_general_508.pdf.

150. Golomb BA, Dang TT, Criqui MH. Peripheral arterial disease: morbidity and mortality implications. Circulation. 2006 Aug 15;114(7):688-99.

151. Dolan NC, Liu K, Criqui MH, et al. Peripheral artery disease, diabetes, and reduced lower extremity functioning. Diabetes Care. 2002 Jan;25(1):113-20.

152. Powell CK, Kripalani S. Brief report: resident recognition of low literacy as a risk factor in hospital readmission. J Gen Intern Med. 2005 Nov;20(11):1042-4.

CHAPTER 26

Eye Disease Related to Diabetes

Szilárd Kiss, MD

Key Concepts

- The population of persons with diabetes is susceptible to a considerable number of eye conditions that can lead to blindness. These generally occur more frequently and at a younger age in people with diabetes than in the general population.

- Early diagnosis and treatment can prevent or delay vision loss from eye disorders.

- Early treatment of diabetic retinopathy can prevent severe vision loss.

- Diabetic retinopathy, the leading cause of blindness among individuals aged 20 to 74 in

the United States,[1] is often present before the person notices any visual changes.

- Tight control of blood glucose levels, blood pressure management, blood lipid control, and smoking cessation help prevent severe vision loss due to diabetic retinopathy.

- Diabetes educators need to encourage persons with diabetes to have annual retinal evaluations, whether or not they are experiencing any visual symptoms.

Introduction

Diabetes is the leading cause of blindness among adults aged 20 to 74 in the United States. The literature suggests that 8000 to 23,000 new cases of legal blindness associated with diabetes present annually.[2–6] Various ocular conditions are 25 times more common among people with diabetes than in the general population.[4] Of people with diabetes who are on work disability, 15% to 20% have some visual impairment.[7]

As people advance in age, they are more at risk for certain eye conditions, such as glaucoma and cataracts. People with diabetes have an even greater risk for these conditions, which often present earlier in age in these individuals than in the general population. Uncontrolled, poorly managed diabetes creates a more serious condition called diabetic retinopathy, which affects the retina.

The retina is the light-sensing tissue lining the inner surface of the eye. The cornea and the lens create an image of the visual world on the retina, which

serves a function analogous to film in a traditional camera or to a charge-coupled device and complementary metal oxide semiconductor image sensor in a digital camera. Light striking the retina initiates a cascade of chemical and electrical events that ultimately trigger nerve impulses that are then sent to various visual centers of the brain via the optic nerve. Disorders of the retina typically affect either central or peripheral vision. Figure 26.1 identifies parts of the eye that are discussed in this chapter.

Diabetic retinopathy is the most severe form of diabetic eye disease. Diabetic retinopathy results from leaky blood vessels and the growth of abnormal blood vessels in the retina. Within 1 year of developing diabetic retinopathy, 5% to 10% of patients will progress to a more advanced stage.[3]

The number of Americans aged 40 years or older with retinopathy is estimated to triple by 2050, to 16.0 million for all diabetic retinopathy and 3.4 million for vision-threatening diabetic retinopathy.[8]

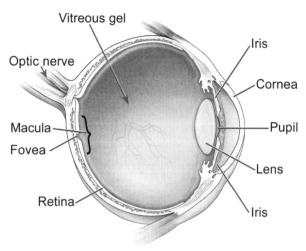

FIGURE 26.1   Normal Eye

Source: National Eye Institute, National Institutes of Health, Reference #NEA08.

This chapter focuses on eye diseases associated with diabetes mellitus. For each ocular condition, the epidemiology, risk factors, clinical findings, stages of the disease, and appropriate treatments are outlined.

◈   *Common eye diseases.* Common eye diseases are discussed first, including cataracts, glaucoma,

and other ocular manifestations that occur more frequently in people with diabetes.

◈   *Diabetic retinopathy.* Information on diabetic retinopathy is presented next. Major clinical studies and current treatment strategies for diabetic retinopathy are outlined. The text emphasizes how appropriate and timely therapy can prevent severe visual loss in up to 90% of cases.[9]

Cataracts

Cataracts are one of the leading causes of reversible blindness in the world today, and at least 300,000 to 400,000 new cases of visually disabling cataracts occur annually in the United States. The rate of cataracts for individuals with diabetes is significantly higher, with faster progression to vision loss, than that of the general population.[8] With early detection, close monitoring, and timely surgical intervention, visual impairment due to cataracts is reversible. Cataracts are a vision-impairing disease characterized by a gradual, progressive thickening and opacification of

---

Case: Reluctance in Self-Care Leads to Vision Loss

MG is a 50-year-old male who was diagnosed with type 2 diabetes 10 years ago. His blood glucose levels have ranged from 100 to 355 mg/dL (5.6 to 19.7 mmol/L) in the last 3 months. He has insisted, however, that he is doing fine because he does not "feel" that his diabetes is causing any problems. He is using oral medications to control his diabetes and lives a sedentary lifestyle; he was referred to the ophthalmologist by his family physician to rule out diabetic retinopathy. Findings from the initial examination were as follows:

- Best-corrected visual acuity was 20/40 in the right eye and 20/20 in the left eye. Since MG had never checked his vision 1 eye at a time before, he had never noticed the difference in visual acuity between both eyes.

- Intraocular pressure (IOP) was 19 mm Hg on the right eye and 22 mm Hg on the left eye.

- Slitlamp biomicroscopy revealed a 2+ posterior subcapsular cataract in the right eye and mild cataract changes in the left eye.

- The fundus examination revealed a 0.5 cup-to-disc (C/D) ratio of the optic nerves.

- A few retinal microaneurysms were also noted without macular edema or neovascularization at this point.

Diagnosis

Because of the fundus examination finding and the IOP measurement, MG was considered a glaucoma suspect. He was diagnosed as follows:

- Mild nonproliferative diabetic retinopathy in both eyes

- Posterior subcapsular cataract in the right eye

- Glaucoma suspect

The findings and the importance of ocular follow-up were explained to MG. The ophthalmologist discussed the presence of cataract changes and explained that since these changes did not interfere with MG's daily activities, they did not warrant surgery at this time. MG was advised to schedule a follow-up visit within 8 to 12 months. He was also referred to a glaucoma specialist for evaluation of possible glaucoma.

the lens. The lens is the eye structure in charge of focusing images on the retina. The lens's transparent intraocular tissue helps bring rays of light to focus on the retina.

The most common patient complaint is of a progressive gradual decrease in visual acuity at distance and at near, but patients may also complain of a decrease in contrast sensitivity in brightly lit environments, disabling glare during the day, and/or glare from the headlights of oncoming cars at night. The progression of cataracts may frequently result in a mild-to-moderate degree of myopic shift or increase in nearsightedness. Consequently, presbyopic patients report an increase in their near vision and less need for reading glasses as they experience the so-called second sight. Patients must be told that this change is temporary and that they will eventually lose the "second sight." In some cases, patients with cataracts may present with monocular diplopia that is not corrected with use of spectacles or prisms. These cases can usually be solved with cataract surgery.

The Eye Disease Prevalence Group (EDPRG) estimates that in the year 2000, 20.5 million people over age 40 in the United States had a cataract in either eye.[10] It predicts this number to increase to 30.1 million by the year 2020. The number of cases of cataracts among African Americans and whites 40 years or older with diabetes is expected to increase 235% by 2050.[8] This increase is significantly more pronounced for minorities, especially those who are older. For example, the number of cataract cases in African-American women 75 years or older who have diabetes is projected to increase by 637% between 2005 and 2050.[8]

How Do Cataracts Form?

When the blood glucose level is high, the aqueous glucose levels are also elevated. The glucose diffuses through the lens capsule and increases its concentration within the crystalline lens. This results in a glycosylation of lens proteins. Some of the glucose is converted by the intracellular enzyme aldose reductase into sorbitol. This causes alterations in lens permeability and results in cataract formation.[11]

Cortical Cataract

A special type of cataract, known as a cortical cataract, is seen in many individuals with diabetes. It has a "snowflake" appearance with bilateral, widespread subcapsular changes. Often, it has an abrupt onset and an acute course. These cataracts are seen most often in the younger person whose diabetes is not controlled. These lens changes mature rapidly and result in total opacification over a period of a few weeks with very significant visual loss. This "true diabetic cataract" is becoming rarer as better programs to control diabetes have been available.

Common Senile Cataract

Common senile cataracts (nuclear sclerotic cataracts and posterior subcapsular cataracts) occur more frequently and at younger ages, and progress more rapidly in persons afflicted with diabetes than in the general population.[12]

What Treatment Options Are Available?

The only treatment option for cataracts is surgical cataract extraction and placement of an intraocular lens implant. Cataract surgery is a very safe and relatively quick procedure in which the patient can have total visual recovery within days if there is no other pathology affecting the vision. With current cataract extraction techniques, this procedure can be done as soon as the person notices any change in visual acuity. Since there is no real visual acuity cutoff at which the surgery is performed, the patient must be told that this is an elective procedure and must also be informed of all possible risks of surgery.

Complications

Diabetes is not a contraindication for cataract surgery. However, cataract surgery can stimulate additional problems for persons with diabetes, especially if the cataract surgery results in a capsulotomy (rupture in the bag that holds the lens). In this case, the angiogenic factors produced by the retina that can cause proliferative diabetic retinopathy flow from the posterior segment forward to reach the iris. This, in turn, may stimulate neovascular glaucoma, a recognized complication of cataract surgery in individuals with diabetes.[11] Proper stabilization of any diabetic retinopathy prior to cataract extraction can significantly reduce the risk of the development of these complications. In some cases, lens extraction may be needed to improve retinal surveillance.[13]

The appropriate management of individuals with diabetes who are undergoing cataract surgery is an evolving task. Cataract surgery with more modern techniques, such as phacoemulsification, may not cause the progression of diabetic retinopathy, as had been suggested by earlier studies using older cataract extraction techniques.[14] More important, it remains unclear whether the progression of diabetic retinopathy in some patients following cataract surgery is a result of the surgery itself or a reflection of the natural progression of the disease.

Recent small case series suggest that adjunctive use of anti-inflammatory (either steroids or non-steroidal anti-inflammatory drugs) or anti-vascular endothelial growth factor (anti-VEGF) agents at the time of cataract surgery may improve visual recovery from surgery, decrease the incidence of postsurgical macular edema, and perhaps even decrease the progression of diabetic retinopathy.[15,16] These data may be most applicable to persons who have poorly controlled diabetes and who require cataract surgery prior to full treatment of their diabetic retinopathy. However, larger prospective clinical trials are still needed to confirm these results and to recommend these medications for all persons with diabetes undergoing cataract surgery.

Glaucoma

Glaucoma is the second-leading cause of blindness in the United States after cataracts, with more than 1.6 million people having significant visual impairment.[17] Glaucoma is the leading cause of blindness in African Americans.[18] There are several categories of glaucoma, which are based on chronology or etiology. Those most commonly associated with diabetes are discussed here:

- Primary open-angle glaucoma
- Neovascular glaucoma

Primary Open-Angle Glaucoma

Primary open-angle glaucoma (POAG) is described as a multifactorial optic neuropathy (optic nerve disease) characterized by a chronic and progressive loss of optic nerve fibers (clinically, this can be evaluated according to the optic nerve C/D ratio, which

usually ranges from 0.1 to 0.4). Such loss develops in the presence of an open anterior chamber angle (the eyes' main drainage system), characteristic visual-field abnormalities, and IOP that is too high for the continued health of the eye (normal IOP ranges from 8 to 22 mm Hg). Because of the silent nature of the disease, patients usually do not present with any visual complaints until late in the course. At this time, patients present with complaints of a constriction in the visual field (decrease in peripheral vision) or a decrease in visual acuity. Although there is still controversy, some epidemiologic studies show that POAG is found more often in individuals with type 2 diabetes than in age-matched individuals without diabetes.[19–21]

Treatment of POAG is limited to the reduction of IOP. This is mainly performed through topical medications (eyedrops) and occasionally via laser or incisional surgery. The US Preventive Services Task Force (USPSTF) concluded in the March 2005 recommendation statement "Screening for Glaucoma" that there is good evidence that screening can detect increased IOP and early POAG in adults.[22] The USPSTF also found good evidence that early treatment of adults with increased IOP detected by screening reduces the number of persons who develop small visual-field defects and allows for early treatment to prevent progression. However, the task force did not find sufficient evidence to determine the extent to which screening, with earlier detection and treatment, would reduce impairment in vision-related function or quality of life. Harms associated with treatment of increased IOP and early POAG include local eye irritation and an increased risk for cataracts. Further research is needed to clarify the balance between the benefit from early treatment and the given known harm of early screening for glaucoma.

Initial evaluation of a patient suspected of having POAG includes measurement of IOP and central corneal thickness, examination of the angle structures via gonioscopy, evaluation and documentation of optic nerve head and retinal nerve fiber layer, and testing of the visual field by automated static threshold perimetry. Medical therapy (eg, eyedrops) is presently the most common initial intervention for treating POAG. Laser trabeculoplasty and filtering surgery are other treatment options and are typically second or third line. These 3 interventions lower

IOP and decrease the progression of the visual field cut. Since glaucoma cannot be cured, patients with POAG require lifetime monitoring and therapy. The monitoring for POAG consists of IOP measurement, visual field testing, and optic nerve head and retinal nerve fiber layer evaluation, typically carried out several times a year. For patients diagnosed with glaucoma, compliance with the treatment plan as well as regular follow-up examinations by an ophthalmologist is essential to maintaining vision.

Among Americans with diabetes, the number of persons with POAG is expected to substantially increase by 2050 for all demographic groups, but particularly for Hispanics in all age groups and African Americans 50 years or older.[8] There is a projected twelvefold increase from 2005 to 2050 in the number of Hispanics with diabetes 65 years or older with glaucoma.

Glaucoma and Diabetes

In addition to POAG, a great visual threat to persons having both glaucoma and diabetes is development of neovascular glaucoma.

Neovascular Glaucoma

Neovascular glaucoma (NVG) is a secondary glaucoma. Retinal ischemia is the most common and important mechanism in NVG. Significantly higher vascular endothelial growth factor (VEGF)[23] levels occur in the ocular fluids of individuals with proliferative diabetic retinopathy than in persons with nonproliferative diabetic retinopathy. Even higher levels of VEGF are found in the ocular fluids of patients with NVG. Patients presenting with NVG may experience ocular pain or redness, multicolored halos, or headache, and some patients may be asymptomatic.

The management of NVG is related to the stage of the disease and the level of diabetic retinopathy. The lasering of the peripheral retina, called panretinal photocoagulation (PRP), remains the primary treatment of both NVG and proliferative diabetic retinopathy. Panretinal photocoagulation is a type of laser surgery delivered in a scatter pattern throughout the peripheral fundus; its intent is to cause a regression of abnormal blood vessels (neovascularization). Panretinal photocoagulation reduces the areas of retinal ischemia, and thus production of VEGF and other angiogenic factors is also reduced. In cases where PRP treatment does not lower the pressure, filtration surgery or the implantation of a drainage device may be necessary to control the pressure and salvage the optic nerve.[24]

Given the prominent role of VEGF in the pathogenesis of NVG, several case series have indicated that the adjunctive use of anti-VEGF drugs, such as ranibizumab or bevacizumab, may be useful for the treatment of NVG either at the time of PRP treatment or even at the time of glaucoma surgery.[25,26] Although the outcomes in these small case series are extremely promising, larger randomized trials are required prior to recommending these medications for all patients with NVG.

Central Retinal Vein Occlusion

Central retinal vein occlusion (CRVO) is a retinal vascular disorder commonly seen in persons with a history of high blood pressure and/or diabetes mellitus.[27] The exact pathogenesis of the occlusion of the central retinal vein is not known. Various local and systemic factors play a role in the pathological closure of the central retinal vein. Clinically, CRVO presents with variable sudden visual loss. The fundus eye exam may show retinal hemorrhages, dilated tortuous retinal veins, cotton-wool spots (soft exudates that represent infarcts of the nerve fiber layer of the retina), macular edema (swelling or thickening in the central part of the retina), and swelling of the optic nerve. Central retinal vein occlusion can be divided into 2 clinical types:

- Nonischemic CRVO
- Ischemic CRVO

Nonischemic CRVO is the milder form of the disease. It may present with good vision, a few retinal hemorrhages and cotton-wool spots, no relative afferent pupillary defect (abnormality in the pupils' reaction to light), and good blood perfusion to the retina. Nonischemic CRVO may resolve fully with good visual prognosis, or it may progress to the ischemic type.

Ischemic CRVO is the severe form of the disease. Usually, ischemic CRVO presents with severe visual loss, extensive retinal hemorrhages and cotton-wool spots, presence of relative afferent pupillary defect, and/or poor blood perfusion to the retina. In addition, the disease may result in NVG and a painful blind eye.

No known effective medical treatment is available for either prevention or treatment of CRVO. If an underlying systemic medical condition is found, treatment may be indicated, but this rarely reverses the vein occlusion.[28] Treatment may, however, help prevent the opposite eye from developing a vascular occlusion. Various medical modalities for the treatment of CRVO have been advocated by multiple authors with varying success in preventing complications and preserving vision. Laser photocoagulation is the treatment of choice in the management of various complications associated with retinal vascular diseases (diabetic retinopathy, branch retinal vein occlusion). That is why PRP has been used in the treatment of neovascular complications of CRVO such as NVG for numerous years. Guidelines on treatment modalities and follow-up care of patients with CRVO were provided by the Central Vein Occlusion Study (CVOS),[29] a multicenter prospective study sponsored by the National Eye Institute.

Implants

The role of intravitreal glucocorticoids is promising. Ozurdex (0.7 mg dexamethasone intravitreal implant) was the first drug approved by the Food and Drug Administration (FDA) that was indicated specifically for the treatment of macular edema secondary to central and branch retinal vein occlusions.[30] Patients receiving this intravitreal implant, which provides a sustained release of dexamethasone over a 6-month period, were not only more likely to gain vision following a CRVO but also more likely to gain more vision. The use of Ozurdex specifically in persons with diabetes is currently under investigation.[31–33]

Antiangiogenic Therapy With Anti-VEGF Agents

Anti-vascular endothelial growth factor agents were more recently approved for the treatment of macular edema secondary to CRVO and branch retinal vein occlusion (BRVO). These agents work by limiting macular edema and improving vision by reducing vascular permeability. In 2 large phase III trials in patients with macular edema following BRVO or CRVO, monthly injections of ranibizumab (Lucentis®, Genentech/Roche) 0.5 mg into the eye were associated with significantly greater improvement in vision compared with sham injections.[34,35] With continued monitoring and frequent injections, the benefits of ranibizumab were sustained for 12 months and beyond.[36]

In September 2012, aflibercept (Eylea®, Regneron; VEGF trap-eye) was also approved by the FDA for treatment of macular edema associated with CRVO. In the phase III pivotal trials, nearly 60% of patients receiving intravitreal injections of aflibercept 2 mg monthly achieved at least a 15-letter improvement in visual acuity from baseline over 6 months compared with less than 20% in the control group. Additionally, patients receiving aflibercept achieved, on average, a 20-letter improvement in vision compared with placebo.[37,38] These gains in vision were sustained with close monitoring and continued injections over 12 months.[39]

Neuropathies

Prolonged diabetes is a risk factor in the development of a number of neuropathies. The mechanism responsible for the observed neurological defects is believed to be an injury that damages the small vessels nourishing the nerves. Defects of this nature that affect the eye include the following:

- ◈ Ischemic optic neuropathy
- ◈ Ocular palsies
- ◈ Diabetic corneal neuropathy

Ischemic Optic Neuropathy

Ischemic optic neuropathy refers to irreversible optic nerve damage due to loss of blood flow to the nerve. Patients present with complaints of loss of central field and/or a characteristic altitudinal visual field defect. This ocular complication occurs more frequently in persons with diabetes than in the general population and can lead to permanent visual loss.

Ocular Palsies

Ocular palsies result from ischemia to the third, fourth, and sixth cranial nerves. Impairment of extraocular muscle function leads to strabismus (crossing of the eyes) or diplopia (double vision). This condition is temporary, and normal function usually returns within a few months.

Diabetic Corneal Neuropathy

Diabetic corneal neuropathy can lead to severe dry eye and corneal ulcers. (The cornea is the transparent front part of the eye that covers the iris, pupil, and anterior chamber and provides most of the eyes' optical power.) In addition to these corneal epithelial problems, the corneal endothelium has an increased incidence of dysfunction in individuals with diabetes.[40,41] Usually, these patients complain of tearing, occasional ocular pain, and blurry vision. This condition needs to be treated with topical lubricants to decrease the occurrence of further complications.

Other Visual Impairments
Blurring of Vision

Blurring of vision due to instability of blood glucose is related to osmotic changes in the lens of the eye. This problem commonly occurs at the onset of diabetes and during periods of fluctuating blood glucose control. The patient needs to be reassured that this condition is transient and should be instructed to delay testing for new refractive lenses until the blood glucose has been stabilized for 6 to 8 weeks.

Temporary Visual Changes

Temporary visual changes such as dimming of vision, bright flashing lights, or double vision may be experienced during periods of hypoglycemia (low blood glucose levels).[2,42,43]

Diabetic Retinopathy

Diabetic retinopathy is the leading cause of legal blindness among working-aged people in the United States. It is the most common and most important eye disease affecting people with diabetes. Symptoms often do not appear until the late stages of this condition. Delay in treatment decreases effectiveness of therapy. Progression of diabetic retinopathy can be rapid once it is identified. Early recognition is imperative to prevent vision loss.

Diabetic retinopathy[3,5,42,44] occurs when the microvasculature that nourishes the retina is damaged. This damage is caused by elevated blood glucose levels as well as high blood pressure. The damage permits leakage of blood components through the vessel walls. The retina is a layer of nerve tissue at the back of the eye that is responsible for converting light into the electrical signals interpreted by our brains. It is analogous to the film in a camera. These images are relayed along the optic nerve to the brain. Any disturbance to the retina can cause visual symptoms, most often decreased visual acuity. Unlike the changes in the lens that may lead to a cataract, which can be removed and replaced with an artificial intraocular lens, once the retina is severely damaged, permanent visual disturbance results. At this time, the retina cannot be replaced by an artificial retina.

There are many theories regarding the pathogenic mechanisms that lead to the development of diabetic eye disorders. The most popular of these theories relate to abnormalities of (1) protein glycosylation, (2) aldose reductase activity, and (3) glycosylated hemoglobin. All of these mechanisms can result in a relative tissue hypoxia, which may be the final common pathway.[11]

The first clinical findings of diabetic retinopathy are abnormalities of the retinal blood vessels. For instance, the first identifiable lesion is a microaneurysm located within 30° of the center of the macula.[45] (The macula is the small central area of the retina surrounding the fovea; it is the area of acute central vision used for reading and discriminating fine detail and color. A microaneurysm is a minute bubble in the wall of a small blood vessel.) After these first abnormalities are detected, more will tend to occur.

Preventing Blindness

Diabetic retinopathy, the most common and most important eye disease affecting persons with diabetes, is the nation's leading cause of legal blindness.

Intervention impedes the leading cause of blindness in persons with diabetes. Without appropriate intervention, diabetic retinopathy can progress from a mild asymptomatic form to a severe, rapidly progressing and blinding condition.

Retinopathy is staged from its mildest form, using the term "nonproliferative" (mild, moderate, and severe), to its most advanced form, called proliferative retinopathy.[46] Table 26.1 summarizes the stages. Retinopathy is often detectable within 5 years of the onset of diabetes.[2,3] Since type 2 diabetes may go undetected for well over 5 years after its onset, 21% of persons with type 2 diabetes already have retinopathy at the time of initial diagnosis.

Ninety percent of people who are diagnosed with either type 1 diabetes or type 2 diabetes and are less than 30 years of age will develop nonproliferative retinopathy within 20 years after the initial diagnosis, and 50% will progress to sight-threatening proliferative retinopathy.[47]

The number of people with diabetic retinopathy and sight-threatening diabetic retinopathy is expected to triple by 2050 to over 16 million people.[8] There's even a larger growth projected for Hispanics and

---

Case—Part 2: Poor Follow-up Prevents Timely Intervention

Three years passed. MG had missed all of his follow-up appointments with the ophthalmologist after the initial exam, but he saw the glaucoma specialist once. The glaucoma specialist had started him on eyedrops to control the eye pressure, but MG stopped using them 2 years ago. He returned to the retina service approximately 3 years after his initial examination. By this time, he noticed his vision had decreased, and he had started seeing several "cobwebs," especially in the right eye.

- On examination, he had a visual acuity of 20/200 in the right eye and 20/40 in the left.

- IOP was 22 and 21 mm Hg, respectively, in the right and left eyes.

- A 2+ posterior subcapsular cataract was noted (unchanged since last visit) on the right eye and mild cataract on the left eye.

- On the fundus exam, the C/D ratio was unchanged from the last visit.

- The retinal evaluation revealed that MG had progressed to a more severe stage of diabetic retinopathy with neovascularization at the disc. Multiple intraretinal hemorrhages, microaneurysms, and cotton-wool spots along with hard exudates were noted within the macular area. There were several areas of retinal thickening (edema) on both eyes.

- Fluorescein angiography, macular optical coherence tomography, and visual field tests were performed. They showed a large amount of dye leakage from both eyes, macular thickening, and visual field defects in both eyes.

Diagnosis

- Proliferative diabetic retinopathy
- Clinically significant macular edema
- Subcapsular cataract in right eye
- Primary open-angle glaucoma

Treatment

- MG was given laser treatment (PRP and focal laser) in both eyes according to standards of care and scheduled for follow-up in 6 to 8 weeks.

- He was also referred to the glaucoma specialist to restart glaucoma treatment.

Follow-up

Six weeks later, MG's visual acuity was 20/80 in the right eye and 20/30 in the left eye, and significant improvement was noted in the retinal exam. There was regression of the neovascularization and improvement of the macular edema. He saw the glaucoma specialist, who restarted him with glaucoma eyedrops. His IOP was reduced to 14 mm Hg on both eyes. For 2 years, MG continued his eye examinations as indicated and remained stable.

The progression of eye disease might have been prevented in this case or at least delayed through continued close treatment and ongoing observation of the patient's eye disease. Application of effective teaching strategies might have helped this man realize the implications of his self-care choices and motivate him to engage in successful comprehensive self-management.

African Americans, especially among those 65 years or older.

Risk Factors

The development and progression of retinopathy correlate strongly with the degree of glycemic control and the duration of diabetes.[5,6,42]

The severity of hyperglycemia is the key alterable risk factor associated with the development and progression of diabetic retinopathy.[48–50] Hyperglycemia and blood pressure are modifiable risk factors. Blood pressure control and blood lipid control are important.

Glucose Control

The relationship of hyperglycemia severity to the development and progression of diabetic retinopathy was demonstrated in the Diabetes Control and Complications Trial (DCCT) for type 1 diabetes and in the UK Prospective Diabetes Study (UKPDS) for type 2 diabetes.[49,51] The data resulting from these studies emphasized the importance of achieving tight blood glucose control in all persons with diabetes in an attempt to decrease the severity of its complications. Once retinopathy is present, duration of diabetes appears to be less of a factor than hyperglycemia; therefore, it must be stressed to the patient and healthcare providers that controlled blood glucose levels will greatly determine progression to the later, more advanced stages of diabetic retinopathy.[50] (See chapter 22, Hyperglycemia.)

Blood Pressure

Another important alterable factor is high blood pressure. Epidemiologic studies and clinical trials have repeatedly implicated hypertension as an important modifiable risk factor for the development of diabetic retinopathy.[52] Each 10-mm Hg increase in systolic blood pressure has been associated with an approximately 10% increased risk of early retinopathy and a 15% increased risk of proliferative diabetic retinopathy or diabetic macular edema (DME). In the UKPDS, patients with hypertension with tight blood pressure control had a 37% reduction in the risk of microvascular disease, a 34% reduction in the rate of progression of retinopathy, and a 47% reduction

in the deterioration of visual acuity in people with type 2 diabetes.[53,54]

Hyperlipidemia

Although there have been several studies on the relationship between lipid abnormalities and the development of diabetic retinopathy, this association, in contrast to other risk factors like hyperglycemia and hypertension, has been somewhat inconsistent.[55] In the Wisconsin Epidemiologic Study of Diabetic Retinopathy (WESDR), total serum cholesterol was not a significant factor in the severity of retinopathy but was significantly associated with the presence (odds ratio 1.65) and severity of hard exudates in subjects with young-onset diabetes.[56] The Australian Diabetes, Obesity and Lifestyle Study reported that cholesterol was not associated with diabetic retinopathy, while the Singapore Malay Eye Study reported that higher body mass index and higher total and LDL cholesterol levels were associated with a lower prevalence of diabetic retinopathy (odds ratio 0.75).[57,58] In the DCCT study, researchers showed that severity of retinopathy was associated with increasing triglycerides and inversely associated with HDL cholesterol.[59] In the Fenofibrate Intervention and Event Lowering in Diabetes (FIELD) trial, treatment with fenofibrate, a lipid-lowering medication taken by mouth, reduced the need for laser treatment in patients with vision-threatening diabetic retinopathy by approximately 30%.[59] Results from the ACCORD-Eye study were similar to those of the FIELD study. Here, too, treatment with fenofibrate was associated with a 40% decrease in retinopathy progression.[60] In both studies, patients with preexisting diabetic retinopathy derived greater benefit from oral fenofibrate therapy.

Other Risk Factors

Smoking has also been linked to the development and progression of vision-threatening diabetic retinopathy.[61] There is less agreement concerning the importance of other factors such as age, clotting factors, renal disease, and use of specific types of high blood pressure medication.[50,62–64]

Evidence Base

Several large clinical studies have provided excellent information on the natural history and effective treatment strategies that can prevent severe vision loss. These studies include 5 major clinical trials: the DCCT,[49,65,66] the Diabetic Retinopathy Study (DRS),[67,68] the Early Treatment Diabetic Retinopathy Study (ETDRS),[69,70] the Diabetic Retinopathy Vitrectomy Study (DRVS),[71,72] and the UKPDS.[51,53,73]

Natural History

In its earliest stages, diabetic retinopathy, termed nonproliferative diabetic retinopathy (NPDR), is characterized by retinal vascular abnormalities. These include microaneurysms (which are seen as sacular outpouchings along weakened vascular walls), intraretinal hemorrhages that may appear as dots or a flame shape, and cotton-wool spots. Increased retinal vascular leakage (permeability) can occur in this or later stages of retinopathy and may result in retinal thickening (edema) and fluid deposits (hard exudates). Clinically significant macular edema (CSME) is a term used frequently for retinal thickening and/ or hard exudates that either involve the center of the macula or threaten to infiltrate it.

As retinopathy progresses, there is a gradual closure of the retinal vessels, which results in decreased perfusion and ischemia. Signs of increased ischemia include vascular abnormalities (eg, beading, loops), intraretinal microvascular abnormalities that appear as dilated capillaries that arise around ischemic areas where there is capillary closure, and increased retinal hemorrhages and exudation.

The more advanced and vision-threatening stage, proliferative diabetic retinopathy (PDR), is characterized by the growth of new blood vessels along the surface of the retina (neovascularization). These vessels may extend to the vitreous cavity using the posterior vitreous surface as a scaffold. (The vitreous is the transparent, colorless, gelatinous mass that fills the rear two thirds of the eyeball, between the lens and the retina.) The blood vessels are fragile and rupture easily. For this reason, neovascularization in the optic disc (NVD) or neovascularization elsewhere (NVE) is prone to bleeding, which ultimately results in a vitreous hemorrhage. (The optic disc is the ocular end of the optic nerve; it denotes the exit of retinal nerve fibers from the eye and entrance of blood vessels to the eye.) This and other fibrous proliferation may result in epiretinal membrane formation, vitreoretinal traction bands, retinal tears, and ultimately retinal detachments.[74] See Tables 26.1 and 26.2 for specific classifications of diabetic retinopathy stages and findings, including macular edema.

TABLE 26.1 Diabetic Retinopathy—International Clinical Disease Severity Scale	
No apparent retinopathy	No abnormalities
Mild nonproliferative diabetic retinopathy	Microaneurysms only
Moderate nonproliferative diabetic retinopathy	More than just microaneurysms but less than severe nonproliferative diabetic retinopathy
Severe nonproliferative diabetic retinopathy	Any of the following: More than 20 intraretinal hemorrhages in each of 4 quadrants Definite venous beading in 2 or more quadrants Prominent intraretinal microvascular abnormalities in 1 or more quadrants And no signs of proliferative diabetic retinopathy
Proliferative diabetic retinopathy	One or both of the following: Neovascularization Vitreous or preretinal hemorrhage

Source: CP Wilkinson, FL Ferris III, RE Klein, et al, Global Diabetic Retinopathy Project Group, "Proposed international clinical diabetic retinopathy and diabetic macular edema disease severity scales (review)," *Ophthalmology* 110, no. 9 (2003), 1677-82.

TABLE 26.2 Diabetic Macular Edema—International Clinical Disease Severity Scale

Diabetic macular edema apparently absent	No apparent retinal thickening or hard exudates in posterior pole
Diabetic macular edema apparently present	Some retinal thickening or hard exudates in posterior pole
Mild diabetic macular edema	Some retinal thickening or hard exudates in posterior pole, but distant from the center of the macula
Moderate diabetic macular edema	Retinal thickening or hard exudates approaching the center of the macula but not involving the center
Severe diabetic macular edema	Retinal thickening or hard exudates involving the center of the macula

Source: CP Wilkinson, FL Ferris III, RE Klein, et al, Global Diabetic Retinopathy Project Group, "Proposed international clinical diabetic retinopathy and diabetic macular edema disease severity scales (review)," *Ophthalmology* 110, no. 9 (2003), 1677-82.

Diabetic Macular Edema

The macula is the specialized portion of the retina responsible for central vision. Macular edema is leakage of fluid and exudate from the vessels into the macula. This is a serious consequence that affects the primary area of focus.[3,5] Macular edema may accompany NPDR or PDR. Table 26.2 outlines the progression and severity of macular edema.

Clinically significant macular edema, as defined by the ETDRS, exists with any of the following findings:

- Retinal thickening within 500 µm of the center of the fovea (the central pit in the macula that produces the sharpest vision)
- Hard exudates within 500 µm of the center of the fovea with adjacent retinal thickening
- At least 1 disc area (1.5 × 1.5 mm) of retinal thickening, any part of which is within 1 disc diameter (~1.5 mm) of the center of the fovea[75]

Focal edema is associated with hard exudate rings that result from leakage of the microaneurysms. Diffuse edema results from the breakdown of the blood-retinal barrier with leakage from microaneurysms, retinal capillaries, and arterioles. Clinically significant macular edema results when retinal thickening and exudates are sufficient enough to threaten or impair the central vision. Visual loss may vary from mild blurring to a visual acuity of 20/200 or less (legal blindness). (The higher the bottom number, the more vision is decreased. Normal visual acuity is 20/20.) The risk for development of CSME is 10% to 15% for all persons having diabetes for 15 to 20 or more years.

Clinically significant macular edema is determined through a dilated pupil, by slitlamp biomicroscopy, and/or by stereoscopic fundus photography. Fluorescein angiography is a study used to evaluate the retinal vessels, and it helps guide treatment and monitor progression and therapeutic results. Macular edema that is not clinically significant may be observed. Clinically significant macular edema was traditionally treated with laser surgery by using focal argon photocoagulation to seal the leaking blood vessels. Focal photocoagulation is a laser technique directed to abnormal blood vessels with specific areas of focal leakage to reduce chronic fluid leakage in patients with macular edema.

More recently, in patients with symptomatic visual loss associated with DME, the treatment paradigm for DME has shifted away from focal/grid laser photocoagulation toward intravitreal pharmacotherapeutics, principally anti-VEGF medications.[76] Six prospective clinical trials examining the effect of intravitreal ranibizumab in the treatment of DME (READ-2, RESOLVE, RESTORE, RISE, RIDE, and DRCR.net protocol I) have all demonstrated improved visual outcomes with anti-VEGF therapy compared with laser treatment alone.[76] In the RISE and RIDE studies, for example, over 40% of patients receiving monthly ranibizumab injections for 2 years gained 15 letters of vision improvement compared with 15% of patients who were treated with laser alone. With continued close monitoring and repeated injections, this gain was sustained for the entire 3-year duration of the study. Ranibizumab 0.3 mg was recently approved by the FDA for the treatment of DME and may be used in combination with focal/grid laser photocoagulation. Although not yet approved by the FDA, pharmacotherapy with longer acting intravitreal corticosteroids also remains a treatment option for many patients, especially in refractory cases of DME.

Eye Examination

The initial diabetic eye examination should include the following components as a minimum:

- Best corrected visual acuity
- Intraocular pressure
- Ocular motility
- Gonioscopy (a test to visualize the anterior chamber angle and help classify glaucoma), when indicated
- Slitlamp biomicroscopy (examining the lens and other structures at the front of the eye)
- Dilated funduscopy including stereoscopic examination of the posterior pole
- Examination of the peripheral retina and vitreous

Other studies such as diagnostic imaging are performed when indicated.

Frequency of Examination

Recommended frequencies of diabetic eye exams, for both type 1 diabetes and type 2 diabetes, are listed in the following sidebar. See chapter 24 for information on progression of retinopathy as a maternal complication in pregnancy; see also the first case study's discussion of preconception care in that chapter.

Recommended Frequency of Diabetic Eye Examination

- *Type 1 diabetes:* Individuals with type 1 diabetes should have a routine diabetic eye exam at puberty, if diabetes is diagnosed by then, and within 3 to 5 years of receiving a diagnosis of diabetes. Thereafter, exams are annual and when pregnant.
- *Type 2 diabetes:* All persons with type 2 diabetes should be referred for an ophthalmic evaluation at the time of diagnosis.[77] Routine diabetic eye exams should be scheduled yearly thereafter as well as when pregnant.

Type 1 Diabetes

Type 1 diabetes usually has an abrupt onset; therefore, one can usually determine how long a person has had diabetes. Diabetic retinopathy usually becomes apparent as early as 6 to 7 years after onset of the disease, but since the development of vision-threatening retinopathy is rare in children prior to puberty,[78,79] ophthalmic examination is recommended to begin 3 to 5 years after the diagnosis of type 1 diabetes and every year thereafter.[74,80] The eye care provider may need to evaluate the patient more often if progression of retinopathy warrants it.

Type 2 Diabetes

At the time an individual is diagnosed with type 2 diabetes, the disease has usually been present for an undetermined period of time. For this reason, up to 3% of those diagnosed with diabetes at age 30 years or older have CSME at the time of the initial diagnosis.[76] Almost 30% of patients will have some manifestation of diabetic retinopathy at diagnosis. Thus, it is imperative that a patient diagnosed with type 2 diabetes get a full eye evaluation shortly after the diagnosis.

The onset and diagnosis of type 1 diabetes typically occur at an earlier age than that of type 2 diabetes. Most people with an initial diagnosis of type 1 diabetes will not show any ocular manifestations at the time of diagnosis. However, a great majority of those individuals will develop diabetic retinopathy at some point during their lifetime.[61] This is in contrast to people with type 2 diabetes, who are typically diagnosed at an older age and may have changes in the eyes due to diabetes at the time of initial diagnosis. Consequently, both persons with type 1 diabetes and those with type 2 diabetes require careful ophthalmic surveillance and management throughout their lifetime to ensure that treatable causes of vision loss are addressed appropriately.

Table 26.3 summarizes the recommended frequency of ophthalmologic examinations based on the stage of retinopathy.

Care Process

The primary purpose of evaluating and managing diabetic retinopathy is to prevent, retard, or reverse loss of vision. Doing so maintains and/or improves

TABLE 26.3 Suggested Schedule for Ophthalmologic Examination

Stage of Retinopathy	Frequency of Examination
No retinopathy	Annually
Mild nonproliferative retinopathy	Annually
Moderate nonproliferative retinopathy	Within 6–12 months
Clinically significant macular edema or proliferative retinopathy	Every 3–4 months
Proliferative retinopathy with high-risk characteristics	Individualized to patient needs

Source: M Bernbaum, T Stich, "Eye Disease and Adaptive Diabetes Education for Visually Impaired Persons," in MJ Franz, ed, *A Core Curriculum for Diabetes Educators: Diabetes and Complications,* 5th ed (Chicago: American Association of Diabetes Educators, 2003), 131.

vision-related quality of life (see sidebar for self-management and self-care strategies). Once diabetic retinopathy is established, treatment is provided according to its severity scale or retinopathy stage (see Tables 26.1 and 26.2).

Early treatment reduces visual loss by 50% after 3 years.[81] Within 1 year of diagnosis of eye disease, 5% to 10% of patients will progress to a more advanced stage.[3] These guidelines are thus imperative:

- Normal-to-mild nonproliferative retinopathy requires observation and should be reexamined annually.[80]
- Moderate nonproliferative retinopathy without macular edema should be reexamined within 6 to 12 months, as disease progression is common.[63]
- Mild-to-moderate nonproliferative retinopathy with CSME should be treated with focal argon photocoagulation to seal leaking blood vessels.

Vision improves in only a minority of patients; for the majority, the goal of laser photocoagulation treatment is to stabilize visual acuity.

Patients with CSME and excellent visual function should be considered for treatment before visual loss occurs. When treatment is deferred because the center of the macula is not involved or imminently threatened, the patient should be observed at least

every 3 to 4 months for progression.[74] Severe NPDR and (non-high-risk) PDR have similar clinical courses. Consequently, subsequent recommendations and treatment are similar, as shown in the ETDRS.

Importance of Self-Management Education and Self-Care

Treatment of retinopathy begins with preventive measures such as optimizing blood glucose, lipids, and blood pressure. Smoking cessation may also be of value. Routine annual screening and follow-up by an ophthalmologist are essential to ensure that any intervention is appropriately timed.[3,5,42,44,75,81,82]

Patient education about the following topics is an important part of the care process[74]:

- Maintaining near-normal glucose levels
- Maintaining near-normal blood pressure
- Lowering serum lipid levels

Laser Surgery

In eyes with severe diabetic retinopathy, the risk of progression to proliferative disease is 50% to 75% within 1 year. The ETDRS also studied the value of laser surgery for these patients. Panretinal photocoagulation should be considered and should not be delayed if the eye has reached the high-risk proliferative stage (if neovascularization of the optic disc is extensive or vitreous/preretinal hemorrhage has occurred recently). Careful follow-up at 3 to 4 months is important. The goal of laser therapy is to reduce the risk of visual loss. The ETDRS protocol provides detailed guidelines for treatment.[83,84] The patient should be seen for a follow-up visit every 1 to 4 weeks until completion of PRP and then every 2 to 4 months thereafter.

When PRP is to be carried out in eyes with macular edema, it is preferable to perform focal photocoagulation before PRP. There is evidence that PRP may exacerbate macular edema and may cause moderate visual loss compared with untreated eyes.[69] Panretinal laser photocoagulation should not be delayed if the diabetic retinopathy is in the high-risk stage. In these cases, panretinal and focal photocoagulation may be performed concomitantly.[74]

Similar to the treatment of DME, pharmacotherapy with intravitreal anti-VEGF treatment will likely have a future role in the therapy and prevention of proliferative diabetic retinopathy.[85] However, while these studies are still ongoing, the standard therapy remains panretinal laser photocoagulation.

Vitreous Surgery

In cases of high-risk PDR, photocoagulation may not be delivered due to cataracts or severe vitreous or preretinal hemorrhage. In other cases, active PDR may persist despite extensive PRP. In these cases, it may be necessary to perform vitreous surgery. Vitreous surgery is frequently indicated in patients with tractional retinal detachment and in nonclearing vitreous hemorrhage precluding PRP. Patients with vitreous hemorrhage and rubeosis iridis (neovascularization of the iris) should also be considered for prompt vitrectomy and intraoperative photocoagulation, as demonstrated in the DRVS.[71,72]

Other Treatments Being Investigated

Currently, there are different drugs being studied for the management of diabetic retinopathy. Some of these drugs include the administration of short- and long-acting corticosteroids for DME. Other drugs with antiangiogenic activity (inhibitors of the vascular endothelial growth factor) are also being studied. Review of the available literature by the American Academy of Ophthalmology indicates that anti-VEGF pharmacotherapy, via repeated intravitreal injection into the eye, either alone or in combination with focal laser photocoagulation, is a safe and effective treatment of DME over several years' time.[76] Further evidence is required to support the long-term safety and comparative efficacy of anti-VEGF agents.

Ancillary Tests

If used appropriately, a number of tests ancillary to the clinical examination may enhance patient care. These include the following:

⬥ *Color fundus photography.* This is a more reproducible technique than a clinical examination for detecting diabetic retinopathy in clinical research studies. However, clinical examination is superior for detecting retinal thickening and identifying fine-caliber neovascularization (NVD or NVE).

⬥ *Fluorescein angiography.* This is a clinically valuable test for selected patients with diabetic retinopathy and can be used as a guide for treating DME.[75] It is also helpful as a means for evaluating areas of retinal ischemia or the cause of unexplained decreased visual acuity.

⬥ *Ultrasonography (echography).* This is a valuable test for diabetic eyes with opaque media. The test should be considered when media opacities preclude exclusion of retinal detachment or retinal masses by indirect ophthalmoscopy.

⬥ *Optical coherence tomography.* Provides high-resolution (5 μm) imaging of vitreoretinal interface, retina, and subretinal space. Optical coherence tomography can be useful for quantifying retinal thickness and macular edema and identifying vitreomacular traction.[86]

Counseling and Referral

The ophthalmologist has the responsibility to not only manage eye disease but also ensure that people with diabetes are referred for appropriate management of their systemic condition.[42]

An important aspect of treatment is meeting the patient's needs in adapting to loss of vision.[71,87–90] An offer of psychosocial counseling should be made before there is actual deterioration of vision to help alleviate anxiety and depression. Chapters 8 (Problem Solving) and 9 (Healthy Coping) can be of value in assessing and addressing anxiety and depression and in learning how to work with a patient to recognize and manage these issues.

Low-vision evaluation is indicated as soon as vision loss impacts normal daily activities. Referral to rehabilitation services as early as possible will allow the person to acquire adaptive skills and maintain participation and independence in work and recreational activities. Patients need information and instruction in adaptive diabetes self-care as soon as vision is compromised, preferably before adaptive equipment is required.

The extent of vision impairment and the individual's ability to adapt to the vision loss must be evaluated before undertaking adaptive education.

The adaptive education and training needs of persons with preexisting eye disease due to other causes may differ from persons experiencing a new onset of diabetic retinopathy. The diabetes educator can play a key role in referring patients with visual impairment to the proper rehabilitative and psychosocial services.

Focus on Education

Teaching Strategies

◈ **Provide hope and support, and prevent vision loss.** Most diabetic eye diseases can be controlled without significant visual loss if they are diagnosed and managed in a timely manner. Visual impairment and blindness do not have to be part of diabetes. The primary purpose in managing retinopathy is to prevent, retard, or reverse loss of vision. In addition, consistent, frequent monitoring of blood pressure, blood glucose, and lipids is needed.

◈ **Prepare adequately for those with visual impairment.** Teaching methods need to include large print, magnifiers, and the option of recording the instructor's information or directions or obtaining prerecorded instructions. Provide hands-on time and extra time for return demonstration when teaching people with varied levels of visual capacity.

◈ **Appropriately assess and reassess patients' needs and capacity for self-care management.** Persons with visual impairment and diabetes face daily challenges that are multifactorial. Their visual limitations significantly impact their daily tasks. Review daily routines and strategize accordingly for modifying the needed activities.

◈ **Focus on one task at a time.** Reevaluate implementation of the task, adjust accordingly, and then add another task. This way, you will minimize confusion or the feeling of being overwhelmed with all that has to be done. Also, each successfully accomplished task will increase the confidence in making the new task a reality!

◈ **Help with adapting to loss of vision.** Anxiety and depression can negatively influence patients' confidence in their ability to manage their diabetes. Reassess their willingness and readiness to self-manage on an ongoing basis, as their attitude and confidence will change with the acceptance and overall perspective of the condition.

◈ **Strategize for timely referrals.** Rehabilitative and psychosocial services are available, and referral needs to be made promptly to prepare patients for vision loss as well as help them adapt to vision already lost. Assisting patients with the task instead of telling them to do it on their own will ensure its implementation.

Messages for Patients

◈ **Maintain good diabetes control.** Keeping blood glucose, blood pressure, and lipids under control, along with smoking cessation, helps preserve vision.

◈ **Use your support network.** A support network is instrumental to successful diabetes care with or without visual impairment. Invite family or significant others to attend education sessions for support and to assist in "helping" roles. Ensure, however, that "helpers" do not take over, for example, when vision is compromised.

◈ **Ask about vision changes.** Blurriness may be temporary due to elevated blood glucose. Wait until blood glucose resolves before considering eye glasses or changes in lenses.

◈ **Discuss eye care.** Be knowledgeable about screening to protect vision and other reasons to consult an eye care specialist. Understand what the recommendations are for diabetic eye examinations, for both initial visits and follow-up. Identify the frequency of eye care visits that will best protect vision for the individual.

⊙ Protect vision through eye examinations. Knowing the current status of eye disease and what symptoms to watch for is important. Schedule a retinal evaluation by an ophthalmologist to assess eye condition. This examination is not just a fitting for glasses; it is a dilated eye exam. Use the appointment to ask questions like these: What condition are my eyes in? What can I do to keep my vision? Is it okay to exercise? and What do I need to change?

⊙ Seek out specialists when help is needed. To help alleviate anxiety and depression and begin the process of adapting to loss of vision, psychosocial counseling is appropriate to include *before* deterioration of vision occurs.

Health Literacy and Numeracy

⊙ There is no "typical" vision-impaired patient. Use different approaches for low-vision patients and blind patients. You can use print with special equipment and materials for low vision. The extent of visual disability within patients who are blind can depend on their eyes' physical sensory impairment, the duration of the onset of vision impairment, and the way in which that impairment occurred. Vision may also fluctuate or may be influenced by factors such as inappropriate lighting, light glare, or fatigue. The best way to know which education approach to use is to ask the patient, "What works best for you?" Individualize strategies based on the patient's preferences and skill of communication (Braille, speed listening).

⊙ Communicate effectively with your patients.
- Identify yourself and your role.
- Call a patient by name if you want his or her attention.
- Use descriptive words such as "straight," "forward," and "left" in relation to the patient's body orientation. Avoid nondescript terms such as "over there," "here," and "this."
- Describe in detail pertinent visual occurrences of the learning activities.
- Offer to read written information.
- Do not speak loudly to people with visual impairments.
- Use a projector to show step-by-step instructions.
- Appropriately label objects used for identification.
- Use an actual object for demonstrations.
- Use a tape recorder.
- Make all handouts available in an appropriate form such as regular print, large print, or Braille, or on cassette, depending on the patient's preferences.
- Enlist the aid of a special education professional, if needed, for teaching the task of taking insulin or monitoring glucose.

⊙ Put a meaning to the task. Motivation to self-manage diabetes among visually impaired patients varies. Explore their health belief system and confidence in their ability to apply the information learned. Use a confidence scale to assess whether they are able, willing, and ready to do a specific task. For example, ask, "What do you think can be done for you to use a meter to test your blood glucose?"

⊙ Minimize the use of "unrealistic optimism"—for example, "Bad things are unlikely to happen when . . ." versus "Good things are likely to happen when . . ."—as patients' perception of their ability to handle things can be very unpredictable. Also, their responses can be defensive, and they can be skeptical of information that is inconsistent with their attitudes or preferences. The best approach is not to make any assumptions about health literacy or patients' ability to do things.

Focus on Practice

Clinician style: Be empathetic, accepting, supportive of self-efficacy, and collaborative.

Skills: Utilize active listening, open-ended questions, and summarizing.

Tools: Use appropriate teaching and behavioral change approaches.

Collaboration: Utilize the expertise of other professionals to help patients realize their full potential in achieving their clinical care goal and enjoying their life.

Ongoing support: People need to be reminded more often than they need to be instructed. Create a series of functional messages and directions that can be used to maintain a healthy routine and tasks.

Program Planning

Anticipate a need for alternatives to traditional patient handouts. As blood glucose levels change, patients may experience short-term blurred vision or reoccurring blurriness, as well as more permanent vision changes. When preparing your teaching materials, plan to accommodate this change by using one or more of the following alternative methods for conveying information:

- Enlarged-print handouts
- Transferring materials from black on white to white on black
- Audio recording
- Schedule a time outside of the scheduled visit/classroom if needed to clarify information and to reinforce and encourage participants

References

1. Fong DS, Aiello LP, Ferris FL III, Klein R. Diabetic retinopathy. Diabetes Care. 2004;27(10):2540-53.

2. Klein R, Klein BEK. Vision disorders in diabetes. In: National Diabetes Data Group, eds. Diabetes in America. 2nd ed. Bethesda, Md: National Institutes of Health; 1995:293-337.

3. Ferris FL III, Davis MD, Aiello LM. Treatment of diabetic retinopathy (review). New Engl J Med. 1999;341:667-78.

4. Javitt JC, Aiello LP. Cost effectiveness of detecting and treating diabetic retinopathy. Ann Intern Med. 1996;124:164-9.

5. Aiello LP, Gardner TW, King GL, et al. Diabetic retinopathy (technical review). Diabetes Care. 1998;21(1):143-56.

6. Aiello LP, Cavallerano J, Bursell SE. Diabetic eye disease. Endocrinol Metab Clin North Am. 1996;25:271-91.

7. Harris MI. Summary. In: National Diabetes Data Group, eds. Diabetes in America. 2nd ed. Bethesda, Md: National Institutes of Health; 1995:1-13.

8. Saaddine JB, Honeycutt AA, Venkat Narayan KM, Zhang X, Klein R, Boyle JP. Projection of diabetic retinopathy and other major eye diseases among people with diabetes mellitus: United States, 2005-2050. Arch Ophthalmol. 2008;126(12):1740-7.

9. Ferris FL III. How effective are treatments for diabetic retinopathy? JAMA. 1993;269:1290-1.

10. Congdon N, Vingerling JR, Klein BE, et al; Eye Diseases Prevalence Research Group. Prevalence of cataract and pseudophakia/aphakia among adults in the United States. Arch Ophthalmol. 2004;122(4):487.

11. Feman SS. Diabetes and the eye. In: Duane's Clinical Ophthalmology on CD-ROM. Philadelphia: Lippincott Williams & Wilkins; 2004.

12. Ederer F, Hiller R, Taylor HR. Senile lens change in diabetes in two population studies. Am J Ophthalmol. 1981; 91:381.

13. Flanagan DW. Current management of established diabetic eye disease. Eye. 1993;7:302.

14. Shah AS, Chen SH. Cataract surgery and diabetes. Curr Opin Ophthalmol. 2010;21(1):4-9.

15. Cheema RA, Al-Mubarak MM, Amin YM, Cheema MA. Role of combined cataract surgery and intravitreal bevacizumab injection in preventing progression of diabetic retinopathy: prospective randomized study. J Cataract and Refractive Surg. 2009 Jan;35(1):18-25.

16. Kim SY, Yang J, Lee YC, Park YH. Effect of a single intraoperative sub-Tenon injection of triamcinolone acetonide

on the progression of diabetic retinopathy and visual outcomes after cataract surgery. J Cataract and Refractive Surg. 2008;34(5):823-6.

17. Leske MC. The epidemiology of open-angle glaucoma: a review. Am J Epidemiol. 1983;118:66.

18. Sommer A, Tielsch JM, Katz J, et al. Racial differences in the cause-specific prevalence of blindness in east Baltimore. N Engl J Med. 1991;325(20):1412.

19. Becker B. Diabetes mellitus and primary open-angled glaucoma. Am J Ophthalmol. 1971;71:1.

20. Klein BE, Klein R, Jensen SC. Open-angle glaucoma in older onset diabetes: the Beaver Dam Eye Study. Ophthalmology. 1994;101:1173.

21. Dielemans I, de Jong PTVM, Stolk R, et al. Primary open-angle glaucoma, intraocular pressure, and diabetes mellitus in the general elderly population: the Rotterdam Study. Ophthalmology. 1996;103:1271.

22. US Preventive Services Task Force. Screening for glaucoma (recommendation statement). Ann Fam Med. 2005;3:171-2.

23. Aiello LP, Avery RL, Arrig PG. Vascular endothelium growth factor in ocular fluid of patients with diabetic retinopathy and other retinal disorders. N Engl J Med. 1994; 331:1480.

24. Molteno ACB, VanRooyen MNB, Bartholomew RS. Implants for draining neovascular glaucoma. Br J Ophthalmol. 1977;61:120.

25. Ciftci S, Bayezit Sakalar Y, Unlu K, Keklikci U, Caca I, Dogan E. Intravitreal bevacizumab combined with panretinal photocoagulation in the treatment of open angle neovascular glaucoma. Eur J Ophthalmol. 2009;19:1029-34. Epub 2009 Jun 25.

26. Chen CH, Lai IC, Wu PC, et al. Adjunctive intravitreal bevacizumab-combined trabeculectomy versus trabeculectomy alone in the treatment of neovascular glaucoma. J Ocul Pharmacol Ther. 2010;26(1):111-8.

27. The Eye Disease Case-Control Study Group. Risk factors for central retinal vein occlusion. Arch Ophthalmol. 1996; 114:545.

28. Schwab PJ, Okun E, Fahey FJ. Reversal of retinopathy in Waldenstrom's macroglobulinemia by plasmapheresis: a report of two cases. Arch Ophthalmol. 1960;64:67.

29. Central Vein Occlusion Study Group. A randomized clinical trial of early panretinal photocoagulation for ischemic central vein occlusion: the Central Vein Occlusion Study Group N report. Ophthalmology. 1995;102(10):1434-44.

30. Kuno N, Fujii S. Biodegradable intraocular therapies for retinal disorders: progress to date. Drugs Aging. 2010 Feb 1;27(2):117-34.

31. Schwartz SG, Flynn HW Jr. Pharmacotherapies for diabetic retinopathy: present and future. Exp Diabetes Res. 2007; 2007:52487.

32. Grover D, Li TJ, Chong CC. Intravitreal steroids for macular edema in diabetes. Cochrane Database Syst Rev. 2008 Jan 23;1:CD005656.

33. Allergan. Safety and efficacy of a new treatment in vitrectomized subjects with diabetic macular edema [study in recruiting stage] (cited 2010 Oct 18). On the Internet at: http://www.clinicaltrials.gov.

34. Brown DM, Campochiaro PA, Singh RP, et al. Ranibizumab for macular edema following central retinal vein occlusion: six-month primary end point results of a phase III study. Ophthalmology. 2010;117(6):1124-33.

35. Campochiaro PA. Ranibizumab for macular edema following branch retinal vein occlusion: six-month primary end point results of a phase III study. Ophthalmology. 2010; 117(6):1102-12.

36. Campochiaro PA. Sustained benefits from ranibizumab for macular edema following central retinal vein occlusion: twelve-month outcomes of a phase III study. Ophthalmology. 2011;118(10):2041-9.

37. Boyer D, Heier J, Brown DM, et al. Vascular endothelial growth factor Trap-Eye for macular edema secondary to central retinal vein occlusion: six-month results of the phase 3 COPERNICUS study. Ophthalmology. 2012; 119(5):1024-32.

38. Holz FG, Roider J, Ogura Y, et al. VEGF Trap-Eye for macular oedema secondary to central retinal vein occlusion: 6-month results of the phase III GALILEO study. Br J Ophthalmol. 2013;97(3):278-84.

39. Brown DM, Heier JS, Clark WL, et al. Intravitreal aflibercept injection for macular edema secondary to central retinal vein occlusion: 1-year results from the phase 3 COPERNICUS study. Am J Ophthalmol. 2013;155(3): 429-37.

40. Schultz RO, Peters MA, Sobocinski K. Diabetic corneal neuropathy. Trans Am Ophthalmol Soc. 1983;81:107.

41. Busted N, Olsen T, Schmitz O. Clinical observations on the corneal thickness and the corneal endothelium in diabetes mellitus. Br J Ophthalmol. 1982;65:687.

42. Frank KJ, Dieckert JP. Diabetic eye disease: a primary care perspective. South Med J. 1996;89:463-70.

43. Cox DJ, Kiernan BD, Schroeder DB, Cowley M. Psychosocial sequelae of visual loss in diabetes. Diabetes Educ. 1998; 24:481-4.

44. Sanders R, Wilson M. Diabetes-related eye disorders. J Natl Med Assoc. 1993;85:104-8.

45. Feman SS. The natural history of the first clinically visible features of diabetic retinopathy. Trans Am Ophthalmol Soc. 1994;92:744.

46. Wilkinson CP, Ferris FL III, Klein RE, et al. Proposed international clinical diabetic retinopathy and diabetic

macular edema disease severity scales. Ophthalmology. 2003;110:1677-82.

47. Deshpande AD, Harris-Hayes M, Schootman M. Epidemiology of diabetes and diabetes-related complications. Phys Ther. 2008 Nov;88(11):1254-64.

48. Klein R, Klein BE, Moss SE, et al. Glycosylated hemoglobin predicts the incidence and progression of diabetic retinopathy. JAMA. 1988;260:2864-71.

49. The Diabetes Control and Complications Trial (DCCT) Research Group. The effect of intensive treatment of diabetes on the development and progression of long-term complications in insulin-dependent diabetes mellitus. N Engl J Med. 1993;329:977-86.

50. Davis MD, Fisher MR, Gangnon RE, et al. Risk factors for high-risk proliferative diabetic retinopathy and severe visual loss: Early Treatment Diabetic Retinopathy Study Report #18. Invest Ophthalmol Vis Sci. 1998;39:233-52.

51. UK Prospective Diabetes Study (UKPDS) Group. Intensive blood-glucose control with sulphonylureas or insulin compared with conventional treatment and risk of complications in patients with type 2 diabetes (UKPDS 33). Lancet. 1998;352:837-53.

52. Mohamed Q, Gillies MC, Wong TY. Management of diabetic retinopathy: a systematic review. JAMA. 2007;298: 902-16.

53. UK Prospective Diabetes Study Group. Tight blood pressure control and risk of macrovascular and microvascular complications in type 2 diabetes (UKPDS 38). BMJ. 1998; 317:703-13.

54. Snow V, Weiss KB, Mottur-Pilson C. The evidence base for tight blood pressure control in the management of type 2 diabetes mellitus. Ann Intern Med. 2003;138:587-92.

55. Lim LS, Wong TY. Lipids and diabetic retinopathy. Expert Opin Biol Ther. 2012;12(1):93-105.

56. Klein BE, Moss SE, Klein R, Surawicz TS. The Wisconsin Epidemiologic Study of Diabetic Retinopathy: XIII. Relationship of serum cholesterol to retinopathy and hard exudate. Ophthalmology. 1991;98:1261-5.

57. Wong TY, Cheung N, Tay WT. Prevalence and risk factors for diabetic retinopathy: the Singapore Malay Eye Study. Ophthalmology. 2008;115:1869-75.

58. Tapp RJ, Shaw JE, Harper CA. The prevalence of and factors associated with diabetic retinopathy in the Australian population. Diabetes Care. 2003;26:1731-7.

59. Lyons TJ, Jenkins AJ, Zheng D, et al. Diabetic retinopathy and serum lipoprotein subclasses in the DCCT/EDIC cohort. Invest Ophthalmol Vis Sci. 2004;45(3):910-8.

60. Keech AC, Mitchell P, Summanen PA, et al. Effect of fenofibrate on the need for laser treatment for diabetic retinopathy (FIELD study): a randomised controlled trial. Lancet. 2007 Nov 17;370(9600):1687-97.

61. Klein R, Lee KE, Gangnon RE, Klein BEK. The 25-year incidence of visual impairment in type 1 diabetes mellitus: the Wisconsin Epidemiologic Study of Diabetic Retinopathy. Ophthalmology. 2010;117(1):63-70.

62. Klein R, Klein BE, Moss SE, et al. The Wisconsin Epidemiologic Study of Diabetic Retinopathy: IX. Four-year incidence and progression of diabetic retinopathy when age at diagnosis is less than 30 years. Arch Ophthalmol. 1989; 107(2):237-43.

63. Klein R, Klein BE, Moss SE, et al. The Wisconsin Epidemiologic Study of Diabetic Retinopathy: X. Four-year incidence and progression of diabetic retinopathy when age at diagnosis is 30 years or more. Arch Ophthalmol. 1989; 107(2):244-9.

64. Klein R, Sharrett AR, Klein BE, et al. The association of atherosclerosis, vascular risk factors, and retinopathy in adults with diabetes: the atherosclerosis risk in communities study. Ophthalmology. 2002;109:1225-34.

65. The Diabetes Control and Complications Trial (DCCT). The relationship of glycemic exposures (HbA1c) to the risk of development and progression of retinopathy. Diabetes. 1995;44:968-83.

66. The Diabetes Control and Complications Trial (DCCT) Research Group. The effect of intensive diabetes treatment on the progression of diabetic retinopathy in insulin dependent diabetes mellitus. Arch Ophthalmol. 1995;113:36-51.

67. The Diabetic Retinopathy Study (DRS) Research Group. Report no. 14. Indications for photocoagulation treatment of diabetic retinopathy. Int Ophthalmol Clin. 1987;27: 239-53.

68. The Diabetic Retinopathy Study (DRS) Research Group. DRS report no. 3. Four risk factors for severe visual loss in diabetic retinopathy. Arch Ophthalmol. 1979;97:654-5.

69. Early Treatment Diabetic Retinopathy Study Research Group. ETDRS report no. 9. Early photocoagulation for diabetic retinopathy. Ophthalmology. 1991;98:766-85.

70. Early Treatment Diabetic Retinopathy Study Research Group. ETDRS report no. 19. Focal photocoagulation treatment of diabetic macular edema: relationship of treatment effect to fluorescein angiographic and other retinal characteristics at baseline. Arch Ophthalmol. 1995;113: 1144-55.

71. The Diabetic Retinopathy Vitrectomy Study Research Group. Diabetic Retinopathy Vitrectomy Study report no. 2. Early vitrectomy for severe vitreous hemorrhage in diabetic retinopathy: two-year results of a randomized trial Arch Ophthalmol. 1985;103:1644-52.

72. The Diabetic Retinopathy Vitrectomy Study Research Group. Diabetic Retinopathy Vitrectomy Study report no. 5. Early vitrectomy for severe vitreous hemorrhage in diabetic retinopathy: four-year results of a randomized trial. Arch Ophthalmol. 1990;108:958-64.

73. UK Prospective Diabetes Study (UKPDS) Group (UKPDS 34). Effect of intensive blood-glucose control with metformin on complications in overweight patients with type 2 diabetes. Lancet. 1998;352:854-65.

74. American Academy of Ophthalmology Quality of Care Committee Retina Panel. Preferred Practice Pattern for Diabetic Retinopathy. San Francisco: American Academy of Ophthalmology; 2003.

75. Early Treatment Diabetic Retinopathy Study Research Group. ETDRS report no. 1. Photocoagulation for diabetic macular edema. Arch Ophthalmol. 1985;103: 1796-806.

76. Ho AC, Scott IU, Kim SJ, et al. Anti-vascular endothelial growth factor pharmacotherapy for diabetic macular edema: a report by the American Academy of Ophthalmology. Ophthalmology. 2012;119(10):2179-88.

77. Klein R, Klein BE, Moss SE, et al. The Wisconsin Epidemiologic Study of Diabetic Retinopathy: III. Prevalence and risk of diabetic retinopathy when age of diagnosis is 30 or more years. Arch Ophthalmol. 1984;102:527-32.

78. Klein R, Klein BE, Moss SE, et al. Retinopathy in young-onset diabetic patients. Diabetes Care. 1985;8:311-5.

79. Krolewski AS, Warram JH, Rand LI, et al. Risk of proliferative diabetic retinopathy in juvenile onset type I diabetes: a 40-year follow-up study. Diabetes Care. 1986;9:443-52.

80. Klein R, Klein BE, Moss SE, et al. The Wisconsin Epidemiologic Study of Diabetic Retinopathy: II. Prevalence and risk of diabetic retinopathy when age at diagnosis is less than 30 years. Arch Ophthalmol. 1984;102:520-6.

81. The Diabetic Retinopathy Study Research Group. Preliminary report on effects of photocoagulation therapy. Am J Ophthalmol. 1976;81:383-96.

82. Ferris F. Early photocoagulation in patients with either type I or type II diabetes. Trans Am Ophthalmol Soc. 1996;94:505-37.

83. Early Treatment Diabetic Retinopathy Study Research Group. ETDRS report no. 2. Treatment techniques and clinical guidelines for photocoagulation of diabetic macular edema. Ophthalmology. 1987;94:761-74.

84. Early Treatment Diabetic Retinopathy Study Research Group. ETDRS report no. 3. Techniques for scatter and local photocoagulation treatment of diabetic retinopathy. Int Ophthalmol Clin. 1987;27:254-64.

85. Tremolada G, Del Turco C, Lattanzio R, et al. The role of angiogenesis in the development of proliferative diabetic retinopathy: impact of intravitreal anti-VEGF treatment. Exp Diabetes Res. 2012;2012:728325.

86. Strom C, Sander B, Larsen N, et al. Diabetic macular edema assessed with optical coherence tomography and stereo fundus photography. Invest Ophthalmol Vis Sci. 2002; 43:241-5.

87. Bernbaum M, Albert SG. Referring patients with diabetes and vision loss for rehabilitation—who is responsible? Diabetes Care. 1996;19:175-7.

88. Bernbaum M, Albert SG, Duckro PN. Psychosocial profiles in patients with visual impairment due to diabetic retinopathy. Diabetes Care. 1988;11:551-7.

89. Jacobson AM. Current concepts: the psychological care of patients with insulin-dependent diabetes mellitus. N Engl J Med. 1996;334:1249-53.

90. Wulsin LR, Jacobson AM, Rand LI. Psychosocial adjustment to advanced proliferative diabetic retinopathy. Diabetes Care. 1993;16:1061-6.

CHAPTER 27

Diabetic Kidney Disease

Amanda Kirpitch, MA, RD, CSSD, LDN, CDE
Sherry Smith-Ossman, MS, ANP, RNCS, RN, CDE

Key Concepts

- Early detection and diagnosis of chronic kidney disease is essential for preventing and/or delaying further disease progression.

- Laboratory parameters and diagnostic tests aid in classifying the stages of chronic kidney disease, the various types of kidney failure, and the presence of nephrotic syndrome.

- Other concomitant health considerations, such as hyperparathyroidism and anemia, require early treatment.

- Cardiovascular disease is a concern. The risk of cardiovascular disease in persons with chronic kidney disease is 30 times the norm.

Introduction

The spectrum of changes in the kidney that occur among individuals diagnosed with diabetes that cannot be ascribed to other causes has been called diabetic nephropathy, or preferably, diabetic kidney disease (DKD).[1] At the mild end of this spectrum is microalbuminuria. At the more severe end is overt DKD, which is characterized by persistent proteinuria, hypertension, and a progressive decline in kidney function, which may lead to renal replacement therapies (RRTs; ie, hemodialysis, peritoneal dialysis, or transplantation) and/or premature mortality from cardiovascular disease (CVD). Appropriate and timely clinical intervention may delay or prevent microalbuminuria from progressing to kidney failure.[2]

Chronic kidney disease (CKD) is a growing public health problem in the United States. Thirty-one percent of the US population is estimated to have CKD.[3,4] Diabetes is the most common primary diagnosis in persons with kidney failure/end-stage renal disease (ESRD), accounting for approximately 45% of new cases.[5] The increased prevalence of diabetes in the CKD population is related to 2 major factors[6]: (1) the increased incidence of type 2 diabetes in the

general population and (2) the innovative therapeutic approaches that have allowed persons diagnosed with diabetes to live longer. The overweight and obesity epidemic continues to be elevated among the nation's youth—for example, 31.8% of 2- to 19-year-olds are above the 85th percentile for body mass index (BMI), of which 17% are obese.[7] It is anticipated that with current trends, the incidence of type 1 diabetes in youth will triple by 2050, and the number of youth diagnosed with type 2 diabetes will quadruple in this time period.[8] The long-term health implications of poor glycemic management will increase the propensity of comorbid conditions such as kidney disease in much younger individuals. These factors likely influence the number of individuals eligible for conservative renal management and/or RRTs.

As measured in the 5-year survival data by disease etiology (diabetes, hypertension, glomerulonephritis), one half of all persons diagnosed with DKD who receive dialysis die within 2 years of initiation of dialysis; this is the highest mortality rate among the 3 leading causes of kidney failure.[5] Regardless of disease etiology, the primary cause of death among

A case study is woven throughout the chapter to show one method for applying the best research evidence to clinical practice. The chapter uses the case of a 55-year-old African-American woman with type 2 diabetes of 15 years' duration and at considerable risk for progressive kidney disease as a tool to examine appropriate screening, assessment, and treatment options. Teachable moments, using the AADE7 Self-Care Behaviors™, are emphasized throughout the chapter as well, and strategies are provided for dealing with the challenges of this complicated condition. This chapter also identifies unanswered clinical questions related to DKD and offers insight into additional topics for scientific inquiry. At the end of the chapter, the reader will find clinical pearls for practice, featuring teaching strategies, messages for patients, health literacy, and practice-related issues.

persons with CKD is CVD. Persons with CKD have an increased risk of CVD that is 30 times higher than that of the general population.[9,10] Thus, the need for a "proactive, comprehensive, integrated intervention and treatment approach to successfully manage diabetes, CKD, and CVD" is appropriate to emphasize.[6]

Kidney Function in Health and Disease

The kidney is an intricate organ. It maintains homeostatic control through regulation of fluid volume, sodium and potassium levels, acid-base ratios, and calcium-phosphorus balance.[11,12] The kidney is one of the main detoxifying organs of the body; it excretes waste products such as excess water, electrolytes, metabolites, drugs, and other potentially harmful toxins. Lastly, it supplies endocrine functions necessary for bone maintenance, blood pressure control, normal metabolism, and red blood cell production.

To fully appreciate all these diverse functions, one must first examine how the kidneys and the entire system work.[11,12] The urinary system is composed of the kidneys, ureters, bladder, and urethra. Each kidney weighs about 6 oz and is approximately the size of a human fist. The outer core of the kidneys is encapsulated by a fibrous, rigid sheath that forms

the renal cortex. Directly underneath this cortex is the medulla. Between these 2 segments, the nephrons and their collecting tubules are housed. The functional unit or "workhorse" of the kidney is the nephron. Each kidney has well over 1 million nephrons. Within each nephron are several components[12,13]:

- *Glomerulus and Bowman's capsule.* Fifty capillaries make up the branches of small arteries in the glomerulus. Through this tuft of afferent and efferent arterioles, blood flows into the kidney. The exchange of waste products occurs at the Bowman's capsule. Approximately 180 L of filtrate pass through the kidneys at the glomerulus, and 1 to 2 L of urine are actually excreted.
- *Proximal convoluted tubule.* This section of the nephron, which is directly connected to the Bowman's capsule, is the main location where glucose, sodium, bicarbonate, potassium, chloride, calcium, phosphate, water, and other solutes are absorbed. The reabsorption of fluid through sodium pumps also occurs in the proximal convoluted tubule.
- *Loop of Henle.* This is the site where urine is concentrated or diluted. The process is largely dictated by the fluid requirements of the body.
- *Distal tubule.* This tubule has 3 parts: the ascending limb of the Loop of Henle, the macula densa, and the distal convoluted tubule. Ninety-nine percent of the water filtered by the kidneys is reabsorbed here.
- *Collecting duct.* Secretion of potassium is a major function of the collecting duct. As urine is produced in the nephrons, it flows from the collecting duct to the main cavity of the renal pelvis, then on to the ureter into the bladder, and then it is expelled through the urethra.

Renal Physiology

Through glomerular filtration, tubular secretion, and reabsorption, the kidneys are able to regulate the chemical composition of the body fluids and eliminate metabolic wastes.[11,12] Homeostatic regulation of the urine osmolality is controlled by the distal convoluted tubules and collecting ducts. Reabsorption and transport of water greatly varies with cellular permeability and is largely affected by secretion of the antidiuretic hormone (ADH). As plasma osmolality increases in a dehydrated condition, ADH secretion increases so that water is conserved by the kidneys; the opposite is true in a hypervolemic state.

The kidneys are also the major site where calcium and phosphorus levels remain in balance. Parathyroid hormone (PTH), secreted by the parathyroid glands, is paramount to achieving this balance. The hormone maintains this balance by enhancing calcium and phosphorus absorption from the gastrointestinal tract and bone. During episodes of increased calcium intake, there is a transitory rise in circulating levels of calcium with a subsequent fall in PTH secretion. This results in more calcium filtered by the kidneys and excess amounts excreted. The inverse occurs during periods of low dietary calcium intake. Parathyroid hormone synthesis and release also responds to variations in circulating levels of serum phosphorus, irrespective of serum calcium or vitamin D levels.[14] The final step in the activation of vitamin D occurs within the kidneys. Vitamin D is essential for assisting with the absorption of calcium from the intestinal lumen as well as augmenting bone resorption. Vitamin D, in concert with calcitonin and PTH, maintains calcium-phosphorus homeostasis and protects overall bone health.

As already described, the kidneys are greatly affected by a number of hormones.[11,12] However, the kidneys are invaluable to the endocrine system as well. For instance, renin and erythropoietin produced by the kidneys are released to stimulate effects elsewhere in the body system. Renin, an enzyme, is vital for maintaining normal blood pressure and is generated by the kidneys in response to decreased blood volume. Renin acts to form angiotensin, which serves as a powerful vasoconstrictor and triggers the release of aldosterone, which enhances sodium and water retention. Erythropoietin, a hormone, is also manufactured by the kidneys. This hormone stimulates the bone marrow to produce red blood cells, which in turn prevents severe anemia from developing. As evident, the kidneys are one of the most vital organs in the body in maintaining homoeostasis and optimal health. Achieving such balance is increasingly difficult during declining kidney function.

Renal Pathophysiology

Kidney failure may be either sudden, causing acute kidney injury, or progressive in nature, as in CKD.[12,13]

Acute Kidney Injury

Persons with acute kidney injury (AKI) have a rapid onset of symptoms, including the following: elevation in blood urea nitrogen (BUN), creatinine, and electrolytes and minimal urinary output. Acute kidney injury is typically caused by ischemic or nephrotoxic injury, multiorgan system failure, sepsis, obstructive uropathy, or acute glomerular nephritis.[15,16] Morbidity and mortality rates can be as high as 80%, depending on etiology. Usually with adequate dialytic support and nutritional intervention, the condition will reverse itself. However, when the AKI is more severe, as when it is superimposed with other illnesses (such as sepsis) or when actual tissue damage to the parenchymal tissue occurs, additional medical and nutritional support will be required.

Chronic Kidney Disease

The National Kidney Foundation–Kidney Disease Outcomes Quality Initiative (NKF-KDOQI) presents evidence-based practice guidelines for the management and treatment of all phases of kidney disease. It was launched in 1995, with routine updates and reviews of the practice guidelines given as necessary. For example, the Clinical Practice Guidelines for Diabetes and Chronic Kidney Disease were released in 2007. Guidelines were updated in 2012 with a focus on hyperglycemia, dyslipidemia, and albuminuria.[1,3,4,17] Additional guidelines continue to be developed. The language associated with kidney disease has been standardized because synonymous terms were easily confused. The stages of CKD replace commonly used terms such as pre-dialysis, pre-ESRD, and chronic renal insufficiency. This system classifies CKD by an at-risk stage and 5 progressive stages as defined by the glomerular filtration rate (GFR).

Chronic kidney disease is the classification for all damage to the kidney irrespective of cause. Persons diagnosed with CKD experience a permanent loss of GFR that occurs over a period of months to years. Eventually, CKD may lead to Stage 5, requiring RRT such as dialysis or transplantation to sustain life. Although RRTs are discussed, the focus of this chapter is on how to delay or prevent further disease progression.

Chronic kidney disease can be identified in 2 ways[18]:

- Presentation of kidney damage for >3 months, with or without elevated GFR as evidenced by
  — structural or functional abnormalities recognized by a biopsy or other imaging tests
  — urine or blood laboratory result abnormalities
- GFR <60 mL/min/1.73 m^2 for ≥3 months, with or without evidence of kidney damage

Stages of CKD   In 2002, a standard for classifying the stages of CKD was outlined by the NKF-KDOQI.[19] This information is summarized in Table 27.1. Kidney function is dependent on the measurement of the GFR through a number of validated equations. Some decreases in kidney function may be secondary to the normal aging process.[12,13] If decline persists, kidney function should be monitored to enable appropriate and timely intervention.

Nephrotic Syndrome

Nephrotic syndrome is considered "one of the most serious challenges of clinical nephrology" (p. 4).[13] The presentation of nephrotic syndrome may occur in many different types of CKD, and it is characterized by changes in the glomerular basement membrane leading to profound proteinuria. Clinical signs present as increased urinary losses of albumin (>3 g per day in adults, proportional in children), decreased circulating serum levels of albumin, high blood pressure, elevated serum lipids, and retained fluid.[12,13]

Medical Management   Proteinuria represents a significant risk factor for CVD and progression to kidney failure. Thus, medical management is directed toward minimizing such losses, controlling blood pressure, and correcting hypervolemia through the use of corticosteroids, immunosuppressants, and angiotensin receptor blockers. To correct dyslipidemia, hydroxymethylglutaryl coenzyme A reductase inhibitors may be prescribed. See chapter 18 for more on pharmacologic therapies for dyslipidemia and hypertension.

TABLE 27.1 **Stages of CKD—A Clinical Action Plan**			
Chronic kidney disease is defined as either kidney damage or GFR <60 mL/min/1.73 m^2 for ≥3 months. Kidney damage is defined as pathologic abnormalities or markers of damage, including abnormalities in blood or urine tests or imaging studies.			
Stage	*Description*	*GFR (mL/min/1.73 m^2)*	*Action**
	At increased risk	≥60 (with CKD risk factors)	Screen Reduce risks for CKD
1	Kidney damage with normal or ↑ GFR	≥90	Diagnose and treat Treat comorbid conditions Slow progression Reduce risk for CVD
2	Kidney damage with mild ↓ GFR	60–89	Estimate progression
3	Moderate ↓ GFR	30–59	Evaluate and treat complications
4	Severe ↓ GFR	15–29	Prepare for kidney replacement therapy
5	Kidney failure	<15 (or dialysis)	Replacement (if uremia present)

*Includes actions from preceding stages

Abbreviations: CVD, cardiovascular disease; GFR, glomerular filtration rate.

Source: Adapted with permission from National Kidney Foundation, "Clinical practice guidelines for chronic kidney disease: evaluation, classification, and stratification," *Am J Kidney Dis* 39, 2 Suppl 1 (2002): S1-266.

Nutritional Management   Dietary manipulation may have minimal impact on serum lipids during episodes of nephrotic syndrome, and hypercholesteremia often requires pharmacologic therapy. Limiting protein intake to 0.8 g per kilogram standard body weight may assist in reversing the proteinuria experienced as long as iatrogenic malnutrition does not result. The protein level may be changed to 1.0 g per kilogram standard body weight in the attempt to achieve adequate nutritional status. More research is needed to establish optimal nutritional management for proteinuria. Sodium restriction should be based on fluid status and the need to control edema. Other electrolytes and minerals should be monitored, with the meal plan individualized accordingly.

Diabetic Kidney Disease

Long-standing and/or poorly controlled diabetes can result in a type of CKD known as diabetic kidney disease. It is defined by the presence of proteinuria and is common in patients with worsening high blood pressure, poor glycemic control, and/or genetic predisposition. It is characterized by structural and functional changes to the kidney. Not all kidney disease that is found in persons with diabetes represents DKD.[18]

Pathogenesis of DKD

Hyperglycemia plays a role in the pathogenesis of DKD. Alteration in tubuloglomerular feedback occurs, resulting in renal vasodilation, increased renal blood flow, and hyperfiltration.[2,20] Accelerated formation of nonenzymatic advanced glycosylation end-products (AGEs) in tissues is directly correlated with hyperglycemia. An increase in circulating AGE peptides parallels the severity of renal dysfunction in diabetic nephropathy. Glycosylation of proteins in the capillary basement membrane may stimulate mesangial expansion. Glycation of albumin can also contribute to its loss across the glomerular basement membrane.

Other hormonal imbalances, aside from insufficient insulin, have been implicated in the pathogenesis of DKD. Growth hormone and glucagon, which are both elevated in poorly controlled diabetes, have been shown to produce glomerular hyperfiltration.[2,20]

Changes in circulating levels of angiotensin II, catecholamines, and prostaglandins, or altered responsiveness to these vasoactive hormones, may also result in hyperfiltration. Angiotensin II may promote cellular and glomerular hypertrophy as well as mesangial expansion.

Renal hemodynamic changes play a role in the pathogenesis of DKD. Glomerular hypertension contributes to increased pressure and flow across the glomerular membrane, resulting in hyperfiltration. Glomerular hypertension and the associated renal vasodilation and hyperfiltration increase glomerular protein filtration, leading to proteinuria and glomerulosclerosis with consequent destruction of nephrons.

Stages of DKD

The stages of nephropathy (DKD), along with the metabolic consequences summarized in Table 27.2, provide a developmental framework. Kidney failure will ensue if the DKD is left untreated or not controlled. The stages of nephropathy seen in Table 27.2 align with those for CKD described in Table 27.1, but provide more detail specific to diabetes.

Individuals may progress through the stages of nephropathy at differing rates. Progression varies according to age and comorbidities such as atherosclerosis, hypertension, or autonomic neuropathy. The first sign of incipient nephropathy (Stage 3) is microalbuminuria (>30 mg/day).[21–23]

Progression of Disease

In the absence of medical intervention, 80% of persons with type 1 diabetes will progress in 10 to 15 years to overt nephropathy (clinical albuminuria >300 mg/day) with hypertension. Research has indicated that the incidence rate of persons diagnosed with type 1 diabetes and risk for ESRD is decreasing, in comparison with previous reports.[23,24] There are wide variations among the study samples cited in the research; however, the following can generally be said:

* *Type 1 diabetes.* At present, the common conception is that kidney failure will develop in 10 to 20 years in approximately 50% of persons diagnosed with type 1 diabetes.[23–25]
* *Type 2 diabetes.* Conversely, in persons diagnosed with type 2 diabetes, only 20% to 40% will develop incipient nephropathy that progresses to overt nephropathy, and within 20 years only 20% will progress to kidney failure.[23]

TABLE 27.2   Stages of Diabetic Kidney Disease
Stage 1
• GFR >90 mL/min; normal or increased GFR with enlarged kidneys. • Hyperglycemia leads to increased kidney filtration due to osmotic load and toxic effects of high blood glucose.
Stage 2
• Mildly decreased GFR 60 to 89 mL/min. • Clinically silent phase, but continued kidney hyperfiltration and hypertrophy. • Concentration of PTH starts to rise.
Stage 3
• Moderately decreased GFR 30 to 59 mL/min. • Microalbuminuria (defined as 30 to 300 mg/d); loss of albumin in urine. • Within 5 years, 20% develop nephropathy or standard care; 50% do not progress. • Microalbuminuria is a better predictor of progression in type 1 than type 2 diabetes. • Microalbuminuria is a predictor of increased cardiovascular disease, particularly in type 2 diabetes. • Microalbuminuria is associated with higher hemoglobin A1C levels (>8.1). • Decrease in calcium absorption (GFR <50 mL/min). • Onset of anemia (erythropoietin deficiency). • Lipoprotein activity falls.
Stage 4
• GFR severely decreased 15 to 29 mL/min. • Overt nephropathy. • Almost always with hypertension, >300 mg/d albumin in urine, about 10% have nephrotic range proteinuria. • TGL concentrations start to rise. • Hyperphosphatemia. • Metabolic acidosis. • Tendency toward hyperkalemia.
Stage 5
• Kidney failure (GFR <15 mL/min) needing renal replacement therapy (dialysis or transplantation). • Over 30 years, >24% of patients with T1DM progress to this stage. • Over 25 years, about 8% of patients with T2DM progress to this stage.

Abbreviations: GFR, glomerular filtration rate; PTH, parathyroid hormone; TGL, triglyceride.

Sources: Data adapted from K Iseki, M Yamazato, M Tozawa, S Takishita, "Hypocholesterolemia is a significant predictor of death in a cohort of chronic hemodialysis patients," *Kidney Int* 61 (2002): 1887-93; CA Maggio, FX Pi-Sunyer, "The prevention and treatment of obesity: application to type 2 diabetes (technical review)," *Diabetes Care* 20 (1997): 1744-66. Cited by L Byham-Gray, J Stover, K Wiesen, *A Clinical Guide to Nutrition Care in Kidney Disease* (Chicago: Academy of Nutrition and Dietetics, 2013), 115.

Early Identification Is Essential

Early identification of DKD facilitates appropriate treatment that may have the following desired effects:

◆ Prevent or delay the progression to ESRD/kidney failure
◆ Improve outcomes of people with DKD

Interventions Are Most Effective When Instituted Early

The onset and course of DKD may be ameliorated by several interventions, including the following[1,23,26–31]:

◆ Attaining and maintaining glycemic, blood pressure, and lipid control
◆ Monitoring protein intake
◆ Attaining and maintaining a healthy body weight through appropriate food choices and physical activity

These interventions are most effective when instituted early. Thus, detecting microalbuminuria and monitoring kidney function before DKD progresses are important strategies.[1,2]

Risk Factors for DKD

Ethnicity and Genetics To deliver the highest-quality care possible to all persons diagnosed with diabetes, the changing demographics among the CKD population must be recognized. Diabetes is the leading cause of kidney failure among all major races (whites, blacks, Native Americans, Hispanics, and Asians) reported in the US Renal Data System (USRDS), with dramatic increases occurring within the Native American, Hispanic, and black cultures.[5] By the mid-1990s, diabetes surpassed hypertension as the leading etiology for kidney failure among black Americans.[5] Blacks have an increased risk incidence and severity of disease that is 36 times that of whites. In the United States, recent data show a plateau in rates of ESRD due to diabetes in the white and Asian populations, while the incidence in black, Native American, and Hispanic populations is climbing, particularly in younger people.

Research evidence also supports a strong genetic predisposition for DKD.[32–35] Familial aggregation of kidney disease has frequently been observed. Researchers have observed similar glomerular involvement in family members in multiple cases. The data seem to span across multiple racial and ethnic groups. Correlations exist but no specific genes have been identified.[32–35]

Age The median age of persons with kidney failure treated with RRTs over the past 3 decades has risen to 64.1 years. The largest increase has been reported in persons over the age of 75 years, with the incidence rate increasing by 10.4% in the last decade.[5] It is important to note that kidney function decreases with age.

Smoking Smoking is a known risk factor for heart disease and also results in poor outcomes in dialysis and transplantation. It is strongly suggested to encourage patients to cease smoking.

Concurrent Complications From Diabetes The presence of existing retinopathy and neuropathy in persons with diabetes may indicate increased risk for also developing DKD. However, this should be evaluated closely, as there is now evidence that this is not always the case. In a study of persons with type 1 diabetes and persons with type 2 diabetes and macroalbuminuria, the incidence of retinopathy was present in the majority of the people. However, 47.5% of persons with type 2 diabetes, hypertension, and macroalbuminuria did not present with retinopathy.[36]

Screening and Detection

Recommended Frequency of Screening for DKD

◆ *Type 1 diabetes:* 5 years after diagnosis; annually thereafter
◆ *Type 2 diabetes:* At diagnosis and annually thereafter; also during pregnancy

In type 2 diabetes, screening should be initiated at the time of diagnosis because the diabetes may have been present but undiagnosed for some time and have had resultant impact on the kidneys for several years. Those with type 1 diabetes have an even greater risk of overt nephropathy and kidney failure as the disease progresses. Annual screening facilitates early detection and reduction in the progression of kidney disease.

The Dialysis Morbidity and Mortality Study (DMMS) found that 30% of all persons with Stage 5 CKD did not see a nephrologist until 3 months before initiating RRT, and 50% never consulted with a dietitian before starting such therapy.[37] Recent statistics indicate that referral mechanisms to specialized nephrology care are not improving. In the latest USRDS data reported, more than 42% of the patients diagnosed with CKD and hypertension were not seen by a nephrologist until they initiated RRT.[5] In the 12 months before initiation of RRT, appropriate and timely medical care for those diagnosed with CKD greatly reduces morbidity and mortality.[38,39]

Screening Tests for CKD/DKD

Urine Tests

The amount of microalbumin in the urine needs to be measured, and various tests are used for this with varying levels of reliability. Spot urine for measurement of urinary albumin to creatinine ratio is the preferred test. For confirmation of albuminuria, 2 additional first-void specimens over the next 3 to 6 months are needed. Two thirds of these samples should fall within micro or macro range to confirm diagnosis. In the absence of infection, strenuous exercise, or hematuria, an elevated level should be confirmed prior to starting drug therapy.[29]

- Microalbuminuria is diagnosed at >30 mg in 24 hours.
- Clinical albuminuria is diagnosed at >300 mg in 24 hours.

Blood Tests

Estimating GFR   An accurate predictor of kidney function is an estimation of the GFR. A number of methods for estimating GFR (eGFR) may be used; 2 validated approaches include the abbreviated Modifications of Diet in Renal Disease (MDRD) Study equation and the Cockcroft-Gault equation. Both take into account a number of factors that may affect kidney function, such as sex, age, race, weight, and

serum creatinine (SCr) levels.[3] A GFR calculator is available on the National Kidney Foundation Web site (http://www.kidney.org), allowing the practitioner to readily predict the level of kidney function. The higher stages of CKD are represented by lower GFR levels (inverse relationship).

Abbreviated MDRD Study Equation

$$\text{GFR (mL/min/1.73 m}^2) = 186.3 \times \text{SCr} - 1.154 \times \text{Age} - 0.203 \times 0.742 \text{ (if female)} \times 1.210 \text{ (if African American)}$$

Cockcroft-Gault Equation

$$\text{Creatinine clearance} = \text{(mL/min)}$$

$$\frac{(140 - \text{Age}) \times \text{Weight in kg} \times 0.85 \text{ if female}}{72 \times \text{SCr}}$$

Regardless of the degree of urine albumin excretion, SCr should be measured at least annually in all adults with diabetes to estimate the GFR. Serum creatinine should not be used alone as a measure of kidney function, but instead should be used to estimate GFR and stage the level of CKD. Serum creatinine may be affected by body shape, size, and dietary intake.

Prevention and Delay of CKD

The following are important parameters to monitor and control in preventing or delaying the progression of CKD. Each is discussed separately below, with targets summarized in a chart.

- Blood glucose control
- Blood pressure control
- Lipid levels, for CVD risk
- Hemoglobin, for anemia
- Serum markers of bone and mineral metabolism

Blood Glucose

Optimizing glycemic control is the mainstay of therapy for preventing or delaying further disease progression. Maintaining the A1C level at <7% reduces risk for complications. The Diabetes Control and Complications Trial (DCCT) demonstrated that tight glycemic control lowered the risk for microalbuminuria in type 1 diabetes by 30%, and among persons with microalbuminuria, the risk for further disease progression was reduced by 50%.[26] The UK Prospective Diabetes Study (UKPDS) indicated that individuals with type 2 diabetes had a 25% risk reduction in DKD when intensive diabetes therapy was initiated.[27,28] Additionally, for every 1% drop in A1C, there was a 35% reduction in risk for complications. It is also now clear that A1C may be underestimated in patients with kidney disease. Increased attention has been given to the risk and occurrence of hypoglycemia in persons with diabetes. People with significantly decreased kidney function (Stages 4 and 5) are at higher risk for hypoglycemia as well. Studies showing intensive treatment for glycemic control have shown evidence of increased hypoglycemia in both people with type 1 diabetes and people with type 2 diabetes. In 2012, KDOQI updated its guidelines to reflect caution in intensifying treatment with respect to hypoglycemia.[17] The recommendation is to keep the A1C target at 7% and not below for people with diabetes and CKD. When evaluating risk-benefit for patients in intensifying treatment, it is also suggested to be mindful of limited life expectancy, comorbid conditions, and risk for hypoglycemia. In some populations, such as the elderly and those at higher risk for falls, it may be prudent to extend targets above 7%. (See the sidebar for blood glucose targets.)

Blood Pressure

Controlling blood pressure slows the decline of GFR in persons with DKD. In fact, the most recent release of USRDS data indicates that the ESRD rate has stabilized, perhaps indicating that adequate screening and preventive measures (eg, angiotensin-converting enzyme [ACE] inhibitors, angiotensin receptor blockers [ARBs], and/or diuretics) are decreasing the incidence of disease progression.[5,8] A number of studies have substantiated the inverse relationship between blood pressure and GFR; that is, as blood pressure rises, the GFR drops.[36]

Recent research has concluded that intensifying blood pressure control may have little influence on reducing cardiac events and in fact may increase this risk. In the ACCORD and INVEST trials, no improvement in tightening systolic blood pressure beyond <140 mm Hg was shown, although there was some benefit with regard to decreasing risk of stroke in ACCORD.[36] General consensus in renal literature is that lowering blood pressure will result in a reduction in deterioration of

GFR. However, in the Ibesartan Diabetic Nephropathy Trial (IDNT), there was evidence for excessive lowering of blood pressure and an increase of cardiac events.[36] In the context of this and in accordance with guidelines set by the American Diabetes Association, a target blood pressure of <140/80 mm Hg is advisable in persons with diabetes; nonetheless, tighter control is necessary with the existence of DKD to <130/80 mm Hg.[36,40] Blood pressure should be measured at every ambulatory care visit. Treatment should include consideration of a number of antihypertensive agents, namely, ACE inhibitors and/or ARBs in the presence of proteinuria. (See sidebar for blood pressure targets.)

Lipids

As suggested earlier, the presence of proteinuria is a significant risk factor for CVD.[9] The relationship between these factors may be related to genetic predisposition, endothelial dysfunction, associated hypertension, insulin resistance, atherogenic dyslipidemias, hyperglycemia, and anemia.[17,41] Statins may be an effective treatment in reducing LDL cholesterol in patients with CKD. Statins are not indicated for patients on dialysis. Combination therapies using statins and ezetimibe may be effective in reducing LDL cholesterol with fewer side effects. Fenofibrates have shown some effect at lower stages of CKD in reducing progression to microalbuminuria from normal levels and potential regression from microalbuminuria to normal levels. More data are expected to come in the treatment of dyslipidemia in CKD. (See sidebar for lipid targets.)

New Risk Calculator for Atherosclerotic Cardiovascular Disease Events[42]

The American College of Cardiology and the American Heart Association in collaboration with the National Heart, Lung, and Blood Institute and some other stakeholders developed a calculator to establish risk for first-time cardiac events within the population. The calculator was developed from extensive research reviews and is intended to use variables that the work group felt had the most evidence to induce risk. These include age, total and HDL cholesterol, systolic blood pressure, diabetes, and smoking status. The calculator is currently intended for use in African-American and white men and women due to the available research data in these populations. The hope is to continue to expand research in this area and expand the use of this calculator as well as improve its use. The calculator provides the 10-year risk for a first-time event in persons who have not had an event. Events are characterized by nonfatal myocardial infarction, coronary heart disease death, or fatal or nonfatal stroke. The calculator is intended to be used in concordance with clinical practice and evaluation.

Hemoglobin

In the RENAAL (Reduction of Endpoints in Non-insulin-Dependent Diabetes Mellitus With the Angiotensin II Antagonist Losartan) trial, baseline hemoglobin predicted kidney failure in type 2 diabetes with nephropathy.[43] Early treatment of anemia is associated with improved outcomes.[1] Symptoms associated with anemia in CKD are decreased exercise tolerance, impaired cognitive function, sexual dysfunction, impaired functional status, anorexia, and decreased quality of life. Reversing the anemia experienced in CKD has been shown to decrease left ventricular hypertrophy and increase survival on dialysis as well as enhance quality of life and improve exercise capacity.

When GFR is <60 mL/min/1.73 m^2 (Stage 3 CKD), the hemoglobin should be evaluated. If hemoglobin is suboptimal, additional lab studies are recommended, inclusive of complete blood count (CBC), reticulocyte count, serum iron, total iron binding capacity (TIBC), serum ferritin, and transferrin saturation (TSAT). Depending on lab values, iron supplementation and possibly erythropoietin administration may be necessary. (See sidebar for hemoglobin targets.)

Summary of Target Values in Preventing or Delaying Progression of CKD

Blood Glucose

Target ranges for fasting plasma glucose levels should be as follows[1,44]:

- 90 to 130 mg/dL (5-7 mmol/L) in CKD
- <140 mg/dL (7.8 mmol/L) in hemodialysis
- <160 mg/dL (8.8 mmol/L) in peritoneal dialysis
- A1C checked twice a year, or quarterly in individuals with poor glycemic control

Blood Pressure

The goals for blood pressure control are similar to those for the general population as outlined by the Joint National Committee (JNC) for Prevention, Detection, Evaluation and Treatment of High Blood Pressure (Eighth Report)[40]:

- Blood pressure <140/80 mm Hg, measured at each healthcare visit
- Blood pressure <130/70 mm Hg in the presence of DKD

Lipids

Since CVD is the leading cause of death in DKD, aggressive management of lipids is suggested. Per the KDOQI Practice Guidelines on Managing Dyslipidemias, serum lipids need to be kept within target ranges similar to the Adult Treatment Panel (ATP) III Guidelines, published by the National Cholesterol Education Program[17,41]:

- Total cholesterol <200 mg/dL
- LDL cholesterol <100 mg/dL (<5.5 mmol/L)
- Triglycerides <150 mg/dL (<8.3 mmol/L)
- HDL cholesterol >40 mg/dL (>2.2 mmol/L)
- Serum lipids monitored at least annually and checked more frequently when abnormalities are detected

Treat the Trio

Diabetes educators must seek to help individuals manage not only their diabetes but also CKD and CVD. A proactive, integrated approach ensures the best outcome.

Hemoglobin

- Hemoglobin between 11 and 12 g/dL

Screening Criteria

- CKD without anemia
    —Stage 3: screen annually
    —Stages 4 and 5: screen twice per year
- CKD with anemia not treated with erythropoietin
    —Stages 3 to 5: every 3 months
- CKD Stage 5 on hemodialysis: monthly

Serum Markers of Bone and Mineral Metabolism

Abnormalities in bone and mineral metabolism are frequently seen in persons diagnosed with CKD.[3] Compromises in bone remodeling occur when the GFR drops below 60 mL/min/1.73 m^2 (ie, when 50% of kidney function is lost), suggesting that by the time an individual is diagnosed at Stage 5 CKD (eg, GFR <15 mL/min/1.73 m^2), severe complications requiring treatment and management have developed.[3] During CKD, the activation of vitamin D to 1,25-dihydroxycholecalciferol (ie, calcitriol) is disrupted, resulting in hyperphosphatemia, hypocalcemia, and secondary hyperparathyroidism.[45] Besides the conditions often associated with bone and mineral disorders (such as muscle and bone pain, and bone fractures), the systemic effects of such imbalances include soft tissue and vascular calcification as well as erythropoietin-resistant anemia.[46-48] Evidence currently exists that identifies the effect of such metabolic derangements on morbidity and mortality among this patient population.[49] Scientific efforts toward reversing these trends or outcomes have been and continue to be supported.[14,50-53] Calcium, phosphorus, and plasma PTH levels should be monitored closely. (See sidebar for targets.)

Serum Markers

The KDOQI Practice Guidelines for Bone Disease and Chronic Kidney Disease recommend the following[49,53]:

- Intact PTH levels: in CKD Stage 3, target is 35 to 70 pg/mL; in CKD Stage 4, target is 70 to 110 pg/mL
- Phosphorus at or above 2.7 mg/dL and no higher than 4.6 mg/dL in CKD Stages 3 and 4
- Serum calcium within normal ranges, preferably 8.4 to 9.5 mg/dL
- PTH, serum calcium, and phosphorus measured annually in CKD Stage 3, quarterly in CKD Stages 4 and 5

Case: A Woman With Type 2 Diabetes of Long Duration

MG is a 55-year-old widowed African-American woman who has had type 2 diabetes for approximately 15 years. She was referred to the diabetes clinic for intensive education and self-management training. Physical findings revealed some shortness of breath upon exertion, blood pressure elevated to 155/90 mm Hg, height 5 ft 3 in, and weight 200 lb.

From the serum biomarker results, it is evident MG is currently at Stage 3 CKD, with an eGFR of 48 mL/min/1.73 m^2, and is experiencing profound microalbuminuria (>30 mg). This diagnosis is substantiated by the noted elevation in the casual glucose level and A1C. MG is anemic (hemoglobin <11.0 g/dL) and showing early signs of mineral and bone metabolism disorders (secondary hyperparathyroidism). MG is also at considerable cardiovascular risk, not only because of the proteinuria but also because she presented with classic dyslipidemia and uncontrolled hypertension. MG is on metformin 1000 mg twice daily and glipizide twice daily at 5 mg.

Test	Results	Target Range
Hemoglobin (g/dL)	9.4	>11.0
Creatinine (mg/dL)	1.9	0.6–1.2
eGFR	(Stage 3) 48 mL/min/1.73 m^2	90–120 mL/min/1.73 m^2
Serum albumin (g/dL)	3.3	≥4.0
A1C (%)	8.5	<7.0
LDL-C (mg/dL)	130	<100
HDL-C (mg/dL)	45	>40
Glucose (casual) mg/dL	175	<140
Albumin (mg/g CR)	283	<30
Calcium (mg/dL)	8.9	8.4–9.5
Phosphorus (mg/dL)	4.0	2.7–4.6
PTH (pg/mL)	75	35–70

Treatment of CKD

Treatment options for those diagnosed with CKD are described below. The individual's right to self-determination is central to the decision to undergo treatment of CKD—whether to choose or not choose RRT in late-stage disease. Proceeding without RRT should be presented as a treatment option to patients and their family or caregivers. If no treatment is administered, death is imminent in less than a year. The patient and family should be encouraged to discuss this decision with clergy, a psychologist, a social worker, the healthcare team, and/or other family members. Plans for supportive care (eg, home care, hospice care) are necessary for the person who wishes to forgo treatment.

CKD Stages 1 through 4

Treatment options for individuals with DKD are dependent on the stage of CKD.

For persons with diabetes in the early stages of CKD (Stages 1 through 3) or with preclinical nephropathy, intervention is geared toward glycemic control, hypertensive management with the use of medications that are active on the renin-angiotensin system, and protein restriction.

To attain A1C goals without undesired hypoglycemia and weight gain, management of DKD must be appropriately balanced according to diet, oral medications, insulin, and activity levels.[1,29] Irregular blood glucose levels may be partially explained by changes in oral intake and appetite. Nonetheless, episodes of hyperglycemia and/or hypoglycemia may also result secondary to alterations in insulin metabolism with changing kidney function. One fourth to one third of injected insulin is catabolized by the kidney.[31] In addition, patients with decreased kidney function are at risk for increased insulin resistance.

Oral Medications

With continued updates and available research, new medications for glycemic control are on the rise. When reviewing options for patients, many factors should be considered. First and foremost is the safety of medications on declining kidney function.[54] Metformin is contraindicated in patients with GFR <60 due to increased risk for lactic acidosis. Glucagon-like peptide-1 receptor agonists are not a good match due to side effects that can mimic or worsen decreased intake or anorexia associated with late-stage DKD. Limited results have also been seen with amylin, alpha-glucosidase inhibitors, bile acid sequestrants, and dopamine 2 agonists. There have been some positive outcomes and reasonable treatment effects from the use of DPP-4 inhibitors as well as sitagliptin and saxagliptin. Thiazolidinediones may also be useful, particularly rosiglitazone, but there is a risk for edema and associated cardiac risk. If endogenous insulin remains present, glimepiride and glipizide would be preferred in terms of sulfonylureas due to their short-acting nature and metabolization by the liver. See Table 27.3 for more specifics on when to consider these medications in practice.

TABLE 27.3 Dose Adjustment for Insulin Compounds and Oral Medicines for Diabetes in CKD	
Medication Class and Agents	*CKD Stages 3, 4, and 5 ND*
Insulin	
Glargine	No advised dose adjustment
Detemir	No advised dose adjustment
Neutral Protamine Hagedorn (NPH)	No advised dose adjustment
Regular	No advised dose adjustment
Aspart	No advised dose adjustment
Lispro	No advised dose adjustment
Glulisine	No advised dose adjustment
First-generation sulfonylureas	
Acetohexamide	Avoid use
Chlorpropamide	GFR 50–80 mL/min/1.73 m^2: reduce dose 50%, GFR <50 mL/min/1.73 m^2: avoid use

TABLE 27.3 Dose Adjustment for Insulin Compounds and Oral Medicines for Diabetes in CKD (continued)	
First-generation sulfonylureas (continued)	
Tolazamide	Avoid use
Tolbutamide	Avoid use
Second-generation sulfonylureas	
Glipizide	No dose adjustment
Glimepiride	Start conservatively at 1 mg daily
Glyburide	Avoid use
Gliclazide	No dose adjustment
Meglitinides	
Repaglinide	If GFR <30 mL/min/1.73 m² start conservatively at 0.5 mg with meals
Nateglinide	If GFR <30 mL/min/1.73 m² start conservatively at 60 mg with meals
Biguanides	
Metformin	United States FDA label states, "do not use if SCr ≥1.5 mg/dL in men, ≥1.4 mg/dL in women" British National Formulary and the Japanese Society of Nephrology recommend cessation if eGFR <30 mL/min/1.73 m²
Thiazolidinediones	
Pioglitazone	No dose adjustment
Rosiglitazone	No dose adjustment
Alpha-glucosidase inhibitors	
Acarbose	Avoid if GFR <30 mL/min/1.73 m²
Miglitol	Avoid if GFR <25 mL/min/1.73 m²
DPP-4 inhibitor	
Sitagliptin	GFR >50 mL/min/1.73 m²: 100 mg daily GFR 30–50 mL/min/1.73 m²: 50 mg daily GFR <30 mL/min/1.73 m²: 25 mg daily
Saxagliptin	GFR >50 mL/min/1.73 m²: 5 mg daily GFR ≤50 mL/min/1.73 m²: 2.5 mg daily
Linagliptin	No dose adjustment
Vildagliptin	GFR ≥50 mL/min/1.73 m²: 50 mg twice daily GFR <50 mL/min/1.73 m²: 50 mg daily
Incretin mimetic	
Exenatide	Not recommended in GFR <30 mL/min/1.73 m²
Liraglutide	Not recommended in GFR <60 mL/min/1.73 m²
Amylin analog	
Pramlintide	No dose adjustment and not recommended for patients with CKD stage 4 or greater
Dopamine receptor agonist	
Bromocriptine mesylate	Not studied in patients with reduced GFR

Source: National Kidney Foundation, "KDOQI Clinical Practice Guideline for Diabetes and CKD: 2012 update," *Am J Kidney Dis* 60, no. 5 (2012; cited 2014 Apr 2): 850-86, on the Internet at: http://www.kidney.org/professionals/KDOQI/guidelines_diabetesUp/diabetes-ckd-update-2012.pdf.

Insulin

As kidney function declines, exogenous insulin acts longer and in an unpredictable manner, characterized by recurrent or severe hypoglycemia in some individuals. The use of multiple daily insulin injections and hypoglycemia awareness training may reduce the frequency and severity of hypoglycemic episodes.

Energy Requirements

Energy requirements should be established between 23 and 35 kcal per kilogram of standard body weight, with 50% to 60% originating from carbohydrates and 20 to 30 g of dietary fiber (see Table 27.4).[44]

Hypertension Medications

Systematic reviews of ACE inhibitors and ARBs on mortality and outcomes in DKD have indicated that these medications are preferable to other antihypertensives in reducing microalbuminuria and slowing decline.[38,55] The KDOQI Practice Guidelines for Hypertension recommend when to seek further treatment and the best way to manage hypertension in CKD.[38] In persons with advanced stages of CKD, potassium levels should be monitored, as both ACE inhibitors and ARBs may cause hyperkalemia. Conversely, if the patient is on a potassium-wasting diuretic, it may have an opposite effect resulting in hypokalemia. Sodium intake should be decreased to less than 2400 mg per day in the presence of hypertension, and fluid restrictions are necessary only in progressive DKD (Stage 4) (Tables 27.2 and 27.3).

Dietary Manipulation

Research studies have demonstrated that a protein-controlled diet may be beneficial in some persons whose DKD appears to be progressing.[23,30,56] With the onset of overt DKD, a protein limitation equal to 0.8 to 1.0 g per kilogram standard body weight (<10% total kilocalories) should be implemented (Table 27.4). Further protein restriction (0.6 g per kilogram standard body weight) has been suggested and may be of minimal benefit in slowing the decline in individuals who are stable, but they must be monitored for clinical signs of malnutrition. Once the GFR drops below 60 mL/min/1.73 m^2, there is a spontaneous decline in appetite and oral intake.[57] Weight loss is an independent risk factor for mortality on dialysis, so an adequate, palatable, and realistic meal plan during the early stages of CKD is very important. High biologic value (HBV) protein sources, or foods that contain a high proportion of essential amino acids, will be helpful in minimizing the nitrogen load and consequent azotemia that may develop once advanced stages of CKD are experienced. Vegetarian meal plans can be used in early as well as later stages of CKD, but the practitioner must ensure that the individual is following the principles of a healthy diet (eg, adequacy, balance, moderation, and variety). Plant proteins, such as soy, are excellent alternatives to animal proteins and may have a heart-protective effect of improving serum lipids if consumed with regularity.[23,31] When soy is used, the practitioner will need to monitor serum phosphorus and potassium levels; soy foods are rich sources of these minerals, and overconsumption may negatively impact homeostasis, especially in CKD Stages 4 and 5. To provide sufficient energy, fats can and should be used in the meal plan, but adjusted according to recommendations from the ATP III Guidelines (Table 27.4).

Other Lifestyle Changes

Dietary manipulation is a major factor in the therapeutic lifestyle changes suggested, but other risk factors for CVD also need to be reduced, such as sedentary activity and cigarette smoking or tobacco use.

Pharmacologic Interventions

Pharmacologic agents may be used in CKD and should be tailored to the individual's lipid profile. For example, a person experiencing an elevation in LDL-C may benefit from a statin medication in addition to therapeutic lifestyle changes. Multiple medical approaches may be used, depending on laboratory results, and the KDOQI Practice Guidelines on Dyslipidemias provide excellent examples and insight for the practitioner.[17,41]

As mentioned, treating the early signs of anemia and osteodystrophy has a significant effect on patient outcomes. Individuals with a low serum hemoglobin may benefit from iron supplementation (200 mg per day) if diagnosed as deficient. If the blood count does not improve with supplemental iron, synthetic erythropoietin may be administered. Evidence is strong that the use of calcitriol (activated vitamin D) is beneficial for retarding or preventing metabolic bone disease in the early stages of CKD with minimal risk

TABLE 27.4 Recommended Dietary Modifications at Various Stages of Diabetic Nephropathy

Nutrient	Pre-Clinical Nephropathy Stages 1, 2, 3	Progressive Nephropathy Stage 4	Hemodialysis	Peritoneal Dialysis	Transplantation
Energy (kcal/kg/d)	23–35; adequate to achieve and/or maintain DBW	23–35; adequate to achieve and/or maintain DBW	30–35; adequate to achieve and/or maintain DBW	30–35; allow for dialysate calories; adequate to achieve and/or maintain DBW	30–35; adequate to achieve and/or maintain DBW
Protein	12%–15% of calories; 0.8–1.0 g/kg/d	10% of calories; 50% HBV; 0.8–0.9 g/kg/d	12%–20% of calories; 50% HBV; 1.2 g/kg/d*	12%–20% of calories; 50% HBV; 1.2–1.3 g/kg/d*	1.3–2.0 g/kg after surgery; 0.8–1.0 g/kg per day in stable patients
Carbohydrate	50%–60% of calories; ↑ fiber to 20–30 g	50%–60% of calories; ↑ fiber to 20–30 g	50%–60% of calories; ↑ fiber to 20–30 g	50%–60% of calories (including dialysate); ↑ fiber to 20–30 g	50%–60% of calories; ↑ fiber to 20–30 g
Fat	25%–35% calories as fat; <7% saturated fat; Emphasis on MUFA; <200 mg cholesterol/d	25%–35% calories as fat; <7% saturated fat; Emphasis on MUFA; <200 mg cholesterol/d	25%–35% calories as fat; <7% saturated fat; Emphasis on MUFA; <200 mg cholesterol/d	25%–35% calories as fat; <7% saturated fat; Emphasis on MUFA; <200 mg cholesterol/d	25%–35% calories as fat; <7% saturated fat; Emphasis on MUFA; <200 mg cholesterol/d
Sodium (mg/d)	No HTN: ≤3,000; HTN: ≤2,400	No HTN: ≤3,000; HTN: ≤2,400	2,000–2,400	No HTN: ≤2,000–4,000; Monitor fluid balance	No HTN: ≤3,000; HTN: ≤2,400
Potassium (g/d)	No restriction	Monitor labs; 2 if hyperkalemic	2–3; adjust to serum levels	Unrestricted if serum levels normal	Unrestricted unless hyperkalemic
Phosphorus	Maintain serum value WNL; 800–1,000 mg/d; adjust for protein	10–12 mg/g protein *or* 10 mg/kg/d; 800–1,000 mg/d	10–12 mg/g protein *or* 800–1,000 mg/d; adjust for protein	10–12 mg/g protein *or* 800–1,000 mg/d; adjust for protein	RDA; supplement as needed
Calcium (g/d)	Maintain serum value WNL; 1.0–1.5	1.0–1.5; daily limit including binder load: <2.0	Daily limit including binder load: <2.0	Daily limit including binder load: <2.0	0.8–1.5; individualize per metabolic needs
Fluid	No restriction	Output plus 1,000 mL	Output plus 1,000 mL; limit interdialytic fluid gain	Maintain balance	Unrestricted unless overloaded

Abbreviations: DBW, desired body weight; HBV, high biological value protein; HTN, hypertension; MUFA, monosaturated fatty acids; RDA, Recommended Dietary Allowance; WNL, within normal limits.

*1.2–1.5 g/kg/d during catabolic stress.

Sources: Data adapted from Expert Panel on Detection, Evaluation, and Treatment of High Blood Cholesterol in Adults, "Executive summary of the Third Report of the National Cholesterol Education Program (NCEP) Expert Panel on Detection, Evaluation, and Treatment of High Blood Cholesterol in Adults (Adult Treatment Panel III)," *JAMA* 285 (2001): 2486–97; K Iseki, M Yamazato, M Tozawa, S Takishita, "Hypocholesterolemia is a significant predictor of death in a cohort of chronic hemodialysis patients," *Kidney Int* 61 (2002): 1887–93; CA Maggio, FX Pi-Sunyer, "The prevention and treatment of obesity: application to type 2 diabetes (technical review)," *Diabetes Care* 20 (1997): 1744–66; JA Rumberger, BH Brundage, DJ Rader, G Kondos, "Electron beam computed tomographic coronary calcium scanning: a review and guidelines for use in asymptomatic persons," *Mayo Clin Proc* 74 (1999): 243–52; GA Block, FK Port, "Re-evaluation of risks associated with hyperphosphatemia and hyperparathyroidism in dialysis patients: recommendations for a change in management," *Am J Kidney Dis* 35 (2000): 1226–37; GM Chertow, SK Burke, MA Dillon, E Slatopolsky, "Long-term effects of sevelamer hydrochloride on the calcium x phosphate product and lipid profile of haemodialysis patients," *Nephrol Dial Transplant* 14 (1999): 2901–14. Cited by L Byham-Gray, J Stover, K Wiesen, *A Clinical Guide to Nutrition Care in Kidney Disease* (Chicago: Academy of Nutrition and Dietetics, 2013), 128.

Use of a 24-hour food recall and diet history revealed that MG was following a high-protein diet 6 months ago and lost 10 lb but was not able to comply with the low-carbohydrate plan. MG had regained over 15 lb. She generally skipped breakfast, ate salad for lunch at her desk, drank diet sodas throughout the day, and sometimes ordered food in or stopped at a local fast-food restaurant for dinner. MG rarely cooked since her husband died last year from cancer. MG remarked that she often ate a lot at night when she was feeling the most "out of sorts." Treatment goals were as follows, and guidance for the application of the AADE7 Self-Care Behaviors™ was provided:

- Tight glycemic control

- Regulation of blood pressure

- Lowered protein intake

Healthy Eating

- The meal plan was geared toward weight loss (current BMI 36), with a lower protein intake, to prevent further damage to the kidneys.

- Meal planning was simplified and incorporates the use of quick meal ideas/recipes and alternatives to the typical fast-food menu options.

- Education was essential to review the macronutrient components of diet as well as how to balance the meal plan throughout the day to achieve optimal glycemic control.

- The concerns with consuming a high-protein intake as well as the need for a more structured rather than erratic eating pattern were emphasized.

- Education focused on substituting healthy mono- and polyunsaturated fats for saturated fats—reduced consumption of fast food and takeout should improve overall quality of diet.

Healthy Coping and Problem Solving

- MG's feelings about the loss of her husband and the frequency of her night binges needed to be considered to determine whether referrals to psychological services might be warranted to enable MG's successful management of her diabetes.

- The educator helped MG examine familial and friends/peer support and available networking opportunities.

- MG needed to be active in her treatment plan, learn how to complete routine blood glucose monitoring, and be empowered to take on the responsibility of adjusting her diet, activity level, and medications as necessary.

Being Active

To further assist with weight loss, the educator discussed the need for MG to engage in physical activity. MG was encouraged to use a pedometer to safely monitor her activity level throughout the day, as long as it was medically advisable.

Taking Medication and Reducing Risks

- *Diabetes.* Because of the poor glycemic control over the last several months, options to intensify treatment were reviewed and evaluated. Due to the contraindication of metformin, it was discontinued, further increasing her need for additional medications. Discussion was held with MG regarding other options for glycemic management, giving pros and cons and involving her in the decision of her care while advising her of the risk of continued elevated blood glucose levels. Insulin therapy was discussed. After careful consideration and understanding of the impact of glycemic control on worsening kidney status and the absence of the support of metformin, MG agreed to insulin. She was educated on technique, titration, hypoglycemia, and the expected outcomes with the new medication.

- *Hypertension.* It was identified that MG required either an ACE inhibitor or an ARB to assist with hypertensive control and to reduce proteinuria.

- *Anemia.* Further testing would determine whether she needed supplemental iron and/or erythropoietin administered to reverse the anemia and its effects on fatigue.

- *Bone health.* Since her PTH was mildly elevated, further assessment of vitamin D status was warranted to determine whether calcitriol should be initiated.

- *CVD.* Statin medication would not need to be started immediately. MG indicated she was able to modify her diet in order to improve the serum lipids.

Monitoring

Lastly, MG was told about the importance of maintaining regular checkups with her diabetes team and how referral to a nephrologist was paramount. The nephrologist would seek to further retard disease progression and, if appropriate, prepare MG for further treatment options in kidney failure.

for the individual.[58] The challenge arises in correcting the imbalance of one serum value but not disturbing the balance of another biomarker. For example, suppressing PTH with activated vitamin D may lead to a concomitant rise in serum calcium level, with consequent effects and additional systemic complications. Finding and maintaining the right balance among the serum markers of bone disease (eg, serum calcium, serum phosphorus, and PTH level) is as much of an art form as it is a scientific intervention. The KDOQI Clinical Practice Guidelines for Bone Metabolism and Disease in CKD strongly encourage the achievement of target values, supported by research evidence and clinical expertise/opinion, for calcium, phosphorus, and PTH levels in the attempt to minimize or reduce renal osteodystrophy complications.[49,53] Close monitoring of serum markers and responding to abnormalities in a timely fashion are required to achieve such target ranges. If the PTH level is above target, the person should be evaluated for serum levels of vitamin D, and activated vitamin D provided if suboptimal levels are identified. Serum phosphorus levels may be controlled with a low-phosphorus diet as well as phosphorus binder medications. The KDOQI Clinical Practice Guidelines for Bone Metabolism have useful treatment algorithms concerning PTH, calcium, and phosphorus in the early stages of CKD.[3]

CKD Stage 5

Once kidney failure results (Stage 5 CKD), a number of options are available as either maintenance dialysis (hemodialysis and peritoneal dialysis) or transplantation:

- *Hemodialysis:* In center or at home
- *Peritoneal dialysis:* Continuous ambulatory, continuous cyclic, or intermittent
- *Transplantation:* Kidney or kidney-pancreas

The person diagnosed with kidney failure and family members need to be involved in treatment decisions. This part of the chapter reviews treatment options in Stage 5 CKD and the effects of such modalities on glycemic control. Since the individual diagnosed with kidney failure will likely be closely followed by a healthcare team (nephrologist, nurse, dietitian, social worker) associated with a dialysis

treatment facility, it is important for the patient and family to discuss issues relating to RRT with the nephrology team, as appropriate.

Hemodialysis

Hemodialysis (HD) is a process of cleansing or filtering the blood of nitrogenous wastes. The blood of the person being treated is circulated and cleansed outside the body.[11,12] With effective dialysis treatments, uremia can be treated and the person can achieve an improved level of health and well-being. The process is described below, with related factors for consideration noted after the description.

Process   The filter used for HD is a semipermeable membrane. The membrane, a thin material with holes, permits passage of small particles but retains larger particles. During dialysis, the patient's blood passes on one side of the membrane while dialysate (prepared dialysis solution) passes on the other side of the membrane. The solution removes fluid and particles (waste products) from the blood by diffusive clearance. Blood is withdrawn through a needle inserted into a specially prepared blood vessel, usually a synthetic graft or an arteriovenous fistula (using the patient's own blood vessels) located in the patient's forearm. The needle is attached by plastic tubing to an HD machine. A pump keeps blood moving through the dialyzer as wastes and fluid are filtered out. The cleansed blood returns to the patient through another needle in the same or an adjacent blood vessel. Hemodialysis can be performed in an ambulatory setting or in the person's home.

Considerations   Treatments are usually 3 to 4 hours long, 3 times per week, on average. Because the blood is not being cleansed 24 hours a day, the person must still follow an individualized meal plan with fluid restriction. The meal plan is designed to minimize azotemia and the buildup of waste products and provide adequate protein, energy, electrolytes, and fluids (Table 27.4).

In comparison with individuals with other types of kidney disease, persons with diabetes, at the initiation of dialysis, generally have increased comorbid conditions, a higher incidence of complications, and are less well-nourished.[23,31]

Blood Glucose Control Factors that can alter glucose levels for the person receiving HD treatment include the glucose concentration in the dialysate bath, appetite alteration on dialysis days and nondialysis days, decreased activity on dialysis days, and emotional stress. Probing the individual about glucose patterns, eating habits, and activity level on dialysis and nondialysis days will help explain fluctuations in blood glucose levels. Because of the lack of glucosuria in DKD, these individuals may experience extreme fluctuations in blood glucose levels.[15,33] Hyperglycemia causes polydipsia, which negatively influences fluid control. Cellular shifts of potassium occur during hyperglycemic episodes, which may result in vacillating serum potassium levels.

Peritoneal Dialysis

Peritoneal dialysis (PD) takes place inside the body, employing the body's own capillary and serosal membranes. Blood is filtered through the peritoneal membrane that lines the abdominal cavity. Surgery is required to place a catheter through an opening in the wall of the abdominal cavity. This opening allows the dialysis solution to be instilled into the peritoneal cavity and waste products to pass from the bloodstream into the dialysis solution. The used solution is drained and replaced with a new solution on a regular basis. Currently, 3 types of PD are used:

⬥ *Continuous ambulatory peritoneal dialysis (CAPD).* This is a manual method of performing PD. The patient exchanges new fluid (dialysate) every 4 to 6 hours during a 24-hour period each day. The dialysate passes from a plastic bag through the catheter and stays in the patient's abdomen with the catheter sealed. The dialysate is drained after several hours, and then the process begins again with fresh dialysate solution.

⬥ *Continuous cyclic peritoneal dialysis (CCPD).* This is like CAPD except a machine that is connected to the catheter automatically fills and drains the dialysate solution from the patient's abdomen.

⬥ *Intermittent peritoneal dialysis (IPD).* This form of dialysis uses the same type of machine as CCPD to fill and drain the dialysate solution from the patient's abdomen. Intermittent peritoneal dialysis treatments take longer than

CCPD, and assistance from a family member, friend, or health professional is required.

Treatment Modality Considerations Peritoneal dialysis is often a preferred treatment modality because of its ability to achieve a steady state in terms of serum chemistries and fluid balance.[23,31] Persons receiving this treatment often report greater satisfaction with PD over HD because of the liberalization in diet that occurs. Peritoneal dialysis allows the removal of uremic toxins on a daily basis, and therefore generally does not require strict potassium or fluid restrictions (Table 27.4). Despite glucose absorption from dialysate, glycemic control can be achieved with intraperitoneal insulin added to the dialysate. Such administration allows for continual delivery of insulin into the portal circulation. There may be some insulin loss due to difficulties with absorption or its adsorption to the dialysate bag; hence, supplemental subcutaneous insulin may still be required. Intraperitoneal insulin can also be an additional source of bacterial contamination for the dialysate, resulting in a higher total insulin dose required.

An additional consideration with the use of PD is the presence of gastroparesis.[59] Gastroparesis is a neuropathic complication often associated with long-standing diabetes and poor control. Patients experience considerable nausea and/or vomiting that can result in malnutrition. In addition, patients often experience erratic glycemic control due to delayed digestion and timing of insulin doses resulting in increases in hyper- and hypoglycemia. This process can be further complicated by the initiation of PD due to additional volume load in the abdominal space. There may be some value, at least in terms of glycemic control, in adding insulin to the dialysate. If optimal management does not occur with CAPD, patients may gain benefit with intermittent PD or by decreasing volume exchanged during the day and increasing volume overnight.

Blood Glucose Control Factors that can affect blood glucose regulation for persons on PD include the following:

⬥ Concentration of the dialysate solution
⬥ Method(s) of insulin delivery (eg, intraperitoneal, subcutaneous, or both)
⬥ Infection (peritonitis)

To understand variability in blood glucose levels, the practitioner should assess the following:

- Glucose concentration used in the dialysate (eg, 1.5%, 2.5%, or 4.25%)
- Type and amount of insulin, as well as the location of insulin injection
- Any clinical signs of infection

In PD patients who need better ultrafiltration due to hypervolemia or in persons with diabetes, an icodextran solution (7.5%) may be substituted for one of the traditional dextrose-containing solutions.[60] Since icodextran is a glucose polymer and produces maltose upon metabolism, there is a potentially deleterious secondary effect when home glucose monitors requiring glucose dehydrogenase pyrroloquinoline quinone (GDH-PQQ) chemistry test strips are used. These nonglucose sugars may be read by such test strips as a falsely high serum glucose level, thereby either masking a hypoglycemic episode or causing aggressive insulin management.[54] The consequences may lead to serious injury or death.[61]

Kidney Transplantation

Kidney transplantation can be performed using a kidney from a living related donor, a living unrelated donor, or a suitable cadaveric donor.[62] Once transplantation has occurred, immunosuppressive medications are required throughout the recipient's life to prevent the body from rejecting the transplanted organ. Persons with diabetes must take additional insulin following transplantation because the newly functioning kidney catabolizes insulin once again, because posttransplant steroid therapy has a hyperglycemic effect, and because the person experiences a notable increase in appetite, which can lead to weight gain.

Blood Glucose Control Following transplantation, blood glucose control may be altered by the following factors[62]:

- Degree of function of the transplanted kidney
- Treatment of transplant rejection
- Changes in steroid dose: Immunosuppressant agents (specifically, corticosteroids, cyclosporine, and tacrolimus) may contribute to posttransplant diabetes
- Patient's increased appetite and ability to consume a more liberal diet with subsequent weight gain
- Diuretic therapy
- Presence of infection: Transplant recipients are more susceptible to infection because of immunosuppression

Simultaneous Transplant: Kidney and Pancreas

Persons with type 1 diabetes may be considered for a simultaneous kidney-pancreas transplantation.[62] A kidney-pancreas transplantation restores both glucose metabolism and kidney function. Criteria for patient selection vary at each transplant center but typically include the criteria listed in Table 27.5. Contraindications and complications are also summarized in the table.

TABLE 27.5 Kidney-Pancreas Transplantation: Criteria, Contraindications, and Complications

Criteria (may include the following)*	*Contraindications* (may include the following)	*Complications* (may include the following)
Diagnosis of type 1 diabetes	Presence of HIV	Cardiac incompetence
Evidence of secondary complications such as renal insufficiency or preproliferative retinopathy	Malignancy	Arterial or venous thrombosis
	Psychosis	Anastomotic leaks, bleeding
Metabolic instability	Any active infection	Side effects of immunosuppression
	Severe neuropathies	Pancreatitis
Adequate financial resources/insurance (insurance carriers review eligibility for payment case by case)	Inoperable cardiovascular disease	Metabolic acidosis related to exocrine pancreatic function

*Criteria for patient selection vary at each transplant center; the above are typical.

Summary

Despite medical advances in DKD, the morbidity and mortality of individuals with diabetes on RRTs are higher than among those who do not have diabetes. Early detection, referral, and treatment are essential to preserve residual kidney function. Although tight glycemic control and hypertensive management focused on minimizing proteinuria seem effective in slowing disease progression, the evidence is not strong to suggest that severe protein restriction is required, even in the earliest stages of CKD (Stages 1 and 2). Malnutrition and weight loss may result from such restrictive diets and will have a significant impact on survival and treatment outcomes. Adequate energy coupled with a palatable diet, and perhaps the availability of ketoacid analogs, may improve the diets prescribed in CKD. The interrelated nature of diabetes, CVD, and CKD complicate treatment and management. Nonetheless, further research into how to best manage these conditions is warranted. Greater understanding of the role of anemia and secondary hyperparathyroidism on CKD and diabetes should not only elucidate the relationship of CKD to CVD but also, perhaps, determine the variability in incidence rates of disease progression in type 1 diabetes and type 2 diabetes.

Focus on Education

Teaching Strategies

⊘ **Screening.** Explain the need to determine kidney function regularly: in type 1 diabetes, annually after 5 years' onset; in type 2 diabetes, annually. Screen annually with a 24-hour urine; screen also for anemia and osteodystrophy. Blood tests are required periodically, as are tests for potassium and cholesterol. Discuss which tests measure which function, define expected and normal lab values, and provide a record-keeping tool to bring to each clinic/education visit.

⊘ **Referrals.** Nephrology is necessary when loss of function is noted. Collaboration with the nephrology team is key to the patient's care and management. Referral to a registered dietitian is necessary for a comprehensive nutrition evaluation. Assistance is appropriate with changes and coping with chronic disease. Individuals may need help with scheduling these appointments. Include family and significant others for support and reinforcement.

⊘ **Eating.** Develop meal plans that are adequate, palatable, and realistic. Protein restriction may be warranted in later stages of CKD to slow disease progression and when RRT is not initiated.

⊘ **Treatment.** Medical management minimizes function loss and complications; this includes control of blood pressure and blood glucose, correction of hypervolemia, and pharmacologic intervention to correct dyslipidemia, hypertension, and elevated glucose. Review the purposes for testing for these, demonstrate tools for home monitoring, and discuss signs for change.

Messages for Patients

⊘ **Make therapeutic lifestyle changes.** Begin making lifestyle changes of value to minimize complications, as good control makes a difference. Modify daily eating patterns and food choices one at a time. Some people like to modify their eating habits one meal or snack at a time. You can keep adding physical activity and other self-management tasks needed to maximize the renal functioning.

⊘ **Actively participate in self-monitoring and record keeping, determining progress toward goal.** Keeping a written record of your eating, physical activity, weight, blood pressure, and blood glucose will allow you to pattern manage. You can identify the cause and effect of what happens when and why. Sometimes whole therapy is modified based on atypical behaviors. Identifying trends will allow changing or modifying medications/food/activity or a self-care routine in order to achieve desirable clinical outcomes.

⊘ **Put medication, activity, and meal plan recommendations into action.** You can choose tasty foods that are low in sodium or potassium, for example. A kidney-friendly lifestyle does not have to be restrictive. You can explore reasonable substitutions or additions to your food preferences or physical activity opportunities. Communicate with your clinicians if the food, activity, or medication recommendations are not realistic to implement.

⊘ **Utilize a healthcare professional and personal support network.** It takes time to implement all of the self-care behaviors. Ask for help when needed. People can relapse and go back to unhealthy behaviors based on social triggers or just be tired with being a perfect patient all of the time.

⊘ **Follow up with clinic visits and laboratory testing to monitor kidney function.** Treatment strategies and approaches change with time; therefore, it is beneficial to reevaluate them on an ongoing basis.

⊘ **Review care options.** Select the best care by learning about the choices, particularly for RRTs. Invite involvement of family and appropriate others for support and clarity.

Health Literacy

⊘ **Educators need to be sensitive to the complexity of the information and directions given to people with diabetes and kidney conditions from multiple clinicians and healthcare providers.** Do patients know how to connect all of the recommendations and put them into action? Here are some meaningful statistics about typical patients:
- 33% are unable to read basic healthcare materials
- 42% cannot comprehend directions for taking medication on an empty stomach
- 26% are unable to understand information on an appointment slip

- 43% do not understand the rights and responsibilities section of a Medicaid application
- 60% do not understand a standard informed consent[63]
- Up to 80% of patients forget what their doctor tells them as soon as they leave the office, and nearly 50% of what they do remember is recalled incorrectly[64]

⊘ **People with low health literacy may be embarrassed to admit they do not understand what they are instructed to do.** They adapt coping mechanisms that effectively mask their challenges, for example, saying they forgot their eyeglasses, to avoid filling out forms; laughing about being forgetful when asked about their medical treatments; nodding politely when being spoken to by educators; and not asking any questions.[65]

⊘ **"People are generally better persuaded by the reasons which they have themselves discovered, than by those which have come into the mind of others" —Blaise Pascal in Pensées, 1670.** Help your patients self-discover their own solutions to your recommendations or suggestions.

⊘ **Locate quality health information.** Provide a list of resources that the patient and caregiver may access to learn more about the disease and its management.

⊘ **Evaluate information for credibility and quality.** Include ways to examine patient education information either on the Internet or in print media for its reliability from a credible source. Provide credible sources of information for the patient.

⊘ **Relative risks and benefits.** Discuss with the patient and caregiver the positive and negative effects of all aspects of treatment in a manner understandable to them. Support informed treatment decisions made.

⊘ **Interpreting test results.** Review laboratory values and blood glucose records with the patient and caregiver and assist them in understanding the factors that impact them.

Focus on Practice

⊘ **The variables of kidney condition and life stage/age will dictate the treatment options and education strategies.** Preventive care versus nephropathy versus dialysis require different clinical interventions and a care system. A careful assessment of the condition and its treatment strategies will outline effective management of the condition and corresponding patient support.

⊘ **"We are made wise not by the recollection of our past, but by the responsibility for our future" —George Bernard Shaw.** Diabetes educators need to be responsible for a chronic condition system change that minimizes dependence on compliance, adherence, and restrictions. Diabetes self-management has evolved to a patient empowerment and a concordance model with focusing on patients' involvement in clinical decision making. Educators can exemplify this practice to other disciplines and systems by making each patient aware of the choices and expectations from his or her own care.

⊘ **Create a system of ongoing communication among primary care providers, nephrologists, dietitians, nurses, social workers, and other healthcare professionals involved in care.** All of the healthcare professionals can be united in supporting patients by sharing consistent information and realistic expectations for self-management.

⊘ **Provide patients with a peer-to-peer support network like a support group or social networking system.** Access to a peer support system will help minimize any overwhelming feelings of frustration that can prevent adequate self-care.

References

1. National Kidney Foundation. Kidney Disease Outcomes Quality Initiative (KDOQI) clinical practice guidelines and clinical practice recommendations for diabetes and chronic kidney disease 2007 (cited 2014 Apr 2). On the Internet at: http://www.kidney.org/professionals/KDOQI/guideline_diabetes.

2. Coonrod B, Ernst KL. Nephropathy. A Core Curriculum for Diabetes Education: Diabetes and Complications. 5th ed. Chicago: American Association of Diabetes Educators; 2003.

3. National Kidney Foundation. Kidney Disease Outcomes Quality Initiative (KDOQI) clinical practice guidelines for chronic kidney disease and clinical practice recommendations for diabetes and chronic kidney disease 2007 (cited 2014 Mar 2). On the Internet at: http://www.kidney.org/professionals/KDOQI/guideline_diabetes.

4. National Kidney Foundation. Kidney Disease Outcomes Quality Initiative (KDOQI) clinical practice guidelines for chronic kidney disease: evaluation, classification, and stratification 2002 (cited 2014 Apr 2). On the Internet at: http://www.kidney.org/professionals/KDOQI/guidelines_ckd/toc.htm.

5. National Institutes of Health. US Renal Data System, USRDS 2009 Annual Data Report: Atlas of End-Stage Renal Disease in the United States. Bethesda, Md: National Institutes of Health, National Institute of Diabetes and Digestive and Kidney Diseases; 2010.

6. Goeddeke-Merickel C. The goals of comprehensive and integrated disease state management for diabetic kidney-disease patients. Adv Chronic Kidney Dis. 2005;12(2):236-42.

7. Ogden CL, Carroll MD, Kit B. Prevalence of childhood and adult obesity in the United States, 2011-2012. JAMA. 2014;311(8):806-14.

8. National Institutes of Health. US Renal Data System, USRDS 2013 Annual Data Report: Atlas of End-Stage Renal Disease in the United States. Bethesda, Md: National Institutes of Health, National Institute of Diabetes and Digestive and Kidney Diseases; 2013.

9. Levey A, Beto JA, Coronado BE, et al. Controlling the epidemic of cardiovascular disease in chronic renal disease: what do we know? what do we learn? where do we go from here? National Kidney Foundation Task Force on Cardiovascular Disease. Am J Kidney Dis. 1998;32:853-906.

10. National Kidney Foundation. KDOQI clinical practice guidelines for managing dyslipidemias in chronic kidney disease 2003 (cited 2014 Apr 2). On the Internet at: http://www.kidney.org/professionals/KDOQI/guidelines_lipids/toc.htm.

11. Byham-Gray L. Medical Nutrition Therapy for Renal Disease: Understanding the Implications. 2nd ed. Clarksville, Md: Wolf Rinke Associates Inc; 2004.

12. Reddi AS, Kuppasani K. Kidney function in health and disease. In: Byham-Gray LD, Burrowes JD, Chertow GS, eds. Nutrition in Kidney Disease. Totowa, NJ: Humana Press, Springer Publications Inc; 2008.

13. Gonyea J, McCarthy M. Overview: pathophysiology of the kidney. In: Byham-Gray LD, Wiesen K, eds. A Clinical Guide to Nutrition Care in Kidney Disease. Chicago: American Dietetic Association; 2004.

14. McCann L. Bone and mineral metabolism and disease. In: Byham-Gray LD, Burrowes JD, Chertow GS, eds. Nutrition in Kidney Disease. Totowa, NJ: Humana Press, Springer Publications Inc; 2008.

15. Mehta RL, Kellum JA, Shah SV, et al. Acute Kidney Injury Network: report of an initiative to improve outcomes in acute kidney injury. Crit Care. 2007;11:R31-9.

16. Gervasio JM, Cotton AB. Nutrition support therapy in acute kidney injury: distinguishing dogma from good practice. Curr Gastroenterol Rep. 2009;11:325-31.

17. National Kidney Foundation. Kidney Disease Outcomes Quality Initiative (KDOQI) clinical practice guidelines for chronic kidney disease and clinical practice recommendations for diabetes and chronic kidney disease: 2012 update (cited 2014 Mar 2). On the Internet at: http://www.kidney.org/professionals/KDOQI/pdf/Diabetes_AJKD_FebSuppl_07.pdf.

18. National Kidney Foundation. Diabetes and Chronic Kidney Disease Handbook (cited 2014 Apr). On the Internet at: http://www.kidney.org/professionals/KDOQI/pdf/Diabetes_AJKD_FebSuppl_07.pdf.

19. National Kidney Foundation. Clinical practice guidelines (cited 2014 Apr 2). On the Internet at: http://www.kidney.org/professionals/KDOQI.

20. Harvey KS. Nutrition and pharmacologic approaches. In: Byham-Gray LD, Burrowes JD, Chertow GS, eds. Nutrition in Kidney Disease. Totowa, NJ: Humana Press, Springer Publications Inc; 2008.

21. McCann L, ed. Pocket Guide to Nutrition Assessment of the Patient with Chronic Kidney Disease: A Concise, Practical Resource for Comprehensive Nutrition Care in CKD. 4th ed. New York: National Kidney Foundation; 2009.

22. American Dietetic Association. Evidence Analysis Library: chronic kidney disease (cited 2014 Apr 2). On the Internet at: http://www.adaevidenceanalysislibrary.com/topic.cfm?cat=3927.

23. Pagenkemper JJ. Nutrition management of diabetes in chronic kidney disease. In: Byham-Gray LD, Wiesen K, eds. A Clinical Guide to Nutrition Care in Kidney Disease. Chicago: American Dietetic Association; 2004.

24. Finne P, Reunanen A, Stenman S, Groop PH, Gronhagen-Riska C. Incidence of end-stage renal disease in patients with type 1 diabetes. JAMA. 2005;294(14):1782-7.

25. DeFronzo R. Diabetic nephropathy. In: Lebovitz H, ed. Therapy for Diabetes Mellitus and Related Disorders. Alexandria, Va: American Diabetes Association; 2004.

26. Diabetes Control and Complications Trial Group. The effect of intensive treatment of diabetes on the development and progression of long-term complications in insulin-dependent diabetes mellitus. N Engl J Med. 1993;329:977-86.

27. UK Prospective Diabetes Study Group. Intensive blood glucose control with sulphonylureas or insulin compared with conventional treatment and risk of complications in patients with type 2 diabetes (UKPDS 33). Lancet. 1998;352:837-53.

28. UK Prospective Diabetes Study Group. Effect of intensive blood glucose control with metformin on complications in overweight patients with type 2 diabetes (UKPDS 34). Lancet. 1998;352:854-62.

29. American Diabetes Association. Position statement: standards of medical care in diabetes—2010. Diabetes Care. 2010;33:S11-61.

30. Robertson LM, Waugh N, Robertson A. Protein restriction for diabetic renal disease. Cochrane Database Syst Rev. 2007 Oct 17;(4):CD002181.

31. Pagenkemper JJ. Diabetes mellitus. In: Byham-Gray LD, Burrowes JD, Chertow GS, eds. Nutrition in Kidney Disease. Totowa, NJ: Humana Press, Springer Publications Inc; 2008.

32. Seaquist E, Goetz FC, Rich S, Barbosa J. Familial clustering of diabetic kidney disease: evidence for genetic susceptibility to diabetic nephropathy. N Engl J Med. 1989;320:1161-5.

33. Sedor J. Frontiers in diabetic nephropathy: can we predict who will get sick? J Am Soc Nephrol. 2006;17:336-8.

34. Rich S. Genetics of diabetes and its complications. J Am Soc Nephrol. 2006;17:353-60.

35. Fioretto F, Caramori ML, Mauer M. The kidney in diabetes: dynamic pathways of injury and repair. The Camillo Colgi Lecture 2007. Diabetologia. 2008;51:1347-55.

36. Stanton R. Clinical challenges in diagnosis and management of diabetic kidney disease. Am J Kidney Dis. 2014;63(2 Suppl 2):S3-21.

37. National Institutes of Health, National Institute of Digestive, Diabetes and Kidney Diseases. USRDS 1997 annual data report (cited 2005 Nov 29 [site no longer accessible]). On the Internet at: http://www.usrds.org/adr_1997.htm.

38. Moore H, Reams SM, Wiesen K, Nolph KD, Khanna R, Laothong C. National Kidney Foundation Council on Renal Nutrition Survey: past-present clinical practices and future strategic planning. J Renal Nutr. 2003;13:233-40.

39. Chronic Kidney Disease: Evidence Analysis Workgroup. Medical nutrition therapy (cited 2010 Mar 29). On the

Internet at: http://www.adaevidenceanalysislibrary.com/topic.cfm?cat=3929.

40. James P, Oparil S, Carter B, et al. 2014 evidence-based guideline for the management of high blood pressure in adults: report from the panel members appointed to the Eighth Joint National Committee (JN8). JAMA. 2014; 11(5):507-20.

41. National Kidney Foundation. K/DOQI clinical practice guidelines for managing dyslipidemias in chronic kidney disease. Am J Kidney Dis. 2003;41 Suppl 3:S1-152.

42. Goff D, Lloyd-Jones D, Bennett G, et al. 2013 ACC/AHA guideline on the assessment of cardiovascular risk: a report of the American College of Cardiology/American Heart Association Task Force on Practice Guidelines. Circulation. 2013 Nov 12:1-50.

43. Mohanram A, Zhang Z, Shahinfar S, Keane WF, Brenner BM, Toto RD. Anemia and end-stage renal disease in patients with type 2 diabetes and nephropathy. Kidney Int. 2004; 66(3):1131-8.

44. Byham-Gray L, Stover J, Wiesen K. A Clinical Guide to Nutrition Care in Kidney Disease. 2nd ed. Chicago: Academy of Nutrition and Dietetics; 2013.

45. Malluche H, Faugere MC. Effects of 1,25(OH)2D3 administration on bone metabolism and disease in patients with renal failure. Kidney Int. 1990;29 Suppl:S48-53.

46. de Francisco A. Secondary hyperparathyroidism: review of the disease and its treatment. Clin Ther. 2004;26:1976-93.

47. Goodman W. The consequences of uncontrolled secondary hyperparathyroidism and its treatment in chronic kidney disease. Semin Dial. 2004;17:209-16.

48. Block G. Prevalence and clinical consequences of elevated Ca x P product in hemodialysis patients. Clin Nephrol. 2000;54:318-24.

49. NKF-KDOQI. K/DOQI clinical practice guidelines for bone metabolism and disease in chronic kidney disease. Am J Kidney Dis. 2003;42 Suppl 3:S1-202.

50. Pisoni R, Greenwood RN. Selected lessons learned from the Dialysis Outcomes and Practice Patterns Study (DOPPS). Contrib Nephrol. 2005;149:58-68.

51. Young E, Akiba T, Albert JM, et al. Magnitude and impact of abnormal mineral metabolism in hemodialysis patients in the Dialysis Outcomes and Practice Patterns Study (DOPPS). Am J Kidney Dis. 2004;44:34-8.

52. Young E, Albert JM, Satayathum S, et al. Predictors and consequences of altered mineral metabolism: the Dialysis Outcomes and Practice Patterns Study (DOPPS). Kidney Int. 2005;67:1179-87.

53. Kidney Disease—Improving Global Outcomes (KDIGO). Clinical practice guideline for the diagnosis, evaluation, prevention, and treatment of chronic kidney disease-mineral and bone disorder (CKD-MBD) (cited 2010 Feb 20). On the Internet at: http://www.kdigo.org/home/mineral-bone-disorder.

54. Williams M, Garg R. Glycemic management in ESRD and earlier stages of CKD. Am J Kidney Dis. 2014;63(2 Suppl 2): S22-38.

55. Strippoli G, Craig M, Deeks JJ, et al. Effects of angiotensin converting enzyme inhibitors and angiotensin II receptor antagonists on mortality and renal outcomes in diabetic nephropathy: systematic review. BMJ. 2004;329:828-939.

56. Yu H, Pedrini MT, Levey AS, et al. Progression of chronic renal failure. Arch Intern Med. 2003;163:1417-29.

57. National Kidney Foundation. Kidney Disease Outcomes Quality Initiative (KDOQI) clinical practice guidelines for nutrition in chronic renal failure. Am J Kidney Dis. 2000;35 Suppl 2:S1-140.

58. McCann L. KDOQI practice guidelines for bone metabolism and disease in CKD: another opportunity for renal dietitians to take a leadership role in improving outcomes for patients with CKD. J Renal Nutr. 2005;15:265-74.

59. DiazBuxo J. Peritoneal dialysis prescriptions for diabetic patients (cited 2014 Mar 4). On the Internet at: http://www.advancesinpd.com/adv99/99-2-Peritoneal.html.

60. Wiesen K. Dialysis. In: Byham-Gray LD, Burrowes JD, Chertow GS, eds. Nutrition in Kidney Disease. Totowa, NJ: Humana Press, Springer Publications Inc; 2008.

61. US Food and Drug Administration. FDA public health notification: potentially fatal errors with GDH-PQQ glucose monitoring technology. MedWatch-FDA Safety Information and Adverse Event Reporting Program (cited 2010 Mar 29). On the Internet at: http://www.fda.gov/safety/medwatch/SafetyInformation/SafetyAlertsforHumanMedicalProducts/ucm177295.htm.

62. Kent PS. Transplantation. In: Byham-Gray LD, Burrowes JD, Chertow GS, eds. Nutrition in Kidney Disease. Totowa, NJ: Humana Press, Springer Publications Inc; 2008.

63. Williams MV, Parker RM, Baker DW, et al. Inadequate functional health literacy among patients at two public hospitals. JAMA. 1995;274(21):1677-82.

64. Kessels RP. Patients' memory for medical information. J Royal Soc Med. 2003;96:219-22.

65. Weiss BD, ed. 20 Common Problems in Primary Care. New York: McGraw-Hill; 1999.

CHAPTER 28

Diabetic Neuropathies

Aaron I. Vinik, MD, PhD, FCP, MACP

Etta J. Vinik, MA (Ed)

Key Concepts

- The specific syndrome guides the treatment. Management of diabetic neuropathy is complex, and the key to success depends on separating out the underlying pathological processes in each particular clinical presentation.

- A careful history and detailed physical examination, together with objective testing, are essential for the diagnosis.

- Preventive strategies and patient education are key in reducing complication rates and mortality.

- Somatic and autonomic neuropathies are among the most common long-term complications of diabetes as well as its precursors—impaired glucose tolerance and the metabolic syndrome.

- Diabetic neuropathy, which includes somatic and autonomic neuropathies, is associated with considerable morbidity and mortality and has a significant impact on quality of life.

- Entrapments occur in one third of patients and can be treated medically or surgically.

- Proximal neuropathy is an inflammatory condition that coexists with diabetic neuropathy and is amenable to anti-inflammatory therapy.

- Focal mononeuropathies involving single nerves occur and, for the most part, resolve spontaneously.

- Diabetic neuropathy is highly prevalent in diabetic populations but often not recognized by physicians.

- Small-fiber neuropathy may lead to foot ulceration and subsequent gangrene and amputation.

- Large-fiber neuropathy produces numbness and ataxia, impairs quality of life, and may lead to falls and fractures.

- A number of simple tests that can be done in the clinic are useful for detecting diabetic neuropathy and predicting complications, such as foot ulcers and gangrene.

- Standard and validated quantitative measures of disease progression are now available and allow better interpretation of responses to different treatments and study results.

- The pathogenesis of neuropathy is still poorly understood. Recent studies on new agents that target the pathophysiological mechanisms have led to a better understanding of the pathogenesis of diabetic neuropathy as well as the pain mechanisms for the different types of pain syndromes.

- The newer symptomatic treatment modalities, based on etiologic factors, have potential for making a significant impact on morbidity and mortality.

Introduction

Translation of the science of neuropathy into clinical care is a major challenge for diabetes care providers. It requires knowledge on the one hand and careful attention to patient histories, symptoms, and signs on the other. The emergence of the study of neuropathy as a science in its own right, enhanced by technological and biological advances, has resulted in more knowledge about neuropathy. However, the scientific and patient community still awaits major research breakthroughs in understanding its pathophysiology and etiology.

Diabetic neuropathy (DN) is not a single entity, but rather a number of different syndromes, each with a range of clinical and subclinical manifestations. Effective management is based on recognizing the particular manifestation and underlying pathogenesis of the particular form of DN in each patient, and using this information to initiate therapy at a level that avoids undesirable side effects. Since different syndromes can now be distinguished by different affected nerve fibers, the artful healthcare provider, by mindful interaction with the patient and a carefully honed skill set, is able to separate out the different and often intertwined neuropathic entities and administer individualized treatment.

State of the Disease

Diabetic neuropathy is the most common form of neuropathy in developed countries and is responsible for 50% to 75% of nontraumatic amputations.[1] These disorders are among the most frequent complications of diabetes mellitus and a significant cause of morbidity and mortality. The major morbidity is foot ulceration, which can lead to gangrene and, ultimately, to limb loss. The true prevalence is not known, and reports vary from 10% to 90%, depending on the criteria and methods used to define neuropathy.[2–8] Each year close to 100,000 amputations are performed on persons with diabetes in the United States, yet up to 75% of them are preventable.[5] The national annual direct cost of foot ulcers in the United States has been estimated at approximately $5 billion.[9] Diabetic neuropathy is clearly a huge global economic burden; on an individual level, it

also has a tremendous impact on a patient's quality of life (QOL).[10,11] Until as recently as 2011, these statistics have been widely quoted. However, in January 2012, the Centers for Disease Control and Prevention (CDC) issued a press release on the results of a study showing a dramatic decline in diabetes-related foot ulcers in the United States by 65%. Importantly, the study also showed that this decline was restricted to those demographic areas where patients had access to diabetes care that included education on foot care.[12] The problem continues in underserved populations in rural and inner-city areas.[13]

This report was published in *Diabetes Care* in the same month (January 24, 2012) and was underscored in an article wherein experts attributed the improvement to better management of risk factors that lead to the loss of feet and legs. The American Diabetes Association's president of medicine and science that year, Vivian Fonseca, MD, stated, "This is very encouraging and important news for people with diabetes. The decline confirms the tremendous progress we have made in translating research into practice."[14]

Meanwhile, healthcare professionals are being confronted by new challenges related to results of recent studies showing that the autonomic system in its cardiovascular form is associated with at least a threefold increased risk for mortality.[2,13,15] More recently, diabetic autonomic neuropathy (DAN) or even autonomic imbalance between the sympathetic and the parasympathetic nervous systems has been implicated as a predictor of cardiovascular risk.[13,15] Once autonomic neuropathy (AN) sets in, life can become quite dismal and the mortality rate can approximate 25% to 50% within 5 to 10 years.[5,6]

Diabetic neuropathy also has a tremendous impact on patients' QOL, predominantly by causing weakness, ataxia, and incoordination predisposing to falls and fractures.[9] Chronic, persistent pain accounts for 40% of patient visits in a primary care setting, and about 20% of the presenting patients attest to enduring pain for more than 6 months.[10] Persistent neuropathic pain significantly interferes with QOL, impairing sleep and recreation; it also significantly impacts emotional well-being and is associated with, if not the cause of, depression, anxiety, loss of sleep, and noncompliance with treatment.[11]

A Problem Diabetes Education Can Address

Educators have a major opportunity to assist in preventing the painful, devastating, and costly complications of DN.

- Although DN is highly prevalent in the diabetes population, healthcare providers often do not recognize it.
- When DN is recognized, most providers regard it as a single disease (rather than a heterogeneous group of disorders) and dismiss it with, "Nothing can be done; learn to live with it." At most, providers will prescribe a palliative for pain or other symptoms.

This chapter offers suggestions for dealing with these problems. Educators have the following opportunities to assist patients affected by these common, painful, and potentially devastating diabetes complications:

- Acquire more information about neuropathy
- Recognize the different components of the disease
- Elicit useful information from patients by asking the right questions
- Use the information to guide interventions
- Explain the importance of controlled blood glucose in preventing and reversing certain neuropathies
- Emphasize meticulous foot care to prevent and reverse certain neuropathies

The diabetes educator can play a significant role in helping to prevent or reverse neuropathy (in some instances) by explaining the importance of controlled blood glucose and meticulous foot care. Blood glucose, blood pressure, lipids, and lifestyle modifications remain essential measures to reduce the risk of macrovascular disease. Diabetes educators can be proud of their role in the dramatic decline of foot amputations as reported by the CDC.

This chapter includes new information on AN and its effect on QOL, and explains the cardiovascular component as a predictor of mortality. It emphasizes the importance of addressing persistent neuropathic pain as a difficult-to-manage clinical problem. Additionally, it exhorts the diabetes educator to counsel patients on the risks of falling and strategies to prevent falls.

This chapter also provides information about new research on different treatment modalities that not only relieve neuropathic symptoms but also provide hope for changing the course of the disease.

Definition

Distal symmetric polyneuropathy (DSP) has recently been defined as a symmetrical, length-dependent sensorimotor polyneuropathy attributable to metabolic and microvascular alterations as a result of chronic hyperglycemia exposure (diabetes) and cardiovascular risk covariates.[7] Its onset is generally insidious, and without treatment, the course is chronic and progressive. The loss of small-fiber-mediated sensation results in the loss of thermal and pain perception, whereas large-fiber impairment results in loss of touch and vibration perception. Sensory fiber involvement may also result in "positive" symptoms, such as paresthesias and pain. Nonetheless, up to 50% of neuropathic patients can be asymptomatic. Distal symmetric polyneuropathy can be associated with the involvement of the autonomic nervous system (ANS) (ie, DAN, which rarely causes severe symptoms[16,17]), but in its cardiovascular form (as mentioned above) it is definitely associated with at least a threefold increased risk for mortality.[2-4] Also, as mentioned above, DAN has recently been implicated as a predictor of cardiovascular risk.[3,4]

Since asymptomatic (subclinical) neuropathy is common, a careful clinical examination is needed for the diagnosis.[17] In fact, absence of symptoms cannot be equated with absence of neuropathy. On the other hand, the importance of excluding nondiabetic causes was emphasized in the Rochester Diabetic Neuropathy Study, in which up to 10% of peripheral neuropathy in persons with diabetes was found to be due to nondiabetic causes.[18]

However, neuropathy still remains underdiagnosed by endocrinologists as well as non-endocrinologists, as shown in the Glycemic Optimization With Algorithms and Labs at Point of Care (GOAL A1C) study.[19]

Identification of neuropathy in 7000 patients in the presence of mild neuropathy was accurate only one third of the time and reached 75% *only* if neuropathy was severe. Clearly, more education for healthcare providers is needed on criteria for neuropathy diagnosis. These criteria will be discussed further in this chapter.

Diagnosis/Clinical Assessment Tools

Scoring Systems

Symptoms of neuropathy can vary markedly from one patient to another, making the correct assessment of these disorders difficult at times. For this reason, standardized, validated symptom questionnaires with similar scoring systems have been developed for measuring severity of symptoms and the degree of reproducible neuropathic deficits. These include the Michigan Neuropathy Screening Instrument (MNSI),[20] the Neuropathy Symptom Score for neuropathic symptoms, and the Neuropathy Disability Score (NDS) or the Nerve Impairment Score (NIS) for neuropathic deficits.[21] The Neurologic Symptom Score[22,23] has 38 items that capture symptoms of muscle weakness, sensory disturbances, and autonomic dysfunction and are useful for patient follow-up and for assessing patient responses to treatment.

The neurological history and examination are central to patient care and should always be performed initially and then at all subsequent visits.

Screening Recommendations

Table 28.1 contains DN screening recommendations from the American Diabetes Association (ADA).

Combinations of more than 1 test have more than 87% sensitivity in detecting chronic sensorimotor neuropathy.[24,25] Longitudinal studies have shown that these simple tests are good predictors of foot-ulcer risk.[26] Numerous composite scores to

---

Case: Neuropathic Pain

CM, a 48-year-old woman with an 18-year history of type 2 diabetes, returned to see her primary care provider after a 2-year absence. Her complaint was numbness and pain in both feet. She has a past medical history of obesity, hypertension, hypertriglyceridemia, and background retinopathy.

Physical Signs

- Blood pressure (BP) 152/88 mm Hg, heart rate 80 beats per minute, body mass index (BMI) 38.9

- Microaneurysms (on ophthalmoscopic examination)

- 2/6 Systolic ejection murmur

- Normal thyroid, carotids, heart, abdomen

- Dorsalis pedis pulses 2+ symmetrically

- Calluses over fifth metatarsal heads and lateral edge of great toes, bilaterally

- Ankle jerks absent

- Vibratory sense absent

- Touch pressure absent (5.07 Semmes-Weinstein monofilament [SWM])

Medications

- Metformin (Glucophage®, Bristol-Myers Squibb) 1 g bid

- Glipizide GITS (Glucotrol XL®, Pfizer Inc) 10 mg/d

- Trandolapril (Mavik®, Abbott Laboratories) 4 mg/d

- Aspirin 81 mg/d, multivitamins

Questions to Consider

- What is the significance of the physical findings (especially the calluses and the absence of ankle jerks, vibratory sense, and touch pressure)?

- How common is the problem of nerve impairment?

- Is this a typical presentation?

- What investigations should be conducted?

TABLE 28.1 DN: Screening Recommendations

Frequency

All persons should be screened for DN at diagnosis of type 2 diabetes and annually thereafter

All persons should be screened for DN 5 years after diagnosis of type 1 diabetes and annually thereafter

Method

Screening must include sensory examination of the feet and ankle reflexes. One or more of the following can be used to assess sensory function:

- Pinprick
- Temperature
- Vibration perception (using 128-Hz tuning fork)
- 10-g monofilament pressure perception on the dorsal surface of the distal halluces

Source: AJ Boulton, AI Vinik, JC Arezzo, et al, "Diabetic neuropathies: a statement by the American Diabetes Association," *Diabetes Care* 28, no. 4 (2005): 956-62.

evaluate clinical signs of DN, such as the NIS, are useful in documenting and monitoring neuropathic deficits.[27]

Objective Devices for the Diagnosis of Neuropathy

The neurological examination should focus on the lower extremities and should always include an accurate foot inspection for deformities, ulcers, fungal infection, muscle wasting, hair distribution or loss, and the presence or absence of pulses. Sensory modalities should be assessed using simple handheld devices such as the following:

- Touch—cotton wool or soft brush
- Vibration—128-Hz tuning fork
- Pressure—1-g and 10-g SWM
- Pinprick—Wartenberg wheel or a pin
- Temperature—testing with cold or warm objects or NeuroQuick (Schweers)[28]

Finally, the Achilles reflexes should be tested[24,29] (Table 28.2).

Quantitative Sensory Testing

Quantitative sensory testing (QST) is of value in detecting subclinical neuropathy, assessing progression, and predicting risk for foot ulceration.[27,30] These standardized measures of vibration and thermal thresholds also play an important role in multicenter clinical trials as primary efficacy end points, as do QOL measures.[9]

Moreover, assessment of thermal thresholds is a key element in the diagnostic pathway of small-fiber polyneuropathy.[17,31] A consensus subcommittee of the American Academy of Neurology stated that QST received a Class II rating as a diagnostic test with a type B strength of recommendation.[32]

Skin Biopsy and Intraepidermal Nerve Fiber Density

Skin biopsy has become a widely used tool to investigate small-caliber sensory nerves including somatic unmyelinated intraepidermal nerve fibers (IENFs), dermal myelinated nerve fibers, and autonomic nerve fibers in peripheral neuropathies and other conditions.[33-35] The importance of the skin biopsy as a diagnostic tool for DSP is increasingly being recognized.[36-38] This technique quantitates small epidermal nerve fibers through antibody staining of the pan-axonal marker protein gene product 9.5 (PGP 9.5). Though minimally invasive (3-mm diameter punch biopsy), it enables a direct study of small fibers, which cannot be evaluated by nerve

TABLE 28.2 Examination—Bedside Sensory Tests

Sensory Modality	*Nerve Fiber*	*Instrument*	*Associated Sensory Receptors*
Vibration	Aβ (large)	128 Hz tuning fork	Ruffini corpuscle mechanoreceptors
Pain (pinprick)	C (small)	Neuro-tips	Nociceptors for pain and warmth
Pressure	Aβ, Aα (large)	1-g and 10-g monofilament	Pacinian corpuscle
Light touch	Aβ, Aα (large)	Wisp of cotton	Meissner's corpuscle
Cold	Aδ (small)	Cold tuning fork	Cold thermoreceptors

conduction velocity studies. It has led to the recognition of small nerve fiber syndrome as part of impaired glucose tolerance and the metabolic syndrome (Figure 28.1). When patients present with "burning foot or hand syndrome," evaluation for glucose tolerance and the metabolic syndrome (including waist circumference, blood pressure, and plasma triglyceride and HDL-C levels) becomes mandatory. Therapeutic lifestyle changes[39] can result in nerve fiber regeneration, reversal of the neuropathy, and alleviation of symptoms. Different techniques for tissue processing and nerve fiber evaluation have been used. For diagnostic purposes in peripheral neuropathies, the recent guidelines from the Joint Task Force of the European Federation of Neurological Societies and the Peripheral Nerve Society should be applied.[40] Quantification of IENF density appears to be more sensitive than sensory nerve conduction study or sural nerve biopsy in diagnosing small-fiber neuropathy.

Corneal Confocal Microscopy

Corneal confocal microscopy is a noninvasive technique used to detect small-nerve-fiber loss in the cornea, which correlates with both increasing neuropathic severity and reduced IENF density in persons with diabetes.[41,42] A novel technique of real-time mapping permits an area of 3.2 mm² to be mapped with a total of 64 theoretically nonoverlapping single 400 μm² images.[43]

Contact Heat-Evoked Potentials

Contact heat-evoked potentials (CHEPs) have been studied in healthy controls, in persons newly diagnosed with diabetes, in persons with established diabetes, and in patients with the metabolic syndrome. It appears that CHEPs is capable of detecting small-fiber neuropathy in the absence of other indices, and that CHEPs correlates with quantitative sensory perception and objective tests of small-fiber function such as the cooling detection threshold and cold pain.[44,45]

Sudomotor Function

Changes in peripheral ANS function are an early manifestation of distal small-fiber neuropathy.[7] Sudomotor dysfunction is one of the earliest detectable neurophysiologic abnormalities in distal small-fiber neuropathies. Sweat glands are innervated by small, unmyelinated sympathetic C-nerve fibers that are responsible for the sweat response. Skin biopsies have confirmed that epidermal C-nerve fibers are reduced in persons with diabetes.[46] Thus, sudomotor function represents an attractive tool to evaluate the peripheral and autonomic nervous systems in people with diabetes mellitus.[47] The various techniques of sudomotor function testing, each with its strengths and weaknesses, are very sensitive and specific in the detection of distal small-fiber neuropathy. Most of these techniques, however, have

IENF Loss in Small Fiber Neuropathy

Control	Metabolic syndrome	Diabetes

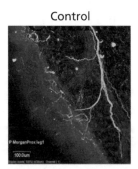 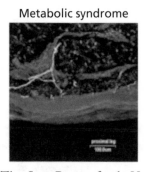 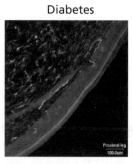

FIGURE 28.1   Loss of Cutaneous Nerve Fibers That Stain Positive for the Neuronal Antigen PGP 9.5 in Metabolic Syndrome and Diabetes

Sources: AI Vinik, J Ullal, HK Parson, CM Casellini, "Diabetic neuropathies: clinical manifestations and current treatment options," *Nat Clin Pract Endocrinol Metab* 2 (2006): 269-81; GL Pittenger, M Ray, NI Burcus, P McNulty, B Basta, AI Vinik, "Intraepidermal nerve fibers are indicators of small-fiber neuropathy in both diabetic and nondiabetic patients," *Diabetes Care* 27 (2004): 1974-79; G Pittenger, A Mehrabyan, K Simmons, et al, "Small fiber neuropathy is associated with the metabolic syndrome," *Metab Syndr* 3 (2005): 113-21.

Diagnosis and Initial Treatment

CM's healthcare provider ordered the following tests and obtained the results noted:

- Electrolytes: normal

- Thyroid function tests, B_{12}: normal

- A1C: 9.5% (4.1%-6.5%)

- Albumin/creatinine ratio: 98 g/mg (normal <30)

- Triglycerides: 298 mg/dL (normal <150)

- Cholesterol: 187 mg/dL (normal <200)

CM had previously mentioned numbness and pain. What other questions are appropriate to ask about the discomfort in her feet?

When CM described her pain, she mentioned 3 kinds:

- Constant, diffused, sharp, burning

- Knifelike lightning episodes that occur occasionally at night

- Dull, gnawing "bone" pain, similar to a toothache

Is there any significance to these descriptions? What do they reveal? Into which of the following categories does her pain fit:

- Distal symmetric polyneuropathy?

- Acute or chronic (greater or less than 6 months)?

- Small- or large-fiber?

What initial approach to the management of her neuropathic discomfort would you have recommended?

In an attempt to improve her glycemic control, NPH insulin at bedtime was added to her current medications, and topical capsaicin (Zostrix®, GenDerm US) 0.025% 4 times per day was suggested. (NPH insulin is still frequently used because of cost issues. However, a long-acting analogue, such as insulin glargine [Lantus®, Sanofi Aventis] or insulin detemir [Levemir®, Novo Nordisk], should be considered.)

Finding Acceptable Pain Relief

One Month Later

CM returned for follow-up. Her NPH insulin had been titrated upward, and her overall glycemic control appeared improved; however, she required further pain relief. In addition to improved glycemic control, what agents would you have suggested?

- Her trandolapril was doubled to 8 mg per day.

- Amitriptyline, 10 mg nightly, was added, with instructions to increase by 10 mg per week until side effects decrease or relief is achieved.

Three Months Later

CM returned for continued follow-up. Her A1C had declined to 7.4% (4.1%-6.5%) with the addition of 70 units of NPH insulin nightly. Although her A1C is still not acceptable—it has come down from 9.5%—that is not the issue here. With 80 mg per day of amitriptyline, she had acceptable relief from the superficial burning symptoms but not from the deep-seated gnawing symptoms. What would you have recommended?

- Clonidine (Catapres®, Boehringer Ingleheim), 0.1 mg at bedtime, was added.

Subsequent Follow-up

CM had acceptable relief from all of her symptoms. But 1 year later, she again complained of burning, superficial (just below the skin) discomfort. She could not tolerate more than 100 mg per day of amitriptyline. She had side effects of dry mouth, blurring of vision, and constipation. What would you have suggested? Was her provider's suggestion likely to be effective?

- Pregabalin (Lyrica®, Pfizer Inc), 300 mg per day, was prescribed, with cessation of amitriptyline.

- Clonidine was discontinued, and duloxetine (120 mg per day) was added.

- Nutrinerve™ had been prescribed but was currently unavailable. Alpha-lipoic acid, 300 mg per day, with food was substituted.

Pain relief was achieved with a combination of pregabalin and duloxetine.

This chapter's section on treatment of DN based on pathogenic mechanisms helps readers consider whether the therapies chosen were appropriate and if there were alternatives. Note the use of the therapies for neuropathic pain: pregabalin, duloxetine, and alpha-lipoic acid.

remained underutilized in clinical practice due to lack of availability, results variability, and technical demands of the tests—most of them being tedious, cumbersome, and time-consuming. SUDOSCAN™ (Impeto Medical) is a new patented device designed to precisely evaluate sweat gland function based on sweat chloride concentrations through reverse iontophoresis and chronoamperometry.[48–50] This is a simple noninvasive test that is easy to perform. Patients place their hands and feet on the electrodes and stand still for 2 to 3 minutes. Neither special subject preparation nor specially trained medical personnel are needed. The reproducibility of this sweat function measurement has been successfully validated in different studies, and inter-device reproducibility has been confirmed through measurements with 2 different devices.[50,51] Sudoscan is being investigated by groups in the United States to measure sudomotor dysfunction. Preliminary data show that persons with diabetes with DSP have significantly worse electrochemical skin conductance of both feet and hands than persons with diabetes without DSP and healthy controls.

Nerve Conduction Velocity

The use of electrophysiologic measures (measures of nerve conduction velocity [NCV]) in both clinical practice and multicenter clinical trials is recommended. In persons with type 2 diabetes,[52] NCV abnormalities in the lower limbs increased from 8% at baseline to 42% after 10 years of disease. A slow progression of NCV abnormalities in type 1 diabetes was observed in the Diabetes Control and Complications Trial (DCCT).[53] In fact, NCV plays a key role in ruling out other causes of neuropathy and is essential for the identification of focal and multifocal neuropathies.[17,54]

Skin Biopsy

It is important to recognize that patients with painful, predominantly small-fiber neuropathy have normal NCV study results. There is consistent evidence that small, unmyelinated fibers are affected early in diabetes mellitus and that these alterations are not diagnosed by routine NCV studies. Therefore, other methods, such as QST or skin biopsy with quantification of IENFs, are needed to detect those patients.[36,55,56] As previously mentioned, the

importance of the skin biopsy as a diagnostic tool for chronic sensorimotor neuropathy is increasingly being recognized.[36–38]

QOL Measures

The effect of neuropathy per se on the QOL of the person with diabetes is widely recognized. A number of instruments have been developed and validated to assess QOL in DN. The Norfolk QOL-DN questionnaire is a validated tool that addresses specific symptoms and the impact of large, small, and autonomic nerve-fiber functions; the tool has been used in clinical trials and is available in 38 validated language versions.[7] The NeuroQol[57] measures patients' perceptions of the impact of neuropathy and foot ulcers.

The diagnosis of distal polyneuropathy is mainly clinical, aided by specific diagnostic tests according to the type and severity of the neuropathy; however, nondiabetic causes of neuropathy must always be excluded, depending on the clinical findings.

The spectrum of clinical neuropathic syndromes described in persons with diabetes includes dysfunction of almost every segment of the somatic peripheral and autonomic nervous systems[58]—thus the adage "Knowing neuropathy means to know the whole of medicine." Distinguishing each syndrome by its pathophysiologic, therapeutic, and prognostic features is feasible. This theme will be reiterated throughout the chapter.

Overview of DNs

This chapter describes different aspects of DN, explains the various nomenclatures, presents a clear and comprehensible classification of this complex disease state, and describes treatment options for specific neuropathic disorders.

As mentioned, DNs are a heterogeneous group of disorders that include abnormalities ranging from subclinical to clinical manifestations. Diabetes-related neuropathies have been classified on the basis of their clinical manifestations as well as anatomical findings[59] (see Table 28.3). Most of the pathology of DN occurs in the peripheral (surrounding) nervous system, although there may be some central nerve involvement. The peripheral nerve system is composed of the ANS (sympathetic and parasympathetic) and the sensorimotor nervous system. Autonomic nerves control *involuntary* functions (eg, breathing, heartbeat), while sensory nerves send information from the skin and internal organs about sensory perception (eg, hot and cold sensation), and motor nerves send commands from the brain to the body (eg, "Remove your hand from the hot stove"), thus controlling voluntary functions.[9]

TABLE 28.3   Clinical DNs: Classification

Rapidly Reversible Neuropathy

• Hyperglycemic neuropathy

Generalized Symmetrical Polyneuropathy

• Acute sensory neuropathy

• Chronic sensorimotor neuropathy (distal diabetic polyneuropathy)

  – Small-fiber neuropathy

  – Large-fiber neuropathy

Autonomic Neuropathy

• Cardiac autonomic neuropathy

• Gastrointestinal disorders related to autonomic neuropathy

• Sexual dysfunction related to autonomic neuropathy

• Bladder dysfunction related to autonomic neuropathy

• Sudomotor dysfunction related to autonomic neuropathy

• Pupillomotor and visceral (metabolic) response related to autonomic neuropathy

Focal and Multifocal Neuropathies

• Focal-limb

• Cranial neuropathy

• Proximal-motor neuropathy (amyotrophy)

• Truncal radiculoneuropathy

• Coexisting chronic inflammatory demyelinating neuropathy

Sources: Adapted from AJ Boulton, AI Vinik, JC Arezzo, et al, "Diabetic neuropathies: a statement by the American Diabetes Association," *Diabetes Care* 28, no. 4 (2005): 956-62; PK Thomas, JD Ward, PJ Watkins, "Diabetic neuropathy," in H Keen, J Jarrett, eds, *Complications of Diabetes* (London: Edward Arnold Publishing Company, 1982): 109-36.

Implications for Diabetes Education and Care

Because of the prevalence of neuropathy, and because it is an insidious and often silent disease, educators are advised to bring even the slightest suspicion of sensory and autonomic neuropathy to the provider's attention for nerve function testing. Table 28.4 lists the evidence-graded recommendations for screening.

Recommendations

◆ All patients should be screened for DSP at diagnosis of type 2 diabetes and 5 years after the diagnosis of type 1 diabetes, and at least annually thereafter using simple clinical tests. (B)

◆ Electrophysiological testing is rarely needed, except in situations where the clinical features are atypical. (E)

◆ Screening for signs and symptoms of cardiac autonomic neuropathy (CAN) should be instituted at diagnosis of type 2 diabetes and 5 years after the diagnosis of type 1 diabetes. Special testing is rarely needed and may not affect management or outcomes. (E)

◆ Medications for the relief of specific symptoms related to DSP and AN are recommended, as they improve the QOL of the patient. (E)

Conditions Mimicking DN

A number of conditions can be mistaken for painful DN:

◆ Intermittent claudication—the pain is exacerbated by walking

◆ Morton's neuroma—the pain and tenderness are localized to the intertarsal space and may be elicited by applying pressure with the thumb in the appropriate intertarsal space

◆ Osteoarthritis—the pain is confined to the joints, made worse with joint movement or exercise, and associated with morning stiffness that improves with ambulation

◆ Radiculopathy—the pain originates in the shoulder, arm, thorax, or back and radiates into the legs and feet

◆ Charcot neuroarthropathy—the pain is localized to the site of the collapse of the bones of

Level of Evidence	Description
TABLE 28.4 ADA Evidence-Grading System for Clinical Practice Recommendations	
A	Clear evidence from well-conducted, generalizable, and randomized controlled trials that are adequately powered, including the following: • Evidence from a well-conducted multicenter trial • Evidence from a meta-analysis that incorporated quality rating in the analysis Compelling nonexperimental evidence (ie, the "all or none" rule developed by the Center for Evidence-Based Medicine at Oxford) Supportive evidence from well-conducted, randomized controlled trials that are adequately powered, including the following: • Evidence from a well-conducted trial at 1 or more institutions • Evidence from a meta-analysis that incorporated quality ratings in the analysis
B	Supportive evidence from well-conducted cohort studies, including the following: • Evidence from a well-conducted cohort study or registry • Evidence from a well-conducted meta-analysis of cohort studies Supportive evidence from a well-conducted case-control study
C	Supportive evidence from poorly controlled or uncontrolled studies, including the following: • Evidence from randomized clinical trials with 1 or more major or 3 or more minor methodological flaws that could invalidate the results • Evidence from observational studies with high potential for bias (such as case series with comparison to historical controls) • Evidence from case series or case reports Conflicting evidence with the weight of evidence supporting the recommendation
E	Expert consensus or clinical experience

Source: "Clinical practice recommendations, 2013," *Diabetes Care* 36 Suppl 1, Jan (2013).

the foot, and the foot is hot rather than cold (as occurs in neuropathy)

◆ Plantar fasciitis—shooting or burning pain in the heel with each step and exquisite tenderness in the sole of the foot

◆ Tarsal tunnel syndrome—pain and numbness radiate from beneath the medial malleolus to the sole and are localized to the inner side of the foot

In contrast, DSP pain is bilateral, symmetrical (covering the whole foot and particularly the dorsum), and worse at night, interfering with sleep.

Implications for Diabetes Education and Care

Educators should take note of the conditions that mimic DN.

Recognize that the most important differential diagnoses from the general medicine perspective include neuropathies caused by alcohol abuse, uremia, hypothyroidism, vitamin B_{12} deficiency, peripheral arterial disease, cancer, inflammatory and infectious diseases, elevated mercury levels, celiac disease, and neurotoxic drugs.[60]

Classification and Diagnostic Assessment of Distal Symmetric Diabetic Polyneuropathies

Because of the lack of agreement on the definition and diagnostic assessment of neuropathy, several consensus conferences were convened to overcome the current problems, the most recent of which has redefined the minimal criteria for the diagnosis of typical distal symmetric diabetic polyneuropathies (DSPN), as summarized below.[7]

Toronto Classification of DSPN[7]

1. *Possible DSPN:* The presence of symptoms or signs of DSPN may include the following: symptoms—decreased sensation, positive neuropathic sensory symptoms (eg, "asleep numbness," prickling or stabbing pain, burning or aching pain) predominantly in the toes, feet, or legs; signs—symmetric decrease of distal sensation or unequivocally decreased or absent ankle reflexes.

2. *Probable DSPN:* The presence of a combination of symptoms and signs of neuropathy including any 2 or more of the following: neuropathic symptoms, decreased distal sensation, or unequivocally decreased or absent ankle reflexes.

3. *Confirmed DSPN:* The presence of an abnormality of nerve conduction and either a symptom (or symptoms) or a sign (or signs) of neuropathy confirm DSPN. If nerve conduction is normal, a validated measure of small-fiber neuropathy (with class 1 evidence) may be used. To assess for the severity of DSPN, several approaches are recommended: the graded approach outlined above and in Table 28.4; various continuous measures of sum scores of neurologic signs, symptoms, or nerve test scores; scores of function of activities of daily living; or scores of predetermined tasks or of disability.

4. *Subclinical DSPN:* The presence of no signs or symptoms of neuropathy is confirmed with abnormal nerve conduction or a validated measure of small-fiber neuropathy (with class 1 evidence). Definition 1, 2, or 3 can be used for clinical practice, and definition 3 or 4 can be used for research studies.

5. *Small-fiber neuropathy:* Small-fiber neuropathy should be graded as follows: (1) possible: the presence of length-dependent symptoms and/or clinical signs of small-fiber damage; (2) probable: the presence of length-dependent symptoms, clinical signs of small-fiber damage, and normal sural nerve conduction; and (3) definite: the presence of length-dependent symptoms, clinical signs of small-fiber damage, normal sural nerve conduction, and altered IENF density at the ankle and/or abnormal thermal thresholds at the foot.[28]

The diagnosis of DSPN should rest on the findings of the clinical and neurological examinations, that is, the presence of neuropathic symptoms (positive and negative, sensory and motor) and signs (sensory deficit, allodynia and hyperalgesia, motor weakness, absence of reflexes)[61]:

1. symptoms alone have poor diagnostic accuracy in predicting the presence of polyneuropathy,
2. signs are better predictors than symptoms,
3. multiple signs are better predictors than a single sign, and
4. relatively simple examinations are as accurate as complex scoring systems.

Thus, both symptoms and signs should be assessed.

The basic neurological assessment comprises the general medical and neurological history, inspection of the feet, and neurological examination of sensation using simple semiquantitative bedside instruments such as the 10-g SWM or Neuropen® (Owen Mumford)[62] (to assess touch/pressure); NeuroQuick (Schweers)[63] or Tip Therm® (tip therm GmbH)[64] (to assess temperature); calibrated Rydel-Seiffer tuning fork (to assess vibration); pinprick (to assess pain); and deep tendon reflexes (to assess the knee and ankle). In addition, assessment of joint position and motor power may be indicated. The normal range for the tuning fork on the dorsal distal joint of the great toe is ≥5/8 scale units in persons 21 to 40 years old, ≥4.5/8 in those 41 to 60 years old, ≥4/8 in individuals 61 to 71 years old, and ≥3.5/8 in those 72 to 82 years old.[65]

The following findings should alert healthcare providers to consider causes for DSPN other than diabetes and referral for a detailed neurological workup: (1) pronounced asymmetry of the neurological deficits; (2) predominant motor deficits, mononeuropathy, or cranial nerve involvement; (3) rapid development or progression of the neuropathic impairments; (4) progression of the neuropathy despite optimal glycemic control; (5) symptoms from the upper limbs; (6) family history of nondiabetic neuropathy; and (7) diagnosis of DSPN cannot be ascertained by clinical examination.[66]

Subtypes of DSPN

Rapidly Reversible Hyperglycemic Neuropathy

Reversible abnormalities of nerve function with distal sensory symptoms may occur in persons with recently diagnosed or poorly controlled diabetes. These are unlikely to be caused by structural abnormalities, as recovery soon follows restoration of euglycemia.[17]

Rapidly reversible hyperglycemic neuropathy usually presents with distal sensory symptoms, and whether these abnormalities result in an increased risk of developing chronic neuropathies in the future remains unknown.[17,67]

Implications for Diabetes Education and Care

In people recently diagnosed with diabetes or those with poorly controlled diabetes, the opportunity exists to reverse neuropathy. A concerted effort to encourage the individual to achieve this goal by tight blood glucose control is essential. The individual must be advised and understand that the pain may get worse with initiation of glycemic control before it gets better. During the early phase of glycemic control, when the blood vessels are constricted, blood is shunted away from the damaged area, exacerbating the pain. Later, the body adapts by dilating the blood vessels and increasing the blood flow.

Acute Sensory Neuropathy

Acute sensory neuropathy (ASN) is a variant of chronic sensorimotor neuropathy that is characterized by severe pain, wasting, weight loss, depression, and in males, erectile dysfunction.[68] Patients report, especially in the feet, unremitting burning, deep pain, and hyperesthesia. Other symptoms include sharp, stabbing, or electric shock–like sensations in the lower limbs that appear more frequently during the night. Signs are usually absent with a relatively normal clinical examination, except for allodynia (interpretation of all stimuli as painful, even light touch). Occasionally, ankle reflexes are absent or reduced.[69] Acute sensory neuropathy is usually associated with

poor glycemic control but may also appear after rapid improvement of glycemia. It has been hypothesized that changes in blood glucose flux produce alterations in epineurial blood flow, leading to ischemia.[70] Other authors propose an immune-mediated mechanism.[56]

Implications for Diabetes Education and Care

The key to management of ASN is achieving blood glucose stability.[30] Most patients also require medication for neuropathic pain.[71] The natural history of this disease is resolution of symptoms within 1 year.[72]

Chronic Sensorimotor Neuropathy

Chronic sensorimotor neuropathy (also referred to as distal diabetic polyneuropathy or distal symmetric polyneuropathy) is the most common form of diffuse neuropathy in diabetes. Chronic sensorimotor neuropathy primarily involves the sensory nerves. Sensory symptoms are more prominent than motor symptoms and usually involve the lower limbs. Symptoms include pain, paresthesia, hyperesthesia, deep aching, and burning and sharp stabbing sensations similar to but less severe than those described in ASN. In addition, patients may experience negative symptoms such as numbness in the feet and legs, leading in time to painless foot ulcers and subsequent amputations if the neuropathy is not promptly recognized and treated. Unsteadiness is also frequently seen due to abnormal proprioception and muscle sensory function.[73,74] Alternatively, some patients may be completely asymptomatic and signs may be discovered only by a detailed neurological examination.

Sensory deficits occur in the distal portions of the limbs, spreading over time from the toes to the legs and then from the fingers to the arms in a "stocking-glove" pattern, involving small nerve fibers, large nerve fibers, or both. Distal symmetric polyneuropathy is frequently accompanied by AN. All patients with DSP are at increased risk of neuropathic complications such as foot ulceration and Charcot neuroarthropathy (see Figure 28.2).

Small-Nerve-Fiber Neuropathy

Small-nerve-fiber neuropathy often presents with pain, but without objective signs or electrophysiologic evidence of nerve damage. Table 28.5 lists clinical manifestations of small-fiber neuropathies.

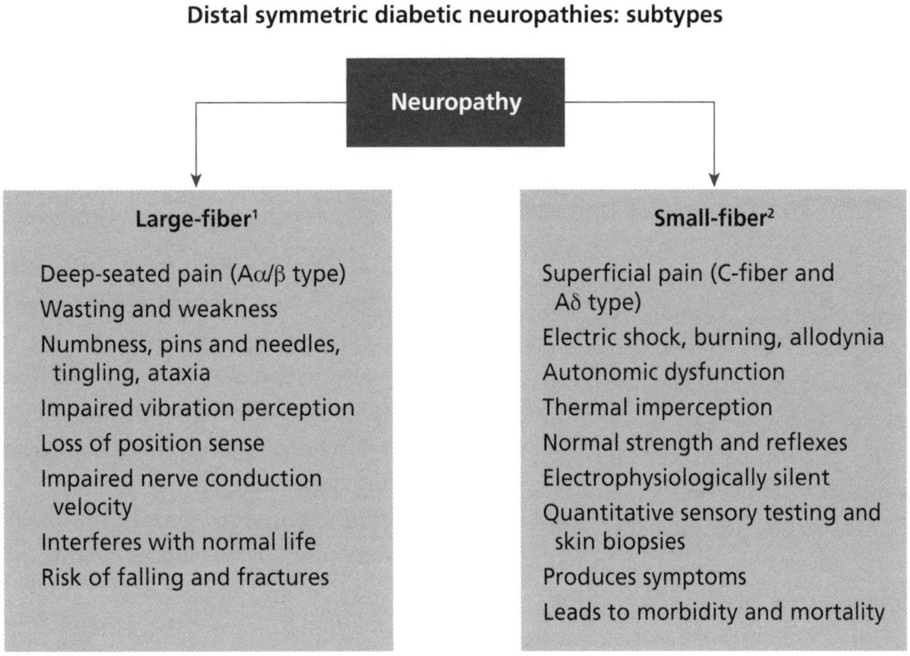

Distal symmetric diabetic neuropathies: subtypes

Neuropathy

Large-fiber[1]

Deep-seated pain (Aα/β type)

Wasting and weakness

Numbness, pins and needles, tingling, ataxia

Impaired vibration perception

Loss of position sense

Impaired nerve conduction velocity

Interferes with normal life

Risk of falling and fractures

Small-fiber[2]

Superficial pain (C-fiber and Aδ type)

Electric shock, burning, allodynia

Autonomic dysfunction

Thermal imperception

Normal strength and reflexes

Electrophysiologically silent

Quantitative sensory testing and skin biopsies

Produces symptoms

Leads to morbidity and mortality

FIGURE 28.2   **Clinical Presentation of Small- and Large-Fiber Neuropathies**

[1]Aα fibers are large myelinated fibers that are in charge of motor functions and muscle control. Aα/β fibers are also large myelinated fibers too, with sensory functions such as perception to touch, vibration, and position.

[2]Aδ fibers are small myelinated fibers responsible for pain stimuli and cold perception. Small C-fibers can be myelinated or unmyelinated and have both sensory (warm perception and pain) and autonomic functions (blood pressure and heart rate regulation, sweating, gastrointestinal tract and genitourinary tract).

Source: Modified from original diagram by A Vinik, C Casellini, A Nakave, C Patel, "Diabetic neuropathies," edited by R Rushakoff. On the Internet at: http://diabetesmanager.pbworks.com/w/page/17680180/Diabetic%20Neuropathies.

TABLE 28.5   **Small-Fiber Neuropathies: Clinical Manifestations**
Small, thinly myelinated Aδ and unmyelinated C fibers are affected
Symptoms are prominent; pain is the C-fiber type: burning, superficial, and associated with allodynia (interpretation of all stimuli—ie, touch—as painful)
Late in the condition, progression to numbness and hypoalgesia (lack of sensation)
Abnormal cold and warm thermal sensation
Defective autonomic function with decreased sweating; dry skin; impaired vasomotion; the vascular responses to vasoconstrictive and vasodilative stimuli, whose net effect acts on blood flow; and the presentation of a cold foot
Reflexes and motor strength are remarkably intact
Nerve conduction velocity studies show no deficit
Loss of cutaneous nerve fibers is shown on skin biopsies using PGP 9.5 staining
Diagnosed clinically by reduced sensitivity to 1-g SWM and pricking sensation using the Wartenberg wheel or similar instrument*
Abnormalities in thresholds for warm thermal perception, neurovascular function, pain, quantitative sudorimetry, and quantitative autonomic function tests
Risk is foot ulceration, subsequent gangrene, and amputation

*Source: AJ Boulton, RA Malik, JC Arezzo, JM Sosenko, "Diabetic somatic neuropathies," *Diabetes Care* 27 (2004): 1458-86.

Ulceration, Gangrene, and Amputation Are Risks With Small-Fiber Neuropathy

With small-fiber neuropathy, the greatest risk is for foot ulceration and subsequent gangrene and amputation.

As previously mentioned, small, unmyelinated nerve fibers are affected early in diabetes and are not reflected in NCV studies. Other methods that do not depend on conduction, such as QST or skin biopsy with quantification of IENFs, are necessary to identify these cases.[56] However, NCV plays a key role in ruling out other causes of neuropathy and is essential for the identification of focal neuropathies and entrapments as well as multifocal neuropathies.[17,54] Also, as mentioned, the importance of the skin biopsy as a diagnostic tool for chronic sensorimotor neuropathy is increasingly being recognized.[36–38]

Pain Mechanism in Small-Fiber Neuropathy

The mechanism for pain in small-fiber neuropathy is not well understood.[75] Hyperglycemia may be a factor in lowering the pain threshold. A striking amelioration of symptoms with the intravenous administration of insulin can be achieved.[76] Disappearance of pain may not necessarily reflect nerve recovery but rather nerve death. When patients volunteer the loss of pain, progression of the neuropathy must be excluded by careful examination.

Implications for Diabetes Education and Care

A comprehensive clinical examination is key to the diagnosis of chronic sensorimotor neuropathy. Examine feet in detail to detect ulcers, calluses, and deformities, and inspect footwear at every visit. Check shoes for stones, buttons, or other loose items that are potentially harmful to insensate feet. All persons with chronic sensorimotor neuropathy are at increased risk of foot ulceration and Charcot neuroarthropathy.

Large-Nerve-Fiber Neuropathies

Large-nerve-fiber neuropathies may involve sensory and/or motor nerves. These tend to be the neuropathies of *signs*, with a lesser degree of *symptoms*. Large fibers mediate motor function, vibration perception, position sense, and cold thermal perception. Unlike the small-nerve fibers, these myelinated, rapidly conducting fibers begin in the toes and have their first synapse in the medulla oblongata. (Myelin is a fatlike substance that forms a sheath around certain nerve fibers.) These fibers tend to be affected first because of their length and the tendency in diabetes for nerves to "die back." Because they are myelinated, they are the fibers represented in the electrophysiologic nerve conduction studies, and subclinical abnormalities in nerve function are readily detected.

The symptoms may be minimal: sensation of walking on cotton, floors feeling strange, or the inability to turn the pages of a book or to discriminate among coins. Large-nerve-fiber neuropathy produces numbness, ataxia, and incoordination, impairing daily living activities and causing falls and fractures.[36] See Table 28.6 for clinical manifestations of large-fiber neuropathies.

TABLE 28.6   Large-Fiber Neuropathies: Clinical Manifestations

Large myelinated Aα/β fibers are affected and may involve sensory and/or motor nerves

Impaired vibration perception and position sense are often the first objective evidence

Abnormal tendon reflexes

Pain is described as deep-seated gnawing, dull, a "toothache" in the bones of the feet, or crushing or cramplike pain (called type A-d nerve fibers)

Sensation of walking on cotton, floors feeling strange, inability to turn pages of a book or to discriminate among coins

Sensory ataxia (waddling like a duck)

Wasting of small muscles of feet with hammertoes

Weakness of hands and feet

Shortening of the Achilles tendon with pes equines (horses' foot)

Increased blood flow (hot foot)

Higher risk of falls, fractures, and development of Charcot neuroarthropathy

Most patients have a mixture of large- and small-nerve-fiber involvement

The Diagnosis of Neuropathic Pain

The diagnosis of neuropathic pain—as opposed to pain from causes other than neuropathy—is made by careful history taking. Patients should be queried at the time of an office visit as to whether they are experiencing tingling, burning, or pain at rest in their feet. A positive response warrants further investigation and screening for painful diabetic peripheral neuropathy (PDPN). Somatosensory, motor, or autonomic bedside evaluation can be done and is complemented by use of one of the pain screening tools (DN4, Pain DETECT, etc).[77] The physician should ensure that all the features of pain, such as distribution, quality, severity, timing, associated symptoms, and exacerbating and relieving factors (if any), are recorded. In particular, the presence of numbness, burning, tingling, lightning pain, stabbing, and prickling should be recorded, as is done in the Norfolk QOL tool,[78] the Neuropathy Total Symptom Score-6 (NTSS-6) questionnaire,[79] and the Pain DETECT.[77] Pain intensity and quality should be assessed using pain intensity scales (Visual Analogue Scale or a numerical rating scale)[80] and pain questionnaires (Brief Pain Inventory [BPI] and the Neuropathic Pain Symptom Inventory [NPSI]). A number of tools and questionnaires have been developed to quantify the impact of pain on sleep, on mood, and on QOL, mainly to be used in clinical trials. In clinical practice, the BPI Interference, the Profile of Moods, or the hospital scale for anxiety and depression (HADS) can provide a simple measure of the impact of pain on QOL. Responses to treatment by self-reporting using a diary can record the course of painful symptoms and their impact on daily life.[81] These questionnaires, pain inventories, and self-reporting diaries are also most useful for outcome measures in clinical trials on drugs used for pain relief. Validated scoring systems for symptoms and signs are available in the form of questionnaires or checklists, such as the Neuropathy Symptom Score and the Michigan Neuropathy Screening Instrument Questionnaire for symptoms, and the Michigan Neuropathy Screening Instrument and the Neuropathy Disability Score for signs.[20,82]

Definition of Neuropathic Pain

A definition of peripheral neuropathic pain in diabetes, adapted from a definition proposed by the International Association for the Study of Pain,[83] is "pain arising as a direct consequence of abnormalities in the peripheral somatosensory system in people with diabetes" (p. 2286)[7] A grading system for the degree of certainty of the diagnosis of neuropathic pain has been proposed. It is based on 4 simple criteria, namely,

1. whether the pain has a distinct neuroanatomical distribution,
2. whether the history of the patient suggests the presence or absence of a lesion or disease of the peripheral or central somatosensory system,
3. whether either of these findings is supported by at least one confirmatory test, and
4. whether there is an abnormality of nerve conduction.[83]

Degree of certainty is defined according to the number of criteria met: 1 to 4 (definite neuropathic pain), 1 and 2 plus 3 or 4 (probable neuropathic pain), or only 1 and 2 (possible neuropathic pain). There is no consensus on their diagnostic validity, since neuropathic pain is a composite of pain and other sensory symptoms associated with nerve injury. For example, sensory deficits, abnormal spontaneous or induced sensations such as paresthesias (eg, tingling), spontaneous attacks of electric shock–like sensations, and allodynia preclude a simple definition (see below).

Distinction Between Nociceptive and Non-nociceptive Pain

Because of its complexity, the presentation of pain poses a diagnostic dilemma for the clinician who needs to distinguish between neuropathic non-nociceptive pain arising as a direct consequence of a lesion or disease of the somatosensory system and nociceptive pain that is due to trauma, inflammation, or injury. It is imperative to try to establish the nature of any predisposing factor, including the pathogenesis of the pain, if one is to be successful in its management. Patients are encouraged to find solutions, using targeted pain-centered strategies such as biofeedback and positive diversions rather than prescription drugs approved for general pain, which do not address the disease process. The inciting injury may be focal or diffuse and may involve single or, more likely, multiple mechanisms such as metabolic disturbances encompassing hyperglycemia, dyslipidemia, glucose fluctuations, or intensification of therapy with insulin. On the other hand, the injury might embrace autoimmune mechanisms, neurovascular insufficiency, deficient neurotrophism, oxidative and nitrosative stress, and inflammation.[71,84] Because pain syndromes in diabetes may be focal or diffuse, proximal or distal, acute or chronic, each has its own pathogenesis, and the treatment must be tailored to the underlying disorder if the outcome is to be successful. The presence of diabetes must be established, if this has not already been done.

A number of self-administered questionnaires have been developed, validated, translated, and subjected to cross-cultural adaptation to both diagnose and distinguish neuropathic as opposed to non-neuropathic pain: Leeds Assessment of Neuropathic Symptoms and Signs (LANSS) Pain Scale, Douleur Neuropathique en 4 questions (DN4), Neuropathic Pain Questionnaire (NPS), Pain DETECT, and ID-Pain.[79,85–90] Assessment questionnaires such as the Short-Form McGill Pain Questionnaire, the BPI, and the Neuropathic Pain Symptom Inventory (NPSI) assess pain quality and intensity (III/B).[85,91,92]

According to IMMPACT (Initiative on Methods, Measurement and Pain Assessment in Clinical Trials), the following pain characteristics should be evaluated to assess the efficacy and effectiveness of chronic pain treatment[93]:

1. pain intensity measured on a 0 to 10 numerical rating scale (NRS);
2. physical functioning, assessed by the Multidimensional Pain Inventory (MPI) and Brief Pain Inventory (BPI) Interferences scale;
3. emotional functioning, assessed by the Beck Depression Inventory (BDI) and Profile of Mood States; and
4. patient rating of overall improvement, assessed by the Patient Global Impression of Change (PGI-C)

Laboratory Tests to Evaluate Neuropathic Pain

Since neuropathic pain is subjective, no tests can objectively quantify this pain in humans. Tests of pain in animal studies are really measures of reaction time to heat or other stimuli, which is one of the reasons for failure of translation of animal studies to man. Thus, laboratory tests do not reflect spontaneous pain but rather the function of the nociceptive system and, ultimately, with QST, the evoked positive sensory phenomena associated with neuropathic pain (ie, hyperalgesia and allodynia). This means that the results of laboratory tests become useful only in the context of a comprehensive clinical examination. Other tests were discussed earlier in the chapter.

Evaluation of pain intensity is essential for monitoring the response to therapy. There are a number of symptom-based screening tools, such as the NTSS-6, BPI, QOL-DN, SF-36 Health Survey (a short-form, 36-question health survey), Visual Analog Scale for Pain Intensity, NeuroQol, and Norfolk Neuropathy Symptoms Score. With the visual analog scale, the patient marks the intensity of his or her pain on a scale from 0 to 10, allowing an assessment of the response to intervention. Simultaneously, the patient should complete a QOL tool, such as the Norfolk QOL-DN, which needs to include comorbidities such as anxiety, depression, and sleep interference.

Pharmacologic Therapeutic Modalities for Diabetic Neuropathic Pain

Treatment Based on Pathogenic Concepts of Pain

Painful symptoms in DSPN may constitute a considerable management problem. The efficacy of a single therapeutic agent is not the rule, and simple analgesics are usually inadequate to control the pain. There is agreement that patients should be offered the available therapies in a stepwise fashion.[94–97] Effective pain treatment considers a favorable balance between pain relief and side effects without implying a maximum effect. The following general considerations in the pharmacotherapy of neuropathic pain require attention:

◆ The appropriate and effective drug has to be tried and identified in each patient by carefully titrating the dose based on efficacy and side effects.
◆ Lack of efficacy should be judged only after 2 to 4 weeks of treatment using an adequate dose.

♦ Because the evidence from clinical trials suggests only a maximum response of ≈50% for any monotherapy, analgesic combinations may be useful.

♦ Potential drug interactions have to be considered given the frequent use of polypharmacy in persons with diabetes.

Two drugs have been approved in the United States for neuropathic pain: pregabalin and duloxetine. A recent meta-analysis in which duloxetine was indirectly compared with pregabalin and gabapentin for the treatment of PDPN concluded that these 2 drugs have comparable efficacy and tolerability.[98] Some studies have analyzed healthcare costs in persons with PDPN treated with pregabalin, duloxetine, or other usually used drugs. In general, all studies showed similar results, with a good cost-effective profile for both drugs.[99–101]

Guard Against Amputation

Recent statistics show that diabetes/foot-care education has proved effective in preventing amputations. Unfortunately, this type of education is not universally accessible and patients still need to be reminded to take care of their feet.

Implications for Diabetes Education and Care

Reinforce information and instruction on foot care so patients routinely inspect and attend to problems affecting their feet. Address the goal of management and prevention of foot complications with patient education and self-management skills. Encourage preventive strategies to emphasize the following:

♦ Proper care of nails, calluses, and injuries
♦ Proper-fitting footwear
♦ Daily inspection of feet and shoes
♦ Follow-up care as recommended
♦ In special populations, such as the visually impaired, the educator should encourage patients to have a family member check their feet once a day if possible, or at least once a week
♦ A visit to the podiatrist for care of nails and to check for calluses and ulcers
♦ Cushioned shoes that fit well and thick, padded socks
♦ Proper cleaning and drying of feet

Combinations of Large- and Small-Fiber Damage

Most patients with chronic sensorimotor neuropathy have a "mixed" variety of neuropathy, with both large-nerve-fiber and small-nerve-fiber damage. Early in the course of the neuropathic process, multifocal sensory loss might also be found. In some individuals, severe distal muscle weakness can accompany the sensory loss, resulting in an inability to stand on the toes or heels. Some grading systems use this as a definition of severity.

Implications for Diabetes Education and Care

Severe weakness is rare and, if present, should raise the question of a possible nondiabetic neuropathy, such as Gullain-Barré syndrome, chronic inflammatory demyelinating polyneuropathy, or monoclonal gammopathies.[13,17,32] Another important point is that chronic sensorimotor neuropathy is frequently accompanied by DAN, which is easily determined by the methods discussed below.

Risk of Falling

There is a heightened awareness of the risk of falling in an older population of people with type 2 diabetes, most of whom show evidence of at least mild to moderate neuropathy as defined by the 1989 San Antonio criteria (2 or more of the following: abnormal signs and symptoms, nerve conduction testing, autonomic function testing, and QST). It would certainly be remiss to exclude this important issue from a chapter on neuropathy.

The normal aging process is associated with an increased risk of falling, fall-related injury, and subsequent loss of functional ability. For older individuals, the chance of falling and injury generally increases if they also develop age-related diseases like type 2 diabetes, often exhibiting greater impairments in balance and altered gait dynamics compared with healthy individuals of a similar age.[102–104] It has been suggested that the risk of falling for older individuals with diabetes is increased because they need to compensate for age as well as disease-related factors that can impact their balance and stability. Age-related physiological changes that potentially affect balance include loss of lower limb muscle strength and power, changes in muscle function, and slower reaction times.[105,106] The person with diabetes also has to compensate for disease processes like DN, with its confounding factors such as proximal muscle weakness and loss of proprioception, as well as the effects of hypoglycemia, which contribute to a loss of stability and balance. Additionally, the person with diabetes is also being treated for hypertension, hyperlipidemia, cardiac disease, and depression. These are additional risk factors for unsteadiness, loss of balance, and falls, and so are the medications used to treat them.[107] Reduced physical activity with aging is a common factor related to the decline in postural stability and is also linked to an increased risk in falls.[102,107,108] It is also well known that the normal process of aging is often associated with a slower speed of cognitive processing (as measured by increased reaction time,[109,110] slower postural reactions,[107,111] and decreased strength and muscle function[112]; all are essential factors for optimal balance control[108]).

The benefits of strength and endurance training on gait, balance, and fall risk have been well established for older, healthy individuals,[112,113] but this approach has now been shown to apply to older individuals with type 2 diabetes.[114] Unfortunately, many older individuals tend to exhibit slower reaction times.[108,109] This slowness in movement responses translates to balance tasks where older individuals at increased risk of falling also respond more slowly to changes in posture.

A recent study in Virginia[108] found that a low-intensity exercise intervention in older individuals with diabetes resulted in a reduction in the risk of falls, with concurrent improvement in a number of physiological and postural assessments. The researchers showed that effective interventions can be easily implemented in this high-risk population to prevent or lower the risk of falls. By following a basic exercise program, a high-risk group demonstrated improved balance, increased lower limb strength, improvements in proprioceptive function, faster reaction times, and, consequently, decreased risk of falling. The results of this study lend strong support for the practice of prescribing supervised exercise, gait, and balance training to older individuals with type 2 diabetes to alleviate some of the risk factors associated with falls.

Implications for Diabetes Education and Care

In general, an exercise program geared toward improving strength, gait, and balance can result in improvements in a range of risk factors for falls, impacting positively on sensory, motor, and cognitive processes. The ability to respond quickly and appropriately to any external perturbation is an essential component for correcting oneself to avoid a possible fall.[111,115]

As with patients entering any exercise program, following guidelines and adhering to caveats are imperative.

- Check feet for ulcers, cuts, sores, or blisters; previous amputations of toes; or partial foot.
- Test sensation in the feet using a monofilament or tuning fork.
- Check that shoes selected for exercise fit well, provide support, and are cushioned.
- Test blood pressure from a lying to a standing position. If blood pressure falls, the patient may have autonomic dysfunction. Refer to physical therapist for training (with caution), using compensatory exercise.
- Test for abnormal cardiovascular response to exercise (refer to section on autonomic neuropathy in this chapter for more information).
- Test whether patient is able to stand on 1 leg for 3 seconds (if not, caution experienced trainer to modify exercise appropriately).
- Test whether patient is able to get up from a chair with no supporting arms (if not, reinforce the need to deal with this deficit and suggest gentle building of gluteus muscles in addition to supervised gait and balance training).
- Encourage helpful interventions such as a cane or walker to patients with balance and gait problems.
- Encourage the use of nonslip bath and shower mats. Recommend that all unattached floor rugs, which may be hazardous for tripping and falling, be removed from the home.
- Check visual and auditory acuity. Deficits in these functions are risk factors for many types of possible accidents.

Caveats for Exercise

Autonomic dysfunction impairs exercise tolerance, reduces response in heart rate and blood pressure, and blunts increases in cardiac output in response to exercise.

Persons with diabetes who are likely to have CAN should be tested for cardiac stress before undertaking an exercise program. Persons with CAN need to rely on their perceived exertion, not heart rate, to avoid hazardous levels of intensity of exercise.[116,117] Presently, there is inadequate evidence to recommend routine screening of asymptomatic persons with diabetes with an exercise EKG test. Emerging data support the futility of stress imaging testing in identifying persons with diabetes with preclinical coronary artery disease, particularly those individuals with high-risk features and comorbidities, such as long-standing disease, CAN, multiple chronic renal failures, resting ECG abnormalities, and peripheral artery disease. Rather, a simple bedside evaluation of heart rate variability (HRV) in response to a Valsalva maneuver has the greatest sensitivity of predicting a major adverse cardiovascular event.[118]

Autonomic Neuropathy

Autonomic neuropathy (AN) is often referred to in the diabetic population as diabetic autonomic neuropathy (DAN).

Autonomic neuropathy significantly impacts survival and QOL:

- Although serious and common, AN (or DAN) is among the least recognized and poorly understood complications of diabetes.[119]
- The reported prevalence of AN varies widely (7.7%-90.0%), depending on the study population and methods used for diagnosis.[120,121]
- Autonomic dysfunction has recently been shown to be a predictor of cardiovascular dysfunction.[51,52]

The ANS supplies all organs in the body and consists of an afferent system and an efferent system, involving both the parasympathetic and the sympathetic nervous systems. Autonomic neuropathy may involve any system in the body. Involvement of the ANS can occur as early as the first year after diagnosis, and major manifestations are cardiovascular, gastrointestinal, and genitourinary system dysfunction.[58,122]

Disturbances in the ANS may be *functional* (eg, gastroparesis with hyperglycemia and ketoacidosis) or

organic, wherein nerve fibers are actually lost. This creates great difficulty in diagnosing and treating as well as establishing true prevalence rates. Many conditions affect the ANS (AN is not unique to diabetes); thus, the diagnosis of DAN rests with excluding other causes. Subclinical involvement may be widespread, whereas clinical symptoms and signs may be focused within a single organ.

Symptoms

The following are some common symptoms of AN:

- Reduced exercise tolerance
- Edema
- Paradoxical supine or nocturnal hypertension
- Intolerance to heat (due to defective thermoregulation)
- Gastrointestinal and genitourinary dysfunction

Table 28.7 lists the most common clinical features, diagnostic methods, and treatment options for AN.

Cardiac Autonomic Neuropathy

Cardiovascular dysfunction is associated with abnormalities in heart rate control and vascular dynamics. Parasympathetic nerves slow the heart rate, and sympathetic nerves increase the speed and force of heart contractions and stimulate the vascular tree to increase the blood pressure. The Consensus Panel on Diabetic Neuropathy, after extensive review of the literature, recently concluded that the prevalence of confirmed CAN in unselected people with type 1 diabetes or type 2 diabetes is approximately 20%, but it can be as high as 65% with increasing age and diabetes duration. Clinical correlates or risk markers for CAN are age, diabetes duration, glycemic control, microvascular complications (peripheral polyneuropathy, retinopathy, and nephropathy), hypertension, and dyslipidemia. Established risk factors for CAN are glycemic control in type 1 diabetes, and a combination of hypertension, dyslipidemia, obesity, and glycemic control in type 2 diabetes.[123]

Additional factors that have emerged as identifying susceptibility to cardiovascular events with intensification of glycemic control include duration of diabetes 12 to 15 years, impaired renal function, coronary artery calcification, a previous cardiovascular

TABLE 28.7 AN: Clinical Features, Diagnosis, and Treatment		
Symptoms	*Tests*	*Treatments*
Cardiac		
Resting tachycardia, exercise intolerance	HRV, MUGA thallium scan, MIBG scan	Graded supervised exercise, ACE inhibitors, β-blockers
Postural hypotension, dizziness, weakness, fatigue, syncope	HRV, supine and standing BP, catecholamines	Mechanical measures, clonidine, midodrine, octreotide, erythropoietin
Gastrointestinal		
Gastroparesis, erratic glucose control	Gastric emptying study, barium study	Frequent small meals, prokinetic agents (metoclopramide, domperidone, erythromycin)
Abdominal pain, early satiety, nausea, vomiting, bloating, belching	Endoscopy, manometry, electrogastrogram	Antibiotics, antiemetics, bulking agents, tricyclic antidepressants, pyloric botox, gastric pacing
Constipation	Endoscopy	High-fiber diet and bulking agents, osmotic laxatives, lubricating agents
Diarrhea (often nocturnal, alternating with constipation)	None	Soluble dietary fiber, gluten and lactose restriction, anticholinergic agents, cholestyramine, antibiotics, somatostatin, pancreatic enzyme supplements
Sexual Dysfunction		
Erectile dysfunction	H&P, HRV, penile-brachial pressure index, nocturnal penile tumescence	Sex therapy; psychological counseling; 5′-phosphodiesterase inhibitors; PG E1 injections, devices, or prostheses
Vaginal dryness	None	Vaginal lubricants
Bladder Dysfunction		
Frequency, urgency, nocturia, urinary retention, incontinence	Cystometrogram, postvoiding sonography	Bethanechol, intermittent catheterization
Sudomotor Dysfunction		
Anhidrosis, heat intolerance, dry skin, hyperhidrosis	Quantitative sudomotor axon reflex, sweat test, skin blood flow	Emollients and skin lubricants, scopolamine, glycopyrrolate, botulinum toxin, vasodilators
Pupillomotor and Visceral Dysfunction		
Visual blurring, impaired adaptation to ambient light, Argyll-Robertson pupil	Pupillometry, HRV	Care with driving at night
Impaired visceral sensation: silent myocardial infarction, hypoglycemia unawareness		Recognition of unusual presentation of myocardial infarction, control of risk factors, control of plasma glucose levels

Abbreviations: ACE, angiotensin-converting enzyme; BP, blood pressure; H&P, history and physical examination; HRV, heart rate variability; MI, myocardial infarction; MIBG, metaiodobenzylguanidine; MUGA, multigated angiography; PG, prostaglandin

Source: Copyright © 2005 American Diabetes Association. Adapted with permission from AJ Boulton, A Vinik, J Arezzo, et al, "Diabetic neuropathies (position statement)," *Diabetes Care* 28, no. 4 (2005): 956-62.

event, being African American, being female, a history of neuropathy or numb feet, and loss in HRV.[4,124,125]

The Cardiovascular Autonomic Neuropathy Subcommittee of the Toronto Consensus Panel on Diabetic Neuropathy recommends CAN screening to all asymptomatic persons with type 2 diabetes at diagnosis and all persons with type 1 diabetes after 5 years of disease—in particular, those at greater risk for CAN because of a history of poor glycemic control (hemoglobin A1C >7%), or the presence of 1 major cardiovascular risk factor (hypertension, dyslipidemia, or smoking), or the presence of macro- or microangiopathic complications (level of evidence B).

The subcommittee also suggested that CAN screening might be required in asymptomatic patients for preoperative risk assessment before major surgical procedures (level of evidence C).[123]

Morbidity and Mortality in CAN

Cardiac autonomic neuropathy is a significant cause of morbidity and mortality and is associated with a high risk of cardiac arrhythmias and sudden death, possibly related to silent myocardial ischemia. Cardiovascular disease remains the main cause of excess mortality among persons with type 1 diabetes or type 2 diabetes. Reduced HRV as a marker of autonomic dysfunction has been shown to have dire consequences in terms of morbidity. The first sign of cardiac impairment is usually resting tachycardia. The 3 major associated syndromes are the following[126]:

◆ Cardiac denervation syndrome
◆ Abnormal cardiovascular response to exercise
◆ Orthostatic (postural) hypotension

Cardiac Denervation Syndrome

Cardiac denervation is defined as a fixed heart rate that does not change in response to stress, exercise, breathing patterns, or sleep. This syndrome results from both parasympathetic and sympathetic system impairment. Initially, parasympathetic tone decreases, which causes a relative increase in sympathetic tone and an increase in heart rate. Progressive impairment of sympathetic tone causes a gradual slowing of the heart. Over time, both parasympathetic and sympathetic tone become impaired.[24] Initially, a fixed heart rate of 100 to 120 beats per minute is common. In the later stages, the fixed heart rate will be in the range of 80 to 100 beats per minute. The heart

rate is unresponsive to stress, exercise, or tilting.[103,104] In the later stages, the person may suffer myocardial ischemia or myocardial infarction (MI) without experiencing pain. The resulting delay or failure to seek treatment contributes to increasing mortality rates. These persons are also at risk for cardiac arrhythmias and sudden death.[24]

Diagnostic Tests Methods of CAN assessment in clinical practice include assessment of symptoms and signs, cardiovascular autonomic reflex tests based on heart rate and blood pressure, and ambulatory blood pressure monitoring.[123]

Cardiovascular autonomic reflex tests assess cardiovascular autonomic function through time-domain heart rate response to deep breathing, Valsalva maneuver, and postural change and by measuring the end-organ response, that is, heart rate and blood pressure changes. Although indirect autonomic measures, they are considered the gold standard in autonomic testing. Heart rate variations during deep breathing, Valsalva maneuver, and lying-to-standing (heart rate tests) are indices mainly of parasympathetic function, whereas the orthostatic hypotension, the blood pressure response to a Valsalva maneuver, and sustained isometric muscular strain provide indices of sympathetic function. These tests are noninvasive, safe, clinically relevant (they correlate with tests of peripheral nervous system function), easy to carry out, sensitive, specific, reproducible, and standardized, and therefore they are considered consolidated gold-standard measures of autonomic function.

There is now strong evidence of inflammation with activation of inflammatory cytokines in persons with diabetes. These changes correlate with abnormalities in sympathetic-vagal balance. Several investigations have shown the neuroregulatory role for the ANS being a key instrument in the inflammatory process.

Patients suffer from severe orthostasis, postural hypotension, exercise intolerance, enhanced intraoperative instability, and an increased incidence of silent MI and ischemia. There are simple bedside tests to diagnose CAN using HRV, responses to breathing, the Valsalva maneuver, and standing. Functional abnormalities and imbalance between the sympathetic and parasympathetic nervous systems are discerned with respiratory modulation of different-frequency oscillations in HRV.

Several agents have become available for the correction of functional defects in the ANS. Restoration of autonomic balance is possible and has been shown with therapeutic lifestyle changes, increased physical activity, diabetes treatment, beta-adrenergic blockers, and potent antioxidants such as alpha-lipoic acid. There are exciting new prospects for pathogenesis-oriented intervention.

Implications for Diabetes Education and Care
Teach patients with cardiac denervation syndrome to avoid heavy exercise, aerobic exercise, and straining themselves. Stress testing is a requirement before initiating any type of exercise program. In addition, these patients should be carefully evaluated prior to initiation of intensive insulin therapy because of the risk of hypoglycemia, which can result in cardiac arrhythmias.[24]

Abnormal Cardiovascular Response to Exercise

Some people with DAN may lose their normal increased cardiac output and vascular tone response to exercise and become hypotensive with aerobic activity.[24] If an individual becomes faint or dizzy while exercising, the individual's blood pressure should be checked immediately. If needed, provide therapy or seek an intervention by a healthcare provider.

Postural Hypotension

Blood pressure is normally maintained upon standing by a sympathetic reflex that increases the heart rate and by peripheral vascular resistance in association with an increase in norepinephrine levels. Orthostatic hypotension is defined as a drop in systolic blood pressure of more than 30 mm Hg or a diastolic drop of more than 10 mm Hg within 2 minutes of changing from a supine position to a standing position. This syndrome occurs late in diabetes and signals advanced autonomic impairment.

Orthostatic hypotension, which results from blood pooling in the feet, can occur without symptoms but is often accompanied by dizziness, light-headedness, weakness, visual impairment, or syncope.[24] This places the patient at risk for injury from falls. All persons with diabetes must have their blood pressure and pulse rates assessed in the lying, sitting, and standing positions. Symptomatic patients

should have this test at each office visit. Greater accuracy in the assessment can be achieved by having the patient rest in a supine position and then stand quietly while the blood pressure is measured at 1-minute intervals for 3 to 5 minutes.[24]

Treatment of symptoms involves raising the head of the bed 30° at night, increasing venous pressure with supportive elastic whole-body stockings (or stockings that go to at least the waist and are applied while the person is supine), and wearing an antigravity suit. Other therapies include correcting hypovolemia, midodrine, octreotide, and erythropoietin (refer to Table 28.7). Florinef is not recommended, because it usually causes hypertension and fluid retention before alleviating orthostasis.

Implications for Diabetes Education and Care
Patients should receive education on the proper application and use of elastic body stockings, which need to be waist high (knee- and thigh-high stockings that cut into the leg are hazardous, as they may restrict the blood supply). Patients should also receive instruction on rising slowly from a recumbent position. Graded, supervised exercise to improve strength and balance is recommended, as well as nutritional counseling on salt intake. Liberalize salt intake to >6 g per day. Silent MI, respiratory failure, amputations, and sudden death are hazards for persons with diabetes with CAN.[127,128] Therefore, it is imperative to make this diagnosis early so that appropriate intervention can be instituted.[129]

Treatment of the Underlying Cause of AN

Treatment of the underlying cause of AN can include management of the following:

- Hyperglycemia
- Lipids
- Blood pressure
- Use of antioxidants[121,130]
- Angiotensin-converting enzyme (ACE) inhibitors[131,132]

These treatments are designed to minimize the effects of hyperglycemia, dyslipidemia, hypertension, oxidative and nitrosative stress, and compromised nerve function.

Gastrointestinal Disorders Related to AN

If the nerves are affected by AN, gastric emptying of both liquids and solids may be delayed. Vagal nerve dysfunction is usually responsible for motility.

Upper Gastrointestinal Dysfunction

Most upper gastrointestinal dysfunction involves the esophagus, stomach, and upper small intestine. Symptoms of gastroparesis (delayed gastric emptying) can include heartburn, reflux, anorexia, early satiety, nausea, abdominal bloating, erratic blood glucose levels due to delayed absorption of food, and vomiting undigested food eaten several hours or days earlier.[133,134] Signs associated with gastroparesis include weight loss and a succussion splash (a splashing sound made during body movement) over the upper left quadrant of the abdomen, although delayed gastric emptying can also occur without symptoms.[133,134]

Diagnosis   A barium series of the upper gastrointestinal tract is useful to rule out obstruction. A solid-phase gastric emptying phase study is the most specific way to diagnose delayed gastric emptying.[112,113] Gastroscopy may be needed to exclude a bezoar. The blood glucose must be normal when the test is performed. The recommended blood glucose level for the test is <240 mg/dL. A blood glucose level >240 mg/dL impairs gastric emptying.

Implications for Diabetes Education and Care   Normalizing blood glucose levels may improve gastric emptying. The presence of gastroparesis complicates balancing insulin doses with food absorption. Frequent monitoring of pre- and postprandial blood glucose levels is required to detect hypoglycemia and hyperglycemia and determine the insulin dose. Rapid-acting insulin is probably not appropriate for some patients with gastroparesis, although some find it useful if taken after the meal.

Treatment includes the following:

- Referral to a dietitian for a low-fat, low-fiber diet
- Use of multiple small and mostly liquid meals eaten throughout the day
- Referral to a gastroenterologist
- Medications to decrease inhibition of gastric motility, such as metoclopramide (Reglan®,

ANI Pharmaceuticals [oral], Baxter Healthcare [injectable]), taken 30 minutes before all meals and snacks and at bedtime
- Other medications that increase the motility of the stomach, such as erythromycin or lubiprostone (Amatiza®, Sucampo Pharmaceuticals), may be useful
- In the most severe stages, jejunostomy tube feedings may be necessary
- Gastric pacing, botox injected into the pyloris, or phosphodiesterase inhibitors, such as sildenafil (Viagra®, Pfizer Inc), vardenafil HCl (Levitra®, Bayer), and tadalafil (Cialis®, Eli Lilly), which increase gastric nitric oxide

Lower Intestinal Tract Dysfunction

Lower intestinal tract dysfunction is the result of damage to the efferent autonomic nerves and leads to hypotonia and poor contraction of the smooth muscles to the gut, which results in constipation.

Constipation   Constipation is fairly common and has been reported in up to 60% of all persons with diabetes. Treatment involves increasing fiber in the diet while avoiding excess fiber (below the normal recommended daily dose*), judicious use of laxatives, adequate hydration, increased activity, stool softeners and bulk laxatives such as psyllium (Metamucil®, Procter and Gamble), and medications such as metoclopramide or neostigmine (Prostigmin®, Valeant Pharmaceuticals) to increase intestinal motility.[133,135]

Diarrhea can also occur as a result of both decreased small intestinal motility and hypermotility without bacterial overgrowth.[133,134] Although constipation is more common, diarrhea is usually more troublesome to patients. Diarrhea may be nocturnal, intermittent with constipation, and associated with fecal incontinence; it may occur without cramping or pain. Treatment involves the use of antibiotics (eg, tetracycline or metronidazole) to decrease the

---

*Normal dietary fiber guidelines are as follows:
- Females: 21 to 26 g per day
- Males: 30 to 38 g per day
- Progressively decrease the number of grams for males and females over the age of 50

The average American consumes only 14 g of fiber per day. The patient's regular fiber intake should be calculated and adjusted accordingly.

bacterial overgrowth. It is better to drive the bowel (eg, with metoclopramide or erythromycin) than to inhibit motility. Nonetheless, medications that may be useful for slowing intestinal motility are loperamide, codeine, diphenoxylate hydrochloride, or atropine sulfate. However, care should be exercised because they may aggravate the situation. Fiber and psyllium may increase stool bulk and consistency. In addition, some patients may benefit from biofeedback, relaxation, and bowel training. Early treatment of diarrhea may help prevent the development of incontinence.[133,134]

Implications for Diabetes Education and Care Include a discussion of how these symptoms are related to diabetes. Stress the need to inform providers of symptoms to allow for early detection and treatment. Explain with care diagnostic tests, test results, and therapies.

Sexual Dysfunction Related to AN

Sexual dysfunction is common among people with diabetes. As many as 75% of men and 35% of women experience sexual problems due to DN.[136] Male sexual dysfunction involves erectile dysfunction and retrograde ejaculation. Retrograde ejaculation is unusual and may respond to use of an antihistamine, desipramine, or phenylephrine.[137]

Male Sexual Dysfunction

Erectile dysfunction (ED) occurs in men with diabetes at an earlier age than in the general population. The incidence of ED in men with diabetes aged 20 to 29 years is 9% and increases to 95% by 70 years of age. Erectile dysfunction may be the presenting symptom of diabetes. More than 50% notice the onset of ED within 10 years of the diagnosis, but it may precede the other complications of diabetes. The etiology of ED in diabetes is multifactorial. Neuropathy, vascular disease, diabetes control, nutrition, endocrine disorders, and psychogenic factors as well as drugs used in the treatment of diabetes and its complications play a role.[136,137] Diagnosis of the cause of ED is made by a logical stepwise progression.[137,138]

Diagnostic Assessments Assessments should include a careful medical and sexual history; physical and psychological evaluations; blood test for diabetes and levels of testosterone, prolactin, and thyroid hormones; a test for nocturnal erections; and tests to assess penile, pelvic, and spinal nerve function, penile blood supply, and blood pressure. A simple test of autonomic function using HRV will exclude a neurologic cause of ED. A flowchart can assist in defining the problem.[136,137]

The healthcare provider must ask questions to help distinguish the various forms of organic ED from those that are psychogenic in origin. Physical examination must include an evaluation of the ANS, vascular supply, and hypothalamic-pituitary-gonadal axis.

Autonomic neuropathy causing ED is almost always accompanied by loss of ankle jerks and absence or reduction of vibration sense over the large toes. More direct evidence of impairment of penile autonomic function can be obtained by demonstrating normal perianal sensation, assessing the tone of the anal sphincter during a rectal exam, and ascertaining the presence of an anal wink. These measurements are easily and quickly done at the bedside and reflect the integrity of sacral parasympathetic divisions.

A test for nocturnal penile tumescence (NPT) distinguishes psychogenic from organic dysfunction. Normal NPT defines psychogenic ED, and a negative response to vasodilators implies vascular insufficiency. However, the NPT test is not so simple. It is much like having a sphygmomanometer cuff inflate over the penis many times during the night while the patient is trying to sleep.

Treatment of ED A number of treatment modalities are available, and each treatment has positive and negative effects. Therefore, patients must be made aware of both aspects before making a therapeutic decision. Before considering any form of treatment, every effort should be made to have the person withdraw from alcohol and eliminate smoking. If possible, the patient should be removed from drugs that are known to cause ED, and metabolic control should be optimized.

Research has revealed that the ability to have and maintain an erection depends on nitric oxide and cyclic guano monophosphate (cGMP). Agents such as sildenafil, vardenafil, and tadalafil exert their effect by increasing nitric oxide and cGMP levels that may be low in men with diabetes. Before any of these agents are prescribed, ischemic heart disease must be excluded. These medications are absolutely contraindicated in persons being treated with nitroglycerine or other nitrate-containing drugs. Severe hypotension and fatal cardiac events can occur.[139]

Direct injection of prostacylin into the corpus cavernosum will induce satisfactory erections in a significant number of men. Also, surgical implantation of a penile prosthesis may be appropriate. The less expensive type of prosthesis is a semirigid, permanently erect type that may be embarrassing and uncomfortable for some men. The inflatable type is 3 times more expensive and subject to mechanical failure, but it avoids the embarrassment caused by other devices.

Implications for Diabetes Education and Care   The advent of therapies such as sildenafil, vardenafil, and tadalafil has created a new era of openness regarding sexual issues. Current recommendations include continuous low-dose therapy rather than as-needed dosing. However, many patients may still be reticent about their sexual function. The diabetes educator should be aware that a problem may exist and alert the physician. When appropriate, including both sexual partners in selecting therapy is extremely important. Review all therapeutic options as well as their costs and benefits. Although these drugs facilitate erections, stimulation is also necessary. This should be explained to both partners.

Female Sexual Dysfunction

Women with diabetes mellitus may experience decreased sexual desire, difficulties in arousal, and pain during sexual intercourse. They also have decreased vaginal lubrication even if stimulated.[140] However, female sexual dysfunction, decreased vaginal lubrication, vaginal flushing, and delayed or absent orgasmic response need further assessment.

Sexual difficulties in women with diabetes that are not related to AN include loss of libido (possibly related to depression as a result of diabetes and its complications), hormonal fluctuations/menopause, and frequent occurrence of yeast and other vaginal infections.

Implications for Diabetes Education and Care   Diabetes educators need to address sexual concerns because these issues may be difficult for patients to discuss. Discuss sexual function, the potential for

diabetes-related problems, and the need to bring problems to the attention of providers. Offer to include patients' partners in the discussion and point out the importance of their inclusion in treatment decisions. Management includes application of estrogen or lubricating vaginal creams and referral to a gynecologist. Offer the patient and her partner referral for counseling with a sex therapist.

Bladder Dysfunction Related to AN

In AN, the motor function of the bladder is unimpaired, but afferent fiber damage results in diminished bladder sensation. Symptoms of a neurogenic bladder are usually insidious and progressive. In the early stages, the sensation of the need to void may be blunted. This infrequent urination may be misinterpreted as decreased polyuria due to improved blood glucose control. In later stages, difficulty in emptying the bladder, dribbling, and overflow incontinence may occur.[24] The urinary bladder can be enlarged to more than 3 times its normal size. Patients are seen with bladders filled to their umbilicus, yet they feel no discomfort. Loss of bladder sensation occurs with diminished voiding frequency, and the person is no longer able to void completely. An untreated neurogenic bladder often leads to urinary tract infections as a result of urinary stasis. These frequent infections may accelerate deterioration of renal function. More than 2 urinary tract infections per year among men and 3 among women indicate the need for further evaluation of bladder function.

Diagnosis

Bladder insensitivity is diagnosed by a cystometrogram. A post-voiding residual of greater than 150 cc confirms bladder dysfunction or cystopathy, which may put the patient at risk for urinary infections.

Treatment of Cystopathy

A patient with cystopathy should be instructed to palpate his or her bladder and, if unable to initiate micturition with a full bladder, use Crede's maneuver (massage or put pressure on the lower portion of the abdomen just above the pubic bone) to start the flow of urine. The principal aim of the treatment should be to improve bladder emptying and reduce the risk of urinary tract infection. Parasympathomimetics such as bethanechol are sometimes helpful, although frequently they do not help to completely empty the bladder. Extended sphincter relaxation can be achieved with an α_1-blocker such as doxazosin (Cardura®, Pfizer Inc). Self-catheterization can be particularly useful, with the risk of infection generally being low.

Implications for Diabetes Education and Care

Stress the need for frequent, complete urination; the signs and symptoms of urinary tract infections; and the importance of early treatment of infections. Teach patients to palpate for bladder fullness.

Sudomotor Dysfunction (Sweating Disturbances) Related to AN

Excessive perspiration (hyperhidrosis) of the upper body, often related to eating (gustatory sweating), and deficiency of sweat (anhidrosis) of the lower body are characteristic features of AN. Gustatory sweating accompanies the ingestion of certain foods, particularly spicy foods and cheeses. The administration of glycopyrrolate (antimuscarinic compound) has been suggested for persons with diabetes who experience gustatory sweating.[70] Symptomatic relief can be obtained by avoiding the specific food irritant.

Emphasize Foot Care

Loss of lower body sweating can cause dry, brittle skin that cracks easily, predisposing one to ulcer formation that can lead to limb loss. Alert patients to pay special attention to foot care, as many individuals do not recognize or treat problems.

Implications for Diabetes Education and Care

Patients rarely think to report abnormal sweating. However, this symptom is a red flag for the potential for heat stroke and foot ulcers. A careful history and examination of the feet for dryness and fissures are important to conduct at each visit.[24] Patient education should include inspection for fissures and lubrication for dry feet; avoidance of hot, spicy, or other offending foods; and prevention of hyperthermia and heat stroke.

Case: Complexities of AN

RK is a 36-year-old white nonobese man (height 5 ft 7 in, weight 142 lb) with a 15-year history of type 1 diabetes. His diabetes has been poorly controlled for many years on a regimen of a single dose of 35 units of 70/30 insulin per day without regular blood glucose monitoring. He has had repeated admissions to hospitals for diabetic ketoacidosis and has resisted attempts at intensification of treatment or improved monitoring.

Over the past few weeks, RK developed intractable burning pain in the feet, which he described as a "dog gnawing at the bones" and like having a "toothache in the feet." He found it unbearable to have his feet come into contact with the bedclothes, and putting on his shoes and socks in the morning was close to impossible. The pain was worse at night, and he was getting little sleep.

Symptoms

- Constantly tired, weak, apathetic, lethargic, and incapable of carrying out his normal daily activities

- Had become significantly depressed by the pain and was not eating well

- Felt bloated and full after eating only little bits of food, and occasionally vomited and could taste food on his breath that he had eaten maybe a day or two before

- Irregular bowels, varied from marked constipation to explosive diarrhea, with episodes sometimes so sudden and forceful he would soil himself

Physical Signs

- A lean individual who displayed signs of weakness

- Resting blood pressure: 80/64 mm Hg; heart rate: 96 beats per minute

- On standing, blood pressure fell to 50/40 mm Hg; heart rate did not change

- Background retinopathy

- No renal disease or clinical evidence of cardiovascular disease

Question to Consider

- What kind of neuropathy did RK have?

Research studies have shown defective blood flow in the small capillary circulation.[141–143] The clinical counterpart is dry, cold skin; loss of sweating; and development of fissures and cracks that are portals of entry for organisms leading to infectious ulcers and gangrene. This is an example of the value of research translating into clinical care. Awareness of the consequences of defective blood flow and education toward behaviors for preventing fissures and cracks can protect against the ravages of foot ulcers and gangrene.

Case—Part 2: Complexities of AN

Diagnosis

RK had clear evidence of mixed sensory motor polyneuropathy with AN. Which tests should be ordered?

The following tests were ordered, with results as noted:

- Gastroparesis: documented with a gastric emptying time of solid foods of 55 minutes (normal <17 minutes)

- Cholesterol: 132 mg/dL (normal 110-200 mg/dL), triglycerides: 101 mg/dL (normal 40-149 mg/dL), A1C: 11.5% (normal <6.05%)

- Urine protein: 500 mg (normal <250 mg for 24 hours), creatinine: 1.7 mg/dL (normal 0.5-1.2 mg/dL), BUN: 40 mg/dL (normal 6-22 mg/dL)

- Supine norepinephrine: 196 pg/mL, rising to 369 pg/mL after standing 15 minutes

- Resting cardiac ejection fraction: 61% (normal >60%), no increase with maximal exercise

- Resting heart rate: 100 beats per minute (normal 60-80 beats per minute)

- Beat-to-beat HRV: 12 beats per minute between deep inspiration; expiration E:I ratio: 1.01 (normal >1.3)

- Valsalva ratio: 1.06 (normal >1.10)

- Heart rate response to standing (the 30:15 ratio): 1.0 (normal >1.0)

- Orthostatic systolic pressure drop: 36 mm Hg (normal <30 mm Hg) and he became quite dizzy

Treatment

What would you suggest to help control RK's hyperglycemia?

- NPH insulin at bedtime was added to his medications at the time he was treated. Now, with choices of insulin therapy available, basal/bolus therapy to treat his hyperglycemia should be considered.

What about his painful neuropathy?

- Topical capsaicin 0.025% 4 times a day was suggested. Other medications to consider for painful neuropathy are gabapentin (Neurontin®, Pfizer Inc) and pregabalin.

How would you address the autonomic neuropathy?

What can be done for the orthostasis?

Is there anything that would improve gastric emptying?

This chapter's section on AN helps readers answer questions raised in this case.

Pupillomotor and Visceral (Metabolic) Response Related to AN

Abnormal Pupillary Response

The iris is innervated by both parasympathetic and sympathetic nerve fibers. Sympathetic nerve fibers cause the pupils to dilate and are generally more severely affected. Abnormal pupillary responses are related to duration of diabetes.[24] Slow dilation of pupils in response to darkness may be observed during clinical examination. Patients may report slow adaptation when entering a dark room.

Implications for Diabetes Education and Care

Stress using caution during night driving, the importance of turning on lights when entering a dark room, and using nightlights in darkened hallways and bathrooms to help prevent injuries.

Hypoglycemia Unawareness

Blood glucose concentration is normally maintained during starvation or increased insulin action by an asymptomatic parasympathetic response with bradycardia and mild hypotension, followed by a sympathetic response with glucagon and epinephrine secretion for short-term glucose counterregulation and growth hormone and cortisol in long-term regulation. The release of catecholamine alerts the person to take the required measures to prevent coma due to low blood glucose. The absence of warning signs of impending neuroglycopenia is known as "hypoglycemic unawareness." Failure of glucose counterregulation can be confirmed by the absence of glucagon and epinephrine responses to hypoglycemia that is induced by a standard, controlled dose of insulin.[144]

In persons with type 1 diabetes mellitus, the glucagon response is impaired with diabetes duration of 1 to 5 years, and after 14 to 31 years of diabetes, the glucagon response is almost undetectable. The glucagon response is not present in those with AN. However, a syndrome of hypoglycemic autonomic failure occurs with intensification of diabetes control and repeated episodes of hypoglycemia. The exact mechanism is not understood, but it does represent a real barrier to physiologic glycemic control. In the absence of severe autonomic dysfunction, hypoglycemic unawareness associated with hypoglycemia is at least partly reversible. It is important to reduce the previous target and goals and to set new levels.[145]

Patients with hypoglycemia unawareness and unresponsiveness pose a significant management problem for the healthcare team. Although AN may improve with intensive therapy and normalization of blood glucose, there is a risk to the patient, who may become hypoglycemic (without being aware of it) and be unable to mount a counterregulatory response. Following are some recommendations:

- In pump therapy, use boluses of smaller-than-calculated amounts, and in intensive conventional therapy, use long-acting insulin with very small boluses.
- In general, modify goals for glucose and A1C levels in these patients to avoid the possibility of hypoglycemia.[146]

Further complicating management for some patients is the development of a functional autonomic insufficiency associated with intensive insulin treatment, which resembles AN in all relevant aspects. In these instances, relaxing therapy, as for the patient with bona fide AN, is prudent. If hypoglycemia occurs in these patients at a certain glucose level, it will take a lower glucose level to trigger the same symptoms in the next 24 to 48 hours. Avoidance of hypoglycemia for a few days will result in recovery of the adrenergic response.

Implications for Diabetes Education and Care

Include prevention of hypoglycemia, appropriate treatment, the value of frequent home blood glucose monitoring, using caution while driving, and wearing appropriate diabetes identification. Teach family members the signs and treatment of hypoglycemia, including glucagon administration. Blood glucose awareness training may improve functional capacity.[121,147] Continuous glucose monitoring is very helpful, as alarms can be set to notify the patient when his or her glucose level drops below the target level.

Focal and Multifocal Neuropathies

The various focal neuropathies are acute and unpredictable. They are not specific to diabetes and are not related to the duration of diabetes. There are no strategies for prevention or early detection. Focal neuropathies are generally classified into the following types:

- Mononeuropathies
- Entrapment syndromes

The primary symptom of focal neuropathies is acute local pain.

Focal Limb Neuropathies

Focal limb neuropathies are usually due to entrapments. Entrapment syndromes start slowly and progress and persist unless intervention is prescribed. Carpal tunnel syndrome (compression or entrapment of the median nerve of the wrist) occurs 3 times as frequently in people with diabetes compared with healthy populations[54,148] and is found in up to one third of people with diabetes.[54] The diagnosis can be made by a careful history and physical and confirmed by electrophysiological studies.

Treatment consists of resting, aided by placement of a wrist splint in a neutral position to avoid repetitive trauma. Anti-inflammatory medications and steroid injections are sometimes useful. Surgery should be considered if weakness appears and medical treatment fails.[17,149]

Mononeuropathies

Mononeuropathies occur primarily in older people; the onset is acute and associated with pain, and their course is self-limiting, resolving within 6 to 8 weeks. They are due to vascular obstruction.[150] Mononeuropathies, characterized by their acute onset, should be distinguished from entrapment syndromes (see Table 28.8).

Cranial Neuropathies

Cranial neuropathies in persons with diabetes are extremely rare (0.05%) and occur in older individuals with a long duration of diabetes.[151] The third cranial nerve is most often affected. The onset is generally abrupt with headache, eye pain, or dysesthesias of the upper lip preceding palsy. The patient is unable to move the eye. After a few weeks the pain subsides and ocular function improves, with full recovery in 3 to 5 months.

Implications for Diabetes Education and Care Assure the patient that this is a temporary situation that will soon resolve. Suggest the use of an eye patch for the affected eye. The physician should rule out ruptured communicating artery aneurysm.

Proximal-Motor Neuropathy (Amyotrophy)

Proximal-motor neuropathy typically occurs in older people (50-60 years of age) with type 2 diabetes and presents with severe pain and unilateral or bilateral muscle weakness and atrophy in proximal thighs. Pathogenesis is still unclear, although immune-mediated epineurial microvasculitis is the culprit in some cases. Immunosuppressive therapy is recommended using high-dose steroids or intravenous immunoglobulin.[152]

Implications for Diabetes Education and Care Treatment of proximal neuropathies can be very rewarding, as 91% are due to the coexistence of chronic inflammatory demyelinating polyneuropathy and respond to intravenous immunoglobulin therapy. For those who fail to respond, immunosuppressive agents may be effective.[153]

Chronic Inflammatory Demyelinating Polyneuropathy

When an unusually severe, predominantly motor and progressive polyneuropathy develops in persons with diabetes, chronic inflammatory demyelinating polyneuropathy should be considered. Progressive motor deficit and progressive sensory neuropathy in spite of optimal glycemic control, together with typical NCV findings and an unusually high cerebrospinal-fluid protein level, suggest the possibility of an underlying demyelinating neuropathy. This neuropathy occurs 11 times more frequently in people with diabetes than in those without diabetes.[153–156]

Implications for Diabetes Education and Care The diagnosis is often overlooked, but it is very important to recognize the condition because it is treatable. Immunomodulatory therapy with intravenous immunoglobulin or immunotherapy can produce a relatively rapid and substantial improvement.[156]

Diabetic Truncal Radiculoneuropathy

Diabetic truncal radiculoneuropathy affects middle-aged to elderly persons, especially males. (Radiculopathy is the disease condition of the nerve roots in spinal nerves.) Pain is the most important symptom, occurring in a girdle-like distribution over the lower thoracic or abdominal wall, unilaterally or bilaterally distributed. Pain and/or loss of sensation is usually worse at night. Motor weakness is rare. Resolution generally occurs within 4 to 6 months.

TABLE 28.8 Mononeuropathies Versus Entrapment Syndrome		
Feature	*Mononeuropathy*	*Entrapment Syndrome*
Onset	Sudden	Gradual
Pattern	Single nerve, but may be multiple	Single nerve exposed to trauma
Nerves involved	Cranial nerves III, VI, VII; ulnar; median; peroneal	Median, ulnar, peroneal, medial and lateral plantar
Natural history	Resolves spontaneously	Progressive
Treatment	Symptomatic	Rest, splints, local steroids, diuretics, surgery

Source: Adapted with permission from Elsevier from A Vinik, A Mehrabyan, "Diabetic neuropathies," *Med Clin North Am* 88, no. 4 (2004): 954.

Implications for Diabetes Education and Care
Nonnarcotics or simple analgesics may help control the pain, which generally subsides in 6 to 24 months. The distribution of pain and sensory disturbance is clinically diagnosed by an experienced clinician.

Treatment of DN Based on Pathogenetic Mechanisms

Glycemic and Metabolic Control

Studies have shown a relationship between hyperglycemia and the development and severity of DN. The DCCT research group reported that clinical and electrophysiological evidence of neuropathy was reduced by 50% in persons with type 1 diabetes treated intensively with insulin.[157] In the UK Prospective Diabetes Study (UKPDS), control of blood glucose was associated with improvement in vibration perception.[158,159]

Vascular Risk Factors and DN

The Steno trial, using multifactorial intervention, reported a reduction in the development of AN in people with type 2 diabetes.[132] The EURODIAB, a prospective study that included 3250 patients across Europe, showed that the incidence of neuropathy is also associated with potentially modifiable cardiovascular risk factors, including a raised triglyceride level, BMI, smoking, and hypertension.[160]

Treatment and Prevention
Treatment and prevention of neuropathy should include measures to reduce both microvascular and macrovascular risk factors (hyperglycemia, blood pressure, and lipid control) and lifestyle modifications (exercise and weight reduction, smoking cessation, a diet rich in omega-3 fatty acids, and avoidance of excess alcohol consumption).[132]

Oxidative Stress

A number of studies have shown that hyperglycemia causes oxidative stress in tissues, including peripheral nerves that are susceptible to complications of diabetes. Studies show that hyperglycemia induces an increased presence of markers of oxidative stress, such as superoxide and peroxynitrite ions, which are now measurable in tissues and in body fluids. Persons with diabetic peripheral neuropathy have a reduced internal antioxidant defense mechanism against free radicals.[161]

Treatment
Therapies known to reduce oxidative stress are recommended.[162] Those under investigation include aldose reductase inhibitors (ARIs), γ-linolenic acid, and alpha-lipoic acid.

◆ *Aldose reductase inhibitors* reduce the flux of glucose through the polyol pathway, inhibiting tissue accumulation of sorbitol and fructose. (Sorbitol is a crystalline alcohol that is the intermediate product in the metabolism of glucose in the nerve and other tissues.) Newer ARIs are currently being explored,[163] but it is becoming clear that these agents may be insufficient per se, and combinations of treatments may be needed.[149]

◆ *γ-Linolenic acid* can cause significant improvement in clinical and electrophysiological tests for neuropathy.[164]

◆ *Alpha-lipoic acid*, or thioctic acid, has been used for its antioxidant properties and for its thiol-replenishing redox-modulating properties. A number of studies show its favorable influence on microcirculation and reversal of some symptoms of neuropathy.[165] Ongoing studies will examine its long-term effects on electrophysiology and clinical assessments.

Inhibition of the enzyme PKC B has been shown in a phase 2 study to reduce symptoms due to DN[166] in patients who had mild neuropathy detectable by the presence of a sural nerve amplitude on nerve electrophysiology.[167] However, the phase 3 study did not meet the end point of symptom relief, so no further studies of the effects of ruboxistaurin on more objective measures of nerve function are being carried out.

Some of the research studies mentioned above could provide models for the translation of the results of clinical trials involving neuropathy into preventive medicine and optimal clinical care. However, the art of a skilled healthcare provider will still be required to interact fully with the patient and maximize the outcomes of translational research.

Controversies in Neuropathy Management

Mechanical Measures

Transcutaneous Electrical Nerve Stimulation

Transcutaneous electrical nerve stimulation (TENS, or electrotherapy) may be helpful and is one of the more benign therapies for painful neuropathy.[168,169] Caveat: It is important to move the electrodes around to identify sensitive areas and obtain maximal relief.

Static Magnetic Field Therapy

Static magnetic field therapy has been reported to be of benefit, but blinding in these studies was difficult.[170] It is very easy to determine when there is a magnet in a patient's shoe. For this reason, it is difficult to do a blinded study.

Frequency-Modulated Electromagnetic Neural Stimulation

Frequency-modulated electromagnetic neural stimulation (FREMS) has been shown to induce a significant reduction in daytime and nighttime pain. In addition, a significant increase in tactile threshold was detected using SWM, lowering of the vibration detection threshold, and improved motor nerve conduction velocity using a biosthesiometer. There was an extra benefit shown in measures of QOL using the SF-36 Health Survey, in terms of general health, physical, and social functioning.[171] This finding suggests that FREMS may be an active, safe method to improve symptoms of neuropathy with the possibility of enhancing neurological function.

Infrared Light

Infrared light had benefits in a study of 27 patients whose extremities were treated for 2 weeks with sham or active infrared. There was reportedly a reduction in the number of insensate sites in patients with mild neuropathy, but not in those with greater sensory loss. Improved balance was also reported but was not quantified objectively. Clearly, these observations need to be extended for longer periods, and more objective measures need to be applied to evaluate responsiveness to treatment.[172]

Implanted Spinal Cord Stimulation

An implanted spinal cord stimulator was used in a series of patients with severe painful neuropathy who were unresponsive to conventional therapy.[173] However, this should be recommended only in very resistant cases, as it is invasive, expensive, and unproven in controlled studies.

Vibration

Vibration on the sole of the foot below the individual's threshold for 30 to 60 seconds has been shown to enhance sensitivity, neurotransmission, and vibration detection threshold.[174] Although monofilament application to the sole of the foot after vibration resulted in enhanced detection, this enhancement did not apply to the big toe. The ability to amplify signals from the neuropathic foot may have relevance for protecting feet from injury and possibly even enhancing postural stability. These studies need to be expanded to longer term to determine the durability of their effects.

Surgical Treatment of Neuropathy

Tarsal Tunnel Release

The role of tarsal tunnel release in the management of the person with diabetes who has a painful foot syndrome remains controversial.[54] The major problem is the application of tarsal tunnel release in patients with diabetic peripheral neuropathy *in general* and not *specifically* for those patients with tarsal tunnel entrapment syndrome (TTS). Tarsal tunnel entrapment syndrome is not difficult to diagnose clinically when DSPN is not severe and NCV is moderately abnormal. Mild symmetric peroneal and tibial NCV abnormality with intact ankle jerks and sensation of the dorsal aspect of the foot with the above-mentioned clinical signs are the most important diagnostic features of TTS. When the neuropathy is severe, diagnosis may be impossible. A positive Tinel sign, tapping just below the medial malleolus, may be helpful but may also simply reflect nerve damage in peripheral neuropathy, a negative sign suggesting that nerve damage predicts a poor outcome of surgery. Caveat: If patients are carefully selected, release of the tibial nerve through the tarsal tunnel in the patient may improve plantar sensibility and help prevent plantar ulceration and ultimate lower extremity amputation. Several studies lend credence to this notion, though some are subject to design flaws.[175,176]

Summary

The following are key issues in DN:

◆ Diabetic neuropathies are among the most common long-term complications of diabetes, although they often are not recognized by healthcare providers.

◆ Management of the disease is complex.

◆ A thorough history and detailed physical examination, together with the aid of simple tests (performed in the clinic), are essential for the diagnosis.

◆ In each particular clinical situation, the best treatment option should be determined on the basis of the underlying pathological process, the clinical presentation, and cost in relation to effectiveness.

◆ There has been increasing understanding of the pathogenesis of DN over the past decades, and new therapies are currently being studied that hold promise for the treatment of this disease.

This chapter addressed the challenges facing diabetes educators and suggested opportunities for dealing with DN. The message is powerful: DN is not a single entity but rather a number of different syndromes, each with a range of clinical and subclinical manifestations. Effective management is based on recognizing the particular manifestation and underlying pathogenesis of the particular form of DN in each patient and using this information to initiate therapy at a level that improves QOL for the person with diabetes.

Focus on Education

Teaching Strategies

↻ **Assess daily neuropathy-related pain management.** Diabetic neuropathy includes somatic and autonomic neuropathies, is associated with considerable morbidity and mortality, and has a significant impact on QOL. Ask patients the following questions:

• How does your pain impact your daily routine?

• What is your pain management strategy?

• How do you navigate the healthcare system to utilize all of the resources and support available to you?

↻ **Focus on prevention.** Help patients see how desirable glucose control can minimize the possibility of neuropathies.

↻ **Reverse neuropathies:**

• Inform the patient about potential treatment options. Offer assurance that treatment of many of the neuropathies can lead to eliminating or minimizing pain and discomfort. Some conditions are due to coexistence of other problems and respond to therapy.

• Diabetic neuropathy is not a single disease (but rather a heterogeneous group of disorders), and it might require multiple treatment approaches.

↻ **Diagnose neuropathies.** Often neuropathies are overlooked or "tolerated" as a natural progression of a disease. The key is screening, early detection, and treatment. Emphasis needs to be placed on routine annual and semiannual exams. Detection can be difficult; thus, clinicians are to inspect feet and skin at every visit to detect changes or symptoms.

↻ **Control neuropathies.** Neuropathies can be controlled by treatment. Associated pain can be treated with nonnarcotics or simple analgesics.

Messages for Patients

↻ **The key is screening, early detection, and treatment.**

• Keep track of your scheduled screening and its follow-up plan.

• Create a daily routine to examine/screen and care for your feet or other neuropathy-impacted system.

- Adhere to the proscribed medication or therapy recommended.
- Keep track of your pain management—what triggers pain, what it takes to relieve it, and how long it takes to manage the symptoms—and communicate with your healthcare providers about it.

⊙ **Keep ABCs (A1C, blood pressure, and cholesterol) under control.** Blood glucose, blood pressure, lipids, and lifestyle modifications are essential measures to reduce the risk of macrovascular disease, which contributes to DN.

⊙ **Manage your pain.** Read about the condition and its treatment, openly describe and talk about pain associated with neuropathies, and use medications (prescription and over-the-counter) appropriately. Relieving pain improves QOL and allows for clearer problem solving.

⊙ **Attend all checkups.** Schedule appointments in advance and note them on the calendar. Make this a priority. Identification and early treatment increase good response and reduction in symptoms. Insist that the healthcare provider look at your skin and feet at every visit and talk about the pain and problems to look for with neuropathies.

⊙ **Follow medication and treatment regimens.** Pay attention to timing of medicines. Use only the supplements advised by the healthcare team. Obtain a routine review of medicines with a pharmacist and the healthcare team; this is advisable to offer the best combination of treatments.

⊙ **Diabetic neuropathies do not have to limit you from enjoying good QOL.** Whether you are experiencing pain or working on minimizing or eliminating it, multiple treatment approaches are available to help you in your efforts. Different healthcare professionals can help in different ways. Ask your doctor to direct you to someone qualified to help with your needs.

⊙ **Diabetic neuropathies can have an impact on your work, your relationships, and your ability to manage your diabetes.** Talk to the diabetes care team about getting support with coping and overcoming challenges that will come with all the changes to your life.

Health Literacy

⊙ **Patients might be embarrassed to talk about some of the symptoms associated with DN.** Request their permission to ask them a few questions about it or tell them why you need to examine them. Explain why you do what you are doing.

⊙ **Demonstrate the treatment strategies when possible or use visuals to outline treatment steps.** Allow people to verbalize or demonstrate back to you what they will do (let them teach you).

⊙ **Create reminders for daily care.** Establish a routine that allows for the treatment to be part of the usual daily tasks and monitor progress.

⊙ **Help patients explore the following:**
- How treatment cost, treatment regimen, and other factors affect their compliance
- The costs and consequences of noncompliance
- Therapy-related problems
- Development of solutions
- Selection of therapies
- Follow-up to assess outcomes

Consider that age, race, gender, income, education, patient intelligence, actual seriousness of the disease, and the efficacy of the treatment may be associated with compliance.

⊙ **Encourage patients to seek social support.** Social support allows patients to be accountable for their care. Also, peer-to-peer support helps patients explore options and validate their feelings and attitudes, and facilitates general discussions about care.

Focus on Practice

⟳ **Establish a network of appropriate referral services for DNs.** Effective management is based on recognizing the particular manifestation and underlying pathogenesis of the particular form of DN. Treatment modalities are very individualized at all care levels to ultimately improve QOL for the person with diabetes.

⟳ **Integrate DN management into the diabetes self-management education.** There has been increasing understanding of the pathogenesis of DN over the past decades, and new therapies are currently being studied that hold promise for the treatment of this disease.

⟳ **Examine access to care for people with DN.** There is a significantly higher direct medical cost for individuals diagnosed with a diabetic complication of neuropathy.

References

1. Holzer SE, Camerota A, Martens L, Cuerdon T, Crystal-Peters J, Zagari M. Costs and duration of care for lower extremity ulcers in patients with diabetes. Clin Ther. 1998;20(1):169-81.

2. Vinik AI, Ziegler D. Diabetic cardiovascular autonomic neuropathy. Circulation. 2007;115:387-97.

3. Vinik AI, Maser RE, Ziegler D. Neuropathy: the crystal ball for cardiovascular disease. Diabetes Care. 2010;33: 1688-90.

4. Vinik AI, Maser RE, Ziegler D. Autonomic imbalance: prophet of doom or scope for hope? Diabet Med. 2011;28: 643-51.

5. Levitt NS, Stansberry KB, Wychanck S, Vinik AI. Natural progression of autonomic neuropathy and autonomic function tests in a cohort of IDDM. Diabetes Care. 1996; 19:751-4.

6. Rathmann W, Ziegler D, Jahnke M, Haastert B, Gries FA. Mortality in diabetic patients with cardiovascular autonomic neuropathy. Diabet Med. 1993;10:820-4.

7. Tesfaye S, Boulton AJ, Dyck PJ, et al. Diabetic neuropathies: update on definitions, diagnostic criteria, estimation of severity, and treatments. Diabetes Care. 2010;33: 2285-93.

8. Vinik AI, Nevoret ML, Casellini C, Parson H. Diabetic neuropathy. Endocrinol Metab Clin North Am. 2013 Dec;42(4):747-87. doi: 10.1016/j.ecl.2013.06.001

9. Frykberg RG, Zgonis T, Armstrong DG, et al. Diabetic foot disorders: a clinical practice guideline. J Foot Ankle Surg. 2006;45(5 Suppl):S1-66.

10. Mantyselka P, Ahonen R, Kumpusalo E, Takala J. Variability in prescribing for musculoskeletal pain in Finnish primary health care. Pharm World Sci. 2001;23:232-6.

11. Jensen MP, Chodroff MJ, Dworkin RH. The impact of neuropathic pain on health-related quality of life: review and implications. Neurology. 2007;68:1178-82.

12. Li Y, Rios Burrows N, Gregg EW, Albright A, Geiss LS. Declining rates of hospitalizations for nontraumatic lower limb-extremity amputation in the diabetic population aged 40 years or older: US, 1988-2008. Diabetes Care. 2012;35:273-7.

13. Dyck PJ, Kratz KM, Karnes JL, et al. The prevalence by staged severity of various types of diabetic neuropathy, retinopathy, and nephropathy in a population-based cohort: The Rochester Diabetic Neuropathy Study. Neurology. 1993;43:817-24.

14. WebMD. CDC: Big drop in diabetes amputations. 2012 Jan 24. On the Internet at: http://www.webmd.com/diabetes/news/20120124/cdc-big-drop-diabetes-amputations.

15. Vinik AI, Mitchell BD, Leichter SB, Wagner AL, O'Brian JT, Georges LP. Epidemiology of the complications of diabetes. In: Leslie RDG, Robbins DC, eds. Diabetes: Clinical Science in Practice. Cambridge, UK: Cambridge University Press; 1995:221-87.

16. Ziegler D. Painful diabetic neuropathy: treatment and future aspects. Diabetes Metab Res Rev. 2008;24 Suppl 1:S52-7.

17. Boulton AJ, Malik RA, Arezzo JC, Sosenko JM. Diabetic somatic neuropathies. Diabetes Care. 2004;27:1458-86.

18. Dyck PJ, Karnes JL, O'Brien PC, Litchy WJ, Low PA, Melton III LJ. The Rochester Diabetic Neuropathy Study: reassessment of tests and criteria for diagnosis and staged severity. Neurology. 1992;42:1164-70.

19. Herman WH, Kennedy L. Underdiagnosis of peripheral neuropathy in type 2 diabetes. Diabetes Care. 2005;28(6): 1480-1.

20. Feldman EL, Stevens MJ, Thomas PK, Brown MB, Canal N, Greene DA. A practical two-step quantitative clinical and electrophysiological assessment for the diagnosis and staging of diabetic neuropathy. Diabetes Care. 1994;17:1281-9.

21. Young MJ, Boulton AJM, MacLeod AF, Williams DRR, Sonksen PH. A multicenter study of the prevalence of diabetic peripheral neuropathy in the United Kingdom hospital clinic population. Diabetologia. 1993;36:150-4.

22. Dyck PJ. Severity and staging of diabetic polyneuropathy. In: Textbook of Diabetic Neuropathy. Stuttgart, Germany: Thieme; 2003:170-5.

23. Dyck PJ. Detection, characterization and staging of polyneuropathy: assessed in diabetes. Muscle Nerve. 1988;11:21-32.

24. Boulton AJ, Vinik AI, Arezzo JC, et al. Diabetic neuropathies: a statement by the American Diabetes Association. Diabetes Care. 2005;28(4):956-62.

25. Vinik AI, Suwanwalaikorn S, Stansberry KB, Holland MT, McNitt PM, Colen LE. Quantitative measurement of cutaneous perception in diabetic neuropathy. Muscle Nerve. 1995;18:574-84.

26. Abbott CA, Carrington AL, Ashe H, et al. The North-West Diabetes Foot Care Study: incidence of, and risk factors for, new diabetic foot ulceration in a community-based patient cohort. Diabetes Med. 2002;19(5):377-84.

27. Dyck PJ, Davies JL, Litchy WJ, O'Brien PC. Longitudinal assessment of diabetic polyneuropathy using a composite score in the Rochester Diabetic Neuropathy Study cohort. Neurology. 1997;49(1):229-39.

28. Haanpaa ML, Backonja MM, Bennett MI, et al. Assessment of neuropathic pain in primary care. Am J Med. 2009;122(10 Suppl):S13-21.

29. Boulton AJ, Gries FA, Jervell JA. Guidelines for the diagnosis and outpatient management of diabetic peripheral neuropathy. Diabet Med. 1998;15:508-14.

30. Yarnitsky D, Sprecher E. Thermal testing: normative data and repeatability for various test algorithms. J Neurol Sci. 1994;125:39-45.

31. Cruccu G, Sommer C, Anand P, et al. EFNS guidelines on neuropathic pain assessment: revised 2009. Eur J Neurol. 2010;17:1010-18.

32. Shy ME, Frohman EM, So Y, Arezzo JC, Cornblath DC, Giuliani MJ; the subcommittee of the American Academy of Neurology. Quantitative sensory testing: report on the Therapeutic and Technology Assessment Subcommittee of the American Academy of Neurology. Neurology. 2003;602:898-906.

33. Pittenger G, Mehrabyan A, Simmons K, et al. Small fiber neuropathy is associated with the metabolic syndrome. Metab Syndr Relat Disord. 2005;3:113-21.

34. Lauria G, Hsieh S, Johansson O, et al. European Federation of Neurological Societies/Peripheral Nerve Society Guideline on the use of skin biopsy in the diagnosis of small fiber neuropathy. Report of a joint task force of the European Federation of Neurological Societies and the Peripheral Nerve Society. Eur J Neurol. 2010;17:903-12.

35. Lauria G, Bakkers M, Schmitz C, et al. Intraepidermal nerve fiber density at the distal leg: a worldwide normative reference study. J Peripher Nerv Syst. 2010;15:202-7.

36. Pittenger GL, Ray M, Burcus NI, McNulty P, Basta B, Vinik AI. Intraepidermal nerve fibers are indicators of small-fiber neuropathy in both diabetic and nondiabetic patients. Diabetes Care. 2004;27:1974-79.

37. Kennedy WR, Wendelschafer-Crabb G, Johnson T. Quantitation of epidermal nerves in diabetic neuropathy. Neurology. 1996;47:1042-8.

38. Polydefkis M, Hauer P, Griffin JW, McArthur JC. Skin biopsy as a tool to assess distal small fiber innervation in diabetic neuropathy. Diabetes Technol Ther. 2001;3(1):23-8.

39. Smith AG, Russell J, Feldman EL, et al. Lifestyle intervention for pre-diabetic neuropathy. Diabetes Care. 2006;29:1294-9.

40. Joint Task Force of the EFNS and the PNS. European Federation of Neurological Societies/Peripheral Nerve Society Guideline on the use of skin biopsy in the diagnosis of small fiber neuropathy. Report of a joint task force of the European Federation of Neurological Societies and the Peripheral Nerve Society. J Periph Nerv Syst. 2010;15:79-92.

41. Quattrini C, Tavakoli M, Jeziorska M, et al. Surrogate markers of small fiber damage in human diabetic neuropathy. Diabetes. 2007;56:2148-54.

42. Tavakoli M, Quattrini C, Abbott C, et al. Corneal confocal microscopy: a novel noninvasive test to diagnose and stratify the severity of human diabetic neuropathy. Diabetes Care. 2010;33:1792-7.

43. Zhivov A, Blum M, Guthoff R, Stachs O. Real-time mapping of the subepithelial nerve plexus by in vivo confocal laser scanning microscopy. Br J Ophthalmol. 2010;94:1133-5.

44. Parson HK, Nguyen VT, Boyd AL, Vinik A. CHEPS detects neuropathic changes earlier than traditional clinical measures. Diabetes. 2009;58(Suppl 1) abstract:A220.

45. Parson HK, Nguyen VT, Orciga MA, Boyd AL, Casellini CM, Vinik AI. Contact heat-evoked potential stimulation for the evaluation of small nerve fiber function. Diabetes Technol Ther. 2013;15:150-7.

46. McArthur JC, Stocks EA, Hauer P, Cornblath DR, Griffin JW. Epidermal nerve fiber density: normative reference range and diagnostic efficiency. Arch Neurol. 1998;55:1513-20.

47. Illigens BM, Gibbons CH. Sweat testing to evaluate autonomic function. Clin Auton Res. 2009;19:79-87.

48. Mayaudon H, Miloche PO, Bauduceau B. A new simple method for assessing sudomotor function: relevance in type 2 diabetes. Diabetes Metab. 2010;36:450-4.

49. Gin H, Baudoin R, Raffaitin CH, Rigalleau V, Gonzalez C. Non-invasive and quantitative assessment of sudomotor function for peripheral diabetic neuropathy evaluation. Diabetes Metab. 2011;37:527-32.

50. Hubert D, Brunswick P, Calvet JH, Dusser D, Fajac I. Abnormal electrochemical skin conductance in cystic fibrosis. J Cyst Fibros. 2011;10:15-20.

51. Calvet JH, Dupin J, Winiecki H, Schwarz PEH. Assessment of small fiber neuropathy through a quick, simple and non invasive method in a German diabetes outpatient clinic. Exp Clin Endocrinol Diabetes. 2012;120:1-4.

52. Partanen J, Niskanen L, Lehtinen J, Mervaala E, Siitonen O, Uusitupa M. Natural history of peripheral neuropathy in patients with non-insulin-dependent diabetes mellitus. N Engl J Med. 1995;333:89-94.

53. DCCT Research Group. The effect of intensive diabetes therapy on the development and progression of neuropathy. Ann Intern Med. 1995;122:561-8.

54. Vinik A, Mehrabyan A, Colen L, Boulton A. Focal entrapment neuropathies in diabetes. Diabetes Care. 2004;27(7):1783-8.

55. Pittenger G, Simmons K, Anandacoomaraswamy D, Rice A, Barlow P, Vinik A. Topiramate improves intraepidermal nerve fiber morphology and quantitative neuropathy measures in diabetic neuropathy patients. J Peripher Nerv Syst. 2005;10 Suppl 1.

56. Sinnreich M, Taylor BV, Dyck PJ. Diabetic neuropathies. Classification, clinical features, and pathophysiological basis. Neurologist. 2005;11:63-79.

57. Vileikyte L, Peyrot M, Bundy C, et al. The development and validation of a neuropathy- and foot ulcer-specific quality of life instrument. Diabetes Care. 2003;26(9):2549-55.

58. Vinik AI, Holland MT, LeBeau JM, Liuzzi FJ, Stansberry KB, Colen LB. Diabetic neuropathies. Diabetes Care. 1992;15:1926-75.

59. Thomas PK, Ward JD, Watkins PJ. Diabetic neuropathy. In: Keen H, Jarrett J, eds. Complications of Diabetes. London, England: Edward Arnold Publishing Company; 1982:109-36.

60. Young RJ, Ewing DJ, Clarke BF. Chronic and remitting painful diabetic polyneuropathy. Correlations with clinical features and subsequent changes in neurophysiology. Diabetes Care. 1988;11:34-40.

61. England JD, Gronseth GS, Franklin G, et al. Distal symmetric polyneuropathy: a definition for clinical research: report of the American Academy of Neurology, the American Association of Electrodiagnostic Medicine, and the American Academy of Physical Medicine and Rehabilitation. Neurology. 2005;64:199-207.

62. Paisley AN, Abbott CA, van Schie CHM, Boulton AJM. A comparison of the Neuropen against standard quantitative sensory threshold measures for assessing peripheral nerve function. Diabet Med. 2002;19:400-5.

63. Ziegler D, Siekierka-Kleiser E, Meyer B, Schweers M. Validation of a novel screening device (NeuroQuick) for quantitative assessment of small nerve fiber dysfunction as an early feature of diabetic polyneuropathy. Diabetes Care. 2005;28:1169-74.

64. Viswanathan V, Snehalatha C, Seena R, Ramachandran A. Early recognition of diabetic neuropathy: evaluation of a simple outpatient procedure using thermal perception. Postgrad Med J. 2002;78:541-2.

65. Martina IS, van Koningsveld R, Schmitz PI, van der Meche FG, van Doorn PA. Measuring vibration threshold with a graduated tuning fork in normal aging and in patients with polyneuropathy. European Inflammatory Neuropathy Cause and Treatment (INCAT) group. J Neurol Neurosurg Psychiatry. 1998;65:743-7.

66. Ziegler D, Hidvegi T, Gurieva I, et al. Efficacy and safety of lacosamide in painful diabetic neuropathy. Diabetes Care. 2010;33:839-41.

67. Boulton AJ, Malik RA. Diabetic neuropathy. Med Clin North Am. 1998;82:909-29.

68. Thomas PK. Classification, differential diagnosis, and staging of diabetic peripheral neuropathy. Diabetes. 1997;46 Suppl 2:S54-7.

69. Oyibo SO, Prasad YD, Jackson NJ, Jude EB, Boulton AJ. The relationship between blood glucose excursions and painful diabetic peripheral neuropathy: a pilot study. Diabet Med. 2002;19(10):870-3.

70. Tesfaye S, Malik R, Harris N, et al. Arterio-venous shunting and proliferating new vessels in acute painful neuropathy of rapid glycaemic control (insulin neuritis). Diabetologia. 1996;39:329-35.

71. Vinik A. The approach to the management of the patient with neuropathic pain. In: Wartofsky L, ed, A Clinical Approach to Endocrine and Metabolic Diseases. Vol. 2. Chevy Chase, Md: The Endocrine Society; 2012;177-94.

72. Archer AG, Watkins PJ, Thomas PK, Sharma AK, Payan J. The natural history of acute painful neuropathy in diabetes mellitus. J Neurol Neurosurg Psychiatry. 1983;46:491-9.

73. Cavanagh PR, Simoneau GG, Ulbrecht JS. Ulceration, unsteadiness, and uncertainty: the biomechanical consequences of diabetes mellitus. J Biomech. 1993;26 Suppl 1:23-40.

74. Katoulis EC, Ebdon-Parry M, Lanshammar H, Vileikyte L, Kulkarni J, Boulton AJ. Gait abnormalities in diabetic neuropathy. Diabetes Care. 1997;20:1904-7.

75. Vinik A, Pittenger G, Barlow P, Mehrabyan A. Diabetic neuropathies: an overview of clinical aspects, pathogenesis, and treatment. In: LeRoith D, Taylor S, Olefsky J, eds. Diabetes Mellitus. 3rd ed. Philadelphia: Lippincott Williams and Wilkins; 2004:1331-63.

76. Vinik A, Mehrabyan A. Understanding diabetic neuropathies. Emerg Med. 2004;36(5):39-44.

77. Bennett MI, Attal N, Backonja MM, et al. Using screening tools to identify neuropathic pain. Pain. 2007;127:199-203.

78. Vinik EJ, Hayes RP, Oglesby A, et al. The development and validation of the Norfolk QOL-DN, a new measure of patients' perception of the effects of diabetes and diabetic neuropathy. Diabetes Technol Ther. 2005;7(3):497-508.

79. Bastyr E, Zhang D, Bril V; the MBBQ Study Group. Neuropathy Total Symptom Score-6 Questionnaire (NTSS-6) Is Valid Instrument for Asessing the Positive Symptoms of Diabetic Peripheral Neuropathy (DPN). *Diabetes.* 2002;51:A199.

80. Scholz J, Mannion RJ, Hord DE, et al. A novel tool for the assessment of pain: validation in low back pain. PLoS Med. 2009;6:e1000047.

81. Spallone V. La neuropatia diabetica dolorosa: approccio alla diagnosi e alla terapia di un problema emergente. Me Dia. 2009;9:1-14.

82. Young RJ. Structural functional interactions in the natural history of diabetic polyneuropathy: a key to the understanding of neuropathic pain? Diabet Med. 1993;10 Suppl 2:89S-90.

83. Treede RD, Jensen TS, Campbell JN, et al. Neuropathic pain: redefinition and a grading system for clinical and research purposes. Neurology. 2008;70:1630-5.

84. Vinik A, Ullal J, Parson HK, Casellini CM. Diabetic neuropathies: clinical manifestations and current treatment options. Nat Clin Pract Endocrinol Metab. 2006;2:269-81.

85. Bouhassira D, Attal N, Fermanian J, et al. Development and validation of the Neuropathic Pain Symptom Inventory. Pain. 2004;108:248-57.

86. Bennett MI, Smith BH, Torrance N, Potter J. The S-LANSS score for identifying pain of predominantly neuropathic origin: validation for use in clinical and postal research. J Pain. 2005;6:149-58.

87. Krause S, Backonja M. Development of a neuropathic pain questionnaire. Clin J Pain. 2003;19:306-4.

88. Bouhassira D, Attal N, Alchaar H, et al. Comparison of pain syndromes associated with nervous or somatic lesions and development of a new neuropathic pain diagnostic questionnaire (DN4). Pain. 2005;114:29-36.

89. Freyhagen R, Baron R, Gockel U. Pain detect: a new screening questionnaire to detect neuropathic components in patients with back pain. Curr Med Res Opin. 2006;22:1911-20.

90. Portenoy R. Development and testing of a neuropathic pain screening questionnaire: ID Pain. Curr Med Res Opin. 2006;22:1555-65.

91. Dworkin RH, Turk DC, Revicki DA, et al. Development and initial validation of an expanded and revised version of the Short-form McGill Pain Questionnaire (SF-MPQ-2). Pain. 2009;144:35-42.

92. Daut RL, Cleeland CS, Flanery RC. Development of the Wisconsin Brief Pain Questionnaire to assess pain in cancer and other diseases. Pain. 1983;17:197-210.

93. Dworkin RH, Turk DC, Wyrwich KW, et al. Interpreting the clinical importance of treatment outcomes in chronic pain clinical trials: IMMPACT recommendations. J Pain. 2008;9:105-21.

94. Finnerup NB, Otto M, McQuay HJ, Jensen TS, Sindrup SH. Algorithm for neuropathic pain treatment: an evidence based proposal. Pain. 2005;118:289-305.

95. Finnerup NB, Sindrup SH, Jensen TS. The evidence for pharmacological treatment of neuropathic pain. Pain. 2010;150:573-81.

96. Dworkin RH, O'Connor AB, Backonja M, et al. Pharmacologic management of neuropathic pain: evidence-based recommendations. Pain. 2007;132:237-51.

97. Dworkin RH, O'Connor AB, Audette J, et al. Recommendations for the pharmacological management of neuropathic pain: an overview and literature update. Mayo Clin Proc. 2010;85:S3-14.

98. Quilici S, Chancellor J, Lothgren M, et al. Meta-analysis of duloxetine vs. pregabalin and gabapentin in the treatment of diabetic peripheral neuropathic pain. BMC Neurol. 2009;9:6-19.

99. Burke J, Sanchez R, Joshi A, Cappelleri J, Kulakodlu M, Halpern R. Health care costs in patients with painful diabetic peripheral neuropathy prescribed pregabalin or duloxetine. Pain Pract. 2012;12:209-18.

100. De Salas-Cansado M, Perez C, Saldana MT, et al. An economic evaluation of pregabalin versus usual care in the management of community-treated patients with refractory painful diabetic peripheral neuropathy in primary care settings. Prim Care Diabetes. 2012;6:303-12.

101. Bellows BK, Dahal A, Jiao T, Biskupiak J. A cost-utility analysis of pregabalin versus duloxetine for the treatment of painful diabetic neuropathy. J Pain Palliat Care Pharmacother. 2012;26:153-64.

102. Lord S, Sherrington C, Menz H, Close J. Falls in Older People: Risk Factors and Strategies for Prevention. 2nd ed. Cambridge, UK: Cambridge University Press; 2007.

103. Maurer MS, Burcham J, Cheng H. Diabetes mellitus is associated with an increased risk of falls in elderly residents of a long-term care facility. J Gerontol A Biol Sci Med Sci. 2005;60(9):1157-62.

104. Schwartz AV, Hillier TA, Sellmeyer DE, et al. Older women with diabetes have a higher risk of falls: a prospective study. Diabetes Care. 2002;25(10):1749-54.

105. Clark RD, Lord SR, Webster IW. Clinical parameters associated with falls in an elderly population. Gerontology. 1993;39(2):117-23.

106. Close JC, Lord SL, Menz HB, Sherrington C. What is the role of falls? Best Pract Res Clin Rheumatol. 2005;19(6): 913-35.

107. Tinetti ME, Kumar C. The patient who falls: "It's always a trade-off." JAMA. 2010;303(3):258-66.

108. Morrison S, Colberg SR, Mariano M, Parson HK, Vinik AI. Balance training reduces falls risk in older individuals with type 2 diabetes. Diabetes Care. 2010;33(4):748-50.

109. Dhesi JK, Bearne LM, Moniz C, et al. Neuromuscular and psychomotor function in elderly subjects who fall and the relationship with vitamin D status. J Bone Miner Res. 2002;17(5):891-7.

110. Welford AT. Between bodily changes and performance: some possible reasons for slowing with age. Exp Aging Res. 1984;10(2):73-88.

111. Tucker MG, Kavanagh JJ, Morrison S, Barrett RS. Voluntary sway and rapid orthogonal transitions of voluntary sway in young adults, and low and high fall-risk older adults. Clin Biomech (Bristol, Avon). 2009;24(8):597-605.

112. Fukagawa NK, Wolfson L, Judget J, Whipple R, King M. Strength is a major factor in balance, gait, and the occurrence of falls. J Gerontol A Biol Sci Med Sci. 1995;50A:64-7.

113. Buckner DM, Cress ME, de Lateur BJ, et al. The effect of strength and endurance training on gait, balance, fall risk, and health services use in community-living older adults. J Gerontol. 1997;52A(4):M218-24.

114. Won-Park S, Goodpaster B, Strotmeyer E, et al. Decreased muscle strength and quality in older adults with type 2 diabetes: the health, aging and body composition study. Diabetes. 2006;55(6):1813-8.

115. Lord S, Fitzpatrick R. Choice stepping reaction time: a composite measure of falls' risk in older people. J Gerontol A Biol Sci Med Sci. 2001;56(10):M627-32.

116. Vinik AI, Ziegler D. Diabetic cardiovascular autonomic neuropathy. Circulation. 2007;115(3):387-97.

117. Maser RE, Mitchell BD, Vinik AI, Freeman R. The association between cardiovascular autonomic neuropathy and mortality in individuals with diabetes: a meta-analysis. Diabetes Care. 2003;26(6):1895-901.

118. Vinik A, Maser RE. Letter to editor: screening for asymptomatic coronary artery disease in patients with type 2 diabetes. JAMA. 2009;302(7):735-6.

119. Boulton A, Vinik A, Arrezzo J, et al. Position statement: diabetic neuropathies. Diabetes Care. 2005;28(4):956-62.

120. Ziegler D, Dannehl K, Muhlen H, Spuler M, Gries FA. Prevalence of cardiovascular autonomic dysfunction assessed by spectral analysis, vector analysis, and standard tests of heart rate variation and blood pressure responses at various stages of diabetic neuropathy. Diabetes Med. 1992;9(9):806-14.

121. Vinik AI, Maser RE, Mitchell BD, Freeman R. Diabetic autonomic neuropathy. Diabetes Care. 2003;26(5): 1553-79.

122. Zola BE, Vinik AI. Effects of autonomic neuropathy associated with diabetes mellitus on cardiovascular function. Coron Artery Dis. 1992;3:33-41.

123. Spallone V, Ziegler D, Freeman R, et al. Cardiovascular autonomic neuropathy in diabetes: clinical impact, assessment, diagnosis, and management. Diabetes Metab Res Rev. 2011;27:639-53.

124. Pop-Busui R, Evans G, Gerstein H, et al; the ACCORD Study Group. Effects of cardiac autonomic dysfunction on mortality risk in the action to control cardiovascular risk in diabetes (ACCORD) trial. Diabetes Care. 2010;33:1578-84.

125. Calles-Escandon J, Lovato L, Simons-Morton D, et al. Effect of intensive compared with standard glycemia treatment strategies on mortality by baseline subgroup characteristics. Diabetes Care. 2010;33:721-7.

126. Tracey KJ. Reflex control of immunity. Nat Rev Immunol. 2009;9:418-28.

127. Ziegler D. Diabetic cardiovascular autonomic neuropathy: prognosis, diagnosis and treatment. Diabetes Metab Rev. 1994;10(4):339-83.

128. Valensi P. Diabetic autonomic neuropathy: what are the risks? Diabetes Metab. 1998;24:66-72.

129. Mancia G, Paleari F, Parati G. Early diagnosis of diabetic autonomic neuropathy: present and future approaches. Diabetologia. 1997;40:482-4.

130. Ziegler D, Gries FA. Alpha-lipoic acid in the treatment of diabetic peripheral and cardiac autonomic neuropathy. Diabetes. 1997;46 Suppl 2:S62-6.

131. Athyros VG, Didangelos TP, Karamitsos DT, Papageorgiou AA, Boudoulas H, Kontopoulos AG. Long-term effect of converting enzyme inhibition on circadian sympathetic and parasympathetic modulation in patients with diabetic autonomic neuropathy. Acta Cardiol. 1998;53(4):201-9.

132. Gaede P, Vedel P, Larsen N, Jensen GV, Parving HH, Pedersen O. Multifactorial intervention and cardiovascular

disease in patients with type 2 diabetes. N Engl J Med. 2003;348(5):383-93.

133. Vinik A, Mehrabyan A. Gastrointestinal disturbances. In: Lebovitz H, ed. Therapy for Diabetes Mellitus and Related Disorders. 4th ed. Alexandria, Va: American Diabetes Association; 2004:424-39.

134. Jones KL, Russo A, Stevens JE, Wishart JM, Berry MK, Horowitz M. Predictors of delayed gastric emptying in diabetes. Diabetes Care. 2001;24(7):1264-9.

135. Horowitz SH, Ginsberg-Fellner F. Ischemia and sensory nerve conduction in diabetes mellitus. Neurology. 1979; 29:695-704.

136. Vinik AI, Richardson D. Erectile dysfunction in diabetes. Diabetes Reviews. 1998;6:16-33.

137. Richardson D, Vinik A. Etiology and treatment of erectile failure in diabetes mellitus. Curr Diab Rep. 2002;2(6): 501-9.

138. Vinik A, Richardson D. Erectile dysfunction. In: Sinclair A, Finucane P, eds. Diabetes in Old Age. 2nd ed. Chichester, UK: John Wiley & Sons; 2001:89-102.

139. Vinik A, Mehrabyan A. Diagnosis and management of diabetic autonomic neuropathy. Compr Ther. 2003; 29(2/3):130-45.

140. Enzlin P, Mathieu C, Vanderschueren D, Demyttenaere K. Diabetes mellitus and female sexuality: a review of 25 years' research. Diabet Med. 1998;15(10):809-15.

141. Stansberry KB, Hill MA, Shapiro SA, McNitt PM, Bhatt BA, Vinik AI. Impairment of peripheral blood flow responses in diabetes resembles an enhanced aging effect. Diabetes Care. 1997;20:1711-6.

142. Stansberry KB, Peppard HR, Babyak LM, Popp G, McNitt PM, Vinik AI. Primary nociceptive afferents mediate the blood flow dysfunction in non-glabrous (hairy) skin of type 2 diabetes: a new model for the pathogenesis of microvascular dysfunction. Diabetes Care. 1999;22:1549-54.

143. Haak ES, Usadel KH, Kohleisen M, Yilmaz A, Kusterer K, Haak T. The effect of alpha-lipoic on the neurovascular reflex arc in patients with diabetic neuropathy assessed by capillary microscopy. Microvasc Res. 1999;58:28-34.

144. Meyer C, Hering BJ, Grossmann R, et al. Improved glucose counterregulation and autonomic symptoms after intraportal islet transplants alone in patients with long-standing type I diabetes mellitus. Transplantation. 1998;66(2): 233-40.

145. Cryer PE, Davis SN, Shamoon H. Hypoglycemia in diabetes. Diabetes Care. 2003;26:1902-12.

146. Vinik A. Diagnosis and management of diabetic neuropathy. Clin Geriatr Med. 1999;15(2):293-319.

147. Cox DJ, Gonder-Frederick L, Julian DM, Clarke W. Long-term follow-up evaluation of blood glucose awareness training. Diabetes Care. 1994;17(1):1-5.

148. Perkins B, Olaleye D, Bril V. Carpal tunnel syndrome in patients with diabetic polyneuropathy. Diabetes Care. 2002;25:565-9.

149. Vinik A, Mehrabyan A. Diabetic neuropathies. Med Clin North Am. 2004;88(4):947-99.

150. Vinik A, Mehrabyan A. Diabetic monoradiculopathy/amyoradiculopathy. In: Lebovitz H, ed. Therapy for Diabetes Mellitus and Related Disorders. 4th ed. Alexandria, Va: American Diabetes Association; 2004:416-23.

151. Watanabe K, Hagura R, Akanuma Y, et al. Characteristics of cranial nerve palsies in diabetic patients. Diabetes Res Clin Pract. 1990;10(1):19-27.

152. James P, Dyck B, Windenbank A. Diabetic and non-diabetic lumbosacral radiculoplexus neuropathy: new insights into pathophysiology. Muscle Nerve. 2002;25: 477-91.

153. Vinik AI, Anandacoomaraswamy D, Ullal J. Antibodies to neuronal structures: innocent bystanders or neurotoxins? Diabetes Care. 2005;28(8):2067-72.

154. Sharma K, Cross J, Farronay O, Ayyar D, Sheber R, Bradley W. Demyelinating neuropathy in diabetes mellitus. Arch Neurol. 2002;59:758-65.

155. Krendel DA, Zacharias A, Younger DS. Autoimmune diabetic neuropathy. Neurol Clin. 1997;15(4):959-71.

156. Ayyar DR, Sharma KR. Chronic inflammatory demyelinating polyradiculoneuropathy in diabetes mellitus. Curr Diab Rep. 2004;4(6):409-12.

157. DCCT Research Group. The effect of intensive treatment of diabetes on the development and progression of long-term complications in insulin dependent diabetes mellitus. N Engl J Med. 1993;329:977-86.

158. UK Prospective Diabetes Study (UKPDS) Group. Effect of intensive blood-glucose control with metformin on complications in overweight patients with type 2 diabetes (UKPDS 34). Lancet. 1998;352:854-65.

159. UK Prospective Diabetes Study Group. Tight blood pressure control and risk of macrovascular and microvascular complications in type 2 diabetes: UKPDS 38. BMJ. 1998;317:703-13.

160. Tesfaye S, Chaturvedi N, Eaton SE, et al. Vascular risk factors and diabetic neuropathy. N Engl J Med. 2005;352(4):341-50.

161. Ziegler D, Sohr CG, Nourooz-Zadeh J. Oxidative stress and antioxidant defense in relation to the severity of diabetic polyneuropathy and cardiovascular autonomic neuropathy. Diabetes Care. 2004;27(9):2178-83.

162. Vincent AM, Russell JW, Low P, Feldman EL. Oxidative stress in the pathogenesis of diabetic neuropathy. Endocr Rev. 2004;25(4):612-28.

163. Bril V, Buchanan RA. Aldose reductase inhibition by AS-3201 in sural nerve from patients with

diabetic sensorimotor polyneuropathy. Diabetes Care. 2004;27(10):2369-75.

164. Keen H, Payan J, Allawi J, et al. Treatment of diabetic neuropathy with linolenic acid. Diabetes Care. 1993;16: 8-15.

165. Ziegler D, Nowak H, Kempler P, Vargha P, Low PA. Treatment of symptomatic diabetic polyneuropathy with the antioxidant alpha-lipoic acid: a meta-analysis. Diabetes Med. 2004;21(2):114-21.

166. Vinik A. The protein kinase C-beta inhibitor, ruboxistaurin, for the treatment of diabetic microvascular complications. Expert Opin Investig Drugs. 2005;14(12):1547-59.

167. Vinik AI, Bril V, Litchy WJ, Price KL, Bastyr EJ III. Sural sensory action potential identifies diabetic peripheral neuropathy responders to therapy. Muscle Nerve. 2005 Nov;32(5):619-25.

168. Somers DL, Somers MF. Treatment of neuropathic pain in a patient with diabetic neuropathy using transcutaneous electrical nerve stimulation applied to the skin of the lumbar region. Phys Ther. 1999;79:767-75.

169. Hamza MA, White PF, Craig WF, et al. Percutaneous electrical nerve stimulation: a novel analgesic therapy for diabetic neuropathic pain. Diabetes Care. 2000;23(3): 365-70.

170. Weintraub MI, Wolfe GI, Barohn RA, et al. Static magnetic field therapy for symptomatic diabetic neuropathy: a randomized, double-blind, placebo-controlled trial. Arch Phys Med Rehabil. 2003;84(5):736-46.

171. Bosi E, Conti M, Vermigli C, et al. Effectiveness of frequency-modulated electromagnetic neural stimulation in the treatment of painful diabetic neuropathy. Diabetologia. 2005;48(5):817-23.

172. Leonard DR, Farooqi MH, Myers S. Restoration of sensation, reduced pain, and improved balance in subjects with diabetic peripheral neuropathy: a double-blind, randomized, placebo-controlled study with monochromatic near-infrared treatment. Diabetes Care. 2004;27(1): 168-72.

173. Tesfaye S, Watt J, Benbow SJ, Pang KA, Miles J, MacFarlane IA. Electrical spinal-cord stimulation for painful diabetic peripheral neuropathy. Lancet. 1996;348: 1698-701.

174. Khaodhiar L, Niemi JB, Earnest R, Lima C, Harry JD, Veves A. Enhancing sensation in diabetic neuropathic foot with mechanical noise. Diabetes Care. 2003;26(12): 3280-3.

175. Wieman TJ, Patel VG. Treatment of hyperesthetic neuropathic pain in diabetics: decompression of the tarsal tunnel. Ann Surg. 1995;221:660-5.

176. Dellon A. Treatment of symptomatic diabetic neuropathy by surgical decompression of multiple peripheral nerves. Plast Reconstr Surg. 1992;89(4):689-97.

INDEX

Note: Tables and exhibits are italicized in the index.

B

C

F

G

education in, 64

problem solving in, 255–256

Growth hormone

elevated levels of, 779

physical activity effects on, *460*

Guided imagery, 625–626

Guidelines for the Practice of Diabetes Education (AADE), 51

Gymnema, *588,* 593–594

H

Health Belief Model (HBM), *94,* 94–96

Health homes, 19

Health insurance

Affordable Care Act and, 274

blood glucose meter coverage by, 201

description of, 5–6

Health insurance exchanges, 19–20

Health literacy skills, 35, 56–57

Health professionals

patient and, collaboration between, 253

problem solving by, 253–254

Healthcare Effectiveness Data and Information Set (HEDIS), 327

Healthcare team, *250*

Healthy coping. *see* Coping

Healthy eating. *see* Nutrition

Healthy eating pattern, 433–434

Healthy Food Choices, 134

Healthy People 2010, 16

Healthy People 2020, 16

Hearing-impaired patients, 68

Heart. *see* Cardiovascular disease (CVD)

Heart rate, 146, 148

HEEADSSS, 37

Helping the Student with Diabetes Succeed, 397

Hemochromatosis, 368

Hemodialysis (HD), 791–792

Hemoglobin, 784

Hemoglobin A1C. *see* A1C

Hepatic glucose, 638

Hepatitis B virus vaccinations, 235, 297

High-density lipoprotein cholesterol (HDL-C)

chronic kidney disease prevention target values, 784

description of, 542

guidelines for, 292

monitoring of, 225

niacin and, 553

High-sensitivity C-reactive protein, 543

Hispanic/Latino populations, 58

depression in, 281

diabetes prevalence in, 4, 358, *358*

diabetic retinopathy in, 762

glaucoma prevalence in, 759

HLA markers, 368

HLA-DQ genotypes, 368

HLA-DR-3 haplotype, 368

HLA-DR-4 haplotype, 368

HMG-CoA reductase inhibitors (statins)

cardiovascular disease and, 731–732

characterization of, 546

contraindications for, 549

dosage information, 547, *547–548*

drug interactions, 549, *550*

dyslipidemia treated with, 778

mechanism of action, 546–547

monitoring of, 549

patient instructions, 549

precautions for, 549

in pregnancy, 549

safety of, 732

Homeopathy, 624

Honeymoon period, 389

Hoorn Screening Study, 664

Hormonal disorders, 368

Hospitalization. *see also* Institutional care settings

adverse events after discharge from, 343

assessments during, 37, *341*

discharge planning, 343–349

glycemic target levels during, 649, *649*

medication history, 341

medication use during, 342

for pregnancy, *691–692*

transitional care during, 340–342

Hydration, 654–655, 657

Hydrochlorothiazide (HydroDIURIL®), *560*

Hyperchloremic acidosis, 645

Hypercholesteremia, 414

Hyperemesis gravidarum, 702

Hyperglycemia. *see also* Blood glucose; Glycemic control

antihyperglycemic management for, 493, 496, 501–504, *502–503*

assessment of, 640–642, 651–652

cardiovascular disease risks, 374, 720

complications of, 670–671

definition of, 635

diabetic kidney disease and, 779

direct instruction and, 249

education regarding, 656

exercise and, 469–471

high-risk individuals for, 655

inpatient concerns, 649–650

in institutional care setting, *657*

laboratory tests, 640–641

markers for, 641

in myocardial infarction, 740

pain threshold and, 812

prevention of, 249, 657

I

N

Q

T